DRUG	INTERACTION	POSSIBLE EFFECT
MISCELLANEOUS DRUGS		
bromocriptine (Chap. 110)		▲ Nausea and abdominal pain
chloral hydrate (Chap. 28)		▲ CNS depression ▲ Flushing, headache, tachycardia ▼ Psychomotor skills
chloramphenicol (Chap. 18)		Disulfiram-type reaction*
cycloserine (Chap. 11)		▲ Convulsions
disulfiram (Chap. 110)		Disulfiram-alcohol reaction*
guanethidine (Chap. 21)		▲ Orthostatic hypotension ▲ Vasodilation
isoniazid (Chap. 11)		▲ Hepatitis ▼ Chronic alcoholism
lincomycin (Chap. 18)	Give patient nothing by mouth—except water—for 1 to 2 hours before and after receiving drug	▼ Blood absorption of drug
meprobamate (Chap. 31)		▲ Metabolism of drug (chronic alcoholism) ▼ Metabolism of drug (acute alcoholism)
metronidazole (Chap. 7)		Disulfiram-type reaction*
nitroglycerin (Chap. 22)		▲ Cardiovascular collapse

*Disulfiram-alcohol reaction can include such signs and symptoms as blurred vision, confusion, dyspnea, flushing, hypotension, nausea and vomiting, sweating, tachycardia, thirst, and vertigo. For more information about the disulfiram-alcohol reaction, see Chapter 110, UNCATEGORIZED DRUGS.

KEY:

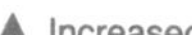 Increased

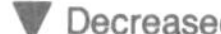 Decreased

Major drug-alcohol reaction; patient should avoid all alcohol and alcohol-based drugs

Moderate drug-alcohol reaction; patient should limit intake of alcohol and alcohol-based drugs

Major drug-food reaction; patient should avoid foods listed in chart

XANAX
Halcion 25mg

Hydroxyzine HCL 10mg

Professional Guide to Drugs™

INTERMED COMMUNICATIONS, INC.
SPRINGHOUSE, PENNSYLVANIA

Second Edition

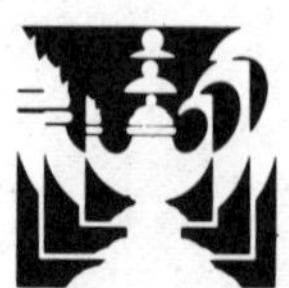

INTERMED COMMUNICATIONS BOOKS

Professional Guide to Drugs

The clinical procedures described and recommended in this publication are based on research and consultation with pharmacists and other health-care professionals. To the best of our knowledge, these procedures reflect currently accepted clinical practice; nevertheless, they can't be considered absolute and universal recommendations. For individual application, treatment recommendations must be considered in light of the patient's clinical condition and, before administration of new or infrequently used drugs, in light of latest package-insert information. The authors and the publisher disclaim responsibility for any adverse effects resulting directly or indirectly from the suggested procedures, from any undetected errors, or from the reader's misunderstanding of the text.

Library of Congress Cataloging in Publication Data
Main entry under title:

PROFESSIONAL GUIDE TO DRUGS
Includes index.
1. Drugs—Handbooks, manuals, etc.
I. Intermed Communications, Inc.
[DNLM: 1. Drugs. QV 55 P964]
RM300.P75 1982 615′.7 82-6120
ISBN 0-916730-51-4 AACR2

Staff for this volume

Associate Editor: June Norris
Assistant Editor: Holly Ann Burdick
Copy Chief: Jill Lasker
Copy Editor: Jo Lennon
Copyediting Assistants: Sandra J. Purrenhage, Hilda Rogers
Production Coordinator: Patricia Hamilton
Associate Designer: Kathaleen Motak Singel
Assistant Designer: Christopher Laird
Design Assistant: Robert Walsh
Illustrator: Robert Jackson
Art Production Manager: Robert J. Perry, III
Art Assistants: Craig T. Siman, Sandra Simms, Joan Walsh
Typography Manager: David C. Kosten
Typography Assistants: Janice Haber, Ethel Halle, Diane Paluba, Nancy Wirs
Production Manager: Wilbur D. Davidson
Quality Control Manager: Robert L. Dean
Editorial Assistant: Sally Johnson

Staff for the preceding edition

Editorial Director: Maryanne Wagner
Clinical Editor: Anne Moraca-Sawicki, RN, MSN
Special Projects Editor: Susan Rossi Williams
Senior Editor: Jerome Rubin
Assistant Editors: Nancy Holmes, Patricia E. McCulla, Debra M. Rosenberg
Copy Editors: Barbara Hodgson, David R. Moreau
Copyediting Assistant: Diane A. Dufresne
Assistant Designer: Jacalyn Bove
Design Assistants: Jacquelyn Diotte, Darcy Feralio, Janet Schmoyer
Illustrators: Jean Gardner, Tom Herbert, Thomas Lewis, Kim Milnazik, John Murphy
Art Assistants: Virginia Crawford, Diane Fox, Don Knauss, Peter Pizzo, Robert Renn, George Retseck, Louise Stamper, Ron Yablon
Editorial Assistants: Maree E. DeRosa, Bernadette Glenn
Researcher: Vonda Heller

Advisory board

At the time of original publication, these advisors, clinical consultants, and contributors held the following positions.

Lillian S. Brunner, RN, MSN, ScD, FAAN, *Consultant in Nursing, Presbyterian–University of Pennsylvania Medical Center, Philadelphia.*

Donald C. Cannon, MD, PhD, *Professor, Pathology and Laboratory Medicine, the Medical School, University of Texas Health Science Center, Houston.*

Luther Christman, RN, PhD, *Dean, Rush College of Nursing; Vice-President, Nursing Affairs, Rush University, Chicago, Ill.*

Kathleen A. Dracup, RN, MN, CCRN, *Research Fellow, Medicine/Cardiology, University of California at Los Angeles.*

Stanley J. Dudrick, MD, *Professor of Surgery, St. Luke's Episcopal Hospital and University of Texas Medical School at Houston.*

Halbert E. Fillinger, MD, *Assistant Medical Examiner, Philadelphia County, Philadelphia, Pa.*

M. Josephine Flaherty, RN, PhD, *Principal Nursing Officer, Department of National Health and Welfare, Ottawa, Ont.*

Joyce LeFever Kee, RN, MSN, *Associate Professor, University of Delaware College of Nursing, Newark.*

Dennis E. Leavelle, MD, *Director, Mayo Medical Laboratories, Department of Laboratory Medicine, Mayo Clinic, Rochester, Minn.*

Roger M. Morrell, MD, PhD, FACP, *Professor, Neurology and Immunology/Microbiology, Wayne State University, School of Medicine, Detroit, Mich.; Chief, Neurology Service, Veterans Administration Medical Center, Allen Park, Mich.*

Ara G. Paul, PhD, *Dean, College of Pharmacy, University of Michigan, Ann Arbor.*

Rose Pinneo, RN, MS, *Associate Professor of Nursing and Clinician II, University of Rochester, N.Y.*

Thomas E. Rubbert, JD, LLB, BSL, *Attorney-at-Law, Los Angeles, Calif.*

Maryanne Schreiber, RN, BA, *Product Manager, Patient Monitoring, Hewlett Packard Co., Waltham Division, Waltham, Mass.*

Frances J. Storlie, RN, PhD, ANP, *Adult Nurse Practitioner, Vancouver, Wash.*

Claire L. Watson, RN, *Supervisor, Systems Support Department, IVAC Corp., San Diego, Calif.*

Clinical consultants

Beverly A. Baldwin, RN, MA, *Assistant Professor, School of Nursing, University of Maryland, Baltimore.*

Heather Boyd-Monk, RN, BSN, *Educational Coordinator, Wills Eye Hospital, Philadelphia, Pa.*

Nancy Burns, RN, PhD, *Assistant Professor, University of Texas School of Nursing, Arlington.*

Carla J. Burton, RN, BSN, *Dermatology Nurse Clinician, Beth Israel Hospital, Boston, Mass.*

Deborah Bussey, RN, BSN, *Head Nurse, Thoracic Oncology Outpatient Clinic, M.D. Anderson Hospital and Tumor Institute, Houston, Tex.*

Priscilla A. Butts, RN, MSN, *Lecturer, University of Pennsylvania, Philadelphia.*

Judy Donlen, RNC, MSN, *Instructor, Perinatal Graduate Program, University of Pennsylvania School of Nursing, Philadelphia.*

Jeanne Dupont, RN, *Head Nurse, Emergency Department, Massachusetts Eye and Ear Infirmary, Boston.*

DeAnn M. Englert, RN, MSN, *Assistant Professor, Louisiana State University Medical Center School of Nursing, New Orleans.*

Margarethe Hawkin, RN, MA, CNRN, *Clinical Nurse Specialist in Neurology and Epilepsy, Seattle (Wash.) Veteran's Administration Medical Center.*

Kathleen M. Hawkins, RN, *Dermatology Nurse Specialist, University of Colorado, Health Sciences Center, Denver.*

Carolyn Holt, RN, BSEd, *Coordinator, Nursing Staff Development, Columbus-Cuneo-Cabrini Medical Center, Chicago, Ill.*

Gail D'Onofrio Long, RN, MSN, *Clinical Nurse Specialist in Medical Intensive Care and Coronary Care, University Hospital, Boston, Mass.*

Elizabeth A. Phillips, RN, BA, BSN, *Administrative Supervisor, Delaware Valley Medical Center, Bristol, Pa.*

Turena Reeves, RN, *Coordinator, Intravenous Therapy, Germantown Hospital and Medical Center, Philadelphia, Pa.*

Despina Seremelis, RN, BSN, *Staff Nurse, Oncology Unit, Temple University Hospital, Philadelphia, Pa.*

Barbara Solomon, RN, MSN, *Clinical Nurse Expert, Division of Arthritis and Metabolism, National Institute of Health, Bethesda, Md.*

Robin Tourigin, RN, MSN, *Nurse Clinician, Thomas Jefferson University Hospital, Philadelphia, Pa.*

Paula Brammer Vetter, RN, BSN, *Clinical Instructor in Coronary Intensive Care, Cleveland (Ohio) Clinic Hospital.*

Carmen Brochu Wohrle, RN, MSN, *Assistant Director of Nursing, Deaconess Hospital, Spokane, Wash.*

Contributors

Ron Ballentine, PharmD, Associate Professor and Chairman, Department of Clinical Pharmacy and Administration, University of Houston; Drug Information Specialist, M.D. Anderson Hospital and Tumor Institute, Houston, Tex.

Alan D. Barreuther, PharmD, Assistant Professor, Pharmacy Practice, College of Pharmacy; Instructor, Department of Pharmacology, College of Medicine, Arizona Health Sciences Center, Tucson.

Peter W. Chan, PharmD, Clinical Pharmacist, Aurora, Colo.

Bruce B. Clutcher, BS, Staff Pharmacist, University of Pennsylvania Hospital, Philadelphia.

Michael R. Cohen, BS, RPH, Director of Pharmacy, Quakertown (Pa.) Community Hospital; Assistant Clincial Professor of Pharmacy, Temple University School of Pharmacy, Philadelphia, Pa.

Lawrence J. Dwork, BS, Clinical Pharmacist, Grant Hospital, Columbus, Ohio.

Bruce M. Frey, PharmD, Clinical Pharmacist in Pediatrics, Thomas Jefferson University Hospital, Philadelphia, Pa.; Clinical Assistant Professor, Philadelphia (Pa.) College of Pharmacy and Science.

Matthew P. Fricker, BS, Clinical Pharmacist, Temple University Hospital, Philadelphia, Pa.

Steven J . Gilbert, BS, Staff Pharmacist, The Graduate Hospital, Philadelphia, Pa.

James R. Hildebrand III, PharmD, Clinical Pharmacist Supervisor, Thomas Jefferson University Hospital, Philadelphia, Pa.

Jay H. Hoffman, BS, Clinical Pharmacist, Thomas Jefferson University Hospital, Philadelphia, Pa.

Alan W. Hopefl, PharmD, Assistant Professor of Clinical Pharmacy, St. Louis (Mo.) College of Pharmacy; Assistant Professor of Pharmacology in Medicine, St. Louis (Mo.) University School of Medicine.

Michael G. Krevitskie, BS, Staff Pharmacist, Lower Bucks Hospital, Bristol, Pa.

Joseph A. Linkewich, PharmD, Associate Professor of Clinical Pharmacy, Philadelphia (Pa.) College of Pharmacy and Science.

Steven Meisel, PharmD, Clinical Coordinator, Pharmacy Department, St. Joseph's Hospital, St. Paul, Minn.

George Melnik, BS, Nutritional Support Service Pharmacist, Philadelphia (Pa.) Veterans Administration Medical Center.

Linda Nelson, PharmD, Instructor in Clinical Pharmacy, Philadelphia (Pa.) College of Pharmacy and Science.

David R. Pipher, PharmD, Clinical Pharmacist, Montefiore Hospital, Pittsburgh, Pa.

Susan Rogers, PharmD, Clinical Pharmacist, Radnor, Pa.

Joel Shuster, PharmD, Director of Pharmacy Services, The Fairmount Institute, Philadelphia, Pa.; Clinical Assistant Professor, Philadelphia (Pa.) College of Pharmacy and Science.

William Simonson, PharmD, Associate Professor of Pharmacy, Oregon State University School of Pharmacy, Corvallis.

Anthony P. Sorrentino, PharmD, Manager, Jefferson Apothecary, Philadelphia, Pa.

Joseph F. Steiner, PharmD, Associate Professor of Clinical Pharmacy; Director of Clinical Pharmacy Program, University of Wyoming, Family Practice Residency Center, Casper.

Janet Louise Wagner, PharmD, Assistant Professor of Clinical Pharmacy, University of Cincinnati (Ohio) College of Pharmacy.

Frank F. Williams, PharmD, Assistant Director, Inpatient Services, Pharmacy Department, Temple University Hospital, Philadelphia, Pa.

Special thanks to those who contributed to past editions: Richard Bailey, BS; Marquette L. Cannon, PharmD; Judith Hopfer Deglin, PharmD; Betty H. Dennis, MS; Dina Dichek, BS; Teresa P. Dowling, PharmD; Dan R. Ford, PharmD; Lee Gardner, PharmD; Marie Gardner, PharmD; Philip P. Gerbino, PharmD; Patricia J. Hedrick, PharmD; Arthur I. Jacknowitz, PharmD; Sandra G. Jue, PharmD; Barbara H. Korberly, PharmD; Sheldon M. Leiman, BS; Lauren F. McKaig, BS; Kathryn Murphy, MSN; David W. Newton, PhD; George David Rudd, MS; Jamshid B. Tehrani, PhD; C. Wayne Weart, PharmD.

We'd like to thank these community pharmacists who helped us obtain the tablets and capsules photographed in the full-color DRUGS OF ABUSE section: William Balas, RPh; Mark Cohen, RPh; John McVan, RPh; Seymour Margolis, RPh.

Contents

I General Information

II Antimicrobial and Antiparasitic Agents

III Cardiovascular System Drugs

IV Central Nervous System Drugs

IX Agents for Fluid and Electrolyte Balance

X Hematologic Agents

XI Antineoplastic Agents

XII Eye, Ear, Nose, and Throat Drugs

Foreword

Comprehensive, accurate, and up-to-date drug information is essential for professionals and patients alike. Health-care professionals are expected to act according to the most current drug information despite the rapid accumulation of knowledge in this continuously expanding field. Patients, too, need reliable drug information to cope effectively with the complexities of drug therapy.

Obviously, health-care professionals need a good working knowledge of the drugs they select, prescribe, dispense, and administer. Those who prescribe must have the latest information to help them choose the most effective drug with the least potential for hazardous effects. Prescribers and those who dispense, administer, and monitor drugs must know correct dosage, recommended frequency and duration of therapy, and potential side effects, as well as relevant information about preparation and storage.

Patients also play important roles in promoting safe and effective drug therapy. Health educators and consumer advocates encourage patients to know the names, dosages, strengths, and frequency of administration of the drugs they are taking; the reasons for their use; and their anticipated benefits and possible adverse effects. Such understanding promotes patients' compliance and enhances their ability to monitor their own drug responses. Clearly, well-informed patients greatly improve the chances for successful drug therapy.

How to meet these needs for information? Obviously, a dependable, comprehensive reference source is indispensable. PROFESSIONAL GUIDE TO DRUGS is just such a reference source, designed to provide rapid access to current and comprehensive information—what you need to know—on over 1,100 drugs. The contents are organized in a format that makes this information easy to find. For example, its index makes each drug accessible by both generic and trade names. Drugs are grouped into 105 classes based on their pharmacologic actions, and into 15 major drug sections by clinical use or by the body system they influence.

In an easy-to-use tabular form, each drug is identified by both generic and trade names. The tables also list explicit dosage instructions, indications, side effects, and clinically significant interactions. Special considerations include contraindications, special cautions, suggestions for administration and patient comfort, and instructions for proper storage and preparation.

Each chapter also covers major uses of drugs; mechanisms of action; absorption, distribution, metabolism, and excretion of drugs; and their onset and duration of action. Selected combination products are also listed. Numerous charts, diagrams, and illustrations help you develop a better understanding of pharmacology and drug therapy.

In the general information section, you will find comprehensive chapters on basic pharmacology; drug therapy in adults, children, and the elderly; and principles of intravenous solution compatibility. An extensive full-color identification section shows nearly 500 photographs of commonly abused drugs; an appendix includes specific instructions for managing drugs that produce acute toxicity.

PROFESSIONAL GUIDE TO DRUGS has been written by experts in their fields—clinical pharmacists and other health-care professionals. Unlike many other drug reference books, it summarizes the latest information available, based on clinical experience. This book is an essential addition to the professional and home library.

NEIL M. DAVIS, MS, PHARMD, and
MICHAEL R. COHEN, BS, RPH
Coauthors of MEDICATION ERRORS: CAUSES AND PREVENTION (Philadelphia: George F. Stickley Co., 1981).

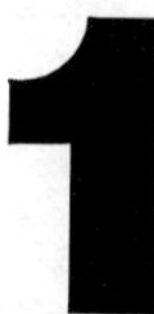

How to use Professional Guide to Drugs

Professional Guide to Drugs is meant to fill a very special need. It represents a joint effort to provide health-care professionals with comprehensive, practical drug information. With this in mind, it emphasizes clinical aspects, not pharmacology, and does not attempt to replace detailed pharmacology texts. For the same reason, the information is arranged in a format designed to make it readily accessible.

Introductory information

Following this chapter are five other preliminary chapters. Chapter 2 explains important general aspects of pharmacology that will be referred to throughout the book. It also tells about side effects and adverse reactions, and gives general guidelines about drug use in pregnancy and the presence of drugs in breast milk. Chapters 3, 4, and 5 summarize the implications of drug therapy in adults, children, and the elderly. Chapter 6 offers information to aid in the effective and safe administration of intravenous drugs, plus an updated I.V. compatibility chart.

In the remaining chapters—except for Chapter 70, which explains the implications of chemotherapy—all drugs are classified according to their common, approved therapeutic use. Each chapter has two parts. The first, an introductory section, summarizes the known pharmacology of the drugs in that chapter. Specifically, this section answers the following questions:

- What are the principal therapeutic uses of these drugs?
- Is their mechanism of action known? If so, what is it?
- How are these drugs absorbed, distributed, metabolized, and excreted?
- How long do they take to act, and how long do their effects last?
- Finally, what are the principal combination products in which these drugs are commonly found?

Carefully selected charts, graphs, and diagrams make this information easier to understand than standard pharmacology texts.

Drug identification section

Twenty full-color pages show photographs of common drugs of abuse, including both controlled substances and others that you will want to identify. These substances are arranged by color for fast identification.

Tabular information

The second part of each chapter consists of tabular information divided into three columns:

In the first column: an alphabetic list of drugs by generic name, immediately followed by an alphabetic list of brand names. (Occasionally, a combination product appears in the tables under the head of its major ingredient.) Brands available in both the United States and Canada are designated with a diamond (♦); those available *only* in Canada with a double diamond (♦♦). A brand name with no symbol after it is available only in the United States. If a drug is a controlled substance, that too is clearly indicated (example: Controlled Substance Schedule II). Products listed, although generally available, may not be approved by the Food and Drug Administration. The mention of a brand name in no way implies endorsement of that product or guarantees its legality.

The first column also includes: major indications and specific dosage instructions for adults and children, as applicable. Children's doses are usually indicated in terms of mg/kg/day. Dosage instructions reflect current clinical trends in therapeutics and can't be considered an absolute and universal recommendation. For individual application, dosage instructions must be considered in context with the patient's clinical condition.

In the second column: a list of each drug's commonly observed side effects (and rare ones, if life-threatening). The most common and life-threatening side effects are italicized for easy reference. An exception to this rule is a side effect that, although normally considered quite hazardous, has been reported to be mild and reversible with the drug in question. For example, thrombocytopenia is considered a life-threatening side effect of mithramycin (a chemotherapeutic drug). However, the thrombocytopenia associated with methyldopa (Aldomet) is generally mild and reversible. Hence, thrombocytopenia listed as a side effect of mithramycin is italicized, whereas the same side effect under methyldopa is not. Side effects are grouped according to the body system in which they appear.

In the third column: each drug's confirmed, *clinically significant* interactions with other drugs, including additive effects, potentiated effects, and antagonistic effects. Also included are specific suggestions for dealing with dangerous drug interaction (for example, reducing doses, or monitoring certain laboratory tests). Drug interactions are listed under the drug that is adversely affected. For example, magnesium trisilicate, an ingredient in antacids, interacts with tetracycline to cause decreased absorption of tetracycline. Therefore, this interaction is listed under tetracycline. To check on the possible effects of using two or more drugs simultaneously, refer to the interaction entry for *each* of the drugs.

The third column also presents: special considerations starting with contraindications and precautions, followed by monitoring techniques and suggestions for prevention and treatment of side effects. Also included are suggestions for promoting patient comfort, for patient teaching, and for preparing, administering, and storing each drug.

Appendix and Index

An appendix offers useful, supplementary information on the recognition and management of acute toxicity. Finally, a comprehensive index lists each drug alphabetically by both generic and brand name and lists the subject of charts, illustrations, and teaching tips. Drugs that do not appear in the index are mainly fillers, preservatives, and drugs that are not used alone.

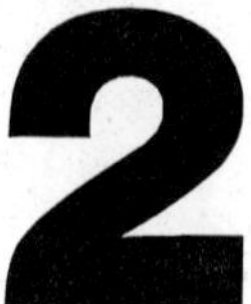

Pharmacology

Administration of any drug provokes a series of physiochemical events within the body. The first event—the *drug action*—occurs when a drug reaches its site of action and combines with cellular drug receptors. The physiologic response to this action is the *drug effect*.

Depending on the number of different cellular drug receptors affected by a given drug, a drug effect can be local or systemic, or both. For example, the anti–peptic ulcer drug cimetidine (Tagamet) acts solely by blocking histamine receptor cells in the parietal cells of the stomach. This is known as a local drug effect because the drug action is sharply limited to one area and doesn't spread to other parts of the body. However, diphenhydramine (Benadryl) produces a systemic effect in that it blocks histamine receptors in widespread areas of the body.

Furthermore, certain drugs may produce either type of effect depending on the route of administration. For example, epinephrine dilates the bronchioles when inhaled as an aerosol. However, I.V. administration of epinephrine produces a systemic effect on all adrenergic receptors.

Mechanisms of drug action

Understanding the principles of pharmacokinetics (the movement of a drug through the body as it is absorbed, distributed, metabolized, and excreted) helps you know the proper drug and dosage form required to produce the desired drug effect. The following summaries explain how each of these pharmacokinetic processes works.

1. *Absorption*

A drug must be absorbed into the bloodstream before it can act within the body. Several factors determine the speed and degree of absorption: various patient characteristics, the drug's physiochemical effects, dosage form, route of administration, and interactions with other substances in the gastrointestinal (GI) tract.

Drugs already in solution—such as syrups, elixirs, and injectables—are usually absorbed more rapidly than other dosage forms. This explains why some drugs, such as digoxin, produce higher blood levels when administered as solutions than they do as tablets.

If the drug is in tablet or capsule form, it must first disintegrate. Smaller particles of the disintegrated drug can dissolve in gastric juices and be absorbed into the bloodstream. When it is absorbed and circulating in the bloodstream, the drug is *bioavailable,* or ready to produce its effect.

Drugs administered intramuscularly are absorbed through the muscle before entering the bloodstream. This relatively fast process can be prolonged by administering the drug in an oil solution, or as a suspension, that is, by decreasing the solubility of the drug. For example, an intramuscular injection of penicillin G potassium is absorbed almost immediately; an intramuscular injection of penicillin G procaine takes several hours to be absorbed because its oily base makes the drug relatively lipid-insoluble.

Drugs administered intravenously are placed directly into the circulation and thus are immediately bioavailable.

For a drug to be absorbed when given other than intravenously, it must first pass through membranes by such methods as *active (carrier) transport* and *passive diffusion*.

- *Active transport* plays a minor role in drug absorption. The drug combines with a "carrier" on one side of the membrane and is taken through to the other side, where it dissociates from the carrier and is deposited in the bloodstream.

• *Passive diffusion* is the more common method of drug absorption. The rate of transfer during passive diffusion depends on the *concentration gradient* and the *lipid solubility* of the drug. If a drug's concentration in the GI tract is greater than its concentration in the bloodstream, this sets up the concentration gradient necessary for passive diffusion. The drug will continue to pass through the GI membrane into the bloodstream until drug concentrations are equal in both areas. The higher concentration of drug in the GI tract maintains the concentration gradient until the drug is completely absorbed.

Lipid solubility also affects passive diffusion. The higher the lipid solubility of the drug, the greater and more rapid the absorption. The lipid solubility of a drug is due to several factors, including the degree of ionization of the drug in solution. Nonionized (uncharged) drugs have greater lipid solubility and are therefore more readily absorbed than ionized (charged) drugs, which are lipid-insoluble. Since most drugs are either weak acids or weak bases, their degree of ionization depends on their location in the GI tract.

Weak acids, such as aspirin, have a higher ratio of nonionized to ionized molecules in the acidic environment of the stomach, and thus are more readily absorbed from this area.

Weak bases, such as quinidine, however, have a higher proportion of nonionized molecules in the alkaline medium of the small intestine. Some nonionized molecules of the drug are present in both the stomach and the intestine, so absorption occurs to some extent in both locations. Only the ratio of nonionized to ionized molecules changes. Another difference is more absorption in the small intestine, because it has a larger surface area than the stomach, a good blood supply, and a pH of 6.0 to 8.0.

Gastric emptying time also affects absorption of medications from the GI tract. For instance, food or antacids in the stomach may prolong gastric emptying time and delay a drug's reaching the small intestine. However, if GI motility is increased, as in diarrhea, drugs may travel through the GI tract so rapidly that they're not completely absorbed. This condition would particularly undermine absorption of sustained-release preparations that are intended to be absorbed over 8 to 12 hours.

2. *Distribution*

As soon as a drug starts to be absorbed, it moves from the bloodstream into body fluids and tissues; this is distribution. Initially, tissues with a high blood flow—highly perfused organs such as the heart, liver, kidneys, and brain—receive most of the drug. Since absorption may take place over several hours, the processes of absorption, distribution, metabolism, and excretion can be occurring simultaneously.

A drug's ability to cross a lipid membrane influences its distribution to various sites in the body (for example, the central nervous system, the placenta, and breast milk). Since some drugs cannot pass through certain cell membranes, their distribution is limited. Other drugs, such as ethyl alcohol, can pass through virtually all cell membranes. Remember these points:

• *Plasma-protein binding* can greatly influence the distribution and therefore the effectiveness and duration of drug action.

Many drugs are insoluble in plasma; these are transported as weak complexes bound to plasma proteins, especially albumin. (Drug binding can occur at sites of absorption, at extravascular sites, or, most commonly, in the blood.) Some drugs are highly bound to plasma proteins, many are moderately bound, and others may not be bound at all. All drugs bound to plasma proteins have a ratio of free, or unbound, drug to bound drug. For example, warfarin is 97% bound to plasma proteins. Only 3% is unbound, or free

HOW IONIZATION AFFECTS ABSORPTION

Why are some drugs more lipid-soluble (and thus more readily absorbed) in the stomach, while others are more lipid-soluble in the intestine? A major reason is the ratio of nonionized to ionized molecules in a drug. This important ratio depends on whether the drug is a weak acid or a weak base, and what the pH of its environment is.

Ionized drug molecules are electrically charged. Since the lipid membrane itself is highly charged, it repels the ionized drug.

WEAK ACIDS (such as aspirin, sulfonamides, and most barbiturates) are more readily absorbed from the acidic environment of the stomach, where a higher percentage of their molecules remains nonionized.

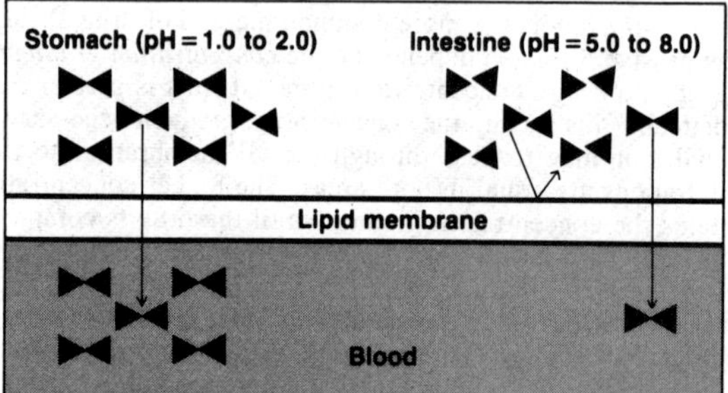

WEAK BASES (such as amphetamine, quinidine, and ephedrine) are more readily absorbed from the alkaline environment of the intestine, where a higher percentage of their molecules remains nonionized.

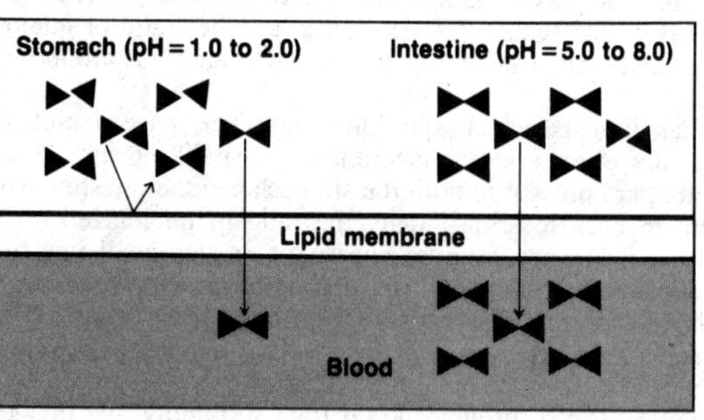

KEY: ⧓ = nonionized (more lipid-soluble) ▶◀ = ionized (less lipid-soluble)

drug. Only free drug is pharmacologically active, or able to produce an effect at the drug receptor site; only free drug can be metabolized or excreted.

Bound drug acts as a reservoir; as free drug is eliminated, bound drug is released from the plasma proteins. Thus, drug binding is reversible. Such binding regulates the amount of free drug in circulation and prevents the drug from reaching its site of action fully concentrated.

• The *volume of distribution*—the total area to which a drug is distributed—depends on the individual characteristics of the patient and the drug. For example, in an edematous patient, a given dose must be distributed to a larger volume than in a nonedematous patient; therefore, the drug amount may have to be increased. (Remember that the dosage should be decreased when edema is corrected.)

Conversely, in an extremely dehydrated patient, the drug is distributed to a much smaller volume, so the dose must be decreased.

Particularly obese patients may present another problem: Some drugs, such as digoxin, gentamicin, and tobramycin, are not well distributed to fatty tissue. For such drugs, therefore, dosage based on actual body weight may lead to overdose and serious toxicity. In some cases, dosage must be based on lean body weight (which may be estimated from actuarial tables that give average weight range for height).

3. *Combination with receptors*
Through absorption and distribution, the drug reaches its site of action and combines with receptors in the cells. Certain drugs have an affinity for certain cells and not for others, so their biologic effect is produced selectively and specifically. When a drug combines with a receptor at a specific site, a series of biochemical and physiologic changes begin in response to the drug. Most receptors are proteins, such as enzymes of the body's metabolic or regulatory pathways or intracellular proteins of infecting bacteria. The receptor for penicillin, for example, is the enzyme transpeptidase. Penicillin renders this enzyme incapable of making the cell walls of the bacteria strong and rigid. Hence, the cell walls break down and the bacteria die.

Proteins also act as receptors for the body's regulatory chemicals, such as hormones and neurotransmitters. Drugs can mimic these chemicals or block their effects at the receptor sites.

A drug's ability to combine with a receptor is called *affinity; efficacy* refers to the drug's ability to activate the receptor. Drugs that have both characteristics are *agonists*. The degree of response to an agonist depends on the drug's affinity for the receptor site and its concentration there.

Drugs called *antagonists* may also combine with a receptor; these produce no pharmacologic response but inhibit actions of agonists for this receptor. An antagonist can be either competitive or noncompetitive. It's competitive if a sufficiently high dose of an agonist can overcome its effects. For example, enough histamine (agonist) can overcome antihistamine (antagonist). The process in this case is reversible.

An antagonist is noncompetitive if an agonist can't overcome it, regardless of dose. For example, organophosphates noncompetitively block cholinergic receptors. The process in this case is irreversible, since the antagonist inactivates the receptor.

Whether a drug is an agonist or antagonist, its affinity for the receptor depends on its specific molecular structure. Relatively small changes in the drug molecule may result in major differences in the pharmacologic effect. This relationship of molecular configuration to pharmacologic effect is called the *structure-activity relationship*. Modification of the drug's molecular structure may still permit the drug to interact with the receptor but may produce changes in the drug's pharmacokinetic or therapeutic effects.

Investigations of the structure-activity relationships of drugs and of endogenous substances such as hormones have led to the discovery of safer drugs and of new or more effective drugs. Good examples of products developed from such research are the nonsteroidal anti-inflammatory drugs. The drug ibuprofen's chemical structure can be manipulated to obtain a compound with similar therapeutic indications but slightly different pharmacokinetic characteristics. Naproxen's one such compound. Naproxen's longer duration of action may suit some patients' needs better than ibuprofen's short duration of action. Both drugs, however, produce the same therapeutic effect.

4. *Metabolism*
Some drugs are excreted virtually unchanged. Most drugs, however, are metabolized (biotransformed) by the liver before they're excreted by the kidneys. Hepatic metabolism usually produces a metabolite of the drug that is less lipid-soluble and more water-soluble, and thus able to be readily excreted by the kidneys.

A metabolite may be pharmacologically active or inactive. An *active* metabolite may produce effects similar to those of the drug itself or other, possibly toxic, effects.

In some cases, the drug being administered is pharmacologically *inactive* and must be metabolized to the active compound to be effective. Examples of this are cyclophosphamide, a cytotoxic drug, and chloral hydrate, a hypnotic. These inactive drugs must then undergo a second biotransformation before they can be excreted.

The liver is the main site of drug metabolism, but other tissues (for example, the lungs, kidneys, blood, and intestine) may also metabolize drugs. Orally administered drugs traverse the liver before reaching the systemic circulation. If they're significantly metabolized in this process, only a fractional amount of unmetabolized drug remains to cause the desired effect. This *first-pass effect* (biotransformation before the drug reaches general circulation) explains why oral doses of many drugs are much higher than parenteral doses. The oral dosage range of propranolol, for example, is 10 to 80 mg; the I.V. dose is 1 to 3 mg.

The rate at which a drug is metabolized varies with the patient. In some patients, drugs are metabolized so quickly that blood and tissue levels prove therapeutically inadequate. In others, metabolism is so slow that ordinary doses can produce toxic results.

Some drugs can alter the metabolism of other drugs. For example, a drug such as phenobarbital can stimulate hepatic-metabolizing enzymes to speed metabolism and change the effect of the other drugs metabolized by the liver.

Hepatic diseases may affect one or more of the liver's functions, resulting in increased, decreased, or unchanged drug metabolism. Patients with hepatic diseases, therefore, must be closely monitored for drug effect and toxicity.

5. *Excretion*

Some slight elimination takes place through perspiration, saliva, tears, feces, and breast milk. Certain volatile anesthetics, such as halothane, are eliminated primarily by exhalation. But most drugs are excreted by the kidneys either as the unchanged drug or as a metabolite. Renal excretion of drugs follows the usual pattern of excretion: passive glomerular filtration, active tubular secretion, and tubular reabsorption.

Some drugs (digoxin, gentamicin) are eliminated practically unchanged by the kidneys. For safe use of such drugs, renal function must be adequate or the drug will accumulate and produce toxic effects. In a patient with renal impairment, the route of drug excretion should be reviewed and dosage modifications made as necessary. Also, if a patient's renal function changes, all current medications in his regimen must be reevaluated.

Some drugs can alter the effect and excretion of other drugs. For example, probenecid can block renal excretion of penicillin, causing it to accumulate and enhancing its effects. Antacids speed excretion and thus diminish the effects of salicylates (aspirin).

A drug's excretion is also affected by its blood concentration, half-life, and accumulation in the body. Here's what you should know about these factors:

- *Blood concentration*. The ongoing processes of absorption, distribution, metabolism, and excretion are continuously affecting blood concentration of a drug. Absorption of an oral drug is greater than its excretion until the peak blood level is reached. After this, more drug is excreted than absorbed, and the blood concentration of the drug falls. A drug administered by I.V. bolus is immediately bioavailable, rapidly distributed, and excreted.
- *Half-life*. This is the time required for the blood concentration of a drug to decrease by 50%. Half-life is an important drug characteristic used to establish optimum dosage regimens, such as loading dose, maintenance dose, and duration between doses. For example, a drug with a short half-life, such as penicillin G, must be given several times daily to maintain therapeutic effects; a drug like digoxin with a long half-life can be given once daily.

The figure opposite shows the half-life of an I.V. injection of gentamicin. Since for every half-life the concentration of the drug is halved, after five half-lives, 95% of the drug will have been eliminated.

- *Accumulation*. Many drugs reach a therapeutic blood level after the same dose is repeated several times. When an immediate response is required, a large or loading dose is given, followed by smaller maintenance doses. The drug will accumulate if each successive dose is given before the previous dose has been completely excreted. This process continues until the dose given is equal to the amount of the drug being excreted. At this time *a steady state* exists, and the blood level will remain in this range as long as consecutive doses are given and no other pharmacokinetic processes (such as renal function, metabolism, or bioavailability) change.

Accumulation explains why the full effects of a drug may not appear for a few days to several weeks after therapy has started. This also explains how toxicity occurs. When a drug is excreted more slowly than it is absorbed, the amount of drug within the blood and organs increases. Unless dosage is decreased, cumulative toxicity results.

Other modifying factors

The patient's age is another important factor that influences a drug's action and effect. For example, elderly patients may have decreased muscle mass and diminished hepatic and renal functions. Consequently, lower doses and longer dosage intervals may be necessary to avoid toxicity in the elderly. (For more information on this subject, see

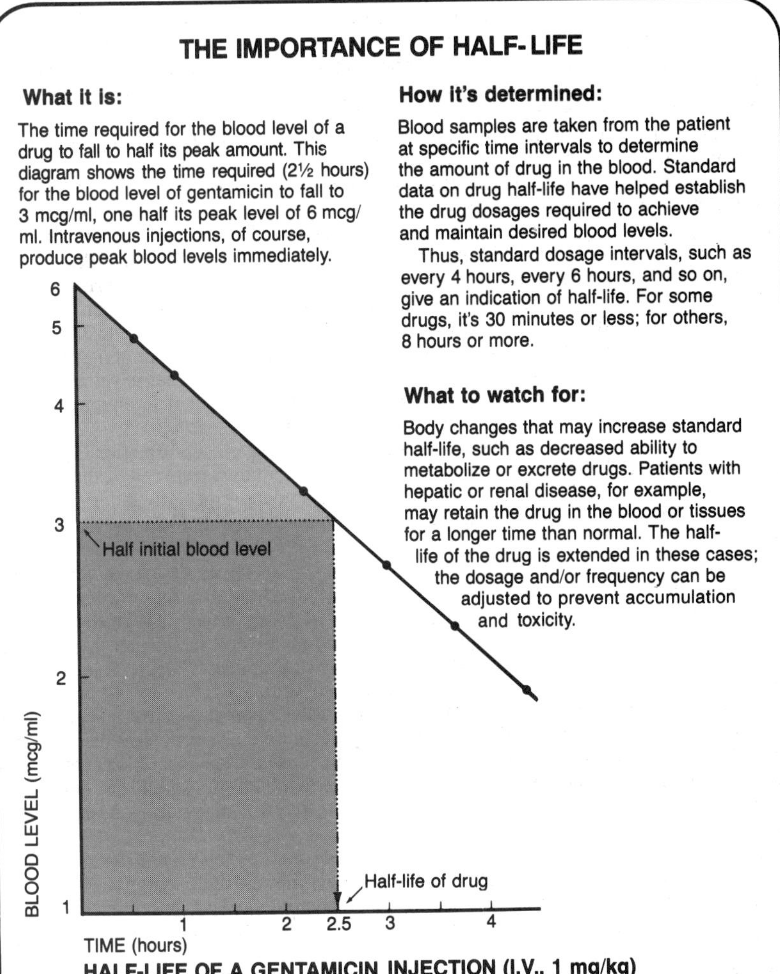

THE IMPORTANCE OF HALF-LIFE
What it is:
The time required for the blood level of a drug to fall to half its peak amount. This diagram shows the time required (2½ hours) for the blood level of gentamicin to fall to 3 mcg/ml, one half its peak level of 6 mcg/ml. Intravenous injections, of course, produce peak blood levels immediately.
How it's determined:
Blood samples are taken from the patient at specific time intervals to determine the amount of drug in the blood. Standard data on drug half-life have helped establish the drug dosages required to achieve and maintain desired blood levels.
Thus, standard dosage intervals, such as every 4 hours, every 6 hours, and so on, give an indication of half-life. For some drugs, it's 30 minutes or less; for others, 8 hours or more.
What to watch for:
Body changes that may increase standard half-life, such as decreased ability to metabolize or excrete drugs. Patients with hepatic or renal disease, for example, may retain the drug in the blood or tissues for a longer time than normal. The half-life of the drug is extended in these cases; the dosage and/or frequency can be adjusted to prevent accumulation and toxicity.
6
5
4
3
2
1
Half initial blood level
Half-life of drug
BLOOD LEVEL (mcg/ml)
1
2
2.5
3
4
TIME (hours)

HALF-LIFE OF A GENTAMICIN INJECTION (I.V., 1 mg/kg)

Chapter 5, DRUG THERAPY IN THE ELDERLY.)

Neonates have underdeveloped metabolic enzyme systems and reduced renal function, both slowing the excretion of some drugs. They need highly individualized doses and careful monitoring. (For more information on this subject, see Chapter 4, DRUG THERAPY IN CHILDREN.)

- *An underlying disease* can also markedly affect drug action. For example, acidosis may cause insulin resistance, and hyperthyroidism may speed the metabolism of some drugs. Genetic diseases—such as glucose-6-phosphate dehydrogenase (G-6-PD) deficiency and hepatic porphyria—may turn drugs into toxins, with serious consequences. A patient with G-6-PD deficiency may develop hemolytic anemia when given sulfonamides or certain other drugs. A genetically susceptible patient can develop an acute attack of porphyria if given a barbiturate or a sulfonamide. When treated with isoniazid, a patient with a highly active hepatic enzyme system (a rapid acetylator, for example) can develop hepatitis from the rapid intrahepatic buildup of a toxic metabolite.
- *Patient noncompliance* to the drug regimen can also affect response to the drug.

What to consider about administration

• *Dosage forms do matter.* Some tablets and capsules are too large for very ill patients to swallow readily. An oral solution or elixir of the same drug may be requested, but the liquid is more easily and completely absorbed and produces higher blood levels than the tablet. When a potentially toxic drug, such as digoxin, is given in solution, the increased amount absorbed can cause toxicity. Also, enteric-coated tablets and sustained-release preparations may affect the degree of absorption of a drug and necessitate a dosage change to produce the desired effect.

• *Routes of administration are not therapeutically interchangeable.* For example, phenytoin (Dilantin) is readily absorbed orally, but slowly and erratically absorbed intramuscularly. Conversely, carbenicillin must be given parenterally because oral administration yields inadequate blood levels to treat systemic infections. Carbenicillin is given orally only to treat urinary tract infections because it concentrates in the urine.

• *The timing of drug administration can be important.* Sometimes, giving an oral drug during or shortly after mealtime decreases the amount of drug absorbed. This is not clinically significant with most drugs and may, in fact, be desirable with irritating drugs such as aspirin or indomethacin (Indocin). Certain penicillins and tetracyclines should not be given with meals because some foods can inactivate them. If in doubt about the effects of foods on a certain drug, check with a pharmacist.

• *The patient's age, height, and weight should be considered.* This information is essential when calculating the dose for many drugs. It should be accurately recorded on the patient's chart. The chart should also include current laboratory data, especially kidney and liver function studies, and whether the patient is edematous or dehydrated so that dosages can be adopted.

• *Metabolic changes may occur.* Physiologic changes, such as depressed respiratory function or the development of acidosis or alkalosis, might alter drug effect.

• *The possibility of pregnancy should be considered.* Many drugs may produce effects that are harmful to a developing fetus. Before a drug is given to a woman in her child-bearing years, she should be asked whether she may be pregnant. (For more information on administering drugs to pregnant patients, see pp. 12 to 13.)

• *The patient's history is important.* Whenever possible, a comprehensive family history should be obtained from the patient or his family, including past or present diseases that contraindicate a drug currently being used. Past reactions to drugs, possible genetic traits that might alter drug response, and the concurrent use of other drugs should be considered. Multiple drug therapy can dramatically change the effects of many drugs or cause drug interactions.

• *Foods in the stomach may speed up, retard, or sometimes even prevent drug absorption.* And some foods may affect one drug on way and another a different way.

Drugs given orally go through several processes before entering systemic circulation. Tablets, for example, must disintegrate and dissolve before they can be absorbed through the intestinal mucosa. But tablet breakdown is affected by the stomach's pH, so when food changes the pH, the rate and degree of breakdown—and of drug absorption—may also change.

Food stimulates various body secretions, including gastric acid and bile. For this reason, acid-labile drugs should be taken on an empty stomach, when gastric acid secretions are minimal. Fat-soluble drugs, however, should be administered with meals because bile helps disolve them.

Food delays stomach emptying, so a drug given with meals may remain in the stomach longer and delay therapeutic effect. So, for a rapid effect, the drug should be administered when the patient's stomach is empty.

But sometimes a food buffer may be useful. It can, for example, reduce the gastrointestinal distress, nausea, and mucosal damage caused by ulcerogenic drugs such as aspirin and indomethacin (Indocin).

Drug interactions

A drug interaction takes place when one drug administered in combination with or shortly after another drug alters the effect of one or both drugs. Usually, the effect of one drug is either increased or decreased. (In rare instances, an effect that cannot be attributed to either drug alone results.)

Drug interactions may result from alterations of the pharmocokinetics of absorption, distribution, metabolism, or excretion of one drug by another or from a combination of the drugs' actions or effects. For instance, one drug may inhibit or stimulate the metabolism or excretion of the other; or it may displace another from plasma-protein binding sites, freeing it for further action. Remember these points:

• *Combination therapy is based on drug interaction.* One drug, for example, may be given to potentiate, or increase, the effects of another. Probenecid, which blocks the excretion of penicillin, is sometimes given with penicillin to maintain adequate blood levels of penicillin for a longer period. Often, two drugs with similar actions are given together precisely because of the *additive effect* that results. For instance, aspirin and codeine, both analgesics, are given in combination because together they provide greater pain relief than either does alone.

• *Drug interactions are sometimes used to prevent or minimize certain side effects.* Hydrochlorothiazide and spironolactone, both diuretics, are administered in combination because the former is potassium-depleting and the latter, potassium-sparing.

• *Harmful drug interactions decrease efficacy or increase toxicity.* A hypertensive patient well controlled with guanethidine may see his blood pressure rise to its former high level if he takes the antidepressant amitriptyline (Elavil) at the same time. Drug combinations that produce antagonism between two drugs should be avoided if possible. Another kind of inhibiting effect occurs when tetracycline is administered with drugs or foods that contain calcium or magnesium (for example, antacids, milk). The calcium and magnesium ions combine with tetracycline in the GI tract and cause inadequate absorption of the tetracycline.

• *Several other factors may contribute to an adverse drug interaction:*

—use of more than one medication to treat a condition
—ingestion of alcohol alone with medication
—self-medication with over-the-counter drugs or another person's prescription
—treatment by more than one doctor for different ailments.

Many adverse drug interactions can be prevented by appropriate modifications in dose, time, or route of administration. Patients receiving drugs that may interact must be monitored closely and taught to look for signs that may indicate adverse interaction.

Side effects

Any drug effect other than what is therapeutically intended is called a side effect. It may be expected and benign, or unexpected and potentially harmful. For example, during hay fever season, a patient may have to contend with the drowsiness caused by an antihistamine, such as chlorpheniramine, to obtain relief from hay fever symptoms. However, the woman who develops thrombophlebitis while taking oral contraceptives faces possible serious complications and hospitalization.

Thus, a side effect may be tolerated for the drug's therapeutic effect, or it may be so unacceptable or hazardous that the drug must be discontinued. Many dose-related side effects lessen or disappear when dosage is reduced (guanethidine-induced orthostatic hypotension is an example). Other side effects subside after continued drug use: Drowsiness associated with methyldopa (Aldomet) and orthostatic hypotension associated with prazosin (Minipress) usually subside after several days as the patient builds up a tolerance to these effects.

Although most side effects are therapeutically undesirable, occasionally one can be put to clinical use. For example, the drowsiness associated with diphenhydramine (Benadryl) makes this drug clinically useful as a mild hypnotic.

To deal with side effects correctly, even minor changes in the patient's clinical status should be noted. Minor changes, such as signs of hypersensitivity and idiosyncratic reactions, may be an early warning of pending toxicity.

Hypersensitivity, a term sometimes used interchangeably with drug allergy, is the result of an antigen-antibody immune reaction that occurs when a drug is given to a susceptible patient. To be susceptible, the patient must have had prior exposure to the drug (or one of its derivatives).

Hypersensitivity can produce a relatively mild reaction such as urticaria, a more severe reaction such as serum sickness with symptoms of fever and lymphadenopathy, or a life-threatening anaphylactic reaction characterized by hypotension, bronchospasm, and laryngeal edema. One of the most common hypersensitivities is penicillin allergy, with patient response ranging from rash to anaphylaxis.

Idiosyncratic reactions occur rarely. These are highly unpredictable, individual, and unusual. Probably the best known is aplastic anemia, caused by the antibiotic chloramphenicol (Chloromycetin). This reaction develops in only 1 in 40,000 patients, but it's usually fatal. A more common idiosyncratic reaction is extreme sensitivity to very low doses of a drug, or insensitivity to higher-than-normal doses.

Recognizing drug allergies or serious idiosyncratic reactions can be lifesaving. The patient should be asked about drugs he is taking or has taken in the past and what, if any, unusual effects he's experienced from taking them. If a patient claims to be allergic to a drug, he should explain exactly what happened when he took it. He may be calling a harmless side effect, such as upset stomach, an allergic reaction, or he may have a true tendency to anaphylaxis. In either case, this information is needed. Of course, any clinical changes throughout the patient's hospital stay must be recorded and reported. If a hazardous side effect is suspected, the drug should be withheld until the effect is evaluated.

The patient's complaints about how a drug makes him feel should be considered objectively. Undesirable side effects may be reduced in several ways. Obviously, reducing dosage helps in many cases, but so may simply rescheduling the same dose. For example, although pseudoephedrine (Sudafed) may stimulate a patient, this may not be a problem if it's given early in the day. Similarly, the drowsiness that occurs with antihistamines or tranquilizers can be acceptable—even desirable—to the patient if the dose is given at bedtime.

Most important, the patient needs to be told what side effects to expect so he won't become worried or stop taking the drug on his own. Of course, he should be reminded to report any unusual or unexpected side effects.

Toxic reactions

Toxic reactions to drugs can be either *acute*, resulting from an excessive dose accidentally or deliberately taken, or *chronic*, from accumulation of the drug in the body. These toxic effects may be extensions of the desired pharmacologic effect. For example, barbiturates produce hypnotic and sedative effects by acting as nonspecific central nervous system (CNS) depressants. Toxic reactions to barbiturates are exhibited by excessive CNS depression, resulting in depressed respirations, decreased deep tendon reflexes, and possibly coma.

Drug toxicities may also result when drug blood levels rise because of impaired metabolism or excretion. For example, blood levels of theophylline rise when hepatic dysfunction impairs metabolism of the drug. Similarly, digoxin toxicity can follow impaired renal function because digoxin is excreted from the body almost exclusively by the kidneys (by glomerular filtration).

Of course, toxic blood levels also result from excessive dosage. Tinnitus (ringing in ears) caused by aspirin, for example, may be a sign that a safe dose has been exceeded. Most drug toxicity is predictable and dose-related; fortunately, most drug toxicity is also readily reversible with dosage adjustment.

Patients should be carefully monitored for physiologic changes, such as impaired hepatic or renal function, that may alter drug effect. The patient should be told the signs of toxicity, and what to do if a toxic reaction occurs. He should take a drug exactly as prescribed: Serious problems may arise if he changes the dose or schedule. For detailed management of drug toxicity, see APPENDIX, *Drug Toxicities*.

Drugs and pregnancy

Ever since the thalidomide tragedy of the late 1950s—when thousands of infants were born malformed after their mothers used this mild sedative-hypnotic during pregnancy—use of drugs during pregnancy has been a source of medical concern and controversy.

To identify drugs that may cause teratogenesis (the production of physical defects in offspring in utero), preclinical drug studies always include tests on pregnant laboratory animals. These tests point out gross teratogenicity but do not clearly establish safety. Different species react to drugs in different ways, and animal studies do not rule out possible teratogenic effects in humans. For example, the preliminary animal studies on thalidomide gave no warning of teratogenic effects, and it was subsequently released for general use in Europe.

To prevent such tragedies, almost all drugs carry a warning on the package insert. Such warnings state that safety in human pregnancy has not been established, and use of the drug in pregnancy requires that the expected therapeutic benefit be weighed against the possible hazard to mother and fetus. With the exception of vitamins and minerals, no drug is approved warning-free for use in pregnancy. Even Bendectin (a combination of the antihistamine doxylamine and the vitamin pyridoxine, for which nausea and vomiting of pregnancy are official indications) carries a warning for cautious use during pregnancy.

At one time, the placenta was thought to protect the fetus from drug effects, but today the idea of a placental barrier is considered a myth. Almost all drugs cross the placental membrane to some extent. Orally administered drugs that can cross the GI membrane can probably cross the placental membrane. Only drugs with exceptionally large molecular structure, such as heparin, will not cross the placenta; nevertheless, their use in pregnancy still requires caution. Just because drugs cross the placenta, however, does not necessarily mean they will harm the fetus.

Actually, only one factor seems clearly related to exaggerated risk in drug therapy during pregnancy: the stage of fetal development. During two stages of pregnancy—the first and third trimesters—the fetus is especially vulnerable to damage from the mother's use of drugs. During these times, *all* drugs should be given with extreme caution. The most sensitive period for drug-induced fetal malformation is the first trimester, when fetal organs are differentiating (organogenesis). During this time, *all* drugs should be withheld unless doing so would jeopardize the mother's health. Theoretically, during this sensitive time, even aspirin could harm the fetus. So patients should be strongly advised to avoid *all* self-prescribed drugs during the first trimester.

The other time of high fetal sensitivity to drugs is the last trimester. At birth, the newborn must rely on his own metabolism to excrete any drug remaining in his body. Since his detoxifying systems are not fully developed, any residual drug may take a long time to be metabolized—and thus may induce prolonged toxic reactions. Consequently, drugs should be used with caution during the last 3 months of pregnancy and only when absolutely necessary at term.

Nevertheless, in many circumstances, pregnant women must continue to take certain drugs. For example, a woman with epilepsy who is well controlled with an anticonvulsant should continue to take it even during pregnancy. Or a pregnant woman with a bacterial infection must receive antibiotics. In such cases, the potential risk to the fetus is outweighed by the mother's need for the drug.

Following these general guidelines can prevent indiscriminate and potentially harmful use of drugs in pregnancy:

- Before a drug is prescribed for a woman of childbearing age, she should indicate the date of her last menstrual period and whether she may be pregnant.
- Especially during the first and third trimesters, a pregnant patient should avoid *all* drugs except those *essential* to maintain the pregnancy or her health.
- Topical drugs are not exempt from the warning against indiscriminate use during pregnancy. Many topically applied drugs can be absorbed in amounts large enough to be harmful to the fetus.
- When a pregnant patient needs *any* drug, the doctor should prescribe the *safest* possible drug in the *lowest* possible dose to minimize any harmful effect to the fetus.
- Every pregnant patient should check with her doctor before taking *any* drug.

Drugs and lactation

Most drugs a breast-feeding mother takes appear in breast milk. Drug levels in breast milk tend to be high when blood levels are high—generally, shortly after taking each dose. Therefore, the mother should breast-feed *before* taking medication, not *after*.

Breast-feeding should be temporarily interrupted and replaced with bottle-feeding when the mother must take tetracyclines, chloramphenicol, sulfonamides (during first 2 weeks postpartum), oral anticoagulants, iodine-containing drugs, antineoplastics, and propylthiouracil.

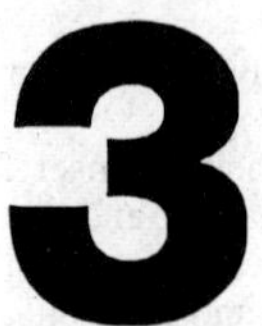

Drug therapy in adults

Since health-care professionals are responsible for prescribing and administering medications, their knowledge of drug therapy and administration must be thorough and up-to-date. What follows is a list of key points.

I. General considerations

- No medicine, not even a placebo, should ever be administered to a patient except under medical supervision. Nevertheless, every member of the health-care team who is directly responsible for patient care should know how a given drug can be expected to act, as well as whatever unpleasant or harmful side effects it can have.
- Before administering a drug, read the label on the bottle three times (when taking it from the shelf, when preparing the dose, and when returning it to the shelf). Remember that the names of different drugs often have similar spellings. If the bottle is without a label, obtain a replacement. Never give a patient anything found in an unlabeled bottle, and properly identify the person receiving the medication.
- Always be sure to replace the cap on any bottle of medication you open. Make sure, too, that it is tightly shut. Do not leave any bottles of medication lying about, and never leave medications at a patient's bedside, except—with caution—antacids, anticholinesterase medications, nonnarcotic cough syrups, inhalants, various lotions and ointments, and nitroglycerin.
- When storing drugs, keep preparations designed for external use only separate and distinct from those designed for internal use. Insist that the pharmacist affix "external use only" labels on drug containers. Of course, keep narcotics and other controlled drugs under double lock.
- Doses of medication should always be administered within at least 30 minutes of the time officially prescribed. This is especially important when administering antibiotics, chemotherapeutic agents, and anticholinesterase agents, as it is essential that a particular level of such drugs be maintained in the bloodstream. Should any dose of medication not be given as scheduled, the reason should be documented.
- Do not give medication that is discolored or in which a precipitate has formed unless the manufacturer's instructions indicate that doing so is not harmful.
- Privacy should be provided as needed when administering certain medications (suppositories, retention enemas, etc.).
- Accurate records should be kept of all doses of medication administered. Also the patient's reactions to medications should be noted, and in the case of narcotics, the patient's pulse and respiration routinely recorded as well.
- Discard needles and syringes into proper containers.
- Store drugs as recommended.
- If large numbers of tablets or capsules are found to be necessary for a single dose, a special dosage form prepared by the pharmacist would be more convenient to the patient.
- Wash your hands thoroughly before preparing or administering any medication.

II. Specific precautions for certain drugs

- *Digitalis preparations.* Before a patient is given any digitalis preparation, his pulse rate should be noted; if the apical pulse is abnormally fast or slow for that patient, or has changed drastically since the previous dose, toxicity may be indicated.
- *Heparin.* 0.1 cubic centimeters of air should be drawn into the syringe before administering heparin subcutaneously. This clears the heparin from the syringe and helps prevent it from leaking into tissue, thus avoiding localized hemorrhaging. The possibility

of hematoma can be reduced by injecting heparin into the subcutaneous tissues of the abdomen above the iliac crest. Drawing back the plunger to check for insertion into a vein *should not be done;* doing so will make the needle waver and precipitate a hematoma. For the same reason, the injection site should never be massaged; doing so could rupture capillaries.

• *Insulin.* Administration of insulin requires a definite plan for rotation of injection sites. The arms, thighs, abdomen, and buttocks together provide at least 56 different injection sites. But care must be taken that the same site is not used more than once every two months; otherwise, changes brought about in the fatty tissue can make the absorption of insulin more difficult.

When mixing regular insulin with a longer-acting type, the regular insulin should be drawn up first to avoid contaminating it with the insoluble longer-acting type. Regular insulin should always be maintained in pure solution, so that, in the event of an emergency, it can be given I.V.

• *Narcotics.* Administration of narcotics requires careful monitoring of the patient's respiration. Narcotics tend to depress the respiratory center, and a respiratory rate of 12 or below is too low for safe administration of narcotic drugs. Also, the patient's pulse rate is an indicator of pain and should be checked and correlated with his respiration rate.

• *Paraldehyde.* Parenteral paraldehyde should always be administered with a glass syringe; it interacts chemically with plastic. For the same reason, oral paraldehyde should never be administered in a Styrofoam cup.

III. Oral medications

• Instructions on a bottle of medicine should always be read and followed carefully.

• Liquid medicine should be poured with the label side up, and the mouth of the bottle should be wiped, so that none of the liquid spills over and obscures the instructions written on the label.

• Holding a graduated medicine cup at eye level ensures accuracy.

• If a dose of medication is to be measured in drops, a medicine dropper should be used and held at a 90° angle.

• Tablets should not be broken unless they are scored.

• Enteric-coated tablets should not be given with milk or antacids. Higher pH causes these tablets to dissolve prematurely in the stomach.

• The patient should not chew, crush, dissolve, or tamper with enteric-coated tablets or sustained-action medication.

• A patient having difficulty swallowing a pill should place it far back in his mouth, since stimulating the back of the tongue activates the swallowing mechanism.

• The patient should be provided with water or another suitable liquid while he takes the medication.

• Diluting a drug usually makes it more palatable and may promote absorption. Liquid medications—except cough syrups, oils, and antacids—should be diluted with water or juice, unless contraindicated (information on label should be checked to determine how compatible the medication is with various juices). Only water should be used for diluting medications for patients with diabetes and for patients on potassium restriction.

IV. Parenteral medications

• The term parenteral, when applied to the administration of drugs, refers to the introduction of drugs into the body by means of injection into the upper layers of the skin, the subcutaneous tissue, the muscles, or the veins.

Intradermal
• Intradermal injections are those made into the upper layers of the skin. Drugs are administered in this way as skin tests.
• The medial surface of the forearm is perhaps the most commonly used site for intradermal injection. Use a tuberculin syringe with a fine, short 26G needle. Cleanse the area, hold the syringe at a 15° angle, and make sure the tip of the needle enters just under the outer layer of the skin. If done properly, a small bleb should form. No more than 0.1 ml should be injected.

Subcutaneous
• Subcutaneous injections are those made beneath the skin. Drugs administered this way are absorbed into the system more slowly than those administered intramuscularly or intravenously. Only nonirritating drugs should be injected subcutaneously, and the amount injected should never exceed 2 ml. Use a hypodermic syringe with a 25G needle.
• Any body surface area where there is loose connective tissue that is located away from the large blood vessels and large muscle groups may be used as a site for subcutaneous injection. Favored areas include the outer surface of the upper arm and the anterior and lateral surfaces of the thigh.
• Clean the injection site with an alcohol sponge beforehand, using a circular motion and moving from the center outward.
• To prevent the needle from entering the muscle, insert it at a 45° angle, and hold the tissue surrounding the injection site in cushion fashion. Release the tissue as soon as the needle is inserted; otherwise, pressure against the nerve endings will cause pain.
• Take care that the needle does not enter a blood vessel; if it does, the solution will be absorbed into the system immediately, and this could prove dangerous. Prevent this by pulling back gently on the plunger after the needle is inserted; if blood appears, withdraw the needle, prepare another dose—using another syringe and needle—then insert it again at a different angle and site. Test again, and if no blood appears, slowly inject the solution.
• Withdraw the needle quickly; this prevents the tissue from pulling, which causes pain. Gentle massage of the injection site with an alcohol sponge stimulates the circulation in the area and facilitates the distribution and absorption of the solution into the system.
• Each injection site should be recorded and a plan for rotation devised.

Intramuscular
• An intramuscular injection introduces into muscular tissue a medicinal solution that is then absorbed into the bloodstream.
• Any body surface area with a significant amount of muscular tissue and located away from large blood vessels and nerves may serve as a site for intramuscular injection. Favored areas include the mid-deltoid area, the gluteus medius, the ventrogluteal area, and the vastus lateralis.
• When injecting into the gluteal region, take care to avoid injecting the needle into either the sciatic nerve or the superior gluteal artery. Have the patient lie on his stomach with his toes pointing inward; this helps the muscles relax and provides maximum exposure.
• Injecting a needle into a tense muscle causes pain. Have the patient relax beforehand by taking several slow, deep breaths.
• Ordinarily, a 1½", 21G needle is used for I.M. injections. A shorter needle should be used if the patient is thin, and a longer one if he is obese. The viscosity of the solution itself must also be taken into consideration when determining what gauge needle to use.
• After drawing up the medication into the syringe, draw up approximately 0.2 or 0.3 ml of air into the syringe as well. The air bubble clears the needle after the drug is injected and prevents leakage into subcutaneous tissue.
• Clean the injection site beforehand, using a circular motion and moving from the center outward. Insert the needle at a 90° angle.
• Take care that the needle does not enter a blood vessel; if it does, the solution will be absorbed more rapidly than intended. To prevent this, pull back gently on the plunger

after the needle is inserted; if blood appears, withdraw the needle, prepare another dose—using another syringe and needle—then insert it again at a different angle and site. Test again, and if no blood appears, slowly inject the solution.

• Withdraw the needle quickly; this prevents the tissue from pulling, which causes pain. Gentle massage of the injection site with an alcohol sponge stimulates the circulation in the area and facilitates distribution and absorption of the solution into the system.

• When injecting substances that stain or are irritating, use the Z-track method. Use a needle that is 2″ long. In addition to the medication, draw up approximately 0.2 ml of air into the syringe. Then change the needle. Before injecting laterally, displace the subcutaneous tissue at the injection site (when using this technique, always inject into the gluteus medius). Upon completing the injection, wait 10 seconds before withdrawing the needle. This delay, the air bubble, and the relaxation of the laterally displaced tissue upon its release, together help ensure that the needle track is properly sealed off. Do not massage the injection site after the needle is withdrawn. Doing so can cause the solution to back into the subcutaneous tissue.

• Each injection site should be recorded and a plan for rotation devised.

Intravenous

• Intravenous therapy involves introducing medication or other parenteral fluids into a patient's vein. A bolus injection introduces a concentrated amount of solution all at once. An intravenous infusion introduces a large amount of fluid over an extended period. Intravenous infusions are used to maintain or replace the body's water, electrolytes, and calories; to restore the body's acid/base balance; to replenish blood volume; and to provide access for the administration of various medications.

• Substances injected intravenously are absorbed into the system immediately. Take special care to prevent or recognize toxic reactions or shock caused by introducing too much solution too quickly or by allergic reactions. The patient's condition, age, the type

REDUCING THE PAIN OF I.M. INJECTIONS

You can reduce the pain of I.M. injections by following these tips:

• *Encourage your patient to relax the muscle you'll be injecting.* Injections into tense muscles cause more pain and bleeding than injections into relaxed muscles. (Give injections into the gluteal muscles while the patient lies face down with his toes pointed in, or on his side with the knee and hip of the upper leg flexed and anterior to the lower leg).

• *Avoid extra-sensitive areas.* When you choose the injection site, roll the muscle mass under your fingers and look for twitching. This indicates an extra-sensitive "trigger" area. Injections in this area may cause referred pain or a sharp pain as if the nerve were hit.

• *Wait until the skin antiseptic is dry.* If the antiseptic is still wet, it clings to the needle, creating pain when it reaches the sensory nerves of the subcutaneous tissues.

• *Always use a new needle.* The point and bevel of the needle can be dulled when they pass through the rubber stoppers in vials. Unless you change the needle, the dulled or rough edge that results causes more friction and pain during injection. Changing the needle also removes another source of pain—irritating medication that adheres to the outside of the needle when you draw the medication out of the vial.

• *Draw about 0.2 cc of air into the syringe.* This clears the needle bore of medication, which could leak out through the needle before or during insertion. When the needle is inverted for the injection, the air bubble rises to the plunger end of the syringe. Injecting this harmless air bubble reduces "tracking"—the leakage of medication from the needle injection path.

• *Dart the needle in rapidly and withdraw it rapidly to minimize puncture pain.*

• *Aspirate to be sure the needle isn't in a blood vessel.* Then, inject the medication slowly to allow it to spread into the tissue under less pressure.

• *Unless contraindicated, massage the relaxed muscle to distribute the medication better and increase its absorption.* This will reduce the pain caused by tissue stretching from a large-volume injection. (Physical exercise of the injected muscle serves the same purpose.)

of fluid or drug being administered, the size of the administration set, and the viscosity of the liquid itself are the principal factors determining the rate of flow, which should (for accuracy) be measured in microdrops (requiring a special solution set), and strictly in accordance with the doctor's instructions.

• The medication should be diluted according to directions, using an unopened, sterile vial of diluent, since diluent used previously for other drugs may well have been contaminated by them. Most drugs prove irritating to the vessel walls, but proper dilution can at least keep such irritation to a minimum. Unit doses are best diluted and prepared by the pharmacist.

• Before any medication is administered intravenously, the possibility of drug incompatibilities should be considered. The infusion site should be cleaned with an alcohol sponge, using a circular motion and moving from the center outward, before insertion of the needle or catheter.

• I.V. tubing and dressings should be changed daily. Apply antimicrobial ointment to the infusion site. The catheter type and the date the needle or catheter was inserted should be recorded on the I.V. dressing and on the patient's chart.

• To administer small amounts (150 ml or less) of I.V. solution or diluted medication, a volume-control I.V. set may be used. Such sets should be changed daily, and the date and time of change should be recorded. Only one medication may be administered via a single volume-control set.

• The piggyback technique, uses minibottles or minibags. Pharmacy prepares a single dose in a 100- to 250-ml bottle. The bottle is attached to a solution set before administration and the line cleared of air. This set is "piggybacked."

• Supplemental drugs may be administered with a needle and syringe into the injection device on the tubing, which should be flushed with 10 ml of sterile normal saline solution immediately before and after each such injection. Supplemental drugs should be administered only one at a time.

• Should the flow of solution stop, signs of infiltration should be checked for first. Then, whether or not the tubing is in any way defective should be determined. Also, holding the bottle below the level of the needle should dislodge backward anything obstructing the flow. The catheter should be irrigated with 1 ml sterile normal saline solution. If a filter is in place, it may need to be changed.

• Before administration of an I.V. bolus, the patient's tolerance should be assessed. How are his vital signs? Is his output sufficient? Medication should be administered slowly. A good rule of thumb is to take not less than 1 minute (the administration rate should be known before injecting). If a particular drug needs to be administered over a period longer than 5 minutes, employing a piggyback infusion or a volume-control set infusion should be considered.

• Adverse reactions to drugs administered I.V. can occur almost immediately. In the event such a reaction does occur, administration should be discontinued immediately. Emergency drugs and equipment should be available at all times.

• When additional fluids are not needed, some medications are injected into a heparin lock, a catheter or cannula inserted into a vein for that purpose. The heparin lock should be flushed immediately before and after with dilute solutions of heparin and/or sterile normal saline.

V. Ophthalmic medications

• The person who is about to instill eye drops should first wash his hands thoroughly.

• When eye drops are instilled, the patient should be positioned with his head back and his eyes open. The lower eyelid should be pulled down in such a way as to form a small pocket with the lid. The patient should roll his eyes upward; then one drop of medication is squeezed onto the lining of the lid. (If more than one drop needs to be administered, the patient should blink before the second is instilled. The part of the dose lost in tears is not a cause for concern.) The medication should be aimed at the lower conjunctiva and not at the cornea, which is very sensitive. Also, no part of the eye should be touched with the eyedropper. The patient should close his eyes immediately upon release of his eyelid; then any excess medication is gently blotted away with a tissue or a cotton ball.

• When eye ointments are instilled, the patient's eyelids are first cleansed with a saline or other irrigating solution. Care should be taken not to contaminate the applicator. After a small amount of medication is squeezed onto the lining of the lower lid, the eyelid should be released, the patient should close his eyes, and excess blotted away.

VI. Ear drops

• Drops should always be administered at room temperature, since cold drops can cause severe pain. The patient should be on his side; the pinna should be gently pulled up and back, and the drops instilled. The patient should lie on his side for several minutes.

VII. Nose drops

• Medication is absorbed into the nostrils more easily if the patient tilts his head backward. The tip of the nostril should be gently raised and the drops instilled. The dropper should not touch the nasal mucosa.

VIII. Topical drugs and suppositories

• Liquid and semisolid topicals should be applied strictly according to directions.
• To administer a rectal suppository, first the tip of the suppository should be lubricated with a small amount of water-soluble jelly. The patient should lie on his left side. The suppository should be inserted with a gloved hand, then the buttocks pressed downward for a few moments until the urge to expel subsides.
• To administer a vaginal suppository, the patient should first assume the lithotomy position. The tip of the suppository should be lubricated with a small amount of water-soluble jelly or water, and the suppository inserted into the vagina with a gloved hand or applicator. The patient should remain with her hips elevated for about 5 minutes.
• When administering a urethral suppository, the perineal area should first be cleansed thoroughly, then the suppository should be inserted, using standard sterile procedures.
• Sublingual tablets should be placed under the patient's tongue, where the rich supply of blood facilitates absorption. The patient should not drink fluids or swallow excessively until the drug is completely absorbed.

PATIENT-TEACHING AID

HOW TO USE NOSE DROPS

Dear Patient:

If the doctor has prescribed nose drops, follow these instructions to instill them correctly:
• position the dropper as shown in this illustration so the medication will flow down the back of your nose, not your throat.
• squeeze the dropper bulb to instill the correct number of drops into the nostril.
• repeat the process in the other nostril, if prescribed.
• breathe through your mouth to avoid sniffing the medication into your sinuses or aspirating into your lungs.

Be sure you know the name of the medication and the prescribed dosage. In addition:
• Follow the doctor's orders exactly. Don't overuse the medication.
• Because nose drops are easily contaminated, don't buy more nose drops than you'll use in a short time. Discard the medication if it contains sediment or looks discolored.
• Don't share your medication with family members. Doing so may spread infection.
• Call the doctor if you notice any side effects.

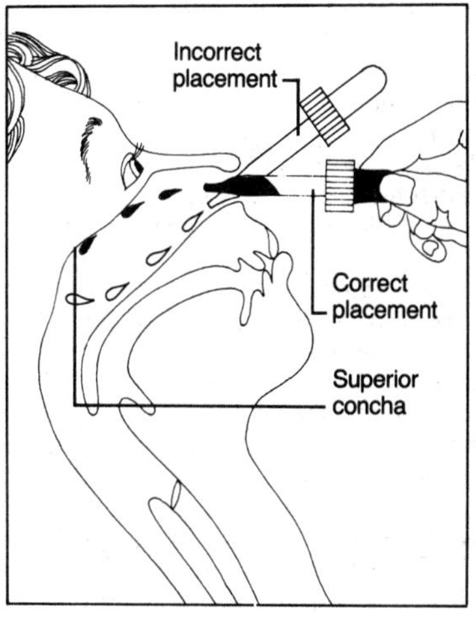

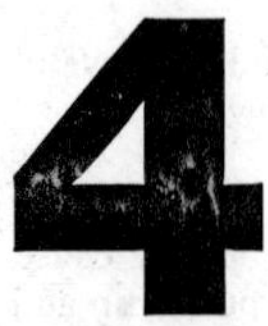

Drug therapy in children

In children, the special characteristics of absorption, distribution, metabolism, and excretion can profoundly affect drug dosage. These factors must be considered when administering drugs to a child to ensure optimal drug effect and minimal toxicity.

Absorption

Drug absorption in children depends on the form of the drug; its physical properties; other drugs or substances, such as food, taken simultaneously; physiologic changes; and concurrent disease.

• The pH of neonatal gastric fluid is neutral or slightly acidic and becomes more acidic as the infant matures. This affects drug absorption. For example, nafcillin and penicillin G, erratically absorbed or malabsorbed in an adult due to degradation by gastric acid, are better absorbed in an infant due to low gastric acidity.

• Various infant formulas or milk products may increase gastric pH and impede absorption of acidic drugs. So, if possible, a child should be given oral medications when his stomach is empty.

• Gastric emptying time and transit time through the small intestine—longer in children than in adults—can affect absorption. Also, intestinal hypermotility (as in diarrhea) can diminish the drug's absorption.

• A child's comparatively thin epidermis allows increased absorption of topical drugs.

Distribution

As with absorption, changes in body weight and physiology during childhood can significantly influence a drug's distribution and effects. In a premature infant, body fluid makes up about 85% of total body weight; in a full-term infant, 55% to 70%; and in an adult, 50% to 55%. Extracellular fluid (mostly blood) comprises 40% of a neonate's body weight, compared with 20% in an adult. Intracellular fluid remains fairly constant throughout life and has little effect on drug dosage.

Since most drugs travel through extracellular fluid to reach their receptors, however, extracellular fluid volume influences a water-soluble drug's concentration and effect. Children have a larger proportion of fluid to solid body weight, so their distribution area is proportionately greater.

Because the proportion of fat to lean body mass increases with age, the distribution of fat-soluble drugs is more limited in children than adults. As a result, a drug's lipid or water solubility affects the dosage for a child.

Binding to plasma proteins

As the result of a decrease in either albumin concentration or intermolecular attraction between drug and plasma protein, many drugs are less bound to plasma proteins in infants than in adults. Furthermore, preparations that bind plasma proteins may displace endogenous compounds, such as bilirubin or free fatty acids. Conversely, an endogenous compound may displace a weakly bound drug. For example, displacement of bound bilirubin can cause a rise in unbound bilirubin, which can lead to increased risk of kernicterus at normal bilirubin levels.

Since only unbound, or free, drug has a pharmacologic effect, any alteration in ratio of protein-bound to unbound active drug can greatly influence effect. Several diseases, such as malnutrition and nephrotic syndrome, can also decrease plasma protein and increase the concentration of unbound drug, intensifying the drug's effect or producing toxicity.

Metabolism

A newborn infant's ability to metabolize a drug depends on the integrity of his hepatic enzyme system, his intrauterine exposure to the drug, and the nature of the drug itself.

Certain metabolic mechanisms are underdeveloped in neonates. Glucuronidation, the mechanism that neutralizes drugs, for example, is insufficiently developed to permit full pediatric doses until the infant is 1 month old. Because of this, the use of chloramphenicol in a newborn infant may cause gray baby syndrome, illustrating the newborn's inability to metabolize the drug. Use of chloramphenicol in neonates, therefore, requires decreased dosage (25 mg/kg/day) and monitoring of blood levels.

Conversely, intrauterine exposure to drugs may induce precocious development of hepatic enzyme mechanisms, increasing the infant's capacity to metabolize potentially harmful substances.

Older children can metabolize some drugs (theophylline, for example) more rapidly than adults. This may be due to their increased hepatic metabolic activity. They may therefore require larger doses than those recommended for adults.

Also, preparations given concurrently to a child may alter hepatic metabolism and induce release of hepatic enzymes. Phenobarbital, for example, can induce hepatic enzyme production and accelerate metabolism of drugs given concurrently.

Excretion

Renal excretion of a drug is the net effect of glomerular filtration, active tubular secretion, and passive tubular reabsorption. Because so many drugs are excreted in the urine, the degree of renal development or presence of renal disease can profoundly affect a child's dosage requirements. If a child is unable to excrete a drug renally, drug accumulation and possible toxicity may result unless dosage is reduced.

Physiologically, an infant's kidneys differ from an adult's in that they have:

- high resistance to blood flow and subsequent decreased renal fraction of cardiac output.
- incomplete glomerular and tubular development and short, incomplete loops of Henle. (A child's glomerular filtration reaches adult values by age 2½ to 5 months; his tubular secretion may reach adult values by age 7 to 12 months.)
- low glomerular filtration rate. (Penicillins are eliminated by this route.)
- decreased ability to concentrate urine or reabsorb various filtered compounds.
- reduced ability by the proximal tubules to secrete organic acids.

Calculating and monitoring pediatric dosages

Formulas that modify adult dosages shouldn't be used for calculating pediatric dosages; a child is not a scaled-down version of an adult. Pediatric dosages should be calculated on the basis of either body weight (mg/kg) or body surface area (mg/m^2).

- Dosages should be reevaluated at regular intervals to ensure necessary adjustments as the child develops.
- Although useful for adults and older children, dosages based on body surface area aren't useful in premature or full-term infants. The body weight method is more reliable.
- The maximum adult dose shouldn't be exceeded when calculating amounts per kilogram of body weight (except with certain drugs, such as theophylline, if indicated).
- An accurate maternal drug history—prescription and nonprescription drugs, vitamins, and herbs or other health foods taken during pregnancy—is necessary because in utero exposure may harm the neonate and hinder subsequent drug therapy.
- Drugs passed through breast milk can also have adverse effects on the nursing infant.

Before a drug is prescribed for a breast-feeding mother, the potential effects on the infant should be investigated. For example, sulfa drugs given to a breast-feeding mother for a urinary tract infection appear in breast milk and may cause kernicterus at lower-than-normal levels of unconjugated bilirubin. Also, high concentrations of isoniazid appear in breast milk. Since this drug is metabolized by the liver, an infant's immature hepatic enzyme mechanisms cannot metabolize the drug, and the infant may suffer central nervous system (CNS) toxicity.

Oral medications

• *When oral medication is given to an infant,* it should be administered in liquid form if possible. For accuracy, a syringe, never a vial or cup, should be used to measure and give the preparation.
• Lifting the infant's head prevents aspiration of the medication, and pressing down on his chin prevents choking.
• The drug may also be placed in a nipple and the infant allowed to suck the contents.
• *If the patient is a toddler,* he should be told how the medication will be given. If possible, the parents should enlist the child's cooperation.
• Even if the medication has a pleasant taste, it shouldn't be mixed with food or called candy.
• The child should drink liquid medication from a calibrated medication cup rather than from a spoon: it's easier and more accurate. If the preparation is available only in tablet form, it can be crushed and mixed with a compatible syrup. (The pharmacist can determine if the tablet can be crushed without losing its effectiveness.)
• *If the patient's an older child* who can swallow a tablet or capsule by himself, he should place the medication on the back of his tongue and swallow it with water or fruit juice. Milk or milk products may interfere with drug absorption.

Intravenous infusions

The following special considerations should be noted when administering I.V. solutions to children.

Protecting the insertion site

In infants, a peripheral vein or a scalp vein in the temporal region should be used for I.V. infusions. The scalp vein is safest since the needle is not likely to be dislodged; however, the head must be shaved around

FLUID AND NUTRITION BALANCE: MEETING INFANTS' AND CHILDREN'S NEEDS

Maintaining proper fluid and electrolyte levels in infants is critical. Why? Because an infant's body is 70% to 75% water, whereas an adult's is only 50% to 60%. Therefore, gastrointestinal upset in an infant may lead to severe dehydration and dangerous disturbance of acid-base and electrolyte balance. Also, administering I.V. fluids too fast can lead to dangerous fluid overload. To help guard against severe dehydration or fluid overload, watch closely for these signs of fluid imbalance when the infant you're caring for is vomiting or has diarrhea.

Fluid overload

• Rapid pulse rate
• Hypertension
• Increased urinary output
• Decreased urine specific gravity
• Edema
• Fine rales

Dehydration

• Rapid pulse rate
• Hypotension
• Decreased urinary output
• Increased urine specific gravity
• Dry mucous membranes
• Depressed fontanelles
• Poor skin turgor
• Lethargy
• Refusal to eat
• Distended abdomen
• Weakness
• Absence of tearing and salivation

Remember, each patient's therapy must be adjusted to his individual needs and tolerance levels. When replacing fluid and electrolytes, the type and amounts you'll use may vary from one age-group to another. Nutritional requirements also change with changing growth patterns.

The tables at right contain some basic guidelines you can follow.

FLUID RECOMMENDATIONS

In Newborn Infants

1st day	60 to 80 ml/kg
2nd day	70 to 90 ml/kg
3rd day	80 to 100 ml/kg
4th day	100 to 120 ml/kg
5th day and thereafter	120 to 140 ml/kg

Note: Patent ductus arteriosus or other congenital cardiac conditions may require that fluids be given with greater caution. Also, increased losses may raise fluid requirements.

In Infants and Children

1 to 10 kg	100 ml/kg/day
10 to 20 kg	1,000 ml plus 50 ml/each kg over 10
20 to 30 kg	1,500 ml plus 20 ml/each kg over 20

Note: Increased losses raise fluid requirements. Also, fluid restriction or concurrent disease may limit fluid intake.

NUTRITIONAL REQUIREMENTS

Protein 1 to 3 g/kg/day

Carbohydrates Enough to supply necessary calories and, in combination with fat, to supply 20 to 50 nonprotein calories for every gram of protein.

Fats 1 to 4 g/kg/day to provide necessary calories in combination with carbohydrates. If patient's fat intake is restricted, supply 2% to 4% of the calories as linoleic acid to prevent essential fatty acid deficiency.

Electrolytes
- Sodium ....3 to 4 mEq/kg/day
- Potassium .....2 to 3 mEq/kg/day
- Chloride ....2 to 4 mEq/kg/day
- Acetate ....1 to 1.5 mEq/kg/day

Vitamins
- Folic acid ......50 to 75 mcg/kg/day
- Vitamin B_{12} ....5 to 10 mcg/kg/day
- Vitamin K ......150 to 200 mcg/kg/day
- MVI ....0.5 ml/kg/day

Minerals
- Phosphate .....1 to 3 millimoles/kg/day
- Calcium ....300 to 800 mg/kg/day as the gluconate salt
- Magnesium ...0.25 to 0.5 mEq/kg/day
- Trace elements
  - *Zinc* ....300 mcg/kg/day in infants less than 3 kg; 100 mcg/kg/day over 3 kg
  - *Chromium* ..0.14 mcg/kg/day
  - *Manganese* 2 mcg/kg/day
  - *Copper* ......20 mcg/kg/day

DAILY CALORIC REQUIREMENTS

0 to 1 year	90 to 120 kcal/kg
1 to 7 years	70 to 100 kcal/kg
7 to 12 years	60 to 75 kcal/kg
12 to 18 years	30 to 60 kcal/kg

Caloric requirements may increase:

- 12% for each degree of fever over 37° C. (98.6° F.)
- 20% to 30% with major surgery
- 40% to 50% with severe sepsis
- 50% to 100% with long-term failure to thrive.

the site. Disfigurement may also result from the needle and infiltrated fluids. For these reasons, the scalp veins are not used as frequently today as they were in the past.

The extremities are the most accessible insertion sites; however, since patients tend to move about, these precautions are necessary:

- The insertion site should be protected to prevent catheter or needle dislodgment.
- A padded arm board should be used to minimize dislodgment.
- The clamp should be placed out of the child's reach; if extension tubing is used to allow the child greater mobility, the connection should be securely taped.
- The child should be restrained only when necessary.
- To allay anxiety, a simple explanation should be given to the child who must be restrained while asleep.

Maintaining flow rate and fluid balance

Administering a continuous I.V. infusion to a child, requires monitoring flow rate and checking the patient's condition and insertion site at least hourly—more frequently when giving medication intermittently.

The flow rate should be adjusted only while the patient is composed; crying and other emotional upset can constrict blood vessels. Flow rate may be retarded if a pump isn't used. Flow should be adequate because some drugs (calcium, for example) can be very irritating at low flow rates.

Making dilutions

Some drugs are hyperosmolar; in infants, these drugs must be diluted to prevent radical changes in fluid that might induce CNS hemorrhage. Sodium bicarbonate, for example, must be diluted to half strength to lower osmolality and lessen the risk of CNS bleeding.

In general, however, the minimum amount of compatible fluid over the shortest recommended period of time is best. Also, the total daily fluid intake and the amount allotted to medication should be checked.

Intramuscular injections

If indicated, intramuscular injections are preferred when the drug cannot be given by other parenteral routes and rapid absorption is necessary.

- In children under 2 years, the vastus lateralis muscle is the preferred injection site; in older children, either the ventrogluteal area or the gluteus medius muscle can be used.
- To determine needle size, the patient's age, muscle mass, and nutritional status, and the drug's viscosity should be considered; injection sites should be recorded and rotated.
- The child who is old enough to understand should be told that the injection will hurt, but that the medication will help him. He should be restrained during the injection and comforted afterward.

Dermatomucosal medications

- Ear drops should be warmed to room temperature; cold drops can cause pain and possible vertigo. To administer, the patient is turned on his side with the affected ear up. If he is younger than 3 years, the pinna is pulled down and back; if he is older than 3 years, the pinna is pulled up and back.
- Inhalants should be avoided in young children, as obtaining cooperation is difficult.
- The inhaler should be explained to an older child before he is given medication through a metered-dose nebulizer. First he holds the nebulizer upside down and closes his lips around the mouthpiece. Then he exhales; pinches his nostrils shut; and when he starts to inhale, releases one dose of medication into his mouth. Finally, he continues inhaling until his lungs feel full.
- Most inhaled agents are not useful if taken orally; therefore, if there is doubt about the patient's ability to use the inhalant correctly, he shouldn't use it.

Parenteral nutrition

Intravenous nutrition is given to patients who can't or won't take adequate food orally and to patients with hypermetabolic conditions who need I.V. supplementation. The latter group includes premature infants and children who have burns or other major trauma, intractable diarrhea, malabsorption syndromes, gastrointestinal abnormalities, emotional disorders such as anorexia nervosa, and congenital abnormalities.

Before fat emulsions are administered to infants and children, however, potential benefits must be weighed against possible risks. Fats—supplied as 10% or 20% emulsions—are administered both peripherally and centrally. Their use is limited by the child's ability to metabolize them. An infant or child with a diseased liver cannot efficiently metabolize fats.

Some fats, however, must be supplied both to prevent essential fatty acid deficiency and to permit normal growth and development. A minimum of calories (2% to 4%) must be supplied as linoleic acid—an essential fatty acid found in lipids. In the infant, fats are essential for normal neurologic development.

Nevertheless, fat solutions may decrease oxygen perfusion and may adversely affect patients with pulmonary disease. This risk can be minimized by supplying only the minimum fat needed for essential fatty acid requirements, not the usual intake of 40% to 50% of the patient's total calories.

Fatty acids can also displace bilirubin bound to serum albumin, causing a rise in free, unconjugated bilirubin and an increased risk of kernicterus. However, fat solutions may interfere with some bilirubin assays and cause falsely elevated levels. To avoid this complication, a blood sample should be drawn 4 hours after infusion of the lipid emulsion; or if the emulsion is introduced over 24 hours, the blood sample should be centrifuged before the assay is performed.

HOW TO GIVE NOSE DROPS TO AN INFANT

Before you begin, wash your hands and gather the bottle of medication, a medication dropper with a protective rubber tip, and tissues.

Important: Warm the medication by running warm water over the bottle for several minutes, or by carrying the bottle in your pocket for 30 minutes.

Now, carefully place the infant with his head tilted back on your arm.

Draw the medication into the dropper.

Then, open the infant's nostrils by gently pushing up the tip of his nose. Instill the ordered number of drops in the nostril. Avoid touching the nostril with the dropper.

Repeat the process in the other nostril, if ordered.

After instilling the drops, keep the infant's head tilted back for 3 to 5 minutes, but be alert for signs of aspiration. If the infant begins to cough, sit him upright and pat his back until he has cleared his lungs.

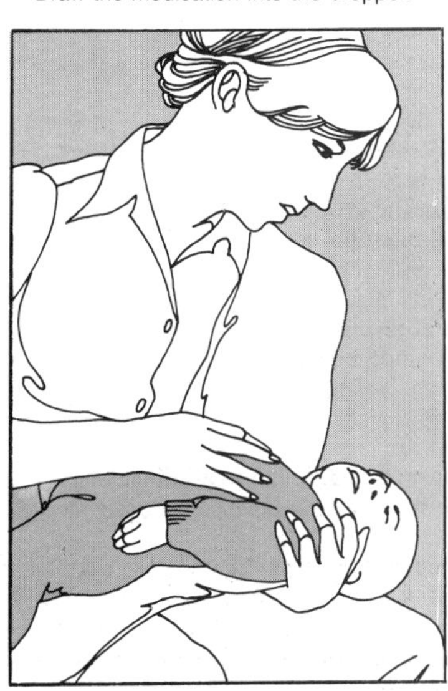

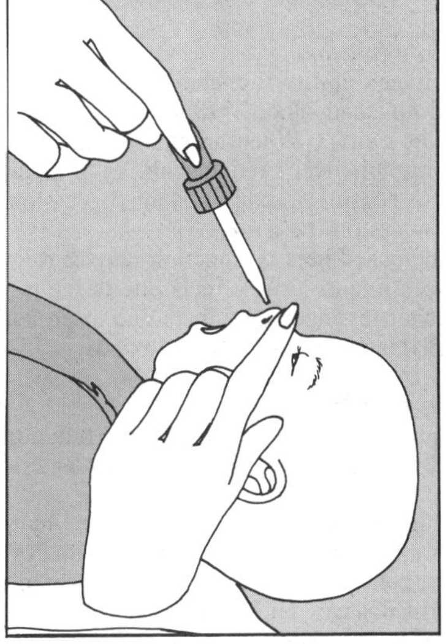

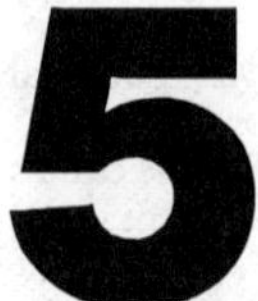

Drug therapy in the elderly

Providing drug therapy for elderly patients requires an understanding of physiologic and pharmacokinetic changes that may alter drug dosage; common adverse reactions; and compliance problems in the elderly.

Physiologic changes affecting drug action

As a person ages, gradual changes occur in his anatomy and physiology. Some of these age-related changes may alter the therapeutic and toxic effects of medications.

Body composition

Proportions of fat, lean tissue, and water in the body change with age. Total body mass and lean body mass tend to decrease; the proportion of body fat tends to increase. Varying from person to person, these changes in body composition affect the relationship between a drug's concentration and solubility in the body. For example, a *water-soluble drug,* such as gentamicin, is *not* distributed to fat. Since there's relatively less lean tissue in an elderly person, more drug remains in the blood, and toxic levels can result. Likewise, pentobarbital, which is distributed *only* to fat, may produce lower blood levels in the elderly patient.

Gastrointestinal function

In the elderly, decreases in gastric acid secretion and gastrointestinal motility slow emptying of stomach contents and movement of intestinal contents through the entire tract. Furthermore, although inconclusive, research shows the elderly may have more difficulty absorbing medications. This is a particularly significant problem with drugs having a narrow therapeutic range, such as digoxin, in which any change in absorption can be crucial.

Hepatic function

The liver's ability to metabolize certain drugs decreases with age. This is probably due to diminished blood flow to the liver, which results from the age-related decrease in cardiac output. When an elderly patient takes certain sleep medications, such as secobarbital, his liver's reduced ability to metabolize the drug may produce a hangover effect due to central nervous system depression. Elimination of these medications is highly dependent on the liver.

Decreased hepatic function may cause:

- more intense drug effects due to higher blood levels
- longer-lasting drug effects due to prolonged blood concentrations
- greater incidence of drug toxicity.

Renal function

Although an elderly person's renal function is usually sufficient to eliminate excess body fluid and waste, his ability to eliminate some medications may be reduced by 50% or more.

Many medications commonly used by the elderly, such as digoxin, are excreted primarily through the kidneys. If the kidneys' ability to excrete the drug is decreased, high blood concentrations may result. Digoxin toxicity, therefore, is relatively common.

Drug dosages can be modified to compensate for age-related decreases in renal function. Aided by laboratory tests, such as BUN and serum creatinine, clinical pharmacists and doctors can adjust medication dosages to provide the expected therapeutic benefits without the risk of toxicity. Patients should be observed for signs of toxicity. A patient taking digoxin, for example, may experience anorexia, nausea, and vomiting.

Adverse drug reactions

As compared with younger people, the elderly reportedly experience twice as many adverse drug reactions, relating to greater drug consumption, poor compliance, and physiologic changes.

Signs and symptoms of adverse drug reactions—confusion, weakness, and lethargy—are often mistakenly attributed to senility or disease. If the adverse reaction isn't identified, the patient may continue to receive the drug. Furthermore, he may receive unnecessary additional medication to treat complications caused by the original medication.

Although any medication can cause adverse reactions, most of the serious reactions in the elderly are caused by relatively few medications: diuretics, digoxin, corticosteroids, sleep medications, and nonprescription drugs. Patients who take these drugs should be carefully observed for toxicities.

Diuretic toxicity

Because total body water decreases with age, normal doses of potassium-wasting diuretics, such as hydrochlorothiazide and furosemide, may result in fluid loss and even dehydration in an elderly patient. These diuretics may deplete serum potassium, causing weakness in the patient; and they may raise blood uric acid and glucose levels, complicating preexisting gout and diabetes mellitus.

Digoxin toxicity

As the body's renal function and rate of excretion decline, digoxin concentrations in the blood may build to toxic levels, causing nausea, vomiting, diarrhea, and most serious, cardiac arrhythmias. Severe toxicity may be prevented by observing the patient for early signs such as appetite loss, confusion, or depression.

Corticosteroid toxicity

Elderly patients on corticosteroids may experience short-term effects including fluid retention and psychological manifestations ranging from mild euphoria to acute psychotic reactions. Long-term toxic effects, such as osteoporosis, can be especially severe in elderly patients who have been taking prednisone or related steroidal compounds for months or even years. To prevent serious toxicity, patients on long-term regimens should be carefully monitored, especially for subtle changes in appearance, mood, and mobility, as well as for signs of impaired healing and fluid and electrolyte disturbances.

Sleep medication toxicity

In some cases, sedatives or sleeping aids, such as flurazepam, cause excessive sedation or residual drowsiness.

Nonprescription drug toxicity

When aspirin and aspirin-containing analgesics are used in moderation, toxicity is minimal, but prolonged use may cause gastrointestinal irritation and gradual blood loss resulting in severe anemia. Although anemia from chronic aspirin consumption can affect all age groups, the elderly are most vulnerable to it because of their already reduced iron stores.

Laxatives may cause diarrhea in elderly patients who are extremely sensitive to drugs such as bisacodyl. Chronic oral use of mineral oil as a lubricating laxative may result in lipid pneumonia due to aspiration of small residual oil droplets in the patient's mouth.

Patient noncompliance
Approximately one third of the elderly fail to comply with their prescribed drug therapy. They may fail to take prescribed doses or to follow the correct schedule; they may take medications prescribed for previous disorders, discontinue medications prematurely, or use p.r.n. medications indiscriminately.

The patient's medication regimen should be reviewed with him. He must clearly understand the dose and the time and frequency of doses. Also, he should know how to take each medication, that is, with food or water, or by itself.

The patient should be given whatever help is necessary to avoid drug therapy problems, and referred to his doctor or pharmacist if he needs further information.

PATIENT-TEACHING AID

TAKING YOUR ORAL MEDICATIONS

Dear Patient:

For your drug therapy to be effective, you must take your medications exactly as your doctor directs, particularly when taking several medications at one time. Here are some helpful hints:

- **Label empty jars,** extra prescription bottles (you can get these from your pharmacist), or envelopes with the times of day or the days of the week you must take medication. Use a separate container for each time. Each morning fill these containers with the appropriate dose of each medication.

Note: Some drugs may deteriorate when exposed to light. Before you remove drugs from their original containers, check with your pharmacist or doctor.

- **Make a medication calendar.** Use a calendar that has enough space to fill in the names of the drugs you need to take each day. Then put a check mark next to the name of the drug after you take each dose.
- **Make a chart.** List:

—name of drug
—what it's for
—what it looks like (shape, color)
—directions for taking the drug
—special cautions or side effects
—time of day to take drug.

Hang this chart near your medicine cabinet.

- **Set your alarm clock** or ask a relative or friend to remind you when to take your medications.

SENILITY OR SIDE EFFECTS?

Myth: *All elderly patients who exhibit symptoms associated with old age (such as drowsiness, forgetfulness, and confusion) are senile.*

Fact: *Many symptoms attributed to senility are actually side effects of drugs commonly prescribed for the elderly.*

Elderly patients themselves may assume that adverse drug reactions are due simply to aging. Thus, if elderly patients aren't warned about side effects, they may ignore them or suffer through them needlessly. Here's what can be done to help distinguish drug effects from senility in the elderly patient:

- The patient's medication should be checked to be sure he's getting the lowest effective dose. Monitoring the patient for therapeutic and adverse effects until steady-state blood concentrations have been attained and documenting observations can help to determine the lowest effective dose.
- The patient should be taught to watch for possible side effects of his medications. He should contact his doctor if they occur.
- He should have a thorough physical examination to rule out undiagnosed conditions, such as cardiac disease and nutritional deficiencies, that can contribute to senility.
- All his medications should be reviewed for possible drug interactions that may cause senilitylike symptoms. Watch for these:

SYMPTOMS	POSSIBLE CAUSES
Confusion	Methyldopa, an antihypertensive agent; digoxin, a cardiac medication; and cimetidine, an antiulcer drug
Depression	Reserpine, an antihypertensive agent
Anorexia	Digoxin
Weakness	Certain diuretics, such as furosemide and hydrochlorothiazide, which can deplete body potassium
Lethargy and drowsiness	Various tranquilizers, analgesics, and sleep medications, including chlorpromazine, meperidine, and pentobarbital
Ataxia	Inappropriately high doses of flurazepam and other sedatives or hypnotics
Forgetfulness	Barbiturates
Constipation	Medications with anticholinergic properties, such as belladonna-containing drugs
Diarrhea	Various oral antacid preparations containing magnesium hydroxide
Gastrointestinal distress	Oral iron preparations or antiarthritic medications, such as aspirin, ibuprofen, or indomethacin

Understanding intravenous solution compatibility

Administering medications by the parenteral route is common today. When parenteral medications are given intermittently, they're best administered using the piggyback method, a volume control burette, or an intermittent infusion device (heparin lock). Thus, multiple venipunctures and possible incompatibilities are avoided when adding medications to a large-volume parenteral solution. However, sometimes medications *must* be administered through a single I.V. line or more than one medication given at a time in a single solution. Then, incompatibility—an undesired physical or chemical reaction between a drug and a solution or another drug—is a significant risk.

Factors affecting compatibility

Many things influence the stability and compatibility of medications—some controllable and some not. Understanding these factors promotes safe and accurate administration of I.V. medications.

- *Concentration of drug:* The higher the concentration of each drug mixed, the greater the chance for ion interaction, which produces incompatibility or instability. Proper dilution of drugs helps minimize this risk.
- *Length of time in solution:* Chemical reactions aren't necessarily instantaneous; reaction rates vary. For example, a reaction may occur in less than 1 second or after many days. However, the longer two drugs remain in contact with each other, the more likely a potential reaction will lead to an undesirable result. The time that drugs are in solution should be minimized by mixing them just before administration.
- *Temperature:* A drug usually remains stable at a low temperature. Reaction rates double for each 10° C. (18° F.) rise in temperature. Many antibiotics in solution are four to eight times more stable under refrigeration (5° C. [41° F.]) than at room temperature (20° to 25° C. [68° to 77° F.]). Refrigerated antibiotics usually may be used for longer periods than those stored at room temperature. Whether the drug can be refrigerated should be determined by checking manufacturer's information or asking the pharmacist.
- *pH:* A drug added to a solution may change the solution's pH or the drug's stability. For example, many antibiotics lose stability in alkaline (pH above 8.0) or acidic (pH below 4.0) solutions. Some solutions decompose if an alkaline drug like calcium, which causes the pH to exceed 7.0, is added.

Physical incompatibility

A drug's physicochemical properties can cause solubility problems that visibly alter the solution: for example, precipitation, altered color, gas formation, turbidity, or cloudiness. Such changes are produced by physical or chemical reactions involving the drug's pH, the solvent, and the container holding the admixture.

Physical incompatibility reactions

- *Color change:* Especially with cephalosporins and phenothiazines, color change or darkening may or may not indicate chemical breakdown. For example, darkened cephalothin solutions may be infused if begun within 6 hours and completed within 24 hours after preparation. Also, chlorpromazine solutions are usable if they're pale yellow but not if they're dark yellow or brown. Nevertheless, any color change of a drug mandates consultation with a pharmacist before administration.
- *Complexation:* This reaction occurs between drugs, inactivating them. For example, tetracycline in the presence of calcium ions forms a complex that inhibits tetracycline's antibacterial action.

• *Adsorption:* Some antibiotics and protein products, such as insulin, adhere to glass or plastic containers, syringes, and administration sets. But, *ad*sorption of insulin varies with its concentration; contact time with tubing or glass; flow rate of insulin solution; and presence of other proteins, such as human serum albumin.
• *Precipitation:* When administered in combination with other drugs or solutions, certain drugs such as phenytoin, diazepam, digoxin, and pentobarbital may form a precipitate.

Chemical incompatibility
Chemical incompatibility causes a drug to degrade to a therapeutically inactive or toxic product. This irreversible breakdown isn't always visible: an example is the interaction of gentamicin and carbenicillin, and ampicillin sodium mixed in 5% dextrose in water stored for 4 hours or more at room temperature before administration.

Chemical incompatibility reactions
• *Oxidation:* A loss of electrons from one drug to another may turn the drug or solution pink, red, brown, or some other color, and make it therapeutically inactive. This reaction occurs especially with epinephrine, morphine, dopamine, and isoproterenol. The risk of oxidation can be minimized by adding an antioxidant (a preservative, such as sodium bisulfite) to the drug, or by packaging the drug in amber glass vials or ampuls.
• *Reduction:* A drug is reduced when it gains electrons from another drug. Penicillins, for example, are reduced when combined with other drugs.
• *Photolysis:* Exposure to light can cause hydrolysis (chemical splitting of a compound by water) or oxidation, discoloring the solution. Photolysis can be minimized in light-sensitive products such as nitroprusside by packaging them in amber glass and covering the container with aluminum foil during administration.

General guidelines
Whenever possible, medications should be administered separately. To minimize incompatibilities, a heparin lock should be used to infuse multiple doses of a drug that's incompatible with other parenteral drugs.

If several incompatible drugs must be infused through the same I.V. line, the tubing should be cleared between doses with a solution compatible with each drug. For example, an order may be given to administer phenytoin I.V. to a patient receiving an infusion of

WHAT BUFFERS DO

Buffers are substances added to drugs or solutions during manufacture to maintain a desired pH. Although a drug may have its own buffer, it is usually too weak to counteract the pH change that occurs when the drug's added to a strongly acidic or alkaline I.V. solution. This change in pH can cause the drug to separate from the primary solution.

Penicillin G potassium, for example, is considered most stable between pH 6.0 and 7.0. But if you add it to a solution of 5% dextrose in water, along with other highly buffered drugs that make the solution alkaline (amphotericin B or cephalothin solution), penicillin G potassium rapidly deteriorates. The ideal pH of I.V. fluids is about 7.4, the pH of blood.

5% dextrose in one half normal saline solution (D_5½ NS); the two are incompatible. First stop the D_5½ NS, then clear the tubing with normal saline solution, administer the phenytoin, clear the tubing again with the normal saline solution, and finally restart the flow of D_5½ NS.

When medications must be administered concurrently or mixed in the same large-volume parenteral solution, the *Intravenous Solution Compatibilities* chart on pp. 34 to 35 and the following guidelines should be considered:

- Chemical analogs or families of drugs react similarly. If one drug in a class is incompatible with the desired solution, others in this class may be incompatible too.
- When preparing a drug, manufacturer's instructions should be followed meticulously because the preservatives used in some diluents may be incompatible with the drug. For example, bacteriostatic normal saline solution contains benzyl alcohol, which is incompatible with a drug such as chloramphenicol sodium succinate.
- When reconstituting I.V. drugs and inspecting for a precipitate, the container shouldn't be shaken; instead it should be rotated or swirled. This action prevents air bubble entrapment and foaming, which impair accurate drug dose measurement in syringes and trigger air exclusion alarms when solutions are administered by infusion pump. Also, air bubbles may be mistaken for particles in the solution.
- When reconstituting a drug, it should be thoroughly mixed before administering or adding it to a solution.
- When mixing drugs in a large-volume parenteral solution, one drug should be added at a time; then the solution should be mixed and examined before adding other drugs. Thorough mixing before adding other drugs prevents layering. Also, adding more than two drugs should be avoided whenever possible.
- Chemical reactions depend on concentration. These reactions may be minimized by adding the most concentrated or most soluble drug to the large-volume parenteral solution first.
- Some precipitates are too fine or too clear to be detected, or are the same color as the

ABBREVIATIONS FOR I.V. SOLUTIONS

AA	Amino acids
D	Dextrose solution (percentage unspecified)
D5LR	Dextrose 5% in Ringer's injection, lactated
D5R	Dextrose 5% in Ringer's injection
D-S	Dextrose-saline combinations
D2.5½NS	Dextrose 2.5% in sodium chloride 0.45%
D2.5NS	Dextrose 2.5% in sodium chloride 0.9%
D5¼NS	Dextrose 5% in sodium chloride 0.225%
D5½NS	Dextrose 5% in sodium chloride 0.45%
D5NS	Dextrose 5% in sodium chloride 0.9%
D10NS	Dextrose 10% in sodium chloride 0.9%
D5W	Dextrose 5% in water
D10W	Dextrose 10% in water
DXN-NS	Dextran 6% in sodium chloride 0.9%
IS	Invert sugar
LR	Ringer's injection, lactated
NS	Sodium chloride 0.9%
PH	Protein hydrolysate
R	Ringer's injection
TPN	Total parenteral nutrition
W	Sterile water for injection

solution. When the container is swirled or rotated, the solution should be inspected for a precipitate in good light against both a dark and light background.

- Color changes in the membrane of any I.V. filter device indicate drug incompatibility not visible in the solution. This reaction becomes visible as the drug is trapped and accumulates in the filter chamber.
- If a physical change, such as a precipitate or discoloration, is detected, the admixture shouldn't be administered and the pharmacist should be notified.
- Administering intermittent medications along with total parenteral nutrition solutions by a central venous catheter should be avoided. Doing so risks contamination and incompatibilities. A secondary line should be used for these drugs.
- Administering medications through the same peripheral venous sites as amino acids and fat emulsions should be avoided; instead, they should be infused through a peripheral site not used for other drug therapy.
- Additives shouldn't be mixed with blood or blood products.
- If no compatibility information is available, drugs shouldn't be mixed. The pharmacist should be consulted.

LAMINAR FLOW HOOD

To reduce the risk of airborne contamination, your hospital pharmacist will probably prepare admixtures under a laminar flow hood such as the one illustrated here. This hood keeps dust particles from entering the work area by providing a constant flow of microfiltered air. The laminar flow hood is one excellent reason why I.V.s should be made up in the pharmacy whenever possible.

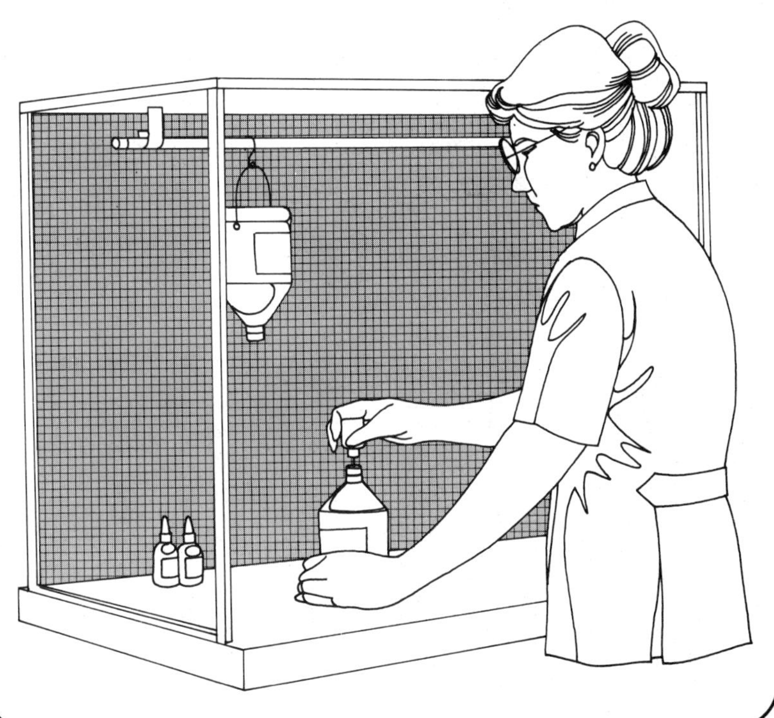

INTRAVENOUS SOLUTION COMPATIBILITIES

Physical compatibility does not exclude the possibility of therapeutic incompatibility.

	albumin	amikacin	aminophylline	amino acid injection	amphotericin B	ampicillin	calcium gluconate	carbenicillin	cefamandole	cefazolin	cefoxitin	cephalothin	chloramphenicol	cimetidine	clindamycin	corticotropin (ACTH)	dexamethasone	dextrose 5% in water	dextrose 5% in lactated Ringer's	dextrose 5% in 0.45% NaCl	dextrose 5% in 0.9% NaCl	diazepam	diazoxide	diphenhydramine
albumin	X	○	○	○		○	○	○	○	○	○	○	○	○	○	○	○	C	C	C	C	●	NR	○
amikacin	○	X	8	○		●	24	8	NR	8	NR	●	24	24	24	○	●	24	24	24	24	●	NR	24
aminophylline	○	8	X	24		●	C	○	○	○	○	●	○	●	●	●	C	C	C	C	C	●	NR	C
amino acid injection	○	○	24	X		12	24	24	○	24	○	24	1	24	24	○	○	C	C	C	C	●	NR	○
amphotericin B						T	O		B	E		P	R	E	P	A	R	E	D		B	Y		P
ampicillin	○	●	●	●		X	●	●	○	○	○	○	1	C	●	○	○	2	4	4	4	●	NR	○
calcium gluconate	○	24	C	24		●	X	C	●	●	○	●	C	○	●	C	C	C	C	C	C	●	NR	C
carbenicillin	○	8	C	24		●	C	X	○	C	○	○	●	○	24	○	○	C	C	C	C	●	NR	○
cefamandole	○	NR	○	○		○	●	○	X	○	○	○	○	○	○	○	○	C	C	C	C	●	NR	○
cefazolin	○	8	○	24		○	●	C	○	X	○	○	24	24	○	○	C	C	C	C	C	●	NR	○
cefoxitin	○	NR	○	○		○	○	○	○	○	X	○	○	○	○	○	○	C	C	C	C	●	NR	○
cephalothin	○	●	●	24		○	●	○	○	○	○	X	C	24	24	○	○	C	C	C	C	●	NR	●
chloramphenicol	○	24	○	○	T	1	C	●	○	24	○	C	X	○	○	C	C	C	C	C	C	●	NR	C
cimetidine	○	24	●	24	O	C	●	○	○	24	○	24	○	X	24	24	○	C	C	C	C	●	NR	○
clindamycin	○	24	●	24		○	○	24	○	○	○	24	○	24	X	○	○	C	C	C	C	●	NR	○
corticotropin (ACTH)	○	○	●	○	B	●	C	○	○	○	○	○	C	○	○	X	○	C	C	C	C	●	NR	○
dexamethasone	○	●	●	○	E	○	C	○	○	C	○	○	C	○	○	○	X	C	C	C	C	●	NR	●
dextrose 5% in water	C	24	C	C		2	C	C	C	C	C	C	C	C	C	C	C	X	○	○	○	●	NR	C
dextrose 5% in lactated Ringer's	C	24	C	C	P	4	C	C	C	C	C	C	C	C	C	C	C	○	X	○	○	●	NR	C
dextrose 5% in 0.45% NaCl	C	24	C	C	R	4	C	C	C	C	C	C	C	C	C	C	C	○	○	X	○	●	NR	C
dextrose 5% in 0.9% NaCl	C	24	C	C	E	4	C	C	C	C	C	C	C	C	C	C	C	○	○	○	X	●	NR	C
diazepam	●	●	●	●	P	●	●	●	●	●	●	●	●	●	●	●	●	●	●	●	●	X	●	●
diazoxide	NR	NR	NR	NR	A	NR	NR	NR	NR	NR	NR	NR	NR	NR	NR	NR	NR	NR	NR	NR	NR	●	X	NR
diphenhydramine	○	24	C	○	R	○	C	○	○	○	○	●	C	○	○	○	●	C	C	C	C	●	NR	X
dopamine	○	○	●	24	E	●	24	24	○	○	○	6	24	○	○	○	○	C	C	C	C	●	NR	○
epinephrine	○	24	●	○	D	○	●	●	○	○	○	●	●	○	○	○	○	C	C	C	C	●	NR	○
erythromycin (I.V.) lactobionate	○	●	C	24		●	C	●	○	●	○	●	●	NR	○	C	○	C	C	C	C	●	NR	24
fat emulsion 10% & 20%	○	●	●	●	B	●	●	●	●	●	●	●	●	●	●	●	●	●	●	●	●	●	●	●
gentamicin	○	NR	NR	24	Y	●	NR	●	NR	NR	NR	●	●	24	24	NR	NR	C	C	C	C	●	NR	NR
heparin sodium	○	●	C	24		●	C	○	○	○	○	8	C	○	24	24	4	C	C	C	C	●	NR	○
hydrocortisone Na succinate	○	○	C	○	P	C	C	24	○	○	○	24	C	○	24	24	4	C	C	C	C	●	NR	●
insulin (regular)	○	○	●	24	H	○	○	○	○	○	○	8	○	24	○	○	○	○	○	○	○	●	NR	○
isoproterenol	○	○	●	24	A	○	C	○	○	○	○	C	○	○	○	○	○	C	C	C	C	●	NR	○
kanamycin	○	○	C	C	R	●	●	●	○	●	24	●	C	○	24	○	C	C	C	C	C	●	NR	○
lactated Ringer's	C	○	C	C	M	8	C	C	C	C	C	C	C	C	C	C	NR	○	○	○	○	●	NR	C
levarterenol (norepinephrine)	○	24	●	24	A	○	C	○	○	○	○	●	○	○	○	C	○	C	C	C	C	●	NR	○
lidocaine	○	○	C	24	C	●	C	C	C	○	○	●	C	○	○	○	C	C	C	C	C	●	NR	C
metaraminol	○	24	○	24	Y	●	○	○	○	○	○	C	C	○	○	○	●	C	C	C	C	●	NR	●
methicillin	○	●	C	24		●	C	○	○	○	○	●	1	○	○	C	C	6	6	6	6	●	NR	C
methylprednisolone	○	○	6	24	O	○	●	○	○	○	○	●	C	○	24	○	○	C	C	C	C	●	NR	●
miconazole	○	NR	NR	NR	N	NR	NR	NR	NR	NR	NR	NR	NR	NR	NR	NR	NR	C	NR	NR	NR	●	NR	NR
multiple vitamin infusion (MVI)	○	○	○	C	L	○	C	○	○	C	24	○	○	○	24	○	○	C	C	C	C	●	NR	○
nafcillin	○	○	12	○	Y	●	○	○	○	○	○	○	C	○	○	○	C	C	C	C	C	●	NR	C
nitroprusside	○	NR	NR	NR		NR	NR	NR	NR	NR	NR	NR	NR	NR	NR	NR	NR	C	NR	NR	NR	●	NR	NR
0.9% NSS	C	24	C	C		8	C	C	C	C	C	C	C	C	C	C	C	○	○	○	○	●	NR	C
oxacillin	○	8	●	24		●	○	○	○	C	○	●	●	○	○	○	○	C	C	C	C	●	NR	○
oxytocin	○	○	○	○		○	○	○	○	C	○	○	C	○	○	○	○	C	C	C	C	●	NR	○
penicillin G	○	8	●	24		●	C	○	○	C	○	●	C	24	24	C	C	C	C	C	C	●	NR	C
phenytoin	●	●	●	●		●	●	●	●	●	●	●	●	●	●	●	●	●	●	●	●	●	●	●
phytonadione	○	24	●	24		●	○	○	○	○	○	●	C	○	○	○	C	C	C	C	C	●	NR	C
polymyxin B	○	24	○	○		●	○	●	○	●	○	●	●	○	○	○	○	C	NR	NR	NR	●	NR	C
potassium chloride	○	4	C	24		C	C	24	○	C	○	C	C	24	24	C	4	C	C	C	C	●	NR	○
procainamide	○	NR	C	○		○	C	○	○	○	○	○	C	○	○	○	○	C	○	○	○	●	NR	C
sodium bicarbonate	○	24	C	○		○	●	24	○	○	24	C	C	C	24	●	○	C	C	C	C	●	NR	○
tetracycline	○	8	●	24		●	●	●	○	●	○	●	●	○	○	C	C	C	C	C	C	●	NR	C
thiamine	○	○	○	○		○	○	○	○	○	○	○	○	○	○	○	○	C	C	C	C	●	NR	○
ticarcillin	○	●	○	○		●	○	○	○	○	○	○	○	○	○	○	○	C	C	C	C	●	NR	○
tobramycin	○	○	○	○		○	●	●	NR	●	NR	●	○	○	●	○	○	C	C	C	C	●	NR	○
vancomycin	○	24	●	○		○	●	○	○	○	○	○	●	○	○	C	●	C	C	C	C	●	NR	C
vitamin B complex with C	○	24	●	○		●	C	●	○	C	24	C	●	24	24	C	4	C	C	C	C	●	NR	C

Key: C = Compatible ● = Incompatible **NR** = Not recommended by the manufacturer

dopamine	epinephrine	erythromycin lactobionate	fat emulsion 10% & 20%	gentamicin	heparin sodium	hydrocortisone Na succinate	insulin (regular)	isoproterenol	kanamycin	lactated Ringer's	levarterenol (norepinephrine)	lidocaine	metaraminol	methicillin	methylprednisolone	miconazole	multiple vitamin infusion (MVI)	nafcillin	nitroprusside	0.9% NSS	oxacillin	oxytocin	penicillin G	phenytoin	phytonadione	polymyxin B	potassium chloride	procainamide	sodium bicarbonate	tetracycline	thiamine	ticarcillin	tobramycin	vancomycin	vitamin B complex with C
○	○	○	○	○	○	○	○	○	○	C	○	○	○	○	○	○	○	○	○	C	○	○	○	●	○	○	○	○	○	○	○	○	○	○	○
●	24	●	●	○	●	○	○	○	○	○	24	○	24	●	○	NR	○	○	NR	24	8	○	8	●	24	24	4	NR	24	8	○	●	○	24	24
○	●	C	●	NR	C	C	●	●	C	C	●	C	○	C	6	NR	○	12	NR	C	●	○	●	●	●	○	C	C	C	●	○	○	○	●	●
24	○	24	●	24	24	○	24	24	C	C	24	24	24	24	24	NR	C	○	NR	C	24	○	24	●	24	○	24	○	○	24	○	○	○	○	○
H	A	R	M	A	C	Y		O	N	L	Y																								
●	○	●	●	●	●	C	○	○	●	8	○	●	●	●	○	NR	○	●	NR	8	●	○	●	●	●	●	C	○	○	●	○	●	○	○	●
24	●	C	●	NR	C	C	○	C	●	C	C	C	○	C	●	NR	C	○	NR	C	○	○	C	●	○	○	C	C	●	●	○	○	●	●	C
24	●	●	●	●	○	24	○	○	●	C	○	C	○	○	○	NR	○	○	NR	C	○	○	○	●	○	●	24	○	24	●	○	○	●	○	●
○	○	○	●	NR	○	○	○	○	○	C	○	C	○	○	○	NR	○	○	NR	C	○	○	○	●	○	○	○	○	○	○	○	○	NR	○	○
○	○	●	●	NR	○	○	○	○	●	C	○	○	○	○	○	NR	C	○	NR	C	C	C	C	●	○	●	C	○	○	●	○	○	●	○	C
○	○	○	●	NR	○	○	○	○	24	C	○	○	○	○	○	NR	24	○	NR	C	○	○	○	●	○	○	○	○	24	○	○	○	NR	○	24
6	●	●	●	●	8	24	8	C	●	C	●	●	C	●	●	NR	○	○	NR	C	●	○	●	●	●	●	C	○	C	●	○	○	●	○	C
24	○	●	●	●	C	C	○	○	C	C	●	C	C	1	C	NR	○	C	NR	C	●	C	C	●	C	●	C	C	C	●	○	○	○	●	●
○	○	NR	●	24	○	○	24	○	○	C	○	○	○	○	○	NR	○	○	NR	C	○	○	24	●	○	○	24	○	C	○	○	○	○	○	24
○	○	○	●	24	24	24	○	○	24	C	○	○	○	○	24	NR	24	○	NR	C	○	○	24	●	○	○	24	○	24	○	○	○	●	○	24
○	○	○	●	NR	24	24	○	○	○	C	C	○	○	C	○	NR	○	○	NR	C	○	○	C	●	○	○	C	○	●	C	○	○	○	C	C
○	○	○	●	NR	4	4	○	○	C	○	NR	C	●	C	○	NR	○	C	NR	C	○	○	C	●	C	○	4	○	○	C	○	○	○	●	4
C	C	C	●	C	C	C	○	C	C	○	C	C	C	6	C	C	C	C	NR	○	C	C	C	●	C	C	C	C	C	C	C	C	C	C	C
C	C	C	●	C	C	C	○	C	C	○	C	C	C	6	C	NR	C	C	NR	○	C	C	C	●	C	NR	C	○	C	C	C	C	C	C	C
C	C	C	●	C	C	C	○	C	C	○	C	C	C	6	C	NR	C	C	NR	○	C	C	C	●	C	NR	C	○	C	C	C	C	C	C	C
C	C	C	●	C	C	C	○	C	C	○	C	C	C	6	C	NR	C	C	NR	○	C	C	C	●	C	NR	C	○	C	C	C	C	C	C	C
●	●	●	●	●	●	●	●	●	●	●	●	●	●	●	●	●	●	●	●	●	●	●	●	●	●	●	●	●	●	●	●	●	●	●	●
NR	NR	NR	●	NR	NR	NR	NR	NR	NR	NR	NR	NR	NR	NR	NR	NR	NR	NR	NR	NR	NR	NR	NR	NR	NR	NR	NR	NR	NR	NR	NR	NR	NR	NR	NR
○	○	24	●	NR	○	●	○	○	○	C	○	C	●	C	●	NR	○	C	NR	C	○	○	C	●	C	C	○	C	○	C	○	○	○	C	C
X	○	○	●	6	24	○	○	○	24	C	○	24	○	○	18	NR	○	○	NR	C	24	○	6	●	○	○	24	○	●	24	○	○	○	○	○
○	X	○	●	NR	○	○	○	○	○	C	○	2	C	○	○	NR	○	○	NR	C	●	○	●	●	●	○	○	○	●	●	○	○	○	●	●
○	○	X	●	NR	●	C	○	○	○	C	○	C	●	C	○	NR	●	○	NR	C	○	○	C	●	○	C	C	○	24	●	●	○	○	○	●
●	●	●	X	●	●	●	●	●	●	●	●	●	●	●	●	●	●	●	●	●	●	●	●	●	●	●	●	●	●	●	●	●	●	●	●
6	NR	NR	●	X	●	NR	NR	NR	NR	C	NR	C	NR	NR	NR	NR	NR	●	NR	C	●	NR	NR	NR	NR	NR	NR	NR	NR	NR	NR	●	NR	NR	●
24	○	●	●	●	X	●	○	8	●	C	●	8	●	●	C	NR	○	C	NR	C	○	○	●	●	●	●	C	C	○	●	○	○	●	●	C
18	○	C	●	NR	●	X	8	○	●	C	C	C	●	●	4	NR	○	●	NR	C	○	○	C	●	○	○	C	C	C	●	○	○	○	●	C
○	○	○	●	NR	○	8	X	○	○	○	○	●	○	○	●	NR	○	○	NR	C	○	○	●	●	○	○	C	●	●	○	○	○	○	○	C
○	○	○	●	NR	8	○	○	X	○	C	○	●	○	○	○	NR	C	○	NR	C	○	○	○	●	○	○	C	○	●	C	○	○	○	○	C
24	○	○	●	NR	●	●	○	○	X	C	○	○	C	●	○	NR	●	NR	NR	C	NR	○	C	●	○	C	○	○	○	C	●	●	NR	NR	●
C	C	C	●	C	C	C	○	C	C	X	C	C	●	6	C	NR	C	C	NR	○	C	C	C	●	C	NR	C	○	C	C	C	C	C	C	C
○	○	○	●	NR	●	C	○	○	○	C	X	●	●	●	C	NR	C	C	NR	NR	●	●	○	●	○	○	C	○	●	●	○	○	○	○	C
24	2	C	●	C	8	C	●	●		C	●	X	C	○	○	NR	○	○	NR	C	○	○	C	●	○	○	C	○	●	C	○	○	○	○	C
○	C	●	●	NR	●	●	○	○	C	●	●	C	X	●	●	NR	●	●	NR	C	●	C	●	●	●	○	C	C	C	C	○	○	○	C	●
○	○	C	●	NR	●	●	○	○	●	6	●	○	●	X	○	NR	○	○	NR	6	○	○	●	●	●	C	C	NR	●	●	○	○	○	●	●
18	○	○	●	NR	C	4	●	○	○	C	C	○	●	○	X	NR	○	●	NR	C	○	○	●	●	○	○	C	○	C	●	○	C	○	○	●
NR	NR	NR	●	NR	NR	NR	NR	NR	NR	NR	NR	NR	NR	NR	NR	X	NR	NR	NR	C	NR	NR	NR	●	NR	NR	NR	NR	NR	NR	NR	NR	NR	NR	NR
○	○	●	●	NR	○	○	○	C	●	C	C	○	●	○	○	NR	X	○	NR	C	○	○	4	●	○	○	C	○	○	●	○	○	○	○	○
○	○	○	●	●	C	●	○	○	○	C	C	○	●	○	●	NR	○	X	NR	C	○	○	○	●	○	○	C	○	C	●	○	○	●	○	●
NR	NR	NR	●	NR	NR	NR	NR	NR	NR	NR	NR	NR	NR	NR	NR	NR	NR	NR	X	NR	NR	NR	NR	●	NR	NR	NR	NR	NR	NR	NR	NR	NR	NR	NR
C	C	C	●	C	C	C	C	C	C	○	NR	C	C	6	C	C	C	C	NR	X	C	C	C	●	C	C	C	○	C	C	C	C	C	C	C
24	●	○	●	●	○	○	○	○	NR	C	●	○	●	○	○	NR	○	○	NR	C	X	○	●	●	●	○	C	○	○	●	○	○	○	○	●
○	○	○	●	NR	○	○	○	○	○	C	●	○	C	○	○	NR	○	○	NR	C	○	X	C	●	C	○	○	○	○	C	○	○	○	○	○
6	●	C	●	NR	●	C	●	○	C	C	●	C	●	●	●	NR	4	○	NR	C	●	C	X	●	C	●	C	C	●	●	○	○	●	●	●
●	●	●	●	●	●	●	●	●	●	●	●	●	●	●	●	●	●	●	●	●	●	●	●	X	●	●	●	●	●	●	●	●	●	●	●
○	●	○	●	NR	●	○	○	○	NR	C	○	○	●	●	○	NR	○	○	NR	C	●	C	C	●	X	○	○	○	○	○	○	○	○	●	○
○	○	C	●	NR	●	C	○	○	C	○	○	○	○	C	○	NR	○	○	NR	C	○	○	●	●	○	X	○	○	○	●	○	○	○	○	C
24	○	C	●	NR	C	C	C	C	○	C	C	C	C	C	C	NR	C	C	NR	C	C	○	C	●	○	○	X	○	○	C	○	○	○	C	C
○	○	○	●	NR	C	C	●	○	○	○	○	○	C	NR	○	NR	○	○	NR	○	○	○	C	●	○	○	○	X	○	C	○	○	○	C	C
●	●	24	●	NR	○	C	●	●	○	C	●	●	C	●	C	NR	○	C	NR	C	○	○	●	●	○	○	○	○	X	●	○	○	○	●	●
24	●	●	●	NR	●	●	○	C	C	C	●	C	C	●	●	NR	●	●	NR	C	●	C	●	●	○	●	C	○	●	X	○	○	○	○	●
○	○	●	●	NR	○	○	○	○	●	C	○	○	○	○	○	NR	○	○	NR	C	○	○	○	●	○	○	○	○	○	○	X	○	○	○	C
○	○	○	●	●	○	○	○	○	●	C	○	○	○	○	C	NR	○	○	NR	C	○	○	○	●	○	○	○	○	○	○	○	X	●	○	○
○	○	○	●	NR	●	○	○	○	NR	C	○	○	○	○	○	NR	○	●	NR	C	○	○	●	●	○	○	○	○	○	○	○	●	X	○	○
○	●	○	●	NR	●	●	○	○	NR	C	○	○	C	●	○	NR	○	○	NR	C	○	○	●	●	●	○	C	C	●	○	○	○	○	X	●
○	●	●	●	●	C	C	C	C	●	C	C	C	●	●	●	NR	○	●	NR	C	●	○	●	●	○	C	C	C	●	●	C	○	○	●	X

○ = Data unavailable **2, 4, 8, 24** = Compatible only for the number of hours indicated **X** = Identical drug

Recognizing common drugs of abuse:

An identification guide and basic facts to help you

In your work, you may encounter addicts more often than you realize. That's because some are difficult—if not impossible—to identify. You should be cautious about basing an identification on only physical signs or abnormal behavior. For one thing, most symptoms suggesting drug abuse are common to various diseases. For another, the current popularity of mixed drug ingestion causes mixed symptoms. Taking stimulants and sedatives simultaneously, for instance, may cause antagonistic effects that defy interpretation. Also, differences in duration of effect may lead to withdrawal symptoms of one drug during the intoxicant phase of another.

Despite the difficulties of identifying drug abusers, you can spot certain signs of addiction and abuse. See the chart below for these and other related effects.

Types of addiction

As you can see in the chart, these drugs may cause physical or psychological dependence, or both. *Physical dependence* (or addiction) oc-

EFFECTS OF SOME COMMON DRUGS OF ABUSE

	CATEGORY/ DRUG	DEPENDENCE: Physical	DEPENDENCE: Psychological	POSSIBLE EFFECTS
Narcotics	**codeine**	Moderate	Moderate	Euphoria; respiratory depression; constricted pupils; nausea; risk of infection and hepatitis from I.V. (mainlined) drugs; wan, undernourished appearance; drowsiness and lethargy—user is on the "nod" (alternately dozing and waking) **Overdose:** Slow, shallow breathing; clammy skin; convulsions; coma; possibly death **Withdrawal:** Watery eyes, runny nose, yawning, anorexia, irritability, tremors, panic, chills and sweating, dilated pupils, piloerection (gooseflesh), cramps, nausea
	heroin	Strong	Strong	
	hydromorphone	Strong	Strong	
	meperidine	Strong	Strong	
	methadone	Strong	Strong	
	morphine	Strong	Strong	
Stimulants	**amphetamine**	Possible	Strong	Increased wakefulness, excitation, euphoria, talkativeness, irritability, dilated pupils, nervousness, increased pulse rate, elevated blood pressure **Overdose:** Agitation, fever, hallucinations, convulsions, possibly death **Withdrawal:** Apathy, long periods of sleep, irritability, depression, disorientation.
	cocaine	Possible	Strong	
	methylphenidate	Possible	Strong	
	phenmetrazine	Possible	Strong	
Depressants	**barbiturates**	Moderate to strong	Moderate to strong	Extreme drowsiness; slurred speech; disorientation; drunken behavior without alcohol use; slow, rapid, or shallow breathing; constricted pupils **Overdose:** Shallow breathing; cold, clammy skin; dilated pupils; weak, rapid pulse; coma; possibly death **Withdrawal:** Anxiety, insomnia, tremors, delirium, convulsions, possibly death
	chloral hydrate	Moderate	Moderate	
	glutethimide	Strong	Strong	
	methaqualone	Strong	Strong	
	other depressants	Moderate	Moderate	
	benzodiazepines	Little	Moderate	No significant effects
Hallucinogens	**lysergic acid diethylamide (LSD)**	None	Degree unknown	Illusions and hallucinations, poor perception of time and distance **Overdose:** Longer, more intense "trip" episodes, psychosis, possibly death **Withdrawal:** Withdrawal syndrome not reported
	mescaline and peyote	None	Degree unknown	
	phencyclidine (PCP)	Degree unknown	Strong	
	marijuana derivatives	Degree unknown	Moderate	Euphoria, increased appetite, disorientation **Overdose:** Fatigue, paranoia, possibly psychosis **Withdrawal:** Occasional insomnia, hyperactivity, and decreased appetite

curs when a person's body gets so accustomed to the drug that he cannot function normally without it. When the drug is withheld, physical and psychic withdrawal symptoms develop. A person may inadvertently become physically addicted, for example, when he takes certain drugs for a long-term illness.

Psychological dependence (or habituation) produces a desire to take drugs to feel good. The user has no physical compulsion to continue taking the drug. He may merely want to escape problems or situations he can't cope with, or he may seek pleasure and want to stimulate his senses.

Drug tolerance occurs when the user needs to take larger and larger doses to achieve the same effects. Accurate determination of tolerance levels is important in treatment programs.

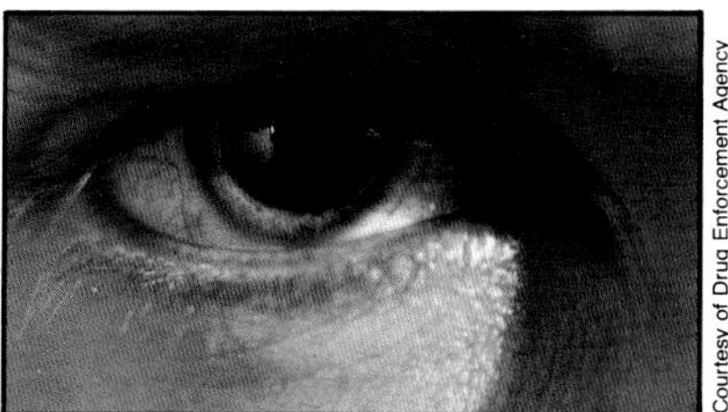

Courtesy of Drug Enforcement Agency

Someone using stimulants (amphetamines, for example) usually has dilated pupils.

Because you may see signs of drug abuse anywhere, you'll want to recognize drugs that can be abused, especially highly controlled substances. If you're working in a health-care

SPECIAL CONSIDERATIONS

Methadone is the drug of choice for withdrawal. As methadone maintenance becomes increasingly popular, more patients receiving methadone therapy are being admitted to general hospitals. This creates special medical and nursing problems. Some patients accurately report the dosage they're taking, but others don't know or exaggerate. A methadone-maintained patient may receive as much as 200 mg/day; the dosage must be verified by contacting the agency treating the patient for addiction. A patient on supervised daily doses of methadone has normal response to pain, so he requires the usual doses of analgesics for pain relief. But not all methadone treatment agencies give supervised daily doses; a patient taking methadone on a less controlled regimen may present all the classic problems of the street addict. So great is his tolerance that he may require massive doses of analgesics to relieve pain.

Abusers quickly develop tolerance, take massive doses, and after days without sleep or food, lapse into the abstinence syndrome. During withdrawal, the amphetamine user needs emotional support. Hospital emergency services would do well to study the crash-pad concept used effectively on college campuses. The crash pad is a haven where withdrawal is eased by generous amounts of kindness and understanding rather than drugs. Where staffing is inadequate for such a method, doctors may prescribe sedatives or tranquilizers to combat agitation and panic. They do so at some risk, because the patient may have already taken a sedative to ease the crash he anticipates when the stimulant wears off. So try to determine if your patient has taken a sedative to bring himself "down."

Patients develop great tolerance for barbiturates—they need to exceed their tolerance only slightly to precipitate a toxic reaction. The reaction poses great risk, because the main effect of barbiturates—CNS depression—is additive and synergistic to that of other sedatives and tranquilizers. Further, abrupt withdrawal from barbiturates poses a risk of major convulsive seizures; in fact, fatalities due to cardiovascular collapse have been reported. Thus, withdrawal must always be carried out under close supervision in a hospital.

In many cases, acute barbiturate intoxication is the result of a dose only slightly higher than the addictive level. After acute poisoning has been relieved, try to learn whether the barbiturates have been taken chronically. If so, gradual withdrawal is indicated. The withdrawal drug of choice is pentobarbital (Nembutal). However, the long-acting barbiturate phenobarbital can also be used.

When managing a patient on a bad "trip," exploit his hypersuggestible state for his own benefit by promising that he is safe from danger and that his reaction will soon pass. To reduce the intensity of the hallucinations, advise him to keep his eyes open. Rarely will you need to restrain him physically. Flashback phenomenon can occur weeks or months after ingestion of a hallucinogen (most commonly LSD, PCP). Once triggered, the flashback produces the same effects as drug ingestion. Medical treatment is symptomatic. If the doctor is reasonably sure the patient's intoxication is caused solely by hallucinogens, he may prescribe a phenothiazine. Doing so runs a risk: The patient may have taken an additional drug—an opiate, for instance—that would be potentiated by the phenothiazine.

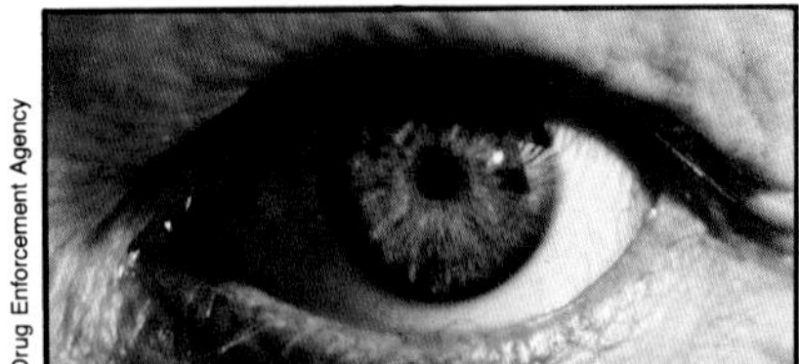
Drug Enforcement Agency

Someone using narcotics (heroin or morphine, for example) has constricted (pinpoint) pupils.

setting, you should be particularly aware of the abuse of prescription drugs, an increasingly serious problem. The health-care professional has to be more alert to the warning signs of abuse among patients and colleagues alike, as well as to drug thefts and substitutions.

To help you verify common drugs that can be abused or misused in tablet and capsule form, a full-color identification section follows. For more information about drug abuse, contact a drug abuse agency. You'll find a list of these agencies in the APPENDIX.

How to use this section

The color photos on the following pages will help you quickly identify almost 500 common drugs. Each drug is shown actual size. Because of printing limitations, colors may vary slightly from the actual tablets or capsules, although every effort has been made to reproduce the colors faithfully.

The section begins with white tablets and capsules, arranged by size, from smallest to largest. Then, beige, gray, yellow, brown, orange, red, pink, violet, blue, green, and multi-colored drugs follow.

The last page of photos contains some over-the-counter preparations that can be abused or misused.

Below each photo a caption gives as much of the following information as applicable: drug's trade name and dosage strength, generic name, controlled-substance schedule number, and manufacturer's name and code number. If the caption doesn't include a generic name, the drug is a combination product.

To identify an unfamiliar drug, turn to the page that contains drugs closest in color to the one you're trying to identify. When you think you've found the correct photo, compare *both* sides of the drug with the photo. In most cases, product markings are shown in the photos for easier identification. Remember, however, that handling may have removed some markings, especially on sugar-coated tablets. Markings and appearance may also have been changed by the manufacturer.

Tablet and capsule colors may vary from one batch of manufacturer's dye to another as well. Some products are sensitive to light and moisture, so their color and/or texture may change if stored for a long time. Color variation may also be affected by the light in which you view the tablets or capsules.

After identifying the drug, consult the index to find more information in this book. For additional details or confirming identification on the drug, please contact the manufacturer.

Except in emergencies, these photos should not be used as a substitute for a comprehensive chemical analysis, because visually similar products may differ markedly in contents.

Schedules of Controlled Substances, USA

Drugs regulated under the jurisdiction of the Controlled Substances Act of 1970 are divided into these five groups, or schedules.

Schedule I: No accepted medical use in the United States, with high potential for abuse. Examples: heroin, lysergic acid diethylamide (LSD), marijuana derivatives, mescaline, peyote, and psilocybin.

Schedule II: High potential for abuse, with severe psychic or physical dependence possible. Includes certain narcotic, stimulant, and depressant drugs. Examples: amobarbital, amphetamine, anileridine, cocaine, codeine, hydromorphone, meperidine, methadone, methamphetamine, methaqualone, methylphenidate, morphine, opium, oxycodone, oxymorphone, pentobarbital, phenmetrazine, and secobarbital.

Schedule III: Less abuse potential than drugs in Schedule II. Includes compounds containing certain narcotic and nonnarcotic drugs. Examples: barbituric acid derivatives (except those listed in another schedule), benzphetamine, chlorphentermine, clortermine, glutethimide, mazindol, methyprylon, Paregoric, and phendimetrazine.

Schedule IV: Less abuse potential than drugs in Schedule III. Examples: barbital, benzodiazepine derivatives, chloral hydrate, diethylpropion, ethchlorvynol, fenfluramine, ethinamate, meprobamate, methohexital, phenobarbital, paraldehyde, and phentermine.

Schedule V: Less abuse potential than drugs in Schedule IV. Consists of preparations containing limited quantities of certain narcotic drugs generally for antidiarrheal or antitussive purposes. Examples: diphenoxylate compound and expectorants with codeine.

Controlled Drugs, Canada

Schedule G: Drugs regulated under the jurisdiction of the Food and Drugs Act of 1952-1953 and regulations issued by the Health Protection Branch, Ottawa, Canada. All salts and derivatives of the following drugs are included: amphetamine, barbituric acid, benzphetamine, butorphanol, chlorphentermine, diethylpropion, methamphetamine, methaqualone, methylphenidate, pentazocine, phendimetrazine, phenmetrazine, phentermine, and thiobarbituric acid.

COMMON DRUGS THAT CAN BE ABUSED

Note: The drugs pictured in this section, although usually prescribed for medicinal and therapeutic purposes, have the potential to be abused or misused under certain circumstances and by certain patients. They include both controlled and noncontrolled substances.

CAPTION KEY:

Trade name (initial letter capitalized) or generic name (initial letter lower cased) and dosage strength
(generic name, when trade name has been listed)
Controlled-substance schedule number, if any
Manufacturer's name and code number, if any

morphine sulfate 10 mg Schedule II Lilly	**morphine sulfate 30 mg** Schedule II Lilly	**Ativan 0.5 mg** *(lorazepam)* Schedule IV Wyeth 81	**Lomotil** Schedule V Searle 61
codeine sulfate 15 mg Schedule II Lilly J09	**codeine sulfate 30 mg** Schedule II Lilly J10	**codeine sulfate 60 mg** Schedule II Lilly J11	**Cytomel 5 mcg** *(liothyronine sodium)* SKF D14
SK-Phenobarbital 15 mg *(phenobarbital)* Schedule IV SKF 136	**SK-Phenobarbital 30 mg** *(phenobarbital)* Schedule IV SKF 137	**Levo-Dromoran 2 mg** *(levorphanol tartrate)* Schedule II Roche 44	**Noludar 50 mg** *(methyprylon)* Schedule III Roche 16
Dolophine 5 mg *(methadone hydrochloride)* Schedule II Lilly J64	**Levothroid 0.05 mg** *(levothyroxine sodium)* Armour LL	**Demerol 50 mg** *(meperidine hydrochloride)* Schedule II Winthrop D35	**Synthroid 0.05 mg** *(levothyroxine sodium)* Flint
Desoxyn 5 mg *(methamphetamine hydrochloride)* Schedule II Abbott	**Haldol 0.5 mg** *(haloperidol)* McNeil	**Periactin 4 mg** *(cyproheptadine hydrochloride)* MSD 62	**Cylert 18.75 mg** *(pemoline)* Schedule IV Abbott TH
phenobarbital 16 mg Schedule IV Rugby	**phenobarbital 32 mg** Schedule IV Various manufacturers	**phenobarbital 65 mg** Schedule IV Various manufacturers	**Mebaral 32 mg** *(mephobarbital)* Schedule IV Breon M31

DRUGS THAT CAN BE ABUSED

Bentyl with phenobarbital 20 mg Merrell 124	**Mysoline 50 mg** *(primidone)* Ayerst	**phenobarbital 100 mg** Schedule IV Philips Roxane	**Plexonal** Schedule III Sandoz 78-57
Sanorex 1 mg *(mazindol)* Schedule III Sandoz 78-71	**Ativan 1 mg** *(lorazepam)* Schedule IV Wyeth 64	**Ativan 2 mg** *(lorazepam)* Schedule IV Wyeth 65	**Lioresal 10 mg** *(baclofen)* Geigy 23
Cytomel 25 mcg *(liothyronine sodium)* SKF D16	**Mebaral 50 mg** *(mephobarbital)* Schedule IV Breon M32	**Mebaral 100 mg** *(mephobarbital)* Schedule IV Breon M33	**Demerol 100 mg** *(meperidine HCl)* Schedule II Winthrop D37
Valium 2 mg *(diazepam)* Schedule IV Roche	**Clonopin 2 mg** *(clonazepam)* Schedule IV Roche 63	**Deaner 25 mg** *(deanol acetamidobenzoate)* Riker	**Doriden 0.125 mg** *(glutethimide)* Schedule III Ciba
Cytomel 50 mcg *(liothyronine sodium)* SKF D17	**Valpin 50-PB** Endo 162	**Hycodan** Schedule III Endo 042	**Donnatal** Robins
Tedral Warner-Lambert 230	**Preludin 25 mg** *(phenmetrazine HCl)* Schedule II Boehringer Ingelheim 42	**Sanorex 2 mg** *(mazindol)* Schedule III Sandoz 78-66	**Dolophine 10 mg** *(methadone HCl)* Schedule II Lilly J72
Norflex 100 mg *(orphenadrine citrate)* Riker	**SK-Bamate 200 mg** *(meprobamate)* Schedule IV SKF 133	**Tegretol 200 mg** *(carbamazepine)* Geigy 67	**Limbitrol 10-25** Schedule IV Roche

DRUGS THAT CAN BE ABUSED

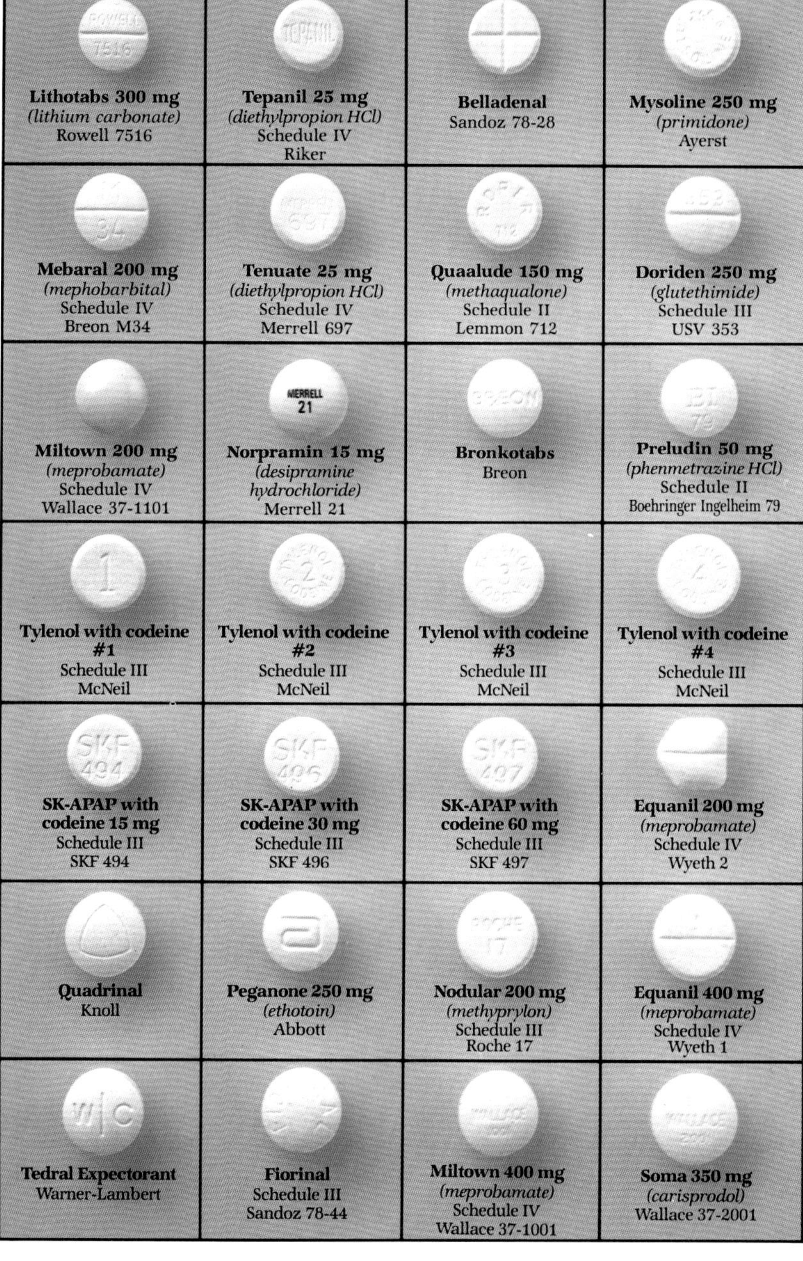

Lithotabs 300 mg
(lithium carbonate)
Rowell 7516

Tepanil 25 mg
(diethylpropion HCl)
Schedule IV
Riker

Belladenal
Sandoz 78-28

Mysoline 250 mg
(primidone)
Ayerst

Mebaral 200 mg
(mephobarbital)
Schedule IV
Breon M34

Tenuate 25 mg
(diethylpropion HCl)
Schedule IV
Merrell 697

Quaalude 150 mg
(methaqualone)
Schedule II
Lemmon 712

Doriden 250 mg
(glutethimide)
Schedule III
USV 353

Miltown 200 mg
(meprobamate)
Schedule IV
Wallace 37-1101

Norpramin 15 mg
(desipramine hydrochloride)
Merrell 21

Bronkotabs
Breon

Preludin 50 mg
(phenmetrazine HCl)
Schedule II
Boehringer Ingelheim 79

Tylenol with codeine #1
Schedule III
McNeil

Tylenol with codeine #2
Schedule III
McNeil

Tylenol with codeine #3
Schedule III
McNeil

Tylenol with codeine #4
Schedule III
McNeil

SK-APAP with codeine 15 mg
Schedule III
SKF 494

SK-APAP with codeine 30 mg
Schedule III
SKF 496

SK-APAP with codeine 60 mg
Schedule III
SKF 497

Equanil 200 mg
(meprobamate)
Schedule IV
Wyeth 2

Quadrinal
Knoll

Peganone 250 mg
(ethotoin)
Abbott

Nodular 200 mg
(methyprylon)
Schedule III
Roche 17

Equanil 400 mg
(meprobamate)
Schedule IV
Wyeth 1

Tedral Expectorant
Warner-Lambert

Fiorinal
Schedule III
Sandoz 78-44

Miltown 400 mg
(meprobamate)
Schedule IV
Wallace 37-1001

Soma 350 mg
(carisprodol)
Wallace 37-2001

DRUGS THAT CAN BE ABUSED

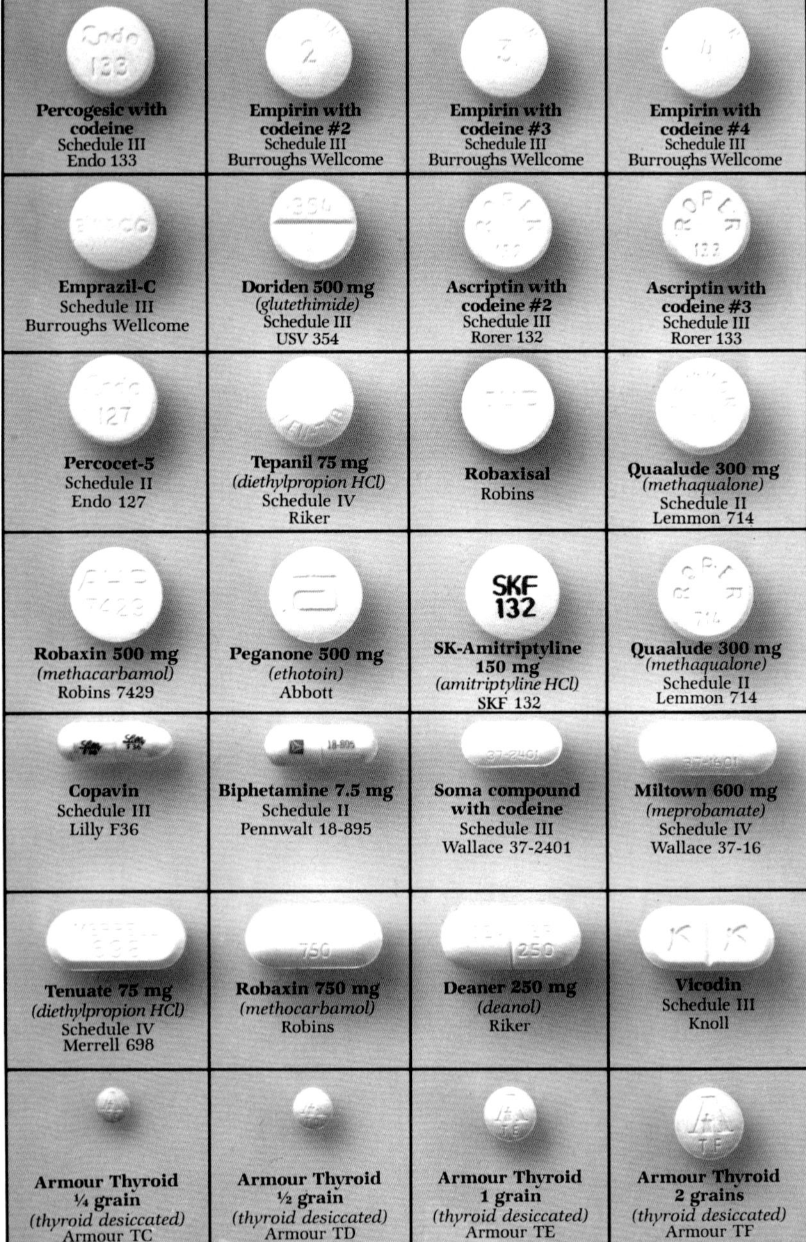

Percogesic with codeine Schedule III Endo 133	**Empirin with codeine #2** Schedule III Burroughs Wellcome	**Empirin with codeine #3** Schedule III Burroughs Wellcome	**Empirin with codeine #4** Schedule III Burroughs Wellcome
Emprazil-C Schedule III Burroughs Wellcome	**Doriden 500 mg** *(glutethimide)* Schedule III USV 354	**Ascriptin with codeine #2** Schedule III Rorer 132	**Ascriptin with codeine #3** Schedule III Rorer 133
Percocet-5 Schedule II Endo 127	**Tepanil 75 mg** *(diethylpropion HCl)* Schedule IV Riker	**Robaxisal** Robins	**Quaalude 300 mg** *(methaqualone)* Schedule II Lemmon 714
Robaxin 500 mg *(methacarbamol)* Robins 7429	**Peganone 500 mg** *(ethotoin)* Abbott	**SK-Amitriptyline 150 mg** *(amitriptyline HCl)* SKF 132	**Quaalude 300 mg** *(methaqualone)* Schedule II Lemmon 714
Copavin Schedule III Lilly F36	**Biphetamine 7.5 mg** Schedule II Pennwalt 18-895	**Soma compound with codeine** Schedule III Wallace 37-2401	**Miltown 600 mg** *(meprobamate)* Schedule IV Wallace 37-16
Tenuate 75 mg *(diethylpropion HCl)* Schedule IV Merrell 698	**Robaxin 750 mg** *(methocarbamol)* Robins	**Deaner 250 mg** *(deanol)* Riker	**Vicodin** Schedule III Knoll
Armour Thyroid ¼ grain *(thyroid desiccated)* Armour TC	**Armour Thyroid ½ grain** *(thyroid desiccated)* Armour TD	**Armour Thyroid 1 grain** *(thyroid desiccated)* Armour TE	**Armour Thyroid 2 grains** *(thyroid desiccated)* Armour TF

DRUGS THAT CAN BE ABUSED

Armour Thyroid 3 grains *(thyroid desiccated)* Armour TG	**Armour Thyroid 5 grains** *(thyroid desiccated)* Armour TI	**Proloid ¼ grain** *(thyroglobulin)* Warner-Lambert	**Proloid ½ grain** *(thyroglobulin)* Warner-Lambert
Proloid 1½ grains *(thyroglobulin)* Warner-Lambert 253	**Proloid 1 grain** *(thyroglobulin)* Warner-Lambert 252	**Proloid 2 grains** *(thyroglobulin)* Warner-Lambert 257	**Proloid 3 grains** *(thyroglobulin)* Warner-Lambert 254
Proloid 5 grains *(thyroglobulin)* Warner-Lambert 255	**Mellaril 50 mg** *(thioridazine hydrochloride)* Sandoz	**Trilafon 2 mg** *(perphenazine)* Schering 705	**Trilafon 4 mg** *(perphenazine)* Schering 940
Trilafon 8 mg *(perphenazine)* Schering 313	**Trilafon 16 mg** *(perphenazine)* Schering 077	**Trilafon 8 mg Repetabs** *(perphenazine)* Schering ADX	**Eskalith 300 mg** *(lithium carbonate)* SKF J09
SK-65 *(propoxyphene hydrochloride)* Schedule IV SKF 463	**Tranxene 3.75 mg** *(clorazepate dipotassium)* Schedule IV Abbott CI	**Tranxene 15 mg** *(clorazepate dipotassium)* Schedule IV Abbott CK	**Euthroid-3** *(liotrix)* Warner-Lambert 263
Vesprin 25 mg *(triflupromazine)* Squibb 922	**Zomax 100 mg** *(zomepirac sodium)* McNeil	**Dilantin Infatabs 50 mg** *(phenytoin sodium)* Parke-Davis 007	**Plegine 35 mg** *(phendimetrazine tartrate)* Schedule III Ayerst
Pro-Banthine with phenobarbital Searle 631	**Percodan** Schedule II Endo 135	**Dilaudid 4 mg** *(hydromorphone HCl)* Schedule II Knoll	**Voranil 50 mg** *(clotermine hydrochloride)* Schedule III USV

DRUGS THAT CAN BE ABUSED

Desoxyn 15 mg *(methamphetamine hydrochloride)* Schedule II Abbott MF	**Levothroid 0.1 mg** *(levothyroxine sodium)* Armour LM	**Amytal 30 mg** *(amobarbital)* Schedule II Lilly T56	**Ritalin 5 mg** *(methylphenidate hydrochloride)* Schedule II Ciba 7
Haldol 1 mg *(haloperidol)* McNeil	**Valium 5 mg** *(diazepam)* Schedule IV Roche	**Synthroid 0.1 mg** *(levothyroxine sodium)* Flint	**Thyrolar 3 grains** *(liotrix)* Armour YH
Zactirin Compound-100 Wyeth 49	**Triavil 4-25** MSD 946	**Luminal 16 mg** *(phenobarbital)* Schedule IV Winthrop	**Prolixin 2.5 mg** *(fluphenazine dihydrochloride)* Squibb 864
Etrafon 2-10 Schering 287	**Meprospan 200 mg** *(meprobamate)* Schedule IV Wallace 37-1401	**Nembutal 30 mg** *(pentobarbital sodium)* Schedule II Abbott	**Nembutal 100 mg** *(pentobarbital sodium)* Schedule II Abbott CH
Mellaril 150 mg *(thioridazine hydrochloride)* Sandoz	**Compazine 5 mg** *(prochlorperazine maleate)* SKF C66	**Compazine 10 mg** *(prochlorperazine maleate)* SKF C67	**Compazine 25 mg** *(prochlorperazine maleate)* SKF C69
Permitil Chronotab 1 mg *(fluphenazine hydrochloride)* Schering WKJ	**Elavil 25 mg** *(amitriptyline hydrochloride)* MSD 45	**Norpramin 25 mg** *(desipramine hydrochloride)* Merrell 11	**Ionamin 30 mg** *(phentermine)* Schedule IV Pennwalt 18-904
Aventyl 10 mg *(nortriptyline hydrochloride)* Lilly H17	**Aventyl 25 mg** *(nortriptyline hydrochloride)* Lilly H19	**Atarax 50 mg** *(hydroxyzine hydrochloride)* Roerig	**Janimine 25 mg** *(imipramine hydrochloride)* Abbott

DRUGS THAT CAN BE ABUSED

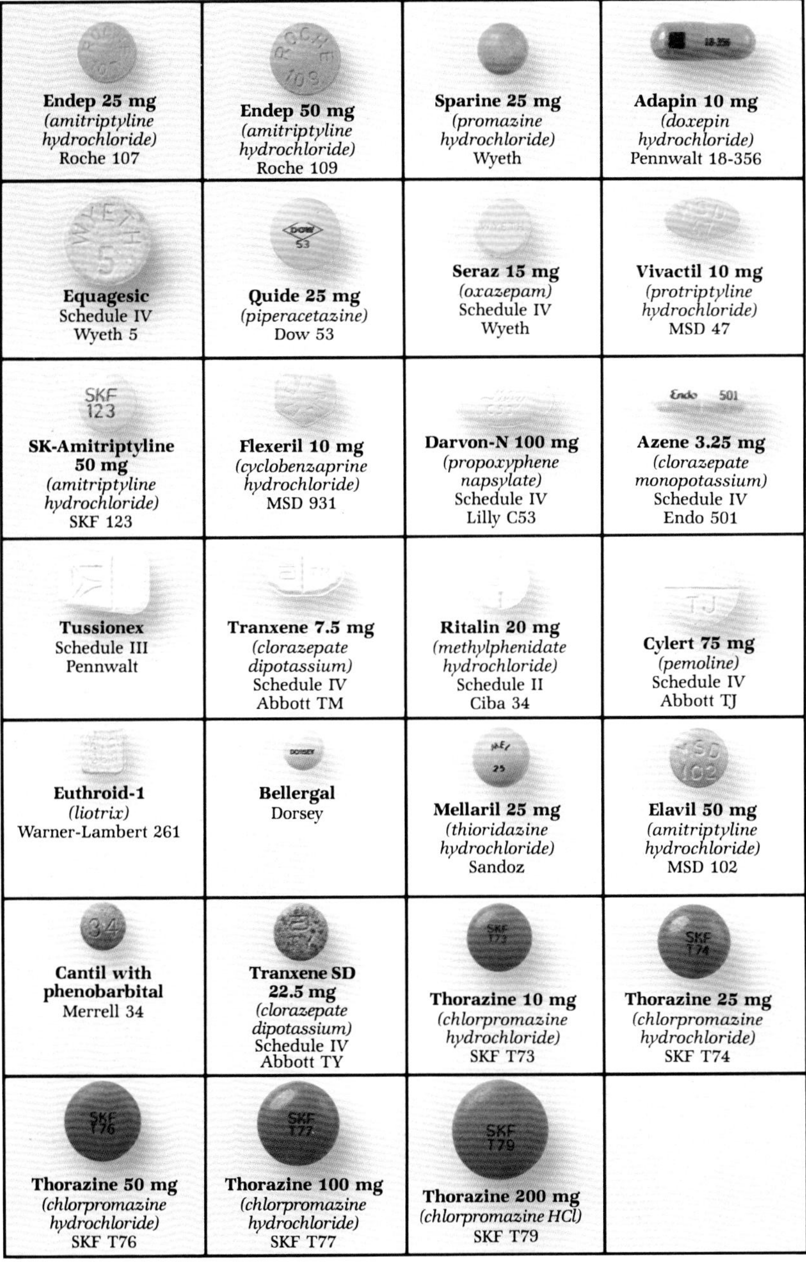

Endep 25 mg *(amitriptyline hydrochloride)* Roche 107	**Endep 50 mg** *(amitriptyline hydrochloride)* Roche 109	**Sparine 25 mg** *(promazine hydrochloride)* Wyeth	**Adapin 10 mg** *(doxepin hydrochloride)* Pennwalt 18-356
Equagesic Schedule IV Wyeth 5	**Quide 25 mg** *(piperacetazine)* Dow 53	**Seraz 15 mg** *(oxazepam)* Schedule IV Wyeth	**Vivactil 10 mg** *(protriptyline hydrochloride)* MSD 47
SK-Amitriptyline 50 mg *(amitriptyline hydrochloride)* SKF 123	**Flexeril 10 mg** *(cyclobenzaprine hydrochloride)* MSD 931	**Darvon-N 100 mg** *(propoxyphene napsylate)* Schedule IV Lilly C53	**Azene 3.25 mg** *(clorazepate monopotassium)* Schedule IV Endo 501
Tussionex Schedule III Pennwalt	**Tranxene 7.5 mg** *(clorazepate dipotassium)* Schedule IV Abbott TM	**Ritalin 20 mg** *(methylphenidate hydrochloride)* Schedule II Ciba 34	**Cylert 75 mg** *(pemoline)* Schedule IV Abbott TJ
Euthroid-1 *(liotrix)* Warner-Lambert 261	**Bellergal** Dorsey	**Mellaril 25 mg** *(thioridazine hydrochloride)* Sandoz	**Elavil 50 mg** *(amitriptyline hydrochloride)* MSD 102
Cantil with phenobarbital Merrell 34	**Tranxene SD 22.5 mg** *(clorazepate dipotassium)* Schedule IV Abbott TY	**Thorazine 10 mg** *(chlorpromazine hydrochloride)* SKF T73	**Thorazine 25 mg** *(chlorpromazine hydrochloride)* SKF T74
Thorazine 50 mg *(chlorpromazine hydrochloride)* SKF T76	**Thorazine 100 mg** *(chlorpromazine hydrochloride)* SKF T77	**Thorazine 200 mg** *(chlorpromazine HCl)* SKF T79	

DRUGS THAT CAN BE ABUSED

Talwin 50 mg *(pentazocine HCl)* Schedule IV Winthrop T21	**Empracet with codeine #3** Schedule III Burroughs Wellcome K9B	**Empracet with codeine #4** Schedule III Burroughs Wellcome L9B	**Desoxyn 10 mg** *(methamphetamine HCl)* Schedule II Abbott ME
Synthroid 0.025 mg *(levothyroxine sodium)* Flint	**Janimine 50 mg** *(imipramine hydrochloride)* Abbott	**Sinequan 75 mg** *(doxepin hydrochloride)* Pfizer 539	**Asendin 150 mg** *(amoxapine)* Lederle
Paraflex 250 mg *(chlorzoxazone)* McNeil	**Soma compound** Wallace 37-2101	**Cylert 37.5 mg** *(pemoline)* Schedule IV Abbott Tl	**Marplan 10 mg** *(isocarboxazid)* Roche
Dilaudid 2 mg *(hydromorphone hydrochloride)* Schedule II Knoll	**Euthroid-½** *(liotrix)* Warner-Lambert 260	**Vivactil 5 mg** *(protriptyline hydrochloride)* MSD 26	**Permitil 2.5 mg** *(fluphenazine hydrochloride)* Schering WDR
Duovent Riker	**Norpramin 100 mg** *(desipramine hydrochloride)* Merrell 20	**Butisol 50 mg** *(butabarbital sodium)* Schedule III McNeil	**Dexedrine 5 mg** *(dextroamphetamine sulfate)* Schedule II SKF E19
Triavil 2-25 MSD 921	**Triavil 4-50** MSD 517	**Kinesed** Stuart 220	**Verequad** Knoll
Asendin 50 mg *(amoxapine)* Lederle	**Tedral-25** Warner-Lambert 238	**Clonopin 0.5 mg** *(clonazepam)* Schedule IV Roche 61	**Moban 5 mg** *(molindone hydrochloride)* Endo 072

DRUGS THAT CAN BE ABUSED

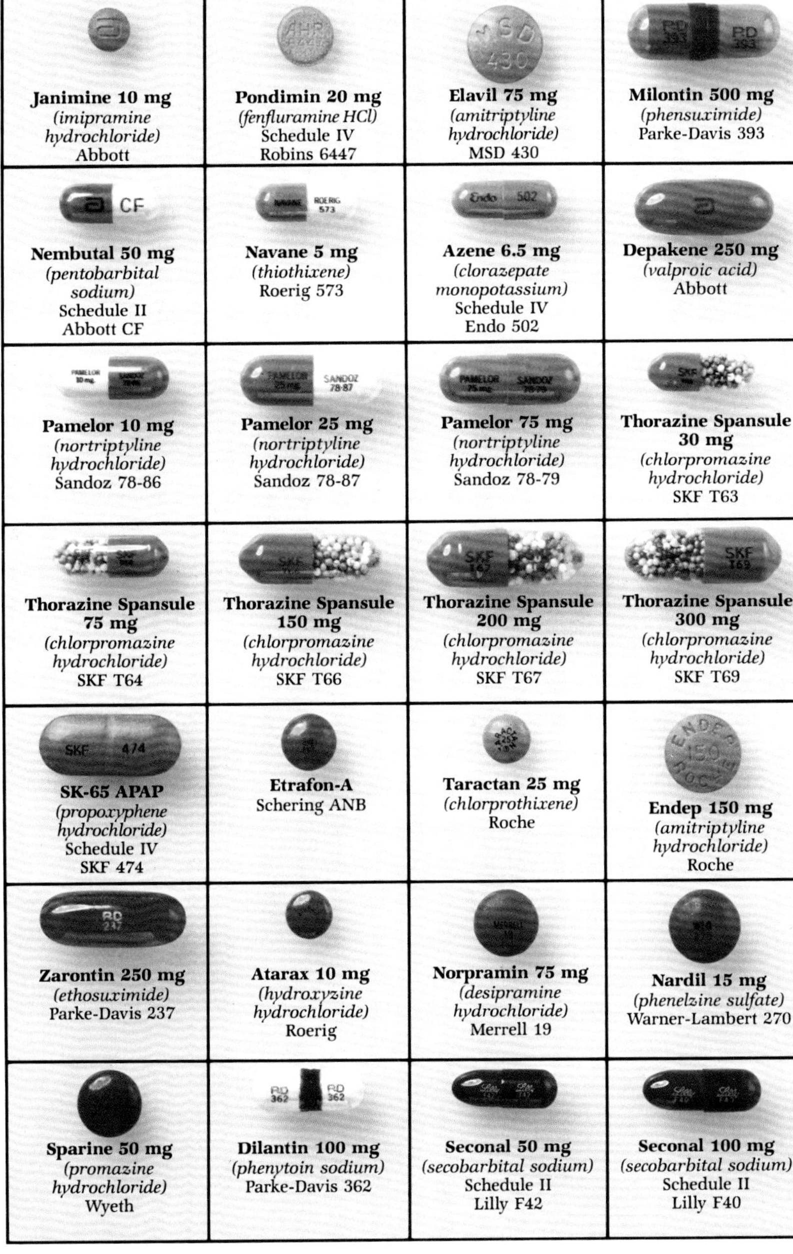

Janimine 10 mg *(imipramine hydrochloride)* Abbott	**Pondimin 20 mg** *(fenfluramine HCl)* Schedule IV Robins 6447	**Elavil 75 mg** *(amitriptyline hydrochloride)* MSD 430	**Milontin 500 mg** *(phensuximide)* Parke-Davis 393
Nembutal 50 mg *(pentobarbital sodium)* Schedule II Abbott CF	**Navane 5 mg** *(thiothixene)* Roerig 573	**Azene 6.5 mg** *(clorazepate monopotassium)* Schedule IV Endo 502	**Depakene 250 mg** *(valproic acid)* Abbott
Pamelor 10 mg *(nortriptyline hydrochloride)* Sandoz 78-86	**Pamelor 25 mg** *(nortriptyline hydrochloride)* Sandoz 78-87	**Pamelor 75 mg** *(nortriptyline hydrochloride)* Sandoz 78-79	**Thorazine Spansule 30 mg** *(chlorpromazine hydrochloride)* SKF T63
Thorazine Spansule 75 mg *(chlorpromazine hydrochloride)* SKF T64	**Thorazine Spansule 150 mg** *(chlorpromazine hydrochloride)* SKF T66	**Thorazine Spansule 200 mg** *(chlorpromazine hydrochloride)* SKF T67	**Thorazine Spansule 300 mg** *(chlorpromazine hydrochloride)* SKF T69
SK-65 APAP *(propoxyphene hydrochloride)* Schedule IV SKF 474	**Etrafon-A** Schering ANB	**Taractan 25 mg** *(chlorprothixene)* Roche	**Endep 150 mg** *(amitriptyline hydrochloride)* Roche
Zarontin 250 mg *(ethosuximide)* Parke-Davis 237	**Atarax 10 mg** *(hydroxyzine hydrochloride)* Roerig	**Norpramin 75 mg** *(desipramine hydrochloride)* Merrell 19	**Nardil 15 mg** *(phenelzine sulfate)* Warner-Lambert 270
Sparine 50 mg *(promazine hydrochloride)* Wyeth	**Dilantin 100 mg** *(phenytoin sodium)* Parke-Davis 362	**Seconal 50 mg** *(secobarbital sodium)* Schedule II Lilly F42	**Seconal 100 mg** *(secobarbital sodium)* Schedule II Lilly F40

DRUGS THAT CAN BE ABUSED

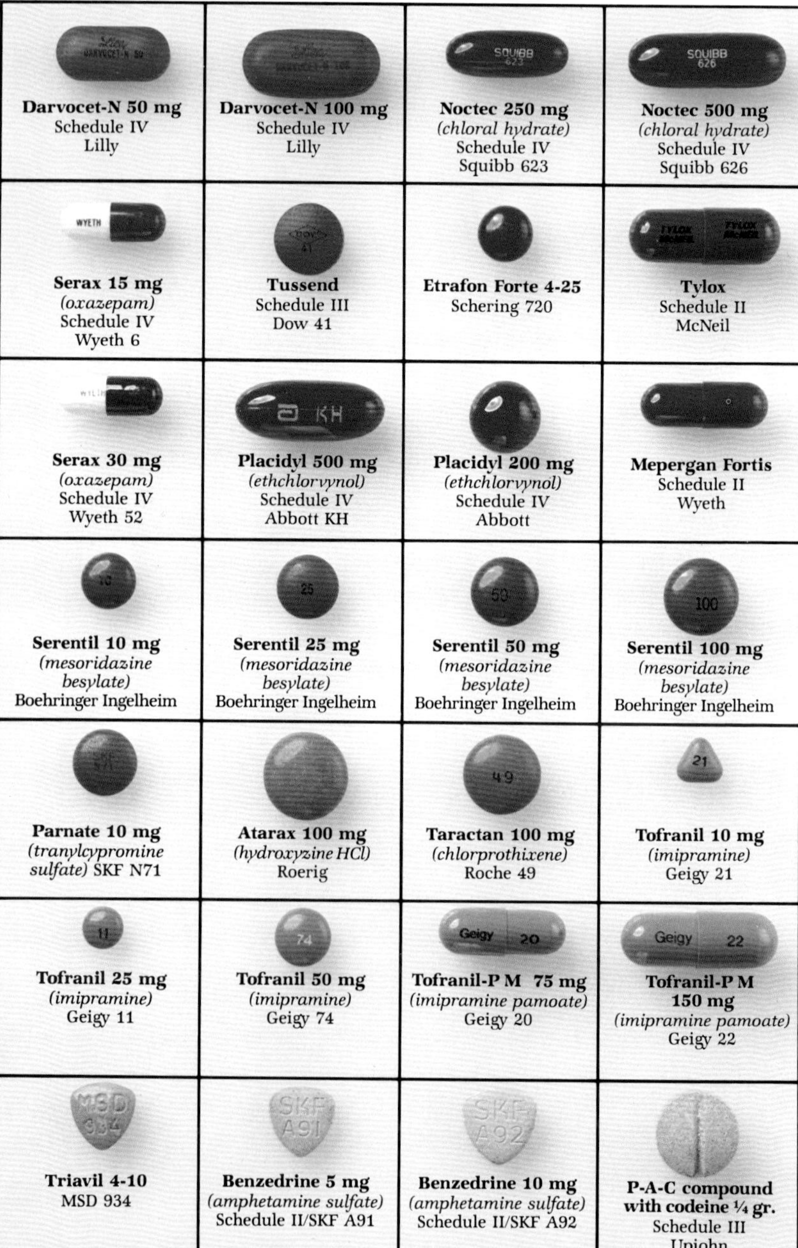

Darvocet-N 50 mg Schedule IV Lilly	**Darvocet-N 100 mg** Schedule IV Lilly	**Noctec 250 mg** *(chloral hydrate)* Schedule IV Squibb 623	**Noctec 500 mg** *(chloral hydrate)* Schedule IV Squibb 626
Serax 15 mg *(oxazepam)* Schedule IV Wyeth 6	**Tussend** Schedule III Dow 41	**Etrafon Forte 4-25** Schering 720	**Tylox** Schedule II McNeil
Serax 30 mg *(oxazepam)* Schedule IV Wyeth 52	**Placidyl 500 mg** *(ethchlorvynol)* Schedule IV Abbott KH	**Placidyl 200 mg** *(ethchlorvynol)* Schedule IV Abbott	**Mepergan Fortis** Schedule II Wyeth
Serentil 10 mg *(mesoridazine besylate)* Boehringer Ingelheim	**Serentil 25 mg** *(mesoridazine besylate)* Boehringer Ingelheim	**Serentil 50 mg** *(mesoridazine besylate)* Boehringer Ingelheim	**Serentil 100 mg** *(mesoridazine besylate)* Boehringer Ingelheim
Parnate 10 mg *(tranylcypromine sulfate)* SKF N71	**Atarax 100 mg** *(hydroxyzine HCl)* Roerig	**Taractan 100 mg** *(chlorprothixene)* Roche 49	**Tofranil 10 mg** *(imipramine)* Geigy 21
Tofranil 25 mg *(imipramine)* Geigy 11	**Tofranil 50 mg** *(imipramine)* Geigy 74	**Tofranil-P M 75 mg** *(imipramine pamoate)* Geigy 20	**Tofranil-P M 150 mg** *(imipramine pamoate)* Geigy 22
Triavil 4-10 MSD 934	**Benzedrine 5 mg** *(amphetamine sulfate)* Schedule II/SKF A91	**Benzedrine 10 mg** *(amphetamine sulfate)* Schedule II/SKF A92	**P-A-C compound with codeine ¼ gr.** Schedule III Upjohn

DRUGS THAT CAN BE ABUSED

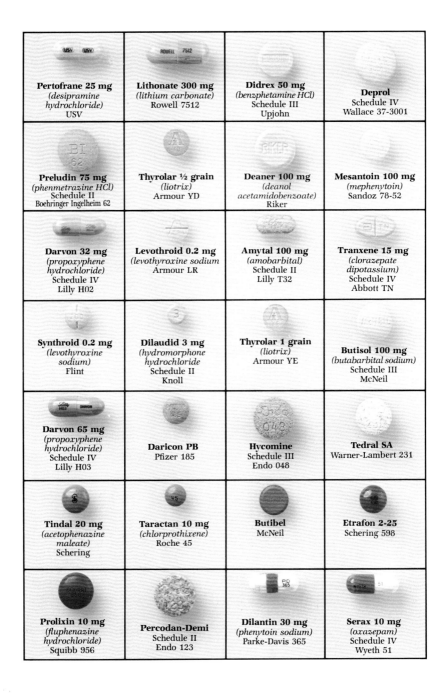

Pertofrane 25 mg *(desipramine hydrochloride)* USV	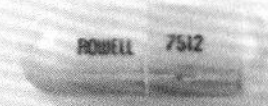 **Lithonate 300 mg** *(lithium carbonate)* Rowell 7512	**Didrex 50 mg** *(benzphetamine HCl)* Schedule III Upjohn	**Deprol** Schedule IV Wallace 37-3001
Preludin 75 mg *(phenmetrazine HCl)* Schedule II Boehringer Ingelheim 62	**Thyrolar ½ grain** *(liotrix)* Armour YD	**Deaner 100 mg** *(deanol acetamidobenzoate)* Riker	**Mesantoin 100 mg** *(mephenytoin)* Sandoz 78-52
Darvon 32 mg *(propoxyphene hydrochloride)* Schedule IV Lilly H02	**Levothroid 0.2 mg** *(levothyroxine sodium* Armour LR	**Amytal 100 mg** *(amobarbital)* Schedule II Lilly T32	**Tranxene 15 mg** *(clorazepate dipotassium)* Schedule IV Abbott TN
Synthroid 0.2 mg *(levothyroxine sodium)* Flint	**Dilaudid 3 mg** *(hydromorphone hydrochloride* Schedule II Knoll	**Thyrolar 1 grain** *(liotrix)* Armour YE	**Butisol 100 mg** *(butabarbital sodium)* Schedule III McNeil
Darvon 65 mg *(propoxyphene hydrochloride)* Schedule IV Lilly H03	**Daricon PB** Pfizer 185	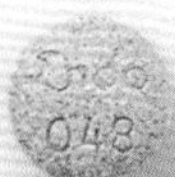 **Hycomine** Schedule III Endo 048	**Tedral SA** Warner-Lambert 231
Tindal 20 mg *(acetophenazine maleate)* Schering	**Taractan 10 mg** *(chlorprothixene)* Roche 45	**Butibel** McNeil	**Etrafon 2-25** Schering 598
Prolixin 10 mg *(fluphenazine hydrochloride)* Squibb 956	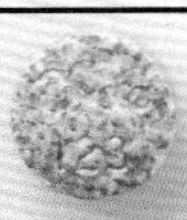 **Percodan-Demi** Schedule II Endo 123	**Dilantin 30 mg** *(phenytoin sodium)* Parke-Davis 365	**Serax 10 mg** *(oxazepam)* Schedule IV Wyeth 51

DRUGS THAT CAN BE ABUSED

Dolene 65 mg
(propoxyphene hydrochloride)
Schedule IV
Lederle
Sparine 100 mg
(promazine hydrochloride)
Wyeth
Haldol 2 mg
(haloperidol)
McNeil
Vesprin
trifluoromazine
Squibb 921
Prolixin 1 mg
(fluphenazine dihydrochloride)
Squibb 863
Mellaril 15 mg
(thioridazine hydrochloride)
Sandoz 78-8
Mellaril 200 mg
(thioridazine hydrochloride)
Sandoz
Noludar 300 mg
(methyprylon)
Schedule III
Roche
Elavil 100 mg
(amitriptyline HCl)
MSD 435
Euthroid-2
(liotrix)
Warner-Lambert 262
Moban 10 mg
(molindone hydrochloride)
Endo 073
Buticaps 15 mg
(butabarbital sodium)
Schedule III
McNeil
Lotusate 120 mg
(talbutal)
Schedule II
Winthrop
Butisol 15 mg
(butabarbital sodium)
Schedule III
McNeil
Ritalin 10 mg
(methylphenidate hydrochloride)
Schedule II
Ciba 3
Valium 10 mg
(diazepam)
Schedule IV
Roche
Synthroid 0.15 mg
(levothyroxine sodium)
Flint
Tranxene 3.75 mg
(clorazepate dipotassium)
Schedule IV
Abbott TL
Pre-Sate 65 mg
(clorphentermine HCl)
Schedule III
Warner-Lambert
Elavil 150 mg
(amitriptyline hydrochloride)
MSD 673
Asendin 100 mg
(amoxapine)
Lederle
Clonopin 1 mg
(clonazepam)
Schedule IV
Roche 62
Carbrital
Schedule III
Parke-Davis 372
Sinequan 150 mg
(doxepin hydrochloride)
Pfizer 537
Bentyl with phenobarbital 100 mg
Merrell
Fastin 30 mg
(phentermine hydrochloride)
Schedule IV
Beecham
Stelazine 1 mg
(trifluoperazine hydrochloride)
SKF S03
Stelazine 2 mg
(trifluoperazine hydrochloride)
SKF S04

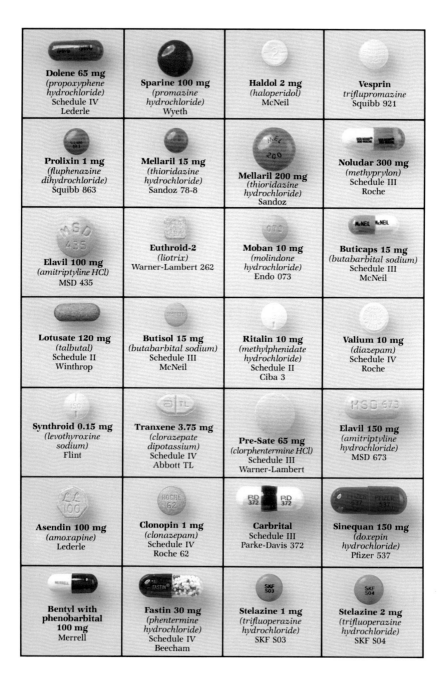

DRUGS THAT CAN BE ABUSED

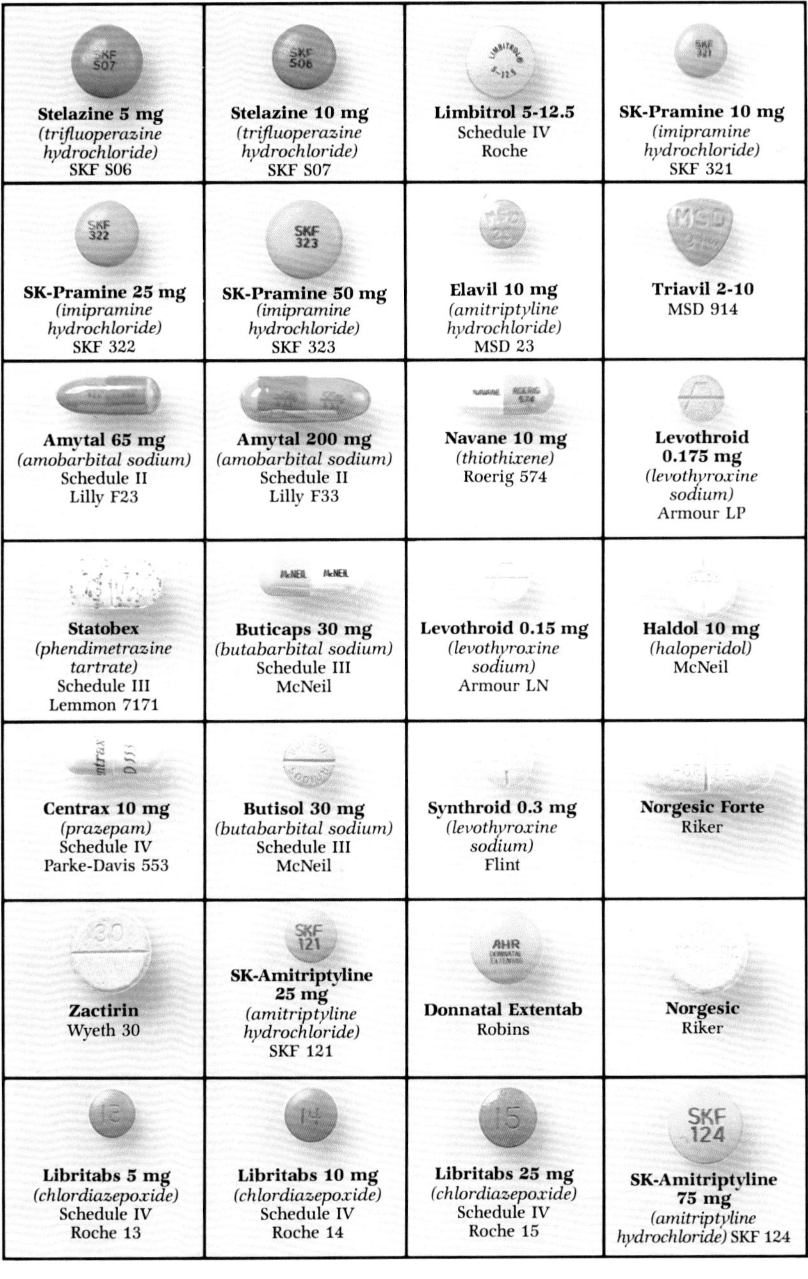

Stelazine 5 mg *(trifluoperazine hydrochloride)* SKF S06	**Stelazine 10 mg** *(trifluoperazine hydrochloride)* SKF S07	**Limbitrol 5-12.5** Schedule IV Roche	**SK-Pramine 10 mg** *(imipramine hydrochloride)* SKF 321
SK-Pramine 25 mg *(imipramine hydrochloride)* SKF 322	**SK-Pramine 50 mg** *(imipramine hydrochloride)* SKF 323	**Elavil 10 mg** *(amitriptyline hydrochloride)* MSD 23	**Triavil 2-10** MSD 914
Amytal 65 mg *(amobarbital sodium)* Schedule II Lilly F23	**Amytal 200 mg** *(amobarbital sodium)* Schedule II Lilly F33	**Navane 10 mg** *(thiothixene)* Roerig 574	**Levothroid 0.175 mg** *(levothyroxine sodium)* Armour LP
Statobex *(phendimetrazine tartrate)* Schedule III Lemmon 7171	**Buticaps 30 mg** *(butabarbital sodium)* Schedule III McNeil	**Levothroid 0.15 mg** *(levothyroxine sodium)* Armour LN	**Haldol 10 mg** *(haloperidol)* McNeil
Centrax 10 mg *(prazepam)* Schedule IV Parke-Davis 553	**Butisol 30 mg** *(butabarbital sodium)* Schedule III McNeil	**Synthroid 0.3 mg** *(levothyroxine sodium)* Flint	**Norgesic Forte** Riker
Zactirin Wyeth 30	**SK-Amitriptyline 25 mg** *(amitriptyline hydrochloride)* SKF 121	**Donnatal Extentab** Robins	**Norgesic** Riker
Libritabs 5 mg *(chlordiazepoxide)* Schedule IV Roche 13	**Libritabs 10 mg** *(chlordiazepoxide)* Schedule IV Roche 14	**Libritabs 25 mg** *(chlordiazepoxide)* Schedule IV Roche 15	**SK-Amitriptyline 75 mg** *(amitriptyline hydrochloride)* SKF 124

DRUGS THAT CAN BE ABUSED

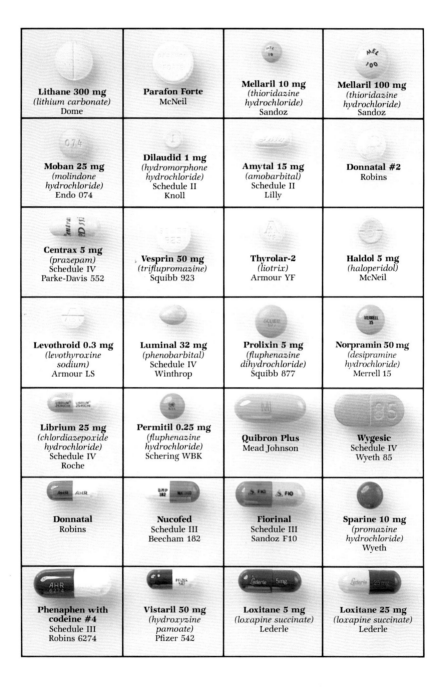

Lithane 300 mg *(lithium carbonate)* Dome	**Parafon Forte** McNeil	**Mellaril 10 mg** *(thioridazine hydrochloride)* Sandoz	**Mellaril 100 mg** *(thioridazine hydrochloride)* Sandoz
Moban 25 mg *(molindone hydrochloride)* Endo 074	**Dilaudid 1 mg** *(hydromorphone hydrochloride)* Schedule II Knoll	**Amytal 15 mg** *(amobarbital)* Schedule II Lilly	**Donnatal #2** Robins
Centrax 5 mg *(prazepam)* Schedule IV Parke-Davis 552	**Vesprin 50 mg** *(triflupromazine)* Squibb 923	**Thyrolar-2** *(liotrix)* Armour YF	**Haldol 5 mg** *(haloperidol)* McNeil
Levothroid 0.3 mg *(levothyroxine sodium)* Armour LS	**Luminal 32 mg** *(phenobarbital)* Schedule IV Winthrop	**Prolixin 5 mg** *(fluphenazine dihydrochloride)* Squibb 877	**Norpramin 50 mg** *(desipramine hydrochloride)* Merrell 15
Librium 25 mg *(chlordiazepoxide hydrochloride)* Schedule IV Roche	**Permitil 0.25 mg** *(fluphenazine hydrochloride)* Schering WBK	**Quibron Plus** Mead Johnson	**Wygesic** Schedule IV Wyeth 85
Donnatal Robins	**Nucofed** Schedule III Beecham 182	**Fiorinal** Schedule III Sandoz F10	**Sparine 10 mg** *(promazine hydrochloride)* Wyeth
Phenaphen with codeine #4 Schedule III Robins 6274	**Vistaril 50 mg** *(hydroxyzine pamoate)* Pfizer 542	**Loxitane 5 mg** *(loxapine succinate)* Lederle	**Loxitane 25 mg** *(loxapine succinate)* Lederle

DRUGS THAT CAN BE ABUSED

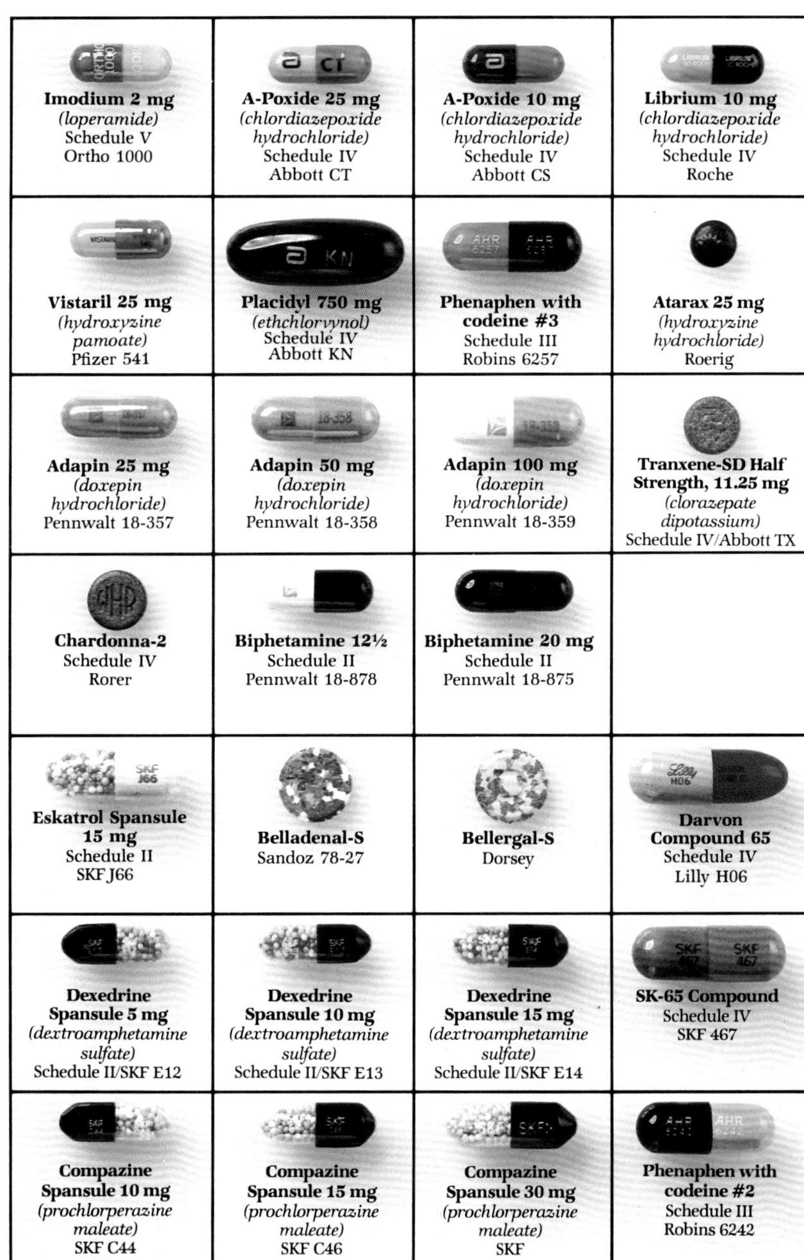

Imodium 2 mg *(loperamide)* Schedule V Ortho 1000	**A-Poxide 25 mg** *(chlordiazepoxide hydrochloride)* Schedule IV Abbott CT	**A-Poxide 10 mg** *(chlordiazepoxide hydrochloride)* Schedule IV Abbott CS	**Librium 10 mg** *(chlordiazepoxide hydrochloride)* Schedule IV Roche
Vistaril 25 mg *(hydroxyzine pamoate)* Pfizer 541	**Placidyl 750 mg** *(ethchlorvynol)* Schedule IV Abbott KN	**Phenaphen with codeine #3** Schedule III Robins 6257	**Atarax 25 mg** *(hydroxyzine hydrochloride)* Roerig
Adapin 25 mg *(doxepin hydrochloride)* Pennwalt 18-357	**Adapin 50 mg** *(doxepin hydrochloride)* Pennwalt 18-358	**Adapin 100 mg** *(doxepin hydrochloride)* Pennwalt 18-359	**Tranxene-SD Half Strength, 11.25 mg** *(clorazepate dipotassium)* Schedule IV/Abbott TX
Chardonna-2 Schedule IV Rorer	**Biphetamine 12½** Schedule II Pennwalt 18-878	**Biphetamine 20 mg** Schedule II Pennwalt 18-875	
Eskatrol Spansule 15 mg Schedule II SKF J66	**Belladenal-S** Sandoz 78-27	**Bellergal-S** Dorsey	**Darvon Compound 65** Schedule IV Lilly H06
Dexedrine Spansule 5 mg *(dextroamphetamine sulfate)* Schedule II/SKF E12	**Dexedrine Spansule 10 mg** *(dextroamphetamine sulfate)* Schedule II/SKF E13	**Dexedrine Spansule 15 mg** *(dextroamphetamine sulfate)* Schedule II/SKF E14	**SK-65 Compound** Schedule IV SKF 467
Compazine Spansule 10 mg *(prochlorperazine maleate)* SKF C44	**Compazine Spansule 15 mg** *(prochlorperazine maleate)* SKF C46	**Compazine Spansule 30 mg** *(prochlorperazine maleate)* SKF	**Phenaphen with codeine #2** Schedule III Robins 6242

DRUGS THAT CAN BE ABUSED

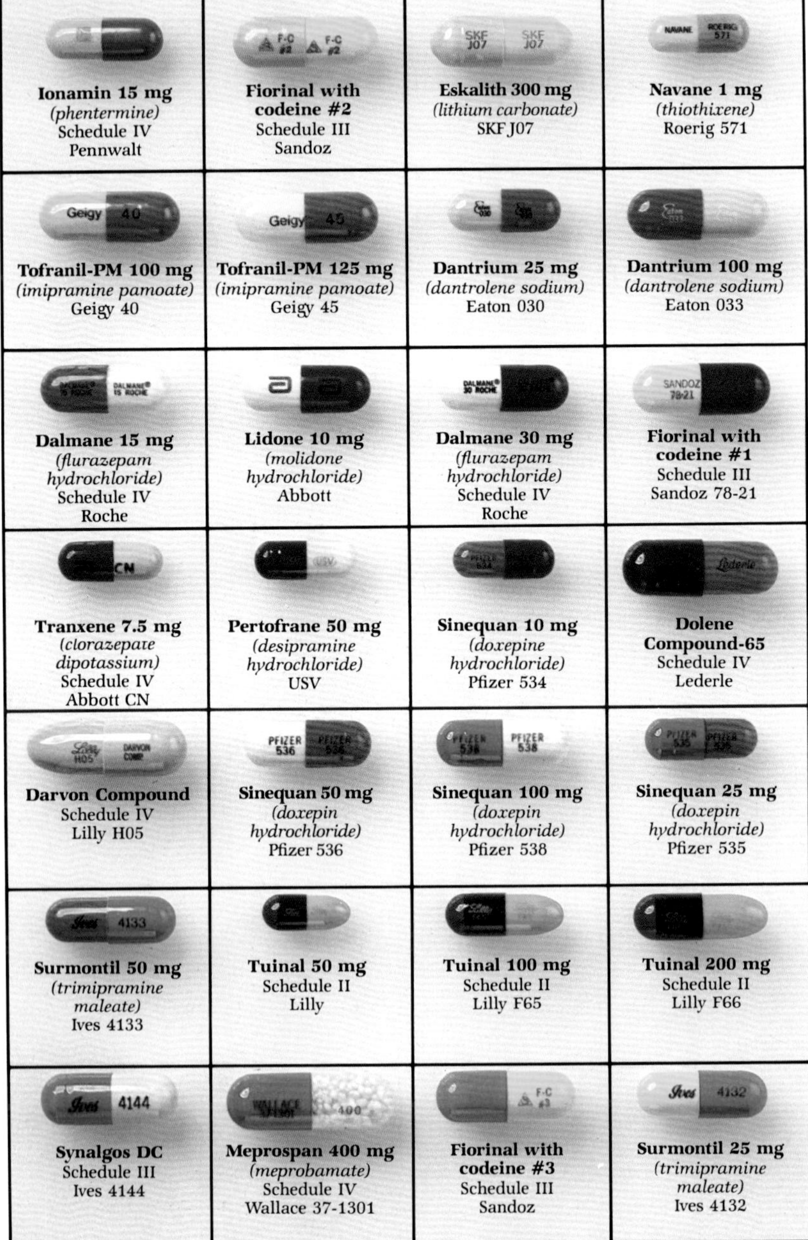

Ionamin 15 mg *(phentermine)* Schedule IV Pennwalt	**Fiorinal with codeine #2** Schedule III Sandoz	**Eskalith 300 mg** *(lithium carbonate)* SKF J07	**Navane 1 mg** *(thiothixene)* Roerig 571
Tofranil-PM 100 mg *(imipramine pamoate)* Geigy 40	**Tofranil-PM 125 mg** *(imipramine pamoate)* Geigy 45	**Dantrium 25 mg** *(dantrolene sodium)* Eaton 030	**Dantrium 100 mg** *(dantrolene sodium)* Eaton 033
Dalmane 15 mg *(flurazepam hydrochloride)* Schedule IV Roche	**Lidone 10 mg** *(molidone hydrochloride)* Abbott	**Dalmane 30 mg** *(flurazepam hydrochloride)* Schedule IV Roche	**Fiorinal with codeine #1** Schedule III Sandoz 78-21
Tranxene 7.5 mg *(clorazepate dipotassium)* Schedule IV Abbott CN	**Pertofrane 50 mg** *(desipramine hydrochloride)* USV	**Sinequan 10 mg** *(doxepine hydrochloride)* Pfizer 534	**Dolene Compound-65** Schedule IV Lederle
Darvon Compound Schedule IV Lilly H05	**Sinequan 50 mg** *(doxepin hydrochloride)* Pfizer 536	**Sinequan 100 mg** *(doxepin hydrochloride)* Pfizer 538	**Sinequan 25 mg** *(doxepin hydrochloride)* Pfizer 535
Surmontil 50 mg *(trimipramine maleate)* Ives 4133	**Tuinal 50 mg** Schedule II Lilly	**Tuinal 100 mg** Schedule II Lilly F65	**Tuinal 200 mg** Schedule II Lilly F66
Synalgos DC Schedule III Ives 4144	**Meprospan 400 mg** *(meprobamate)* Schedule IV Wallace 37-1301	**Fiorinal with codeine #3** Schedule III Sandoz	**Surmontil 25 mg** *(trimipramine maleate)* Ives 4132

DRUGS THAT CAN BE ABUSED

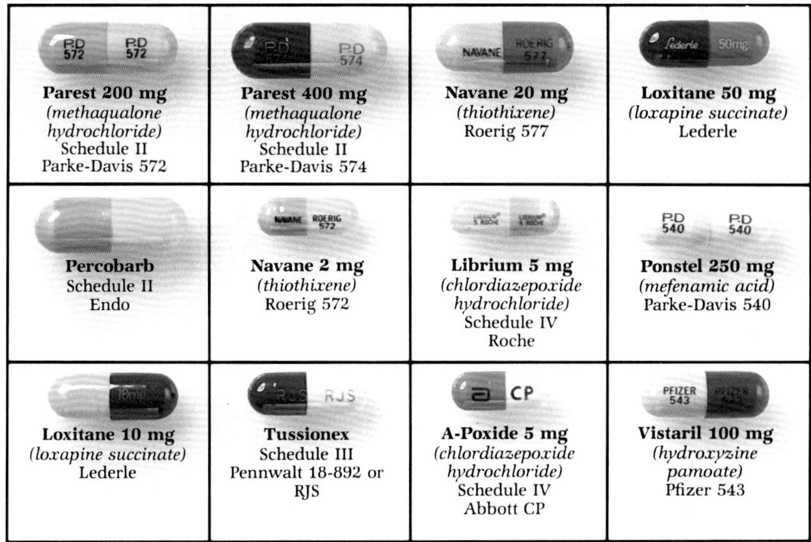

Parest 200 mg
(methaqualone hydrochloride)
Schedule II
Parke-Davis 572
Parest 400 mg
(methaqualone hydrochloride)
Schedule II
Parke-Davis 574
Navane 20 mg
(thiothixene)
Roerig 577
Loxitane 50 mg
(loxapine succinate)
Lederle
Percobarb
Schedule II
Endo
Navane 2 mg
(thiothixene)
Roerig 572
Librium 5 mg
(chlordiazepoxide hydrochloride)
Schedule IV
Roche
Ponstel 250 mg
(mefenamic acid)
Parke-Davis 540
Loxitane 10 mg
(loxapine succinate)
Lederle
Tussionex
Schedule III
Pennwalt 18-892 or RJS
A-Poxide 5 mg
(chlordiazepoxide hydrochloride)
Schedule IV
Abbott CP
Vistaril 100 mg
(hydroxyzine pamoate)
Pfizer 543

MANAGING DRUG OVERDOSE EMERGENCIES

In a drug overdose emergency, proper respiratory management and quick treatment of complications are essential. Follow these guidelines:

- To establish ventilation and maintain an open airway, extend the patient's head and pull his lower jaw forward. Then clear his airway of foreign material. If necessary, use suctioning to clear the airway of mucus or secretions.
- Insert an oral airway. If the patient's level of consciousness is high and he's having no apparent respiratory problems, place him in semi-Fowler's position and keep him under close observation. You may administer oxygen by nasal cannula.
- When ordered, administer a narcotic antagonist to reverse drug-induced respiratory depression. Onset of antagonism and reversal of narcotic depression is rapid, generally occurring within 2 to 3 minutes. Observe the patient closely for several hours for relapse of narcosis symptoms. Repeat administration of an antagonist may be necessary, depending on the amount, route of administration, and type of narcotic being antagonized. Be alert for withdrawal symptoms following administration of a narcotic antagonist.

If respiratory depression is severe and persistent (patient's gag and cough reflexes remain absent and respiratory rate is inadequate), an endotracheal tube may be inserted and a respirator used to achieve adequate ventilation. You may draw samples for arterial blood gas analysis to assess respiratory status, blood pH, and acid-base balance.

When the patient's respiratory status is stable, ingested drugs should be removed from his stomach as soon as possible. Therapies for this vary according to the type of drug taken. See APPENDIX, *Drug Toxicities,* for specific guidelines.

After the acute toxic emergency phase of the overdose has passed, continue maintenance and stabilization of the patient. Close observation of vital signs and level of consciousness is essential. Monitoring techniques and support therapy vary according to patient condition and the type of substance that produced the overdose. Be alert for withdrawal symptoms, especially if the patient is a narcotic abuser or addict.

OVER-THE-COUNTER DRUGS THAT CAN BE ABUSED
with major active ingredients listed

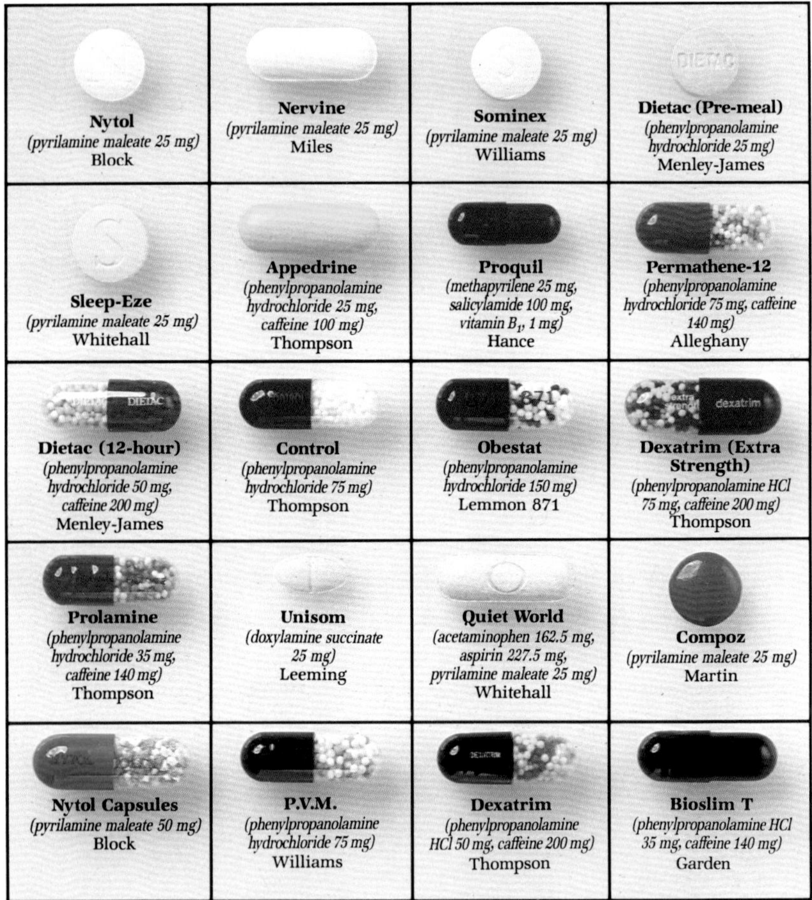

A FINAL CAUTION ON DRUG IDENTIFICATION

As a health-care professional, you're probably aware of the many look-alike products available today. In emergency situations, identification has to be accurate because overdose treatments for controlled substances are different from those for look-alike drugs.

As long as these drugs are properly labeled—that is, comply with current labeling requirements—they can be legally sold and are easily available in drugstores. The same drugs might be sold on the street, however—repackaged without proper labeling. Street buyers might take several of these look-alike tablets or capsules without much effect. At another time, they might get the authentic controlled substance and unknowingly take an overdose.

The federal government has begun to enforce postal regulations to curtail direct-mail advertising of look-alikes, and many states are enacting legislation to strictly curb deceptive marketing of these substances. The Drug Enforcement Agency (DEA) is recommending a model state law against drugs that may mislead consumers either by dosage-unit appearance or by misrepresentations about the drugs.

STREET NAMES TO KNOW

DRUG	STREET NAMES
Amphetamines, amphetamine (Benzedrine), methamphetamine (Desoxyn, Methedrine), dextroamphetamine (Dexedrine)	Beans, bennies, black beauties, black mollies, copilots, crank, crossroads, crystal, dexies, double cross, hearts, love drug, meth, minibennies, peaches, pep pills, speed, rosas, roses, thrusters, truck drivers, uppers, wake-ups, whites
Barbiturates, amobarbital (Amytal), pentobarbital (Nembutal), phenobarbital (Luminal), secobarbital (Seconal)	Barbs, blockbusters, bluebirds, blue devils, blues, Christmas trees, downers, green dragons, Mexican reds, pink ladies, pinks, rainbows, red and blues, redbirds, red devils, reds, sleeping pills, yellow jackets, yellow
Camphorated tincture of opium (Paregoric)	"Blue velvet" when mixed with pyribenzamine and taken I.V.
Cannabis (marijuana)	Acapulco gold, Colombian, grass, hash, herb, J, jay, joint, Mary Jane, Panama red, pot, reefer, smoke, tea, weed
Cocaine	Blow, C, coca, coke, flake, girl, heaven, dust, lady, mujer, nose candy, paradise, perico, rock, snow, stardust, upper, white
Diacetylmorphine (heroin)	Big H, boy, brown, brown sugar, crap, estuffa, H, heroina, hombre, horse, junk, Mexican mud, scag, smack, stuff, thing
Dimethyltryptamine (DMT)	Businessman's special
Lysergic acid diethylamide (LSD)	Acid, big D, blotter acid, brown dot, California sunshine, cubes, haze, microdots, paper acid, purple haze, sugar, sunshine, trips
Meperidine (Demerol)	Dollies
Methadone (Dolophine)	Dollies
Methaqualone (Quaalude)	Ludes, quads, quas, soapers, sopes, sopor
Methylphenidate (Ritalin)	California sunshine
Morphine	Cube, first line, goma, morf, morfina, morpho
Pentazocine (Talwin)	Dollies
Phencyclidine (PCP, Sernylan)	Angel dust, crystal, crystal joint, cyclone, elephant, hog, KJs, peace pill, rocket fuel
3, 4, 5-trimethoxyphenethylamine (Mescaline, Peyote)	Big chief, buttons, cactus, mesc, mescal, mescal buttons
2,5-dimethoxy-4-methylamphetamine (STP, DOM)	Serenity-tranquility-peace pill
3-(2-dimethylaminoethyl) Indol-4-ol dihydrogen phosphate (Psilocybin)	Silly putty, the mushrooms, magic Mexican mushrooms

ADDITIONAL RESOURCES

For a list of drug abuse treatment centers, see APPENDIX, p.1330.

In communities without local treatment facilities, narcotic addicts can be referred to the U.S. District Attorney, who will arrange for civil commitment under provision of the Federal Narcotic Addict Rehabilitation Act. Eligible patients will be treated in federal facilities and returned to their home communities for supervised aftercare.

For further information on drug abuse, contact the National Clearinghouse for Drug Abuse Information, P.O. Box 416, Kensington, Md. 20795, (301) 443-6500.

7

Amebicides and trichomonacides

carbarsone
chloroquine hydrochloride
chloroquine phosphate
diiodohydroxyquin
emetine hydrochloride
metronidazole
metronidazole hydrochloride
oxamniquine
paromomycin sulfate

Amebicides and trichomonacides cure or control diseases caused by amebic or trichomonal infection, such as amebiasis, primary amebic meningoencephalitis, and trichomoniasis. Amebiasis, or amebic dysentery, is an intestinal disorder caused by the parasite *Entamoeba histolytica*. The condition is now being reported more often than it was in the past, particularly among homosexual males.

Primary amebic meningoencephalitis, commonly transmitted through infected swimming pools, is caused by the ameba *Naegleria monocytogenes* and is almost always fatal.

Trichomoniasis is a relatively common vaginal infection caused by *Trichomonas vaginalis*. The infection spreads through sexual activity; infected males and about 70% of infected females are usually asymptomatic.

Major uses

• Metronidazole is the drug of choice for amebic dysentery and trichomonal infections; it may also be useful in treating gram-negative anaerobic infections. Alternate drugs are usually administered in combination with at least one other drug and are not always efficacious.

• The drug of choice for amebic meningoencephalitis is amphotericin B. (See Chapter 9, ANTIFUNGALS, for complete information about amphotericin B.)

Mechanism of action

• Carbarsone is an organic arsenic derivative with amebicidal activity in the intestinal lumen, possibly due to inhibition of sulfhydryl enzymes.

• Chloroquine is mainly an antimalarial. Its mechanism of action as an amebicide is unknown, but it's useful in treating extraintestinal amebiasis.

• Diiodohydroxyquin is an iodine derivative with amebicidal activity in the intestinal lumen. Its precise mechanism of action is unknown.

• Emetine kills *E. histolytica* by indirectly inhibiting protein synthesis.

• Metronidazole is a direct-acting trichomonacide and amebicide that works at both intestinal and extraintestinal sites.

• Oxamniquine reduces the egg load of *Schistosoma mansoni;* mechanism unknown.

• Paromomycin is an aminoglycoside antibiotic that acts as an amebicide in intestinal sites, effective in the presence or absence of bacteria. Its specific mechanism of action is unknown.

Absorption, distribution, metabolism, and excretion

• Carbarsone is readily absorbed from the gastrointestinal (GI) tract after oral and rectal administration but is excreted slowly in urine. The drug may accumulate, causing toxicity.

• Chloroquine is almost completely absorbed in the small intestine after oral administration. About 55% of the drug is bound to plasma proteins, and high concentrations are found in body tissues. It is excreted slowly in urine; small amounts are detectable after therapy is stopped—sometimes even years later.

• Diiodohydroxyquin is poorly absorbed from GI tract; most is eliminated in feces.

• Emetine is absorbed from parenteral sites, slowly detoxified by the liver, and excreted primarily by the kidneys. Detectable in urine 40 to 60 days after treatment, emetine concentrates in the liver, kidneys, and spleen.
• Metronidazole is well absorbed after oral administration, primarily in the small intestine. Limited data suggest wide distribution, with significant concentration in abscesses, bile, cerebrospinal fluid, and many tissues. From 60% to 70% is excreted in the urine unchanged; the remainder is metabolized in the liver.
• Oxamniquine, well absorbed when administered orally, is metabolized to inactive metabolites and excreted in the urine.
• Paromomycin is poorly absorbed from the GI tract after oral administration; almost all the drug is eliminated unchanged in the stool.

Onset and duration
• Chloroquine: Daily doses of 50 mg result in peak blood levels of 125 mcg/ml within 2 to 4 hours; half-life is about 3 days.
• Diiodohydroxyquin, emetine, and paromomycin: Onset is generally within 4 to 8 hours; effects can last 4 to 7 days.
• Metronidazole: Single oral doses of 750 mg cause peak blood levels of 10 to 15 mcg/ml within 2 to 4 hours; half-life is 6 to 12 hours.
• Oxamniquine: After doses of 12 to 15 mg/kg, blood levels peak in 1 to 1½ hours; half-life is 1 to 2½ hours.

PREVENTING AMEBIASIS

Amebic invasion of intestinal mucosa occurs most commonly in the cecum and rectosigmoid area, causing diarrhea and possibly abdominal pain, moderate leukocytosis, dehydration, or intermittent fever. After being carried into the bloodstream, the amebic infection may affect other parts of the body. For example, passage through the diaphragm may result in secondary pulmonary abscess formation.

To avoid contracting the infection, all nurses and visitors in contact with the patient with amebiasis must wear a gown and gloves, and wash their hands on entering and leaving the room. Private rooms are necessary only for children or confused patients. Masks are not needed at all.

Articles contaminated with the patient's urine and feces should be disinfected or discarded. Extreme caution should be used in handling and disposing of stool specimens.

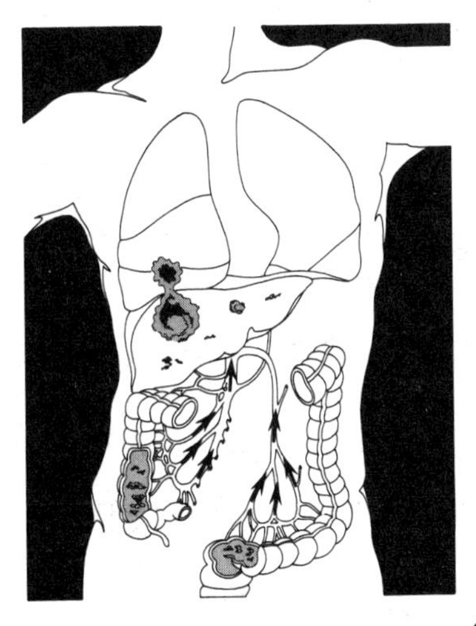

NAMES, INDICATIONS AND DOSAGES	SIDE EFFECTS
carbarsone **Intestinal amebiasis:** ADULTS: 250 mg P.O. b.i.d. or t.i.d. for 10 days. Rectal (as retention enema): 2 g dissolved in 200 ml warm 2% sodium bicarbonate solution, every other night for 5 doses. Discontinue oral therapy when enema is given. CHILDREN: average total dose is 75 mg/kg P.O. daily in 3 divided doses over 10-day period. Recommended total varies according to age—2 to 4 years, 2 g total; 5 to 8 years, 3 g total; 9 to 12 years, 4 g total; and over 12 years, 5 g total.	**Blood:** *agranulocytosis.* **CNS:** neuritis, convulsions, *hemorrhagic encephalitis.* **EENT:** sore throat, retinal edema, visual disturbances. **GI:** epigastric pain and burning, irritation, *nausea, vomiting,* diarrhea, anorexia, constipation, increased motility, abdominal cramps. **GU:** polyuria, albuminuria, kidney damage. **Hepatic:** hepatomegaly, jaundice, hepatitis. **Skin:** eruptions, *exfoliative dermatitis,* pruritus. **Other:** edema of wrists, ankles, and knees; weight loss; splenomegaly.
chloroquine hydrochloride Aralen HCl **chloroquine phosphate** Aralen Phosphate♦, Chlorocon, Roquine **Extraintestinal amebiasis:** ADULTS: 160 to 200 mg chloroquine (hydrochloride) base I.M. daily for no more than 10 to 12 days. As soon as possible, substitute 1 g (600 mg base) chloroquine phosphate P.O. daily for 2 days; then 500 mg (300 mg base) daily for at least 2 to 3 weeks. Treatment is usually combined with an effective intestinal amebicide. **Rheumatoid arthritis:** 250 mg chloroquine phosphate daily with evening meal.	**Blood:** *agranulocytosis.* **CNS:** mild and transient headache, neuromyopathy, psychic stimulation, fatigue, irritability, nightmares, convulsions, dizziness. **EENT:** *visual disturbances* (blurred vision; difficulty in focusing; reversible corneal changes; generally irreversible, sometimes progressive or delayed retinal changes, e.g., narrowing of arterioles; macular lesions; pallor of optic disk; optic atrophy; patchy retinal pigmentation, often leading to blindness), ototoxicity, nerve deafness, vertigo, tinnitus. **GI:** anorexia, abdominal cramps, diarrhea, nausea, vomiting. **Skin:** pruritus, lichen planus-like eruptions, skin and mucosal pigmentary changes, pleomorphic skin eruptions.
diiodohydroxyquin Gynovules♦♦, Inserfem, Yodoxin **Intestinal amebiasis:** ADULTS: 630 to 650 mg P.O. t.i.d. for 20 days. Total daily dose should not exceed 2 g. CHILDREN (USUAL DOSE): 30 to 40 mg/kg of body weight daily in 2 to 3 divided doses for 20 days. Additional courses of diiodohydroxyquin therapy should not be repeated before a resting interval of 2 to 3 weeks.	**Blood:** *agranulocytosis.* **CNS:** neurotoxicity, dysesthesia, weakness, vertigo, malaise, headache, agitation, retrograde amnesia, ataxia, peripheral neuropathy. **EENT:** optic neuritis, optic atrophy, loss of vision. **GI:** anorexia, nausea, vomiting, abdominal cramps, diarrhea, increased motility, constipation, epigastric burning and pain, gastritis, anal irritation and itching. **Skin:** pruritus, hives, papular and pustular eruptions, urticaria, discoloration of hair and nails. **Other:** thyroid enlargement, fever, chills, generalized furunculosis, hair loss.

INTERACTIONS AND SPECIAL CONSIDERATIONS

No significant interactions.

Special considerations:

• Contraindicated as initial treatment in patients with hepatic or renal disease; in patients with contracted visual or color fields; and in patients with known hypersensitivity or intolerance to any arsenical treatment.

• Toxicity may result if recommended dose is exceeded. If second treatment is needed, at least 10 days between courses should be allowed.

• To obtain required dose, carbarsone capsule should be divided. Should be given in ½ glass orange juice or milk, in small amount of 1% sodium bicarbonate solution, or in jelly or other food.

• Should be discontinued at first sign of intolerance or toxicity. Fatal exfoliative dermatitis and hemorrhagic encephalitis have been reported.

• Patient should report any unusual symptoms, even posttreatment.

• Liver function studies should precede therapy. Careful inspection of skin, vision testing, and palpation of liver and spleen should be repeated regularly.

• Intake and output should be monitored, and number, frequency, and character of stools reported.

• A cleansing enema should precede a carbarsone enema.

• Stool specimen should be sent to laboratory promptly; movements of parasites are seen only when stool is warm. Amebic cysts in stool indicate need for additional therapy. Stool specimen should be studied 1 week after stopping therapy and monthly for 1 year. Meticulous personal hygiene helps prevent reinfestation.

No significant interactions.

Special considerations:

• Contraindicated in patients with retinal or visual field changes, porphyria. Use with extreme caution in patients with severe GI, neurologic, or blood disorders. Drug concentrates in liver; use cautiously in patients with hepatic disease or alcoholism. Use with caution in patients with G-6-PD deficiency or psoriasis; drug may exacerbate these conditions.

• Complete blood cell counts, including liver function studies, should be made periodically during prolonged therapy; if severe blood disorder appears that is not attributable to disease under treatment, drug may need to be discontinued.

• Overdosage can quickly lead to toxic symptoms: headache, drowsiness, visual disturbances, cardiovascular collapse, and convulsions, followed by respiratory and cardiac arrest. Children are extremely susceptible to toxicity; long-term treatment should be avoided.

• Baseline and periodic ophthalmologic examinations needed. Blurred vision, increased sensitivity to light, or muscle weakness should be reported. After long-term use, patient should be checked periodically for muscular weakness. Audiometric examinations recommended before, during, and after therapy, especially if long-term.

• To avoid exacerbated drug-induced dermatoses, patient should avoid excessive exposure to sun.

• Each ml parenteral solution containing 50 mg dihydrochloride salt = 40 mg chloroquine base; each 500 mg tablet phosphate = 300 mg chloroquine base.

No significant interactions.

Special considerations:

• Contraindicated in patients with known hypersensitivity to 8-hydroxyquinoline derivatives or iodine-containing preparations. Diiodohydroxyquin causes hepatic damage in such patients. Also contraindicated in patients with hepatic or renal disease, or preexisting optic neuropathy.

• Patient should have periodic ophthalmologic examinations during treatment.

• Should be taken after meals. Crush tablets and mix with applesauce or chocolate syrup.

• Intake and output, and color and amount of stool should be monitored. Warm specimens should be sent to the laboratory frequently.

• Diarrhea possible during the first 2 to 3 days of treatment. Should be reported if it continues past 3 days.

• Patient should not discontinue the medication prematurely but should notify doctor if skin rash occurs.

NAMES, INDICATIONS AND DOSAGES	SIDE EFFECTS

emetine hydrochloride

Acute fulminating amebic dysentery:

ADULTS: 1 mg/kg daily up to 65 mg daily (1 or 2 doses) deep S.C. or I.M. 3 to 5 days to control symptoms. Give another antiamebic drug simultaneously.

CHILDREN OVER 8 YEARS: no more than 20 mg daily deep S.C. or I.M. for 3 to 5 days.

CHILDREN UNDER 8 YEARS: no more than 10 mg daily for 3 to 5 days.

Amebic hepatitis and abscess:

ADULTS: 65 mg daily (1 or 2 doses) deep S.C. or I.M. for 10 days.

CHILDREN OVER 8 YEARS: no more than 20 mg daily for 10 days.

CHILDREN UNDER 8 YEARS: no more than 10 mg daily for 10 days.

CNS: dizziness, headache, mild sensory disturbances, central or peripheral nerve function changes, neuromuscular symptoms (weakness, aching, stiffness, tenderness, pain, tremors).
CV: *acute toxicity*—can occur at any dose (hypotension, tachycardia, precordial pain, dyspnea, *EKG abnormalities*, gallop rhythm, cardiac dilatation, severe acute degenerative myocarditis, pericarditis, congestive failure).
GI: *nausea, vomiting, diarrhea,* abdominal cramps, loss of sense of taste.
Metabolic: decreased serum potassium levels.
Skin: eczematous, urticarial purpuric lesions.
Local: skeletal muscle stiffness, aching, tenderness, muscle weakness at injection site.
Other: edema.

---

metronidazole
Flagyl♦, Neo-Tric♦♦, Novonidazol♦♦, Trikacide♦♦
metronidazole hydrochloride
Flagyl I.V.

Amebic hepatic abscess:

ADULTS: 500 to 750 mg P.O. t.i.d. for 5 to 10 days.

CHILDREN: 35 to 50 mg/kg daily (in 3 doses) for 10 days.

Intestinal amebiasis:

ADULTS: 750 mg P.O. t.i.d. for 5 to 10 days.

CHILDREN: 35 to 50 mg/kg daily (in 3 doses) for 10 days. Follow this therapy with oral diiodohydroxyquin.

Trichomoniasis:

ADULTS (BOTH MALE AND FEMALE): 250 mg P.O. t.i.d. for 7 days or 2 g P.O. in single dose; 4 to 6 weeks should elapse between courses of therapy.

Refractory trichomoniasis:

WOMEN: 250 mg P.O. b.i.d. for 10 days.

Treatment of bacterial infections caused by anaerobic microorganisms:

ADULTS: Loading dose is 15 mg/kg I.V. infused over 1 hour (approximately 1 g for a 70-kg adult). Maintenance dose is 7.5 mg/kg I.V. or P.O. q 6 hours (approximately 500 mg for a 70-kg adult). First maintenance dose should be administered 6 hours following loading dose.

Blood: leukopenia, neutropenia.
CNS: vertigo, headache, ataxia, incoordination, confusion, irritability, depression, restlessness, weakness, fatigue, drowsiness, insomnia, sensory neuropathy, paresthesias of extremities, psychic stimulation, neuromyopathy.
CV: EKG change (flattened T wave).
EENT: blurred vision, difficulty in focusing, nasal congestion.
GI: abdominal cramping, stomatitis, *nausea, vomiting, anorexia,* diarrhea, constipation, proctitis, dry mouth.
GU: darkened urine, polyuria, dysuria, pyuria, incontinence, cystitis, decreased libido, dyspareunia, dryness of vagina and vulva, sense of pelvic pressure.
Skin: pruritus, flushing.
Local: *thrombophlebitis after I.V. infusion.*
Other: overgrowth of nonsusceptible organisms, especially *Candida* (glossitis, furry tongue), metallic taste, fever.

INTERACTIONS AND SPECIAL CONSIDERATIONS

No significant interactions.

Special considerations:

• Contraindicated in patients with cardiac or renal disease, except those with amebic abscess or hepatitis not controlled by chloroquine; patients who have received a course of emetine less than 6 to 8 weeks previously; in children, except for those with severe dysentery unresponsive to other amebicides; and in those with polyneuropathy or muscle disease. Use with caution in aged, debilitated, or preoperative patients, and patients with hypotension.

• Pulse rate and blood pressure should be checked 2 to 3 times daily and use discontinued if drug produces tachycardia, precipitous fall in blood pressure, neuromuscular symptoms, marked gastrointestinal effects, or considerable weakness. Weakness and muscle symptoms usually precede more serious symptoms, and serve as a guide for avoiding toxicity.

• Recommended dose should not be exceeded or therapy extended beyond 10 days. Patient should be confined to bed during treatment and for several days thereafter.

• Drug may alter EKG tracings for 6 weeks. EKG should be taken before therapy, after fifth dose, upon completion, and 1 week after therapy. Patterns can resemble those of myocardial infarction. First and most consistent change is T wave inversion.

• Deep S.C. administration is preferred; I.M. acceptable; I.V. route is dangerous and contraindicated. Injections cause necrosis and edema. Sites should be rotated and warm soaks applied.

• Intake and output; odor and consistency of stools; and presence of mucus, blood, or other foreign matter should be monitored. Warm specimens should be sent to the laboratory frequently, and fecal examinations repeated at 3-month intervals to assure elimination of amebae. Patients with acute amebic dysentery often become asymptomatic carriers. Family members and suspected contacts should be checked.

• Suspect emetine-induced reaction if number of stools increases after initial relief of diarrhea.

• Correct patient hygiene can help prevent reinfection.

• Drug is very irritating: avoid contact with eyes and mucous membranes.

• Restoration of body fluids and nutrients is important adjunct to therapy.

Interactions:

ALCOHOL: disulfiram-like reaction (nausea, vomiting, headache, cramps, flushing). Don't use together.

DISULFIRAM: acute psychoses and confusional states. Don't use together.

Special considerations:

• *Warning:* This drug has been shown to be carcinogenic in mice and possibly rats. Unnecessary use should be avoided.

• Contraindicated in patients with a history of blood dyscrasia or CNS disorder, and in patients with retinal or visual field changes. Use with caution in patients with hepatic disease or alcoholism; in conjunction with known hepatotoxic drugs.

• Patients should avoid alcohol or alcohol-containing medications.

• Should be taken with meals to minimize GI distress.

• Metallic taste and dark or reddish-brown urine are possible.

• When used in the treatment of amebiasis, number and character of stools should be monitored. Metronidazole should be used only after *Trichomonas vaginalis* has been confirmed by wet smear or culture or *Entamoeba histolytica* has been identified. Asymptomatic sexual partners of patients being treated for *T. vaginalis* infection should be treated simultaneously to avoid reinfection. Correct patient hygiene can prevent reinfection.

• Has been used to treat anaerobic infections.

NAMES, INDICATIONS AND DOSAGES	SIDE EFFECTS
oxamniquine Vansil **Treatment of schistosomiasis caused by *Schistosoma mansoni:*** ADULTS: 12 to 15 mg/kg given as a single oral dose. CHILDREN (UNDER 30 KG): 20 mg/kg given in two equally divided oral doses at 2- to 8-hour intervals.	**CNS:** *convulsions, dizziness, drowsiness,* headache. **GI:** nausea, vomiting, abdominal pain, anorexia. **Skin:** urticaria.
paromomycin sulfate Humatin **Intestinal amebiasis, acute and chronic:** ADULTS AND CHILDREN: 25 to 35 mg/kg daily P.O. in 3 doses for 5 to 10 days after meals.	**Blood:** eosinophilia. **CNS:** headache, vertigo. **EENT:** ototoxicity. **GI:** anorexia, nausea, vomiting, epigastric pain and burning, abdominal cramps, diarrhea, constipation, increased motility, steatorrhea, pruritus ani, malabsorption syndrome. **GU:** hematuria, nephrotoxicity. **Skin:** rash, exanthema, pruritus. **Other:** overgrowth of nonsusceptible organisms.

♦ Available in U.S. and Canada. ♦♦ Available in Canada only.
All other products (no symbol) available in U.S. only. Italicized side effects are common or life-threatening.

OBTAINING UNAPPROVED AMEBICIDAL DRUGS

To obtain an amebicidal drug that is not commercially available, call the Center for Disease Control.

With a doctor's order for one of these investigational drugs, you can contact:

Parasitic Disease Drug Service
Center for Infectious Diseases
Center for Disease Control
Atlanta, Ga. 30333
(404) 329-3670

Here's a list of investigational amebicides and the infections they're used to treat:

INTERACTIONS AND SPECIAL CONSIDERATIONS

No significant interactions.

Special considerations:
- There are no known contraindications.
- Use cautiously in patients with a history of convulsive conditions. Epileptiform convulsions have rarely been observed within the first few hours after ingestion. Patients with history of convulsions should be kept under medical supervision.
- Patient should avoid driving and other hazardous activities if he's dizzy or drowsy.
- Gastrointestinal tolerance is improved if the drug is taken after meals.
- Although *S. mansoni* infection is rare in the United States and Canada, travelers or immigrants from such areas as Puerto Rico, Latin America, and Africa may have contracted the infection from contaminated water.

No significant interactions.

Special considerations:
- Contraindicated in impaired renal function or intestinal obstruction. Use with caution in ulcerative lesions of the bowel to avoid inadvertent absorption and resulting renal toxicity. Poorly absorbed orally but will accumulate with renal impairment or ulcerative lesions.
- History of sensitivity to this drug should be considered before first dose.
- Should be taken after meals.
- Personal hygiene should be emphasized, particularly handwashing before eating and after defecation.
- Criterion of cure is absence of amebae in stools examined weekly for 6 weeks after treatment and thereafter at monthly intervals for 2 years. Feces of family members or suspected contacts should be examined.
- High doses or prolonged therapy should be avoided.
- Superinfection (continued fever and other signs of new infections, especially monilial infections) is possible.

INVESTIGATIONAL DRUG	AMEBIC INFECTION
bithionol	Sheep liver fluke infection
cycloguanil pamoate	Leishmaniasis
dehydroemetine	Amebiasis
diloxanide furoate	Amebiasis
melarsoprol	African trypanosomiasis
metrifonate	Schistosomiasis
niclosamide	Tapeworm infection
pentamidine isethionate	*Pneumocystis carinii*
sodium antimony dimercaptosuccinate	Schistosomiasis
stibogluconate sodium	Leishmaniasis
suramin	African trypanosomiasis

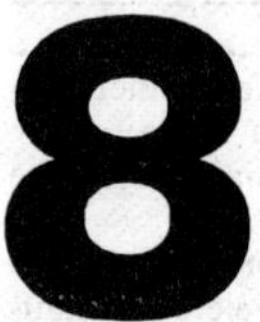

Anthelmintics

antimony potassium tartrate
diethylcarbamazine citrate
gentian violet
mebendazole
piperazine adipate
piperazine citrate
piperazine phosphate
piperazine tartrate
pyrantel pamoate
pyrvinium pamoate
quinacrine hydrochloride
thiabendazole

Anthelmintics rid the body of helminths, or parasitic worms. Although helmintic infections are usually confined to the intestines, dissemination to the genitalia, peritoneum, and hematopoietic system may occur.

Major uses
Anthelmintics eradicate various helminths, including tapeworms, pinworms, hookworms, roundworms, and schistosomes.

Mechanism of action
- Antimony potassium tartrate inhibits phosphofructokinase, and therefore glucose utilization, in schistosomes.
- Diethylcarbamazine appears to sensitize the worms to phagocytosis by the reticuloendothelial system.
- Mebendazole appears to selectively and irreversibly inhibit uptake of glucose and other nutrients in susceptible helminths.
- Piperazine and pyrantel block neuromuscular action, paralyzing the worm and causing its expulsion by normal peristalsis.
- Pyrvinium, a cyanine dye, appears to destroy parasites by preventing them from using exogenous carbohydrates.
- Quinacrine inhibits deoxyribonucleic acid metabolism.
- Mechanism of action of gentian violet and thiabendazole is unknown.

Absorption, distribution, metabolism, and excretion
- Antimony potassium tartrate is extensively bound within erythrocytes after parenteral administration. Excretion is primarily by the kidneys.
- Diethylcarbamazine is readily absorbed from the gastrointestinal (GI) tract, distributed to all body tissues except fat, and excreted in the urine.
- Piperazine is readily absorbed from the GI tract. Some piperazine is metabolized in the liver; the remainder is excreted unchanged in the urine.
- Pyrantel is poorly absorbed from the GI tract. It is metabolized primarily in the liver; the rest is eliminated unchanged in urine and feces. Rates of excretion vary greatly among patients.
- Quinacrine is readily absorbed from the GI tract and is highly concentrated in the liver. Its metabolism and excretion are unknown.
- Thiabendazole is rapidly absorbed from the GI tract; it's metabolized, then excreted in the urine.
- Other anthelmintics—gentian violet, mebandazole, and pyrvinium—are poorly absorbed from the GI tract and are mainly eliminated in the feces.

Onset and duration
Anthelmintics have a rapid onset and short duration.

PARENT-TEACHING AID

HOW TO PREVENT AND CONTROL PINWORMS

Dear Parents:

Pinworms are small, threadlike worms, ⅓″ to ⅔″ (0.8 to 1.7 cm) long. They're found throughout the world, most frequently in preschool age and school-age children. The infection usually spreads in the family.

To help prevent and control pinworms, make sure your child:

- washes his hands carefully after using lavatory facilities and before handling food
- avoids nail-biting
- bathes and changes underwear daily.

If you suspect a household member has pinworms, have the doctor treat the whole family at the same time. Have all family members avoid bathing in or drinking water that may be contaminated. Also:

- Cook meat thoroughly to kill any infectious larvae.
- During pinworm treatment, disinfect clothing and bed linens by washing in hot water (55.5° C. [132° F.]).

THE PINWORM CYCLE

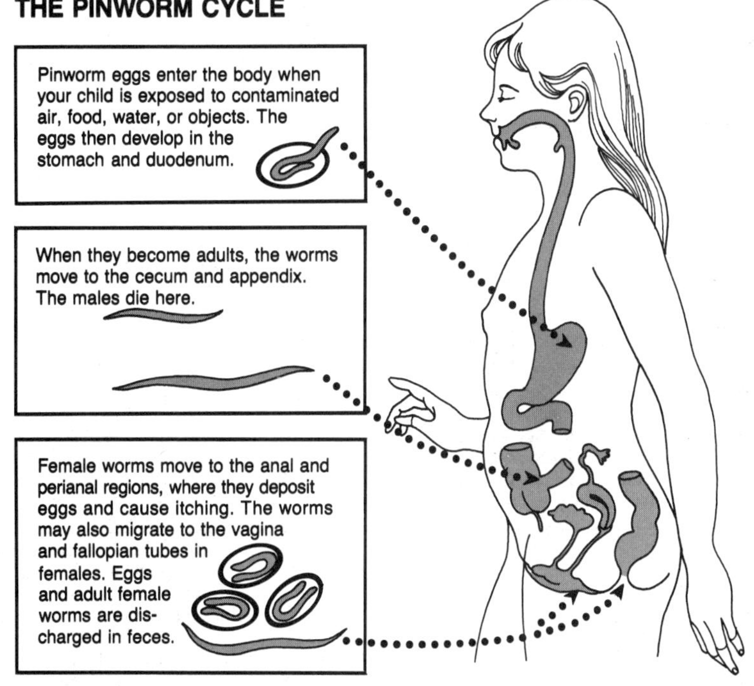

Pinworm eggs enter the body when your child is exposed to contaminated air, food, water, or objects. The eggs then develop in the stomach and duodenum.
When they become adults, the worms move to the cecum and appendix. The males die here.
Female worms move to the anal and perianal regions, where they deposit eggs and cause itching. The worms may also migrate to the vagina and fallopian tubes in females. Eggs and adult female worms are discharged in feces.

NAMES, INDICATIONS AND DOSAGES	SIDE EFFECTS
antimony potassium tartrate (not commercially available; must be compounded) ***Schistosoma japonicum* infection:** ADULTS: initially, 8 ml of 0.5% solution in sterile water for injection or 5% dextrose solution given slow I.V. Increase each subsequent dose 4 ml until 11th day, when 28 ml are given. Give 28 ml on alternate days until a total of 360 ml (1.8 g) is given.	**Blood:** thrombocytopenia. **CV:** hypotension, syncope, bradycardia, EKG changes. **GI:** nausea, vomiting, diarrhea, colic. **Hepatic:** jaundice, *hepatic necrosis.* **Local:** pain at I.V. injection site. **Other:** dyspnea, severe arthralgia, albuminuria, fever, dermatitis.
diethylcarbamazine citrate Hetrazan **Ascariasis (roundworm):** ADULTS: 13 mg/kg P.O. daily for 7 days. CHILDREN: 6 to 10 mg/kg P.O. t.i.d. for 7 to 10 days. **Loiasis, dipetalonemiasis, onchocerciasis, Bancroftian or Malayan filariasis:** ADULTS AND CHILDREN: 2 mg/kg P.O. t.i.d. for 3 to 4 weeks. Repeat if necessary. **Tropical (pulmonary) eosinophilia:** ADULTS AND CHILDREN: 13 mg/kg P.O. daily for 4 to 7 days.	**Blood:** leukocytosis, eosinophilia. **CNS:** *headache, malaise, weakness,* lassitude, syncope. **CV:** tachycardia, tachypnea, hypotension. **GI:** anorexia, nausea, vomiting. **Skin:** pruritus, dermatitis, bullous eruptions. **Other:** arthralgia, myalgia, joint pain, swelling and edema of face, severe pedal edema, fever, lymphadenitis, sweating, cough.
gentian violet **Pinworms:** ADULTS: 60 mg P.O. t.i.d. 7 to 10 days. CHILDREN: 2 mg/kg P.O. daily in 2 to 3 doses for 8 to 10 days, not to exceed 90 mg/day. Discontinue treatment after 7 to 10 days. Resume if needed.	**CNS:** headache, dizziness, lassitude. **GI:** nausea, diarrhea, vomiting (purple), abdominal cramps.
mebendazole Vermox♦ **Pinworms:** ADULTS AND CHILDREN OVER 2 YEARS: 100 mg P.O. as a single dose. If infection persists 3 weeks later, repeat treatment. **Roundworm, whipworm, hookworm:** ADULTS AND CHILDREN OVER 2 YEARS: 100 mg P.O. b.i.d. for 3 days. If infection persists 3 weeks later, repeat treatment.	**GI:** occasional, transient abdominal pain and diarrhea in massive infection and expulsion of worms.
piperazine adipate Entacyl♦♦ **piperazine citrate** Antepar♦, Bryrel, Pin-Tega Tabs, Pipril, Ta-Verm, Vermazine **piperazine phosphate** Antepar Phosphate **piperazine tartrate** Razine Tartrate	**CNS:** ataxia, tremors, choreiform movements, muscular weakness, myoclonus, hyporeflexia, paresthesias, convulsions, sense of detachment, EEG abnormalities, memory defect, headache, vertigo. **EENT:** nystagmus, blurred vision, paralytic strabismus, cataracts with visual impairment, lacrimation, difficulty in focusing, rhinorrhea. **GI:** *nausea, vomiting,* diarrhea, abdominal cramps.

INTERACTIONS AND SPECIAL CONSIDERATIONS

No significant interactions.

Special considerations:
- Treatment of choice for *S. japonicum.*
- Not for use in other worm infestations; toxicity with this agent is high.
- Solutions must be freshly prepared.
- Doses should be given 2 hours after a light meal.
- Patient should lie down for 1 hour after treatment.
- Antiemetics should not be given, since they mask nausea and vomiting, which are signs of hepatic toxicity.
- Extravasation may cause painful cellulitis.
- Rapid injection may lead to severe cough, vomiting, or even death.

No significant interactions.

Special considerations:
- Use with caution in patients with hypertension; severe hepatic, renal, or cardiac disease; and in children under 1 year of age. Patients with recent history of malaria should be treated with an antimalarial agent first to prevent relapse in asymptomatic malarial infections.
- Should be administered carefully to avoid or control allergic or other untoward reactions. Concomitant corticosteroids, antihistamines, or aspirin can minimize allergic reactions.
- Side effects usually minor and transient.
- Good hygiene can help prevent reinfestation.
- Should be taken immediately after meals. Drug has sweet but unpleasant taste.

No significant interactions.

Special considerations:
- Use with caution in patients with cardiac, hepatic, renal, or GI disease.
- Tablets must be taken whole with water at mealtime.
- Patient should abstain from alcohol during treatment.
- If nausea and vomiting occur, stop treatment for 1 to 2 days; resume at reduced dosage. Skin, clothing, vomitus, and feces will be stained purple.
- Good hygiene can help prevent reinfestation.

No significant interactions.

Special considerations:
- Tablets may be chewed, swallowed, or crushed and mixed with food.
- No dietary restrictions, laxatives, or enemas necessary.
- To avoid reinfestation, perianal area should be washed daily; undergarments and bedclothes changed daily; and hands washed and fingernails cleaned after bowel movements and before meals. All family members should be treated.

No significant interactions.

Special considerations:
- Contraindicated in patients with hepatic and/or renal impairment, or convulsive disorders. Use with caution in patients with severe malnutrition or anemia.
- Should be discontinued if CNS or significant GI reactions occur.
- Because of potential neurotoxicity, prolonged or repeated treatment, especially in children, should be avoided.
- No dietary restrictions, laxatives, or enemas necessary.
- May be taken with food.
- To avoid reinfestation, perianal area should be washed daily; undergarments and bedclothes changed daily; and hands washed and fingernails cleaned after bowel movements and before meals. All family members should be treated.

(continued on following page)

NAMES, INDICATIONS AND DOSAGES	SIDE EFFECTS
piperazine *(continued)* **Pinworms:** ADULTS AND CHILDREN: 65 mg/kg P.O. daily 7 to 8 days. Maximum daily dose is 2.5 g. **Roundworm:** ADULTS: 3.5 g P.O. in single doses for 2 consecutive days. CHILDREN: 75 mg/kg P.O. daily in single dose for 2 consecutive days. Maximum daily dose: 3.5 g.	**Skin:** urticaria, photodermatitis, *erythema multiforme*, purpura, eczematous skin reactions. **Other:** arthralgia, fever, bronchospasm.
pyrantel pamoate Antiminth, Combantrin♦♦ **Roundworm and pinworm:** ADULTS AND CHILDREN OVER 2 YEARS: single dose of 11 mg/kg P.O. Maximum dose 1 g. For pinworm, dose should be repeated in 2 weeks.	**CNS:** headache, dizziness, drowsiness, insomnia. **GI:** anorexia, nausea, vomiting, gastralgia, cramps, diarrhea, tenesmus. **Hepatic:** transient elevation of SGOT. **Skin:** rashes. **Other:** fever, weakness.
pyrvinium pamoate Pamovin♦♦, Povan, Pyr-Pam♦♦, Vanquin♦♦ **Pinworm:** ADULTS AND CHILDREN: 5 mg/kg P.O. single dose (maximum 350 mg). Repeat in 2 weeks if needed.	**GI:** nausea, vomiting, cramping, diarrhea (vomiting more common with suspension than with tablets). **Skin:** photosensitivity, *erythema multiforme*.
quinacrine hydrochloride Atabrine **Treatment of giardiasis:** ADULTS: 100 mg P.O. for 5 to 7 days. CHILDREN: 7 mg/kg/day P.O. given in 3 divided doses after meals for 5 days. Maximum 300 mg/day. If necessary, the dosage may be repeated in 2 weeks. **Treatment of tapeworm:** ADULTS AND CHILDREN OVER 14 YEARS: Administer a cleansing enema. Then administer 4 doses of 200 mg P.O. every 10 minutes (total 800 mg). CHILDREN 11 TO 14 YEARS: Total 600 mg P.O. in 3 to 4 doses at 10-minute intervals. CHILDREN 5 TO 10 YEARS: Total 400 mg P.O. in 3 to 4 doses at 10-minute intervals.	**CNS:** *headache, dizziness,* nervousness, vertigo, mood shifts, nightmares. **GI:** *diarrhea, anorexia, nausea, abdominal cramps,* vomiting. **Skin:** pleomorphic skin eruptions.

INTERACTIONS AND SPECIAL CONSIDERATIONS	
• Protect from air, light, and moisture.	
No significant interactions. *Special considerations:* • Use cautiously in severe malnutrition or anemia, or in hepatic dysfunction. Patient should be treated for anemia, dehydration, or malnutrition before taking drug. • No dietary restrictions, laxatives, or enemas necessary. • May be taken with food. Shake well before pouring.	• Careful perianal hygiene can help prevent reinfestation. All family members should be treated. • Protect from light. Store below 30° C. (86° F.).
No significant interactions. *Special considerations:* • Safe use in children who weigh less than 36 kg not established. • Tablets must be swallowed whole to avoid staining teeth. May be taken with food. • Drug stains materials, skin, vomitus, and stools bright red. • No dietary restrictions, laxatives, or enemas necessary.	• Careful perianal hygiene can help prevent reinfestation. All family members should be treated. • Protect from light.
No significant interactions. *Special considerations:* • Contraindicated if primaquine is being given concurrently since primaquine toxicity could be increased. • Use with extreme caution in patients with porphyria or psoriasis; may exacerbate these conditions. • Use with caution in patients with hepatic disease, alcoholism, severe renal or cardiac disease, psychosis, G-6-PD deficiency, and in those over 60 years or under 1 year. • Saline cathartic is necessary after treatment to dispel worms. • Should be taken after meals with large glass of water, tea, or fruit juice to reduce GI irritation. Bitter taste may be disguised by jam or honey. • Nausea and vomiting after large doses may be lessened by taking sodium bicarbonate with each dose. • All of stool should be collected after treatment. Toilet paper should not be put in bedpan.	Scolex (attachment organ) will be stained yellow from drug. • Temporary yellow color of skin and urine is not jaundice. • Patient should be on a bland, nonfat, semisolid diet for 24 hours, and should fast after the evening meal before treatment. • Keep out of reach of children; drug is highly toxic. • Emesis should be induced for overdose.

NAMES, INDICATIONS AND DOSAGES	SIDE EFFECTS
thiabendazole Mintezol♦ **Systemic infection with pinworm, roundworm, threadworm, whipworm, cutaneous larva migrans, and trichinosis:** ADULTS OR CHILDREN OVER 70 KG: 1.5 g P.O. ADULTS OR CHILDREN UNDER 70 KG: 25 mg/kg P.O. in 2 doses daily. Maximum dose is 3 g daily. **Cutaneous infestations with larva migrans (creeping eruption):** ADULTS AND CHILDREN: dose depends on patient's weight. 70 kg or over, 1.5 g P.O./dose; under 70 kg, 4.6 mg/kg/dose. 2 doses daily for 2 successive days. If active lesions still present 2 days after therapy, give second course. *Pinworm*—2 doses daily for 1 day; repeat in 7 days. *Roundworm, threadworm, whipworm*—2 doses daily for 2 successive days. *Trichinosis*—2 doses daily for 2 to 4 successive days.	**CNS:** impaired mental alertness, impaired physical coordination, *drowsiness, giddiness,* headache, dizziness. **GI:** anorexia, nausea, vomiting, diarrhea, epigastric distress. **Skin:** rash, pruritus, *erythema multiforme.* **Other:** lymphadenopathy, fever, flushing, chills.

♦ Available in U.S. and Canada. ♦♦ Available in Canada only.
All other products (no symbol) available in U.S. only. Italicized side effects are common or life-threatening.

BASIC FACTS ABOUT COMMON HELMINTH INFECTIONS

CONDITION	CAUSE	SOURCE OF INFECTION
Tapeworm infection	Tapeworm *(Hymenolepis nana, Taenia saginata, Taenia solium, Diphyllobothrium latum)*	Poorly cooked or infected beef, pork, or fish
Enterobiasis	Pinworm *(Enterobius vermicularis)*	Eggs from contaminated objects (books, clothes, toys, wooden objects)
Hookworm infection	Hookworm *(Necator americanus, Ancylostoma duodenale)*	Contaminated feces
Roundworm infection	Roundworm *(Ascaris lumbricoides)*	Contaminated feces
Schistosomiasis	Schistosome *(Schistosoma japonicum, Schistosoma mansoni, Schistosoma haematobium)*	Infested water containing larvae from snail vector

INTERACTIONS AND SPECIAL CONSIDERATIONS

No significant interactions.

Special considerations:

- Use with caution in patients with hepatic or renal dysfunction, severe malnutrition, anemia, and in patients who are vomiting. Supportive therapy indicated for anemic, dehydrated, or malnourished patients. In children under 15 kg, benefits should be weighed against risks.
- Medication may cause drowsiness and dizziness.
- Should be taken after meals. Shake suspension before measuring; tablets should be chewed before swallowing.
- Laxatives, enemas, and diet restrictions not needed.
- To avoid reinfestation, perianal area should be washed daily; undergarments and bedclothes changed daily; and hands washed and fingernails cleaned after bowel movements and before meals. All family members should be treated.

ENTRY SITE	SYMPTOMS	DRUG
Mouth	• Diarrhea • Abdominal discomfort • Dizziness • Anemia	quinacrine
Mouth (embryonated eggs)	• Perianal pruritus • Perineal irritation, superinfection, and vulvovaginitis • Salpingitis and abdominal pain (females)	pyrvinium, gentian violet, mebendazole, piperazine, pyrantel, thiabendazole
Feet, mouth, skin (filariform larvae)	• Iron deficiency anemia • Abdominal pain • Diarrhea • Urticaria	mebendazole
Mouth (embryonated eggs)	• Colicky abdominal pain • Nausea and vomiting • Malnutrition	piperazine, diethylcarbamazine citrate, mebendazole, pyrantel, thiabendazole
Skin (cercariae)	• Dermatitis, urticaria • Abdominal pain, bloody diarrhea, hematuria • Lymphadenopathy • Hepatomegaly • Fever • Cough	antimony potassium tartrate, oxamniquine

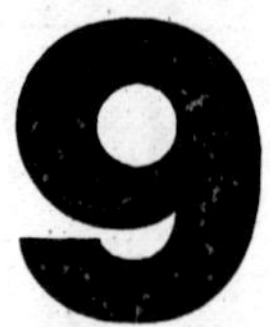

Antifungals

amphotericin B
flucytosine
griseofulvin microsize
griseofulvin ultramicrosize
ketoconazole
miconazole
nystatin

Fungi resist most antibiotics at therapeutic levels; only the antifungals are currently effective against them. Amphotericin B has been the most widely used antifungal, although others have recently been developed. The new drug ketoconazole (Nizoral) shows great promise.

Much of the recent increase in systemic fungal infections is related to cancer chemotherapy's compromise of the immune system.

Major uses

Besides systemic fungal infections, antifungals are effective against meningitis, severe fungal infections caused by *Candida* and *Cryptococcus* organisms, and yeast infections.

• Amphotericin B is useful in the treatment of central nervous system (CNS), pulmonary, cardiac, renal, and other systemic fungal infections. It is effective against blastomycosis, histoplasmosis, cryptococcosis, candidiasis, sporotrichosis, aspergillosis, phycomycosis (mucormycosis), and coccidioidomycosis. It is of no value in treatment of topical fungal infections.

• Flucytosine is effective, usually in combination with amphotericin B, in the treatment of systemic candidiasis, cryptococcosis, and aspergillosis.

• Griseofulvin is used systemically in the treatment of tinea capitis and other tinea infections that don't respond to topical agents.

• Ketoconazole is given orally to treat a wide variety of systemic and mucocutaneous fungal infections.

• Miconazole is administered intravenously to treat systemic coccidioidomycosis, candidiasis, cryptococcosis, and paracoccidioidomycosis. It is usually less effective than amphotericin B.

• Nystatin is used topically to treat superficial candidal infections of the oral mucosa and esophagus.

Mechanism of action

• Amphotericin B and nystatin probably act by binding to sterols in the fungal cell membrane, altering cell permeability and allowing leakage of intracellular components. They may also inhibit glycolysis and protein synthesis.

• Flucytosine appears to penetrate fungal cells, where it is converted to fluorouracil, a known metabolic antagonist. Flucytosine is incorporated into fungal ribonucleic acid (RNA) and causes defective protein synthesis.

• Griseofulvin arrests fungal cell activity by disrupting its mitotic spindle structure.

• Ketoconazole and miconazole inhibit purine transport, and deoxyribonucleic acid, RNA, and protein synthesis; and it increases cell wall permeability, making the fungus more susceptible to osmotic pressure.

Absorption, distribution, metabolism, and excretion

• Amphotericin B is poorly absorbed from the gastrointestinal (GI) tract, so is generally administered by I.V. infusion. It is 90% bound to plasma proteins. It diffuses poorly into body cavities, eyes, and cerebrospinal fluid (CSF), and is slowly excreted by the kidneys.

• Flucytosine is rapidly absorbed from the GI tract, reaching peak levels in about 6 hours. About 90% is excreted unchanged in the urine. The drug is well distributed to all body tissues and to the CNS.
• Griseofulvin, although almost completely absorbed through the duodenum in ultramicrosize formulation, is absorbed unpredictably in microsize formulation. Administration with a high-fat meal, however, may enhance absorption.

The drug concentrates in skin, hair, nails, liver, fat, and skeletal muscles. The highest concentration is found in the outermost horny layer of the skin, the lowest in the deep layers.

Metabolized in the liver, griseofulvin is eliminated in urine, feces, and perspiration, mostly as inactive metabolite and unchanged drug.
• Ketoconazole is absorbed from the GI tract and is distributed poorly into the cerebrospinal fluid. The drug is extensively metabolized in the liver. Inactive metabolites are excreted through the bile and feces.
• Miconazole is poorly absorbed from the GI tract, rapidly metabolized in the liver, and excreted mainly as inactive metabolites. Miconazole penetrates joints but not the CNS.
• Nystatin's oral absorption is negligible. The drug is not absorbed through intact skin or mucous membranes, and blood levels are not measurable at therapeutic doses. The drug is eliminated unchanged in the stool.

Onset and duration
• Amphotericin B has an average peak blood level of 1 mcg/ml after I.V. infusion of 30 mg. Immediately after infusion, no more than 10% of the dose appears in blood; the half-life is 24 hours.

Amphotericin B can be detected in blood and urine 4 weeks after therapy is discontinued.
• Flucytosine is well absorbed from the GI tract. It reaches peak blood levels of 30 to 45 mcg/ml within 6 hours of a single 2-g oral dose in patients with normal renal function.

The dose must be altered, however, for patients with renal impairment. Flucytosine has a half-life of 6 hours and is eliminated unchanged, primarily in the urine.
• Griseofulvin blood levels peak in 4 hours. It is undetectable in skin 2 days—and in blood 4 days—after drug is discontinued. Drug concentrations in skin are highest in warm climates.
• Ketoconazole is well absorbed following oral administration. Peak blood levels are reached within 1 to 2 hours. The half-life is approximately 8 hours.
• Miconazole, with I.V. infusion of 9 mg/kg, reaches blood levels of at least 1 mcg/ml, but they fall rapidly within 30 minutes. The half-life of miconazole is unchanged in patients with renal impairment.
• Nystatin products vary in onset and duration.

Combination products
ACHROSTATIN-V: nystatin 250,000 units and tetracycline HCl 250 mg.
DECLOSTATIN TABS: nystatin 500,000 units and demeclocycline HCl 300 mg.
MYSTECLIN-F CAPS: tetracycline HCl 250 mg and amphotericin B 50 mg buffered with potassium metaphosphate.
MYSTECLIN-F SYRUP:tetracycline HCl 125 mg and amphotericin B 25 mg/5 ml buffered with potassium metaphosphate.
TERRASTATIN CAPS: nystatin 250,000 units and oxytetracycline 250 mg.

NAMES, INDICATIONS AND DOSAGES	SIDE EFFECTS

amphotericin B
Fungizone♦

Systemic fungal infections (histoplasmosis, coccidioidomycosis, blastomycosis, cryptococcosis, disseminated moniliasis, aspergillosis, phycomycosis), meningitis:

ADULTS AND CHILDREN: initially, 1 mg in 250 ml of 5% dextrose in water infused over 2 to 4 hours; or 0.25 mg/kg daily by slow infusion over 6 hours. Increase gradually as patient tolerance develops to maximum 1 mg/kg daily. Therapy must not exceed 1.5 mg/kg. If drug is discontinued for 1 week or more, administration must resume with initial dose and again increase gradually.

Topical (3% cream, lotion, ointment): apply liberally and rub well into affected area b.i.d. to q.i.d.

Intrathecal: 25 mcg/0.1 ml diluted with 10 to 20 ml of cerebrospinal fluid and administered by barbotage 2 or 3 times weekly. Initial dose should not exceed 50 mcg.

Coccidioidal arthritis:

ADULTS: 5 to 15 mg into joint spaces.

Blood: normochromic, normocytic anemia.
CNS: headache, peripheral neuropathy; with intrathecal administration—peripheral nerve pain, paresthesias.
GI: anorexia, weight loss, nausea, vomiting, dyspepsia, diarrhea, epigastric cramps.
GU: abnormal renal function with *hypokalemia, azotemia, hyposthenuria,* renal tubular acidosis, nephrocalcinosis; with large doses—permanent renal impairment, anuria, oliguria.
Local: burning, stinging, irritation, tissue damage with extravasation, *thrombophlebitis,* pain at site of injection.
Other: arthralgia, myalgia, muscle weakness secondary to hypokalemia, *fever, chills,* malaise, generalized pain.

---

flucytosine
Ancobon, Ancotil♦♦

For severe fungal infections caused by susceptible strains of *Candida* (including septicemia, endocarditis, urinary tract and pulmonary infections) and *Cryptococcus* (meningitis, pulmonary infection, and possible urinary tract infections):

ADULTS AND CHILDREN WEIGHING MORE THAN 50 KG: 50 to 150 mg/kg daily q 6 hours P.O.

CHILDREN WEIGHING LESS THAN 50 KG: 1.5 to 4.5 g/m²/day in 4 divided doses P.O.

Severe infections such as meningitis may require doses up to 250 mg/kg.

Blood: anemia, leukopenia, bone marrow depression, thrombocytopenia.
CNS: dizziness, drowsiness, confusion, headache.
GI: *nausea, vomiting, diarrhea,* abdominal bloating.
Hepatic: elevated SGOT, SGPT.
Metabolic: elevated serum alkaline phosphatase, BUN, serum creatinine.
Skin: occasional rash.

---

griseofulvin microsize
Fulvicin-U/F♦, Grifulvin V, Grisactin, Grisovin-FP♦♦, Grisowen
griseofulvin ultramicrosize
Fulvicin P/G, Gris-PEG

Ringworm infections of skin, hair, nails (tinea corporis, tinea pedis, tinea cruris, tinea barbae, tinea capitis, and tinea unguium) when caused by *Trichophyton, Microsporum,* or *Epidermophyton:*

Blood: leukopenia, *granulocytopenia (requires discontinuation of drug).*
CNS: headaches (in early stages of treatment), fatigue with large doses, occasional mental confusion, impaired performance of routine activities, psychotic symptoms.
GI: nausea, vomiting, excessive thirst, flatulence, diarrhea.
Metabolic: porphyria.
Skin: rash, urticaria, photosensitive reactions (may aggravate lupus erythematosus).

♦ Available in U.S. and Canada. ♦♦ Available in Canada only.
All other products (no symbol) available in U.S. only. Italicized side effects are common or life-threatening.

INTERACTIONS AND SPECIAL CONSIDERATIONS

No significant interactions.

Special considerations:

• Use cautiously in patients with impaired renal function.
• Use parenterally only in hospitalized patients, under close supervision, when diagnosis of potentially fatal fungal infection has been confirmed.
• Vital signs should be monitored; fever may appear 1 to 2 hours after start of I.V. infusion and should subside within 4 hours of discontinuation.
• Intake and output should be monitored for change in appearance or volume. Renal damage usually reversible if drug stopped promptly.
• Liver and kidney function tests should be performed weekly. If BUN exceeds 40 mg/100 ml, or if serum creatinine exceeds 3 mg/100 ml, drug may be reduced or stopped until renal function improves. CBC should be monitored weekly and drug stopped if Bromsulphalein, alkaline phosphatase, or bilirubin levels become elevated. Potassium levels should be monitored for signs of hypokalemia; and calcium and magnesium levels checked periodically.
• Potentially ototoxic; patient should report hearing loss, tinnitus, dizziness.
• In the dry state, store at 2° to 8° C. (35.6° to 46.4° F.). Protect from light. Expires 2 years after date of manufacture. Should be reconstituted with 10 ml sterile water only. Mixing with solutions containing sodium chloride, other electrolytes, or bacteriostatic agents such as benzyl alcohol causes precipitation. Solution containing precipitate or foreign matter should not be used. Aseptic technique necessary.
• Appears to be compatible with limited amounts of heparin sodium, hydrocortisone sodium succinate, and methylprednisolone sodium succinate.
• Reconstituted solution is stable for 1 week under refrigeration or 24 hours at room temperature. Should be protected from light and bottle and tubing wrapped in aluminum foil.
• Recommended infusion solution is 10 mg/100 ml of 5% dextrose in water.
• Severity of some side effects can be reduced by premedication with aspirin, antihistamines, antiemetics, or small doses of corticosteroids; addition of phosphate buffer and heparin to the solution; and alternate-day dose schedule. For severe reactions, drug may have to be stopped for varying periods.
• For I.V. infusion, an in-line membrane with mean pore diameter larger than 1 micron can be used. Should be infused very slowly; rapid infusion may result in cardiovascular collapse. Discomfort at infusion site and other potential side effects.
• Antibiotics should be given separately; should not be mixed or piggybacked with amphotericin.
• Several months of therapy may be needed to assure adequate response.
• Topical preparations may stain clothing.

No significant interactions.

Special considerations:

• Use with extreme caution in patients with impaired hepatic or renal function, or bone marrow depression.
• Hematologic, and kidney and liver function studies should precede therapy and should be repeated at frequent intervals thereafter. Before treatment, susceptibility tests should establish that organism is flucytosine-sensitive. Tests should be repeated weekly to monitor drug resistance.
• Flucytosine is well absorbed from the GI tract. Nausea, vomiting, stomach upset are reduced if capsules are given over a 15-minute period.
• Intake and output should be monitored.
• Serum level assays of drug should be performed regularly to maintain flucytosine at therapeutic level (25 to 120 mcg/ml).
• Drug is often combined with amphotericin B; use may be synergistic; but may increase toxic effects.
• Store in light-resistant containers.
• Adequate response may take weeks or months.

Interactions:

BARBITURATES: decreased griseofulvin absorption. Divide into 3 doses of griseofulvin per day.

Special considerations:

• Contraindicated in patients with porphyria or hepatocellular failure. Since griseofulvin is a penicillin derivative, cross-sensitivity is possible. Use cautiously in penicillin-sensitive patients. Use only when topical treatment fails to arrest mycotic disease.
• Blood studies, and kidney and liver function studies should be repeated regularly.
• A long period of treatment may be needed to control infection and prevent relapse, even if symptoms abate in first few days of therapy. Patient should keep skin clean and dry, maintain good hygiene, and avoid intense sunlight.
• Most effectively absorbed and causes least GI distress when taken after high-fat meal.
• Effective treatment of tinea pedis may require concomitant topical agent.

(continued on following page)

NAMES, INDICATIONS AND DOSAGES	SIDE EFFECTS
griseofulvin *(continued)* ADULTS: 500 mg (microsize) P.O. daily in single or divided doses. Severe infections may require up to 1 g daily. CHILDREN OVER 22 KG: 250 to 500 mg P.O. daily. CHILDREN 13 TO 22 KG: 125 to 250 mg daily. ADULTS: 125 mg tablet (ultramicrosize) P.O. b.i.d. or 250 mg daily. Resistant fungal infections of tinea pedis and tinea unguium may require divided daily dose of 500 mg. CHILDREN OVER 22 KG: 125 mg to 250 mg P.O. daily. CHILDREN 13 TO 22 KG: 62.5 mg to 125 mg P.O. daily.	**Other:** estrogen-like effects in children, oral thrush.
ketoconazole Nizoral **Treatment of systemic candidiasis, chronic mucocandidiasis, oral thrush, candiduria, coccidioidomycosis, histoplasmosis, chromomycosis, and paracoccidioidomycosis:** ADULTS AND CHILDREN OVER 40 KG: Initially, 200 mg P.O. daily single dose. Dosage may be increased to 400 mg once daily in patients who don't respond to lower dosage. CHILDREN (LESS THAN 20 KG): 50 mg (¼ tablet) daily single dose. CHILDREN (20 TO 40 KG): 100 mg (½ tablet) daily single dose.	**CNS:** headache, nervousness, dizziness. **GI:** *nausea, vomiting,* abdominal pain, diarrhea, constipation. **Hepatic:** mild, reversible hepatitis. **Skin:** itching.
miconazole Monistat I.V. **Treatment of systemic fungal infections (coccidioidomycosis, candidiasis, cryptococcosis, paracoccidioidomycosis), chronic mucocutaneous candidiasis:** ADULTS: 200 to 3,600 mg/day. Doses may vary with diagnosis and with infective agent. May divide daily dose over 3 infusions, 200 to 1,200 mg/infusion. Repeated courses may be needed due to relapse or reinfection. CHILDREN: 20 to 40 mg/kg/day. Do not exceed 15 mg/kg/infusion.	**Blood:** transient decreases in hematocrit, thrombocytopenia. **CNS:** dizziness, drowsiness. **GI:** *nausea, vomiting,* diarrhea. **Metabolic:** *transient decrease in serum sodium.* **Skin:** *pruritic rash.* **Local:** *phlebitis at injection site.*
nystatin Mycostatin♦, Nadostine♦♦, Nilstat♦, O-V Statin **Gastrointestinal infections:** ADULTS: 500,000 to 1,000,000 units as oral tablets, t.i.d. **Treatment of oral, vaginal, and intestinal infections caused by *Candida albicans (Monilia)* and other *Candida* species:** ADULTS: 400,000 to 600,000 units oral suspension q.i.d. for oral candidiasis. CHILDREN AND INFANTS OVER 3 MONTHS:	**GI:** transient nausea, vomiting, diarrhea (usually with large oral dosage).

♦ Available in U.S. and Canada. ♦♦ Available in Canada only.
All other products (no symbol) available in U.S. only. Italicized side effects are common or life-threatening.

INTERACTIONS AND SPECIAL CONSIDERATIONS

• Diagnosis of infecting organism should be verified in laboratory. Drug should be continued until clinical and laboratory examinations confirm complete eradication.
• Because griseofulvin ultramicrosize is dispersed in polyethylene glycol (PEG), it is absorbed more rapidly and completely than microsize preparations, and is effective at one half the usual griseofulvin dose.

Interactions:
ANTACIDS, ANTICHOLINERGICS, CIMETIDINE: decreased absorption of ketoconazole. Wait at least 2 hours after ketoconazole dose before administering these drugs.

Special considerations:
• Contraindicated in patients with fungal meningitis since ketoconazole penetrates poorly into the cerebrospinal fluid.
• Ketoconazole is not effective in patients with achlorhydria. The drug requires acidity for dissolution and absorption.
• Patient should dissolve each tablet in 4 ml aqueous solution of 0.2 N hydrochloric acid; and, to avoid contact with teeth, should sip the mixture through a straw (glass or plastic). Patient should follow with a glass of water.
• Patient should continue treatment until all clinical and laboratory tests indicate that active fungal infection has subsided. If drug is discontinued too soon, infection will reoccur. Minimum treatment for candidiasis is 7 to 14 days. Minimum treatment for other systemic fungal infections is 6 months.
• Ketoconazole represents a major advance since it is the most effective oral antifungal drug available and it produces the least side effects.

No significant interactions.

Special considerations:
• Rapid injection of undiluted miconazole may produce arrhythmia.
• Premedication with antiemetic may lessen nausea and vomiting.
• Administration should be avoided at mealtime in order to lessen GI side effects.
• Lesser incidence and severity of side effects with this drug may offer a significant advantage over other antifungals.
• In treatment of fungal meningitis and urinary bladder infections, must be supplemented with intrathecal administration and bladder irrigation, respectively.
• I.V. infusion should be given over 30 to 60 minutes.
• Adequate response may take weeks or months.
• Levels of hemoglobin, hematocrit, electrolytes and lipids should be monitored regularly. Transient elevations in serum cholesterol and triglycerides may be due to castor oil vehicle.

No significant interactions.

Special considerations:
• Nystatin is virtually nontoxic and nonsensitizing when used orally, vaginally, or topically; but patient should report any redness, swelling, or irritation.
• Vaginal tablets can be used by pregnant women up to 6 weeks before term to prevent thrush in newborn. Therapy should be continued during menstruation, and applicator washed thoroughly after each use.
• Use of antibiotics, oral contraceptives, and corticosteroids; diabetes; pregnancy; reinfection by sexual partner; and tight-fitting panty hose are predisposing factors for vaginal infection.
• For treatment of oral candidiasis (thrush): Be sure the mouth is clean of food debris before medication is given; then suspension should be held in mouth for several minutes before swallowing. For treatment in infants, medication should be swabbed on oral mucosa. Patient should observe good mouth hygiene. Overuse of mouthwash or poorly fitting dentures, especially in older patients, may alter flora and promote infection.
• After consultation for exact length of therapy, patient should continue medication for 1 to 2

(continued on following page)

NAMES, INDICATIONS AND DOSAGES	SIDE EFFECTS
nystatin *(continued)* 250,000 to 500,000 units oral suspension q.i.d. NEWBORN AND PREMATURE INFANTS: 100,000 units oral suspension q.i.d. **Vaginal infections:** ADULTS: 100,000 units, as vaginal tablets, inserted high into vagina, daily or b.i.d. for 14 days.	

♦ Available in U.S. and Canada. ♦♦ Available in Canada only.
All other products (no symbol) available in U.S. only. Italicized side effects are common or life-threatening.

DRUG ALERT

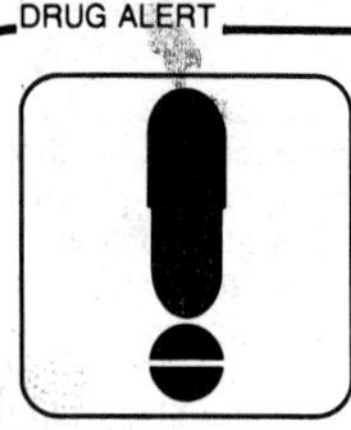

PREVENTING AMPHOTERICIN B TOXICITY

Amphotericin B (Fungizone) is usually prescribed for progressive and life-threatening fungal infections. But the drug can have toxic side effects:

- Fever, chills, nausea, vomiting, and headache commonly occur within minutes after the infusion begins. Side effects may be prevented or minimized by giving the patient 600 to 900 mg of aspirin or acetaminophen and 50 mg of diphenhydramine 1 hour before the infusion. Doses may be repeated every 3 to 4 hours, if necessary. Adding hydrocortisone to the infusion may also help reduce these side effects.
- Thrombophlebitis develops at the I.V. site in about 70% of patients receiving amphotericin B. Signs of thrombophlebitis should be reported so heparin or hydrocortisone may be added to the infusion to control inflammation.
- Hypokalemia is serious and possibly life-threatening, especially to patients taking digitalis. The patient should be closely watched for neuromuscular disturbances, such as weakness, decreased reflexes, or tingling in fingers and toes; EKG abnormalities, such as flat T waves, depressed ST segments, or widened QRS complexes; GI symptoms, such as nausea or paralytic ileus; and CNS symptoms, such as irritability and stupor.

  Hypokalemia can be corrected with potassium supplements, but large amounts may be needed.
- Renal tubular acidosis results from decreased renal excretion of acids after several weeks of amphotericin B therapy. The drug may also decrease the patient's glomerular filtration rate and may possibly precipitate azotemia. Serum creatinine and BUN should be monitored frequently.

  If the renal function indicators are too high (serum creatinine greater than 3 mg/100 ml and BUN greater than 40 mg/100 ml), the drug usually must be stopped to prevent permanent renal damage.

INTERACTIONS AND SPECIAL CONSIDERATIONS

weeks after symptomatic improvement to ensure against reinfection.
- Patient should observe careful hygiene for affected areas.
- Store in tightly closed, light-resistant containers in cool place.
- Immunosuppressed patients sometimes take vaginal tablets (100,000 units) by mouth to provide prolonged contact with oral mucosa.
- Not effective against systemic infections.

DRUG ADVANCES

KNOW THE ADVANTAGES OF KETOCONAZOLE— A NEW ORAL ANTIFUNGAL

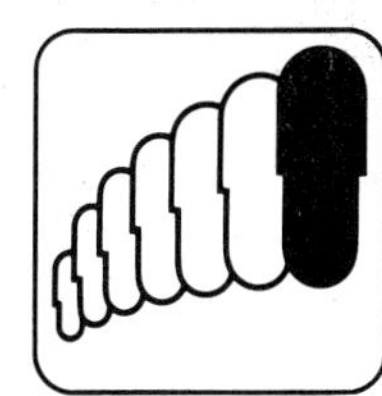

Ketoconazole (Nizoral) represents an important advance in antifungal drug development because it:
- shows none of the serious side effects that usually occur with other antifungal drugs.
- shows impressive cure rates for fungal infections previously resistant to other drugs.
- provides new therapeutic options for long-term treatment and maintenance of severe fungal infections, as well as for prophylaxis in high-risk patients.
- can be administered orally with a once-daily dosage. (This should encourage patient compliance.)
- is effective for a broad range of acute and chronic fungal infections.

Like other antifungals, ketoconazole is particularly useful in treating deep systemic fungal infections and lesions affecting subcutaneous tissue layers. It's also highly effective in treating oral and genitourinary monilial infections, particularly in patients with cancer since chemotherapeutic drugs make them vulnerable to such infections.

Ketoconazole effectively combats these other infections as well:
- systemic candidiasis
- chronic mucocutaneous candidiasis
- oral thrush
- candiduria
- coccidioidomycosis
- histoplasmosis
- chromomycosis
- paracoccidioidomycosis.

Side effects of ketoconazole include headache, dizziness, constipation, diarrhea, somnolence, and nervousness.

Note: Ketoconazole should not be used for fungal meningitis because it penetrates poorly into the cerebrospinal fluid.

10

Antimalarials

chloroquine hydrochloride
chloroquine phosphate
hydroxychloroquine sulfate
primaquine phosphate
pyrimethamine
quinine sulfate

Quinine, the bitter alkaloid obtained from the bark of the cinchona tree; the 4-aminoquinoline derivatives (chloroquine and hydroxychloroquine); and related drugs are used in prophylaxis and treatment of malarial infections.

In many areas of the world, malaria is a common infectious disease with a high mortality. Transmitted by the bite of the anopheles mosquito, malaria is most commonly contracted in Asia, Africa, and Latin America. In the United States, however, malarial infections are usually nonepidemic.

Major uses

- Chloroquine, hydroxychloroquine, primaquine, and pyrimethamine suppress susceptible strains of *Plasmodium—P. vivax, P. malariae, P. ovale,* and *P. falciparum.*
- Chloroquine and hydroxychloroquine are also used in the treatment of systemic lupus erythematosus and rheumatoid arthritis. Chloroquine is used in combination with emetine to treat amebic hepatic abscesses as well as certain fluke infections.
- Quinine may relieve nocturnal leg cramps.
- Pyrimethamine is used in combination with sulfonamides to treat toxoplasmosis.

Mechanism of action

- The 4-aminoquinoline compounds bind to, and alter the properties of, both microbial and mammalian deoxyribonucleic acid.
- Primaquine phosphate is a gametocidal drug that destroys exoerythrocytic forms and prevents delayed primary attack. Its precise mechanism of action is unknown.
- Pyrimethamine inhibits the enzyme dihydrofolate reductase, thereby impeding reduction of folic acid.
- Quinine's exact mechanism of action is unknown, but the drug is often referred to as a generalized protoplasmic poison.

Absorption, distribution, metabolism, and excretion

All the antimalarials are rapidly absorbed from the gastrointestinal tract.

- The 4-aminoquinoline compounds, bound to plasma proteins, achieve very high levels in the liver, spleen, kidneys, and lungs. They are metabolized in the liver and slowly excreted in the urine for months after treatment.
- Primaquine is rapidly metabolized in the liver. Only a small amount of unchanged drug is excreted in the urine; the rest is excreted as metabolite.
- Pyrimethamine is metabolized in the liver and excreted in the urine.
- Quinine, highly protein-bound, is excreted in the urine—mostly as inactive metabolite.

Onset and duration

- The 4-aminoquinolines and primaquine reach peak blood concentrations 6 hours after oral administration. Levels fall rapidly; only very small quantities are detectable after 24 hours. Minute amounts may still, however, be detectable in the urine months after therapy ends.
- Pyrimethamine is eliminated slowly and has a half-life of 4 days. Therapeutic con-

centrations may remain in the blood for as long as 2 weeks.

• Quinine sulfate achieves peak blood levels within 1 to 3 hours; only a negligible concentration can be measured 24 hours after therapy ends.

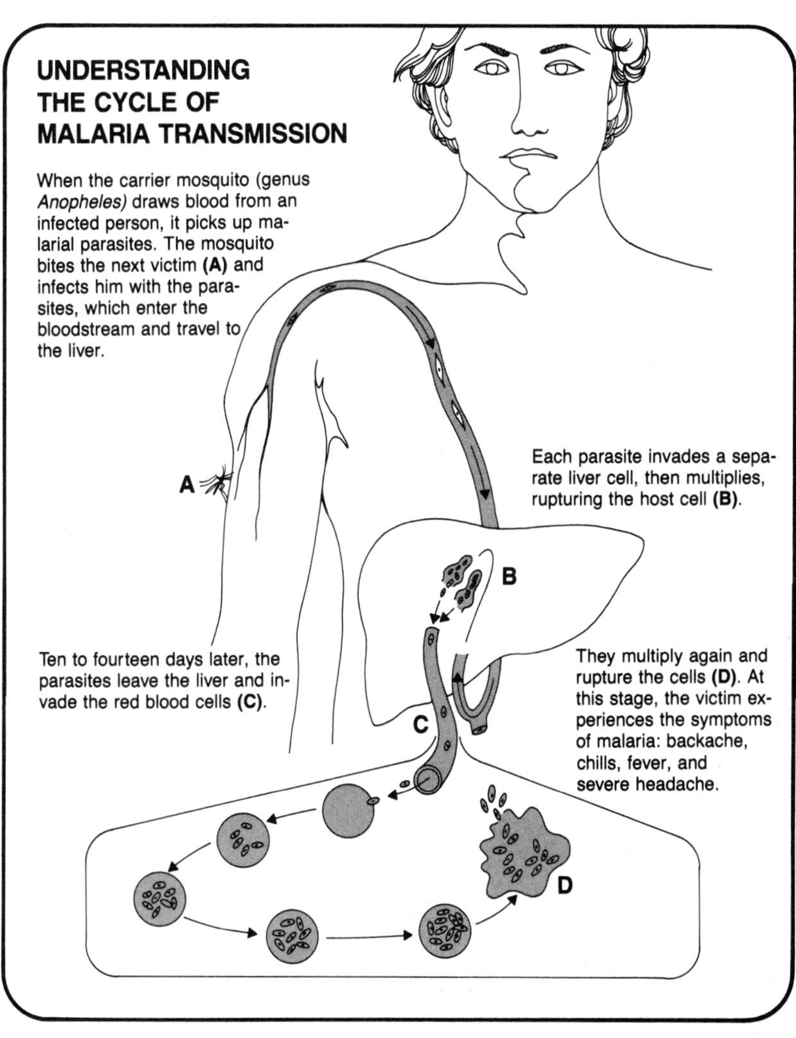

UNDERSTANDING THE CYCLE OF MALARIA TRANSMISSION
When the carrier mosquito (genus *Anopheles)* draws blood from an infected person, it picks up malarial parasites. The mosquito bites the next victim **(A)** and infects him with the parasites, which enter the bloodstream and travel to the liver.
A
Each parasite invades a separate liver cell, then multiplies, rupturing the host cell **(B)**.
B
Ten to fourteen days later, the parasites leave the liver and invade the red blood cells **(C)**.
C
They multiply again and rupture the cells **(D)**. At this stage, the victim experiences the symptoms of malaria: backache, chills, fever, and severe headache.
D

NAMES, INDICATIONS AND DOSAGES

chloroquine hydrochloride
Aralen HCl, Roquine
chloroquine phosphate
Aralen Phosphate♦, Chlorocon

Suppressive prophylaxis and treatment of acute attacks of malaria due to *Plasmodium vivax, Plasmodium malariae, Plasmodium ovale,* and susceptible strains of *Plasmodium falciparum:*
ADULTS: initially, 600 mg (base) P.O., then 300 mg P.O. at 6, 24, and 48 hours. Or 160 to 200 mg (base) I.M. initially; repeat in 6 hours if needed. Switch to oral therapy as soon as possible.
CHILDREN: initially, 10 mg (base)/kg P.O., then 5 mg (base)/kg dose P.O. at 6, 24, and 48 hours (do not exceed adult dose). Or 5 mg (base)/kg I.M. initially; repeat in 6 hours if needed. Switch to oral therapy as soon as possible.

Malaria suppressive treatment:
ADULTS AND CHILDREN: 5 mg (base)/kg P.O. (not to exceed 300 mg) weekly on same day of the week (begin 2 weeks before entering endemic area and continue for 8 weeks after leaving). If treatment begins after exposure, double the initial dose (600 mg for adults, 10 mg/kg for children) in 2 divided doses, P.O. 6 hours apart.

SIDE EFFECTS

Blood: *agranulocytosis.*
CNS: mild and transient headache, neuromyopathy, psychic stimulation, fatigue, irritability, nightmares, convulsions, dizziness.
EENT: *visual disturbances* (blurred vision; difficulty in focusing; reversible corneal changes; generally irreversible, sometimes progressive or delayed, retinal changes, e.g., narrowing of arterioles; macular lesions; pallor of optic disk; optic atrophy; patchy retinal pigmentation, often leading to blindness), ototoxicity (nerve deafness, vertigo, tinnitus).
GI: anorexia, abdominal cramps, diarrhea, nausea, vomiting.
Skin: pruritus, lichen planus–like eruptions, skin and mucosal pigmentary changes, pleomorphic skin eruptions.

hydroxychloroquine sulfate
Plaquenil Sulfate♦

Suppressive prophylaxis of attacks of malaria due to *Plasmodium vivax, Plasmodium malariae, Plasmodium ovale,* and susceptible strains of *Plasmodium falciparum:*
ADULTS AND CHILDREN: for suppression: 5 mg (base)/kg body weight P.O. (not to exceed 310 mg) weekly on same day of the week (begin 2 weeks prior to entering and continue for 8 weeks after leaving endemic area). If not started prior to exposure, double initial dose (620 mg for adults, 10 mg/kg for children) in 2 divided doses P.O. 6 hours apart.

Treatment of acute malarial attacks:
ADULTS AND CHILDREN OVER 15 YEARS: initially, 800 mg (sulfate) P.O., then 400 mg after 6 to 8 hours, then 400 mg daily for 2 days (total 2 g sulfate salt).
CHILDREN 11 TO 15 YEARS: 600 mg (sulfate) P.O. stat, then 200 mg 8 hours later, then 200 mg 24 hours later (total 1 g sulfate salt).
CHILDREN 6 TO 10 YEARS: 400 mg (sulfate) P.O. stat, then 2 doses of 200 mg at 8-hour intervals (total 800 mg sulfate salt).
CHILDREN 2 TO 5 YEARS: 400 mg (sulfate) P.O. stat, then 200 mg 8 hours later (total 600 mg sulfate salt).
CHILDREN UNDER 1 YEAR: 100 mg (sulfate)

Blood: *agranulocytosis, leukopenia,* thrombocytopenia, *aplastic anemia.*
CNS: irritability, nightmares, ataxia, convulsions, psychic stimulation, toxic psychosis, vertigo, tinnitus, nystagmus, lassitude, fatigue, dizziness, hypoactive deep-tendon reflexes, skeletal muscle weakness.
EENT: visual disturbances (blurred vision; difficulty in focusing; reversible corneal changes; generally irreversible, sometimes progressive or delayed, retinal changes, e.g., narrowing of arterioles; macular lesions; pallor of optic disk; optic atrophy; visual field defects; patchy retinal pigmentation, often leading to blindness), ototoxicity (irreversible nerve deafness, tinnitus, labyrinthitis).
GI: anorexia, abdominal cramps, diarrhea, nausea, vomiting.
Skin: pruritus, lichen planus–like eruptions, skin and mucosal pigmentary changes, pleomorphic skin eruptions.
Other: weight loss, bleaching of hair.

♦ Available in U.S. and Canada. ♦♦ Available in Canada only.
All other products (no symbol) available in U.S. only. Italicized side effects are common or life-threatening.

INTERACTIONS AND SPECIAL CONSIDERATIONS

No significant interactions.

Special considerations:

• Contraindicated in patients with retinal or visual field changes, porphyria. Use with extreme caution in presence of severe GI, neurologic, or blood disorders. Drug concentrates in liver; use cautiously in patients with hepatic disease or alcoholism. Use with caution in patients with G-6-PD deficiency or psoriasis; drug may exacerbate these conditions.

• Complete blood cell counts, including liver function studies, should be made periodically during prolonged therapy; if severe blood disorder appears that is not attributable to disease under treatment, drug may need to be discontinued.

• Overdosage can quickly lead to toxic symptoms: headache, drowsiness, visual disturbances, cardiovascular collapse, and convulsions, followed by respiratory and cardiac arrest. Children are extremely susceptible to toxicity; long-term treatment should be avoided.

• Baseline and periodic ophthalmologic examinations needed. Patient should report blurred vision, increased sensitivity to light, or muscle weakness. After long-term use, patient should be checked periodically for ocular muscle weakness. Audiometric examinations recommended before, during, and after therapy, especially if long-term.

• Drug should be taken immediately before or after meals on same day each week.

• To avoid exacerbated drug-induced dermatoses, patient should avoid excessive exposure to sun.

• Each ml parenteral solution containing 50 mg dihydrochloride salt = 40 mg chloroquine base; each 500 mg tablet phosphate = 300 mg base.

No significant interactions.

Special considerations:

• Contraindicated in patients with retinal or visual field changes, porphyria. Use with extreme caution in presence of severe GI, neurologic, or blood disorders. Drug concentrates in the liver; use cautiously in patients with hepatic disease or alcoholism. Use with caution in patients with G-6-PD deficiency or psoriasis; drug may exacerbate these conditions.

• Complete blood cell counts, including liver function studies, should be made periodically during prolonged therapy; if severe blood disorder appears which is not attributable to disease under treatment, medication may need to be discontinued.

• Overdosage can quickly lead to toxic symptoms: headache, drowsiness, visual disturbances, cardiovascular collapse, and convulsions, followed by respiratory and cardiac arrest. Children are extremely susceptible to toxicity; long-term treatment should be avoided.

• Baseline and periodic ophthalmologic examinations needed. Patient should report blurred vision, increased sensitivity to light, or muscle weakness. After long-term use, patient should be checked periodically for ocular muscle weakness. Audiometric examinations recommended before, during, and after therapy, especially if long-term.

• Drug should be taken immediately before or after meals on same day of each week.

• 100 mg sulfate salt = 77.5 mg hydroxychloroquine base.

(continued on following page)

NAMES, INDICATIONS AND DOSAGES	SIDE EFFECTS
hydroxychloroquine sulfate *(continued)* P.O. stat; then 3 doses of 100 mg 6 to 9 hours apart (total 400 mg sulfate salt). **Lupus erythematosus (chronic discoid and systemic):** ADULTS: 400 mg P.O. daily or b.i.d., continued for several weeks or months, depending on response. Prolonged maintenance—200 to 400 mg P.O. daily. **Rheumatoid arthritis:** ADULTS: initially, 400 to 600 mg P.O. daily. When good response occurs (usually in 4 to 12 weeks), cut dosage in half.	
primaquine phosphate **Radical cure of relapsing vivax malaria, eliminating symptoms and infection completely; prevention of relapse:** ADULTS: 15 to 30 mg (base) P.O. daily for 14 days. (26.3 mg tablet = 15 mg of base).	**Blood:** leukopenia, hemolytic anemia in G-6-PD deficiency, methemoglobinemia in NADH methemoglobin reductase deficiency, leukocytosis, acute intravascular hemolysis, mild anemia, *granulocytopenia, agranulocytosis.* **EENT:** disturbances of visual accommodation. **GI:** nausea, vomiting, epigastric distress, abdominal cramps. **Skin:** urticaria.
pyrimethamine Daraprim♦ **Malaria prophylaxis and transmission control:** ADULTS AND CHILDREN OVER 10 YEARS: 25 mg P.O. weekly. CHILDREN 4 TO 10 YEARS: 12.5 mg P.O. weekly. CHILDREN UNDER 4 YEARS: 6.25 mg P.O. weekly. Continue in all age groups at least 10 weeks after leaving endemic areas. **Acute attacks of malaria:** Not recommended alone in nonimmune persons; use with faster-acting antimalarials, such as chloroquine, for 2 days to initiate transmission control and suppressive cure. ADULTS AND CHILDREN OVER 15 YEARS: 25 mg P.O. daily for 2 days. CHILDREN UNDER 15 YEARS: 12.5 mg P.O. daily for 2 days. **Toxoplasmosis:** ADULTS: initially, 100 mg P.O., then 25 mg P.O. daily for 4 to 5 weeks; during same time give 1 g sulfadiazine P.O. q 6 hours. CHILDREN: initially, 1 mg/kg P.O., then 0.25 mg/kg daily for 4 to 5 weeks, along with 100 mg sulfadiazine/kg P.O. daily, divided q 6 hours.	**Blood:** megaloblastic anemia, bone marrow suppression, leukopenia, thrombocytopenia, pancytopenia. **CNS:** stimulation and convulsions (acute toxicity). **GI:** anorexia, vomiting, diarrhea, atrophic glossitis. **Skin:** rashes.

INTERACTIONS AND SPECIAL CONSIDERATIONS

No significant interactions.

Special considerations:

• Contraindicated in patients with lupus erythematosus, rheumatoid arthritis; in patients taking bone marrow suppressants and potentially hemolytic drugs.

• Use with a fast-acting blood schizonticide, such as chloroquine, and use full dose to reduce possibility of drug-resistant strains.

• Caucasians taking more than 30 mg daily, dark-skinned patients taking more than 15 mg (base) daily, and patients with severe anemia or suspected sensitivity should have frequent blood studies and urine examinations. Sudden fall in hemoglobin concentration, erythrocyte or leukocyte count, or marked darkening of the urine suggests impending hemolytic reactions.

• Patients with previous idiosyncrasy (manifested by hemolytic anemia, methemoglobinemia, or leukopenia); family or personal history of favism; erythrocytic G-6-PD deficiency of NADH methemoglobin reductase deficiency should be observed closely for tolerance.

• Drug should be taken with meals or with antacids.

Interactions:

FOLIC ACID AND PARA-AMINOBENZOIC ACID: decreased antitoxoplasmic effects. May require dosage adjustment.

Special considerations:

• Contraindicated in chloroguanide-resistant malaria. Use cautiously in patients with convulsive disorders; smaller doses may be needed. Also use cautiously following treatment with chloroguanide.

• Dosages required to treat toxoplasmosis approach toxic levels. Twice-weekly blood counts, including platelets, are required. If signs of folic or folinic acid deficiency develop, dosage should be reduced or discontinued while patient receives parenteral folinic acid (leucovorin) until blood counts become normal.

• Recommended dosage should not be exceeded.

• Should be taken with meals to minimize GI distress.

NAMES, INDICATIONS AND DOSAGES	SIDE EFFECTS
quinine sulfate Coco-Quinine, Quinamm **Malaria due to *Plasmodium falciparum* (chloroquine-resistant):** ADULTS: 650 mg P.O. q 8 hours for 10 days, with 25 mg pyrimethamine q 12 hours for 3 days, and with 500 mg sulfadiazine q.i.d. for 5 days.	**Blood:** hemolytic anemia, thrombocytopenia, agranulocytosis, hypoprothrombinemia. **CNS:** severe headache, apprehension, excitement, confusion, delirium, syncope, hypothermia, convulsions (with toxic doses). **CV:** hypotension, cardiovascular collapse with overdosage or rapid I.V. administration. **EENT:** altered color perception, photophobia, blurred vision, night blindness, amblyopia, scotoma, diplopia, mydriasis, optic atrophy, tinnitus, impaired hearing. **GI:** epigastric distress, diarrhea, nausea, vomiting. **GU:** renal tubular damage, anuria. **Skin:** rashes, pruritus. **Local:** thrombosis at infusion site. **Other:** asthma, flushing.

INTERACTIONS AND SPECIAL CONSIDERATIONS

Interactions:
SODIUM BICARBONATE: elevates quinine levels by decreasing quinine excretion. Use together cautiously.

Special considerations:
• Contraindicated in patients with G-6-PD deficiency. Use with caution in patients with cardiovascular conditions.
• Should be discontinued if any signs of idiosyncrasy or toxicity occur.
• I.V. therapy must be used cautiously, as marked fall in blood pressure often follows. Blood pressure should be monitored frequently.
• I.V. route is preferred to I.M. route. Extravasation should be avoided.
• Has been used as a treatment for nocturnal leg cramps.
• Quinine is no longer used for acute attacks of malaria due to *Plasmodium vivax* or for suppression of malaria due to organism resistance.
• Should be taken after meals to minimize GI distress.
• May interfere with laboratory determinations of urine catecholamines and steroids.

BASIC FACTS ABOUT MALARIA

Malaria is uncommon outside of Asia, Africa, and South America, but you can't rule out the possibility of dealing with it in one of your patients. Here are some facts to bring your knowledge about malaria up to date.

Cause:	Protozoa are introduced into the human body through the bite of an infected anopheles mosquito, transfusion of blood from an infected donor, or use of a common syringe by drug addicts.
Incubation:	This period usually lasts 10 to 35 days, followed by a 2- to 3-day prodrome of irregular low-grade fever, malaise, headache, and myalgia.
Symptoms:	Clinical effects include periodic attacks of chills and fever without apparent cause, especially with spleen enlargement, in a person who has been in a malarious area within the year, as well as headache, nausea, and vomiting.
Diagnosis:	A blood smear is obtained to check for hepatosplenomegaly cells and Kupffer's cells distended with parasites. (Since intensity of the parasites may vary, more than one blood smear is required.)
Prevention:	Because malarial parasites have shown increasing resistance to antimalarial drugs, these preventive measures are important: control of mosquito breeding places; use of residual insecticide sprays in homes and public buildings, screens on windows and doors, and mosquito netting where screens are unsuitable; personal use of mosquito repellents; and sufficient clothing, particularly after sundown, to protect as much skin as possible.
Special consideration:	Disqualify from blood donation for 3 years persons on suppressive antimalarial therapy and those exposed to malaria (anyone who has visited a region where malaria is prevalent).

11

Antituberculars and antileprotics

capreomycin sulfate
cycloserine
dapsone
ethambutol hydrochloride
ethionamide
isoniazid (INH)
para-aminosalicylic acid
sodium aminosalicylate
pyrazinamide
rifampin
streptomycin sulfate
sulfoxone sodium

Antitubercular agents combat the different types of tuberculosis. Once known as the white plague or consumption, tuberculosis is an infectious disease that can attack any body organ but most commonly compromises the lungs.

Although this disease was usually fatal in the past, medical progress over the last few decades has rendered tuberculosis both controllable and curable. Becoming less prevalent in the United States, tuberculosis nevertheless remains a significant disease among alcoholics; in thickly populated, impoverished communities; on southwestern Indian reservations; and in parts of Asia, Africa, and Europe.

Antileprotics (dapsone and sulfoxone sodium) are therapeutically effective against leprosy (Hansen's disease), a chronic, intracellular, nonfatal disease unique to humans. Uncommon in the United States (overall incidence of reported cases is about 0.06/100,000 population), leprosy claims an estimated 12 to 15 million victims in the world today. Lepers may become severely disfigured and be isolated from the rest of society. Although the precise mechanism and routes of transmission are unknown, leprosy is thought to be transmitted directly from person to person.

Major uses

- Dapsone and sulfoxone are used to treat all forms of leprosy.
- Ethambutol, isoniazid, para-aminosalicylic acid, rifampin, and streptomycin are first-line drugs in the treatment of all forms of tuberculosis.
- Capreomycin, cycloserine, ethionamide, and pyrazinamide are second-line antitubercular agents, used in cases of drug resistance or in retreatment programs.
- Isoniazid is used prophylactically in susceptible persons exposed to tuberculosis.
- Rifampin is used prophylactically in meningococcal infections and *Hemophilus influenzae* meningitis. (It may be used with dapsone or sulfoxone in the initial management of lepromatous leprosy.)

Mechanism of action

- Cycloserine and isoniazid inhibit cell wall biosynthesis by a mechanism that's not well understood.
- Dapsone and sulfoxone are thought to inhibit folic acid biosynthesis.
- Para-aminosalicylic acid inhibits the enzymes responsible for folic acid biosynthesis.
- Rifampin inhibits DNA-dependent RNA polymerase, thus impairing ribonucleic acid synthesis.
- Streptomycin inhibits protein synthesis by binding to 30S ribosomal subunits.
- The mechanism of capreomycin, ethambutol, ethionamide, and pyrazinamide is unknown.

Absorption, distribution, metabolism, and excretion

- Capreomycin sulfate is not significantly absorbed when given orally. Given I.M., it quickly reaches peak blood levels and is excreted in the urine essentially unchanged.
- Cycloserine is rapidly absorbed when given orally. It is distributed throughout body fluids and tissues, including the cerebrospinal fluid (CSF). It is partially metabolized in the liver and excreted in the urine.
- Dapsone is almost completely absorbed orally; it is metabolized in the liver and slowly excreted in the urine. Sulfoxone sodium is hydrolyzed and absorbed mainly as its parent compound, dapsone.
- Ethambutol is well absorbed from the gastrointestinal (GI) tract (75% to 80%). Distribution is unknown, but the drug is detoxified in the liver. Most is recovered unchanged from the urine and as much as 25% from the feces.
- Ethionamide is rapidly absorbed when given orally and widely distributed; significant levels appear in CSF. Most of the drug is metabolized slowly in the liver and is subsequently excreted in the urine.
- Isoniazid is readily absorbed when given orally or I.M., diffusing into all body fluids and tissues. About half the drug is metabolized in the liver and is excreted, together with unchanged drug (about 40%), in the urine.
- Pyrazinamide is well absorbed from the GI tract. It is widely distributed, detoxified in the liver, and excreted in the urine.
- Rifampin is well absorbed and widely distributed. Partially metabolized in the liver, rifampin is eliminated as both metabolite and unchanged drug in urine and feces.
- Salicylates are readily absorbed from the GI tract, distributed throughout most body fluids and tissues, and excreted in the urine as both metabolite and free acid.
- Streptomycin is well absorbed and widely distributed in most body tissues after I.M. injection. It is rapidly excreted, mostly unchanged, in the urine.

Onset and duration

- Capreomycin sulfate reaches peak blood levels in 1 to 2 hours; duration is about 24 hours.
- Cycloserine reaches peak blood levels in 4 to 8 hours; duration is about 12 hours.
- Dapsone produces peak levels within 1 to 3 hours; duration is about 8 to 12 days.
- Ethambutol reaches peak levels in 2 to 4 hours; duration is about 24 hours.
- Ethionamide produces peak levels in 3 hours; since it's metabolized slowly, blood levels are prolonged.
- Isoniazid reaches peak levels within 1 to 2 hours; levels decline to about 50% within either 50 minutes (rapid acetylators) or 3 hours (slow acetylators).
- Para-aminosalicylates reach peak levels within 1 hour; duration is about 10 to 12 hours.
- Pyrazinamide levels peak in 2 hours; duration is about 15 hours.
- Rifampin produces peak levels within 1½ to 4 hours; duration is about 24 hours.
- Streptomycin's peak level occurs within 30 minutes to 2 hours; duration is about 8 to 12 hours.
- Sulfoxone sodium levels peak rapidly (15 to 30 minutes); duration is about 8 hours.

NAMES, INDICATIONS AND DOSAGES	SIDE EFFECTS
capreomycin sulfate Capastat Sulfate **Adjunctive treatment in pulmonary tuberculosis:** ADULTS: 15 mg/kg/day up to 1 g I.M. daily injected deeply into large muscle mass for 60 to 120 days; then 1 g 2 to 3 times weekly for a period of 18 to 24 months. Maximum dose should not exceed 20 mg/kg daily. Must be given in conjunction with another antitubercular drug.	**Blood:** eosinophilia, leukocytosis, leukopenia. **CNS:** headache. **EENT:** *ototoxicity* (tinnitus, vertigo, hearing loss). **GU:** *nephrotoxicity* (elevated BUN and nonprotein nitrogen, proteinuria, casts, red blood cells, leukocytes; tubular necrosis, decreased creatinine clearance). **Local:** pain, induration, excessive bleeding and sterile abscesses at injection site.
cycloserine Seromycin **Adjunctive treatment in pulmonary or extrapulmonary tuberculosis:** ADULTS: initially, 250 mg P.O. every 12 hours for 2 weeks; then, if blood levels are below 25 to 30 mcg/ml and there are no clinical signs of toxicity, dose is increased to 250 mg P.O. q 8 hours for 2 weeks. If optimum blood levels are still not achieved, and there are no signs of clinical toxicity, then dose is increased to 250 mg P.O. q 6 hours. Maximum dose 1 g/day. If CNS toxicity occurs, drug is discontinued for 1 week, then resumed at 250 mg daily for 2 weeks. If no serious toxic effects occur, dose is increased by 250 mg increments every 10 days until blood level of 25 to 30 mcg/ml is obtained.	**CNS:** drowsiness, headache, tremor, dysarthria, vertigo, confusion, loss of memory, *possible suicidal tendencies and other psychotic symptoms, nervousness, hallucinations, depression,* hyperirritability, paresthesias, paresis, hyperreflexia. **Other:** hypersensitivity (allergic dermatitis).
dapsone Avlosulfon♦ **Lepromatous leprosy:** ADULTS: weeks 1 to 4: 25 mg P.O. 2 times a week; weeks 5 to 8: 50 mg 2 times a week; weeks 9 to 12: 75 mg 2 times a week; weeks 13 to 16: 100 mg 2 times a week; weeks 17 to 20: 100 mg 3 times a week; weeks 21 to 24: 100 mg 4 times a week. CHILDREN: reduced dosage, but not necessarily by body weight; usually approximately ½ of adult dose using same schedule. **Tuberculoid leprosy:** ADULTS: same as for lepromatous leprosy in adults, but maximum dosage is 200 mg P.O. weekly (i.e., 100 mg 2 times a week). **Alternate dosage schedule:** ADULTS: 10 to 15 mg P.O. daily for 6 days a week, slowly increased to 62.5 mg daily for 6 days a week over a 6-month period.	**Blood:** anemia, especially hemolytic; methemoglobinemia; possible leukopenia. **CNS:** psychosis, headache, dizziness, lethargy, severe malaise, paresthesias. **EENT:** tinnitus, allergic rhinitis. **GI:** anorexia, abdominal pain, nausea, vomiting. **Hepatic:** hepatitis. **Skin:** allergic dermatitis (generalized or fixed maculopapular rash).

♦ Available in U.S. and Canada. ♦♦ Available in Canada only.
All other products (no symbol) available in U.S. only. Italicized side effects are common or life-threatening.

INTERACTIONS AND SPECIAL CONSIDERATIONS

No significant interactions.

Special considerations:
• Contraindicated in patients receiving other ototoxic or nephrotoxic drugs. Use cautiously in patients with impaired renal function, history of allergies, or hearing impairment.
• Considered a "second-line" drug in the treatment of tuberculosis.
• Drug is never given I.V.; may cause neuromuscular blockade.
• Patient's hearing should be evaluated before and during therapy; he should report tinnitus, vertigo, or hearing impairment.
• Renal function (output, specific gravity, BUN, urinalysis, serum creatinine) should be monitored before and during therapy. Dose must be reduced in renal impairment.
• Serum potassium levels and hepatic function should be monitored periodically.
• Reconstituted solutions can be stored for 48 hours at room temperature or 14 days if refrigerated. Straw- or dark-colored solution does not indicate a loss in potency.

Interactions:
ISONIAZID: monitor for CNS toxicity (dizziness or drowsiness).

Special considerations:
• Contraindicated in patients with seizure disorders, depression or severe anxiety, severe renal insufficiency, or chronic alcoholism. Use cautiously in patients with impaired renal function; reduced dosage required.
• Considered a "second-line" drug in the treatment of tuberculosis.
• Specimen for culture and sensitivity tests should be obtained before therapy begins and periodically thereafter to detect possible resistance.
• Cycloserine blood levels should be obtained at least weekly. Toxic reactions may occur with blood levels above 30 mcg/ml.
• Pyridoxine, anticonvulsants, tranquilizers, or sedatives may help to relieve side effects.
• Patient may develop personality changes.
• Hematologic tests and renal and liver function studies should be monitored.
• Patient should take drug exactly as prescribed; should not discontinue use without doctor's advice.

Interactions:
PROBENECID: elevates levels of dapsone. Use together with extreme caution.

Special considerations:
• Contraindicated in renal amyloidosis. Use cautiously in chronic renal, hepatic, or cardiovascular disease; refractory types of anemia.
• Therapy should be interrupted if generalized, diffuse dermatitis occurs.
• Dapsone dosage should be reduced or temporarily discontinued if hemoglobin falls below 9 g/dl; if leukocyte count falls below 5,000/ mm^3; if erythrocyte count falls below 2.5 million/mm^3; or if it remains persistently low.
• Patient should receive hematinics during dapsone therapy.
• Antihistamines may help to combat dapsone-induced allergic dermatitis.
• Erythema nodosum type of lepra reaction may occur during therapy as a result of *Mycobacterium leprae* bacilli (malaise, fever, painful inflammatory induration in the skin and mucosa, iritis, neuritis). In severe cases, therapy should be stopped and glucocorticoids given cautiously.
• Twice-a-week dosage schedule reduces toxic effects.
• CBC should be monitored frequently (weekly for the first month, monthly for six months, and semiannually thereafter).

NAMES, INDICATIONS AND DOSAGES	SIDE EFFECTS
ethambutol hydrochloride Etibi♦♦, Myambutol♦ **Adjunctive treatment in pulmonary tuberculosis:** ADULTS AND CHILDREN OVER 13 YEARS: initial treatment for patients who have not received previous antitubercular therapy 15 mg/kg P.O. daily single dose. Re-treatment: 25 mg/kg P.O. daily single dose for 60 days with at least 1 other antitubercular drug; then decrease to 15 mg/kg P.O. daily single dose.	**CNS:** headache, dizziness, mental confusion, possible hallucinations, peripheral neuritis (numbness and tingling of extremities). **EENT:** optic neuritis (vision loss and loss of color discrimination, especially red and green). **GI:** anorexia, nausea, vomiting, abdominal pain. **Metabolic:** elevated uric acid. **Skin:** dermatitis, pruritus. **Other:** anaphylactoid reactions, joint pain, fever, malaise, bloody sputum.
ethionamide Trecator SC **Adjunctive treatment in pulmonary or extrapulmonary tuberculosis (when primary therapy with streptomycin, isoniazid, and paraaminosalicylic acid cannot be used or has failed):** ADULTS: 500 mg to 1 g P.O. daily in divided doses. Concomitant administration of other effective antitubercular drugs and pyridoxine recommended. CHILDREN: 12 to 15 mg/kg P.O. daily in 3 to 4 doses. Maximum dose 750 mg.	**Blood:** thrombocytopenia. **CNS:** *peripheral neuritis,* psychic disturbances (especially mental depression). **CV:** postural hypotension. **GI:** *anorexia,* metallic taste in mouth, nausea, vomiting, sialorrhea, *epigastric distress,* diarrhea, stomatitis, weight loss. **Hepatic:** jaundice, hepatitis, elevated SGOT and SGPT. **Skin:** rash, *exfoliative dermatitis.*
isoniazid (INH) Hyzyd, Isotamine♦♦, Laniazid, Rimifon♦♦, Rolazid, Teebaconin **Primary treatment against actively growing tubercle bacilli:** ADULTS: 5 mg/kg P.O. or I.M. daily single dose, up to 300 mg/day, continued for 18 months to 2 years. INFANTS AND CHILDREN: 10 to 20 mg/kg P.O. or I.M. daily single dose, up to 300 to 500 mg/day, continued for 18 months to 2 years. Concomitant administration of at least one other effective antitubercular drug is recommended. **Preventive therapy against tubercle bacilli of those closely exposed or those with positive skin test whose chest X-rays and bacteriologic studies are consistent with nonprogressive tuberculous disease:** ADULTS: 300 mg P.O. daily single dose, continued for 1 year. INFANTS AND CHILDREN: 10 mg/kg P.O. daily single dose, up to 300 mg/day, continued for 1 year.	**Blood:** *agranulocytosis,* hemolytic anemia, *aplastic anemia,* eosinophilia, leukopenia, neutropenia, thrombocytopenia, methemoglobinemia, pyridoxine-responsive hypochromic anemia. **CNS:** *peripheral neuropathy* (especially in the malnourished, alcoholics, diabetics, and slow acetylators), usually preceded by paresthesias of hands and feet. **GI:** nausea, vomiting, epigastric distress, constipation, dryness of the mouth. **Hepatic:** *hepatitis, occasionally severe and sometimes fatal, especially in the elderly.* **Metabolic:** hyperglycemia, metabolic acidosis. **Local:** irritation at injection site. **Other:** rheumatic syndrome and systemic lupus erythematosus–like syndrome; hypersensitivity (fever, rash, lymphadenopathy, vasculitis).

INTERACTIONS AND SPECIAL CONSIDERATIONS

No significant interactions.

Special considerations:
• Contraindicated in patients with optic neuritis, and children under 13 years. Use cautiously in patients with impaired renal function, cataracts, recurrent eye inflammations, gout, and diabetic retinopathy.
• Dose must be reduced in renal impairment.
• Visual acuity and color discrimination tests should be performed before and during therapy.
• Renal, hematopoietic, and hepatic functions should be monitored in long-term use.
• Patient should be observed for symptoms of gout.
• Patient should take this drug exactly as prescribed; should not discontinue use without doctor's advice.
• Serum uric acid should be monitored.

No significant interactions.

Special considerations:
• Contraindicated in patients with severe hepatic damage. Use cautiously in patients with diabetes mellitus.
• Culture and sensitivity tests should be performed before starting therapy.
• Stop drug if skin rash occurs; may progress to exfoliative dermatitis.
• Hepatic, hematopoietic, and renal function should be monitored.
• Should be taken with meals or antacids to minimize GI effects.
• Patient may require antiemetic.
• Pyridoxine may be ordered to prevent neuropathy.
• Patient should take this drug exactly as prescribed; should not discontinue drug without doctor's advice.
• Excess alcohol ingestion should be avoided because it may make patient more vulnerable to hepatic damage.

Interactions:
ALUMINUM-CONTAINING ANTACIDS AND LAXATIVES: may decrease the rate and amount of isoniazid absorbed. Give isoniazid at least 1 hour before antacid or laxative.
DISULFIRAM: neurologic symptoms, including changes in behavior and coordination, may develop with concomitant isoniazid use. Avoid concomitant use.

Special considerations:
• Contraindicated in patients with acute hepatic disease, or isoniazid-associated hepatic damage. Use cautiously in patients with chronic non–isoniazid-associated hepatic disease, seizure disorders, severe renal impairment, chronic alcoholism; in elderly patients; in slow acetylator phenotypes (approximately 50% of Blacks and Caucasians).
• Hepatic function should be monitored if clinical signs of hepatic dysfunction occur during therapy. Patient should report immediately symptoms of hepatic impairment (loss of appetite, fatigue, malaise, jaundice, dark urine).
• Alcohol may be associated with increased incidence of isoniazid-related hepatitis. Use should be discouraged.
• Pyridoxine may be given to prevent peripheral neuropathy, especially in malnourished patients.
• Patient should take this drug exactly as prescribed; should not discontinue drug without doctor's advice.
• Store drug at room temperature.
• Excessive laxative use should be avoided.
• Patient should avoid cheese. May precipitate hypertensive crisis.
• Patient should take with food if GI irritation occurs.

NAMES, INDICATIONS AND DOSAGES	SIDE EFFECTS
para-aminosalicylic acid PAS, Nemasol Sodium♦♦ **sodium aminosalicylate** Parasal Sodium, Pasdium **Treatment of tuberculosis:** ADULTS: 10 to 12 g P.O. daily, divided in 2 or 3 doses. CHILDREN: 200 to 300 mg/kg P.O. daily, divided in 3 or 4 doses. **Treatment of tuberculosis:** ADULTS: 14 to 16 g P.O. daily, divided in 3 or 4 doses. CHILDREN: 200 to 300 mg/kg P.O. daily, divided in 3 or 4 doses.	**Blood:** *leukopenia, agranulocytosis,* eosinophilia, thrombocytopenia, hemolytic anemia. **CNS:** encephalopathy. **CV:** vasculitis. **GI:** *nausea, vomiting,* diarrhea, abdominal pain. **GU:** albuminuria, hematuria, crystalluria. **Hepatic:** *jaundice, hepatitis.* **Metabolic:** goiter, with or without myxedema; acidosis; hypokalemia. **Skin:** rash. **Other:** infectious mononucleosis–like syndrome, fever, lymphadenopathy.
pyrazinamide Tebrazid♦♦ **Hospitalized patients seriously ill with tuberculosis (when primary and secondary antitubercular drugs cannot be used or have failed):** ADULTS: 20 to 35 mg/kg P.O. daily, divided in 3 to 4 doses. Maximum dose 3 g daily.	**Blood:** hemolytic anemia, possible bleeding tendency due to altered clotting mechanism or vascular integrity. **GI:** anorexia, nausea, vomiting. **GU:** dysuria. **Hepatic:** *hepatitis.* **Metabolic:** interference with control in diabetes mellitus, hyperuricemia. **Other:** malaise, fever, arthralgia.
rifampin Rifadin♦, Rimactane♦ **Primary treatment in pulmonary tuberculosis:** ADULTS: 600 mg P.O. daily single dose 1 hour before or 2 hours after meals. CHILDREN OVER 5 YEARS: 10 to 20 mg/kg P.O. daily single dose 1 hour before or 2 hours after meals. Maximum dose 600 mg daily. Concomitant administration of other effective antitubercular drugs is recommended. **Meningococcal carriers:** ADULTS: 600 mg P.O. daily for 2 days. CHILDREN OVER 5 YEARS: 10 to 20 mg/kg/day P.O., not to exceed 600 mg/day.	**Blood:** eosinophilia, thrombocytopenia, transient leukopenia, hemolytic anemia, decreased hemoglobin. **CNS:** headache, fatigue, *drowsiness,* ataxia, dizziness, mental confusion, generalized numbness. **EENT:** visual disturbances, exudative conjunctivitis. **GI:** epigastric distress, anorexia, nausea, vomiting, abdominal pain, diarrhea, flatulence, sore mouth and tongue. **GU:** menstrual disturbances. **Metabolic:** hyperuricemia. **Hepatic:** *serious hepatotoxicity as well as transient abnormalities in liver function studies.* **Skin:** pruritus, urticaria, rash.

♦ Available in U.S. and Canada. ♦♦ Available in Canada only.
All other products (no symbol) available in U.S. only. Italicized side effects are common or life-threatening.

INTERACTIONS AND SPECIAL CONSIDERATIONS

Interactions:
ASCORBIC ACID, AMMONIUM CHLORIDE: acidify urine, increasing possibility of para-aminosalicylic acid crystalluria. Avoid if possible.
PROBENECID: may increase levels of para-aminosalicylic acid. Use together cautiously.
RIFAMPIN: para-aminosalicylic acid may interfere with absorption of rifampin. Give these drugs 8 to 12 hours apart.
DIPHENHYDRAMINE: inhibits absorption of para-aminosalicylic acid. Monitor for decreased para-aminosalicylic acid effect.

Special considerations:
• Use cautiously in patients with impaired renal function, decreased hepatic function, and gastric ulcers.
• Sodium aminosalicylate should not be given to patients on sodium-restricted diets. A 15 g dose provides 1.6 g sodium.
• Should be taken with meals or antacid to reduce gastrointestinal distress. Patient should swallow enteric-coated tablets whole and not with antacids.
• Renal, hematopoietic, hepatic functions, and serum electrolytes should be monitored.
• Patient should report immediately symptoms of hepatic impairment (loss of appetite, fatigue, malaise, jaundice, dark urine), fever, sore throat, or skin rash.
• Patient should take any of these drugs exactly as prescribed; should not discontinue drug without doctor's advice.
• Protect from water, heat, sun. If drug turns brown or purple, don't use.
• Concomitant administration of at least one other effective antitubercular drug is recommended.

No significant interactions.

Special considerations:
• Contraindicated in patients with severe hepatic disease. Use cautiously in patients with diabetes mellitus or gout.
• Nearly 100% excreted in urine; reduced dose needed in renal impairment.
• Liver function studies and examination for jaundice, liver tenderness or enlargement should be done before and frequently during therapy.
• Patient may develop gout and hepatic impairment (loss of appetite, fatigue, malaise, jaundice, dark urine, liver tenderness).
• Hematopoietic studies and serum uric acid levels should be monitored.
• Due to serious hepatotoxic effects, this drug is not recommended for initial therapy or long-term use.
• When used with surgical management of tuberculosis, pyrazinamide should be started 1 to 2 weeks preoperatively and continued for 4 to 6 weeks postoperatively.

Interactions:
PARA-AMINOSALICYLIC ACID: may interfere with absorption of rifampin. Give these drugs 8 to 12 hours apart.
PROBENECID: may increase rifampin levels. Use cautiously.

Special considerations:
• Use cautiously in patients with hepatic disease or in those receiving other hepatotoxic drugs.
• Hepatic function, hematopoietic studies, and serum uric acid levels should be monitored.
• Drowsiness and red-orange discoloration of urine, feces, saliva, sweat, sputum, and tears are possible. Soft contact lenses may be permanently stained.
• Patient should take this drug exactly as prescribed and report side effects. Should not discontinue use without doctor's advice.
• Should be taken 1 hour before or 2 hours after meals for optimal absorption.
• Increases enzyme activity of liver; may necessitate increased doses of warfarin, corticosteroids, oral contraceptives, and oral hypoglycemics. See each drug entry for specific drug interactions.

NAMES, INDICATIONS AND DOSAGES	SIDE EFFECTS
streptomycin sulfate **Primary treatment in tuberculosis:** ADULTS: with normal renal function, 1 g I.M. daily for 2 to 3 months, then 1 g 2 or 3 times a week. Inject deeply into upper outer quadrant of buttocks. CHILDREN: with normal renal function, 20 mg/kg daily in divided doses injected deeply into large muscle mass. Give concurrently with other antitubercular agents, but *not* with capreomycin, and continue until sputum specimen becomes negative.	**Blood:** eosinophilia, leukopenia, neutropenia, pancytopenia, hemolytic anemia. **CNS:** *transient paresthesias,* especially circumoral; lassitude; muscle weakness. **CV:** myocarditis. **EENT:** *ototoxicity* (damage to vestibular and auditory portions of 8th cranial nerve, severe headache, *nausea, vomiting, vertigo,* ataxia, *tinnitus, roaring and sense of fullness in the ears,* hearing loss), optic nerve dysfunction (blurred vision, amblyopia). **GI:** stomatitis. **GU:** *nephrotoxicity* (transient proteinuria, increase in BUN and serum creatinine levels); nephrotoxicity less common than with other aminoglycosides. **Local:** pain, irritation at injection site. **Other:** respiratory depression, muscle weakness, systemic lupus erythematosus syndrome, *hypersensitivity* (rash, fever, urticaria, pruritus, angioneurotic edema).
sulfoxone sodium Diasone Sodium♦ **Lepromatous and tuberculoid leprosy:** ADULTS: weeks 1 and 2: 330 mg P.O. 2 times a week; weeks 3 and 4: 330 mg 4 times a week; week 5 and following weeks: 330 mg daily for 6 days, skip a day and continue. CHILDREN 4 YEARS AND OLDER: give ½ the adult dose.	**Blood:** possible leukopenia, *anemia, especially hemolytic;* methemoglobinemia. **CNS:** psychosis, headache, dizziness, lethargy, severe malaise, paresthesias. **EENT:** tinnitus, allergic rhinitis. **GI:** anorexia, *abdominal pain,* nausea, vomiting. **Skin:** allergic dermatitis (generalized or fixed maculopapular rash). **Other:** hepatitis, drug fever, lepra reaction.

♦ Available in U.S. and Canada. ♦♦ Available in Canada only.
All other products (no symbol) available in U.S. only. Italicized side effects are common or life-threatening.

INTERACTIONS AND SPECIAL CONSIDERATIONS

Interactions:
OTHER AMINOGLYCOSIDES, METHOXYFLURANE: may increase streptomycin's ototoxic and nephrotoxic effects. Use cautiously.
ETHACRYNIC ACID, FUROSEMIDE: may increase streptomycin's ototoxic effects. Monitor carefully.
DIMENHYDRINATE: may mask symptoms of ototoxicity. Use together cautiously.

Special considerations:
- Contraindicated in patients with labyrinthine disease; hypersensitivity to any of the aminoglycosides; those receiving other ototoxic or nephrotoxic drugs, neuromuscular blocking agents, and general anesthetics. Use cautiously in elderly patients and in those with impaired renal function.
- Renal function studies should be monitored and dosage reduced in renal impairment.
- Patient's hearing should be tested before, during, and 6 months after therapy. Patient should report tinnitus, roaring noises, and fullness in ears.
- Patient may develop respiratory depression.
- To minimize renal damage, patient should be well hydrated.
- Superinfection (continued fever and other signs of new infections, especially of the upper respiratory tract) is possible.
- Very sensitizing topically. Hands should be protected when preparing drug.
- In primary treatment of tuberculosis, streptomycin is discontinued when sputum becomes negative.

No significant interactions.

Special considerations:
- Contraindicated in renal amyloidosis. Use cautiously in chronic renal, hepatic, or cardiovascular disease, or refractory anemias.
- Therapy should be interrupted if generalized, diffuse dermatitis occurs.
- Sulfoxone sodium should be reduced or temporarily discontinued if hemoglobin falls below 9 g/dl; if leukocyte count falls below 5,000/mm^3; if erythrocyte count falls below 2.5 million/mm^3; or if it remains persistently low.
- Patient should receive hematinics during sulfoxone sodium therapy.
- Antihistamines may help combat sulfoxone sodium-induced allergic dermatitis.
- Erythema nodosum type of lepra reaction may occur during sulfoxone sodium therapy as a result of circulating antigens caused by disintegrating *Mycobacterium leprae* bacilli (malaise, fever, painful areas of inflammatory induration in the skin and mucosa, iritis, neuritis). In severe cases, therapy should be interrupted and glucocorticoids given cautiously.
- CBC should be monitored frequently.
- If drug fever is severe or frequent, therapy should be interrupted or dosage reduced.
- To minimize stomach upset, drug should be taken with meals.
- Protect drug from light.

12

Aminoglycosides

amikacin sulfate
gentamicin sulfate
kanamycin sulfate
neomycin sulfate
streptomycin sulfate
tobramycin sulfate

Aminoglycosides are broad-spectrum antibiotics that act against both gram-positive and gram-negative bacteria as well as some strains of mycobacteria. Because of the risk of serious nephrotoxicity and ototoxicity (auditory and vestibular effects), their systemic use is generally reserved for infections caused by gram-negative organisms resistant to less toxic agents.

Major uses

Aminoglycosides combat serious bacterial infection and provide presurgical bacteriostatic and bactericidal action in the intestine.

All aminoglycosides (except neomycin) may be used alone or in combination with penicillin to treat infections caused by group D streptococcus (enterococcus).

- Amikacin, gentamicin, kanamycin, and tobramycin may be used to treat serious infections caused by susceptible strains of *Escherichia coli, Klebsiella, Proteus, Enterobacter,* and *Pseudomonas aeruginosa*. They may also be used in combination with other antibiotics in serious infections when the organism has not been identified.
- Neomycin may be administered orally as adjunctive treatment in hepatic encephalopathy. It may also be used as an antimicrobial irrigating agent of the urinary tract or peritoneum.
- Neomycin and kanamycin may be used orally to promote bowel sterility before gastrointestinal surgical procedures.

Mechanism of action

Aminoglycosides act directly on the ribosomes of susceptible organisms. By binding directly to the 30S ribosomal subunit, they inhibit protein synthesis. Generally, they are bactericidal in high concentrations and bacteriostatic in low concentrations.

Absorption, distribution, metabolism, and excretion

Aminoglycosides are not well absorbed from the gastrointestinal tract, so they must be given parenterally for systemic effect. Given orally, these antibiotics produce only a local effect (bowel sterilization).

They are distributed uniformly to most body fluids and tissues; penetration into cerebrospinal fluid, however, is inadequate.

Since aminoglycosides accumulate in the kidneys, nephrotoxicity is possible.

All aminoglycosides are rapidly excreted, mostly unchanged, in the urine by normal kidneys.

Onset and duration

Aminoglycoside blood levels peak within 30 minutes after I.V. infusion and within 60 minutes after I.M. injection.

The half-life of all aminoglycosides is from 2 to 4 hours but is significantly prolonged in patients with impaired renal function.

Combination products
None.

PREVENT NEPHROTOXICITY IN AMINOGLYCOSIDE THERAPY

Since aminoglycosides are excreted unchanged in urine, renal tissue is exposed to high concentrations of these drugs.

Impaired renal function, or nephrotoxicity, may result. Fortunately, it can be reversed if it's detected early and the dosage is immediately decreased.

To help prevent this adverse effect, the patient's renal status should be closely watched and these guidelines followed:

- The patient should be weighed and baseline renal function studies performed before therapy begins. Any change in the patient's renal function may be noted by assessing his daily weight in terms of fluid retention.
- During therapy, blood urea nitrogen (BUN) and serum creatinine levels should be monitored regularly.
- The patient should be encouraged to drink plenty of fluids.
- Urinary output should be monitored regularly and recorded in milliliters instead of vague measures such as "urine quantity sufficient (q.s.)."

The following should be reported immediately:

- cells or casts in urine
- oliguria
- proteinuria
- decreased creatinine clearance (or elevated serum creatinine)
- elevated BUN.

Of the currently available aminoglycosides, streptomycin is thought to be the least nephrotoxic. But streptomycin is not very effective in treating gram-negative bacterial infections such as those caused by *Pseudomonas.* Tobramycin, amikacin, and gentamicin are the most effective of these drugs against such organisms. Studies show that of these three, tobramycin is probably the least nephrotoxic (see the illustration below).

New aminoglycosides that will have even less nephrotoxicity than these drugs may soon be available.

Administration of the most nephrotoxic drugs requires careful observation of patients with a history of renal disease or concurrent renal disease not induced by aminoglycosides.

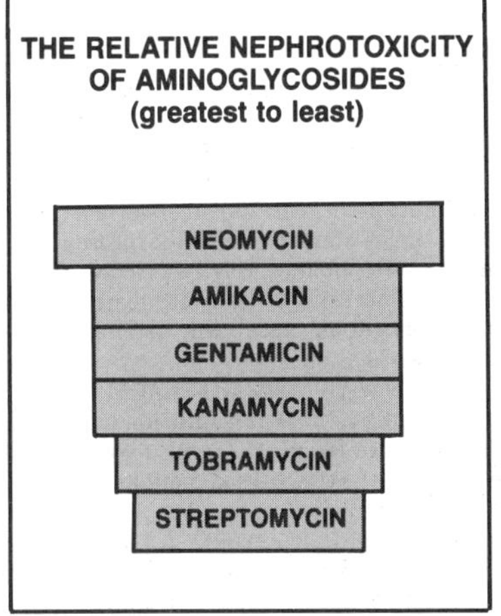

THE RELATIVE NEPHROTOXICITY OF AMINOGLYCOSIDES (greatest to least)
NEOMYCIN
AMIKACIN
GENTAMICIN
KANAMYCIN
TOBRAMYCIN
STREPTOMYCIN

NAMES, INDICATIONS AND DOSAGES | SIDE EFFECTS

amikacin sulfate
Amikin♦

Serious infections caused by sensitive *Pseudomonas aeruginosa, Escherichia coli, Proteus, Klebsiella, Serratia, Enterobacter, Acinetobacter, Providencia, Citrobacter, Staphylococcus:*

ADULTS AND CHILDREN WITH NORMAL RENAL FUNCTION: 15 mg/kg/day divided q 8 to 12 hours I.M. or I.V. infusion (in 100 to 200 ml 5% dextrose in water run in over 30 to 60 minutes). May be given by direct I.V. push if necessary.

NEONATES WITH NORMAL RENAL FUNCTION: initially, 10 mg/kg I.M. or I.V. infusion (in 5% dextrose in water run in over 1 to 2 hours), then 7.5 mg/kg q 12 hours I.M. or I.V. infusion.

Meningitis:

ADULTS: systemic therapy as above; may also use up to 4 mg intrathecally or intraventricularly daily.

CHILDREN: systemic therapy as above; may also use 1 to 2 mg intrathecally daily.

Serious urinary tract infections:

ADULTS: 250 mg I.M. b.i.d.

ADULTS WITH IMPAIRED RENAL FUNCTION: initially, 7.5 mg/kg. Subsequent doses and frequency determined by blood amikacin levels and renal function studies.

CNS: headache, lethargy.
EENT: *ototoxicity (tinnitus, vertigo, hearing loss).*
GI: nausea, vomiting.
GU: *nephrotoxicity (cells or casts in the urine, oliguria, proteinuria, decreased creatinine clearance, increased BUN and serum creatinine levels).*
Skin: rash, urticaria.

---

gentamicin sulfate
Apagen, Bristagen, Cidomycin♦♦, Garamycin♦, U-Gencin

Serious infections caused by sensitive *Pseudomonas aeruginosa, Escherichia coli, Proteus, Klebsiella, Serratia, Enterobacter, Citrobacter, Staphylococcus:*

ADULTS WITH NORMAL RENAL FUNCTION: 3 mg/kg/day in divided doses q 8 hours I.M. or I.V. infusion (in 50 to 200 ml of normal saline solution or 5% dextrose in water infused over 30 minutes to 2 hours). May be given by direct I.V. push if necessary. For life-threatening infections, patient may receive up to 5 mg/kg/day in 3 to 4 divided doses.

CHILDREN WITH NORMAL RENAL FUNCTION: 2 to 2.5 mg/kg I.M. or I.V. infusion q 8 hours.

INFANTS AND NEONATES OVER 1 WEEK WITH NORMAL RENAL FUNCTION: 2.5 mg/kg q 8 hours I.M. or I.V. infusion.

NEONATES UNDER 1 WEEK: 2.5 mg/kg I.V. q 12 hours. For I.V. infusion, dilute in normal saline solution or 5% dextrose in water and infuse over 30 minutes to 2 hours.

Meningitis:

ADULTS: systemic therapy as above; may also use 4 to 8 mg intrathecally daily.

CHILDREN: systemic therapy as above; may

CNS: headache, lethargy.
EENT: *ototoxicity (tinnitus, vertigo, hearing loss).*
GI: nausea, vomiting.
GU: *nephrotoxicity (cells or casts in the urine, oliguria, proteinuria, decreased creatinine clearance, increased BUN, nonprotein nitrogen, and serum creatinine levels).*
Skin: rash, urticaria.

INTERACTIONS AND SPECIAL CONSIDERATIONS

Interactions:

I.V. ETHACRYNIC ACID, I.V. FUROSEMIDE: increase ototoxicity. Use cautiously.

DIMENHYDRINATE: may mask symptoms of ototoxicity. Use with caution.

CARBENICILLIN: amikacin antagonism. Don't mix together in I.V. Schedule 1 hour apart.

OTHER AMINOGLYCOSIDES, METHOXYFLURANE: increase ototoxicity and nephrotoxicity. Use together cautiously.

Special considerations:

- Use cautiously in patients with impaired renal function; in neonates, infants, and elderly patients.
- Specimen for culture and sensitivity should be obtained before first dose. Therapy may begin pending test results.
- Patient should be weighed and baseline renal function studies obtained before therapy begins.
- Renal function (output, specific gravity, urinalysis, BUN, creatinine levels, and creatinine clearance) should be monitored.
- Patient should be well hydrated while taking this drug to minimize chemical irritation of the renal tubules.
- Patient's hearing should be evaluated before and during therapy. Patient should report tinnitus, vertigo, and hearing loss.
- Superinfection (continued fever and other signs of new infections, especially of upper respiratory tract) is possible.
- Usual duration of therapy is 7 to 10 days. If no response after 3 to 5 days, therapy should be stopped and new specimens obtained for culture and sensitivity.
- Peak blood levels above 35 mcg/ml are associated with higher incidence of toxicity.
- Amikacin is usually reserved for gentamicin-resistant organisms.

Interactions:

I.V. ETHACRYNIC ACID, I.V. FUROSEMIDE: increase ototoxicity. Use cautiously.

DIMENHYDRINATE: may mask symptoms of ototoxicity. Use with caution.

CARBENICILLIN: gentamicin antagonism. Don't mix together in I.V. Schedule 1 hour apart.

CEPHALOSPORINS: increase nephrotoxicity. Use together cautiously.

OTHER AMINOGLYCOSIDES, METHOXYFLURANE: increase ototoxicity and nephrotoxicity. Use together cautiously.

Special considerations:

- Use cautiously in patients with impaired renal function; in neonates, infants, and elderly patients.
- Specimen for culture and sensitivity should be obtained before first dose. Therapy may begin pending test results.
- Patient should be weighed and baseline renal function studies obtained before therapy begins.
- Renal function (output, specific gravity, urinalysis, BUN, creatinine levels, and creatinine clearance) should be monitored.
- Patient should be well hydrated while taking this drug to minimize chemical irritation of the renal tubules.
- Patient's hearing should be evaluated before and during therapy. Patient should report tinnitus, vertigo, and hearing loss.
- Superinfection (continued fever and other signs of new infections, especially of upper respiratory tract) is possible.
- For peak gentamicin level, blood should be drawn 1 hour after I.M. injection and 1 hour after I.V. infusion begins; for trough levels, blood should be drawn just before next dose.
- Usual duration of therapy is 7 to 10 days. If no response in 3 to 5 days, therapy should be stopped and new specimens obtained for culture and sensitivity.
- Peak blood levels above 12 mcg/ml and trough levels (those drawn just before next dose) above 2 mcg/ml are associated with higher incidence of toxicity.
- Hemodialysis (8 hours) removes up to 50% of drug from blood.
- Endocarditis prophylaxis is recommended for all patients with rheumatic or congenital heart disease or prosthetic heart valve.
- Intrathecal form (without preservatives) should be used when intrathecal administration is indicated.

(continued on following page)

NAMES, INDICATIONS AND DOSAGES	SIDE EFFECTS

gentamicin sulfate
(continued)

also use 1 to 2 mg intrathecally daily.

Endocarditis prophylaxis for GI or GU procedure or surgery:
ADULTS: 1.5 mg/kg I.M. or I.V. 30 to 60 minutes before procedure or surgery and q 8 hours after, for 2 doses. Given with aqueous penicillin G or ampicillin.
CHILDREN: 2 mg/kg I.M. or I.V. 30 to 60 minutes before procedure or surgery and q 8 hours after, for 2 doses. Given with aqueous penicillin G or ampicillin.
PATIENTS WITH IMPAIRED RENAL FUNCTION: initial dose is same as for those with normal renal function. Subsequent doses and frequency determined by renal function studies.

Posthemodialysis to maintain therapeutic blood levels:
ADULTS: 1 to 1.7 mg/kg I.M. or I.V. infusion after each dialysis.
CHILDREN: 2 mg/kg I.M. or I.V. infusion after each dialysis.

---

kanamycin sulfate
Kantrex♦, Klebcil

Serious infections caused by sensitive *Escherichia coli, Proteus, Enterobacter aerogenes, Klebsiella pneumoniae, Serratia marcescens, Acinetobacter:*
ADULTS AND CHILDREN WITH NORMAL RENAL FUNCTION: 15 mg/kg/day divided q 8 to 12 hours deep I.M. into upper outer quadrant of buttocks or I.V. infusion (diluted 500 mg/200 ml of normal saline solution or 5% dextrose in water infused at 60 to 80 drops/minute). Maximum daily dose 1.5 g.
NEONATES: 15 mg/kg/day I.M. or I.V. divided q 12 hours.

Adjunctive treatment in hepatic coma:
ADULTS: 8 to 12 g/day P.O. in divided doses.

Preoperative bowel sterilization:
ADULTS: 1 g P.O. q 1 hour for 4 doses, then q 4 hours for 4 doses; or 1 g P.O. q 1 hour for 4 doses, then q 6 hours for 36 to 72 hours.

Intraperitoneal irrigation:
500 mg in 20 ml sterile distilled water instilled via catheter into wound after patient fully recovered from anesthesia and neuromuscular blocking agent effects.
Wound irrigation—up to 2.5 mg/ml in normal saline irrigation solution.

CNS: headache, lethargy.
EENT: *ototoxicity (tinnitus, vertigo, hearing loss).*
GI: nausea, vomiting.
GU: *nephrotoxicity (cells or casts in the urine, oliguria, proteinuria, decreased creatinine clearance, increased BUN and serum creatinine levels).*
Skin: rash, urticaria.

♦ Available in U.S. and Canada. ♦♦ Available in Canada only.
All other products (no symbol) available in U.S. only. Italicized side effects are common or life-threatening.

INTERACTIONS AND SPECIAL CONSIDERATIONS

Interactions:
ETHACRYNIC ACID, FUROSEMIDE: increase ototoxicity. Use cautiously.
DIMENHYDRINATE: may mask symptoms of ototoxicity. Use with caution.
OTHER AMINOGLYCOSIDES, METHOXYFLURANE: increase ototoxicity and nephrotoxicity. Don't use together.

Special considerations:
- Oral use contraindicated in intestinal obstruction; in treatment of systemic infection. Use cautiously in impaired renal function and in the elderly.
- Specimen for culture and sensitivity should be obtained before first dose. Therapy may begin pending test results.
- Patient should be weighed and baseline renal function studies obtained before therapy begins.
- Renal function (output, specific gravity, urinalysis, BUN, creatinine levels, and creatinine clearance) should be monitored.
- Patient should be well hydrated while taking this drug to minimize chemical irritation of the renal tubules.
- Patient's hearing should be evaluated before and during therapy. Patient should report tinnitus, vertigo, and hearing loss.
- Superinfection (continued fever and other signs of new infection, especially of upper respiratory tract) is possible.
- If no response in 3 to 5 days, therapy should be stopped and new specimens obtained for culture and sensitivity.
- Peak blood levels over 30 mcg/ml are associated with increased incidence of toxicity.

NAMES, INDICATIONS AND DOSAGES	SIDE EFFECTS
neomycin sulfate Mycifradin Sulfate♦, Neobiotic **Infectious diarrhea caused by enteropathogenic *Escherichia coli:*** ADULTS: 50 mg/kg/day P.O. in 4 divided doses for 2 to 3 days. CHILDREN: 50 to 100 mg/kg/day P.O. divided q 4 to 6 hours for 2 to 3 days. **Suppression of intestinal bacteria preoperatively:** ADULTS: 1 g P.O. q 1 hour for 4 doses, then 1 g q 4 hours for the balance of the 24 hours. CHILDREN: 40 to 100 mg/kg/day P.O. divided q 4 to 6 hours. First dose should be preceded by saline cathartic. **Adjunctive treatment in hepatic coma:** ADULTS: 1 to 3 g P.O. q.i.d. for 5 to 6 days; or 200 ml of 1% or 100 ml of 2% solution as enema retained for 20 to 60 minutes q 6 hours.	**CNS:** headache, lethargy. **EENT:** *ototoxicity (tinnitus, vertigo, hearing loss).* **GI:** nausea, vomiting. **GU:** *nephrotoxicity (cells or casts in the urine, oliguria, proteinuria, decreased creatinine clearance, increased BUN and serum creatinine levels).* **Skin:** rash, urticaria.
streptomycin sulfate **Nonhemolytic streptococcal endocarditis:** ADULTS: 1 g I.M. deep into upper outer quadrant of buttocks q 12 hours for 1 week, then 500 mg I.M. q 12 hours for 1 week with penicillin. **Treatment of tuberculosis:** ADULTS: initially, 0.75 to 1 g I.M. daily for 60 to 90 days, then 1 g 2 to 3 times weekly. **Endocarditis prophylaxis for dental and upper respiratory tract procedures:** ADULTS: 1 g I.M. 30 to 60 minutes before procedure. Used with penicillin. CHILDREN: 20 mg/kg I.M. 30 to 60 minutes before procedure. Used with penicillin. **Endocarditis prophylaxis for GI or GU procedures or surgery:** ADULTS: 1 g I.M. 30 to 60 minutes before procedure and q 12 hours for 2 doses after. Used with penicillin or ampicillin. CHILDREN: 20 mg/kg I.M. 30 to 60 minutes before procedure and q 12 hours for 2 doses after. Used with penicillin or ampicillin. PATIENTS WITH IMPAIRED RENAL FUNCTION: initial dose same as for normal renal function; others determined by renal function tests. **Enterococcal endocarditis:** ADULTS: 1 g I.M. q 12 hours for 2 weeks, then 500 mg I.M. q 12 hours for 4 weeks with penicillin. **Tularemia:** ADULTS: 1 to 2 g I.M. daily in divided doses injected deep into upper outer quadrant of buttocks until patient is afebrile for 5 to 7 days.	**EENT:** *ototoxicity (tinnitus, vertigo, hearing loss).* **GU:** some nephrotoxicity (not nearly as frequent as with other aminoglycosides). **Local:** pain, irritation, and sterile abscesses at injection site. **Skin:** *exfoliative dermatitis.* **Other:** *hypersensitivity* (rash, fever, urticaria, and angioneurotic edema).

♦ Available in U.S. and Canada. ♦♦ Available in Canada only.
All other products (no symbol) available in U.S. only. Italicized side effects are common or life-threatening.

INTERACTIONS AND SPECIAL CONSIDERATIONS

Interactions:
ETHACRYNIC ACID, FUROSEMIDE: increase ototoxicity. Use cautiously.
DIMENHYDRINATE: may mask symptoms of ototoxicity. Use with caution.
OTHER AMINOGLYCOSIDES, METHOXYFLURANE: increase ototoxicity and nephrotoxicity. Use together cautiously.

Special considerations:
- Contraindicated in intestinal obstruction. Use cautiously in impaired renal function, ulcerative bowel lesions, and in the elderly.
- Oral therapy not recommended for systemic infection; parenteral dosage form available for I.M. use but not recommended because of extreme ototoxicity and nephrotoxicity.
- Patient should be weighed and baseline renal function studies obtained before therapy begins.
- Renal function (output, specific gravity, urinalysis, BUN, creatinine levels, and creatinine clearance) should be monitored.
- Patient should be well hydrated while taking this drug to minimize chemical irritation of the renal tubules.
- Respiratory depression, especially in renal disease, hypocalcemia, or neuromuscular diseases such as myasthenia gravis, is possible.
- Hearing of patient with hepatic or renal disease should be evaluated before and during prolonged therapy. Patient should report tinnitus, vertigo, and hearing loss. Onset of deafness may occur several weeks after drug is stopped.
- Superinfection (continued fever and other signs of new infections, especially of upper respiratory tract) is possible.
- Sometimes used in the treatment of high blood cholesterol.
- Nonabsorbable at recommended dosage. However, more than 4 g of neomycin per day may be systemically absorbed and lead to nephrotoxicity.
- Available in combination with polymyxin B as a urinary bladder irrigant.

Interactions:
DIMENHYDRINATE: may mask symptoms of streptomycin-induced ototoxicity. Use together cautiously.
ETHACRYNIC ACID, FUROSEMIDE: increase ototoxicity. Use cautiously.
OTHER AMINOGLYCOSIDES, METHOXYFLURANE: may increase streptomycin's ototoxic and nephrotoxic effects. Use cautiously.

Special considerations:
- Contraindicated in labyrinthine disease. Use cautiously in patients with impaired renal function and in the elderly.
- Specimen for culture and sensitivity should be obtained before first dose. Therapy may begin pending test results.
- Patient should be well hydrated while taking this drug to minimize chemical irritation of the renal tubules.
- Patient's hearing should be evaluated before, during, and 6 months after therapy. Patient should report tinnitus, roaring noises, or fullness in ears.
- Superinfection (continued fever and other signs of new infections, especially of upper respiratory tract) and respiratory depression are possible.
- Peak blood concentrations over 25 mcg/ml are associated with increased incidence of toxicity.
- Endocarditis prophylaxis is recommended for all patients with rheumatic or congenital heart disease or with prosthetic heart valve. Patients should receive prophylactic antibiotics during GI or GU procedures or surgery, or during upper respiratory tract procedures.

NAMES, INDICATIONS AND DOSAGES	SIDE EFFECTS
tobramycin sulfate Nebcin♦ **Serious infections caused by sensitive strains of *Escherichia coli, Proteus, Klebsiella, Enterobacter, Serratia, Staphylococcus aureus, Pseudomonas, Citrobacter, Providencia:*** ADULTS AND CHILDREN WITH NORMAL RENAL FUNCTION: 3 mg/kg I.M. or I.V. daily divided q 8 hours. Up to 5 mg/kg I.M. or I.V. daily divided q 6 to 8 hours for life-threatening infections. NEONATES UNDER 1 WEEK: up to 4 mg/kg I.M. or I.V. daily divided q 12 hours. For I.V. use, dilute in 50 to 100 ml normal saline solution or 5% dextrose in water for adults and less volume for children. Infuse over 20 to 60 minutes. PATIENTS WITH IMPAIRED RENAL FUNCTION: initial dose is same as for those with normal renal function. Subsequent doses and frequency determined by renal function study results.	**CNS:** headache, lethargy. **EENT:** *ototoxicity (tinnitus, vertigo, hearing loss).* **GI:** nausea, vomiting. **GU:** *nephrotoxicity (cells or casts in the urine, oliguria, proteinuria, decreased creatinine clearance, increased BUN and serum creatinine levels).* **Skin:** rash, urticaria.

INTERACTIONS AND SPECIAL CONSIDERATIONS

Interactions:

I.V. ETHACRYNIC ACID, I.V. FUROSEMIDE: increase ototoxicity. Use cautiously.

DIMENHYDRINATE: may mask symptoms of ototoxicity. Use with caution.

CARBENICILLIN: tobramycin antagonism. Don't mix together in I.V. Schedule 1 hour apart.

CEPHALOSPORINS: increase nephrotoxicity. Use together cautiously.

OTHER AMINOGLYCOSIDES, METHOXYFLURANE: increase ototoxicity and nephrotoxicity. Use together cautiously.

Special considerations:

- Use cautiously in patients with impaired renal function and in the elderly.
- Specimen for culture and sensitivity should be obtained before first dose. Therapy may begin pending test results.
- Patient should be weighed and baseline renal function studies should be obtained before starting therapy.
- Usual duration of therapy is 7 to 10 days.
- Renal function (output, specific gravity, urinalysis, BUN, creatinine levels, and creatinine clearance) should be monitored.
- Patient should be well hydrated while taking this drug to minimize chemical irritation of the renal tubules.
- Patient's hearing should be evaluated before and during therapy. Patient should report tinnitus, vertigo, or hearing loss.
- Superinfection (continued fever and other signs of new infections, especially of upper respiratory tract) is possible.
- Peak blood levels over 12 mcg/ml are associated with increased incidence of toxicity.
- For peak tobramycin level, blood should be drawn 1 hour after I.M. injection and 1 hour after I.V. infusion begins; for trough level, blood should be drawn just before next dose.
- Recent studies indicate tobramycin is less nephrotoxic than gentamicin.

WATCH FOR OTOTOXICITY

Ototoxicity, a significant adverse reaction to aminoglycosides, causes damage to the vestibular and the cochlear portions of the auditory nerve. Watch for these symptoms: headache, vertigo, nausea and vomiting with motion, tinnitus, and high-frequency hearing loss. (*Note:* Patients scheduled for aminoglycoside therapy should have a baseline audiogram as well as testing for high-frequency hearing loss during therapy.)

Ototoxicity occurs most often when peak blood levels of aminoglycosides are in the toxic range. This usually happens when the aminoglycoside is administered I.V. too rapidly; in elderly patients; and in patients with: impaired renal function, prior aminoglycoside therapy, concurrent therapy using other ototoxic drugs, abnormal baseline audiogram, history of excessive noise exposure, or history of ear infections.

13

Penicillins

amoxicillin trihydrate
ampicillin
ampicillin sodium
bacampicillin
carbenicillin disodium
carbenicillin indanyl sodium
cloxacillin sodium
cyclacillin
dicloxacillin sodium
hetacillin
hetacillin potassium
methicillin sodium
mezlocillin sodium
nafcillin sodium
oxacillin sodium
penicillin G benzathine
penicillin G potassium
penicillin G procaine
penicillin G sodium
penicillin V
penicillin V potassium
ticarcillin disodium

More than 5 decades after their discovery, penicillins remain the most popular class of antibiotic in clinical use. Chemical modifications of the original penicillin molecule have enhanced its activity against most gram-positive and gram-negative organisms.

Major uses

Penicillins are highly effective against infections due to gram-positive cocci, such as *Streptococcus pneumoniae* and nonpenicillinase-producing staphylococci; they are also effective against some gram-negative cocci, such as *Neisseria meningitidis* and *Neisseria gonorrhoeae*.

They're effective in varying degrees against *Bacillus anthracis, Bacteroides* species, *Clostridium perfringens, Treponema pallidum, Actinomyces,* and *Corynebacterium diphtheriae*.

Penicillins are *not* effective against viruses, mycobacteria, yeasts, plasmodia, fungi, or rickettsiae.

• Amoxicillin, ampicillin, bacampicillin, cyclacillin, and hetacillin are also active against strains of *Escherichia coli, Hemophilus influenzae, Proteus mirabilis, Salmonella* species, and *Shigella* species.

• Carbenicillin, mezlocillin, and ticarcillin have a broader activity than other penicillins against strains of *E. coli, Proteus* species, and *Pseudomonas aeruginosa*.

• Cloxacillin, dicloxacillin, methicillin, nafcillin, and oxacillin are resistant to penicillinase and thus are extremely useful in the treatment of infections due to *Staphylococcus aureus*. They may be used prophylactically before orthopedic and cardiac surgery.

Mechanism of action

Penicillins are thought to be bactericidal against microorganisms by inhibiting cell wall synthesis during active multiplication. They inhibit dipeptidoglycan, a substance that is necessary for cell wall rigidity. Penicillins are more effective against young and rapidly dividing organisms than they are against mature resting cells that are not undergoing the process of cell wall formation.

Bacteria resist penicillin by producing penicillinases—enzymes that convert penicillin to inactive penicilloic acid. The penicillinase-resistant penicillins (cloxacillin, dicloxacillin, methicillin, nafcillin, and oxacillin) resist these enzymes.

Absorption, distribution, metabolism, and excretion

Oral absorption occurs primarily in the duodenum; a small percentage of penicillin is absorbed in the stomach. Penicillins are widely distributed in body fluids and in such tissues as kidneys, liver, lungs, heart, spleen, skin, and intestine. Adequate penetration into cerebrospinal fluid and the brain occurs only with meningeal inflammation.

Penicillins except nafcillin are excreted mostly unchanged in urine (nafcillin is extensively metabolized in the liver). Excretion is delayed in infants, elderly patients, and persons with impaired renal function.

- Ampicillin, cloxacillin, dicloxacillin, hetacillin, nafcillin, oxacillin, penicillin G, and penicillin V are all acid-labile, that is, broken down by gastric and duodenal acid. Therefore, they are best taken on an empty stomach 30 to 60 minutes before or 2 hours after meals. Parenteral administration results in higher but more transient blood levels.
- Bacampicillin is well absorbed from the gastrointestinal tract even when taken with meals. Soon after absorption, the drug is hydrolyzed to ampicillin.
- Carbenicillin disodium, methicillin, mezlocillin, nafcillin, and ticarcillin disodium are very poorly absorbed orally and should be reserved for parenteral use.
- Penicillin G benzathine is slowly absorbed from I.M. injection sites, and therapeutic levels for certain organisms (pneumococcus, *T. pallidum*) may be observed as long as 30 days after a dose.
- Penicillin G procaine is more rapidly absorbed than penicillin G benzathine, but therapeutic levels may be observed as long as 24 hours after administration.
- Carbenicillin indanyl sodium given orally reaches therapeutic levels only in the urine, so it can't be used for systemic infections.

Onset and duration

- Peak blood level for oral penicillins is usually reached within 1 to 2 hours. Because the half-lives of all penicillins are very short (30 to 60 minutes), frequent doses are necessary.
- After parenteral administration, ampicillin, carbenicillin, methicillin, mezlocillin, nafcillin, oxacillin, and penicillin G rapidly reach peak blood levels (immediately with I.V. infusion). The more insoluble procaine and benzathine salts of penicillin G are slowly absorbed from I.M. injection sites.
- Duration of action is generally 3 to 6 hours in patients with normal renal function.

In patients with impaired renal function, the drug may remain in the blood as long as 24 hours after administration.

NAMES, INDICATIONS AND DOSAGES	SIDE EFFECTS

amoxicillin trihydrate
Amoxil♦, Larotid, Polymox♦, Robamox, Sumox, Trimox, Utimox

Systemic infections and chronic urinary tract infections caused by susceptible strains of gram-positive and gram-negative organisms:
ADULTS: 750 mg to 1.5 g P.O. daily, divided into doses given q 8 hours.
CHILDREN: 20 to 40 mg/kg P.O. daily, divided into doses given q 8 hours.

Uncomplicated gonorrhea:
ADULTS: 3 g P.O. with 1 g probenecid given as a single dose.

Uncomplicated urinary tract infections due to susceptible organisms:
ADULTS: 3 g P.O. given as a single dose.

Blood: anemia, thrombocytopenia, thrombocytopenic purpura, eosinophilia, leukopenia.
GI: *nausea*, vomiting, *diarrhea.*
Other: *hypersensitivity (erythematous maculopapular rash, urticaria, anaphylaxis),* overgrowth of nonsusceptible organisms.

---

ampicillin
Amcill♦, Ampilean♦♦, Omnipen, Pfizerpen A, Roampicillin
ampicillin sodium
Omnipen-N, Pen A/N, Polycillin-N, Principen/N, Totacillin-N

Systemic infections caused by susceptible strains of gram-positive and gram-negative organisms:
ADULTS: 1 to 4 g P.O. daily, divided into doses given q 6 hours; 2 to 12 g I.M. or I.V. daily, divided into doses given q 6 hours.
CHILDREN: 50 to 100 mg/kg P.O. daily, divided into doses given q 6 hours; or 100 to 200 mg/kg I.M. or I.V. daily, divided into doses given q 6 hours.

Meningitis:
ADULTS: 8 to 14 g I.V. daily for 3 days, then I.M. divided q 3 to 4 hours.
CHILDREN: up to 300 mg/kg I.V. daily for 3 days, then I.M. divided q 4 hours.

Uncomplicated gonorrhea:
ADULTS: 3.5 g P.O. with 1 g probenecid given as a single dose.

Blood: anemia, thrombocytopenia, thrombocytopenic purpura, eosinophilia, leukopenia.
GI: *nausea*, vomiting, *diarrhea*, glossitis, stomatitis.
Local: pain at injection site, vein irritation, thrombophlebitis.
Other: *hypersensitivity (erythematous maculopapular rash, urticaria, anaphylaxis),* overgrowth of nonsusceptible organisms.

---

bacampicillin
Spectrobid

Upper and lower respiratory tract infections due to streptococci, pneumococci, staphylococci, and *Hemophilus influenzae;* urinary tract infections due to *Escherichia coli, Proteus mirabilis,* and *Streptococcus faecalis;* skin infections due to streptococci and susceptible staphylococci:
ADULTS AND CHILDREN WEIGHING MORE THAN 25 KG: 400 to 800 mg P.O. q 12 hours.

Blood: anemia, thrombocytopenia, thrombocytopenic purpura, eosinophilia, leukopenia.
GI: *nausea*, vomiting, *diarrhea*, glossitis, stomatitis.
Other: *hypersensitivity (erythematous maculopapular rash, urticaria, anaphylaxis),* overgrowth of nonsusceptible organisms.

♦ Available in U.S. and Canada. ♦♦ Available in Canada only.
All other products (no symbol) available in U.S. only. Italicized side effects are common or life-threatening.

INTERACTIONS AND SPECIAL CONSIDERATIONS

Interactions:

PROBENECID: increases blood levels of penicillin. Probenecid is often used for this purpose.
CHLORAMPHENICOL, ERYTHROMYCIN, TETRACYCLINES: antibiotic antagonism. Give penicillins at least 1 hour before bacteriostatic antibiotics.

Special considerations:

• Use cautiously in patients with other drug allergies, especially to cephalosporins (possible cross-allergenicity); and in patients with mononucleosis—high incidence of maculopapular rash in those receiving amoxicillin.
• Cultures for sensitivity tests should be obtained before first dose. Not necessary to wait for results before beginning therapy.
• Before taking penicillin, patient should report any previous allergic reactions to this drug. However, a negative history of penicillin allergy is no guarantee against a future allergic reaction.
• Patient should take medication exactly as prescribed, even after he feels better. Entire quantity prescribed should be taken.
• Should be taken with food to prevent GI distress.
• Large doses may promote yeast growths.
• With prolonged therapy, bacterial and fungal superinfection may occur, especially in the elderly, debilitated, or those with low resistance to infection due to immunosuppressors or irradiation. Close observation is essential.
• Check expiration date. Patient should never use leftover penicillin for a new illness or share penicillin with family and friends.
• Patient should report rash, fever, or chills. A rash is the most common allergic reaction.
• Amoxicillin and ampicillin have similar clinical applications.
• For symptoms and treatment of anaphylaxis, see APPENDIX.

Interactions:

PROBENECID: increases blood levels of penicillin. Probenecid is often used for this purpose.
CHLORAMPHENICOL, ERYTHROMYCIN, TETRACYCLINES: antibiotic antagonism. Give penicillins at least 1 hour before bacteriostatic antibiotics.

Special considerations:

• Use cautiously in patients with other drug allergies, especially to cephalosporins (possible cross-allergenicity); in patients with mononucleosis; high incidence of maculopapular rash in those receiving ampicillin.
• Cultures for sensitivity tests should be obtained before first dose. Not necessary to wait for results before beginning therapy.
• Before taking penicillin, patient should report any previous allergic reactions to this drug. However, a negative history of penicillin allergy is no guarantee against a future allergic reaction.
• Patient should take medication exactly as prescribed, even after he feels better. Entire quantity prescribed should be taken.
• Patient should report rash, fever, or chills. A rash is the most common allergic reaction.
• Taken orally, drug may cause GI disturbances. Food may interfere with absorption, so should be taken 1 to 2 hours before meals or 2 to 3 hours after.
• Should not be given I.M. or I.V. unless infection is severe or patient can't take oral dose.
• Dosage should be altered in patients with impaired hepatic and renal functions.
• For I.V. administration, should be mixed with 5% dextrose in water or a saline solution. Might be incompatible with other drugs or solutions.
• Should be given I.V. intermittently to prevent vein irritation. Site should be changed every 48 hours.
• Large doses may promote yeast growths.
• With prolonged therapy, bacterial or fungal superinfection may occur, especially in the elderly, debilitated, or those with low resistance to infection due to immunosuppressors or irradiation. Close observation is essential.
• Check expiration date. Patient should never use leftover penicillin for a new illness or share penicillin with family and friends.
• Initial dilution in vial is stable for 1 hour. Manufacturer's direction for stability data should be followed when ampicillin is further diluted for I.V. infusion.
• For symptoms and treatment of anaphylaxis, see APPENDIX.

Interactions:

PROBENECID: increased blood levels of bacampicillin or other penicillins. Probenecid is often used for this purpose.
CHLORAMPHENICOL, ERYTHROMYCIN, TETRACYCLINES: antibiotic antagonism. Administer penicillins at least 1 hour before bacteriostatic antibiotics.

Special considerations:

• Use cautiously in patients with other drug allergies, especially to cephalosporins (possible cross-allergenicity).
• Cultures for sensitivity tests should be obtained before first dose. Unnecessary to wait for results before beginning therapy.
• Before taking bacampicillin or any other penicillin, patient should report any allergic reactions to the drug. However, a negative history of penicillin allergy is no guarantee against a future allergic reaction.
• Bacampicillin is especially formulated to produce high blood levels of antibiotic when administered twice daily.

(continued on following page)

NAMES, INDICATIONS AND DOSAGES	SIDE EFFECTS

bacampicillin
(continued)

Gonorrhea:
Usual dosage is 1.6 g plus 1 g probenecid given as a single dose.
Not recommended for children under 25 kg.

---

carbenicillin disodium
Geopen, Pyopen♦

Systemic infections caused by susceptible strains of gram-positive and especially gram-negative organisms *(Proteus, Pseudomonas aeruginosa):*
ADULTS: 30 to 40 g daily I.V. infusion, divided into doses given q 4 to 6 hours.
CHILDREN: 300 to 500 mg/kg daily I.V. infusion, divided into doses given q 4 to 6 hours.

Urinary tract infections:
ADULTS: 200 mg/kg daily I.M. or I.V. infusion, divided into doses given q 4 to 6 hours.
CHILDREN: 50 to 200 mg/kg daily I.M. or I.V. infusion, divided into doses given q 4 to 6 hours.

Blood: *bleeding with high doses,* neutropenia, eosinophilia, leukopenia, *thrombocytopenia.*
CNS: *convulsions,* neuromuscular irritability.
GI: nausea.
Local: pain at injection site, vein irritation, phlebitis.
Metabolic: *hypokalemia.*
Other: *hypersensitivity (edema, fever, chills, rash, pruritus, urticaria, anaphylaxis),* overgrowth of nonsusceptible organisms.

---

carbenicillin indanyl sodium
Geocillin, Geopen Oral♦♦

Urinary tract infection and prostatitis caused by susceptible strains of gram-negative organisms:
ADULTS: 382 to 764 mg P.O. q.i.d.
Not recommended for children.

Blood: leukopenia, neutropenia, eosinophilia, anemia, thrombocytopenia.
GI: *nausea,* vomiting, *diarrhea, flatulence, abdominal cramps, unpleasant taste.*
Other: *hypersensitivity (rash, chills, fever, urticaria, pruritus, anaphylaxis),* overgrowth of nonsusceptible organisms.

♦ Available in U.S. and Canada. ♦♦ Available in Canada only.
All other products (no symbol) available in U.S. only. Italicized side effects are common or life-threatening.

INTERACTIONS AND SPECIAL CONSIDERATIONS

- Diarrhea may occur less frequently with bacampicillin than with ampicillin.
- Patient should take medication even after he feels better. Entire quantity prescribed should be taken.
- Patient should report rash, fever, or chills. A rash is the most common allergic reaction.
- With prolonged therapy, bacterial or fungal superinfection may occur, especially in the elderly or the debilitated, and in those with low resistance to infection due to immunosuppressors or irradiation. Close observation is essential.
- Check expiration date. Patient should never use leftover penicillin products for a new illness or share penicillin with family and friends.
- Unlike ampicillin, bacampicillin may be taken with meals without fear of diminished drug absorption. Should be taken with food to prevent G.I. distress.

Interactions:

PROBENECID: increases blood levels of penicillin. Probenecid is often used for this purpose.
GENTAMICIN, TOBRAMYCIN: chemically incompatible. Don't mix together in I.V. Give 1 hour apart.
CHLORAMPHENICOL, ERYTHROMYCIN, TETRACYCLINES: antibiotic antagonism. Give penicillins at least 1 hour before bacteriostatic antibiotics.

Special considerations:

- Use cautiously in patients with other drug allergies, especially to cephalosporins (possible cross-allergenicity); those with bleeding tendencies, uremia, hypokalemia. Use cautiously in sodium-restricted patients; contains 4.7 mEq sodium/g.
- Cultures for sensitivity tests should be obtained before starting therapy. However, it's not necessary to wait for culture and sensitivity results before beginning therapy.
- Before taking penicillin, patient should report any previous allergic reactions to this drug. However, a negative history of penicillin allergy is no guarantee against a future allergic reaction.
- Dosage should be altered in patients with impaired hepatic and renal function. Patients with impaired renal function are susceptible to nephrotoxicity. Intake and output should be monitored.
- CBC should be checked frequently. Drug may cause thrombocytopenia.
- Serum potassium should be monitored. Patients may develop hypokalemia due to large amount of sodium in the preparation.
- If patient has high blood level of this drug, he may have convulsions. In preparation, side rails should be kept up on bed.
- For I.V. administration, should be mixed with 5% dextrose in water or other suitable I.V. fluids.
- Should be given I.V intermittently to prevent vein irritation and site changed every 48 hours.
- Almost always used with another antibiotic, such as gentamicin.
- Large doses may cause increased yeast growths.
- With prolonged therapy, other superinfections may occur, especially in the elderly, debilitated, or those with low resistance to infection due to immunosuppressors or irradiation. Close observation is essential.
- Check expiration date.
- For symptoms and treatment of anaphylaxis, see APPENDIX.

No significant interactions.

Special considerations:

- Use cautiously in patients with other drug allergies, especially to cephalosporins (possible cross-allergenicity).
- Cultures for sensitivity tests should be obtained before first dose. Unnecessary to wait for test results before starting therapy.
- Before taking penicillin, patient should report any previous allergic reactions to this drug. However, a negative history of penicillin allergy is no guarantee against a future allergic reaction.
- Patient should take medication exactly as prescribed, even after he feels better. Entire quantity prescribed should be taken.
- Patient should report rash (most common allergic reaction), fever, chills.
- When taken orally, drug may cause GI disturbances. Food may interfere with absorption; should be taken 1 to 2 hours before meals or 2 to 3 hours after.
- Large doses may promote yeast growths.
- With prolonged therapy, other superinfections may occur, especially in the elderly, debilitated, or those with low resistance to infection due to immunosuppressors or irradiation. Close observation is essential.
- Check expiration date. Patient should never use leftover penicillin for a new illness or share penicillin with family and friends.
- Should be used only in patients whose creatinine clearance is 10 ml/minute or more.
- Excellent treatment for *Pseudomonas* urinary tract infections in ambulatory patients.
- May be useful in treatment of cystitis, but not pyelonephritis.
- Not effective for any systemic infection because blood levels are nil.
- For symptoms and treatment of anaphylaxis, see APPENDIX.

NAMES, INDICATIONS AND DOSAGES	SIDE EFFECTS
cloxacillin sodium Bactopen♦♦, Cloxapen♦, Novocloxin♦♦, Orbenin♦♦, Tegopen♦ **Systemic infections caused by penicillinase-producing staphylococci:** ADULTS: 2 to 4 g P.O. daily, divided into doses given q 6 hours. CHILDREN: 50 to 100 mg/kg P.O. daily, divided into doses given q 6 hours.	**Blood:** eosinophilia. **GI:** *nausea,* vomiting, *epigastric distress, diarrhea.* **Other:** *hypersensitivity (rash, urticaria, chills, fever, sneezing, wheezing, anaphylaxis),* overgrowth of nonsusceptible organisms.
cyclacillin Cyclapen-W **Systemic and urinary tract infections caused by susceptible strains of gram-positive and gram-negative organisms:** ADULTS: 250 to 500 mg P.O. q.i.d. in equally spaced doses. CHILDREN: 50 to 100 mg/kg/day in equally divided doses.	**Blood:** anemia, thrombocytopenia, thrombocytopenic purpura, leukopenia, neutropenia, eosinophilia. **GI:** *nausea,* vomiting, *diarrhea.* **Other:** *hypersensitivity (edema, fever, chills, rash, pruritus, urticaria, anaphylaxis),* overgrowth of nonsusceptible organisms.
dicloxacillin sodium Dycill, Dynapen♦, Pathocil, Veracillin **Systemic infections caused by penicillinase-producing staphylococci:** ADULTS: 1 to 2 g daily P.O. or I.M., divided into doses given q 6 hours. CHILDREN: 25 to 50 mg/kg P.O. or I.M. daily, divided into doses given q 6 hours.	**Blood:** eosinophilia. **GI:** *nausea,* vomiting, *epigastric distress,* flatulence, *diarrhea.* **Other:** *hypersensitivity (pruritus, urticaria, rash, anaphylaxis),* overgrowth of nonsusceptible organisms.

♦ Available in U.S. and Canada. ♦♦ Available in Canada only.
All other products (no symbol) available in U.S. only. Italicized side effects are common or life-threatening.

INTERACTIONS AND SPECIAL CONSIDERATIONS

Interactions:
PROBENECID: increases blood levels of penicillin. Probenecid is often used for this purpose.
CHLORAMPHENICOL, ERYTHROMYCIN, TETRACYCLINES: antibiotic antagonism. Give penicillins at least 1 hour before bacteriostatic antibiotics.

Special considerations:
- Use with caution in patients with other drug allergies, especially to cephalosporins (possible cross-allergenicity).
- Cultures for sensitivity tests should be obtained before first dose. Unnecessary to wait for test results before starting therapy.
- Before taking penicillin, patient should report any previous allergic reactions to this drug. However, a negative history of penicillin allergy is no guarantee against a future allergic reaction.
- Patient should take medication exactly as prescribed, even if he feels better. Entire quantity prescribed should be taken.
- Patient should report rash, fever, or chills. A rash is the most common allergic reaction.
- When taken orally, drug may cause GI disturbances. Food may interfere with absorption; should be taken 1 to 2 hours before meals or 2 to 3 hours after.
- Large doses may promote yeast growths. With prolonged therapy, other superinfections may occur, especially in the elderly, debilitated, or those with low resistance to infection due to immunosuppressors or irradiation. Close observation is essential.
- Check expiration date. Patient should never use leftover penicillin for a new illness or share penicillin with family and friends.
- For symptoms and treatment of anaphylaxis, see APPENDIX.

Interactions:
PROBENECID: increases blood levels of penicillin. Probenecid is often used for this purpose.
CHLORAMPHENICOL, ERYTHROMYCIN, TETRACYCLINES: antibiotic antagonism. Give penicillins at least 1 hour before bacteriostatic antibiotics.

Special considerations:
- Contraindicated in patients allergic to other penicillins.
- Cultures for sensitivity tests should be obtained before starting therapy. However, it's not necessary to wait for culture and sensitivity results before beginning therapy.
- Before taking penicillin, patient should report any previous hypersensitive reactions to it. However, a negative history of penicillin allergy is no guarantee against a future allergic reaction.
- Patient must take all medication exactly as prescribed, for as long as ordered, even after he feels better.
- Patients with renal insufficiency should receive less drug in accordance with their creatinine clearance level.
- Large doses of penicillin may promote yeast growths.
- With prolonged therapy, bacterial and fungal superinfection may occur, especially in the elderly, debilitated, or those with low resistance to infection due to immunosuppressors or irradiation. Close observation is essential.
- Check expiration date. Patient should never use leftover penicillin for a new illness or share his penicillin with family and friends.
- Patient should report rash, fever, or chills. A rash is the most common allergic reaction.
- For symptoms and treatment of anaphylaxis, see APPENDIX.

Interactions:
CHLORAMPHENICOL, ERYTHROMYCIN, TETRACYCLINES: antibiotic antagonism. Give penicillins at least 1 hour before bacteriostatic antibiotics.
PROBENECID: increases blood levels of penicillin. Probenecid is often used for this purpose.

Special considerations:
- Use cautiously in patients allergic to cephalosporins (possible cross-allergenicity).
- Cultures for sensitivity tests should be obtained before first dose. Unnecessary to wait for test results before starting therapy.
- Before taking penicillin, patient should report any previous allergic reactions to this drug. However, a negative history of penicillin allergy is no guarantee against a future allergic reaction.
- Patient should take medication exactly as prescribed, even if he feels better. Entire quantity prescribed should be taken.
- Patient should report rash, fever, or chills. A rash is the most common allergic reaction.
- When taken orally, it may cause GI disturbances. Food may interfere with absorption; should be taken 1 to 2 hours before meals or 2 to 3 hours after.
- Should not be given I.M. unless infection is severe or patient can't take oral dose.
- Large doses may promote yeast growths.
- With prolonged therapy, other superinfections may occur, especially in the elderly, debilitated, or those with low resistance to infection due to immunosuppressors or irradiation. Close observation is essential.
- Check expiration date. Patient should never use leftover penicillin for a new illness or share penicillin with family and friends.
- For treatment of anaphylaxis, see APPENDIX.

NAMES, INDICATIONS AND DOSAGES	SIDE EFFECTS
hetacillin Versapen **hetacillin potassium** Versapen K **Systemic infections caused by susceptible strains of gram-positive and gram-negative organisms:** ADULTS: 225 to 450 mg P.O. q.i.d. CHILDREN: 22.5 to 45 mg/kg P.O. daily, divided into doses given q 6 hours.	**Blood:** thrombocytopenia, thrombocytopenic purpura, eosinophilia, leukopenia. **GI:** vomiting, *nausea, epigastric distress, diarrhea,* glossitis, stomatitis. **Local:** pain at injection site, vein irritation, phlebitis. **Other:** *hypersensitivity (chills, fever, anaphylaxis, maculopapular rash, urticaria),* overgrowth of nonsusceptible organisms.
methicillin sodium Azapen, Celbenin, Staphcillin♦ **Systemic infections caused by penicillinase-producing staphylococci:** ADULTS: 4 to 12 g I.M. or I.V. daily, divided into doses given q 4 to 6 hours. CHILDREN: 100 to 200 mg/kg I.M. or I.V. daily, divided into doses given q 4 to 6 hours.	**Blood:** *eosinophilia,* hemolytic anemia, transient neutropenia. **CNS:** neuropathy, convulsions with high doses. **GI:** glossitis, stomatitis. **GU:** interstitial nephritis. **Local:** *vein irritation, thrombophlebitis.* **Other:** *hypersensitivity (chills, fever, edema, rash, urticaria, anaphylaxis),* overgrowth of nonsusceptible organisms.
mezlocillin sodium Mezlin **Systemic infections caused by susceptible strains of gram-positive and especially gram-negative organisms *(Proteus, Pseudomonas aeruginosa):*** ADULTS: 200 to 300 mg/kg daily I.V. or I.M. given in 4 to 6 divided doses. Usual dose is 3 g q 4 h or 4 g q 6 h. For very serious infections, up to 24 g daily may be administered. CHILDREN TO AGE 12: 50 mg/kg q 4 by I.V. infusion or direct I.V. injection.	**Blood:** *bleeding with high doses,* neutropenia, eosinophilia, leukopenia, *thrombocytopenia.* **CNS:** *convulsions,* neuromuscular irritability. **GI:** nausea, diarrhea. **Local:** pain at injection site, vein irritation, phlebitis. **Metabolic:** *hypokalemia.* **Other:** *hypersensitivity (edema, fever, chills, rash, pruritus, urticaria, anaphylaxis),* overgrowth of nonsusceptible organisms.

INTERACTIONS AND SPECIAL CONSIDERATIONS

Interactions:
CHLORAMPHENICOL, ERYTHROMYCIN, TETRACYCLINES: antibiotic antagonism. Give penicillins at least 1 hour before bacteriostatic antibiotics.
PROBENECID: increased blood levels of penicillin. Probenecid is often used for this purpose.

Special considerations:
• Contraindicated in patients with mononucleosis. Use cautiously in patients with other drug allergies, especially to cephalosporins (possible cross-allergenicity); gastrointestinal disturbances.
• Cultures for sensitivity tests should be obtained before first dose. Not necessary to wait for culture and sensitivity results before beginning therapy.
• Before taking penicillin, patient should report any previous allergic reactions to this drug. However, a negative history of penicillin allergy is no guarantee against a future allergic reaction.
• Patient should take medication exactly as prescribed, even if he feels better. Entire quantity prescribed should be taken.
• Patient should report rash, fever, or chills. A rash is the most common allergic reaction.
• When taken orally, drug may cause GI disturbances. Food may interfere with absorption; should be taken 1 to 2 hours before meals or 2 to 3 hours after.
• Large doses may promote yeast growths.
• With prolonged therapy, other superinfections may occur, especially in the elderly, debilitated, or those with low resistance to infection due to immunosuppressors or irradiation. Close observation is essential.
• Check expiration date. Patient should never use leftover penicillin for a new illness or share penicillin with family and friends.
• Very similar to ampicillin.
• For treatment of anaphylaxis, see APPENDIX.

Interactions:
CHLORAMPHENICOL, ERYTHROMYCIN, TETRACYCLINES: antibiotic antagonism. Give penicillins at least 1 hour before bacteriostatic antibiotics.
PROBENECID: increases blood levels of penicillin. Probenecid is often used for this purpose.

Special considerations:
• Use cautiously in patients with other drug allergies, especially to cephalosporins (possible cross-allergenicity), and in infants.
• Cultures for sensitivity tests should be obtained before first dose. Unnecessary to wait for test results before starting therapy.
• Before penicillin is given, patient should report any previous allergic reactions to this drug. However, a negative history of penicillin allergy is no guarantee against a future allergic reaction.
• If ordered 4 times a day, should be given every 6 hours—even during the night.
• Urinalysis should be done frequently to monitor renal function.
• If patient has high blood level of this drug, he may have convulsions. In preparation, side rails should be kept up on bed.
• For I.V. administration, should be mixed with a normal saline solution. Other solutions may inactivate methicillin. Initial dilution must be made with sterile water for injection.
• Should be given I.V. intermittently to prevent vein irritation and site changed every 48 hours.
• With prolonged therapy and large doses, yeast growths and other superinfections may occur, especially in the elderly, debilitated, or those with low resistance to infection due to immunosuppressors or irradiation. Close observation is essential.
• Check expiration date.
• For symptoms and treatment of anaphylaxis, see APPENDIX.

Interactions:
GENTAMICIN, TOBRAMYCIN: chemically incompatible. Don't mix together in I.V. solution. Give 1 hour apart.
CHLORAMPHENICOL, ERYTHROMYCIN, TETRACYCLINES: antibiotic antagonism. Give penicillins at least 1 hour before bacteriostatic antibiotics.

Special considerations:
• Use cautiously in patient hypersensitive to drugs, especially to cephalosporins (possible cross-hypersensitivity), and those with bleeding tendencies, uremia, hypokalemia.
• Cultures for sensitivity tests should be obtained before starting therapy. Unnecessary to wait for culture and sensitivity results before starting therapy.
• Before penicillin is given, patient should report allergic reactions to this drug. A negative history of penicillin allergy, however, is no guarantee against future allergic reaction.
• Dosage should be altered in patients with impaired hepatorenal functions.
• CBC should be checked frequently. Drug may cause thrombocytopenia.
• Serum potassium level should be monitored.
• Patient with high serum level of this drug may have convulsions; seizure precautions should be taken.
• For I.V.: mix with 5% dextrose in water or other suitable I.V. fluids; give intermittently to prevent vein irritation; change site every 48 hours.
• Large doses may cause increased yeast growths. Symptoms should be reported.

(continued on following page)

NAMES, INDICATIONS AND DOSAGES	SIDE EFFECTS
mezlocillin sodium *(continued)*	
nafcillin sodium Nafcil, Unipen♦ **Systemic infections caused by penicillinase-producing staphylococci:** ADULTS: 2 to 4 g P.O. daily, divided into doses given q 6 hours; 2 to 12 g I.M. or I.V. daily, divided into doses given q 4 to 6 hours. CHILDREN: 50 to 100 mg/kg P.O. daily, divided into doses given q 4 to 6 hours; or 100 to 200 mg/kg I.M. or I.V. daily, divided into doses given q 4 to 6 hours.	**Blood:** transient leukopenia, neutropenia, granulocytopenia, thrombocytopenia with high doses. **GI:** *nausea,* vomiting, diarrhea. **Local:** *vein irritation, thrombophlebitis.* **Other:** *hypersensitivity (chills, fever, rash, pruritus, urticaria, anaphylaxis).*
oxacillin sodium Bactocill, Prostaphilin♦ **Systemic infections caused by penicillinase-producing staphylococci:** ADULTS: 2 to 4 g P.O. daily, divided into doses given q 6 hours; 2 to 12 g I.M. or I.V. daily, divided into doses given q 4 to 6 hours. CHILDREN: 50 to 100 mg/kg P.O. daily, divided into doses given q 6 hours; 100 to 200 mg/kg I.M. or I.V. daily, divided into doses given q 4 to 6 hours.	**Blood:** granulocytopenia, thrombocytopenia, eosinophilia, hemolytic anemia, transient neutropenia. **CNS:** neuropathy. **GI:** oral lesions. **GU:** interstitial nephritis. **Hepatic:** hepatitis. **Local:** *thrombophlebitis.* **Other:** *hypersensitivity (fever, chills, rash, urticaria, anaphylaxis),* overgrowth of nonsusceptible organisms.

INTERACTIONS AND SPECIAL CONSIDERATIONS

• Almost always used with another antibiotic, such as gentamicin.
• With prolonged therapy, superinfections may occur, especially in the elderly or debilitated, or those with low resistance to infection due to immunosuppressors or irradiation. Patient should be monitored closely.
• Check drug expiration date.
• Compared with similar antibiotics such as carbenicillin and ticarcillin, mezlocillin is less likely to cause hypokalemia.
• Drug may be better suited to patients on salt-free diets than carbenicillin and ticarcillin (contains 1.85 mEq Na^+/g of mezlocillin).
• For treatment of anaphylaxis, see APPENDIX.

Interactions:
CHLORAMPHENICOL, ERYTHROMYCIN, TETRACYCLINES: antibiotic antagonism. Give penicillins at least 1 hour before bacteriostatic antibiotics.
PROBENECID: increases blood levels of penicillin. Probenecid is often used for this purpose.

Special considerations:
• Use cautiously in patients with other drug allergies, especially to cephalosporins (possible cross-allergenicity); and GI distress.
• Cultures for sensitivity tests should be obtained before first dose. Unnecessary to wait for test results before starting therapy.
• Before penicillin is given, patient should report any previous allergic reactions to this drug. However, a negative history of penicillin allergy is no guarantee against a future allergic reaction.
• Patient should take medication exactly as prescribed, even if he feels better. Entire quantity prescribed should be taken.
• Patient should report development of rash, fever, or chills. A rash is the most common allergic reaction.
• When taken orally, drug may cause GI disturbances. Food may interfere with absorption, so should be taken 1 to 2 hours before meals or 2 to 3 hours after.
• Should not be given I.M. or I.V. unless infection is severe or patient can't take oral dose.
• For I.V. administration, should be mixed with 5% dextrose in water or a saline solution. Might be incompatible with other solutions.
• Should be given I.V. intermittently to prevent vein irritation and site changed every 48 hours.
• Large doses may promote yeast growths.
• With prolonged therapy, other superinfections may occur, especially in the elderly, debilitated, or those with low resistance to infection due to immunosuppressors or irradiation. Close observation is essential.
• Check expiration date. Patient should never use leftover penicillin for a new illness or share penicillin with family and friends.
• For symptoms and treatment of anaphylaxis, see APPENDIX.

Interactions:
PROBENECID: increases blood levels of penicillin. Probenecid is often used for this purpose.
SULFAMETHOXYPYRIDAZINE: decreases blood levels of oxacillin. Avoid if possible.
CHLORAMPHENICOL, ERYTHROMYCIN, TETRACYCLINES: antibiotic antagonism. Give penicillins at least 1 hour before bacteriostatic antibiotics.

Special considerations:
• Use cautiously in patients with other drug allergies, especially to cephalosporins (possible cross-allergenicity), and in premature newborns, and in infants.
• Cultures for sensitivity tests should be obtained before first dose. Unnecessary to wait for test results before starting therapy.
• Before taking penicillin, patient should report any previous allergic reactions to this drug. However, a negative history of penicillin allergy is no guarantee against a future allergic reaction.
• Patient should take medication exactly as prescribed, even if he feels better. Entire quantity prescribed should be taken.
• Patient should report rash, fever, or chills. A rash is the most common allergic reaction.
• When taken orally, it may cause GI disturbances. Food may interfere with absorption, so should be taken 1 to 2 hours before meals or 2 to 3 hours after.
• Should not be given I.M. or I.V. unless infection is severe or patient can't take oral dose.
• Periodic liver function studies are indicated; elevated SGOT and SGPT are possible.
• For I.V. administration, should be mixed with 5% dextrose in water or a saline solution.
• Should be given I.V. intermittently to prevent vein irritation and site changed every 48 hours.
• Large doses may promote yeast growths.
• With prolonged therapy, other superinfections may occur, especially in the elderly, debilitated, or those with low resistance to infection due to immunosuppressors or irradiation. Close observation is essential.
• Check expiration date. Patient should never use leftover penicillin for a new illness or share penicillin with family and friends.
• For symptoms and treatment of anaphylaxis, see APPENDIX.

NAMES, INDICATIONS AND DOSAGES	SIDE EFFECTS
penicillin G benzathine Bicillin L-A♦, Megacillin Suspension♦♦, Permapen **Congenital syphilis:** CHILDREN UNDER AGE 2: 50,000 units/kg I.M. as a single dose. **Group A streptococcal upper respiratory infections:** ADULTS: 1.2 million units I.M. in a single injection. CHILDREN OVER 27 KG: 900,000 units I.M. in a single injection. CHILDREN UNDER 27 KG: 300,000 to 600,000 units I.M. in a single injection. **Prophylaxis of poststreptococcal rheumatic fever or glomerulonephritis:** ADULTS AND CHILDREN: 1.2 million units I.M. once a month or 600,000 units twice a month. **Syphilis of less than 1 year's duration:** ADULTS: 2.4 million units I.M. in a single dose. **Syphilis of more than 1 year's duration:** ADULTS: 2.4 million units I.M. weekly for 3 successive weeks.	**Blood:** eosinophilia, hemolytic anemia, thrombocytopenia, leukopenia. **CNS:** neuropathy, convulsions with high doses. **Local:** pain and sterile abscess at injection site. **Other:** *hypersensitivity (maculopapular and exfoliative dermatitis, chills, fever, edema, anaphylaxis).*
penicillin G potassium Arcocillin, Biotic-T, Burcillin-G, Cryspen, Deltapen, Falapen♦♦, Hyasorb, Hylenta♦♦, K-Cillin, Ka-Pen♦♦, Lanacillin, Megacillin♦♦, Novopen-G♦, Parcillin, Pensorb, Pentids, P-50♦♦, Pfizerpen **Moderate-to-severe systemic infections:** ADULTS: 1.6 to 3.2 million units P.O. daily, divided into doses given q 6 hours (1 mg = 1,600 units); 1.2 to 24 million units I.M. or I.V. daily, divided into doses given q 4 hours. CHILDREN: 25,000 to 100,000 units/kg P.O. daily, divided into doses given q 6 hours; or 25,000 to 300,000 units/kg I.M. or I.V. daily, divided into doses given q 4 hours.	**Blood:** hemolytic anemia, leukopenia, thrombocytopenia. **CNS:** neuropathy, convulsions with high doses. **Metabolic:** possible severe potassium poisoning with high doses (hyperreflexia, convulsions, coma). **Local:** *thrombophlebitis, pain at injection site.* **Other:** *hypersensitivity (rash, urticaria, maculopapular eruptions, exfoliative dermatitis, chills, fever, edema, anaphylaxis),* overgrowth of nonsusceptible organisms.

INTERACTIONS AND SPECIAL CONSIDERATIONS

Interactions:
CHLORAMPHENICOL, ERYTHROMYCIN, TETRACYCLINES: antibiotic antagonism. Give penicillins at least 1 hour before bacteriostatic antibiotics.
PROBENECID: increases blood levels of penicillin. Probenecid is often used for this purpose.

Special considerations:
- Use cautiously in patients with other drug allergies, especially to cephalosporins (possible cross-allergenicity).
- Cultures for sensitivity tests should be obtained before first dose. Not necessary to wait for culture and sensitivity results before beginning therapy.
- Before penicillin is given, patient should report any previous allergic reactions to this drug. However, a negative history of penicillin allergy is no guarantee against a future allergic reaction.
- Patient should report rash, fever, or chills. Fever and eosinophilia are the most common allergic reactions.
- Should never be given I.V. Inadvertent I.V. administration has caused cardiac arrest and death.
- Very slow absorption time makes allergic reactions difficult to treat.
- Should be injected deeply into upper outer quadrant of buttocks in adults; in midlateral thigh in infants and small children.
- Check expiration date.
- For treatment of anaphylaxis, see APPENDIX.

Interactions:
CHLORAMPHENICOL, ERYTHROMYCIN, TETRACYCLINES: antibiotic antagonism. Give penicillins at least 1 hour before bacteriostatic antibiotics.
PROBENECID: increases blood levels of penicillin. Probenecid is often used for this purpose.

Special considerations:
- Use cautiously in patients with other drug allergies, especially to cephalosporins (possible cross-allergenicity).
- Cultures for sensitivity tests should be obtained before first dose. Not necessary to wait for culture and sensitivity results before beginning therapy.
- Before taking penicillin, patient should report any previous allergic reactions to this drug. However, a negative history of penicillin allergy is no guarantee against a future allergic reaction.
- Patient should take medication exactly as prescribed, even if he feels better.
- Patient should report rash, fever, or chills. A rash is the most common allergic reaction.
- When taken orally, drug may cause GI disturbances. Food may interfere with absorption, so should be taken 1 to 2 hours before meals or 2 to 3 hours after.
- Should not be given I.M. or I.V. unless infection is severe or patient can't take oral dose. Extremely painful when given I.M. Should be injected deep into large muscle.
- If patient has high serum level of this drug, he may have convulsions. In preparation, side rails should be kept up on bed.
- For I.V. administration, should be mixed with 5% dextrose in water or a saline solution. Might be incompatible with other solutions.
- Should be given I.V. intermittently to prevent vein irritation and site changed every 48 hours.
- Large doses may cause increased yeast growths.
- With prolonged therapy, other superinfections may occur, especially in the elderly, debilitated, or those with low resistance to infection due to immunosuppressors or irradiation. Close observation is essential.
- Check expiration date. Patient should never use leftover penicillin for a new illness or share penicillin with family and friends.
- For treatment of anaphylaxis, see APPENDIX.

NAMES, INDICATIONS AND DOSAGES	SIDE EFFECTS
penicillin G procaine Ayercillin♦♦, Crysticillin A.S., Duracillin A.S., Pfizerpen A.S., Wycillin♦ **Moderate-to-severe systemic infections:** ADULTS: 600,000 to 1.2 million units I.M. daily given as a single dose. CHILDREN: 300,000 units I.M. daily given as a single dose. **Uncomplicated gonorrhea:** ADULTS AND CHILDREN OVER 12 YEARS: give 1 g probenecid; then 30 minutes later give 4.8 million units of penicillin G procaine I.M., divided into 2 injection sites. **Pneumococcal pneumonia:** ADULTS AND CHILDREN OVER 12 YEARS: 300,000 to 600,000 units I.M. daily q 6 to 12 hours.	**Blood:** thrombocytopenia, hemolytic anemia, leukopenia. **CNS:** arthralgia, convulsions. **Other:** *hypersensitivity (rash, urticaria, chills, fever, edema, prostration, anaphylaxis),* overgrowth of nonsusceptible organisms.
penicillin G sodium Crystapen♦♦ **Moderate-to-severe systemic infections:** ADULTS: 1.2 to 24 million units daily I.M. or I.V., divided into doses given q 4 hours. CHILDREN: 25,000 to 300,000 units/kg daily I.M. or I.V., divided into doses given q 4 hours.	**Blood:** hemolytic anemia, leukopenia, thrombocytopenia. **CNS:** arthralgia, neuropathy, convulsions. **CV:** *congestive heart failure with high doses.* **Local:** *vein irritation, pain at injection site, thrombophlebitis.* **Other:** *hypersensitivity (chills, fever, edema, maculopapular rash, exfoliative dermatitis, urticaria, anaphylaxis),* overgrowth of nonsusceptible organisms.
penicillin V Biotic Powder, Ledercillin VK♦, Pfizerpen VK♦, Robicillin-VK, SK-Penicillin VK, Uticillin VK, V-Cillin Drops, V-Pen **penicillin V potassium** Betapen VK, Biotic-V-Powder, Bopen V-K, Cocillin V-K, Lanacillin VK, Ledercillin VK♦, LV, Nadopen-V♦♦, Novopen-V♦♦, Penapar VK, Penbec-V♦♦, Pen-Vee-K♦, Pfizerpen VK, PVF K♦♦, Uticillin VK, V-Cillin K♦ **Mild-to-moderate systemic infections:** ADULTS: 250 to 500 mg (400,000 to 800,000 units) P.O. q 6 hours. CHILDREN: 15 to 50 mg/kg (25,000 to 90,000 units/kg) P.O. daily, divided into doses given q 6 to 8 hours.	**Blood:** eosinophilia, hemolytic anemia, leukopenia, thrombocytopenia. **CNS:** neuropathy. **GI:** *epigastric distress,* vomiting, diarrhea, *nausea.* **Other:** *hypersensitivity (rash, urticaria, chills, fever, edema, anaphylaxis),* overgrowth of nonsusceptible organisms.

♦ Available in U.S. and Canada. ♦♦ Available in Canada only.
All other products (no symbol) available in U.S. only. Italicized side effects are common or life-threatening.

INTERACTIONS AND SPECIAL CONSIDERATIONS

Interactions:
CHLORAMPHENICOL, ERYTHROMYCIN, TETRACYCLINES: antibiotic antagonism. Give penicillins at least 1 hour before bacteriostatic antibiotics.
PROBENECID: increases blood levels of penicillin. Probenecid is often used for this purpose.

Special considerations:
• Contraindicated in patients with hypersensitivity to procaine. Use cautiously in patients with other drug allergies, especially to cephalosporins (possible cross-allergenicity).
• Cultures for sensitivity tests should be obtained before first dose. Not necessary to wait for culture and sensitivity results before beginning therapy.
• Before penicillin is given, patient should report any previous allergic reactions to this drug. However, a negative history of penicillin allergy is no guarantee against a future allergic reaction.
• Patient should report rash, fever, or chills. A rash is the most common allergic reaction.
• Should be given deep I.M. in upper outer quadrant of buttocks in adults; in midlateral thigh in small children.
• Should never be given I.V. Inadvertent I.V. use has caused death due to CNS toxicity from procaine.
• Due to slow absorption rate, allergic reactions are hard to treat.
• Large doses may promote yeast growths.
• With prolonged therapy, other superinfections may occur, especially in the elderly, debilitated, or those with low resistance to infection due to immunosuppressors or irradiation. Close observation is essential.
• Periodic evaluations of renal and hematopoietic function are recommended.
• Check expiration date.
• For treatment of anaphylaxis, see APPENDIX.

Interactions:
CHLORAMPHENICOL, ERYTHROMYCIN, TETRACYCLINES: antibiotic antagonism. Give penicillins at least 1 hour before bacteriostatic antibiotics.
PROBENECID: increases blood levels of penicillin. Probenecid is often used for this purpose.

Special considerations:
• Contraindicated in patients on sodium restriction. Use cautiously in patients with other drug allergies, especially to cephalosporins (possible cross-allergenicity).
• Cultures for sensitivity tests should be obtained before first dose. Not necessary to wait for culture and sensitivity results before beginning therapy.
• Before penicillin is given, patient should report any previous allergic reactions to this drug. However, a negative history of penicillin allergy is no guarantee against a future allergic reaction.
• If patient has high blood level of this drug, he may have convulsions. In preparation, side rails should be kept up on bed.
• For I.V. administration, should be mixed with 5% dextrose in water or a saline solution. Might be incompatible with other solutions.
• I.V. should be given intermittently to prevent vein irritation and site changed every 48 hours.
• Large doses may promote yeast growths.
• With prolonged therapy, other superinfections may occur, especially in the elderly, debilitated, or those with low resistance to infection due to immunosuppressors or irradiation. Close observation is essential.
• Vital signs should be monitored frequently.
• Serum sodium should be monitored.
• Check expiration date.
• For treatment of anaphylaxis, see APPENDIX.

Interactions:
CHLORAMPHENICOL, ERYTHROMYCIN, TETRACYCLINES: antibiotic antagonism. Give penicillins at least 1 hour before bacteriostatic antibiotics.
NEOMYCIN: decreases absorption of penicillin. Give penicillin by injection.
PROBENECID: increases blood levels of penicillin. Probenecid is often used for this purpose.

Special considerations:
• Use cautiously in patients with other drug allergies, especially to cephalosporins (possible cross-allergenicity) and GI disturbances.
• Cultures for sensitivity tests should be obtained before first dose. Not necessary to wait for culture and sensitivity results before beginning therapy.
• Before taking penicillin, patient should report any previous allergic reactions to this drug. However, a negative history of penicillin allergy is no guarantee against a future allergic reaction.
• Patient should take medication exactly as prescribed, even if he feels better. Entire quantity prescribed should be taken.
• Patient should report rash, fever, or chills. A rash is the most common allergic reaction.
• When taken orally, drug may cause GI disturbances. Food may interfere with absorption, so should be taken 1 to 2 hours before meals or 2 to 3 hours after.
• Large doses may promote yeast growths.
• With prolonged therapy, other superinfections may occur, especially in the elderly, debilitated, or those with low resistance to infection due to immunosuppressors or irradiation. Close observation is essential.
• Periodic renal and hematopoietic function

(continued on following page)

NAMES, INDICATIONS AND DOSAGES	SIDE EFFECTS
penicillin V *(continued)*	
ticarcillin disodium Ticar **Severe systemic infections caused by susceptible strains of gram-positive and especially gram-negative organisms *(Pseudomonas, Proteus):*** ADULTS: 18 g I.V. or I.M. daily, divided into doses given q 4 to 6 hours. CHILDREN: 200 to 300 mg/kg I.V. or I.M. daily, divided into doses given q 4 to 6 hours.	**Blood:** leukopenia, neutropenia, eosinophilia, *thrombocytopenia,* hemolytic anemia. **CNS:** convulsions, neuromuscular excitability. **GI:** nausea. **Metabolic:** *hypokalemia.* **Local:** pain at injection site, vein irritation, phlebitis. **Other:** *hypersensitivity (rash, pruritus, urticaria, chills, fever, edema, anaphylaxis),* overgrowth of nonsusceptible organisms.

♦ Available in U.S. and Canada. ♦♦ Available in Canada only.
All other products (no symbol) available in U.S. only. Italicized side effects are common or life-threatening.

INTERACTIONS AND SPECIAL CONSIDERATIONS

studies are recommended in patients receiving prolonged therapy.
• Check expiration date. Patient should never use leftover penicillin for a new illness or share penicillin with family and friends.
• For treatment of anaphylaxis, see APPENDIX.

Interactions:
CHLORAMPHENICOL, ERYTHROMYCIN, TETRACYCLINES: antibiotic antagonism. Give penicillins at least 1 hour before bacteriostatic antibiotics.
PROBENECID: increases blood levels of penicillin. Probenecid is often used for this purpose.
GENTAMICIN, TOBRAMYCIN: chemically incompatible. Don't mix together in I.V. Give 1 hour apart.

Special considerations:
• Use cautiously in patients with other drug allergies, especially to cephalosporins (possible cross-allergenicity); impaired renal function; hemorrhagic conditions; hypokalemia; in sodium-restricted patients (contains 5.2 mEq sodium/g).
• Cultures for sensitivity tests should be obtained before first dose. Not necessary to wait for culture and sensitivity results before beginning therapy.
• Before penicillin is given, patient should report any previous allergic reactions to this drug. However, a negative history of penicillin allergy is no guarantee against a future allergic reaction.
• Dosage should be decreased in patients with impaired hepatic and renal functions.
• CBC should be checked frequently. Drug may cause thrombocytopenia.
• If patient has high blood level of this drug, he may develop convulsions. In preparation, side rails should be kept up on bed.
• For I.V. administration, should be mixed with 5% dextrose in water or other suitable I.V. fluids.
• Should be given I.V. intermittently to prevent vein irritation and site changed every 48 hours.
• If given I.M., should be administered deep into large muscle.
• Large doses may promote yeast growths.
• With prolonged therapy, other superinfections may occur, especially in the elderly, debilitated, or those with low resistance to infection due to immunosuppressors or irradiation. Close observation is essential.
• Serum potassium should be monitored.
• Almost always used with another antibiotic such as gentamicin.
• Check expiration date.
• For symptoms and treatment of anaphylaxis, see APPENDIX.

14

Cephalosporins

cefaclor
cefadroxil monohydrate
cefamandole naftate
cefazolin sodium
cefotaxime sodium
cefoxitin sodium
cephalexin monohydrate
cephaloglycin dihydrate
cephaloridine
cephalothin sodium
cephapirin sodium
cephradine
moxalactam disodium

Structurally related to penicillins, cephalosporins are broad-spectrum antibiotics active against a variety of aerobic gram-positive and gram-negative microorganisms. They all contain 7-aminocephalosporanic acid (beta-lactam ring).

Third generation cephalosporins, such as cefotaxime and moxalactam, have recently been introduced. These cephalosporins have expanded utility against gram-negative microorganisms.

Major uses

Cephalosporins are used to treat infections caused by gram-positive cocci (except enterococci), penicillinase-producing staphylococci, and some gram-negative bacilli, including *Pseudomonas, Escherichia coli, Proteus mirabilis,* and *Klebsiella*. Although these drugs may be used for patients allergic to penicillin, a small percentage of such patients subsequently develop allergies to cephalosporins.

As penicillin alternatives, parenteral and oral cephalosporins combat infections of the respiratory tract, skin, soft tissues, and genitourinary tract. In addition, parenteral cephalosporins are effective against osteoarticular infections, septicemia, and endocarditis. Oral cephalosporins are also therapeutic for otitis media.

When the identity of the organism is unknown in serious infections, cephalosporins may be therapeutic in combination with other antimicrobial drugs (aminoglycosides, for example).

Cephalosporins may be used prophylactically before orthopedic, cardiac, bowel, and gynecologic surgery.

• Cefamandole and cefaclor are active against some ampicillin-resistant strains of *Hemophilus influenzae*.

• Cefamandole, cefotaxime, cefoxitin, and moxalactam are more active than other cephalosporins against strains of the Enterobacteriaceae.

• Cefoxitin and moxalactam are antibiotics that may be useful against infections due to *Bacteroides fragilis*.

Mechanism of action
Cephalosporins are either bactericidal or bacteriostatic, depending on organism susceptibility and reproduction rate, drug dose, and blood and tissue concentrations. They inhibit cell wall synthesis, thereby making the wall less osmotically stable. They are more effective against young, rapidly dividing organisms than against mature, resting cells that are not in the process of cell wall formation.

Absorption, distribution, metabolism, and excretion
- The presence of food in the gastrointestinal (GI) tract retards absorption of oral cephalosporins, causing lower and delayed peak blood levels; it doesn't, however, diminish the total amount of drug absorbed.
- Cefaclor, cefadroxil, cephalexin, cephaloglycin, and cephradine are given orally because they are well absorbed from the GI tract.
- Cefamandole, cefazolin, cefotaxime, cefoxitin, cephaloridine, cephalothin, cephapirin and moxalactam are administered parenterally because they are not well absorbed from the GI tract.
- Most cephalosporins are widely distributed in body tissues and fluid but enter cerebrospinal fluid in only small amounts. Therapeutic levels of these antibiotics are achieved in most tissues. Cefotaxime and moxalactam are well distributed in the cerebrospinal fluid.
- Cefaclor, cefadroxil, cefamandole, cefazolin, cefoxitin, cephalexin, cephaloridine, cephradine, and moxalactam are excreted unchanged in the urine and accumulate in patients with renal insufficiency.
- Cefotaxime, cephaloglycin, cephalothin, and cephapirin are partially metabolized in the liver.

Onset and duration
Onset and duration depend on route of administration and the patient's renal function.
- After oral administration, peak blood levels occur within 1 to 2 hours.
- Peak levels after I.V. administration depend on the rate of infusion; they occur when the infusion is finished.
- Blood levels reach a peak between 30 minutes and 2 hours after intramuscular administration.

Combination products
None.

NAMES, INDICATIONS AND DOSAGES	SIDE EFFECTS
cefaclor Ceclor **Treatment of infections of respiratory or urinary tracts, skin, and soft tissue; and otitis media due to *Hemophilus influenzae, Streptococcus pneumoniae, Streptococcus pyogenes, Escherichia coli, Proteus mirabilis, Klebsiella* species, and *staphylococci:*** ADULTS: 250 to 500 mg P.O. q 8 hours. Total daily dose should not exceed 4 g. CHILDREN: 20 mg/kg/day P.O. in divided doses q 8 hours. In more serious infections, 40 mg/kg/day are recommended, not to exceed 1 g/day.	**Blood:** transient leukopenia, lymphocytosis, anemia, eosinophilia. **CNS:** dizziness, headache, somnolence. **GI:** *nausea,* vomiting, diarrhea, anorexia. **GU:** red and white cells in urine, vaginal moniliasis, vaginitis. **Skin:** *maculopapular rash,* dermatitis. **Other:** hypersensitivity, fever.
cefadroxil monohydrate Duricef, Ultracef **Treatment of urinary tract infections caused by *Escherichia coli, Proteus mirabilis,* and *Klebsiella* species; infections of skin and soft tissue; and streptococcal pharyngitis:** ADULTS: 500 mg to 2 g P.O./day, depending on the infection being treated. Usually given in once-daily or b.i.d. dosage. CHILDREN: 30 mg/kg/day in 2 divided doses.	**Blood:** transient neutropenia, eosinophilia, leukopenia, anemia. **CNS:** dizziness, headache, malaise, paresthesias. **GI:** *nausea,* anorexia, vomiting, *diarrhea,* glossitis, *dyspepsia,* abdominal cramps, anal pruritus, tenesmus, oral candidiasis (thrush). **GU:** genital pruritus, moniliasis. **Skin:** *maculopapular and erythematous rashes.* **Other:** dyspnea.
cefamandole naftate Mandol **Treatment of serious infections of respiratory and genitourinary tracts, skin and soft tissue infections, bone and joint infections, septicemia, and peritonitis due to *Escherichia coli* and other coliform bacteria, *Staphylococcus aureus* (penicillinase- and nonpenicillinase-producing), *Staphyloccus epidermidis,* group A beta-hemolytic streptococci, *Klebsiella, Hemophilus influenzae, Proteus mirabilis,* and *Enterobacter* species:** ADULTS: 500 mg to 1 g q 4 to 8 hours. In life-threatening infections, up to 2 g q 4 hours may be needed. INFANTS AND CHILDREN: 50 to 100 mg/kg/day in equally divided doses q 4 to 8 hours. May be increased to total daily dose of 150 mg/kg (not to exceed maximum adult dose) for severe infections. Total daily dosage is same for I.M. or I.V. administration. In impaired renal function, doses or frequency of administration depend on degree of renal impairment, severity of infection, susceptibility of organism, and blood levels of drug. Should be injected deep I.M. into a large muscle mass, such as gluteus or lateral aspect of thigh.	**Blood:** transient neutropenia, eosinophilia, hemolytic anemia. **CNS:** headache, malaise, paresthesias, dizziness. **GI:** nausea, anorexia, vomiting, diarrhea, glossitis, dyspepsia, abdominal cramps, tenesmus, anal pruritus, oral candidiasis (thrush). **GU:** nephrotoxicity, genital pruritus and moniliasis. **Skin:** *maculopapular and erythematous rashes, urticaria.* **Local:** *at injection site—pain, induration, sterile abscesses,* temperature elevation, tissue sloughing; *phlebitis and thrombophlebitis with I.V. injection.* **Other:** *hypersensitivity,* dyspnea.

INTERACTIONS AND SPECIAL CONSIDERATIONS

Interactions:
PROBENECID: may inhibit excretion and increase blood levels of cefaclor. Use together cautiously.

Special considerations:
• Contraindicated in hypersensitivity to other cephalosporins. Use cautiously in impaired renal status and in patients with history of sensitivity to penicillin. Consider any reaction to previous cephalosporin or penicillin therapy before administering first dose.
• Prolonged use may result in overgrowth of nonsusceptible organisms. Careful observation of patient for superinfection is essential.
• Cultures for sensitivity tests should be obtained before therapy, but therapy may begin pending results of culture and sensitivity tests.
• Major clinical use appears to be in treating otitis media caused by *H. influenzae* when resistant to ampicillin or amoxicillin.
• Mostly used in ambulatory setting.
• Patient should take medication as prescribed, even though he may feel better.
• Patient should notify doctor if skin rash develops.
• Store reconstituted solution in refrigerator. Stable for 14 days if refrigerated. Shake well before using.
• Drug may be taken with meals.
• Cefaclor is a relatively expensive antibiotic and should be used only when the organism is resistant to other agents.

Interactions:
PROBENECID: may inhibit excretion and increase blood levels of cefadroxil. Use together cautiously.

Special considerations:
• Contraindicated in hypersensitivity to other cephalosporins. Use cautiously in impaired renal status and in patients with history of sensitivity to penicillin. Consider any reaction to previous cephalosporin or penicillin therapy before administering first dose.
• Prolonged use may result in overgrowth of nonsusceptible organisms. Careful observation of patient for superinfection is essential.
• Cultures for sensitivity tests should be obtained before therapy, but therapy may begin pending results of cultures and sensitivity tests.
• If creatinine clearance is below 50 ml/min, dosage interval should be increased so drug doesn't accumulate.
• Patient should take medication as prescribed, even though he may feel better.
• Patient should notify doctor if skin rash develops.
• Absorption not delayed by presence of food.
• Longer half-life permits twice-daily dosing.

Interactions:
PROBENECID: may inhibit excretion and increase blood levels of cefamandole. Use together cautiously.

Special considerations:
• Contraindicated in hypersensitivity to other cephalosporins. Use cautiously in impaired renal status and in history of sensitivity to penicillin. Consider reaction to previous cephalosporin or penicillin therapy before first dose.
• Prolonged use may result in overgrowth of nonsusceptible organisms. Careful observation of patient for superinfection is essential.
• Cultures for sensitivity tests should be obtained before therapy, but therapy may begin pending results of cultures and sensitivity tests.
• Cephalosporin of choice for treatment of *Enterobacter* sepsis. Not as effective as cefoxitin in treating anaerobic infections.
• For most cephalosporin-sensitive organisms, cefamandole offers little advantage over previously available agents.
• For I.V. use, 1 g can be reconstituted with 10 ml of sterile water for injection, 5% dextrose or 0.9% sodium chloride for injection. May be combined with the following intravenous fluids: 0.9% sodium chloride injection, 5% dextrose injection, 10% dextrose injection, 5% dextrose and 0.9% sodium chloride injection, 5% dextrose and 0.45% sodium chloride injection, 5% dextrose and 0.2% sodium chloride injection, or sodium lactate injection.
• I.M. cefamandole not as painful as cefoxitin. Does not require addition of lidocaine.
• After reconstitution, remains stable for 24 hours at room temperature or 96 hours under refrigeration.

NAMES, INDICATIONS AND DOSAGES	SIDE EFFECTS

cefazolin sodium

Ancef♦, Kefzol♦

Treatment of serious infections of respiratory and genitourinary tracts, skin and soft tissue infections, bone and joint infections, septicemia, and endocarditis due to *Escherichia coli, Enterobacteriaceae, gonococci, Hemophilus influenzae, Klebsiella, Proteus mirabilis, Staphylococcus aureus, Streptococcus pneumoniae,* and group A *beta-hemolytic streptococci;* and before, during, and after surgery:

ADULTS: 250 mg I.M. or I.V. q 8 hours to 1 g q 6 hours.

CHILDREN OVER 1 MONTH: 8 to 16 mg/kg I.M. or I.V. q 8 hours, or 6 to 12 mg/kg q 6 hours.

Total daily dosage is same for I.M. or I.V. administration and depends on susceptibility of organism and severity of infection.

In patients with impaired renal function, doses or frequency of administration must be modified according to degree of renal impairment, severity of infection, susceptibility of organism, and serum levels of drug. Should be injected deep I.M. into a large muscle mass, such as gluteus or lateral aspect of thigh.

Blood: transient neutropenia, leukopenia, eosinophilia, anemia.
CNS: dizziness, headache, malaise, paresthesias.
GI: nausea, anorexia, vomiting, diarrhea, glossitis, dyspepsia, abdominal cramps, anal pruritus, tenesmus, oral candidiasis (thrush).
GU: nephrotoxicity, genital pruritus and moniliasis, vaginitis.
Skin: *maculopapular and erythematous rashes, urticaria.*
Local: *at injection site—pain, induration, sterile abscesses,* tissue sloughing; *phlebitis and thrombophlebitis with I.V. injection.*
Other: *hypersensitivity,* dyspnea.

cefotaxime sodium

Claforan

Treatment of serious infections of the lower respiratory and urinary tracts, gynecological infections, bacteremia, septicemia, and skin infections.
Among susceptible microorganisms are streptococci, including *Streptococcus pneumoniae* and *Staphylococcus pyogenes; Staphylococcus aureus* (penicillinase- and nonpenicillinase-producing); *Staphylococcus epidermidis; Escherichia coli; Klebsiella* species; *Hemophilus influenzae; Enterobacter* species; *Proteus* species; and *Peptostreptococcus* species:

ADULTS: usual dose is 1 g I.V. or I.M. q 6 to 8 hours. Up to 12 g daily can be administered in life-threatening infections.

Total daily dosage is same for I.M. or I.V. administration. In patients with impaired renal function, doses or frequency of administration must be modified according to degree of renal impairment, severity of infection, susceptibility of organism, and blood levels of drug. Should be injected deep I.M. into a large muscle mass, such as gluteus or lateral aspect of thigh.

Blood: transient neutropenia, eosinophilia, hemolytic anemia.
CNS: headache, malaise, paresthesias, dizziness.
GI: nausea, anorexia, vomiting, diarrhea, glossitis, dyspepsia, abdominal cramps, tenesmus, anal pruritus, oral candidiasis (thrush).
GU: nephrotoxicity, genital pruritus and moniliasis.
Skin: *maculopapular and erythematous rashes, urticaria.*
Local: *at injection site–pain, induration, sterile abscesses, temperature elevation, tissue slough; phlebitis and thrombophlebitis with I.V. injection.*
Other: hypersensitivity, dyspnea.

INTERACTIONS AND SPECIAL CONSIDERATIONS

Interactions:
PROBENECID: may increase blood levels of cephalosporins. Use together cautiously.

Special considerations:
- Use cautiously in impaired renal status and in patients with history of sensitivity to penicillin. Consider reaction to previous cephalosporin or penicillin therapy before administering first dose.
- Prolonged use may result in overgrowth of nonsusceptible organisms. Observation for superinfection essential.
- Cultures for sensitivity tests should be obtained before therapy, but therapy may begin pending results of cultures and sensitivity tests.
- In severe renal impairment, doses should not exceed 4 g/day.
- Because of long duration of effect, most infections can be treated with a single dose q 8 hours.
- For I.M. administration, should be reconstituted with sterile water, bacteriostatic water, or 0.9% sodium chloride solution: 2 ml to 250 mg vial; 2 ml to 500 mg vial; 2.5 ml to 1 g vial. Should be shaken well until dissolved. Resultant concentration: 125 mg/ml, 225 mg/ml, 330 mg/ml, respectively.
- Not as painful as other cephalosporins when given I.M.
- Injection sites should be alternated if I.V. therapy lasts longer than 3 days. Use of small I.V. needles in larger available veins preferable.
- For I.V. administration, reconstituted cefazolin sodium is diluted in 50 to 100 ml of 0.9% sodium chloride injection, 5% or 10% dextrose injection, 5% dextrose in lactated Ringer's, 5% dextrose and 0.9% sodium chloride, 5% dextrose and 0.45% or 0.2% sodium chloride, lactated Ringer's injection, Normosol-M in 5% dextrose in water, Ionosol B with 5% dextrose, or Plasma-lyte with 5% dextrose.
- Reconstituted cefazolin sodium is stable for 24 hours at room temperature and for 96 hours under refrigeration.
- About 40% to 75% of patients receiving cephalosporins show a false positive direct Coombs' test, but only a few indicate hemolytic anemia.
- Urine glucose tests with Benedict's Qualitative Reagent, Clinitest, or Fehling's solution may cause false positive reaction during cephalosporin therapy. Clinistix, Diastix, and Tes-Tape are not affected.

Interactions:
PROBENECID: may inhibit excretion and increase blood levels of cefotaxime. Use together cautiously.

Special considerations:
- Contraindicated in hypersensitivity to other cephalosporins. Use cautiously in patients with impaired renal function and in those with history of sensitivity to penicillin. Before first dose patient should report any reaction to previous cephalosporin or penicillin therapy.
- Prolonged use may result in overgrowth of nonsusceptible organisms. Careful observation of patient for superinfection is essential.
- Cultures for sensitivity tests should be obtained before therapy, but therapy may begin pending test results.
- Cefotaxime is the first of the so-called third-generation cephalosporins. It's said to have increased antibacterial activity against gram-negative microorganisms.
- Some doctors may prescribe cefotaxime in clinical situations in which they formerly prescribed aminoglycosides. However, this drug is not effective against infections caused by *Pseudomonas* organisms.
- For I.V. use, drug should be reconstituted with at least 10 ml sterile water for injection. Reconstituted solutions may be further diluted with sterile water for injection; 0.9% sodium chloride; 5% or 10% dextrose and 0.9% sodium chloride; 5% dextrose and 0.45% sodium chloride injection; 5% dextrose and 0.2% sodium chloride injection and lactated Ringer's solution.

NAMES, INDICATIONS AND DOSAGES	SIDE EFFECTS
cefoxitin sodium Mefoxin **Treatment of serious infection of respiratory and genitourinary tracts, skin and soft tissue infections, bone and joint infections, bloodstream and intra-abdominal infections resulting from *Escherichia coli* and other coliform bacteria, *Staphylococcus aureus* (penicillinase- and nonpenicillinase-producing), *Staphylococcus epidermidis*, *streptococci, Klebsiella, Hemophilus influenzae*, and *Bacteroides* species, including *B. fragilis:*** ADULTS: 1 to 2 g q 6 to 8 hours for uncomplicated forms of infection. Up to 12 g/day in life-threatening infections. CHILDREN: 80 to 160 mg/kg/day. Total daily dosage is same for I.M. or I.V. administration and depends on susceptibility of organism and severity of infection. In patients with impaired renal function, doses or frequency of administration must be modified according to degree of renal impairment, severity of infection, susceptibility of organism, and blood levels of drug. Should be injected deep I.M. into a large muscle mass, such as gluteus or lateral aspect of thigh.	**Blood:** transient neutropenia, eosinophilia, hemolytic anemia. **CNS:** headache, malaise, paresthesias, dizziness. **GI:** nausea, anorexia, vomiting, diarrhea, glossitis, dyspepsia, abdominal cramps, tenesmus, anal pruritus, oral candidiasis (thrush). **GU:** nephrotoxicity, genital pruritus and moniliasis. **Skin:** *maculopapular and erythematous rashes, urticaria.* **Local:** *at injection site—pain, induration, sterile abscesses, tissue sloughing; phlebitis and thrombophlebitis with I.V. injection.* **Other:** *hypersensitivity*, dyspnea, elevated temperature.
cephalexin monohydrate Ceporex♦♦, Keflex♦ **Treatment of infections of respiratory or genitourinary tract, skin and soft tissue infections, bone and joint infections, and otitis media due to *Escherichia coli* and other coliform bacteria, group A beta-hemolytic streptococci, *Hemophilus influenzae, Klebsiella, Proteus mirabilis, Streptococcus pneumoniae*, and *staphylococci:*** ADULTS: 250 mg to 1 g P.O. q 6 hours. CHILDREN: 6 to 12 mg/kg P.O. q 6 hours. Maximum 25 mg/kg q 6 hours.	**Blood:** transient neutropenia, eosinophilia, anemia. **CNS:** dizziness, headache, malaise, paresthesias. **GI:** *nausea, anorexia,* vomiting, *diarrhea,* glossitis, dyspepsia, abdominal cramps, anal pruritus, tenesmus, oral candidiasis (thrush). **GU:** genital pruritus and moniliasis, vaginitis. **Skin:** *maculopapular and erythematous rashes, urticaria.* **Other:** *hypersensitivity*, dyspnea.
cephaloglycin dihydrate Kafocin **Treatment of acute and chronic urinary tract infections, including cystitis, pyelitis, pyelonephritis, and asymptomatic bacteriuria when due to susceptible strains of *Escherichia coli, Klebsiella, Enterobacter, Proteus, staphylococci*, and *enterococci:*** ADULTS: 250 to 500 mg P.O. q 6 hours.	**Blood:** transient neutropenia, eosinophilia, anemia. **CNS:** dizziness, headache, malaise, paresthesias. **GI:** *nausea, anorexia, vomiting, diarrhea,* glossitis, dyspepsia, abdominal cramps, anal pruritus, tenesmus, oral candidiasis (thrush). **GU:** genital pruritus and moniliasis, vaginitis. **Skin:** *maculopapular and erythematous rashes, urticaria.* **Other:** *hypersensitivity*, dyspnea.

♦ Available in U.S. and Canada. ♦♦ Available in Canada only.
All other products (no symbol) available in U.S. only. Italicized side effects are common or life-threatening.

INTERACTIONS AND SPECIAL CONSIDERATIONS

Interactions:
PROBENECID: may inhibit excretion and increase blood levels of cefoxitin. Use together cautiously.

Special considerations:
- Contraindicated in hypersensitivity to other cephalosporins. Use cautiously in impaired renal status and in patients with history of sensitivity to penicillin. Consider reaction to previous cephalosporin or penicillin therapy before administering first dose.
- Prolonged use may result in overgrowth of nonsusceptible organisms. Superinfection is possible.
- Cultures for sensitivity tests should be obtained before therapy, but therapy may begin pending results of cultures and sensitivity tests.
- A very useful cephalosporin when anaerobic or mixed aerobic-anaerobic infection is suspected, especially *Bacteroides fragilis*.
- For most cephalosporin-sensitive organisms, cefoxitin offers little advantage over previously available agents.
- For I.V. use, 1 g should be reconstituted with at least 10 ml of sterile water for injection, and 2 g with 10 to 20 ml. Solutions of 5% dextrose and 0.9% sodium chloride for injection can also be used. These primary solutions can be further diluted with the following solutions: Ringer's injection, lactated Ringer's injection, 5% dextrose in lactated Ringer's injection, 5% or 10% invert sugar in water, 10% invert sugar in saline, 5% sodium bicarbonate injection, Aminosol 5% solution, Normosol-M in 5% dextrose in water, Ionosol B with 5% dextrose, Polyonic M 56 in 5% dextrose.
- I.M. injection can be reconstituted with 0.5% or 1% lidocaine HCl (without epinephrine) to minimize pain on injection.
- May cause false positive for urine glucose with Clinitest tablets.
- May be useful in the treatment of resistant gonorrhea.
- After reconstitution, remains stable for 24 hours at room temperature or 1 week under refrigeration.

Interactions:
PROBENECID: may increase blood levels of cephalosporins. Use together cautiously.

Special considerations:
- Use cautiously in impaired renal status and in patients with history of sensitivity to penicillin. Consider any reaction to previous cephalosporin or penicillin therapy before administering first dose.
- Prolonged use may result in overgrowth of nonsusceptible organisms. Careful observation for superinfection essential.
- Cultures for sensitivity tests should be obtained before therapy, but therapy may begin pending results of cultures and sensitivity tests.
- Patient should take medication for as long as ordered, even after he feels better. Group A beta-hemolytic streptococci infections should be treated for a minimum of 10 days.
- Patient should notify doctor if skin rash develops.
- Preparation of oral suspension: add required amount of water to powder in two portions. Shake well after each addition. After mixing, store in refrigerator. Stable for 14 days without significant loss of potency. Keep tightly closed and shake well before using.
- About 40% to 75% of patients receiving cephalosporins show a false positive direct Coombs' test, but only a few of these indicate hemolytic anemia.
- Urine glucose tests with Benedict's Qualitative Reagent, Clinitest, or Fehling's solution may give false positive during cephalosporin therapy. Clinistix, Diastix, Tes-Tape not affected.

Interactions:
PROBENECID: may increase blood levels of cephalosporins. Use together cautiously.

Special considerations:
- Use cautiously in impaired renal function and sensitivity to penicillin. Consider reaction to cephalosporin or penicillin therapy before first dose.
- Cephaloglycin blood levels are low; used only for urinary tract infections.
- Prolonged use may result in overgrowth of nonsusceptible organisms. Careful observation for superinfection essential.
- Cultures for sensitivity tests should be obtained before beginning therapy, but therapy may begin pending test results.
- Patient should take medication as prescribed, even after he feels better.
- About 40% to 75% of patients receiving cephalosporins show a false positive direct Coombs' test, but only a few of these indicate hemolytic anemia.
- Urine glucose tests with Benedict's Qualitative Reagent, Clinitest, or Fehling's solution may give false positive during cephalosporin therapy. Clinistix, Diastix, Tes-Tape not affected.

NAMES, INDICATIONS AND DOSAGES	SIDE EFFECTS

cephaloridine

Ceporan♦♦, Loridine♦

Treatment of serious infections of respiratory tract, central nervous system, genitourinary tract, bones and joints, bloodstream, skin, and soft tissue due to *Escherichia coli* and other coliform bacteria, gonococci, *Hemophilus influenzae, Klebsiella, Proteus mirabilis, pneumococci, staphylococci* (coagulase-positive and coagulase-negative), beta-hemolytic and other streptococci; also, gonorrhea and early syphilis when penicillin is contraindicated:

ADULTS: 250 mg to 1 g I.M. or I.V. q 6 to 12 hours. Not to exceed 4 g daily.

CHILDREN: 7 to 12 mg/kg I.M. or I.V. q 6 hours.

Severe infections: up to 25 mg/kg q 6 hours. Not recommended for children under 1 month or for premature infants.

Total daily dosage is same for I.M. or I.V. administration and depends on susceptibility of organism and severity of infection. Initial loading dose (usually 500 mg) recommended. In patients with impaired renal function, doses and frequency of administration must be modified according to degree of renal impairment, severity of infection, susceptibility of causative organism, and blood levels of drug. Inject deep I.M. into large muscle mass, such as gluteus or lateral aspect of thigh. I.V. is preferable in severe or life-threatening infections.

Blood: transient neutropenia, eosinophilia, anemia.
CNS: headache, malaise, paresthesias.
GI: nausea, anorexia, vomiting, diarrhea, glossitis, dyspepsia, abdominal cramps, tenesmus, anal pruritus, oral candidiasis (thrush).
GU: *nephrotoxicity (especially in doses greater than 4 g daily or in patients with renal impairment),* genital pruritus and moniliasis.
Skin: *maculopapular and erythematous rashes, urticaria.*
Local: at injection site—pain, induration, sterile abscesses, tissue sloughing; phlebitis and thrombophlebitis with I.V. injection.
Other: *hypersensitivity,* dyspnea.

cephalothin sodium

Keflin Neutral♦

Treatment of serious infections of respiratory, genitourinary, or gastrointestinal tract; skin and soft tissue infections (including peritonitis); bone and joint infections; septicemia; endocarditis; and meningitis due to *Escherichia coli* and other coliform bacteria, Enterobacteriaceae, enterococci, gonococci, group A beta-hemolytic streptococci, *Hemophilus influenzae, Klebsiella, Proteus mirabilis, Salmonella, Staphylococcus aureus, Shigella, Streptococcus pneumoniae,* staphylococci, and *Streptococcus viridans:*

ADULTS: 500 mg to 1 g I.M. or I.V. (or intraperitoneally) q 4 to 6 hours; in life-threatening infections, up to 2 g q 4 hours.

CHILDREN: 14 to 27 mg/kg I.V. q 4 hours, or 20 to 40 mg/kg q 6 hours; dose should be proportionately less in accordance with age, weight, and severity of infection.

Dosage schedule determined by degree of renal impairment, severity of infection, and susceptibility of organism. Should be injected deep I.M. into large muscle mass, such as gluteus or lateral aspect of thigh. I.V. route preferable in severe or life-threatening infections.

Blood: transient neutropenia, eosinophilia, hemolytic anemia.
CNS: headache, malaise, paresthesias, dizziness.
GI: nausea, anorexia, vomiting, diarrhea, glossitis, dyspepsia, abdominal cramps, tenesmus, anal pruritus, oral candidiasis (thrush).
GU: nephrotoxicity, genital pruritus and moniliasis.
Skin: maculopapular and erythematous rashes, urticaria.
Local: *at injection site—pain, induration, sterile abscesses, tissue sloughing; phlebitis and thrombophlebitis with I.V. injection.*
Other: *hypersensitivity,* dyspnea, temperature elevation.

INTERACTIONS AND SPECIAL CONSIDERATIONS

Interactions:
PROBENECID: may increase blood levels of cephalosporins. Use together cautiously.
ETHACRYNIC ACID, FUROSEMIDE: may enhance nephrotoxicity of cephaloridine. Use cautiously.

Special considerations:
• Contraindicated in renal impairment, since drug causes a relatively high incidence of dose-related nephrotoxicity. Use cautiously in patient with history of sensitivity to penicillin. Consider any reaction to previous cephalosporin or penicillin therapy before administering first dose. Safe use not established in patients with proteinuria, falling urinary output, rising BUN or serum creatinine, decreasing creatinine clearance, and those receiving other antibiotics with nephrotoxic potential.
• Prolonged use may result in overgrowth of nonsusceptible organisms. Careful observation for superinfection essential.
• Cultures for sensitivity tests should be obtained before beginning therapy, but therapy may begin pending results of cultures and sensitivity tests.
• Drug causes relatively little pain when given I.M.
• Good CNS penetration makes cephaloridine useful in treating meningitis.
• When this drug given I.V., patient should be checked frequently for vein irritation and phlebitis, and injection sites alternated if I.V. therapy lasts longer than 3 days. Use of small I.V. needles in the larger available veins may be preferable.
• Excreted in urine. Renal function should be monitored for signs of impairment: casts in urine, proteinuria, decreased creatinine clearance of urine/plasma creatinine ratio. Doses greater than 4 g daily should be avoided.
• About 40% to 75% of patients receiving cephalosporins show a false-positive direct Coombs' test, but only a few indicate hemolytic anemia.
• Urine glucose tests with Benedict's Qualitative Reagent, Clinitest, or Fehling's solution may give false-positive results during cephalosporin therapy. Clinistix, Diastix, and Tes-Tape are not affected.

Interactions:
PROBENECID: may increase blood levels of cephalosporins. Use together cautiously.

Special considerations:
• Use cautiously in impaired renal function and in patients with history of sensitivity to penicillin. Consider any reaction to previous cephalosporin or penicillin therapy before administering first dose.
• Cultures for sensitivity tests should be obtained before beginning therapy, but therapy may begin pending test results.
• Prolonged use may result in overgrowth of nonsusceptible organisms. Careful observation for superinfection essential.
• This drug causes severe pain when given I.M.; avoid this route if possible.
• When this drug given I.V., patient should be checked frequently for vein irritation and phlebitis and injection sites alternated if I.V. therapy lasts longer than 3 days. Use of small I.V. needles in the larger available veins may be preferable. Addition of a small concentration of heparin (100 units) may reduce incidence of phlebitis.
• For I.M. administration, each gram of cephalothin sodium should be reconstituted with 4 ml of sterile water for injection, providing 500 mg in each 2.2 ml. If vial contents do not dissolve completely, an additional 0.2 to 0.4 ml diluent may be added and contents warmed slightly.
• For I.V. administration, contents of 4 g vial should be diluted with at least 20 ml of sterile water for injection, 5% dextrose injection, or 0.9% sodium chloride injection and added to one of following I.V. solutions: acetated Ringer's injection; 5% dextrose injection; 5% dextrose in lactated Ringer's injection; Ionosol B in 5% dextrose in water; lactated Ringer's injection; Normosol-N in 5% dextrose in water; Plasma-Lyte injection; Plasma-Lyte-N injection in 5% dextrose; Ringer's injection or 0.9% sodium chloride injection. Solution and fluid volume should be chosen according to patient's fluid and electrolyte status.
• About 40% to 75% of patients receiving cephalosporins show a false-positive direct Coombs' test, but only a few of these indicate hemolytic anemia.
• Urine glucose tests with Benedict's Qualitative Reagent, Clinitest, or Fehling's solution may give false-positive during cephalosporin therapy. Clinistix, Diastix, and Tes-Tape are not affected.

NAMES, INDICATIONS AND DOSAGES	SIDE EFFECTS

cephapirin sodium

Cefadyl♦

Serious infections of respiratory, genitourinary, or gastrointestinal tract; skin and soft tissue infections; bone and joint infections (including osteomyelitis); septicemia; endocarditis due to *Streptococcus pneumoniae, Escherichia coli,* group A beta-hemolytic streptococci, *Hemophilus influenzae, Klebsiella, Proteus mirabilis, Staphylococcus aureus,* and *Streptococcus viridans:*

ADULTS: 500 mg to 1 g I.V. or I.M. q 4 to 6 hours up to 12 g daily.

CHILDREN OVER 3 MONTHS: 10 to 20 mg/kg I.V. or I.M. q 6 hours; dose depends on age, weight, and severity of infection.

Should be injected deep I.M. into a large muscle mass, such as gluteus or lateral aspect of thigh. Depending upon causative organism and severity of infection, patients with reduced renal function may be treated adequately with a lower dose (7.5 to 15 mg/kg q 12 hours). Patients with severely reduced renal function and who are to be dialyzed should receive same dose just before dialysis and q 12 hours thereafter.

Blood: transient neutropenia, eosinophilia, anemia.
CNS: dizziness, headache, malaise, paresthesias.
GI: nausea, anorexia, vomiting, diarrhea, glossitis, dyspepsia, abdominal cramps, tenesmus, anal pruritus, oral candidiasis (thrush).
GU: nephrotoxicity, genital pruritus and moniliasis, vaginitis.
Skin: *maculopapular and erythematous rashes, urticaria.*
Local: *at injection site—pain, induration, sterile abscesses, tissue sloughing; phlebitis and thrombophlebitis with I.V. injection.*
Other: *hypersensitivity,* dyspnea.

cephradine

Anspor, Velosef♦

Serious infection of respiratory, genitourinary, or gastrointestinal tract; skin and soft tissue infections; bone and joint infections; septicemia; endocarditis; and otitis media due to *Escherichia coli* and other coliform bacteria, group A beta-hemolytic streptococci, *Hemophilus influenzae, Klebsiella, Proteus mirabilis, Staphylococcus aureus, Streptococcus pneumoniae,* staphylococci, and *Streptococcus viridans:*

ADULTS: 500 mg to 1 g I.M. or I.V. 2 to 4 times daily; do not exceed 8 g daily. Or 250 to 500 mg P.O. q 6 hours. Severe or chronic infections may require larger and/or more frequent doses (up to 1 g P.O. q 6 hours).

CHILDREN OVER 1 YEAR: 6 to 12 mg/kg P.O. q 6 hours. 12 to 25 mg/kg I.M. or I.V. q 6 hours.

Otitis media—19 to 25 mg/kg P.O. q 6 hours. Do not exceed 4 g daily.

All patients, regardless of age and weight: larger doses (up to 1 g q.i.d.) may be given for severe or chronic infections. Parenteral therapy may be followed by oral. Injections should be given deep I.M. into a large muscle mass, such as gluteus or lateral aspect of thigh.

Blood: transient neutropenia, eosinophilia.
CNS: dizziness, headache, malaise, paresthesias.
GI: *nausea, anorexia,* vomiting, heartburn, glossitis, dyspepsia, abdominal cramping, *diarrhea,* tenesmus, anal pruritus, oral candidiasis (thrush).
GU: genital pruritus and moniliasis, vaginitis.
Skin: *maculopapular and erythematous rashes, urticaria.*
Local: *at injection site—pain, induration, sterile abscesses, tissue sloughing; phlebitis and thrombophlebitis with I.V. injection.*
Other: *hypersensitivity,* dyspnea.

INTERACTIONS AND SPECIAL CONSIDERATIONS

Interactions:
PROBENECID: may increase blood levels of cephalosporins. Use together cautiously.

Special considerations:
• Use cautiously in impaired renal function and in patients with a history of sensitivity to penicillin. Consider any reaction to previous cephalosporin or penicillin therapy before administering first dose.
• Prolonged use may result in overgrowth of nonsusceptible organisms. Superinfection is possible.
• Cultures for sensitivity tests should be obtained before beginning therapy, but therapy may begin pending results of cultures and sensitivity tests.
• I.M. injection may be painful.
• For I.M. administration, 1 g vial should be reconstituted with 2 ml sterile water for injection or bacteriostatic water for injection so that 1.2 ml contains 500 mg of cephapirin.
• With I.V. administration, patient should be checked frequently for vein irritation and phlebitis and injection sites alternated if I.V. therapy lasts over 3 days. Use of small I.V. needles in larger veins may be preferable.
• I.V. infusion should be prepared using dextrose injection, sodium chloride injection, or bacteriostatic water for injection, as diluent: 20 ml yields 1 g/10 ml; 50 ml yields 1 g/25 ml; 100 ml yields 1 g/50 ml.
• I.V. infusion with Y-tube: during infusion of cephapirin solution, it is desirable to stop other solution. Volume of cephapirin solution should be checked carefully so that calculated dose is infused. When Y-tube is used, 4 g vial should be diluted with 40 ml of diluent.
• Compatible with following infusion solutions: sodium chloride injection; 5% dextrose in water; sodium lactate injection; 5% dextrose in normal saline; 10% invert sugar in normal saline; 10% invert sugar in water; 5% dextrose and 0.2% sodium chloride injection; lactated Ringer's with 5% dextrose; 5% dextrose and 0.45% sodium chloride injection; Ringer's injection; lactated Ringer's; 10% dextrose injection; sterile water for injection; 20% dextrose injection; 5% sodium chloride in water; and 5% dextrose in Ringer's injection.
• Reconstituted cephapirin is stable and compatible for 10 days under refrigeration and for 24 hours at room temperature.
• About 40% to 75% of patients receiving cephalosporins show a false positive direct Coombs' test, but only a few indicate hemolytic anemia.
• Urine glucose tests with Benedict's Qualitative Reagent, Clinitest, or Fehling's solution may give false positive during cephalosporin therapy. Clinistix, Diastix, and Tes-Tape are not affected.

Interactions:
PROBENECID: may increase blood levels of cephalosporins. Use together cautiously.

Special considerations:
• Use cautiously in impaired renal function and in patients with a history of sensitivity to penicillin. Consider any reaction to previous cephalosporin or penicillin therapy before administering first dose.
• Cultures for sensitivity tests should be obtained before beginning therapy, but therapy may begin pending results of cultures and sensitivity tests.
• Prolonged use may result in overgrowth of nonsusceptible organisms. Superinfection is possible.
• When this drug given I.V., patient should be checked frequently for vein irritation and phlebitis, and injection sites alternated if I.V. therapy lasts over 3 days. Use of small I.V. needles in larger veins may be preferable.
• Patient should take medication for as long as ordered, even after he feels well. Group A beta-hemolytic streptococci infections should be treated for a minimum of 10 days.
• I.M. injection painful.
• For I.M. administration, should be reconstituted with sterile water for injection or with bacteriostatic water for injection: 1.2 ml to 250 mg vial; 2 ml to 500 mg vial; 4 ml to 1 g vial. I.M. solutions must be used within 2 hours stored at room temperature; within 24 hours, refrigerated. Solutions vary from light straw to yellow without affecting potency. When preparing cephradine for intravenous administration, when available, preparation specifically supplied for infusion should be used. When reconstituting, specific product directions should be followed.
• About 40% to 75% of patients receiving cephalosporins show a false positive direct Coombs' test, but only a few indicate hemolytic anemia.
• Urine glucose tests with Benedict's Qualitative Reagent, Clinitest, or Fehling's solution may give false positive during cephalosporin therapy. Clinistix, Diastix, and Tes-Tape are not affected.

NAMES, INDICATIONS AND DOSAGES

moxalactam disodium
Moxam

Treatment of serious infections of lower respiratory and urinary tracts, gynecologic infections, bacteremia, septicemia, and skin infections.
Susceptible microorganisms include *Streptococcus pneumoniae* and *Staphylococcus pyogenes; Staphylococcus aureus* (penicillinase- and nonpenicillinase-producing); *Staphylococcus epidermidis; Escherichia coli; Klebsiella; Hemophilus influenzae; Enterobacter; Proteus;* some *Pseudomonas* species; and *Peptostreptococcus*

ADULTS: Usual daily dose is 2 to 6 g I.M. or I.V. administered in divided doses q 8 h for 5 to 10 days, or up to 14 days. Up to 12 g/day may be needed in life-threatening infections or in-infections due to less susceptible organisms.

CHILDREN: 50 mg/kg I.M. or I.V. q 6 to 8 hours.

NEONATES: 50 mg/kg I.M. or I.V. q 8 to 12 hours.

Total daily dosage is same for temperature. I.M. or I.V. administration and depends on susceptibility of organism and severity of infection. In patients with impaired renal function, doses or frequency of administration must be modified according to degree of impairment, severity of infection, susceptibility of organism, and blood levels of drug. Should be injected deep I.M. into a large muscle mass, such as gluteus or lateral aspect of thigh.

SIDE EFFECTS

Blood: transient neutropenia, eosinophili, hemolytic anemia.
CNS: headache, malaise, paresthesias, dizziness.
GI: nausea, anorexia, vomiting, diarrhea, glossitis, dyspepsia, abdominal cramps, tenesmus, pruritus ani, oral candidiasis (thrush).
GU: nephrotoxicity, genital pruritus, moniliasis.
Skin: *maculopapular and erythematous rashes, urticaria.*
Local: *pain at injection site, induration, sterile abscesses, tissue sloughing; phlebitis and thrombophlebitis with I.V. injection.*
Other: *hypersensitivity,* dyspnea, elevated temperature.

INTERACTIONS AND SPECIAL CONSIDERATIONS

Interactions:

ETHYL ALCOHOL: may cause a disulfiram-like reaction. Warn patients not to drink alcohol for several days after discontinuing moxalactam.

PROBENECID: may inhibit excretion and increase blood levels of moxalactam. Use together cautiously.

Special considerations:

- Contraindicated in hypersensitivity to other cephalosporins. Use cautiously in patients with impaired renal function and in those with history of sensitivity to penicillin. Before first dose, patient should report any reaction to previous cephalosporin or penicillin therapy.
- Prolonged use may result in overgrowth of nonsusceptible organisms. Careful observation of patient for superinfection is essential.
- Cultures for sensitivity tests should be obtained before therapy. Unnecessary to wait for test results before starting therapy.
- Moxalactam is one of the third generation cephalosporins. It's said to have increased antibacterial activity against gram-negative organisms.
- Some doctors may prescribe moxalactam in clinical situations in which they formerly prescribed aminoglycosides. However, the drug is not as potent against *Pseudomonas* infections.
- For direct intermittent I.V. administration: add 10 ml of sterile water for injection, 5% dextrose injection, or 0.990 NaCl injection/g of moxalactam.

DRUG ALERT

WATCH FOR CEPHALOSPORIN AND PENICILLIN CROSS-SENSITIVITY

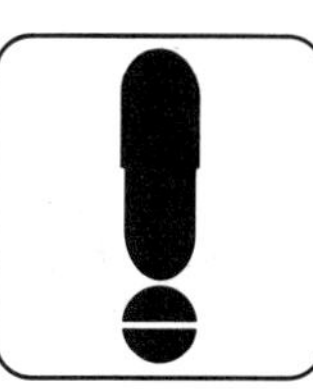

Before a cephalosporin is administered, the patient should be asked whether he's allergic to penicillin. Allergic reactions to cephalosporins are about five times more common in patients with a history of penicillin allergy than in other patients.

Why? Cephalosporins and penicillins are similar in structure. This may explain why cephalosporins are capable of forming an antigenic complex resembling the one formed by penicillin.

Cephalosporins shouldn't be administered to a patient who has recently experienced a severe, immediate reaction to penicillin. And when a cephalosporin is administered, all the necessary supplies to deal with an adverse reaction immediately should be on hand.

15

Tetracyclines

demeclocycline hydrochloride
doxycycline hyclate
methacycline hydrochloride
minocycline hydrochloride
oxytetracycline hydrochloride
tetracycline hydrochloride
tetracycline phosphate complex

The tetracyclines are bacteriostatic antibiotics with broad activity against gram-positive and gram-negative bacteria, *Mycoplasma, Chlamydia,* and *Rickettsia*. Since chlortetracycline was first isolated in 1948, the pharmacologic and microbiologic effects of tetracyclines have been modified. However, because of widespread microbial resistance (*Proteus* and *Pseudomonas* infection, for example), the tetracyclines are the drugs of choice in only a few clinical situations.

Major uses
The tetracyclines are used in prophylaxis and therapy of numerous bacterial diseases, especially of the mixed type, such as chronic bronchitis and peritonitis. They're drugs of choice in treatment of bubonic plague, brucellosis, cholera, mycoplasmosis, trachoma, lymphogranuloma venereum, and Rocky Mountain spotted fever.

They're alternative therapeutic agents for syphilis, gonorrhea, anthrax, nocardiosis, and *Hemophilus influenzae* respiratory infections. They're effective against uncomplicated urinary tract infections from susceptible strains of *Escherichia coli, Klebsiella, Enterobacter,* and *Citrobacter* and in exacerbations of chronic bronchitis.

- Tetracyclines may also be useful as single-dose therapy for shigellosis.
- Oral or topical tetracyclines are therapeutic against acne vulgaris.
- Minocycline is prophylactic in meningococcal infections when rifampin is contraindicated.
- Demeclocycline is a useful adjunct for treating syndrome of inappropriate antidiuretic hormone (SIADH).

Mechanism of action
Tetracyclines are thought to exert bacteriostatic effect by binding to the 30S ribosomal subunit of microorganisms, thus inhibiting protein synthesis.

Absorption, distribution, metabolism, and excretion
- Tetracyclines are readily absorbed after oral administration—some better than others.
- I.M. administration produces lower blood levels than oral administration. Local anesthetic agents are added to I.M. preparations; be sure patient has no hypersensitivity to these agents before administering.
- I.V. administration may produce rapid, high blood levels. Be sure to dilute the dose and give it slowly: phlebitis of the injected vein is common. Avoid extravasation.
- Tetracyclines are widely distributed in most body fluids, including bile, sinus secretions, and synovial, pleural, and ascitic fluids. Cerebrospinal fluid levels vary, but the drugs tend to diffuse well when the meninges are inflamed; the drugs accumulate in bones, liver, spleen, and teeth.
- Doxycycline and minocycline partly metabolized by the liver; elimination routes unclear. Other tetracyclines eliminated unchanged in feces (through bile) and urine.

Onset and duration

• Blood levels after oral administration peak in 2 to 4 hours.
• Blood levels of 1 to 3 mcg/ml persist for 6 or more hours. (Doxycycline and minocycline give the most prolonged blood levels.)
• Peak levels occur 1 hour after I.M. administration; drug is detectable in the blood for as long as 12 hours.
• Half-lives—hence blood levels—of all tetracyclines except doxycycline are prolonged in patients with severe renal impairment.

Combination products

MYSTECLIN-F CAPS: tetracycline HCl 125 mg and amphotericin B 25 mg buffered with potassium metaphosphate.
MYSTECLIN-F CAPS: tetracycline HCl 250 mg and amphotericin B 50 mg buffered with potassium metaphosphate.
MYSTECLIN-F SYRUP: tetracycline HCl 125 mg and amphotericin B 25 mg/5 ml, buffered with potassium metaphosphate.
For more combinations, see Chapter 17.

HALF-LIFE AND ABSORPTION OF TETRACYCLINES

DRUG	HALF-LIFE Normal Kidneys	HALF-LIFE Severe Renal Failure	% ABSORBED*
demeclocycline	15 hr	50 hr	66
doxycycline	15 hr†	15 hr†	93
methacycline	12 hr	44 hr	80
minocycline	19 hr	24 hr	100
oxytetracycline	9 hr	55 hr	58
tetracycline	10 hr	75 hr	77

*On an empty stomach. The administration of tetracyclines with food, iron, calcium, phosphates, or antacids significantly impairs absorption.

†The elimination route for this drug is unclear, but independent of the kidneys.

Note: Since tetracyclines accumulate in the teeth and bones, avoid using them in children younger than 8 years.

NAMES, INDICATIONS AND DOSAGES	SIDE EFFECTS
demeclocycline hydrochloride Declomycin♦, Ledermycin **Infections caused by susceptible gram-negative and gram-positive organisms, trachoma, amebiasis:** ADULTS: 150 mg P.O. q 6 hours or 300 mg P.O. q 12 hours. CHILDREN OVER 8 YEARS: 6 to 12 mg/kg P.O. daily, divided q 6 to 12 hours. **Gonorrhea:** ADULTS: 600 mg P.O. initially, then 300 mg P.O. q 12 hours for 4 days (total 3 g). **Syndrome of inappropriate ADH (hyposmolarity):** ADULTS: 600 to 1200 mg P.O. daily in divided doses.	**Blood:** neutropenia, eosinophilia. **CV:** pericarditis. **EENT:** dysphagia, glossitis. **GI:** anorexia, *nausea, vomiting, diarrhea,* enterocolitis, anogenital inflammation. **Metabolic:** *increased BUN,* diabetes insipidus syndrome (polyuria, polydipsia, weakness). **Skin:** *maculopapular and erythematous rashes, photosensitivity, increased pigmentation, urticaria.* **Other:** hypersensitivity.
doxycycline hyclate Doxychel, Vibramycin♦, Vibra Tabs **Infections caused by sensitive gram-negative and gram-positive organisms, trachoma, amebiasis:** ADULTS: 100 mg P.O. q 12 hours on first day, then 100 mg P.O. daily; or 200 mg I.V. on first day in 1 or 2 infusions, then 100 to 200 mg I.V. daily. CHILDREN OVER 8 YEARS (UNDER 45 KG): 4.4 mg/kg P.O. or I.V. daily, divided q 12 hours first day, then 2.2 to 4.4 mg/kg daily. Over 45 kg, same as adults. Give I.V. infusion slowly (minimum time 1 hour). Infusion must be completed within 12 hours (within 6 hours in lactated Ringer's solution or 5% dextrose in lactated Ringer's solution). **Gonorrhea in patients allergic to penicillin:** ADULTS: 200 mg P.O. initially, followed by 100 mg P.O. at bedtime, and 100 mg P.O. b.i.d. for 3 days; or 300 mg P.O. initially and repeat dose in 1 hour. **Primary or secondary syphilis in patients allergic to penicillin:** ADULTS: 300 mg P.O. daily in divided doses for 10 days.	**Blood:** neutropenia, eosinophilia. **CNS:** benign intracranial hypertension. **CV:** pericarditis. **EENT:** sore throat, glossitis, dysphagia. **GI:** anorexia, *epigastric distress, nausea,* vomiting, *diarrhea,* enterocolitis, anogenital inflammation. **Skin:** *maculopapular and erythematous rashes, photosensitivity, increased pigmentation, urticaria.* **Local:** thrombophlebitis. **Other:** hypersensitivity.
methacycline hydrochloride Rondomycin **Infections caused by sensitive gram-negative**	**Blood:** neutropenia, eosinophilia. **CV:** pericarditis. **EENT:** dysphagia, glossitis. **GI:** anorexia, *epigastric distress, nausea,* vom-

♦ Available in U.S. and Canada. ♦♦ Available in Canada only.
All other products (no symbol) available in U.S. only. Italicized side effects are common or life-threatening.

INTERACTIONS AND SPECIAL CONSIDERATIONS

Interactions:

ANTACIDS (INCLUDING $NaHCO_3$) AND LAXATIVES CONTAINING ALUMINUM, CALCIUM, AND MAGNESIUM; FOOD, MILK, OR OTHER DAIRY PRODUCTS: decrease antibiotic absorption. Give antibiotic 1 hour before or 2 hours after any of the above.

FERROUS SULFATE AND OTHER IRON PRODUCTS, ZINC: decrease antibiotic absorption. Give demeclocycline 3 hours after or 2 hours before iron administration.

METHOXYFLURANE: may cause nephrotoxicity with tetracyclines. Monitor carefully.

Special considerations:

- Use with extreme caution in patients with impaired renal or hepatic function. Use of these drugs during last half of pregnancy and in children younger than 8 years may cause permanent discoloration of teeth, enamel defects, and retardation of bone growth.
- Cultures should be obtained before starting therapy.
- Check expiration date. Outdated or deteriorated demeclocycline may cause nephrotoxicity.
- Do not expose these drugs to light or heat; store in tight container.
- Overgrowth of nonsusceptible organisms, such as monilia, is possible, especially on the tongue. Good oral hygiene may minimize superinfection. If superinfection occurs, drug should be discontinued.
- Observe for diarrhea, which may result from local irritation or superinfection.
- May cause false-positive reading of Clinitest; false-negative reading of Clinistix or Tes-Tape.
- Patient should avoid direct sunlight and ultraviolet light. A sunscreen may help prevent photosensitivity reaction. Photosensitivity persists for some time after discontinuation of drug.
- Effectiveness is reduced when taken with milk or other dairy products, food, antacids, or iron products. Patient should take each dose with a full glass of water on an empty stomach, at least 1 hour before meals or 2 hours afterward. Should be taken at least 1 hour before bedtime to prevent esophagitis.
- Patient should take medication for as long as prescribed, exactly as prescribed, even after he feels better. Streptococcal infections should be treated for at least 10 days.
- For symptoms and treatment of anaphylaxis, see APPENDIX.

Interactions:

ANTACIDS (INCLUDING $NaHCO_3$) AND LAXATIVES CONTAINING ALUMINUM, MAGNESIUM, OR CALCIUM: decrease antibiotic absorption. Give antibiotic 1 hour before or 2 hours after any of the above.

FERROUS SULFATE AND OTHER IRON PRODUCTS, ZINC: decrease antibiotic absorption. Give doxycycline 3 hours after or 2 hours before iron administration.

PHENOBARBITAL, CARBAMAZEPINE, ALCOHOL: decrease antibiotic effect. Avoid if possible.

Special considerations:

- Use of these drugs during last half of pregnancy and in children younger than 8 years may cause permanent discoloration of teeth, enamel defects, and retardation of bone growth.
- Patient may develop thrombophlebitis with I.V. administration.
- Cultures should be obtained before starting therapy.
- Check expiration date.
- Don't expose to light or heat. Protect from sunlight during infusion.
- Overgrowth of nonsusceptible organisms, such as monilia, is possible, especially on the tongue. Good oral hygiene may minimize superinfection. If superinfection occurs, drug should be discontinued.
- Observe for diarrhea, which may result from local irritation or superinfection.
- May be taken with milk or food if GI side effects develop.
- Should not be taken with antacids.
- Patient should take medication exactly as prescribed, even after he feels better. Streptococcal infections should be treated for at least 10 days.
- Reconstitute powder for injection with sterile water for injection. Use 10 ml for 100-mg vial and 20 ml in 200-mg vial. Dilute solution to 100 to 1,000 ml before giving. Maximum concentration for infusion, 1 mg/ml.
- Reconstituted solution is stable for 72 hours refrigerated.
- Doxycycline may be used in patients with renal impairment; does not accumulate in or cause a significant rise in BUN.
- May cause false-positive reading of Clinitest; false-negative reading of Clinistix or Tes-Tape.
- Should not be taken within 1 hour of bedtime because of increased incidence of dysphagia.
- For symptoms and treatment of anaphylaxis, see APPENDIX.

Interactions:

ANTACIDS (INCLUDING $NaHCO_3$) AND LAXATIVES CONTAINING ALUMINUM, MAGNESIUM, OR CALCIUM; FOOD, MILK, OR OTHER DAIRY PRODUCTS: decrease antibiotic absorption. Give antibiotic 1 hour before or 2 hours after any of the above.

FERROUS SULFATE AND OTHER IRON PROD-

(continued on following page)

NAMES, INDICATIONS AND DOSAGES | SIDE EFFECTS

methacycline hydrochloride

(continued)

and gram-positive organisms, trachoma, amebiasis:

ADULTS: 150 mg P.O. q 6 hours or 300 mg q 12 hours.

CHILDREN OVER 8 YEARS: 6 to 12 mg/kg P.O. daily, divided q 6 hours to q 12 hours.

Gonorrhea in patients sensitive to penicillin:

ADULTS: 900 mg P.O. initially, then 300 mg P.O. q.i.d. for total of 5.4 g.

Syphilis in patients sensitive to penicillin:

ADULTS: total dose of 18 to 24 g in equally divided doses over 10 to 15 days.

iting, *diarrhea*, enterocolitis, anogenital inflammation.

Metabolic: increased BUN.

Skin: *maculopapular and erythematous rashes, photosensitivity, urticaria.*

Other: hypersensitivity.

minocycline hydrochloride

Minocin♦, Ultramycin♦♦

Infections caused by sensitive gram-negative and gram-positive organisms, trachoma, amebiasis:

ADULTS: initially, 200 mg P.O., I.V.; then 100 mg q 12 hours or 50 mg P.O. q 6 hours.

CHILDREN OVER 8 YEARS: initially, 4 mg/kg P.O., I.V.; then 4 mg/kg P.O. daily, divided q 12 hours. Give I.V. in 500 to 1,000 ml solution without calcium, over 6 hours.

Gonorrhea in patients sensitive to penicillin:

ADULTS: initially, 200 mg, then 100 mg q 12 hours for 4 days.

Syphilis in patients sensitive to penicillin:

ADULTS: initially, 200 mg, then 100 mg q 12 hours for 10 to 15 days.

Meningococcal carrier state:

100 mg P.O. q 12 hours for 5 days.

Blood: neutropenia, eosinophilia.

CNS: *light-headedness, dizziness from vestibular otxicity.*

CV: pericarditis.

EENT: dysphagia, glossitis.

GI: *anorexia*, epigastric distress, *nausea*, vomiting, *diarrhea*, enterocolitis, inflammatory lesions in anogenital region.

Metabolic: increased BUN.

Skin: *maculopapular and erythematous rashes, photosensitivity, increased pigmentation, urticaria.*

Local: *thrombophlebitis.*

Other: hypersensitivity.

oxytetracycline hydrochloride

Dalimycin, Oxlopar, Oxy-Kesso-Tetra, Oxytetraclor, Terramycin♦, Uri-tet

Infections caused by sensitive gram-negative and gram-positive organisms, trachoma, amebiasis:

ADULTS: 250 mg P.O. q 6 hours; 100 mg I.M. q 8 to 12 hours; 250 mg I.M. q 12 hours; or 250 to 500 mg I.V. q 6 to 12 hours.

CHILDREN OVER 8 YEARS: 25 to 50 mg/kg P.O. daily, divided q 6 hours; 15 to 25 mg/kg I.M. daily, divided q 8 to 12 hours; or 10 to 20 mg/kg I.V. daily, divided q 12 hours.

Blood: neutropenia, eosinophilia.

CNS: benign intracranial hypertension.

CV: pericarditis.

EENT: dysphagia, glossitis.

GI: *anorexia, nausea*, vomiting, *diarrhea*, enterocolitis, anogenital inflammation.

Metabolic: *increased BUN.*

Skin: *maculopapular and erythematous rashes, urticaria, photosensitivity, increased pigmentation.*

Local: *irritation after I.M. injection, thrombophlebitis.*

Other: hypersensitivity.

INTERACTIONS AND SPECIAL CONSIDERATIONS

UCTS, ZINC: decrease antibiotic absorption. Give tetracyclines 3 hours after or 2 hours before iron administration.

Special considerations:
- Use with extreme caution in patients with impaired renal or hepatic function. Use during last half of pregnancy and in children younger than 8 years may cause permanent discoloration of teeth, enamel defects, and retardation of bone growth.
- Cultures should be obtained before starting therapy.
- Check expiration date. Outdated or deteriorated methacycline may cause nephrotoxicity.
- Do not expose these drugs to light or heat.
- Overgrowth of nonsusceptible organisms, such as monilia, is possible, especially on the tongue. Good oral hygiene may minimize superinfection. If superinfection occurs, drug should be discontinued.
- Observe for diarrhea, which may result from local irritation or superinfection.
- Patient should avoid direct sunlight and ultraviolet light. A sunscreen may help prevent photosensitivity reaction. Photosensitivity persists for considerable time after discontinuation of drug.
- Effectiveness is reduced when taken with milk or other dairy products, food, antacids, or iron products. Patient should take each dose with a full glass of water on an empty stomach, at least 1 hour before meals or 2 hours afterward. Dose should be taken at least 1 hour before bedtime to prevent esophagitis.
- Patient should take medication exactly as prescribed, even after he feels better. Streptococcal infections should be treated for at least 10 days.
- May cause false-positive reading of Clinitest; false-negative reading of Clinistix or Tes-Tape.
- For symptoms and treatment of anaphylaxis, see APPENDIX.

Interactions:
ANTACIDS (INCLUDING $NaHCO_3$) OR LAXATIVES CONTAINING ALUMINUM, MAGNESIUM, OR CALCIUM: decrease antibiotic absorption. Give antibiotic 1 hour before or 2 hours after any of the above.
FERROUS SULFATE AND OTHER IRON PRODUCTS, ZINC: decrease antibiotic absorption. Tetracyclines should be given 3 hours after or 2 hours before iron administration.
METHOXYFLURANE: may cause severe nephrotoxicity with tetracyclines. Monitor carefully.

Special considerations:
- Use with extreme caution in patients with impaired renal or hepatic function. Use during last half of pregnancy and in children younger than 8 years may cause permanent discoloration of teeth, enamel defects, and retardation of bone growth.
- Patient may develop thrombophlebitis with I.V. administration of this drug. Extravasation should be avoided.
- Cultures should be obtained before starting therapy.
- Check expiration date.
- Do not expose these drugs to light or heat. Keep cap tightly closed.
- Overgrowth of nonsusceptible organisms, such as monilia, is possible, especially on the tongue. Good oral hygiene may minimize superinfection. If superinfection occurs, drug should be discontinued.
- Observe for diarrhea, which may result from local irritation or superinfection.
- Effectiveness is reduced when taken with antacids or iron products. Patient should take medication exactly as prescribed, even after he feels better. Streptococcal infections should be treated for at least 10 days, syphilis for 10 to 15 days, gonorrhea for at least 4 days, and meningococcal carriers for 5 days.
- Reconstitute 100 mg powder with 5 ml sterile water for injection with further dilution of 500 to 1,000 ml for I.V. infusion. Stable for 24 hours at room temperature.
- May cause false-positive reading of Clinitest; false-negative reading of Clinistix or Tes-Tape.
- Vestibular toxicity resulting in dizziness can occur with this drug.
- For symptoms and treatment of anaphylaxis, see APPENDIX.

Interactions:
ANTACIDS (INCLUDING $NaHCO_3$) AND LAXATIVES CONTAINING ALUMINUM, MAGNESIUM, OR CALCIUM; FOOD, MILK, OR OTHER DAIRY PRODUCTS: decrease antibiotic absorption. Give antibiotic 1 hour before or 2 hours after any of the above.
FERROUS SULFATE AND OTHER IRON PRODUCTS, ZINC: decrease antibiotic absorption. Give tetracyclines 3 hours after or 2 hours before iron administration.
METHOXYFLURANE: may cause severe nephrotoxicity with tetracyclines. Monitor carefully.

Special considerations:
- Use with extreme caution in patients with impaired renal or hepatic function. Use during last half of pregnancy and in children younger than 8 years may cause permanent discoloration of teeth, enamel defects, and retardation of bone growth.
- Patient may develop thrombophlebitis with I.V. administration. Extravasation should be avoided.
- Cultures should be obtained before starting therapy.
- Check expiration date. Outdated or deteriorated oxytetracycline may cause nephrotoxicity.

(continued on following page)

NAMES, INDICATIONS AND DOSAGES	SIDE EFFECTS

oxytetracycline hydrochloride
(continued)

Brucellosis:
ADULTS: 500 mg P.O. q.i.d. for 3 weeks with streptomycin 1 g I.M. q 12 hours first week, once daily second week.

Syphilis in patients sensitive to penicillin:
ADULTS: 30 to 40 g total dose P.O., divided equally over 10 to 15 days.

Gonorrhea in patients sensitive to penicillin:
ADULTS: initially, 1.5 g P.O. followed by 0.5 g q.i.d. for a total of 9 g.

---

tetracycline hydrochloride
Achromycin♦, Cefracycline♦♦, Maso-Cycline, Medicycline♦♦, Neo-Tetrine♦♦, Novotetra♦♦, Panmycin, Robitet, SK-Tetracycline, Sumycin♦, Tetrachel, Tetracrine♦♦, Tetracyn♦, Tetralean♦♦, Triacycline♦♦
tetracycline phosphate complex
Tetrex♦

Infections caused by sensitive gram-negative and gram-positive organisms, trachoma, amebiasis, *Mycoplasma*, *Rickettsia*, and *Chlamydia*:
ADULTS: 250 to 500 mg P.O. q 6 hours; 250 mg I.M. daily or 150 mg I.M. q 12 hours; or 250 to 500 mg I.V. q 8 to 12 hours (I.M. and I.V. hydrochloride salt only).
CHILDREN OVER 8 YEARS: 25 to 50 mg/kg P.O. daily, divided q 6 hours; 15 to 25 mg/kg/day (maximum 250 mg) I.M. single dose or divided q 8 to 12 hours; or 10 to 20 mg/kg I.V. daily, divided q 12 hours.

Brucellosis:
ADULTS: 500 mg P.O. q 6 hours for 3 weeks with streptomycin 1 g I.M. q 12 hours week 1 and daily week 2.

Gonorrhea in patients sensitive to penicillin:
ADULTS: initially,1.5 g P.O., then 500 mg q 6 hours for total of 9 g.

Syphilis in patients sensitive to penicillin:
ADULTS: 30 to 40 g total in equally divided doses over 10 to 15 days.

Acne:
ADULTS AND ADOLESCENTS: initially, 250 mg P.O. q 6 hours, then 125 to 500 mg P.O. daily or every other day.

Shigellosis:
ADULTS: 2.5 g P.O. in 1 dose.

Blood: neutropenia, eosinophilia.
CNS: dizziness, headache.
CV: pericarditis.
EENT: sore throat, glossitis, dysphagia.
GI: anorexia, *epigastric distress, nausea,* vomiting, *diarrhea,* stomatitis, enterocolitis, inflammatory lesions in anogenital region.
Hepatic: hepatotoxicity with doses given I.V.
Metabolic: *increased BUN.*
Skin: *maculopapular and erythematous rashes, urticaria, photosensitivity, increased pigmentation.*
Local: *irritation after I.M. injection, thrombophlebitis.*

♦ Available in U.S. and Canada. ♦♦ Available in Canada only.
All other products (no symbol) available in U.S. only. Italicized side effects are common or life-threatening.

INTERACTIONS AND SPECIAL CONSIDERATIONS

• Do not expose these drugs to light or heat.
• Inject I.M. dosage deeply; may be painful. Sites should be rotated. I.M. preparations contain a local anesthetic; patient should report hypersensitivity to local anesthetics.
• Overgrowth of nonsusceptible organisms, such as monilia, is possible, especially on the tongue. Good oral hygiene may minimize superinfection. If superinfection occurs, drug should be discontinued.
• Observe for diarrhea, which may result from local irritation or superinfection.
• Patient should avoid direct sunlight and ultraviolet light. A sunscreen may help prevent photosensitivity reactions. Photosensitivity persists for considerable time after discontinuation.
• Less effective when taken with milk or other dairy products, food, antacids, or iron products. Each dose should be taken with a full glass of water on an empty stomach, at least 1 hour before or 2 hours after meals. Take at least 1 hour before bedtime to prevent esophagitis.
• Patient should take medication exactly as prescribed, even after he feels better.
• For I.V. use: Reconstitute 250 mg and 500 mg powder for injection with 10 ml sterile water. Dilute to at least 100 ml in 5% dextrose in water, normal saline, or Ringer's solution. Don't mix with any other drug. Store reconstituted solutions in refrigerator. Stable for 48 hours.
• May cause false-positive reading of Clinitest; false-negative reading of Clinistix or Tes-Tape.
• For symptoms and treatment of anaphylaxis, see APPENDIX.

Interactions:
ANTACIDS (INCLUDING $NaHCO_3$) AND LAXATIVES CONTAINING ALUMINUM, MAGNESIUM, OR CALCIUM; FOOD, MILK, OR OTHER DAIRY PRODUCTS: decrease antibiotic absorption. Give antibiotic 1 hour before or 2 hours after any of the above.
FERROUS SULFATE AND OTHER IRON PRODUCTS, ZINC: decrease antibiotic absorption. Give tetracyclines 3 hours after or 2 hours before iron administration.
METHOXYFLURANE: may cause severe nephrotoxicity with tetracyclines. Monitor carefully.

Special considerations:
• Use with extreme caution in patients with impaired renal or hepatic function. Use during last half of pregnancy and in children younger than 8 years may cause permanent discoloration of teeth, enamel defects, and retardation of bone growth.
• Cultures should be obtained before starting therapy.
• Effectiveness reduced when taken with milk or other dairy products, food, antacids, or iron products. Patient should take each dose with a full glass of water on an empty stomach, at least 1 hour before meals or 2 hours afterward. Should be taken at least 1 hour before bedtime to prevent esophagitis.
• Patient may develop thrombophlebitis with I.V. administration. Extravasation should be avoided.
• Check expiration date. Outdated or deteriorated tetracycline may cause nephrotoxicity.
• I.M. solutions should be discarded after 24 hours because they deteriorate. Exception: Achromycin solution should be discarded in 12 hours.
• Do not expose these drugs to light or heat.
• I.M. dosage should be injected deeply and it may be painful. Sites should be rotated. I.M. preparations often contain a local anesthetic; patient should report hypersensitivity to local anesthetics.
• Overgrowth of nonsusceptible organisms, such as monilia, is possible, especially on the tongue. Good oral hygiene may minimize superinfection. If superinfection occurs, drug should be discontinued.
• Observe for diarrhea, which may result from local irritation or superinfection.
• Patient should take medication exactly as prescribed, even after he feels better. Streptoccocal infections should be treated for at least 10 days.
• For I.V. use, 100 mg and 250 mg powder for injection should be reconstituted with 5 ml sterile water; with 10 ml for 500 mg. Should be diluted in 100 to 1,000 ml volume of 5% dextrose in 0.9% saline, and dilute solution refrigerated for I.V. use and used within 24 hours. Exception: Achromycin solution should be used immediately.
• Do not mix tetracycline solution with any other I.V. additive.
• For I.M. use, 100 mg powder for injection should be reconstituted with 2 ml sterile water. Concentration will be 50 mg/ml. Amount of diluent for 250 mg injection varies according to brand. Check with pharmacy or follow manufacturer's instructions.
• May cause false-positive readings of Clinitest; false-negative reading of Clinistix or Tes-Tape.
• For symptoms and treatment of anaphylaxis, see APPENDIX.

16

Sulfonamides

co-trimoxazole
sulfacytine
sulfadiazine
sulfamerazine
sulfamethizole
sulfamethoxazole
sulfapyridine
sulfasalazine
sulfisoxazole

Sulfonamides were the first drugs to be used systemically for the treatment of bacterial infections in humans. First used clinically in the mid-1930s, they significantly reduced incidence of morbidity and mortality of the treatable infectious diseases.

Major uses

Although increased microbial resistance in recent years has limited their utility, sulfonamides are still the drugs of choice for urinary tract infections, otitis media, conjunctivitis, toxoplasmosis, and trachoma.

- Co-trimoxazole is a primary prophylactic and therapeutic drug for acute and chronic urinary tract infections. It is therapeutic for bacterial prostatitis, shigellosis, otitis media, and *Pneumocystis carinii* pneumonia. It may also combat infections caused by organisms resistant to the simple sulfonamides (*Escherichia coli,* for example, which is resistant to sulfisoxazole).
- Sulfacytine, sulfadiazine, sulfamerazine, sulfamethizole, sulfamethoxazole, and sulfisoxazole are useful in the treatment of cystitis and pyelonephritis caused by susceptible strains of *E. coli, Klebsiella, Staphylococcus aureus,* and *Proteus mirabilis.* They are also indicated in the treatment of chancroid, trachoma, and nocardiosis. They are effective against *Hemophilus influenzae* otitis media when combined with penicillin, and against toxoplasmosis when combined with pyrimethamine.
- Sulfadiazine may be prophylactic for rheumatic heart disease in patients allergic to penicillin.
- Sulfapyridine is therapeutic for dermatitis herpetiformis.
- Sulfasalazine is useful in the treatment of mild-to-moderate cases of ulcerative colitis.

Mechanism of action

Sulfonamides have a broad spectrum of antibacterial action and are bacteriostatic. Chemically similar to para-aminobenzoic acid (PABA), these drugs competitively inhibit dihydropteroate synthetase, a bacterial enzyme responsible for incorporation of PABA into dihydrofolic acid (folic acid). This mechanism blocks folic acid synthesis. Hence, nucleic acids—essential building blocks of the bacterial cell—cannot be synthesized. Susceptible bacteria are those that must synthesize their own folic acid.

Absorption, distribution, metabolism, and excretion

These drugs rapidly and adequately absorbed from the GI tract, except sulfasalazine, which produces a local effect in the bowel and is absorbed at a rate of only 10% to 15%.

All sulfonamides are readily distributed throughout the body, largely metabolized in the liver, and excreted in the urine (excretion rate increases with alkaline urine).

Onset and duration

Peak blood levels of the sulfonamides usually appear 2 to 8 hours after oral administration and within minutes after I.V. administration.

• Co-trimoxazole and sulfamethoxazole have half-lives of 12 hours and may be administered twice daily.
• Sulfacytine, sulfadiazine, sulfamerazine, sulfamethizole, sulfapyridine, and sulfisoxazole have half-lives of 4 to 6 hours and are usually administered four times daily.
• Sulfasalazine, usually administered several times daily, has a half-life of 4 to 10 hours.

Combination products
AZO GANTANOL: sulfamethoxazole 500 mg and phenazopyridine hydrochloride 100 mg.
AZO GANTRISIN: sulfisoxazole 500 mg and phenazopyridine hydrochloride 50 mg.
AZOTREX: sulfamethizole 250 mg, tetracycline phosphate complex equivalent to 125 mg tetracycline HCl activity, and phenazopyridine hydrochloride 50 mg.
SULADYNE: sulfamethizole 125 mg, sulfadiazine 125 mg, and phenazopyridine hydrochloride 75 mg.
THIOSULFIL-A: sulfamethizole 250 mg and phenazopyridine hydrochloride 50 mg.
TRIPLE SULFA: sulfadiazine 167 mg, sulfamerazine 167 mg, and sulfamethazine 167 mg.
UROBIOTIC-250: sulfamethizole 250 mg, oxytetracycline 250 mg, and phenazopyridine hydrochloride 50 mg.

DRUG ALERT

BE PREPARED FOR STEVENS-JOHNSON SYNDROME

One side effect of sulfonamides is Stevens-Johnson syndrome, the most common serious skin disorder in hospitalized patients. Onset may be sudden; symptoms include lesions on the skin and mucous membranes, severe pain in mucosal areas (accompanied by secondary photophobia), fever, malaise, and inability to eat and drink.

The characteristic bullous lesions of Stevens-Johnson syndrome produce a thick hemorrhagic crusting on the lips. The patient's eyelids and genitalia may also erode. His temperature may hover around 39° C. (102.2° F.), then begin to fall after 7 to 9 days, as the lesions dry and heal. However, the disease sometimes becomes life-threatening, and large areas of the skin may slough off. Stevens-Johnson syndrome has a mortality of 15% to 20%.

To care for the patient with Stevens-Johnson syndrome:
• Skin and blood cultures should be obtained daily.
• Possible fluid and electrolyte imbalance should be monitored and may require I.V. therapy.
• Aspirin or acetaminophen may be used to suppress fever.
• The denuded areas of the skin should be sponged four times a day with a 1:1 mixture of povidone-iodine skin cleanser in water.
• Prednisone P.O. or prednisolone I.M. may be prescribed to help decrease inflammation.

NAMES, INDICATIONS AND DOSAGES	SIDE EFFECTS
co-trimoxazole (sulfamethoxazole-trimethoprim) Bactrim♦, Bactrim DS♦, Bactrim I.V. Infusion, Septra♦, Septra DS♦, Septra I.V. Infusion **Urinary tract infections and shigellosis:** ADULTS: 160 mg trimethoprim/800 mg sulfa q 12 hours for 10 to 14 days in urinary tract infections and for 5 days in shigellosis. CHILDREN: 8 mg/kg trimethoprim/40 mg/kg sulfa per 24 hours, in 2 divided doses q 12 hours (10 days for urinary tract infections; for 5 days in shigellosis). **Otitis media:** CHILDREN: 8 mg/kg trimethoprim/40 mg/kg sulfa per 24 hours, in 2 divided doses q 12 hours for 10 days. **Pneumocystis carinii pneumonitis:** ADULTS: 20 mg/kg trimethoprim/ 100 mg/kg sulfa per 24 hours, in equally divided doses q 6 hours for 14 days. CHILDREN UP TO 36 KG: 160 mg trimethoprim/800 mg sulfa q 6 hours for 14 days. **Chronic bronchitis:** ADULTS: 160 mg trimethoprim/800 mg sulfa q 12 hours for 10 to 14 days. Not recommended for infants less than 2 months old. Available as tablets or suspension only.	**Blood:** *agranulocytosis, aplastic anemia,* megaloblastic anemia, thrombocytopenia, leukopenia, hemolytic anemia. **CNS:** headache, mental depression, convulsions, hallucinations. **GI:** *nausea, vomiting, diarrhea,* abdominal pain, anorexia, stomatitis. **GU:** toxic nephrosis with oliguria and anuria, crystalluria, hematuria. **Hepatic:** jaundice. **Skin:** *erythema multiforme (Stevens-Johnson syndrome), generalized skin eruption, epidermal necrolysis, exfoliative dermatitis,* photosensitivity, urticaria, pruritus. **Other:** *hypersensitivity, serum sickness, drug fever, anaphylaxis.*
sulfacytine Renoquid **Urinary tract infections:** ADULTS: initially, 500 mg P.O., then 250 mg P.O. q.i.d. for 10 days.	**Blood:** *agranulocytosis, aplastic anemia,* megaloblastic anemia, thrombocytopenia, leukopenia, hemolytic anemia. **CNS:** headache, mental depression, convulsions, hallucinations. **GI:** *nausea, vomiting, diarrhea,* abdominal pain, anorexia, stomatitis. **GU:** toxic nephrosis with oliguria and anuria, crystalluria, hematuria. **Hepatic:** jaundice. **Skin:** *erythema multiforme (Stevens-Johnson syndrome), generalized skin eruption, epidermal necrolysis, exfoliative dermatitis,* photosensitivity, urticaria, pruritus. **Other:** *hypersensitivity, serum sickness, drug fever, anaphylaxis.*
sulfadiazine Microsulfon **Urinary tract infection:** ADULTS: initially, 2 to 4 g P.O., then 500 mg to 1 g P.O. q 6 hours. CHILDREN: initially, 75 mg/kg or 2 g/m^2 P.O., then 150 mg/kg or 4 g/m^2 P.O. in 4 to 6 divided doses daily. Maximum daily dose 6 g. **Rheumatic fever prophylaxis, as an alternative to penicillin:**	**Blood:** *agranulocytosis, aplastic anemia,* megaloblastic anemia, thrombocytopenia, leukopenia, hemolytic anemia. **CNS:** headache, mental depression, convulsions, hallucinations. **GI:** *nausea, vomiting, diarrhea,* abdominal pain, anorexia, stomatitis. **GU:** toxic nephrosis with oliguria and anuria, crystalluria, hematuria. **Hepatic:** jaundice. **Skin:** *erythema multiforme (Stevens-Johnson syndrome), generalized skin eruption, epidermal*

INTERACTIONS AND SPECIAL CONSIDERATIONS

Interactions:
AMMONIUM CHLORIDE, ASCORBIC ACID, PARALDEHYDE: doses sufficient to acidify urine may cause precipitation of sulfonamide and crystalluria. Don't use together.
PABA-CONTAINING LOCAL ANESTHETICS AND OTHER PABA DRUGS: inhibit antibacterial action. Don't use together.

Special considerations:
- Contraindicated in patients with porphyria. Use cautiously and in reduced dosages in patients with impaired hepatic or renal function and in those with severe allergy or bronchial asthma, G-6-PD deficiency, blood dyscrasias.
- Patient should drink a full glass of water with each dose and drink plenty of water during the day to prevent crystalluria. Fluid intake and urinary output should be monitored.
- I.V. infusion must be diluted in 5% dextrose in water prior to administration. Should not be mixed with other drugs or solutions.
- I.V. infusion must be infused slowly over 60 to 90 minutes. Should not be given by rapid infusion or bolus injection.
- This combination is often used in extremely ill immunosuppressed patients when prescribed for treatment of *Pneumocystis* pneumonia.
- Oral suspension available for patients who cannot swallow large tablets.
- "DS" product means "double strength."
- Skin rash, sore throat, fever, or mouth sores may be early signs of blood dyscrasias.
- Should be taken 1 hour before or 2 hours after meals for best absorption.
- Used effectively for treatment of chronic bacterial prostatitis.
- Used prophylactically for recurrent urinary tract infections in women.
- Most side effects develop within 2 weeks of onset of therapy.
- For treatment of anaphylaxis, see APPENDIX.

Interactions:
AMMONIUM CHLORIDE, ASCORBIC ACID, PARALDEHYDE: doses sufficient to acidify urine may cause precipitation of sulfonamide and crystalluria. Don't use together.
PABA-CONTAINING LOCAL ANESTHETICS AND OTHER PABA DRUGS: inhibit antibacterial action. Don't use together.

Special considerations:
- Contraindicated in porphyria. Use cautiously and in reduced dosages in patients with impaired hepatic or renal function, bronchial asthma, history of multiple allergies, G-6-PD deficiency, blood dyscrasias.
- Patient should drink a full glass of water with each dose and drink plenty of water throughout the day to prevent crystalluria. Fluid intake and urinary output should be monitored. Intake should be sufficient to produce output of 1,500 ml daily (between 3,000 and 4,000 ml daily for adults).
- To aid in prevention of crystalluria, sodium bicarbonate may be administered to alkalinize urine. Urine pH should be monitored daily.
- Patient should take medication for as long as prescribed, even after he feels better. Patient should avoid direct sunlight and ultraviolet light to prevent photosensitivity reaction.
- Urinary cultures, CBCs, and urinalyses should be monitored before and during therapy.
- Early signs of blood dyscrasias (sore throat, fever, pallor, or jaundice) require both immediate discontinuation of drug and reevaluation of therapy.
- For treatment of anaphylaxis, see APPENDIX.

Interactions:
AMMONIUM CHLORIDE, ASCORBIC ACID, PARALDEHYDE: doses sufficient to acidify urine may cause precipitation of sulfonamide and crystalluria. Don't use together.
PABA-CONTAINING LOCAL ANESTHETICS AND OTHER PABA DRUGS: inhibit antibacterial action. Don't use together.

Special considerations:
- Contraindicated in patients with porphyria or in infants younger than 2 months (except in congenital toxoplasmosis). Use cautiously and in reduced dosages in patients with impaired hepatic or renal function, bronchial asthma, history of multiple allergies, G-6-PD deficiency, blood dyscrasias.
- Patient should drink a full glass of water with each dose and drink plenty of water throughout the day to prevent crystalluria. Fluid intake and urinary output should be monitored. Intake should be sufficient to produce output of 1,500 ml daily (between 3,000 and 4,000 ml daily for adults). To aid in prevention of crystalluria, so-

(continued on following page)

NAMES, INDICATIONS AND DOSAGES	SIDE EFFECTS
sulfadiazine *(continued)* CHILDREN OVER 30 KG: 1 g P.O. daily. CHILDREN UNDER 30 KG: 500 mg P.O. daily. **Adjunctive treatment in toxoplasmosis:** ADULTS: 4 g P.O. in divided doses q 6 hours for 3 to 4 weeks, discontinued for 1 week, then repeated; given with pyrimethamine 75 mg P.O. daily for 1 to 3 days, then 25 mg P.O. daily for 3 to 4 weeks, discontinued for 1 week, then repeated using 25 mg P.O. daily. CHILDREN: 100 mg/kg P.O. in divided doses q 6 hours for 3 to 4 weeks, discontinued for 1 week, then repeated; given with pyrimethamine, 1 mg/kg P.O. daily for 1 to 3 days, then 0.5 mg/kg P.O. daily for 3 to 4 weeks, discontinued for 1 week, then repeated using 0.5 mg/kg P.O. daily.	*necrolysis, exfoliative dermatitis,* photosensitivity, urticaria, pruritus. **Local:** irritation, extravasation. **Other:** *hypersensitivity, serum sickness, drug fever, anaphylaxis.*
sulfamerazine **Antibacterial (rarely used alone):** ADULTS: initially, 2 to 4 g P.O., then 500 mg to 1 g P.O. q 6 hours. CHILDREN OVER 2 MONTHS: initially, 75 mg/kg or 2 g/m², then 150 mg/kg or 4 g/m² P.O. daily in 4 to 6 equally divided doses. Maximum daily dose 6 g.	**Blood:** *agranulocytosis, aplastic anemia,* megaloblastic anemia, thrombocytopenia, leukopenia, hemolytic anemia. **CNS:** headache, mental depression, convulsions, hallucinations. **GI:** *nausea, vomiting, diarrhea,* abdominal pain, anorexia, stomatitis. **GU:** toxic nephrosis with oliguria and anuria, crystalluria, hematuria. **Hepatic:** jaundice. **Skin:** *erythema multiforme (Stevens-Johnson syndrome), generalized skin eruption, epidermal necrolysis, exfoliative dermatitis,* photosensitivity, urticaria, pruritus. **Other:** *hypersensitivity, serum sickness, drug fever, anaphylaxis.*
sulfamethizole Bursul, Microsul, Proklar-M, Sulfasol, Sulfstat, Sulfurine, Thiosulfil♦, Unisul, Uri-Pak, Urifon, Utrasul **Urinary tract infections only:** ADULTS: 500 mg to 1 g P.O. t.i.d. to q.i.d. CHILDREN OVER 2 MONTHS: 30 to 45 mg/kg P.O. daily, divided into doses given q 6 hours.	**Blood:** *agranulocytosis, aplastic anemia,* megaloblastic anemia, thrombocytopenia, leukopenia, hemolytic anemia. **CNS:** headache, mental depression, convulsions, hallucinations. **GI:** *nausea, vomiting, diarrhea,* abdominal pain, anorexia, stomatitis. **GU:** toxic nephrosis with oliguria and anuria, crystalluria, hematuria. **Hepatic:** jaundice. **Skin:** *erythema multiforme (Stevens-Johnson syndrome), generalized skin eruption, epidermal necrolysis, exfoliative dermatitis,* photosensitivity, urticaria, pruritus. **Other:** *hypersensitivity, serum sickness, drug fever, anaphylaxis.*

INTERACTIONS AND SPECIAL CONSIDERATIONS

dium bicarbonate may be administered to alkalinize urine. Urine pH should be monitored daily.

• Patient should take medication for as long as prescribed, even if he feels better. Patient should avoid direct sunlight and ultraviolet light to prevent photosensitivity reaction.

• Drug should be taken on schedule to maintain constant blood level.

• Purpura, ecchymosis, sore throat, fever, pallor or jaundice may be signs of blood dyscrasias.

• For I.V. administration, drug should be well diluted and I.V. dosages infused slowly. If extravasation occurs, infusion should be stopped. I.V. should be restarted at another site.

• Urinary cultures, CBCs, and urinalyses should be monitored before and during therapy.

• Should be mixed with dextrose 5% in normal saline or Ringer's solution for I.V. infusion; any acidic solution (especially with pH below 9.0) causes precipitation. Diluent should be used cautiously and solution discarded if precipitation occurs.

• Sulfadiazine with pyrimethamine for treatment of toxoplasmosis may be continued for life. Therapy controls but does not cure toxoplasmosis.

• Folic or folinic acid may be used during rest periods in toxoplasmosis therapy to reverse hematopoietic depression and/or anemia associated with pyrimethamine and sulfadiazine.

• Protect drug from light.

• For treatment of anaphylaxis, see APPENDIX.

Interactions:

AMMONIUM CHLORIDE, ASCORBIC ACID, PARALDEHYDE: doses sufficient to acidify urine may cause precipitation of sulfonamide and crystalluria. Don't use together.

PABA-CONTAINING LOCAL ANESTHETICS AND OTHER PABA DRUGS: inhibit antibacterial action. Don't use together.

Special considerations:

• Contraindicated in infants younger than 2 months (except in congenital toxoplasmosis) and in patients with porphyria. Use cautiously in impaired hepatic or renal function, asthma, blood dyscrasias, G-6-PD deficiency, history of multiple allergies.

• Although drug has low incidence of crystalluria, patient should drink a full glass of water with each dose and drink plenty of water throughout the day to prevent crystalluria. Fluid intake and urinary output should be monitored. Intake should be sufficient to produce output of 1,500 ml daily (between 3,000 to 4,000 ml daily for adults). To help prevent crystalluria, sodium bicarbonate may be given to alkalinize urine. Urine pH should be monitored daily.

• Patient should take medication for as long as prescribed, even after he feels better. Patient should avoid direct sunlight and ultraviolet light to prevent photosensitivity reaction. Early signs of blood dyscrasias (sore throat, fever, pallor, or jaundice) require immediate discontinuation of drug and reevaluation of therapy.

• Urinary cultures, CBCs, and urinalyses should be monitored before and during therapy.

• Used in combination sulfonamide preparations such as Triple Sulfa in conjunction with pyrimethamine to treat toxoplasmosis.

• GI superinfection is possible during long-term therapy.

• When given preoperatively, the patient should receive a low-residue diet and a minimum of enemas and cathartics.

• For treatment of anaphylaxis, see APPENDIX.

Interactions:

AMMONIUM CHLORIDE, ASCORBIC ACID, PARALDEHYDE: doses sufficient to acidify urine may cause precipitation of sulfonamide and crystalluria. Don't use together.

PABA-CONTAINING LOCAL ANESTHETICS AND OTHER PABA DRUGS: inhibit antibacterial action. Don't use together.

Special considerations:

• Contraindicated in porphyria. Use cautiously and in reduced dosages in patients with impaired hepatic or renal function, blood dyscrasias, G-6-PD deficiency, asthma, history of multiple allergies.

• Patient should drink a full glass of water with each dose and drink plenty of water throughout the day to prevent crystalluria. Fluid intake and urinary output should be monitored. Intake should be sufficient to produce output of 1,500 ml daily (between 3,000 and 4,000 ml daily for adults). To aid in prevention of crystalluria, sodium bicarbonate may be given to alkalinize urine. Urine pH should be monitored daily.

• Patient should take medication for as long as prescribed, even after he feels better. Patient should avoid direct sunlight and ultraviolet light to prevent photosensitivity reaction. Early signs of blood dyscrasias (sore throat, fever, pallor, or jaundice) require immediate discontinuation of drug and reevaluation of therapy.

• Urinary cultures, CBCs, and urinalyses should be monitored before and during therapy.

• For treatment of anaphylaxis, see APPENDIX.

NAMES, INDICATIONS AND DOSAGES	SIDE EFFECTS
sulfamethoxazole Gantanol♦, Urobak **Urinary tract and systemic infections:** ADULTS: initially, 2 g P.O., then 1 g P.O. b.i.d. up to t.i.d. for severe infections. CHILDREN OVER 2 MONTHS: initially, 50 to 60 mg/kg P.O., then 25 to 30 mg/kg b.i.d. Maximum dose should not exceed 75 mg/kg daily.	**Blood:** *agranulocytosis, aplastic anemia,* megaloblastic anemia, thrombocytopenia, leukopenia, hemolytic anemia. **CNS:** headache, mental depression, convulsions, hallucinations. **GI:** *nausea, vomiting, diarrhea,* abdominal pain, anorexia, stomatitis. **GU:** toxic nephrosis with oliguria and anuria, crystalluria, hematuria. **Hepatic:** jaundice. **Skin:** *erythema multiforme (Stevens-Johnson syndrome), generalized skin eruption, epidermal necrolysis, exfoliative dermatitis,* photosensitivity, urticaria, pruritus. **Other:** *hypersensitivity, serum sickness, drug fever, anaphylaxis.*
sulfapyridine Dagenan♦♦ **Dermatitis herpetiformis:** ADULTS: 500 mg P.O. q.i.d. until improvement noted, then decrease dose by 500 mg every 3 days until minimum effective maintenance dose achieved.	**Blood:** *agranulocytosis, aplastic anemia,* megaloblastic anemia, thrombocytopenia, leukopenia, hemolytic anemia. **CNS:** headache, mental depression, convulsions, hallucinations. **GI:** *nausea, vomiting, diarrhea,* abdominal pain, anorexia, stomatitis. **GU:** toxic nephrosis with oliguria and anuria, crystalluria, hematuria. **Hepatic:** jaundice. **Skin:** *erythema multiforme (Stevens-Johnson syndrome), generalized skin eruption, epidermal necrolysis, exfoliative dermatitis,* photosensitivity, urticaria, pruritus. **Other:** *hypersensitivity, serum sickness, drug fever, anaphylaxis.*
sulfasalazine Azulfidine, Azulfidine En-Tabs, SAS-500 **Mild-to-moderate ulcerative colitis, adjunctive therapy in severe ulcerative colitis:** ADULTS: initially, 3 to 4 g P.O. daily in evenly divided doses; usual maintenance dose is 1.5 to 2 g P.O. daily in divided doses q 6 hours. May need to start with 1 to 2 g initially, with a gradual increase in dose to minimize side effects. CHILDREN OVER 2 YEARS: initially, 40 to 60 mg/kg P.O. daily, divided into 3 to 6 doses; then 30 mg/kg daily in 4 doses. May need to start at lower dose if gastrointestinal intolerance occurs.	**Blood:** *agranulocytosis, aplastic anemia,* megaloblastic anemia, thrombocytopenia, leukopenia, hemolytic anemia. **CNS:** headache, mental depression, convulsions, hallucinations. **GI:** *nausea, vomiting, diarrhea,* abdominal pain, anorexia, stomatitis. **GU:** toxic nephrosis with oliguria and anuria, crystalluria, hematuria. **Hepatic:** jaundice. **Skin:** *erythema multiforme (Stevens-Johnson syndrome), generalized skin eruption, epidermal necrolysis, exfoliative dermatitis,* photosensitivity, urticaria, pruritus. **Other:** *hypersensitivity, serum sickness, drug fever, anaphylaxis.*

♦ Available in U.S. and Canada. ♦♦ Available in Canada only.
All other products (no symbol) available in U.S. only. Italicized side effects are common or life-threatening.

INTERACTIONS AND SPECIAL CONSIDERATIONS

Interactions:
AMMONIUM CHLORIDE, ASCORBIC ACID, PARALDEHYDE: doses sufficient to acidify urine may cause precipitation of sulfonamide and crystalluria. Don't use together.
PABA-CONTAINING LOCAL ANESTHETICS AND OTHER PABA DRUGS: inhibit antibacterial action. Don't use together.

Special considerations:
- Contraindicated in patients with porphyria or in infants younger than 2 months (except in congenital toxoplasmosis). Use cautiously and in reduced dosages in patients with impaired hepatic or renal function and in severe allergy or bronchial asthma, G-6-PD deficiency, blood dyscrasias.
- Patient should drink a full glass of water with each dose and drink plenty of water during the day to prevent crystalluria. Fluid intake and urinary output should be monitored. Intake should be sufficient to produce output of 1,500 ml daily (between 3,000 and 4,000 ml daily for adults). To aid in prevention of crystalluria, sodium bicarbonate may be administered to alkalinize urine. Urine pH should be monitored daily.
- Patient should take medication for as long as prescribed, even after he feels better. Patient should avoid direct sunlight and ultraviolet light to prevent photosensitivity reaction.
- Urinary cultures, CBCs, and urinalyses should be monitored before and during therapy.
- Sulfamethoxazole is also used in adjunctive therapy for treatment of toxoplasmosis following therapy with other first-line agents.
- Early signs of blood dyscrasias (sore throat, fever, pallor, or jaundice) require immediate discontinuation of drug and reevaluation of therapy.
- For treatment of anaphylaxis, see APPENDIX.

Interactions:
AMMONIUM CHLORIDE, ASCORBIC ACID, PARALDEHYDE: doses sufficient to acidify urine may cause precipitation of sulfonamide and crystalluria. Don't use together.
PABA-CONTAINING LOCAL ANESTHETICS AND OTHER PABA DRUGS: inhibit antibacterial action. Don't use together.

Special considerations:
- Contraindicated in porphyria. Use cautiously and in reduced dosages in patients with impaired hepatic or renal function, G-6-PD deficiency, history of multiple allergies, asthma, or blood dyscrasias.
- Patient should drink a full glass of water with each dose and drink plenty of water during the day to prevent crystalluria. Fluid intake and urinary output should be monitored. Intake should be sufficient to produce output of 1,500 ml daily (between 3,000 and 4,000 ml daily for adults).
- Alkalinization of the urine may decrease the danger of crystalluria but may greatly increase renal tubular reabsorption of the drug, sustained blood levels, and risk of toxicity.
- Patient should take medication for as long as prescribed, even after he feels better. Patient should avoid direct sunlight and ultraviolet light to prevent photosensitivity reaction.
- Urinary cultures, CBCs, and urinalyses should be monitored before and during therapy.
- Sulfapyridine is an intermediate-acting sulfonamide with a high potential for toxicity; its use is restricted to treatment of dermatitis herpetiformis when sulfone therapy is contraindicated.
- Occurrence of side effects requires both immediate discontinuation of drug and reevaluation of therapy.
- For treatment of anaphylaxis, see APPENDIX.

Interactions:
AMMONIUM CHLORIDE, ASCORBIC ACID, PARALDEHYDE: doses sufficient to acidify urine may cause precipitation of sulfonamide and crystalluria. Don't use together.
PABA-CONTAINING LOCAL ANESTHETICS AND OTHER PABA DRUGS: inhibit antibacterial action. Don't use together.

Special considerations:
- Contraindicated in porphyria. Use cautiously and in reduced dosages in patients with impaired hepatic or renal function and in those with severe allergy or bronchial asthma, or G-6-PD deficiency.
- Patient should drink a full glass of water with each dose and drink plenty of water during the day to prevent crystalluria. Fluid intake and urinary output should be monitored. Intake should be sufficient to produce output of 1,500 ml daily (betweem 3,000 and 4,000 ml daily for adults).
- Patient should take medication for as long as prescribed, even after he feels better. Patient should avoid direct sunlight and ultraviolet light to prevent photosensitivity reaction.
- Urinary cultures, CBCs, and urinalyses should be monitored before and during therapy.
- Colors alkaline urine orange-yellow.
- Side effects are usually those affecting the GI tract. Spacing doses evenly and administering after food intake should minimize symptoms.
- For treatment of anaphylaxis, see APPENDIX.

NAMES, INDICATIONS AND DOSAGES	SIDE EFFECTS
sulfisoxazole Barazole, Gantrisin♦, G-Sox, J-Sul, Lipo Gantrisin, Novosoxazole♦♦, Rosoxol, SK-Soxazole, Sosol, Soxa, Soxomide, Sulfagan, Sulfizin, Sulfizole♦♦, Urisoxin, Urizole, Velmatrol **Urinary tract and systemic infections:** ADULTS: initially, 2 to 4 g P.O., then 1 to 2 g P.O. q.i.d.; extended-release suspension 4 to 5 g P.O. q 12 hours. CHILDREN OVER 2 MONTHS: initially, 75 mg/kg P.O. daily or 2 g/m^2 P.O. daily in divided doses q 6 hours, then 150 mg/kg or 4 g/m^2 P.O. daily in divided doses q 6 hours; extended-release suspension 60 to 70 mg/kg P.O. q 12 hours. ADULTS AND CHILDREN OVER 2 MONTHS: parenteral dosages (sulfisoxazole diolamine) initially, 50 mg/kg or 1.125 g/m^2 by slow I.V. injection, then 100 mg/kg daily or 2.25 g/m^2 daily in divided doses q 6 hours by slow I.V. injection. 40% solution must be diluted to a concentration of 5% for I.V. use.	**Blood:** *agranulocytosis, aplastic anemia,* megaloblastic anemia, thrombocytopenia, leukopenia, hemolytic anemia. **CNS:** headache, mental depression, convulsions, hallucinations. **GI:** *nausea, vomiting, diarrhea,* abdominal pain, anorexia, stomatitis. **GU:** toxic nephrosis with oliguria and anuria, crystalluria, hematuria. **Hepatic:** jaundice. **Skin:** *erythema multiforme (Stevens-Johnson syndrome), generalized skin eruption, epidermal necrolysis, exfoliative dermatitis,* photosensitivity, urticaria, pruritus. **Other:** *hypersensitivity, serum sickness, drug fever, anaphylaxis.*

INTERACTIONS AND SPECIAL CONSIDERATIONS

Interactions:

AMMONIUM CHLORIDE, ASCORBIC ACID, PARALDEHYDE: doses sufficient to acidify urine may cause crystalluria and precipitation of sulfonamide. Don't use together.

PABA-CONTAINING LOCAL ANESTHETICS AND OTHER PABA DRUGS: inhibit antibacterial action. Don't use together.

Special considerations:

- Contraindicated in patients with porphyria and in infants younger than 2 months (except in congenital toxoplasmosis). Use cautiously in patients with impaired hepatic or renal function, severe allergy or bronchial asthma, G-6-PD deficiency.
- Patient should drink a full glass of water with each dose and drink plenty of water throughout the day to prevent crystalluria. Fluid intake and urinary output should be monitored. Intake should be sufficient to produce output of 1,500 ml daily (between 3,000 and 4,000 ml daily for adults). To aid in prevention of crystalluria, sodium bicarbonate may be administered to alkalinize urine. Urine pH should be monitored daily.
- Patient should take medication for as long as prescribed, even after he feels better. Patient should avoid direct sunlight and ultraviolet light to prevent photosensitivity reaction.
- Urinary cultures, CBCs, and urinalyses should be monitored before and during therapy.
- Parenteral form can be given I.M. or subcutaneously, but these routes are discouraged. Administration of this form with parenteral fluids is not recommended. Diluents other than sterile distilled water may cause precipitation.
- Gantrisin suspension and Lipo Gantrisin suspension cannot be interchanged, since the latter is an extended-release preparation.
- Sulfisoxazole/pyrimethamine combination used to treat toxoplasmosis.
- Early signs of blood dyscrasias (sore throat, fever, pallor, or jaundice) require both immediate discontinuation of drug and reevaluation of therapy.
- GI superinfection is possible during long-term therapy.
- When given preoperatively, the patient should receive a low-residue diet and a minimum of enemas and cathartics.
- Although often given, initial loading dose is not pharmacologically necessary.
- For treatment of anaphylaxis, see APPENDIX.

17

Urinary tract antiseptics

cinoxacin
methenamine hippurate
methenamine mandelate
methylene blue
nalidixic acid
nitrofurantoin
nitrofurantoin macrocrystals

Urinary tract antiseptics concentrate in the renal parenchyma, including the uriniferous tubules and bladder. Because they don't achieve blood levels high enough to treat systemic infections, they act only locally for urinary tract infections.

Though rarely used except in combination with other agents, these drugs cause few adverse reactions. They can be effective in urinary tract infections that resist other modes of therapy.

Major uses

• Methenamine and nitrofurantoin are prophylactic for recurrent urinary tract infections.
• Methylene blue may occasionally be of use in treating mild cystitis and urethritis. It is also effective in idiopathic and drug-induced methemoglobinemia and in cyanide poisoning.
• Cinoxacin, nalidixic acid, and nitrofurantoin are also therapeutic for cystitis and pyelonephritis caused by susceptible strains of *Escherichia coli, Proteus mirabilis, Klebsiella,* and *Enterobacter*. Cinoxacin and nalidixic acid also are effective against *Proteus vulgaris;* nitrofurantoin is effective against *Staphylococus aureus* and enterococci.

Mechanism of action

• In acid urine, methenamines are hydrolyzed to ammonia and to formaldehyde, which is responsible for antibacterial action against gram-positive and gram-negative organisms. Mandelic and hippuric acids, with which methenamines are combined, are also antibacterial.

Methylene blue is a mildly antiseptic dye. High concentrations convert the ferrous iron of reduced hemoglobin to ferric iron to form methemoglobin. This mechanism is the basis for its use as an antidote in cyanide poisoning. Low concentrations of methylene blue can hasten conversion of methemoglobin to hemoglobin.
• Cinoxacin and nalidixic acid are bacteriostatic, inhibiting DNA biosynthesis in microorganisms.
• Nitrofurantoin's bacteriostatic in low concentration and may be bactericidal in high concentration. It may interfere with bacterial enzyme systems.

Absorption, distribution, metabolism, and excretion

• Methenamines are rapidly absorbed and excreted in the urine (90% within 24 hours). Inactive in the blood, they are converted to ammonia and formaldehyde in the urine (at pH 5.5 or less).
• Methylene blue is poorly absorbed orally, but once in the tissues it is rapidly metabolized. It slowly passes into the bile and urine.
• Cinoxacin and nalidixic acid are readily absorbed after oral administration. They're partially metabolized in the liver and rapidly excreted by the kidneys.
• Nitrofurantoin is usually well absorbed from the gastrointestinal tract in either crystalline or macrocrystalline form. Various products may not be bioequivalent. Rapidly metabolized, the drug reaches therapeutic concentration only in the urine, where it is promptly excreted.

Onset and duration

• With methenamine, methylene blue, and nitrofurantoin, antibacterial activity begins within 30 minutes; cinoxacin and nalidixic acid begin to act within 4 hours.

• Antibacterial levels are sustained with twice-daily dosing of cinoxacin and methenamine hippurate. The other urinary tract antiseptics require more frequent dosing.

Combination products

AZO GANTANOL: sulfamethoxazole 500 mg and phenazopyridine HCl 100 mg.
AZO GANTRISIN: sulfisoxazole 500 mg and phenazopyridine HCl 50 mg.
AZO-MANDELAMINE: methenamine mandelate 500 mg and phenazopyridine HCl 50 mg.
AZOTREX: tetracycline phosphate complex equivalent to 125 mg tetracycline HCl activity, sulfamethizole 250 mg, and phenazopyridine HCl 50 mg.
CYSTEX: methenamine 162 mg, salicylamide 65 mg, sodium salicylate 97 mg, and benzoic acid 32 mg.
CYSTISED IMPROVED: methenamine 40.8 mg, phenyl salicylate 18.1 mg, atropine sulfate 0.03 mg, hyoscyamine 0.03 mg, benzoic acid 4.5 mg, methylene blue 5.4 mg, and gelsemium 6.1 mg.
HEXALOL: methenamine 40.8 mg, phenyl salicylate 18.1 mg, atropine sulfate 0.03 mg, hyoscyamine 0.03 mg, benzoic acid 4.5 mg, and methylene blue 5.4 mg.
METHENAMINE AND SODIUM BIPHOSPHATE: methenamine 325 mg and sodium biphosphate 325 mg.
PROSED: methylene blue 5.4 mg, methenamine 40.8 mg, phenyl salicylate 18.1 mg, atropine sulfate 0.03 mg, hyoscyamine 0.03 mg, and benzoic acid 4.5 mg.
SULADYNE: sulfamethizole 125 mg, sulfadiazine 125 mg, and phenazopyridine HCl 75 mg.
THIOSULFIL-A: sulfamethizole 250 mg and phenazopyridine HCl 50 mg.
URO-PHOSPHATE: methenamine 300 mg and sodium acid phosphate 500 mg. Sugar coated.
UROQID-ACID: methenamine mandelate 350 mg and sodium acid phosphate 200 mg.
UROQID-ACID NO. 2: methenamine mandelate 500 mg and sodium acid phosphate 500 mg.

QUESTIONS & ANSWERS

COPING WITH NITROFURANTOIN NAUSEA

What can be done to minimize gastrointestinal upset in a patient taking nitrofurantoin?

Here are several alternatives:

• Reducing the dose may ease nausea and vomiting, especially in small persons. But keep in mind that the minimum effective dose of nitrofurantoin is 5 mg/kg/day.
• The macrocrystalline form of the drug (Macrodantin) is better tolerated because it's absorbed more slowly than the crystalline form. Although effective urine concentrations of the macroscrystalline form may be delayed, this doesn't hinder effective nitrofurantoin treatment.
• The drug should be administered with milk or meals. This also slows drug absorption, reducing nausea.
• Another drug may be substituted.

NAMES, INDICATIONS AND DOSAGES	SIDE EFFECTS
cinoxacin Cinobac **Treatment of initial and recurrent urinary tract infections caused by susceptible strains of *Escherichia coli, Klebiella, Enterobacter, Proteus mirabilis, Proteus vulgaris,* and *Proteus morgani, Serratia,* and *Citrobacter:*** ADULTS AND CHILDREN 12 YEARS OR OLDER: 1 g daily, in two to four divided doses for 7 to 14 days. Not recommended for children under 12 years.	**CNS:** *dizziness, headache,* drowsiness, insomnia, convulsions. **EENT:** sensitivity to light. **GI:** *nausea, vomiting, abdominal pain,* diarrhea. **Skin:** rash, urticaria, pruritis.
methenamine hippurate Hiprex, Hip-Rex♦♦, Urex **methenamine mandelate** Mandacon, Mandelamine♦, Mandelets, Mandelurine♦♦, Methandine♦♦, Prov-U-Sep, Sterine♦♦ **Long-term prophylaxis or suppression of chronic urinary tract infections:** ADULTS AND CHILDREN OVER 12 YEARS: 1 g P.O. q 12 hours. CHILDREN 6 TO 12 YEARS: 500 mg to 1 g P.O. q 12 hours. **Urinary tract infections, infected residual urine in patients with neurogenic bladder:** ADULTS: 1 g P.O. q.i.d. after meals. CHILDREN 6 TO 12 YEARS: 500 mg P.O. q.i.d. after meals. CHILDREN UNDER 6 YEARS: 50 mg/kg divided in 4 doses after meals.	**GU:** with high doses, urinary tract irritation, dysuria, frequency, albuminuria, hematuria. **Hepatic:** elevated liver enzymes. **Skin:** rashes.
methylene blue MG-Blue, Urolene Blue, Wright's Stain **Cystitis, urethritis:** ADULTS: 65 mg P.O. b.i.d. or t.i.d. after meals with glass of water. **Methemoglobinemia and cyanide poisoning:** ADULTS AND CHILDREN: 1 to 2 mg/kg of 1% sterile solution slow I.V.	**Blood:** anemia (long-term use). **GI:** nausea, vomiting, diarrhea. **GU:** dysuria, bladder irritation. **Other:** fever (large doses).
nalidixic acid NegGram♦ **Acute and chronic urinary tract infections caused by susceptible gram-negative organisms *(Proteus, Klebsiella, Enterobacter,* and *Escherichia coli):*** ADULTS: 1 g P.O. q.i.d. for 7 to 14 days; 2 g daily for long-term use. CHILDREN OVER 3 MONTHS: 55 mg/kg P.O. daily divided q.i.d. for 7 to 14 days; 33 mg/kg/day for long-term use.	**Blood:** eosinophilia. **CNS:** drowsiness, weakness, headache, dizziness, vertigo, convulsions in epileptics. **EENT:** sensitivity to light, change in color perception, diplopia, blurred vision. **GI:** *abdominal pain, nausea, vomiting,* diarrhea. **Skin:** pruritus, photosensitivity, urticaria, rash. **Other:** angioedema, fever, chills, increased intracranial pressure and bulging fontanelles in infants and children.

INTERACTIONS AND SPECIAL CONSIDERATIONS

Interactions:
PROBENECID: may decrease urinary levels of cinoxacin by inhibiting renal tubular secretion. Monitor for increased toxicity and reduced antibacterial effectiveness.

Special considerations:
• Contraindicated in patients who are hypersensitive to nalidixic acid. Use cautiously in patients with impaired renal and hepatic function.
• Not effective against *Pseudomonas*, enterococci, or staphylococci.
• A clean-catch urine specimen for culture and sensitivity tests should be obtained before starting therapy and repeated p.r.n.
• High urine levels permit twice-daily dosing.
• CNS side effects should be reported immediately. They indicate serious toxicity and usually mean that administration of drug should be stopped.
• Cinoxacin should be taken with meals to help decrease GI side effects.
• Resistant bacteria may emerge with this drug.
• Photophobic effects are possible; patient should avoid very bright sunlight.

Interactions:
ALKALINIZING AGENTS: inhibit methenamine action. Don't use together.
ACETAZOLAMIDE: antagonizes methenamine effect. Use together cautiously.

Special considerations:
• Contraindicated in patients with renal insufficiency, severe hepatic disease, or severe dehydration.
• Ineffective against *Candida* infection.
• Oral suspension contains vegetable oil. Should be administered cautiously to elderly or debilitated patients because aspiration could cause lipid pneumonia.
• Intake and output should be monitored. Intake should be at least 1,500 to 2,000 ml/day.
• Clean-catch urine specimen should be obtained for culture and sensitivity tests before starting therapy, and repeated p.r.n.
• Patient should limit intake of alkaline foods, such as vegetables, milk, peanuts, fruits, and fruit juices, except cranberry, plum, and prune juices. These juices or ascorbic acid may be used to acidify urine.
• Patient should not take antacids, including Alka-Seltzer and sodium bicarbonate.
• Urine pH should be maintained at 5.5 or less and Nitrazine paper used to check pH.
• *Proteus* and *Pseudomonas* tend to raise urine pH; urinary acidifiers are usually necessary when treating these infections.
• Periodic liver function studies recommended during long-term therapy.
• Administration after meals lessens GI upset.
• Drug should be discontinued at once and therapy reevaluated if rash appears.

No significant interactions.

Special considerations:
• Contraindicated in patients with renal insufficiency.
• Intake and output should be monitored carefully. Intake should be at least 2,000 ml/day.
• Hemoglobin should be monitored; possibility of anemia from accelerated destruction of erythrocytes.
• Turns urine and stool blue-green.
• Seldom used as urinary antiseptic.
• I.V. form has been used to treat nitrite intoxication.

Interactions:
NITROFURANTOIN: may antagonize nalidixic acid effect. Use together cautiously.

Special considerations:
• Contraindicated in patients with convulsive disorders. Use with caution in impaired hepatic or renal function, epilepsy, or severe cerebral arteriosclerosis.
• Not effective against *Pseudomonas*.
• Patient should report visual disturbances; usually disappear with reduced dose.
• Clean-catch urine specimen should be obtained for culture and sensitivity tests before starting therapy, and repeated p.r.n.
• CBC and renal and hepatic function studies should be obtained during long-term therapy.
• Resistant bacteria may emerge within the first 48 hours of therapy.
• May cause a false-positive Clinitest reaction. Clinistix or Tes-Tape should be used to monitor urine glucose. Also gives false elevations in urinary vanillylmandelic acid and 17-ketosteroids. Tests should be repeated after therapy completed.
• Patient should avoid undue exposure to sunlight due to photosensitivity. Patient may continue to be photosensitive up to 3 months after drug is discontinued.

NAMES, INDICATIONS AND DOSAGES	SIDE EFFECTS
nitrofurantoin Furadantin, Furalan, Furantoin, Furatine♦♦, Ivadantin, J-Dantin, Nephronex♦♦, Nifuran♦♦, Nitrex, Novofuran♦♦, Sarodant **nitrofurantoin macrocrystals** Macrodantin♦ **Pyelonephritis, pyelitis, and cystitis due to susceptible *Escherichia coli, Staphylococcus aureus,* enterococci; certain strains of *Klebsiella, Proteus,* and *Enterobacter:*** ADULTS AND CHILDREN OVER 12 YEARS: 50 to 100 mg P.O. q.i.d. with meals. Or, 180 mg I.M. or I.V. b.i.d. in patients over 55 kg; 5 to 7 mg/kg daily I.M. or I.V. in patients under 55 kg. CHILDREN 1 MONTH TO 12 YEARS: 5 to 7 mg/kg P.O. daily, divided q.i.d.	**Blood:** hemolysis in patients with G-6-PD deficiency (reversed after stopping drug). **CNS:** peripheral neuropathy, headache, dizziness, drowsiness, ascending polyneuropathy with high doses or renal impairment. **GI:** anorexia, *nausea, vomiting,* abdominal pain, *diarrhea.* **Hepatic:** hepatitis. **Skin:** maculopapular, erythematous, or eczematous eruption; pruritus; urticaria. **Other:** asthmatic attacks in patients with history of asthma; *anaphylaxis;* drug fever; overgrowth of nonsusceptible organisms in the urinary tract; *pulmonary sensitivity reactions (cough, chest pains, fever, chills, dyspnea).*

♦ Available in U.S. and Canada. ♦♦ Available in Canada only.
All other products (no symbol) available in U.S. only. Italicized side effects are common or life-threatening.

INTERACTIONS AND SPECIAL CONSIDERATIONS

No significant interactions.

Special considerations:
- Contraindicated in patients with moderate to severe renal impairment, anuria, oliguria, creatinine clearance under 40 ml/minute; in patients with G-6-PD deficiency.
- Clean-catch urine specimen should be obtained for culture and sensitivity before starting therapy, and repeated p.r.n.
- Should be taken with food or milk to minimize GI distress.
- I.M. route painful and should not be used for more than 5 days.
- I.V. nitrofurantoin should be diluted to 500 ml of suitable I.V. solution before administering, and reconstituted in sterile water without preservatives.
- Intake and output should be monitored carefully. May turn urine brown or darker.
- Store in amber container. Keep away from metals other than stainless steel or aluminum to avoid precipitate formation. Patient should not use pillboxes made of these materials.
- Treatment should be continued for 3 days after sterile urines obtained.
- Pulmonary status should be monitored.
- For symptoms and treatment of anaphylaxis, see APPENDIX.

18

Miscellaneous anti-infectives

amantadine hydrochloride
bacitracin
chloramphenicol
chloramphenicol palmitate
chloramphenicol sodium succinate
clindamycin hydrochloride
clindamycin palmitate hydrochloride
clindamycin phosphate
colistimethate sodium
erythromycin base
erythromycin estolate
erythromycin ethylsuccinate
erythromycin gluceptate
erythromycin lactobionate
erythromycin stearate
furazolidone
lincomycin hydrochloride
novobiocin calcium
novobiocin sodium
polymyxin B sulfate
spectinomycin dihydrochloride
trimethoprim
troleandomycin phosphate
vancomycin hydrochloride
vidarabine monohydrate

By inhibiting or destroying bacteria or viruses, these miscellaneous anti-infectives provide broad protection against several infectious diseases.

Major uses

- Amantadine is prophylactic in epidemic influenza A viral infections.
- Bacitracin is occasionally used parenterally to treat infants with staphylococcal pneumonia when it's resistant to other drugs. As a bladder irrigating agent, bacitracin protects against gram-positive bacteria.
- Chloramphenicol has broad activity against rickettsia and many gram-positive and gram-negative bacteria. It's the drug of choice in both salmonella infections and infections caused by ampicillin-resistant strains of *Hemophilus influenzae*.
- Clindamycin and lincomycin are effective against respiratory tract, skin, and soft tissue infections caused by susceptible strains of staphylococci, streptococci, and pneumococci.
- Parenteral colistimethate may be used to treat serious infections caused by susceptible strains of *Pseudomonas aeruginosa, Escherichia coli,* and *Klebsiella pneumoniae*. Oral preparations are occasionally used to treat infants with diarrhea due to enterotoxigenic strains of *E. coli*.
- Erythromycins are the drugs of choice in Legionnaires' disease, *Mycoplasma pneumoniae* pneumonia, *Campylobacter fetus* enteritis, and acute diphtheria and its carrier state. As alternatives to penicillin, they're therapeutic in streptococcal, pneumococcal, staphylococcal, gonococcal, and syphilitic diseases, and prophylactic in rheumatic fever. They may also be used for chronic bronchitis, otitis media, and nongonococcal urethritis.
- Furazolidone is now used rarely for intestinal infections caused by susceptible strains of *E. coli, Staphylococcus aureus, Proteus,* and *Giardia lamblia*.
- Novobiocin is used rarely in the treatment of serious infections caused by strains of *S. aureus* and *Proteus* that resist other antibiotics.
- Polymyxin B is usually combined with bacitracin or neomycin in topical creams and ointments and in bladder-irrigating solutions to protect against *P. aeruginosa, E. coli, Enterobacter,* and *Klebsiella*. It is rarely used systemically for serious infections caused by *P. aeruginosa*.
- Spectinomycin is used in the treatment of penicillin-resistant strains of gonorrhea.
- Trimethoprim is most commonly combined with sulfamethoxazole. It is also therapeutic when used alone for urinary tract infections caused by susceptible strains of *E. coli, Enterobacter,* and *K. pneumoniae*.

THE ROLE OF ORAL VANCOMYCIN IN PSEUDOMEMBRANOUS ENTEROCOLITIS

Pseudomembranous enterocolitis is a serious and possibly fatal disease. It occurs when long-term, high-dose antibiotic therapy (such as with clindamycin) kills most normal bowel flora, allowing *Clostridium difficile* to overgrow and produce an endotoxin that damages the bowel wall. Once the bowel wall is damaged, a pseudomembrane composed of creamy white or yellow fibrous patches, fibrin debris, and white cells forms over the damaged area (see illustration).

Symptoms of pseudomembranous enterocolitis include severe diarrhea, fever, chills, abdominal distention with crampy pain, and loss of appetite. Patients with this disorder also have clostridial toxin in the stool and lesions in the bowel wall.

If these symptoms appear, the patient will probably be treated with oral vancomycin for 7 to 14 days. Given orally, vancomycin reaches high levels in the stool, decreasing toxin concentrations there and gradually alleviating diarrhea. Because vancomycin's not absorbed systemically, it probably won't cause unpleasant side effects.

After oral vancomycin therapy, relapse is unlikely but if it occurs, is responsive to retreatment. Because pseudomembranous enterocolitis has responded to retreatment, researchers believe that relapse isn't due to the development of a resistant strain.

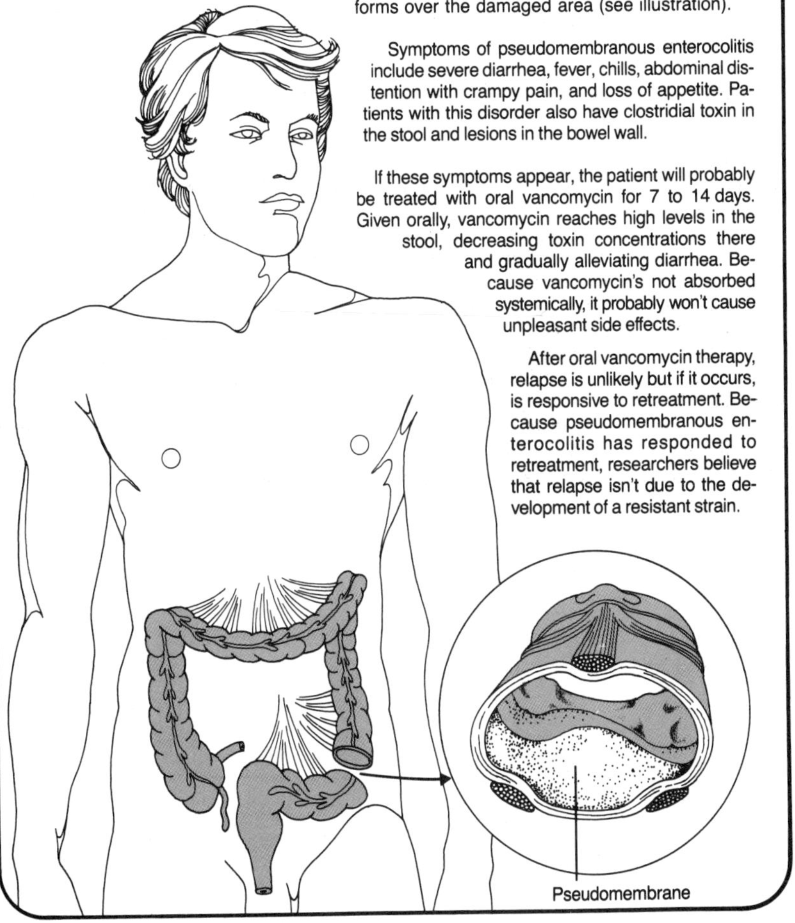

Pseudomembrane

• Troleandomycin may be used to treat infections caused by *Streptococcus pyogenes* and *Streptococcus pneumoniae,* but it's less potent than erythromycin. It may also be used as a steroid-sparing drug in the management of steroid-dependent asthma.
• Vancomycin is used primarily for severe staphylococcal infections resistant to the semisynthetic penicillins and cephalosporins. It may also be used as a prophylactic and therapeutic alternative to penicillins for streptococcal endocarditis. The oral form is the drug of choice for the treatment of antibiotic-induced pseudomembranous enterocolitis.
• Vidarabine is used systemically for serious viral infections caused by herpes simplex and herpes zoster.

Mechanism of action
• Amantadine may interfere with influenza A virus penetration into susceptible cells.
• Bacitracin, colistimethate, polymyxin B, and vancomycin all hinder bacterial cell wall synthesis, damaging the bacterial plasma membrane and making the cell more vulnerable to osmotic pressure.
• Chloramphenicol, clindamycin, lincomycin, erythromycin, and troleandomycin inhibit bacterial protein synthesis by binding to the 50S subunit of the ribosome.
• Furazolidone's mechanism of action is unknown.
• Novobiocin interferes with bacterial cell wall, protein, and nucleic acid synthesis.
• Trimethoprim interferes with the action of dihydrofolate reductase, inhibiting bacterial synthesis of folic acid.
• Vidarabine, as its phosphorylated metabolite, becomes incorporated into viral deoxyribonucleic acid and inhibits viral multiplication.

Absorption, distribution, metabolism, and excretion
• Amantadine is well absorbed from the gastrointestinal (GI) tract. More than 90% is excreted unchanged in the urine within 4 days.
• Bacitracin is not absorbed orally but is absorbed quickly and completely after I.M. administration. It is widely distributed to the tissues and slowly excreted by the kidneys.
• Chloramphenicol, readily absorbed from the GI tract, is distributed rapidly; highest concentrations occur in the liver and kidneys. Cerebrospinal fluid (CSF) levels reach approximately half the blood level. About 90% is metabolized in the liver and excreted by the kidneys; the remainder is excreted unchanged in the urine.
• Clindamycin is almost completely absorbed in both capsule and solution forms. Food can delay but not decrease its absorption. The drug is widely distributed to most body tissues but doesn't cross the blood-brain barrier unless the meninges are inflamed. Most clindamycin is metabolized by the liver and passed into the bile for ultimate elimination in the feces.
• Colistimethate is not absorbed orally. It is excreted unchanged, mainly in the urine.
• Erythromycin absorption varies greatly, depending on the salt and the dosage form (absorption of erythromycin estolate is greatest). The free base and the estolate, ethyl-

succinate, and stearate salts are given orally, whereas lactobionate and gluceptate salts are reserved for parenteral use. Widely distributed except in the brain and CSF, the drug is partially metabolized in the liver and passed into the bile for elimination in the feces.

• Furazolidone, when given orally, is poorly absorbed and doesn't reach therapeutic blood levels. About 5% is excreted in the urine.

• Lincomycin absorption is impaired by food; patients in the fasting state, however, may absorb as much as 30%. Widely distributed except in CSF, it is partly metabolized by the liver and passed into the bile for elimination primarily in the feces.

• Novobiocin diffuses well into pleural, joint, and ascitic fluids but poorly or not at all into CSF, unless the meninges are inflamed; the drug is eliminated in bile, urine, and feces.

• Polymyxin B is not absorbed from the GI tract; blood levels are low, as the drug loses 50% of its activity in blood. It diffuses poorly into tissues and is excreted slowly by the kidneys.

• Spectinomycin is not absorbed from the GI tract but is well absorbed after I.M. administration. It is widely distributed and excreted unchanged by the kidneys.

• Trimethoprim is well absorbed after oral administration. It is widely distributed to most body tissues, except the central nervous system. About 50% is excreted unchanged by the kidneys; the rest is metabolized to inactive compounds and excreted in the urine.

• Troleandomycin is more readily absorbed orally than is erythromycin; 18% to 24% is excreted in the urine, 60% to 70% in the bile.

• Vancomycin is not absorbed orally. After I.V. administration, it is widely distributed, except in CSF, and excreted in urine virtually unchanged.

• Vidarabine is poorly absorbed from the GI tract. It is extensively metabolized to the active metabolite arabinosylhypoxanthine, which is widely distributed in all tissues, including the CSF. It is excreted by the kidneys over 24 hours.

Onset and duration

• Orally administered drugs (amantadine, chloramphenicol, clindamycin, erythromycin, lincomycin, novobiocin, trimethoprim, and troleandomycin) give peak blood levels usually within 2 hours.

• Drugs given I.M. (bacitracin, clindamycin, colistimethate, lincomycin, novobiocin, polymyxin B, and spectinomycin) give peak blood levels usually within 1 hour.

• Drugs given I.V. give peak blood levels almost immediately, so they should be given by this route in acute, life-threatening situations.

• Duration of effect varies from 2 to 6 hours for most of these drugs. The effects of amantadine, novobiocin, polymyxin B, and vancomycin last up to 24 hours; trimethoprim is active for about 12 hours.

Combination products

None.

NAMES, INDICATIONS AND DOSAGES	SIDE EFFECTS
amantadine hydrochloride Symmetrel♦ **Prophylaxis or symptomatic treatment of influenza type A virus, respiratory tract illnesses:** ADULTS AND CHILDREN OVER 9 YEARS: 200 mg P.O. daily in a single dose or divided b.i.d. CHILDREN 1 TO 9 YEARS: 4.4 to 8.8 mg/kg P.O. daily, divided b.i.d. or t.i.d. Don't exceed 150 mg daily. Treatment should continue for 24 to 48 hours after symptoms disappear. Prophylaxis should start as soon as possible after initial exposure and continue for at least 10 days after exposure. May continue prophylactic treatment up to 90 days for repeated or suspected exposures if influenza vaccine unavailable. If used with influenza vaccine, continue dose for 2 to 3 weeks until protection from vaccine develops.	**CNS:** depression, fatigue, confusion, dizziness, psychosis, hallucinations, anxiety, irritability, ataxia, insomnia, weakness, headache. **CV:** peripheral edema, orthostatic hypotension, congestive heart failure. **GI:** anorexia, nausea, constipation, vomiting, dry mouth. **GU:** urinary retention.
bacitracin **Pneumonia or empyema caused by susceptible staphylococci:** INFANTS OVER 2.5 KG: 1,000 units/kg I.M. daily, divided q 8 to 12 hours. INFANTS UNDER 2.5 KG: 900 units/kg I.M. daily, divided q 8 to 12 hours. Although the FDA approves the use of bacitracin in infants only, adults with susceptible staphylococcal infections may receive 10,000 to 25,000 units I.M. q 6 hours (maximum 25,000 units/dose, 100,000 units/day).	**Blood:** blood dyscrasias, eosinophilia. **GI:** nausea, vomiting, anorexia, diarrhea, rectal itching or burning. **GU:** nephrotoxicity *(albuminuria,* cylindruria, oliguria, anuria, increased BUN, tubular and glomerular necrosis). **Skin:** urticaria, rash. **Local:** *pain at injection site.* **Other:** superinfection, fever, *anaphylaxis.*
chloramphenicol **chloramphenicol palmitate** **chloramphenicol sodium succinate** Chloromycetin♦, Mychel, Novochlorocap♦♦ ***Hemophilus influenzae* meningitis, acute *Salmonella typhi* infection, severe infections caused by sensitive *Salmonella* species, *Rickettsia,* lymphogranuloma, psittacosis, various sensitive gram-negative organisms causing meningitis, bacteremia, or other serious infections:** ADULTS AND CHILDREN: 50 to 100 mg/kg P.O. or I.V. daily, divided q 6 hours. Maximum dose is 100 mg/kg/day. PREMATURE INFANTS AND NEONATES 2 WEEKS OR YOUNGER: 25 mg/kg P.O. or I.V. daily, divided q 6 hours. I.V. route must be used to treat meningitis.	**Blood:** *aplastic anemia,* hypoplastic anemia, *granulocytopenia,* thrombocytopenia. **CNS:** headache, mild depression, confusion, delirium, peripheral neuropathy with prolonged therapy. **EENT:** optic neuritis (in patients with cystic fibrosis), glossitis, decreased visual acuity. **GI:** nausea, vomiting, stomatitis, diarrhea, enterocolitis. **Other:** infections by nonsusceptible organisms, hypersensitivity reaction (fever, rash, urticaria, *anaphylaxis), gray baby syndrome in premature and newborn infants (abdominal distention, gray cyanosis, vasomotor collapse, respiratory distress, death within a few hours of onset of symptoms).*

♦ Available in U.S. and Canada. ♦♦ Available in Canada only.
All other products (no symbol) available in U.S. only. Italicized side effects are common or life-threatening.

INTERACTIONS AND SPECIAL CONSIDERATIONS

No significant interactions.

Special considerations:

• Use cautiously in patients with history of epilepsy, congestive heart failure, peripheral edema, hepatic disease, mental illness, eczematoid rash, renal impairment, orthostatic hypotension, cardiovascular disease, and in elderly patients.
• For best absorption, drug should be taken after meals.
• Patient should report side effects to the doctor, especially dizziness, depression, anxiety, nausea, and urinary retention.
• Electrolyte balance and urinary output should be monitored.
• If orthostatic hypotension occurs, patient should not stand or change positions abruptly.
• If insomnia occurs, dose should be taken several hours before bedtime.
• Prophylactic use recommended for patients who can't receive influenza virus vaccine.

No significant interactions.

Special considerations:

• Contraindicated in patients with impaired renal function. Use cautiously in superinfections or neuromuscular disease.
• Culture and sensitivity tests should be done initially and p.r.n.
• For I.M. administration only. Should be given deep I.M.; injection may be painful; should be diluted in solution containing sodium chloride and 2% procaine hydrochloride. Should not be given if patient is sensitive to procaine or PABA derivatives.
• Fluid intake and urinary output should be monitored closely. If intake or output decreases, the doctor should be notified.
• Baseline renal function studies should be obtained before starting therapy. Renal function (BUN, serum creatinine, creatinine clearance) should be monitored daily during therapy.
• Concentration of bacitracin should be between 5,000 and 10,000 units/ml. Should be stored in refrigerator. Drug is inactivated at room temperature.
• Side effects should be reported immediately.
• May be used with neomycin as a bowel preparation, or in solution as a wound irrigant.
• Urine pH should be kept above 6.0.
• Prolonged therapy may result in overgrowth of nonsusceptible organisms, especially *Candida albicans*.
• For treatment of anaphylaxis, see APPENDIX.

Interactions:

PENICILLINS: antagonize antibacterial effect. Give penicillin at least 1 hour before.
ACETAMINOPHEN: elevates chloramphenicol levels. Monitor for chloramphenicol toxicity.

Special considerations:

• Use cautiously in patients with impaired hepatic or renal function, with other drugs causing bone marrow depression or blood disorders. *Don't use for infections caused by organisms susceptible to other agents or for trivial infections such as colds; use only when clearly indicated for severe infection.*
• Culture and sensitivity tests should be done concurrently with first dose and p.r.n.
• CBC, platelets, serum iron, and reticulocytes should be monitored before and every 2 days during therapy. Drug should be stopped immediately if anemia, reticulocytopenia, leukopenia, or thrombocytopenia develops.
• Patient should report side effects, especially nausea, vomiting, diarrhea, fever, confusion, sore throat, or mouth sores.
• Patient should take medication for as long as prescribed, exactly as directed, even after he feels better.
• Should be given I.V. slowly over 1 minute, and injection site checked daily for phlebitis and irritation.
• 1-g vial of powder for injection should be reconstituted with 10 ml sterile water for injection. Concentration will be 100 mg/ml. Stable for 30 days at room temperature but refrigeration recommended. Cloudy solutions should not be used.
• Superinfection by nonsusceptible organisms possible.
• For treatment of anaphylaxis, see APPENDIX.

NAMES, INDICATIONS AND DOSAGES	SIDE EFFECTS
clindamycin hydrochloride **clindamycin palmitate hydrochloride** **clindamycin phosphate** Cleocin, Dalacin C♦♦ **Infections caused by sensitive staphylococci, streptococci, pneumococci, *Bacteroides, Fusobacterium, Clostridium perfringens,* and other sensitive aerobic and anaerobic organisms:** ADULTS: 150 to 450 mg P.O. q 6 hours; or 300 mg I.M. or I.V. q 6, 8, or 12 hours. Up to 2,700 mg I.M. or I.V. daily, divided q 6, 8, or 12 hours. May be used for severe infections. CHILDREN OVER 1 MONTH: 8 to 25 mg/kg P.O. daily, divided q 6 to 8 hours; or 15 to 40 mg/kg I.M. or I.V. daily, divided q 6 hours.	**Blood:** transient leukopenia, eosinophilia, thrombocytopenia. **GI:** *nausea,* vomiting, abdominal pain, *diarrhea, pseudomembranous enterocolitis,* esophagitis, flatulence, anorexia, *bloody or tarry stools.* **Hepatic:** elevated SGOT, alkaline phosphatase, bilirubin. **Skin:** maculopapular rash, urticaria. **Local:** *pain,* induration, *sterile abscess with I.M. injection;* thrombophlebitis, erythema, and pain after I.V. administration. **Other:** unpleasant or bitter taste, *anaphylaxis.*
colistimethate sodium Colistin Sulfate, Coly-Mycin M♦, Coly-Mycin S Oral **Enterocolitis caused by sensitive *Escherichia coli,* sensitive *Shigella,* gastroenteritis:** INFANTS AND CHILDREN: 5 to 15 mg/kg P.O. daily, divided q 6 to 8 hours. **Severe infections, especially of urinary tract, caused by sensitive *Pseudomonas, Enterobacter, E. coli,* and *Klebsiella:*** ADULTS AND CHILDREN: 2.5 to 5 mg/kg I.M. or I.V. daily, divided q 6 to 12 hours. Maximum daily dose not to exceed 5 mg/kg/day in patients with normal renal function.	**CNS:** *circumoral and lingual paresthesias;* paresthesias of extremities; neuromuscular blockage with respiratory arrest, especially in patients with impaired renal function; dizziness; slurring of speech. **GI:** nausea, vomiting, discomfort. **GU:** *nephrotoxicity* (decreased urine output, increased BUN and serum creatinine). **Skin:** pruritus, urticaria. **Local:** pain at I.M. site. **Other:** "drug fever," overgrowth of nonsusceptible organisms.
erythromycin base E-Mycin♦, Ery-Tab, Erythromid♦♦, Ethril 500, Ilotycin♦, Novorythro♦♦, Robimycin♦, Staticin **erythromycin estolate** Ilosone♦, Novorythro♦♦ **erythromycin ethylsuccinate** E.E.S., Erythrocin♦, Pediamycin, Wyamycin Liquid **erythromycin gluceptate** Ilotycin♦ **erythromycin lactobionate** Erythrocin♦ **erythromycin stearate** Bristamycin, E-Biotic, Erypar, Erythrocin♦, Ethril, Novorythro♦♦, Pfizer E, SK-Erythromycin, Wintrocin, Wyamycin **Acute pelvic inflammatory disease caused by *Neisseria gonorrhoeae:*** WOMEN: 500 mg I.V. (erythromycin gluceptate, lactobionate) q 6 hours for 3 days, then 250 mg (erythromycin base, estolate, stearate) or 400 mg (erythromycin ethylsuccinate) P.O. q 6 hours for 7 days.	**EENT:** hearing loss with high doses I.V. **GI:** *abdominal pain and cramping, nausea, vomiting, diarrhea.* **Hepatic:** cholestatic jaundice (with erythromycin estolate). **Skin:** urticaria, rashes. **Local:** *venous irritation, thrombophlebitis following I.V. injection.* **Other:** overgrowth of nonsusceptible bacteria or fungi; *anaphylaxis;* fever.

♦ Available in U.S. and Canada. ♦♦ Available in Canada only.
All other products (no symbol) available in U.S. only. Italicized side effects are common or life-threatening.

INTERACTIONS AND SPECIAL CONSIDERATIONS

Interactions:
ERYTHROMYCIN: antagonist that may block access of clindamycin to its site of action; don't use together.

Special considerations:
• Contraindicated in patients with known hypersensitivity to the antibiotic congener lincomycin; also in history of patients with GI disease, especially colitis. Use cautiously in newborns and in patients with renal or hepatic disease, asthma, or significant allergies.
• Renal, hepatic and hematopoietic functions should be monitored during prolonged therapy.
• Culture and sensitivity tests should be performed initially and p.r.n.
• Should not be used in meningitis. Drug does not penetrate cerebrospinal fluid.
• Don't refrigerate reconstituted oral solution, as it will thicken. Drug is stable for 2 weeks at room temperature.
• Patient should report side effects, especially diarrhea. Patient should not treat diarrhea himself.
• Diphenoxylate (Lomotil) should not be given to treat drug-induced diarrhea. May prolong and worsen diarrhea.
• Should be given deep I.M., and sites rotated. I.M. injection may be painful. Doses greater than 600 mg/injection are not recommended.
• When given I.V., site should be checked daily for phlebitis and irritation. For I.V. infusion, each 300 mg should be diluted in 50 ml solution, and given no faster than 30 mg/minute.
• I.M. injection may cause CPK levels to rise due to muscle irritation.
• Topical form is now available to treat acne.
• For treatment of anaphylaxis, see APPENDIX.

No significant interactions.

Special considerations:
• Contraindicated in patients with known hypersensitivity to the antibiotic congener polymyxin B. Use cautiously in renal impairment.
• Should be given deep I.M. and sites rotated; injection may be painful.
• Sterile water for injection should be used to reconstitute. When mixing, solution should be swirled gently to avoid frothing. I.V. infusion should always be prepared fresh and used within 24 hours.
• I.V. administration site should be checked daily for phlebitis and irritation. For direct I.V. administration, ½ daily dose should be injected over 3 to 5 minutes at 12-hour intervals.
• For continuous I.V. infusion, ½ daily dose should be directly injected over 3 to 5 minutes; the remaining ½ should be added to 5% dextrose, 5% dextrose in 0.9% sodium chloride, 5% dextrose in 0.45% sodium chloride, 5% dextrose in 0.225% sodium chloride, 10% invert sugar, lactated Ringer's injection, or 0.9% sodium chloride solution; then infuse 1 to 2 hours later at rate of 5mg/hour. 1 to 2 hours later at 5 mg/hour.
• Renal function (BUN, creatinine clearance, urinary output) should be closely monitored.
• Side effects may develop, especially speech impairment or paresthesias. Superinfection is possible.
• Store reconstituted oral suspension at 2° to 15° C. (35.6° to 59° F.) and use within 7 days.

Interactions:
CLINDAMYCIN, LINCOMYCIN: may be antagonistic. Don't use together.
PENICILLINS: antagonize antibacterial effect. Give penicillin at least 1 hour before.

Special considerations:
• Erythromycin estolate contraindicated in hepatic disease. Use other erythromycin salts cautiously in patients with impaired hepatic function.
• Culture and sensitivity test should be performed initially and p.r.n.
• For best absorption, patient should take oral form of drug with a full glass of water 1 hour before or 2 hours after meals. If tablets are coated, they may be taken with meals. Patient should not drink fruit juice with medication. Chewable erythromycin tablets should not be swallowed whole.
• Concentration should be noted when administering suspension.
• May cause an overgrowth of nonsusceptible bacteria or fungi. Superinfection is possible.
• Patient should take medication for as long as prescribed, exactly as directed, even if he feels better. Streptococcal infections should be treated for 10 days.
• Patient should report side effects, especially nausea, abdominal pain, or fever.
• Erythromycin estolate may cause serious hepatotoxicity in adults (reversible cholestatic hepatitis). Hepatic function (increased levels of bilirubin, SGOT, SGPT, alkaline phosphatase) should be monitored. Other erythromycin salts cause hepatotoxicity to a lesser degree.
• I.V. dose should be administered over 20 to 60 minutes. Should be reconstituted according to manufacturer's directions and each 250 mg should be diluted in at least 100 ml 5% dextrose in water or 0.9% normal saline solution.
• Erythromycin lactobionate should not be administered with other drugs.
• Has been used successfully in the treatment of Legionnaire's disease.
• Topical form now available to treat acne.
• For treatment of anaphylaxis, see APPENDIX.

(continued on following page)

NAMES, INDICATIONS AND DOSAGES	SIDE EFFECTS

erythromycin
(continued)

Endocarditis prophylaxis for dental procedures:
ADULTS: 1 g (erythromycin base, estolate, stearate) P.O. before procedure, followed by 250 mg P.O. q 6 hours for 8 doses afterward; or 1,200 mg (erythromycin ethylsuccinate) P.O. before procedure, followed by 400 mg P.O. q 6 hours for 8 doses afterward.
CHILDREN: 20 mg/kg (oral erythromycin salts) P.O. 1½ to 2 hours before procedure, then 10 mg/kg q 6 hours for 8 doses.

Intestinal amebiasis:
ADULTS: 250 mg (erythromycin base, estolate, stearate) P.O. q 6 hours for 10 to 14 days.
CHILDREN: 30 to 50 mg/kg (erythromycin base, estolate, stearate) P.O. daily, divided q 6 hours for 10 to 14 days.

Mild-to-moderately severe respiratory tract, skin, and soft tissue infections caused by sensitive group A beta-hemolytic streptococci, *Diplococcus pneumoniae, Mycoplasma pneumoniae, Corynebacterium diphtheriae, Bordetella pertussis, Listeria monocytogenes:*
ADULTS: 250 to 500 mg (erythromycin base, estolate, stearate) P.O. q 6 hours; or 400 to 800 mg (erythromycin ethylsuccinate) P.O. q 6 hours; or 15 to 20 mg/kg I.V. daily, as continuous infusion or divided q 6 hours.
CHILDREN: 30 mg/kg to 50 mg/kg (oral erythromycin salts) P.O. daily, divided q 6 hours; or 15 to 20 mg/kg I.V. daily, divided q 4 to 6 hours.

Syphilis:
ADULTS: 500 mg (erythromycin base, estolate, stearate) P.O. q.i.d. for 15 days.

---

furazolidone
Furoxone

Gastroenteritis, adjunctive therapy in cholera:
ADULTS: 100 mg P.O. q.i.d.
CHILDREN 5 TO 12 YEARS: 25 to 50 mg P.O. q.i.d.
CHILDREN 1 TO 4 YEARS: 17 to 25 mg P.O. q.i.d.
INFANTS 1 MONTH TO 1 YEAR: 8 to 17 mg P.O. q.i.d. Dosage based on 5 mg/kg daily; maximum dose 8.8 mg/kg daily.

Blood: hemolytic anemia in infants under 1 month and patients with G-6-PD deficiency; *agranulocytosis.*
CNS: headache, malaise.
GI: nausea, vomiting, abdominal pain, diarrhea.
Other: hypersensitivity reaction (arthralgia, fever, hypotension, rash, urticaria, angioedema), hypoglycemia.

---

lincomycin hydrochloride
Lincocin♦

Respiratory tract, skin and soft tissue, and urinary tract infections; osteomyelitis, septicemia, caused by sensitive group A beta-hemolytic streptococci, pneumococci, and

Blood: *neutropenia, leukopenia,* thrombocytopenia, purpura.
CNS: dizziness, headache.
CV: hypotension with rapid I.V. infusion.
EENT: glossitis, tinnitus.
GI: nausea, vomiting, *persistent diarrhea,* abdominal cramps, enterocolitis, stomatitis, and

INTERACTIONS AND SPECIAL CONSIDERATIONS

Interactions:
SYMPATHOMIMETICS: hypertensive crisis. Don't use together.

Special considerations:
• Patient should take medication exactly as directed, even if he feels better.
• Side effects should be reported, especially fever, rash, abdominal pain.
• Store medication in dark place at 2° to 15° C. (36.5° to 59° F.).
• Patient should not use over-the-counter nasal sprays or cold and hay fever products.
• Drug may turn urine brown. Flushing, nausea, sweating may occur following ethanol ingestion. Patient should not drink alcohol or use alcohol-containing medication.
• Patient taking drug more than 5 days should avoid eating broad beans, cheese, pickled herring, chicken livers, yeast extracts, or fermented products. Drug is similar to monoamine oxidase inhibitor.
• May cause false-positive urine glucose with Benedict's Reagent.
• Frequent blood and urine studies should be performed on patients with G-6-PD deficiency to detect homolysis.

Interactions:
ANTIDIARRHEAL MEDICATION (KAOLIN, PECTIN, ATTAPULGITE): reduce oral absorption of lincomycin by as much as 90%. Antidiarrheals should be avoided or given at least 2 hours before lincomycin.

Special considerations:
• Contraindicated in known hypersensitivity to clindamycin. Use cautiously in patients with history of GI disorders (especially colitis); asthma or significant allergies; hepatic or renal disease; and endocrine or metabolic disorders.
• Culture and sensitivity tests should be done

(continued on following page)

NAMES, INDICATIONS AND DOSAGES	SIDE EFFECTS

lincomycin hydrochloride
(continued)

staphylococci:
ADULTS: 500 mg P.O. q 6 to 8 hours (not to exceed 8 g daily); or 600 mg I.M. daily or q 12 hours; or 600 mg to 1 g I.V. q 8 to 12 hours (not to exceed 8 g daily).
CHILDREN OVER 1 MONTH: 30 to 60 mg/kg P.O. daily, divided q 6 to 8 hours; or 10 mg/kg I.M. daily or divided q 12 hours; or 10 to 20 mg/kg I.V. daily, divided q 6 to 8 hours. For I.V. infusion, dilute to 100 ml; infuse over 1 hour to avoid hypotension.

pruritus ani.
GU: vaginitis.
Hepatic: cholestatic jaundice.
Skin: rashes, urticaria.
Local: pain at injection site.
Other: hypersensitivity, angioedema.

---

novobiocin calcium
novobiocin sodium
Albamycin

Serious infections from sensitive *Staphylococcus aureus* and *Proteus* when other antibiotics are contraindicated:
ADULTS: 250 to 500 mg P.O. q 6 hours, or 500 mg to 1 g q 12 hours (not to exceed 2 g daily).
CHILDREN: 15 to 45 mg/kg P.O. daily, divided q 6 hours.

Blood: pancytopenia, *leukopenia, agranulocytosis,* anemia, thrombocytopenia, eosinophilia.
GI: nausea, vomiting, anorexia, diarrhea, intestinal hemorrhage.
Hepatic: jaundice, hepatitis.
Skin: urticaria, *maculopapular dermatitis.*
Local: pain at injection site.
Other: *erythema multiforme,* fever in hypersensitivity reactions, swollen joints, overgrowth of nonsusceptible organisms.

---

polymyxin B sulfate
Aerosporin♦

Acute urinary tract infections or septicemia caused by sensitive *Pseudomonas aeruginosa,* or when other antibiotics are ineffective or contraindicated; bacteremia caused by sensitive *Enterobacter aerogenes* and *Klebsiella pneumoniae,* or acute urinary tract infections caused by *Escherichia coli:*
ADULTS AND CHILDREN: 15,000 to 25,000 units/kg/day I.V. infusion, divided q 12 hours; or 25,000 to 30,000 units/kg/day, divided q 4 to 8 hours. I.M. not advised due to severe pain at injection site.

Meningitis caused by sensitive *P. aeruginosa* or *Hemophilus influenzae* when other antibiotics ineffective or contraindicated:
ADULTS AND CHILDREN OVER 2 YEARS: 50,000 units intrathecally once daily for 3 to 4 days, then 50,000 units every other day for at least 2 weeks after cerebrospinal fluid tests are negative and cerebrospinal fluid sugar is normal.
CHILDREN UNDER 2 YEARS: 20,000 units intrathecally once daily for 3 to 4 days, then 25,000 units every other day for at least 2 weeks after cerebrospinal fluid tests are negative and cerebrospinal fluid sugar is normal.

CNS: irritability, drowsiness, facial flushing, weakness, ataxia, respiratory paralysis, headache and meningeal irritation with intrathecal administration, peripheral and perioral paresthesias, convulsions, *coma.*
EENT: blurred vision.
GU: nephrotoxicity (albuminuria, cylindruria, hematuria, proteinuria, decreased urine output, increased BUN).
Skin: urticaria.
Local: *pain at I.M. injection site.*
Other: hypersensitivity reactions with fever, *anaphylaxis.*

INTERACTIONS AND SPECIAL CONSIDERATIONS

initially and p.r.n.
- For best absorption, patient should take drug with a full glass of water 1 hour before or 2 hours after meals.
- Patient should take medication exactly as directed, even if he feels better.
- Patient should report side effects, especially diarrhea, and not treat diarrhea himself. Superinfection is possible, especially when therapy exceeds 10 days.
- Drug-induced diarrhea should never be treated with diphenoxylate compound (Lomotil); it may prolong or worsen diarrhea.
- Should be given deep I.M., and sites rotated. I.M. injection may be painful.
- Site of I.V. administration should be checked daily for phlebitis and irritation.
- Blood pressure in patients receiving drug parenterally should be monitored.
- Hepatic function (alkaline phosphatase, SGOT, SGPT, bilirubin) should be monitored.
- CBC and platelets should be monitored. Development of neutropenia, leukopenia, or other blood disorders requires immediate discontinuation of drug and reevaluation of therapy.

No significant interactions.

Special considerations:
- Use cautiously in patients with hepatic disease or blood disorders. Do not use in infants, as it may cause kernicterus.
- Culture and sensitivity tests should be done initially and p.r.n.
- For best absorption, patient should take drug with a full glass of water 1 hour before or 2 hours after meals.
- Patient should take medication for as long as prescribed and exactly as directed, even after he feels better.
- Side effects, especially skin rash, fever, jaundice, or GI distress, may indicate blood dyscrasia, which requires immediate discontinuation of drug and reevaluation of therapy.
- Liver function (bilirubin, SGOT, SGPT, alkaline phosphatase) should be monitored.
- CBC and platelet and reticulocyte counts should be monitored before and during therapy.

No significant interactions.

Special considerations:
- Use cautiously in patients with impaired renal function or myasthenia gravis.
- Should be given only to hospitalized patients under constant medical supervision.
- For meningitis, must be given intrathecally to achieve adequate cerebrospinal fluid levels.
- Should be given deep I.M. Injection may be painful. If patient isn't allergic to procaine, 1% procaine should be used as diluent to decrease pain, and sites rotated.
- Solution containing local anesthetics should not be given I.V. or intrathecally.
- When given I.V., site should be checked daily for phlebitis and irritation. Each 500,000 unit should be diluted in 300 to 500 ml 5% dextrose in water and infused over 60 to 90 minutes.
- Parenteral solutions should be refrigerated and used within 72 hours.
- Renal function (BUN, serum creatinine, creatinine clearance, urinary output) should be monitored before and during therapy. Intake should be sufficient to maintain output at 1,500 ml/day (between 3,000 and 4,000 ml/day for adults).
- Fever, CNS side effects, rash, or symptoms of nephrotoxicity are serious side effects and doctor should be notified immediately.
- If patient is scheduled for surgery, anesthesiologist should be notified of preoperative treatment with this drug since neuromuscular blockade can occur.
- For treatment of anaphylaxis, see APPENDIX.

NAMES, INDICATIONS AND DOSAGES	SIDE EFFECTS
spectinomycin dihydrochloride Trobicin♦ **Gonorrhea:** ADULTS: 2 to 4 g I.M. single dose injected deeply into the upper outer quadrant of the buttock.	**CNS:** insomnia, dizziness. **GI:** nausea. **GU:** decreased urine output. **Skin:** urticaria. **Local:** pain at injection site. **Other:** fever, chills (may mask or delay symptoms of incubating syphilis).
trimethoprim Proloprim, Trimpex **Treatment of uncomplicated urinary tract infections caused by susceptible strains of *Escherichia coli, Proteus mirabilis, Klebsiella,* and *Enterobacter* species:** ADULTS: 100 mg P.O. q 12 hours for 10 days. Not recommended for children under 12 years.	**Blood:** thrombocytopenia, leukopenia, megaloblastic anemia, methemoglobinemia. **GI:** epigastric distress, nausea, vomiting, glossitis. **Skin:** *rash, pruritus, exfoliative dermatitis.* **Other:** fever.
troleandomycin phosphate Tao **Sensitive pneumococcal pneumonia or group A beta-hemolytic streptococcal respiratory tract infection:** ADULTS: 250 to 500 mg P.O. q 6 hours. CHILDREN: 6.6 to 11 mg/kg P.O. daily, q 6 hours.	**GI:** *nausea,* vomiting, diarrhea, discomfort. **Hepatic:** cholestatic jaundice. **Skin:** urticaria and rashes in hypersensitivity reactions. **Other:** *anaphylaxis.*
vancomycin hydrochloride Vancocin♦ **Severe staphylococcal infections when other antibiotics ineffective or contraindicated:** ADULTS: 500 mg I.V. q 6 hours, or 1 g q 12 hours. CHILDREN: 44 mg/kg I.V. daily, divided q 6 hours. NEONATES: 10 mg/kg I.V. daily, divided q 6 to 12 hours. **Antibiotic-associated pseudomembranous and staphylococcal enterocolitis:** ADULTS: 500 mg P.O. in 30 ml water q 6 hours. CHILDREN: 44 mg/kg P.O. daily, divided q 6 hours with 30 ml water.	**Blood:** transient eosinophilia. **EENT:** tinnitus, ototoxicity (deafness). **GI:** nausea. **GU:** nephrotoxicity (hyaline casts in urine, albuminuria, increased BUN). **Local:** *pain or thrombophlebitis with I.V. administration, necrosis.* **Other:** chills, fever, *anaphylaxis,* overgrowth of nonsusceptible organisms.
vidarabine monohydrate Vira-A **Herpes simplex virus encephalitis:** ADULTS AND CHILDREN INCLUDING NEWBORNS: 15 mg/kg/day for 10 days. Slowly infuse the total daily dose by I.V. infusion at a constant rate over 12- to 24-hour period. Avoid rapid or bolus injection.	**Blood:** anemia, neutropenia, thrombocytopenia. **CNS:** tremor, dizziness, hallucinations, confusion, psychosis, ataxia. **GI:** *anorexia, nausea,* vomiting, diarrhea. **Hepatic:** elevated SGOT, bilirubin. **Skin:** pruritus, rash. **Local:** pain at injection site. **Other:** weight loss.

INTERACTIONS AND SPECIAL CONSIDERATIONS	
No significant interactions. *Special considerations:* • Not effective in the treatment of syphilis. • Serologic test for syphilis done before treatment and 3 months after. • 20G needle should be used to administer drug.	The 4-g dose (10 ml) should be divided into two 5-ml injections—one in each buttock. • Shake vial vigorously after reconstitution and before withdrawing dose. Store at room temperature after reconstitution; use within 24 hours. • Should be reserved for penicillin-resistant strains of gonorrhea.
No significant interactions. *Special considerations:* • Contraindicated in documented megaloblastic anemia due to folate deficiency. • Clinical signs such as sore throat, fever, pallor, or purpura may be early indications of serious blood disorders. Complete blood counts should be done routinely. Prolonged use of trimethoprim at high doses may cause bone marrow depression.	• Dose should be decreased in patients with severely impaired renal function. Trimethoprim should be administered cautiously to patients with impaired hepatic function. • To be of benefit, full course of therapy must be completed.
No significant interactions. *Special considerations:* • Use cautiously in patients with hepatic impairment. • Drug is not recommended for routine use. • For best absorption, patient should take drug with a full glass of water 1 hour before or 2 hours after meals.	• Patient should take medication for as long as prescribed and exactly as directed, even after he feels better. Streptococcal infections should be treated for at least 10 days. • Liver function (bilirubin, SGOT, SGPT, alkaline phosphatase) should be monitored. • Side effects, especially abdominal pain, nausea, or jaundice, may occur. • For treatment of anaphylaxis see APPENDIX.
Interactions: ORAL CONTRACEPTIVES: cholestatic jaundice. Monitor bilirubin values. *Special considerations:* • Contraindicated in patients receiving other neurotoxic, nephrotoxic, or ototoxic drugs. Use cautiously in patients with impaired liver and kidney function; also in those with preexisting hearing loss; in patients over 60 years; and in patients with allergies to other antibiotics. • Patient should take medication exactly as directed, even if he feels better. Staphylococcal endocarditis should be treated for at least 3 weeks. • Patients should receive auditory function tests before and during therapy. • Dizziness, fullness or ringing in ears requires immediate discontinuation of drug.	• Drug should not be given I.M. • For I.V. infusion, should be diluted in 200 ml sodium chloride injection or 5% glucose solution and infused over 20 to 30 minutes. Site should be checked daily for phlebitis and irritation. Pain at infusion site should be reported. Extravasation should be avoided. Severe irritation and necrosis can result. • Renal function (BUN, serum creatinine, urinalysis, creatinine clearance, urinary output) should be monitored before and during therapy. Superinfection is possible. • Refrigerate I.V. solution after reconstitution and use within 96 hours. • Oral preparation stable for 2 weeks if refrigerated. • Used recently to treat pseudomembranous colitis caused by clindamycin. • For treatment of anaphylaxis, see APPENDIX.
No significant interactions. *Special considerations:* • Will reduce mortality caused by herpes simplex virus encephalitis from 70% to 28%. No evidence that vidarabine is effective in encephalitis due to other viruses. • Should not be given I.M. or subcutaneously because of low solubility and poor absorption. • Hematologic tests such as hemoglobin, hematocrit, WBC, and platelets should be monitored during therapy. Kidney and liver function studies should also be monitored. • Patient with impaired renal function may need dosage adjustment.	• Once in solution, vidarabine is stable at room temperature for at least 2 weeks. • Should be used with an I.V. filter. • Must be diluted to a concentration of less than 0.5 mg/ml. • Any intravenous solution is suitable as a diluent.

19

Cardiotonic glycosides

deslanoside
digitalis leaf
digitoxin
digoxin
gitalin
lanatoside C
ouabain

The cardiotonic (cardiac or digitalis) glycosides, which are extracted from plants of the genus *Digitalis* or chemically synthesized from the plant extract, are used to treat congestive heart failure and tachyarrhythmias. All the cardiotonic glycosides act similarly on the cardiovascular system; however, they differ in extent of absorption, metabolism, and excretion. These differences ultimately affect their onset and duration.

The range between therapeutic and toxic doses is extremely narrow. Toxicity may be due to altered absorption, serum electrolyte concentrations, renal or hepatic dysfunction, drug interactions, or other factors. The choice of cardiotonic glycoside and route of administration depend on the disorder and the desired onset of activity.

Major uses
Cardiotonic glycosides increase cardiac output in acute or chronic congestive heart failure. They control the rate of ventricular contraction in atrial flutter or fibrillation. Cardiotonic glycosides are also used to prevent or treat paroxysmal atrial tachycardia and angina

THERAPEUTIC ACTIVITY

THERAPEUTIC ACTIVITY OF CARDIOTONIC GLYCOSIDES

DRUG	ONSET	PEAK	HALF-LIFE	DURATION
deslanoside	10 to 30 min	1 to 2 hr	1½ days	2 to 5 days
digitalis leaf	15 to 120 min	4 to 12 hr	5 to 7 days	2 to 3 wk
digitoxin	30 to 120 min	4 to 12 hr	5 to 7 days	2 to 3 wk
digoxin	15 to 30 min	1½ to 5 hr	1½ days	2 to 3 days
gitalin	30 to 120 min	12 to 20 hr	8 to 12 days	10 to 12 days
lanatoside C	15 to 30 min	1½ to 5 hr	1½ days	2 to 3 days
ouabain	5 to 10 min	½ to 2 hr	21 hr	1 to 2½ days

associated with congestive heart failure.
• Ouabain, a fast-acting cardiotonic glycoside for I.V. use only, is effective in emergencies such as acute left-sided heart failure with pulmonary edema, cardiogenic shock, or atrial arrhythmias.

Mechanism of action
• Cardiotonic glycosides act directly on the myocardium to increase the force of contraction (produce a positive inotropic effect) by two mechanisms:
They promote movement of calcium from extracellular to intracellular cytoplasm. The force of contraction is directly related to the concentration of calcium in the myocardial cytoplasm.
They also inhibit adenosinetriphosphatase (ATPase), the enzyme that regulates potassium and sodium electrolyte concentrations in myocardial cells. Inhibition of ATPase increases intracellular sodium concentration, which in turn increases the force of contraction.
• They decrease conduction velocity through the atrioventricular (AV) node to slow heart rate.
• They prolong the effective refractory period of the AV node by both direct and sympatholytic effects on the sinoatrial (SA) node.

Absorption, distribution, metabolism, and excretion
• Deslanoside is given I.V. or I.M. only because absorption from the gastrointestinal (GI) tract is erratic or incomplete. It is primarily excreted unchanged in the urine. Use with caution in patients with renal dysfunction.
• Digitalis leaf, when given orally, is 20% to 40% absorbed. It's hydrolyzed in the GI tract to form several cardiotonic glycosides, including digitoxin.
• Digitoxin is 90% to 100% absorbed after oral administration. Passing through the enterohepatic circulation, the drug is extensively metabolized in the liver to inactive metabolites and is excreted by the kidneys. Neither the drug nor its metabolites accumulate in the renal parenchyma when renal function is impaired, since biliary and fecal elimination increase.
• Digoxin is 60% to 85% absorbed after oral administration. (Absorption varies with manufacturer.) Although 80% is absorbed after I.M. administration, this route may cause pain and irritation at the injection site.
Digoxin is excreted primarily unchanged in the urine. Use with caution in patients with renal dysfunction.
• Gitalin is a combination of various cardiotonic glycosides. It is well absorbed after oral administration and excreted primarily in the urine.
• Lanatoside C is converted to digoxin by acid and bacterial hydrolysis in the GI tract.
• Oubain is a fast-acting cardiotonic glycoside for I.V. use only. It is not metabolized but is eliminated as unchanged drug in urine and feces.
• None of the cardiotonic glycosides are distributed to adipose tissues. In obese patients, dosage should be based on ideal body weight.

Onset and duration
See table on p. 180.

NAMES, INDICATIONS AND DOSAGES	SIDE EFFECTS
deslanoside Cedilanid-D **Congestive heart failure, paroxysmal atrial tachycardia, atrial fibrillation and flutter:** ADULTS: loading dose 1.2 to 1.6 mg I.M. or I.V. in 2 divided doses over 24 hours; for maintenance, use another glycoside. Not recommended for children.	*The following are signs of toxicity that may occur with all cardiotonic glycosides:* **CNS:** *fatigue, generalized muscle weakness, agitation, hallucinations,* headache, malaise, dizziness, vertigo, stupor, paresthesias. **CV:** *increased severity of congestive heart failure, arrhythmias (most commonly conduction disturbances with or without AV block, premature ventricular contractions, and supraventricular arrhythmias),* hypotension. *Toxic effects on heart may be life-threatening and require immediate attention.* **EENT:** *yellow-green halos around visual images, blurred vision,* light flashes, photophobia, diplopia. **GI:** *anorexia, nausea,* vomiting, diarrhea.
digitalis leaf Pil-Digis **Congestive heart failure, paroxysmal atrial tachycardia, atrial fibrillation and flutter:** ADULTS: loading dose 1.2 to 1.8 g P.O. in divided doses over 24 hours; usual maintenance 100 mg P.O. daily. Not recommended for children.	*The following are signs of toxicity that may occur with all cardiotonic glycosides:* **CNS:** *fatigue, generalized muscle weakness, agitation, hallucinations,* headache, malaise, dizziness, vertigo, stupor, paresthesias. **CV:** *increased severity of congestive heart failure, arrhythmias (most commonly conduction disturbances with or without AV block, premature ventricular contractions, and supraventricular arrhythmias),* hypotension. *Toxic effects on heart may be life-threatening and require immediate attention.* **EENT:** *yellow-green halos around visual images, blurred vision,* light flashes, photophobia, diplopia. **GI:** *anorexia, nausea,* vomiting, diarrhea.

INTERACTIONS AND SPECIAL CONSIDERATIONS

Interactions:

AMPHOTERICIN B, CARBENICILLIN, TICARCILLIN, CORTICOSTEROIDS, AND DIURETICS, INCLUDING CHLORTHALIDONE, ETHACRYNIC ACID, FUROSEMIDE, METOLAZONE, AND THIAZIDES: hypokalemia, predisposing patient to digitalis toxicity. Serum potassium should be monitored.

PARENTERAL CALCIUM AND THIAZIDES: hypercalcemia and hypomagnesemia, predisposing patient to digitalis toxicity. Monitor serum calcium and serum magnesium.

Special considerations:

- Contraindicated in presence of any digitalis-induced toxicity; ventricular fibrillation; ventricular tachycardia unless caused by congestive heart failure. Administering calcium salts to digitalized patient is contraindicated. Calcium affects cardiac contractility and excitability in much the same way as glycosides do and may lead to serious arrhythmias in digitalized patient. Use with extreme caution in patients with acute myocardial infarction, incomplete AV block, chronic constrictive pericarditis, idiopathic hypertrophic subaortic stenosis, renal insufficiency, severe pulmonary disease, hypothyroidism, and in the elderly.
- Hypothyroid patients are very sensitive to glycosides; hyperthyroid patients may need larger doses.
- Baseline data (heart rate and rhythm, blood pressure, electrolytes, BUN, serum creatinine) should be obtained before first dose is given.
- Patient should report recent use of cardiotonic glycosides (within the previous 2 to 3 weeks) before a loading dose is administered. Loading dose should always be divided over first 24 hours unless clinical situation indicates otherwise.
- Should be used only for rapid digitalization, not maintenance.
- Dose is adjusted to patient's clinical condition and is monitored by serum levels of cardiotonic glycoside, calcium, potassium, magnesium, and by EKG.
- Apical-radial pulse should be taken for a full minute. Any significant changes (sudden increase or decrease in rate, pulse deficit, irregular beats, and particularly regularization of a previously irregular rhythm) should be recorded and reported. Blood pressure should be checked and a 12-lead EKG should be taken if these changes occur.
- Observe eating pattern. Patient should report nausea, vomiting, anorexia, visual disturbances, and other symptoms of toxicity.
- I.M. injection is painful; should be given I.V. if possible.
- Serum potassium should be monitored carefully and corrective action taken *before* hypokalemia occurs.
- For symptoms and treatment of toxicity, see APPENDIX.

Interactions:

PARA-AMINOSALICYLIC ACID, ANTACIDS, CHOLESTYRAMINE, KAOLIN-PECTIN, NEOMYCIN AND COLESTIPOL: decreased absorption of digitoxin, the main active component of the digitalis leaf. Schedule doses as far as possible from administration of digitalis leaf.

AMPHOTERICIN B, CARBENICILLIN, TICARCILLIN, CORTICOSTEROIDS, AND DIURETICS, INCLUDING CHLORTHALIDONE, ETHACRYNIC ACID, FUROSEMIDE, METOLAZONE, AND THIAZIDES: hypokalemia, predisposing patient to digitalis toxicity. Monitor serum potassium.

PARENTERAL CALCIUM AND THIAZIDES: hypercalcemia and hypomagnesemia, predisposing patient to digitalis toxicity. Monitor serum calcium and serum magnesium.

PHENYLBUTAZONE, PHENOBARBITAL, PHENYTOIN AND RIFAMPIN: faster metabolism and shorter duration of action of digitoxin. Observe for underdigitalization.

Special considerations:

- Contraindicated in presence of any digitalis-induced toxicity; ventricular fibrillation; ventricular tachycardia unless caused by congestive heart failure. Administering calcium salts to digitalized patient is contraindicated. Calcium affects cardiac contractility and excitability in much the same way as glycosides do and may lead to serious arrhythmias in digitalized patient. Use with extreme caution in patients with acute myocardial infarction, incomplete AV block, chronic constrictive pericarditis, idiopathic hypertrophic subaortic stenosis, renal insufficiency, severe pulmonary disease, hypothyroidism, and in the elderly.
- Hypothyroid patients are very sensitive to glycosides; hyperthyroid patients may need larger doses.
- Baseline data (heart rate and rhythm, blood pressure, electrolytes, BUN, serum creatinine) should be obtained before first dose is given.
- Patient should report recent use of cardiotonic glycosides (within the previous 2 to 3 weeks) before a loading dose is administered. Loading dose should always be divided over first 24 hours unless clinical situation indicates otherwise.
- Dose is adjusted to patient's clinical condition and is monitored by serum levels of cardiotonic glycoside, calcium, potassium, magnesium, and by EKG.
- Apical-radial pulse should be taken for a full minute. Any significant changes (sudden increase or decrease in rate, pulse deficit, irregular beats, and particularly regularization of a previously irregular rhythm) should be recorded and reported. Blood pressure should be checked and a 12-lead EKG should be taken if these changes occur.

(continued on following page)

NAMES, INDICATIONS AND DOSAGES	SIDE EFFECTS

digitalis leaf
(continued)

digitoxin
Crystodigin, De-Tone, Purodigin♦

Congestive heart failure, paroxysmal atrial tachycardia, atrial fibrillation and flutter:
ADULTS: loading dose 1.2 to 1.6 mg I.V. or P.O. in divided doses over 24 hours; maintenance 0.1 mg daily.
CHILDREN 2 TO 12 YEARS: loading dose 0.03 mg/kg or 0.75 mg/m² I.M., I.V., or P.O. in divided doses over 24 hours; maintenance 1/10 loading dose or 0.003 mg/kg or 0.075 mg/m² daily. Monitor closely for toxicity.
CHILDREN 1 TO 2 YEARS: loading dose 0.04 mg/kg over 24 hours in divided doses; maintenance 0.004 mg/kg daily. Monitor closely for toxicity.
CHILDREN 2 WEEKS TO 1 YEAR: loading dose 0.045 mg/kg I.M., I.V., or P.O. in divided doses over 24 hours; maintenance 0.0045 mg/kg daily. Monitor closely for toxicity.
PREMATURE INFANTS, NEONATES, SEVERELY ILL OLDER INFANTS: loading dose 0.022 mg/kg I.M., I.V., or P.O. in divided doses over 24 hours; maintenance 0.0022 mg/kg daily. Monitor closely for toxicity.

The following are signs of toxicity that may occur with all cardiotonic glycosides:
CNS: *fatigue, generalized muscle weakness, agitation, hallucinations,* headache, malaise, dizziness, vertigo, stupor, paresthesias.
CV: *increased severity of congestive heart failure, arrhythmias (most commonly conduction disturbances with or without AV block, premature ventricular contractions, and supraventricular arrhythmias),* hypotension.
Toxic effects on heart may be life-threatening and require immediate attention.
EENT: *yellow-green halos around visual images, blurred vision,* light flashes, photophobia, diplopia.
GI: *anorexia, nausea,* vomiting, diarrhea.

digoxin
Lanoxin♦, Masoxin

Congestive heart failure, atrial fibrillation and flutter, paroxysmal atrial tachycardia:
ADULTS: loading dose 0.5 to 1 mg I.V. or P.O. in divided doses over 24 hours; maintenance 0.125 to 0.5 mg I.V. or P.O. daily (average 0.25 mg). Larger doses are often needed for

The following are signs of toxicity that may occur with all cardiotonic glycosides:
CNS: *fatigue, generalized muscle weakness, agitation, hallucinations,* headache, malaise, dizziness, vertigo, stupor, paresthesias.
CV: *increased severity of congestive heart failure, arrhythmias (most commonly conduction disturbances with or without AV block, premature ventricular contractions, and supraventric-*

♦ Available in U.S. and Canada. ♦♦ Available in Canada only.
All other products (no symbol) available in U.S. only. Italicized side effects are common or life-threatening.

INTERACTIONS AND SPECIAL CONSIDERATIONS

• Observe eating pattern. Patient should report nausea, vomiting, anorexia, visual disturbances, and other symptoms of toxicity.
• Serum potassium should be monitored carefully and corrective action taken *before* hypokalemia occurs.
• Digitalis leaf is a long-acting drug; cumulative effects possible.
• Should be withheld for 1 to 2 days before elective electrocardioversion and dosage adjusted after cardioversion.
• Patient and responsible family member should be instructed about drug action, dosage regimen, how to take pulse, reportable signs, and follow-up plans.
• Therapeutic blood levels of serum digitoxin (the active agent in the leaf) range from 25 to 35 ng/ml.
• For symptoms and treatment of toxicity, see APPENDIX.

Interactions:
PARA-AMINOSALICYLIC ACID, ANTACIDS, CHOLESTYRAMINE, COLESTIPOL, KAOLIN-PECTIN AND NEOMYCIN: decreased absorption of oral digitoxin. Schedule doses as far as possible from oral digitoxin administration.
AMPHOTERICIN B, CARBENICILLIN, TICARCILLIN, CORTICOSTEROIDS, AND DIURETICS, INCLUDING CHLORTHALIDONE, ETHACRYNIC ACID, FUROSEMIDE, METOLAZONE, AND THIAZIDES: hypokalemia, predisposing patient to digitalis toxicity. Monitor serum potassium.
PARENTERAL CALCIUM AND THIAZIDES: hypercalcemia and hypomagnesemia, predisposing patient to digitalis toxicity. Monitor serum calcium and serum magnesium.
PHENYLBUTAZONE, PHENOBARBITAL, PHENYTOIN, AND RIFAMPIN: faster metabolism and shorter duration of digitoxin. Observe for underdigitalization.

Special considerations:
• Contraindicated in presence of any digitalis-induced toxicity; ventricular fibrillation; ventricular tachycardia unless caused by congestive heart failure. Administering calcium salts to digitalized patient is contraindicated. Calcium affects cardiac contractility and excitability in much the same way as glycosides do and may lead to serious arrhythmias in digitalized patient. Use with extreme caution in patients with acute myocardial infarction, incomplete AV block, chronic constrictive pericarditis, idiopathic hypertrophic subaortic stenosis, renal insufficiency, severe pulmonary disease, hypothyroidism, and in the elderly.
• Hypothyroid patients are very sensitive to glycosides; hyperthyroid patients may need larger doses.
• Baseline data (heart rate and rhythm, blood pressure, electrolytes, BUN, serum creatinine) should be obtained before first dose is given.
• History of recent use of cardiotonic glycosides (within the previous 2 to 3 weeks) should be obtained before a loading dose is administered. Divide loading dose over first 24 hours unless clinical situation indicates otherwise.
• Dose is adjusted to patient's clinical condition and is monitored by serum levels of cardiotonic glycoside, calcium, potassium, magnesium, and by EKG.
• Apical-radial pulse should be taken for a full minute. Any significant changes (sudden increase or decrease in rate, pulse deficit, irregular beats, and particularly regularization of a previously irregular rhythm) should be recorded and reported. Blood pressure should be checked and a 12-lead EKG should be taken if these changes occur.
• Observe eating pattern. Patient should report nausea, vomiting, anorexia, visual disturbances, and other symptoms of toxicity.
• Toxicity possible, especially in children and the elderly.
• Serum potassium should be monitored carefully and corrective action taken *before* hypokalemia occurs.
• I.M. injection painful; I.V. administration preferable if parenteral route necessary.
• Digitoxin is a long-acting drug; cumulative effects possible.
• Should be withheld for 1 to 2 days before elective electrocardioversion and dosage adjusted after cardioversion.
• Protect solution from light.
• Patient and responsible family member should be instructed about drug action, dosage regimen, how to take pulse, reportable signs, and follow-up plans.
• Therapeutic blood levels of digitoxin range from 25 to 35 ng/ml.
• For symptoms and treatment of toxicity, see APPENDIX.

Interactions:
PARA-AMINOSALICYLIC ACID, ANTACIDS, CHOLESTYRAMINE, COLESTIPOL, KAOLIN-PECTIN, AND NEOMYCIN: decreased absorption of oral digoxin. Schedule doses as far as possible from oral digoxin administration.
QUINIDINE: increased digoxin blood levels. Monitor for toxicity.
AMPHOTERICIN B, CARBENICILLIN, TICARCILLIN, CORTICOSTEROIDS, AND DIURETICS, INCLUDING CHLORTHALIDONE, ETHACRYNIC ACID, FUROSEMIDE, METOLAZONE, AND THIAZIDES: hypokalemia, predisposing patient to digitalis toxicity. Monitor serum potassium.
PARENTERAL CALCIUM AND THIAZIDES: hypercalcemia and hypomagnesemia, predisposing patient to digitalis toxicity. Monitor serum calcium and serum magnesium.

(continued on following page)

NAMES, INDICATIONS AND DOSAGES	SIDE EFFECTS
digoxin *(continued)* treatment of arrhythmias, depending on patient response. CHILDREN OVER 2 YEARS: loading dose 0.04 to 0.06 mg/kg P.O. divided q 8 hours over 24 hours; I.V. loading dose 0.025 to 0.04 mg/kg; maintenance 0.02 mg/kg P.O. daily divided q 12 hours. CHILDREN 1 MONTH TO 2 YEARS: loading dose 0.06 to 0.075 mg/kg P.O. divided into three doses over 24 hours; I.V. loading dose 0.035 to 0.05 mg/kg; maintenance 0.02 to 0.025 mg/kg P.O. daily divided q 12 hours. NEONATES UNDER 1 MONTH: loading dose 0.05 mg/kg P.O. divided q 8 hours over 24 hours; I.V. loading dose 0.015 to 0.04 mg/kg; maintenance 0.0167 mg/kg P.O. daily divided q 12 hours. PREMATURE INFANTS: loading dose 0.04 mg/kg I.V. divided into 3 doses over 24 hours; maintenance 0.0133 mg/kg I.V. daily divided q 12 hours.	*ular arrhythmias),* hypotension. *Toxic effects on heart may be life-threatening and require immediate attention.* **EENT:** *yellow-green halos around visual images, blurred vision,* light flashes, photophobia, diplopia. **GI:** *anorexia, nausea,* vomiting, diarrhea.
gitalin Gitaligin **Congestive heart failure, atrial fibrillation and flutter, paroxysmal atrial tachycardia:** ADULTS: loading dose 2.5 mg P.O. initially, then 0.75 mg q 6 hours until therapeutic effect is attained (not to exceed 6 mg total in 24 hours); maintenance 0.25 to 1.25 mg daily. Not recommended for children.	*The following are signs of toxicity that may occur with all cardiotonic glycosides:* **CNS:** *fatigue, generalized muscle weakness, agitation, hallucinations,* headache, malaise, dizziness, vertigo, stupor, paresthesias. **CV:** *increased severity of congestive heart failure, arrhythmias (most commonly conduction disturbances with or without AV block, premature ventricular contractions, and supraventricular arrhythmias),* hypotension. *Toxic effects on heart may be life-threatening and require immediate attention.* **EENT:** *yellow-green halos around visual images, blurred vision,* light flashes, photophobia, diplopia. **GI:** *anorexia, nausea,* vomiting, diarrhea.

INTERACTIONS AND SPECIAL CONSIDERATIONS

Special considerations:
• Contraindicated in presence of any digitalis-induced toxicity; ventricular fibrillation; ventricular tachycardia unless caused by congestive heart failure. Administering calcium salts to digitalized patient is contraindicated. Calcium affects cardiac contractility and excitability in much the same way as glycosides do and may lead to serious arrhythmias in digitalized patient. Use with extreme caution in patients with acute myocardial infarction, incomplete AV block, chronic constrictive pericarditis, idiopathic hypertrophic subaortic stenosis, renal insufficiency, severe pulmonary disease, hypothyroidism, and in the elderly. Dose must be reduced in renal impairment.
• Hypothyroid patients are very sensitive to glycosides; hyperthyroid patients may need larger doses.
• Baseline data (heart rate and rhythm, blood pressure, electrolytes, BUN, serum creatinine) should be obtained before first dose is given.
• Patient should report recent use of cardiotonic glycosides (within the previous 2 to 3 weeks) before a loading dose is administered. Loading dose should always be divided over first 24 hours unless clinical situation indicates otherwise.
• Dose is adjusted to patient's clinical condition and is monitored by serum levels of cardiotonic glycoside, calcium, potassium, magnesium, and by EKG.
• Apical-radial pulse should be taken for a full minute. Any significant changes (sudden increase or decrease in rate, pulse deficit, irregular beats, and particularly regularization of a previously irregular rhythm) should be recorded and reported. Blood pressure should be checked and a 12-lead EKG should be taken if these changes occur.
• Observe eating pattern. Patient should report nausea, vomiting, anorexia, visual disturbances, and other symptoms of toxicity.
• Serum potassium should be monitored carefully and corrective action taken *before* hypokalemia occurs.
• Should be withheld for 1 to 2 days before elective electrocardioversion and dose adjusted after cardioversion.
• Patient and responsible family member should be instructed about drug action, dosage regimen, how to take pulse, reportable signs, and follow-up plans.
• One brand should not be substituted for another.
• Therapeutic blood levels of digoxin range from 0.5 to 2.5 ng/ml.
• For symptoms and treatment of toxicity, see APPENDIX.

Interactions:
PARA-AMINOSALICYLIC ACID, ANTACIDS, CHOLESTYRAMINE, COLESTIPOL, KAOLIN-PECTIN, AND NEOMYCIN: decreased absorption of oral gitalin. Schedule doses as far as possible from oral gitalin administration.
AMPHOTERICIN B, CARBENICILLIN, TICARCILLIN, CORTICOSTEROIDS, AND DIURETICS (CHLORTHALIDONE, ETHACRYNIC ACID, FUROSEMIDE, METOLAZONE, AND THIAZIDES): hypokalemia, predisposing patient to digitalis toxicity. Monitor serum potassium.
PARENTERAL CALCIUM AND THIAZIDES: hypercalcemia and hypomagnesemia, predisposing patient to digitalis toxicity. Monitor serum calcium and serum magnesium.

Special considerations:
• Contraindicated in digitalis-induced toxicity; ventricular fibrillation; ventricular tachycardia unless caused by congestive heart failure. Administering calcium salts to digitalized patient is contraindicated. Calcium affects cardiac contractility and excitability in much the same way as glycosides do and may lead to serious arrhythmias in digitalized patient. Use with caution in acute myocardial infarction, incomplete AV block, chronic constrictive pericarditis, idiopathic hypertrophic subaortic stenosis, renal insufficiency, severe pulmonary disease, hypothyroidism, and in the elderly.
• Hypothyroid patients sensitive to glycosides; hyperthyroid patients may need larger doses.
• Baseline data (heart rate and rhythm, blood pressure, electrolytes, BUN, serum creatinine) should be obtained before first dose is given.
• History of recent use of cardiotonic glycosides (within the previous 2 to 3 weeks) should be obtained before loading dose is given. Loading dose should always be divided over first 24 hours unless clinical situation indicates otherwise.
• Adjust dose to patient's condition and monitor by serum levels of cardiotonic glycoside, calcium, potassium, magnesium, and by EKG.
• Apical-radial pulse should be taken for a full minute. Changes (sudden increase or decrease in rate, pulse deficit, irregular beats, and particularly regularization of a previously irregular rhythm) should be recorded and reported. Blood pressure should be checked and a 12-lead EKG taken if these changes occur.
• Observe eating pattern. Patient should report nausea, vomiting, anorexia, visual disturbances, and other symptoms of toxicity.
• Monitor serum potassium; take corrective action *before* hypokalemia occurs.
• Long-acting; cumulative effects possible.
• Withhold for 1 to 2 days before elective electrocardioversion; adjust dose after cardioversion.
• Patient and family member should be told about drug action, dosage regimen, how to take pulse, reportable signs, and follow-up plans.
• For treatment of toxicity, see APPENDIX.

NAMES, INDICATIONS AND DOSAGES	SIDE EFFECTS

lanatoside C

Congestive heart failure, atrial fibrillation and flutter, paroxysmal atrial tachycardia:
ADULTS: average total dose for digitalization is 10 mg P.O. given as follows: loading dose. First day, 3.5 mg; second day, 2.5 mg; third day, 2 mg; thereafter 1.5 mg/day until digitalization obtained; maintenance 0.5 to 1.5 mg daily.
Not recommended for children.

The following are signs of toxicity that may occur with all cardiotonic glycosides:
CNS: *fatigue, generalized muscle weakness, agitation, hallucinations,* headache, malaise, dizziness, vertigo, stupor, paresthesias.
CV: *increased severity of congestive heart failure, arrhythmias (most commonly conduction disturbances with or without AV block, premature ventricular contractions, and supraventricular arrhythmias),* hypotension.
Toxic effects on heart may be life-threatening and require immediate attention.
EENT: *yellow-green halos around visual images, blurred vision,* light flashes, photophobia, diplopia.
GI: *anorexia, nausea,* vomiting, diarrhea.

ouabain

Congestive heart failure, atrial fibrillation and flutter, paroxysmal atrial tachycardia:
ADULTS: loading dose 0.25 to 0.5 mg by slow I.V. injection. Additional 0.1 mg doses may be given every hour until a therapeutic effect is achieved or a total of 1 mg is given. For maintenance, use another glycoside.
Not recommended for children.

The following are signs of toxicity that may occur with all cardiotonic glycosides:
CNS: *fatigue, generalized muscle weakness, agitation, hallucinations,* headache, malaise, dizziness, vertigo, stupor, paresthesias.
CV: *increased severity of congestive heart failure, arrhythmias (most commonly conduction disturbances with or without AV block, premature ventricular contractions, and supraventricular arrhythmias),* hypotension.
Toxic effects on heart may be life-threatening and require immediate attention.
EENT: *yellow-green halos around visual images, blurred vision,* light flashes, photophobia, diplopia.
GI: *anorexia, nausea,* vomiting, diarrhea.

INTERACTIONS AND SPECIAL CONSIDERATIONS

Interactions:
PARA-AMINOSALICYLIC ACID, ANTACIDS, CHOLESTYRAMINE, KAOLIN-PECTIN, NEOMYCIN, AND COLESTIPOL: decreased absorption of digoxin formed in stomach from lanatoside C. Schedule doses as far as possible from lanatoside C administration.
AMPHOTERICIN B, CARBENICILLIN, TICARCILLIN, CORTICOSTEROIDS, AND DIURETICS, (CHLORTHALIDONE, ETHACRYNIC ACID, FUROSEMIDE, METOLAZONE, AND THIAZIDES): hypokalemia, predisposing patient to digitalis toxicity. Monitor serum potassium.
PARENTERAL CALCIUM, AND THIAZIDES: hypercalcemia and hypomagnesemia, predisposing patient to digitalis toxicity. Monitor serum calcium and serum magnesium.

Special considerations:
• Contraindicated in digitalis-induced toxicity; ventricular fibrillation; ventricular tachycardia unless caused by congestive heart failure. Administering calcium salts to digitalized patient is contraindicated. Calcium affects cardiac contractility and excitability in much the same way as glycosides do and may lead to serious arrhythmias in digitalized patient. Use with caution in patients with acute myocardial infarction, incomplete AV block, chronic constrictive pericarditis, idiopathic hypertrophic subaortic stenosis, renal insufficiency, severe pulmonary disease, hypothyroidism, and in the elderly. Dose should be reduced in renal impairment.
• Hypothyroid patients sensitive to glycosides; hyperthyroid patients may need larger doses.
• Baseline data (heart rate and rhythm, blood pressure, electrolytes, BUN, serum creatinine) should be obtained before first dose is given.
• History of recent use of cardiotonic glycosides (within the previous 2 to 3 weeks) should be obtained before a loading dose is given. Loading dose should always be divided over first 24 hours unless clinical situation indicates otherwise.
• Dose is adjusted to patient's clinical condition and is monitored by serum levels of cardiotonic glycoside, calcium, potassium, magnesium, and by EKG.
• Apical-radial pulse should be taken for a full minute. Changes (sudden increase or decrease in rate, pulse deficit, irregular beats, and particularly regularization of a previously irregular rhythm) should be recorded and reported. Blood pressure should be checked and a 12-lead EKG taken if these changes occur.
• Observe eating pattern. Patient should report nausea, vomiting, anorexia, visual disturbances, and other symptoms of toxicity.
• Monitor serum potassium; take corrective action before hypokalemia occurs.
• Should be withheld for 1 to 2 days before elective electrocardioversion and dose adjusted after cardioversion.
• Patient and family member should be told about drug action, dosage regimen, how to take pulse, reportable signs, and follow-up plans.
• For treatment of toxicity, see APPENDIX.

Interactions:
AMPHOTERICIN B, CARBENICILLIN, TICARCILLIN, CORTICOSTEROIDS, AND DIURETICS, (CHLORTHALIDONE, ETHACRYNIC ACID, FUROSEMIDE, METOLAZONE, AND THIAZIDES): hypokalemia, predisposing patient to toxicity. Monitor serum potassium.
PARENTERAL CALCIUM, THIAZIDES: hypercalcemia and hypomagnesemia, predisposing patient to toxicity. Monitor serum calcium and serum magnesium.

Special considerations:
• Contraindicated in digitalis-induced toxicity; ventricular fibrillation; ventricular tachycardia unless caused by congestive heart failure. Administering calcium salts to digitalized patient is contraindicated. Calcium affects cardiac contractility and excitability in much the same way as glycosides do and may lead to serious arrhythmias in digitalized patient. Use with caution in patients with acute myocardial infarction, incomplete AV block, chronic constrictive pericarditis, idiopathic hypertrophic subaortic stenosis, renal insufficiency, severe pulmonary disease, hypothyroidism, and in the elderly. Dose should be reduced in renal impairment.
• Hypothyroid patients sensitive to glycosides; hyperthyroid patients may need larger doses.
• Baseline data (heart rate and rhythm, blood pressure, electrolytes, BUN, serum creatinine) should be obtained before first dose is given.
• History of recent use of cardiotonic glycosides (within the previous 2 to 3 weeks) should be obtained before a loading dose is given. Loading dose should always be divided over first 24 hours unless clinical situation indicates otherwise.
• For rapid digitalization, not maintenance.
• Adjust dose to patient's condition and monitor by serum levels of cardiotonic glycoside, calcium, potassium, magnesium, and by EKG.
• Apical-radial pulse should be taken for a full minute. Changes (sudden increase or decrease in rate, pulse deficit, irregular beats, and particularly regularization of a previously irregular rhythm) should be recorded and reported. Blood pressure should be checked and a 12-lead EKG taken if these changes occur.
• Observe eating pattern. Patient should report nausea, vomiting, anorexia, visual disturbances, and other symptoms of toxicity.
• I.M. route is painful; absorption is unpredictable. Not recommended.
• Monitor serum potassium; take corrective action before hypokalemia occurs.
• For treatment of toxicity, see APPENDIX.

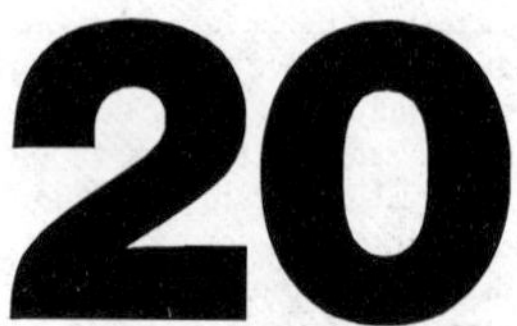

Antiarrhythmics

atropine sulfate
bretylium tosylate
disopyramide
disopyramide phosphate
lidocaine hydrochloride
nifedipine
phenytoin
phenytoin sodium
procainamide hydrochloride
propranolol hydrochloride
quinidine bisulfate
quinidine gluconate
quinidine polygalacturonate
quinidine sulfate
verapamil

Antiarrhythmics are used to prevent or treat atrial and ventricular arrhythmias, including those secondary to myocardial infarction (MI) or digitalis toxicity.

Bradycardia can be due to decreased generation of atrial impulses or to conduction of fewer atrial impulses to the ventricles. Similarly, ventricular tachycardia can develop from an increased number of impulses from either atrial or ventricular areas.

As a group, the antiarrhythmics have a narrow therapeutic index (the toxic dose is not much greater than the therapeutic dose). Careful monitoring of therapy is imperative, since side effects of these drugs are usually serious.

Before therapy begins, underlying conditions, such as electrolyte imbalances, should be corrected.

If drug therapy fails, synchronized cardioversion and electrical pacemakers are effective antiarrhythmic alternatives.

Major uses

Antiarrhythmics are therapeutic for atrial and ventricular arrhythmias of various causes. They're both prophylactic and therapeutic for post-MI arrhythmias.

Verapamil represents a new class of antiarrhythmic agents called *calcium antagonists* or slow channel blockers. Verapamil is effective in managing supraventricular arrhythmias, premature ventricular beats, and Prinzmetal's angina. The overall incidence of side effects has been lower with the calcium antagonists than with the conventional antiarrhythmics.

Mechanism of action

• Group I drugs (disopyramide, procainamide, and quinidine) decrease sodium transport through cardiac tissues, slowing conduction through the atrioventricular (AV) node. These drugs also prolong the effective refractory period and decrease automaticity.

• Group II drugs (lidocaine and phenytoin) increase conduction block against reentry impulses, but have little effect on conduction velocity. They stabilize reentry ventricular arrhythmias associated with MI; phenytoin may also combat arrhythmias due to digitalis toxicity.

• Group III drugs (beta blockers) decrease conduction of impulses through the AV node and increase the effective refractory period. In addition to their beta blockade, group III drugs also have reentry blocking effects similar to those of group II. Propranolol, the only beta blocker approved for use as an antiarrhythmic, is effective for supraventricular arrhythmias and, to a lesser extent, for ventricular arrhythmias.

• The group IV drug bretylium was originally thought to act as an antiadrenergic agent whose action is mediated through the sympathetic division of the autonomic nervous system. Bretylium initially exerts short-lived adrenergic stimulatory effects (caused by

HOW ARRHYTHMIAS AFFECT THE CARDIOVASCULAR SYSTEM

ARRHYTHMIA	EFFECTS
Paroxysmal tachycardia	• Reduced cardiac output, with associated symptoms • Increased oxygen demands on myocardium • Decreased coronary blood supply • Possible progression to atrial fibrillation, ventricular tachycardia, and ventricular fibrillation
Atrial fibrillation with rapid ventricular response	• Compromised cardiac output • Decreased coronary blood supply • Increased oxygen consumption • Loss of "atrial kick"
Ventricular tachycardia	• Decreased ventricular filling • Rapid fall in cardiac output • Development of dyspnea, angina, hypotension, oliguria, syncope • Possible progression to ventricular fibrillation
Ventricular fibrillation	• Failure of normal cardiac contraction sequence • Loss of consciousness, seizures, apnea, death

release of norepinephrine) on the cardiovascular system. When norepinephrine is depleted, the adrenergic blocking actions predominate. Recent pharmacologic studies indicate that bretylium's action may be due to its large quaternary ammonium structure.

• The group V agents, nifedipine and verapamil, selectively inhibit the myocardial cell membrane transport of calcium by blocking the inward current (slow channel) of calcium into cardiac muscle. Impulse transmission through the AV node is delayed, and the spontaneous rhythmicity of the sinoatrial (SA) node is depressed.

• Among the unclassified drugs in this category, atropine blocks the vagal effects on the SA node, relieving severe nodal or sinus bradycardia, or AV block. Increased conduction through the AV node speeds heart rate.

Absorption, distribution, metabolism, and excretion

After oral administration, most antiarrhythmic drugs are well absorbed from the gastrointestinal tract. Bretylium, however, is poorly absorbed and must be given parenterally.

All antiarrhythmics are widely distributed in body tissues and are metabolized primarily in the liver.

• Procainamide is metabolized to an active metabolite, N-acetylprocainamide, which accumulates in patients with impaired renal function. (The other drugs are excreted partly as inactive metabolites and partly as unchanged drug by the kidneys.)

• Propranolol and lidocaine, although well absorbed when administered by mouth, enter the hepatic portal circulation immediately and are quickly metabolized. This is known as the "first-pass effect" (see Chapter 2, PHARMACOLOGY). However, the first-pass effect

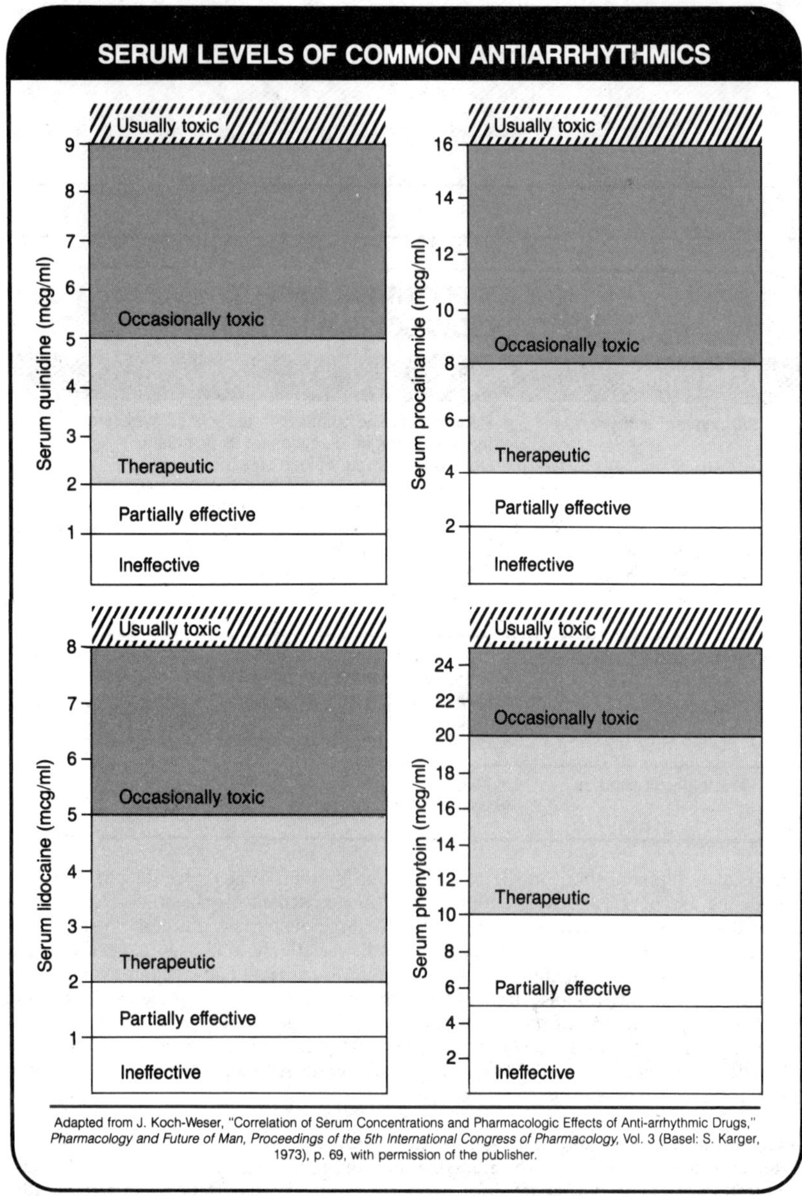

Adapted from J. Koch-Weser, "Correlation of Serum Concentrations and Pharmacologic Effects of Anti-arrhythmic Drugs," *Pharmacology and Future of Man, Proceedings of the 5th International Congress of Pharmacology,* Vol. 3 (Basel: S. Karger, 1973), p. 69, with permission of the publisher.

of propranolol may be nullified by administering large oral doses (relative to parenteral doses). Therefore, propranolol is commonly used both orally and parenterally.

Onset and duration
See chart on opposite page.

Combination products
None.

THERAPEUTIC ACTIVITY OF ANTIARRHYTHMICS

DRUG	ROUTE OF ADMINIS-TRATION	ONSET	PEAK	DURATION	THERA-PEUTIC BLOOD LEVELS
atropine	I.V.	immediate	within minutes	4 to 6 hr	†
bretylium	I.M.	up to 2 hr	6 to 9 hr	up to 10 hr	†
	I.V.	within minutes	within 20 min	up to 10 hr	†
disopyramide	P.O.	30 min	2 hr	6 to 8 hr	3 to 8 mcg/ml
lidocaine	I.M.	5 to 15 min	20 to 30 min	60 to 90 min	2 to 5 mcg/ml
	I.V.	immediate	immediate (after I.V. bolus)	10 to 20 min	2 to 5 mcg/ml
nifedipine	P.O.	10 min	30 min	3 to 6 hr	†
phenytoin	I.V.	immediate	immediate	up to 24 hr	10 to 20 mcg/ml
	P.O.	2 hr	6 hr	up to 24 hr	10 to 20 mcg/ml
procainamide	I.V.	immediate	25 to 60 min	3 to 4 hr	4 to 8 mcg/ml*
	P.O.	30 min	1 hr	3 to 4 hr	4 to 8 mcg/ml*
propranolol	I.V.	immediate	2 to 4 hr	3 to 6 hr	†
	P.O.	30 min	60 to 90 min	3 to 6 hr	†
quinidine	I.M.	30 min	30 to 90 min	6 to 8 hr	2 to 5 mcg/ml
	I.V.	30 min	immediate	6 to 8 hr	2 to 5 mcg/ml
	P.O.	30 min	1 to 3 hr	6 to 8 hr	2 to 5 mcg/ml
verapamil	I.V.	immediate	3 to 5 min	10 to 20 min	†

*N-acetylprocainamide (active metabolite of procainamide): 2 to 8 mcg/ml

† Not established

NAMES, INDICATIONS AND DOSAGES	SIDE EFFECTS
atropine sulfate **Bradycardia, bradyarrhythmia (junctional or escape rhythm):** ADULTS: usually 0.5 to 1 mg I.V. push; repeat q 5 minutes, to maximum 2 mg. Lower doses (less than 0.5 mg) can cause bradycardia. CHILDREN: 0.01 mg/kg dose up to maximum 0.4 mg; or 0.3 mg/m² dose; may repeat q 4 to 6 hours.	**Blood:** leukocytosis. **CNS:** *with doses greater than 5 mg—headache, restlessness,* ataxia, disorientation, hallucinations, delirium, coma, *insomnia, dizziness.* **CV:** *1 to 2 mg—tachycardia, palpitations; greater than 2 mg—extreme tachycardia, angina.* **EENT:** *1 mg—slight mydriasis,* photophobia; *2 mg—blurred vision, mydriasis.* **GI:** *dry mouth (common even at low doses),* thirst, *constipation,* nausea, vomiting. **GU:** *urinary retention.* **Skin:** 2 mg—flushed, dry skin; 5 mg or more—hot, dry, reddened skin.
bretylium tosylate Bretylol **Ventricular fibrillation:** ADULTS: 5 mg/kg by rapid I.V. injection. If necessary, increase dose to 10 mg/kg and repeat q 15 to 30 minutes until 30 mg/kg have been given. **Other ventricular arrhythmias:** ADULTS: initially, 500 mg diluted to 50 ml with 5% dextrose in water or normal saline solution and infused I.V. over more than 8 minutes at 5 to 10 mg/kg. Dose may be repeated in 1 to 2 hours. Thereafter, dose q 6 to 8 hours. **I.V. maintenance:** ADULTS: infused in diluted solution of 500 ml 5% dextrose in water or normal saline solution at 1 to 2 mg/minute. **I.M. injection:** ADULTS: 5 to 10 mg/kg undiluted. Repeat in 1 to 2 hours if needed. Thereafter, repeat q 6 to 8 hours. Not recommended for children.	**CNS:** *vertigo, dizziness, light-headedness, syncope* (usually secondary to hypotension). **CV:** *severe hypotension (especially orthostatic), bradycardia,* anginal pain. **GI:** severe nausea, vomiting (with rapid infusion).
disopyramide Rythmodan♦ **disopyramide phosphate** Norpace♦ **Premature ventricular contractions (unifocal, multifocal, or coupled); ventricular tachycardia not severe enough to require electrocardioversion:** ADULTS: Usual maintenance dose 150 to 200 mg P.O. q 6 hours; for patients who weigh less than 50 kg or those with renal, hepatic, or cardiac impairment—100 mg P.O. q 6 hours. Recommended doses in advanced renal insufficency: creatinine clearance 15 to 40 ml/minute: 100 mg q 10 hours; creatinine clearance 5 to 15 ml/minute: 100 mg q 20 hours; creatinine clearance 1 to 5 ml/minute: 100 mg q 30 hours.	**CNS:** dizziness, agitation, depression, fatigue, muscle weakness, syncope. **CV:** *hypotension, congestive heart failure, heart block.* **EENT:** *blurred vision, dry eyes, dry nose.* **GI:** nausea, vomiting, anorexia, bloating, abdominal pain, *constipation, dry mouth.* **GU:** *urinary retention and hesitancy.* **Hepatic:** cholestatic jaundice. **Skin:** rash in 1% to 3% of patients.

INTERACTIONS AND SPECIAL CONSIDERATIONS

Interactions:
METHOTRIMEPRAZINE: may produce extrapyramidal symptoms. Monitor patient carefully.

Special considerations:
• Side effects vary considerably with dose. Most common are dry mouth (which can be treated with pilocarpine syrup) and thirst. Sucking sour hard candy is recommended.
• In cardiac patients, tachycardia possible.
• Antidote for atropine overdose is physostigmine salicylate.
• Other anticholinergic drugs may increase vagal blockage.
• For symptoms and treatment of toxicity, see APPENDIX.

Interactions:
ALL ANTIHYPERTENSIVES: may potentiate hypotension. Monitor blood pressure.

Special considerations:
• Contraindicated in digitalis-induced arrhythmias. Use cautiously in patients with fixed cardiac output to avoid severe and sudden drop in blood pressure.
• Blood pressure and heart rate and rhythm should be monitored frequently. If supine systolic blood pressure falls below 75 mm Hg, treatment with norepinephrine, dopamine, or volume expansion to raise blood pressure may be required.
• Patient should remain supine until tolerance to hypotension develops.
• Dosage directions should be followed carefully to avoid nausea and vomiting.
• I.V. injections for ventricular fibrillation should be given as rapidly as possible. Should not be diluted.
• I.M. injection sites should be rotated to prevent tissue damage; 5-ml volume should not be exceeded.
• To be used with other cardioresuscitative measures such as CPR, countershock, epinephrine, sodium bicarbonate, and lidocaine.
• Subtherapeutic doses (less than 5 mg/kg) should be avoided, since such doses may cause hypotension.
• Ventricular tachycardia and other ventricular arrhythmias respond less rapidly to treatment than does ventricular fibrillation.
• Dosage should be decreased in renal impairment.
• Should be carefully monitored if pressor amines (sympathomimetics) are given to correct hypotension, as bretylium potentiates pressor amines.
• Ineffective treatment for atrial arrhythmias.
• Has been used investigationally to treat hypertension.
• Increased anginal pain possible in susceptible patients.
• Patient should be observed for side effects.

Interactions:
PHENYTOIN: increases disopyramides metabolism. Monitor for decreased antiarrhytmic effect.

Special considerations:
• Contraindicated in cardiogenic shock or in second- or third-degree heart block with no pacemaker. Use very cautiously, and avoid, if possible, in congestive heart failure. Use cautiously in underlying conduction abnormalities, urinary tract diseases (especially prostatic hypertrophy), hepatic or renal impairment, myasthenia gravis, narrow-angle glaucoma. Adjust dosage in renal insufficiency.
• Discontinue if heart block develops, if QRS complex widens by more than 25%, or if Q-T interval lengthens by more than 25% above baseline.
• Underlying electrolyte abnormalities should be corrected before use.
• Recurrence of arrhythmias possible.
• Apical pulse should be checked before drug is administered. If pulse rate slower than 60 bpm or faster than 120 bpm, doctor should be notified.
• Patient should take drug on time and exactly as prescribed, including night dosages.
• Dry mouth may be relieved with chewing gum or sugarless hard candy.
• Constipation should be managed with proper diet or bulk laxatives.
• Use of disopyramide with other antiarrhythmics may cause further myocardial depression.

NAMES, INDICATIONS AND DOSAGES	SIDE EFFECTS

lidocaine hydrochloride

Lido Pen Auto-Injector, Xylocaine♦

Ventricular arrhythmias from myocardial infarction, cardiac manipulation, or cardiotonic glycosides; ventricular tachycardia:

ADULTS: 50 to 100 mg (1 to 1.5 mg/kg) I.V. bolus at 25 to 50 mg/minute. Give half this amount to elderly or lightweight patients, and to those with congestive heart failure or hepatic disease. Repeat bolus q 3 to 5 minutes until arrhythmias subside or side effects develop. Don't exceed 300 mg total bolus during a 1-hour period. Simultaneously, begin constant infusion: 1 to 4 mg/minute. Use lower dose in elderly patients, those with congestive heart failure or hepatic disease, or patients who weigh less than 50 kg. If single bolus has been given, repeat smaller bolus 15 to 20 minutes after start of infusion to maintain therapeutic serum level. After 24 hours continuous infusion, decrease rate by half.

I.M. administration:

200 to 300 mg in deltoid muscle only.

CNS: *confusion, tremors,* lethargy, *stupor, restlessness,* slurred speech, euphoria, depression, *light-headedness,* muscle twitching, convulsions, coma.
CV: *hypotension,* bradycardia, further arrhythmias.
EENT: *tinnitus, blurred or double vision.*
Other: *anaphylaxis,* soreness at injection site.

nifedipine

Procardia

Management of vasospastic (also called Prinzmetals or variant angina) and classic chronic stable angina pectoris:

ADULTS: Starting dose is 10 mg P.O. t.i.d. Usual effective dose range is 10 to 10 mg t.i.d. Some patients may require up to 30 mg q.i.d. Maximum daily dose is 180 mg.

CNS: *dizziness, lightheadedness, flushing, headache,* weakness, syncope.
CV: peripheral edema, hypotension, palpitations.
EENT: nasal congestion.
GI: *nausea, heartburn,* diarrhea.
Other: muscle cramps, dyspnea.

phenytoin

Dilantin Infatab♦, Dilantin Pediatric

phenytoin sodium

Dantoin♦♦, Dihycon, Dilantin♦, Di-Phen, Diphenylan Sodium, Toin Unicelles

Ventricular arrhythmias unresponsive to lidocaine or procainamide; supraventricular and ventricular arrhythmias induced by cardiotonic glycosides:

ADULTS: loading dose 1 g P.O. divided over first 24 hours, followed by 500 mg daily for 2 days, then maintenance dose 300 mg P.O. daily; 250 mg I.V. over 5 minutes until arrhythmias subside, side effects develop, or 1 g has been given. Infusion rate should never exceed 50 mg/minute (slow I.V. push).

Alternate method:

100 mg I.V. q 15 minutes until side effects develop, arrhythmias are controlled, or 1 g has been given. I.M. dose not recommended because of pain and erratic absorption.

Blood: thrombocytopenia, leukopenia, *agranulocytosis, pancytopenia, lymphadenopathy,* megaloblastic anemia.
CNS: *ataxia,* slurred speech, insomnia, headache, muscle twitching, *lethargy.*
CV: *severe hypotension, vascular collapse (with rapid I.V. infusions greater than 50 mg/minute),* vasodilation, asystole, ventricular fibrillation, AV block.
EENT: *nystagmus, diplopia,* blurred vision.
GI: *gingival hyperplasia, nausea, vomiting,* constipation.
Metabolic: hyperglycemia.
Skin: rash (*morbilliform* most common), dermatitis (bullous, *exfoliative,* purpuric), lupus erythematosus, Stevens-Johnson syndrome.

♦ Available in U.S. and Canada. ♦♦ Available in Canada only.
All other products (no symbol) available in U.S. only. Italicized side effects are common or life-threatening.

INTERACTIONS AND SPECIAL CONSIDERATIONS

Interactions:

BARBITURATES: may decrease patient's response to lidocaine. Adjust dose.

PHENYTOIN: additive cardiac depressant effects. Monitor carefully.

PROCAINAMIDE: may increase neurologic side effects. Monitor carefully.

Special considerations:

• Contraindicated in complete or second-degree heart block. Use of lidocaine with epinephrine (for local anesthesia) to treat arrhythmias contraindicated. Use with caution in elderly patients, those with congestive heart failure, renal or hepatic disease, or in patients who weigh less than 50 kg. Such patients will need a reduced dose.

• Signs of toxicity (dizziness) require immediate discontinuation of drug. Continued infusion could lead to convulsions and coma. Oxygen should be given via nasal cannula, if not contraindicated. Oxygen and CPR equipment should be kept handy.

• Patients receiving infusions must be *attended at all times*. An infusion pump or a microdrip system and timer should be used for monitoring infusion precisely. An infusion rate of 4 mg/minute should never be exceeded, if possible. A faster rate greatly increases the risk of toxicity.

• Patient's response, especially blood pressure, serum electrolytes, BUN, and creatinine, should be monitored for possible abnormalities.

• A bolus dose not followed by infusion will have a short-lived effect.

• A patient who has received lidocaine I.M. will show a sevenfold increase in serum CPK level. Such CPK originates in the skeletal muscle, not the heart. Isoenzymes should be tested if using I.M. route.

• Used investigationally to treat refractory status epilepticus.

• For treatment of anaphylaxis, see APPENDIX.

Interactions:

PROPRANOLOL (AND OTHER BETA BLOCKERS): may cause heart failure. Use together cautiously.

Special considerations:

• Use cautiously in patient with congestive heart failure or hypotension.

• Blood pressure should be checked regularly, especially of patient who is also taking beta blockers or antihypertensives.

• Patient may briefly develop angina exacerbation when beginning drug therapy or at times of dosage increase. This symptom is temporary.

• Although rebound effect hasn't been observed when drug is stopped, dosage should still be reduced slowly under doctor's supervision.

• Patient who is kept on nitrate therapy while drug dosage is being titrated, should continue his compliance. Sublingual nitroglycerin, especially, may be taken as needed when anginal symptoms are acute.

• Nifedipine is the first oral calcium blocker commerically available.

Interactions:

ALCOHOL, BARBITURATES, FOLIC ACID, LOXAPINE SUCCINATE: monitor for decreased phenytoin activity.

ORAL ANTICOAGULANTS, ANTIHISTAMINES, CHLORAMPHENICOL, DIAZEPAM, DIAZOXIDE, DISULFIRAM, ISONIAZID, PHENYLBUTAZONE, PHENYRAMIDOL, SALICYLATES, SULFAMETHIZOLE, VALPROATE: monitor for increased phenytoin activity.

Special considerations:

• Contraindicated in heart block, sinus bradycardia, Stokes-Adams attacks. Use cautiously in patients with congestive heart failure, hepatic or renal dysfunction, hypotension, myocardial insufficiency, respiratory depression, and in elderly or debilitated patients. Cardiac patients on thyroid replacement therapy should be given I.V. phenytoin cautiously to prevent supraventricular tachycardia.

• Drug should be administered slow I.V. push, not to exceed 50 mg/minute in adults.

• Blood pressure and EKG should be monitored for possible abnormalities.

• Should not be mixed with 5% dextrose I.V. fluids, as crystallization will occur. I.V. line should be flushed with saline before and after administration.

• Patients on phenytoin and other antiarrhythmics (disopyramide, quinidine, procainamide, propranolol) should be monitored closely for signs of additive cardiac depression.

• Phenytoin can be diluted in normal saline solution and infused without precipitation. Such infusions should take no longer than 1 hour.

• Oral suspensions should be shaken well to make dosage uniform. After suspension given by nasogastric tube, tube should be flushed with water to facilitate passage to stomach.

• Drug should be given with food or large glass of water to minimize gastric irritation.

• I.M. route of administration should be avoided.

• Patient should take drug on time, exactly as prescribed.

• Dose should be decreased in hepatic dys-

(continued on following page)

NAMES, INDICATIONS AND DOSAGES	SIDE EFFECTS

phenytoin
(continued)

CHILDREN: 3 to 8 mg/kg P.O. or slow I.V. daily or 250 mg/m² daily given as single dose or divided in 2 doses.

---

procainamide hydrochloride
Procan, Procan SR, Pronestyl♦, Sub-Quin

Premature ventricular contractions, ventricular tachycardia, atrial arrhythmias unresponsive to quinidine, paroxysmal atrial tachycardia:
ADULTS: 100 mg q 5 minutes slow I.V. push, no faster than 25 to 50 mg/minute until arrhythmias disappear, side effects develop, or 1 g has been given. When arrhythmias disappear, give continuous infusion of 2 to 6 mg/minute. Usual effective dose 500 to 600 mg. If arrhythmias recur, repeat bolus as above and increase infusion rate; 0.5 to 1 g I.M. q 4 to 8 hours until oral therapy begins.

Loading dose for atrial fibrillation or paroxysmal atrial tachycardia:
ADULTS: 1 to 1.25 g P.O. If arrhythmias persist after 1 hour, give additional 750 mg. If no change occurs, give 500 mg to 1 g q 2 hours until arrhythmias disappear or side effects occur. Maintenance 0.5 to 1 g q 4 to 6 hours.

Loading dose for ventricular tachycardia:
ADULTS: 1 g P.O. Maintenance 50 mg/kg daily given at 3-hour intervals; average 250 to 500 mg q 3 hours.
Note: Sustained-release tablet may be used for maintenance dosing when treating ventricular tachycardia, atrial fibrillation, and paroxysmal atrial tachycardia. Dose is 500 mg to 1 g q 6 hours.

Blood: thrombocytopenia, *agranulocytosis*, hemolytic anemia, *increased ANA titer*.
CNS: hallucinations, confusion, convulsions, depression.
CV: *severe hypotension, bradycardia*, AV block, ventricular fibrillation (after parenteral use).
GI: *nausea, vomiting, anorexia, diarrhea, bitter taste*.
Skin: *maculopapular rash*.
Other: *fever, lupus erythematosus syndrome (especially after prolonged administration)*, myalgia.

---

propranolol hydrochloride
Inderal♦

Supraventricular, ventricular, and atrial arrhythmias; tachyarrhythmias due to excessive catecholamine action during anesthesia, hyperthyroidism, and pheochromocytoma; angina:
ADULTS: 1 to 3 mg I.V. diluted in 50 ml 5% dextrose in water or normal saline solution infused slowly, not to exceed 1 mg/minute. After 3 mg have been infused, another dose may be given in 2 minutes; subsequent doses no sooner than q 4 hours. Maintenance 10 to 80 mg P.O. t.i.d. or q.i.d.

CNS: *fatigue, lethargy*, vivid dreams, hallucinations.
CV: *bradycardia, hypotension, congestive heart failure*, peripheral vascular disease.
GI: nausea, vomiting, diarrhea.
Metabolic: hypoglycemia without tachycardia.
Skin: rash.
Other: *increased airway resistance*, fever.

INTERACTIONS AND SPECIAL CONSIDERATIONS

function.
• Blood levels greater than 20 mcg/ml may be toxic. The difference between therapeutic and toxic levels of phenytoin in the blood is very slight. If toxic symptoms occur, blood should be drawn to determine drug level.
• Good oral hygiene important to minimize gingival hyperplasia.
• Patients with uremia may require dose adjustment for stabilization.
• Patients concurrently on phenytoin and barbiturates, prednisone, or isoniazid should have phenytoin blood levels checked frequently. Patient should be observed for phenytoin toxicity and for failure to respond adequately to phenytoin.
• Patients concurrently on digitoxin and phenytoin may need larger doses.
• Patient should not drink alcohol, as control of previously stable antiarrhythmic effects may be lost.

No significant interactions.

Special considerations:
• Contraindicated in patients with hypersensitivity to procaine and related drugs; in those with complete, second-, or third-degree heart block unassisted by electrical pacemaker, or in those with myasthenia gravis. Use with caution in congestive heart failure or other conduction disturbances, such as bundle branch block or cardiotonic glycoside intoxication, or with hepatic or renal insufficiency.
• Patients receiving infusions must be *attended at all times.* An infusion pump or a microdrip system and timer should be used to monitor infusion precisely.
• Blood pressure and EKG should be monitored continuously during I.V. administration. Possible prolonged Q-T and Q-R intervals, heart block, or increased arrhythmias. If these occur, drug should be withheld, rhythm strip obtained, and doctor notified immediately.
• Patient should remain in supine position for I.V. administration.
• Patient should report fever, rash, muscle pain, diarrhea, or pleuritic chest pain.
• Dose should be decreased in hepatic and renal dysfunction, and given over 6 hours. Half-life of procainamide is increased as much as threefold in these states.
• Patient with congestive heart failure has a lower volume of distribution and can be treated with lower doses.
• Positive antinuclear antibody titer common in about 60% of patients who don't have symptoms of lupus erythematosus syndrome. This response seems related to prolonged use, not dosage.
• After long-standing atrial fibrillation, restoration of normal rhythm may result in thromboembolism, due to dislodgement of thrombi from atrial wall. Anticoagulation usually advised before restoration of normal sinus rhythm.
• Patient should take drug exactly as prescribed. Patient may have to set an alarm clock for night dosage.

Interactions:
INSULIN, HYPOGLYCEMIC DRUGS (ORAL): can alter requirements for these drugs in previously stabilized diabetics. Monitor for hypoglycemia.
CARDIOTONIC GLYCOSIDES: cause excessive bradycardia and increased depressant effect on myocardium. Use together cautiously.
AMINOPHYLLINE: antagonizes beta-blocking effects of propranolol. Use together cautiously.
ISOPROTERENOL, GLUCAGON: antagonizes propranolol effect. May be used therapeutically and in emergencies.
CINETIDINE: inhibits propranolol's metabolism. Monitor for greater beta-blocking effect.
EPINEPHRINE: Severe vasocontriction. Monitor blood pressure and observe patient carefully.

Special considerations:
• Contraindicated in asthma or allergic rhinitis; during ethyl ether anesthesia; in sinus bradycardia and in heart block greater than first degree; in cardiogenic shock; in right ventricular failure secondary to pulmonary hypertension. Use with caution in patients with congestive heart failure, diabetes mellitus, or respiratory disease.
• Drug should always be withdrawn slowly. Abrupt withdrawal might precipitate myocardial infarction or aggravate angina, thyrotoxicosis, or pheochromocytoma. Abrupt withdrawal in thyrotoxicosis may exacerbate hyperthyroidism or precipitate thyroid storm. In thyrotoxicosis, propranolol may mask clinical signs of hyper-

(continued on following page)

NAMES, INDICATIONS AND DOSAGES	SIDE EFFECTS

propranolol hydrochloride
(continued)

quinidine bisulfate
(66% quinidine base)
Biquin Durules♦♦
quinidine gluconate
(62% quinidine base)
Duraquin, Quinaglute Dura-Tabs♦, Quinate♦♦
quinidine polygalacturonate
(60.5% quinidine base)
Cardioquin♦
quinidine sulfate
(83% quinidine base)
CinQuin, Quine, Quinidex Extentabs♦, Quinora, SK-Quinidine Sulfate

Atrial flutter or fibrillation:
ADULTS: 200 mg quinidine sulfate or equivalent base P.O. q 2 to 3 hours for 5 to 8 doses with subsequent daily increases until sinus rhythm is restored or toxic effects develop. Administer quinidine only after digitalization to avoid increasing AV block. Maximum 3 to 4 g daily.

Paroxysmal supraventricular tachycardia:
ADULTS: 400 to 600 mg I.M. gluconate q 2 to 3 hours until toxic side effects develop or arrhythmia subsides.

Premature atrial and ventricular contractions; paroxysmal atrioventricular junctional rhythm; paroxysmal atrial tachycardia; paroxysmal ventricular tachycardia; maintenance after cardioversion of atrial fibrillation or flutter:
ADULTS: test dose 50 to 200 mg P.O., then monitor vital signs before beginning therapy. Quinidine sulfate or equivalent base 200 to 400 mg P.O. q 4 to 6 hours; or initially, quinidine gluconate 600 mg I.M., then up to 400 mg q 2 hours, p.r.n.; or quinidine gluconate 800 mg I.V. diluted in 40 ml 5% dextrose in water, infused at 1 mg/minute.
CHILDREN: test dose 2 mg/kg; 3 to 6 mg/kg q 2 to 3 hours for 5 doses P.O. daily.

Blood: *hemolytic anemia, thrombocytopenia, agranulocytosis.*
CNS: *vertigo, headache, light-headedness,* confusion, restlessness, cold sweat, pallor, fainting.
CV: *premature ventricular contractions; severe hypotension; SA and AV block; ventricular fibrillation, tachycardia; aggravated congestive heart failure; EKG changes (particularly widening of QRS complex, notched P waves, widened Q-T interval, ST segment depression).*
EENT: *tinnitus,* excessive salivation, blurred vision.
GI: *diarrhea, nausea, vomiting,* anorexia, abdominal pains.
Skin: rash, petechial hemorrhage of buccal mucosa, pruritus.
Other: angioedema, acute asthmatic attack, respiratory arrest, *fever, cinchonism.*

verapamil
Calan, Isoptin

Treatment of atrial arrhythmias:
ADULTS: 0.075 to 0.15 mg/kg (5 to 10 mg)

CNS: dizziness, headache.
CV: *transient hypotension, heart failure,* bradycardia, AV block, ventricular asystole.

♦ Available in U.S. and Canada. ♦♦ Available in Canada only.
All other products (no symbol) available in U.S. only. Italicized side effects are common or life-threatening.

INTERACTIONS AND SPECIAL CONSIDERATIONS

thyroidism.

• *Should not be discontinued before surgery for pheochromocytoma*. Before any surgical procedure, anesthesiologist should be notified that patient is receiving propranolol.

• I.V. doses much smaller than oral doses.

• Apical pulse rate and blood pressure should be checked before drug is given. Extremes in pulse rate require immediate discontinuation of drug and reevaluation of cardiac status. Severe bradycardia may be treated with atropine 0.25 to 1 mg I.V.

• After long-standing atrial fibrillation, restoration of normal sinus rhythm may result in thromboembolism due to dislodgement of thrombi from atrial wall. Anticoagulation often advised before restoration of normal atrial rhythm.

• Blood pressure, EKG, and heart rate and rhythm should be monitored frequently, especially during I.V. administration. When propranolol is used with other antihypertensives, blood pressure should be monitored in both sitting and standing positions.

• Patient's lungs should be auscultated for rales and heart for gallop rhythm or for third or fourth heart sounds.

Interactions:

ACETAZOLAMIDE, ANTACIDS, SODIUM BICARBONATE: may increase quinidine blood levels due to alkaline urine. Monitor for increased effect.

BARBITURATES, PHENYTOIN: may antagonize quinidine activity. Monitor for decreased quinidine effect.

Special considerations:

• Contraindicated in cardiotonic glycoside toxicity when AV conduction is grossly impaired; complete AV block with AV nodal or idioventricular pacemaker. Use with caution in myasthenia gravis. Anticholinergic drug doses may have to be increased.

• May increase toxicity of digitalis derivatives. Should be used with caution in patients previously digitalized. Digoxin levels should be monitored.

• Dosage varies—some patients may require drug q 4 hours, others q 6 hours. Dose should be titrated by both clinical response and blood levels.

• When route of administration is changed, dosage should be altered to compensate for variations in quinidine base content.

• Dose should be decreased in congestive heart failure and hepatic disease.

• Apical pulse rate and blood pressure should be checked before starting therapy. Extremes in pulse rate require immediate discontinuation of drug and reevaluation of cardiac status.

• Lidocaine may be effective in treating quinidine-induced arrhythmias, since it increases AV conduction.

• GI side effects, especially diarrhea, are signs of toxicity. Quinidine blood levels, which are toxic when greater than 8 mcg/ml, should be checked. GI symptoms may be decreased by giving with meals. Drug response should be monitored carefully.

• After long-standing atrial fibrillation, restoration of normal sinus rhythm may result in thromboembolism due to dislodgement of thrombi from atrial wall. Anticoagulation often advised before restoration of normal atrial rhythm.

• Discolored (brownish) quinidine solution should never be used.

Interactions:

PROPRANOLOL (AND OTHER BETA BLOCKERS) DISOPYRAMIDE: may cause heart failure. Use together cautiously.

Special considerations:

• Contraindicated in patients with advanced heart failure, AV block, cardiogenic shock, sinus node disease, and severe hypotension.

• Use cautiously in patients with myocardial

(continued on following page)

NAMES, INDICATIONS AND DOSAGES	SIDE EFFECTS
verapamil *(continued)* I.V. push over 60 seconds with EKG and blood pressure monitoring. Repeat dose in 30 minutes if no response. Follow bolus injection with maintenance infusion of 0.005 mg/kg/minute.	

♦ Available in U.S. and Canada. ♦♦ Available in Canada only.
All other products (no symbol) available in U.S. only. Italicized side effects are common or life-threatening.

CALCIUM BLOCKERS: CARDIAC BREAKTHROUGH?

Verapamil and nifedipine, and the even newer diltiazem and lidoflazine, belong to the new breed of cardiac drugs—the calcium blockers. Used for several years, these drugs prevent calcium transport across the cell membrane so the cardiac muscle and the smooth muscle of the coronary arteries won't contract as forcefully.

1. Under normal conditions, a protein complex prevents muscle contraction by keeping actin and myosin (the contractile proteins) apart. Actin and myosin must interact for a muscle to contract. When the muscle cell is stimulated, calcium ions enter the cell.

This influx of calcium releases more calcium from the sarcoplasmic reticulum inside the muscle cell.

2. When enough calcium is released, it binds with the protein complex. Hence, the actin and myosin can interact and the muscle contracts.

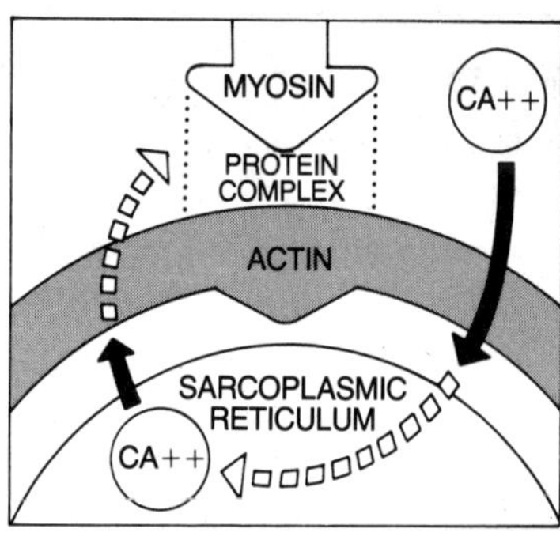

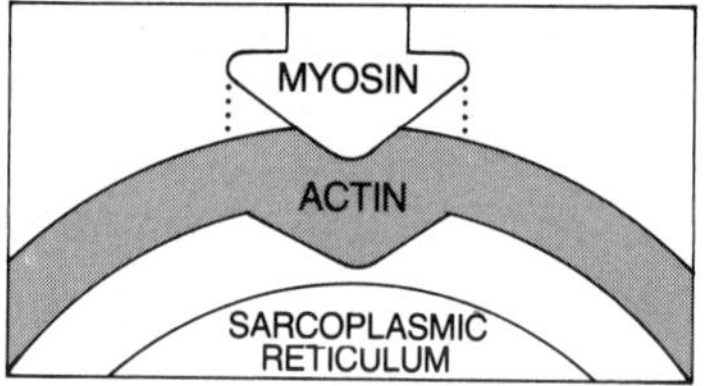

INTERACTIONS AND SPECIAL CONSIDERATIONS

infarction followed by coronary occlusion, sick sinus syndrome, impaired AV conduction, and heart failure with atrial tachyarrhythmia.

• Patients with severely compromised cardiac function or those receiving beta blockers should receive lower doses of verapamil. These patients should be monitored very closely.

• A new and very effective drug for treatment of supraventricular arrhythmias. Not very effective for ventricular arrhythmias.

• Oral form of verapamil is investigational. Being used in treatment of both Prinzmetal's (variant) angina and classic angina pectoris.

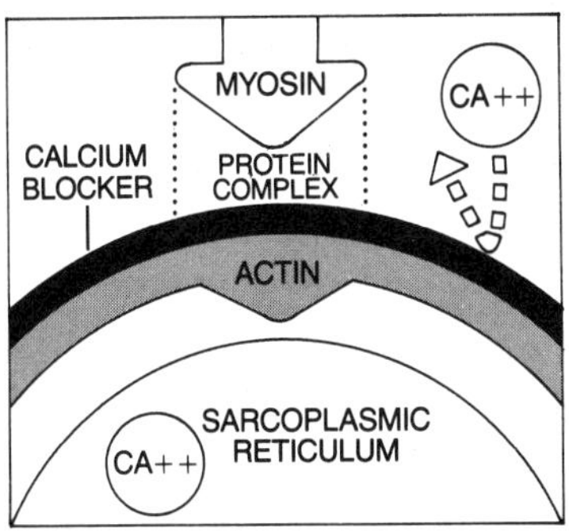

3. Calcium blockers prevent calcium from entering the cell, thereby preventing calcium release from the sarcoplasmic reticulum.

Although all the calcium blockers exert this effect on cardiac muscle, one compound may prove to be more effective for a specific heart condition than another. In general, however, calcium blockers can:

• *reduce electrical excitation and mechanical contraction of the heart.* Arrhythmias, especially those of atrial origin, can be relieved and perhaps even prevented.
• *relieve excruciating anginal pain* caused by spasms of the coronary arteries.
• *allow more rest for damaged tissue.*
• *reduce peripheral arterial resistance and myocardial oxygen demand.*

In addition, calcium blockers *present relatively mild side effects;* headache, dizziness, and constipation are the most common. Unlike beta blockers, these drugs can be used by patients with asthma and those with congestive heart failure that's not too severe.

Some researchers believe calcium blockers have several exciting potential uses, and are speculating that these drugs may eventually be used to treat high blood pressure, prevent recurrent heart attacks, limit damage from attacks, and delay or even eliminate the need for coronary bypass operations. The research continues.

21

Antihypertensives

Sympatholytics
alkavervir
alseroxylon
atenolol
captopril
clonidine hydrochloride
cryptenamine acetate
cryptenamine tannate
deserpidine
guanethidine sulfate
mecamylamine hydrochloride
methyldopa
metoprolol tartrate
metyrosine
nadolol
pargyline hydrochloride
phenoxybenzamine hydrochloride
phentolamine hydrochloride
phentolamine methanesulfonate
propranolol hydrochloride
rauwolfia serpentina
rescinnamine
reserpine
timolol maleate
trimethaphan camsylate

Vasodilaors
diazoxide
hydralazine hydrochloride
minoxidil
nitroprusside sodium
prazosln hydrochloride

(All drugs are listed in alphabetical order in the tables that follow.)

Antihypertensives are used to lower blood pressure in patients whose diastolic blood pressure averages 90 to 95 mmHg or more. To control blood pressure effectively with minimal side effects, two or more antihypertensive agents—with different modes of action—may be needed.

About 15% of adults are hypertensive. About half these people don't realize they're ill because they remain asymptomatic until complications occur. Untreated hypertension can lead to stroke and cardiac or renal disease.

Hypertension is now one of the few chronic diseases for which effective therapy exists. However, treatment depends on accurate diagnosis.

Compliance with prescribed drug regimens is one of the biggest problems in the treatment of this disorder because, to the patient, the side effects from the drugs may seem worse than the disease.

Major uses

Antihypertensives are used primarily to treat mild-to-severe essential hypertension (about 90% of all cases of hypertension). Virtually all parenteral drugs are reserved for treatment of hypertensive emergencies such as hypertensive encephalopathy or malignant hypertension.

Antihypertensives can also be used to control hypertension in the 10% of patients who have secondary hypertension until a surgical cure can be obtained.

• Two alpha blockers—phenoxybenzamine and phentolamine—and the tyrosine hydroxylase inhibitor metyrosine can be used to diagnose and manage pheochromocytoma until surgery, if feasible, can be performed.

• Some vasodilating antihypertensives can also be used in chronic refractory congestive heart failure (CHF) to decrease the arterial resistance (afterload) that the heart must pump against. This decrease in arterial impedance causes an increase in cardiac output. Minoxidil and hydralazine affect mainly the arterial bed, whereas prazosin and nitroprusside affect both the arterial and venous sides.

A vasodilator affecting the arterial bed (afterload) may be used alone or in combination with a nitrate affecting the venous bed (preload) to treat refractory CHF. Preload and

afterload agents are used in combination with standard therapy for CHF (salt reduction, diuretics, and digoxin) to achieve maximal results. Also, see Chapter 22, VASODILATORS.
• Timolol and other beta blockers are used for long-term prophylaxis in survivors of acute myocardial infarction.

Mechanism of action
The chart on pp. 206 to 207 summarizes the neuromuscular and enzymatic mechanisms of the major classes of antihypertensive agents. (See Chapter 62, DIURETICS, for more information on the diuretic effects of the antihypertensives.)

Absorption, distribution, metabolism, and excretion
Given orally, most antihypertensives are rapidly absorbed from the gastrointestinal (GI) tract. Alkavervir and methyldopa, however, are erratically absorbed. All antihypertensives are widely distributed in body tissues, and most are excreted predominately through the kidneys. Prazosin, however, is eliminated through bile and feces.
• Captopril: Well absorbed from the GI tract, distributed to most body tissues, and partially metabolized in the liver. Both metabolite and unchanged drug excreted in urine.
• Hydralazine: Some patients acetylate (metabolize) hydralazine at a faster rate than others. Since acetylation inactivates the drug, rapid acetylators may require doses up to 60% larger than the usual dose to control their blood pressure.
• Methyldopa: Absorption varies from day to day but averages 50% of dose. Onset delayed about 12 to 24 hours after oral dose because methyldopa biotransformed in the liver to the metabolite alpha-methylnorepinephrine, producing antihypertensive effect.

Onset and duration
The chart on pp. 206 to 207 describes the onset and duration of antihypertensives.

Combination products
ALDORIL-15♦: hydrochlorothiazide 15 mg and methyldopa 250 mg.
ALDORIL D30: hydrochlorothiazide 30 mg and methyldopa 50 mg.
APRESAZIDE 25/25: hydrochlorothiazide 25 mg and hydralazine HCl 25 mg.
COMBIPRES 0.1♦: chlorthalidone 15 mg and clonidine HCl 0.1 mg.
DIUPRES-250♦: chlorothiazide 250 mg and reserpine 0.125 mg.
DIUTENSEN: methyclothiazide 2.5 mg and cryptenamine 2 mg (as tannate).
ENDURONYL: methyclothiazide 5 mg and deserpidine 0.25 mg.
ESIMIL: hydrochlorothiazide 25 mg and guanethidine monosulfate 10 mg.
HYDROPRES-25♦: hydrochlorothiazide 25 mg and reserpine 0.125 mg.
HYDROSERP: hydrochlorothiazide 50 mg and reserpine 0.125 mg.
INDERIDE 40/25: propranolol HCl 40 mg and hydrochlorothiazide 25 mg.
ORETICYL 25: hydrochlorothiazide 25 mg and deserpidine 0.125 mg.
RAUZIDE: bendroflumethiazide 4 mg and powdered rauwolfia serpentina 50 mg.
REGROTON: chlorthalidone 50 mg and reserpine 0.25 mg.
RENESE-R: polythiazide 2 mg and reserpine 0.25 mg.
SALUTENSIN♦: hydroflumethiazide 50 mg and reserpine 0.125 mg.
SER-AP-ES♦: hydrochlorothiazide 15 mg, reserpine 0.1 mg, and hydralazine HCl 25 mg.
SERPASIL-APRESOLINE #1: reserpine 0.1 mg and hydralazine HCl 25 mg.
SERPASIL-ESIDRIX #1♦: hydrochlorothiazide 25 mg and reserpine 0.1 mg.

THERAPEUTIC ACTIVITY

THERAPEUTIC ACTIVITY OF ANTIHYPERTENSIVES

DRUG	ROUTE	ONSET	DURATION	SITE AND MECHANISM OF ACTION
Sympatholytics				
alkavervir	P.O.	2 hr	4 to 6 hr	Veratrum alkaloids; alkavervir and cryptenamine stimulate pressor receptors in the heart and the carotid sinus.
cryptenamine	I.M. I.V. P.O.	30 to 40 min 2 to 3 min 2 hr	3 to 6 hr 1 to 2 hr 4 to 6 hr	
alseroxylon, deserpidine, rauwolfia, and rescinnamine	P.O.	days to weeks	days	Peripherally acting antihypertensives; they deplete stores of norepinephrine by inhibiting its uptake.
reserpine	I.M. I.V. P.O.	2 hr 4 to 60 min days to weeks	10 to 12 hr 6 to 8 hr days	
captopril	P.O.	1 hr	6 to 12 hr	Enzyme inhibitors; captopril inhibits angiotensin-converting enzyme and prevents conversion of angiotensin I to angiotensin II in the lungs: metyrosine inhibits tyrosine hydroxylase; and pargyline inhibits monoamine oxidase.
metyrosine	P.O.	1 to 2 days	3 to 4 days	
pargyline	P.O.	days to weeks	weeks	
clonidine	P.O.	30 to 60 min	8 hr	Centrally acting drug: decreases central sympathetic outflow.
guanethidine	P.O.	1 to 3 wk	1 to 3 wk	Peripherally acting drug; directly inhibits release of norepinephrine and depletes stores of norepinephrine in adrenergic nerve endings.
mecamylamine	P.O.	½ to 2 hr	6 to 12 hr	Ganglionic blockers; mecamylamine competes with acetylcholine for cholinergic receptors; trimethanphan stabilizes postsynaptic membranes.
trimethaphan	I.V.	immediate	10 min after infusion is stopped	

DRUG	ROUTE	ONSET	DURATION	SITE AND MECHANISM OF ACTION
methyldopa	I.V. P.O.	4 to 6 hr 12 to 24 hr	24 to 48 hr 24 to 48 hr	Centrally acting drug; activates inhibitory alpha-adrenergic receptors, reducing central sympathetic output.
atenolol	P.O.	days to weeks	24 to 36 hr	Beta blockers: all three drugs block response to beta stimulation; they also depress renin output.
metoprolol	P.O.	days to weeks*	12 to 24 hr	
nadolol	P.O.	days to weeks*	24 to 36 hr	
propranolol	I.V. P.O.	1 to 5 min days to weeks*	4 to 6 hr 12 to 24 hr	
timolol	P.O.	days to weeks	12 to 24 hr	
phenoxybenzamine	P.O.	up to 4 days*	24 to 36 hr	Alpha blockers; both drugs competitively inhibit alpha-adrenergic receptors.
phentolamine	I.M. I.V. P.O.	2 to 5 min 30 to 60 sec up to 4 days*	30 to 45 min 15 to 30 min 24 to 36 hr	
Vasodilators				
diazoxide	I.V.	5 min	3 to 12 hr	Directly relaxes arteriolar smooth muscle.
hydralazine	I.M. I.V. P.O.	10 to 30 min 5 to 20 min 20 to 30 min	2 to 6 hr 2 to 6 hr 3 to 8 hr‡	
minoxidil	P.O.	30 min	24 hr	
nitroprusside	I.V.	immediate	1 to 10 min after infusion is stopped (effect dissipates rapidly)	Relaxes both arteriolar and venous smooth muscle.
prazosin	P.O.	2 hr	less than 24 hr	

* Depending on dosage † Depending on acetylator status

NAMES, INDICATIONS AND DOSAGES	SIDE EFFECTS
alkavervir **Essential, renal, or malignant hypertension; toxemia of pregnancy—** ADULTS: 3 to 5 mg P.O. daily, given in 3 to 4 divided doses not less than 4 hours apart. Give after meals. Initial recommended dose is 8 to 9 mg. No dosing recommendations for children.	**CNS:** mental confusion. **CV:** *orthostatic hypotension,* cardiac arrhythmias, *bradycardia.* **EENT:** blurred vision, excessive salivation, unpleasant taste. **GI:** *nausea, vomiting,* epigastric burning, hiccups. **Other:** respiratory depression, bronchial constriction, sweating.
alseroxylon Raudolfin, Rauwiloid **Mild, labile hypertension:** ADULTS: initially, 4 mg P.O. daily as a single dose or divided in 2 doses for 1 to 3 weeks. Maintenance dose: 2 mg or less daily. No dosing recommendations for children.	**CNS:** mental confusion, *depression, drowsiness, nervousness, anxiety,* insomnia, *nightmares,* sedation. **CV:** *orthostatic hypotension, bradycardia.* **EENT:** *mouth dryness, nasal stuffiness,* glaucoma. **GI:** *hypersecretion of gastric acid, nausea, vomiting,* gastrointestinal bleeding. **Skin:** pruritus, rash. **Other:** *impotence, weight gain.*
atenolol Tenormin **Treatment of hypertension:** ADULTS: initially, 50 mg P.O. daily single dose. Dosage may be increased to 100 mg once daily after 7 to 14 days. Dosages greater than 100 mg are unlikely to produce further benefit.	**CNS:** *fatigue, lethargy,* vivid dreams, hallucinations. **CV:** *bradycardia, hypotension, congestive heart failure,* peripheral vascular disease. **GI:** nausea, vomiting, diarrhea. **Metabolic:** hypoglycemia without tachycardia. **Skin:** rash. **Other:** fever.

♦ Available in U.S. and Canada. ♦♦ Available in Canada only.
All other products (no symbol) available in U.S. only. Italicized side effects are common or life-threatening.

INTERACTIONS AND SPECIAL CONSIDERATIONS

Interactions:

ANESTHETIC AGENTS: may cause additive hypotensive effect. Observe patient carefully.

TRICYCLIC ANTIDEPRESSANTS: may diminish hypotensive response. Avoid if possible.

Special considerations:

- Contraindicated in patients with pheochromocytoma. Use cautiously in patients with angina, cerebrovascular disease, or bronchial asthma, or in those receiving other antihypertensive drugs.
- Rarely used to treat hypertension because of unsatisfactory response and high incidence of side effects.
- The range between therapeutic and toxic doses of this drug is narrow.
- Blood pressure and pulse rate should be monitored closely. Treatment with phenylephrine or ephedrine may be needed for severe hypotension; atropine for bradycardia.
- Patient should understand his disease and therapy. He should take this drug exactly as prescribed, even when he's feeling well. Patient should not stop this drug suddenly, but report unpleasant side effects.
- Orthostatic hypotension can be minimized by rising slowly and avoiding sudden position changes. Unpleasant taste can be relieved with sugarless chewing gum, sour hard candy, or ice chips; nausea and vomiting can be prevented by not eating for at least 4 hours after each dose.
- In very hot weather, patient may require smaller doses.
- This drug should be taken after meals.

Interactions:

MAO INHIBITORS: may cause excitability and hypertension. Avoid if possible.

Special considerations:

- Use cautiously in patients with severe cardiac or cerebrovascular disease, peptic ulcer, ulcerative colitis, renal disease, gallstones, or mental depressive disorders, or in those undergoing surgery.
- Use cautiously in patients taking other antihypertensive drugs.
- Patient's blood pressure and pulse rate should be monitored frequently.
- Patient should understand his disease and therapy. He should take this drug exactly as prescribed, even when he's feeling well. Patient should not discontinue this drug suddenly, but report unpleasant side effects, such as mental depression, nightmares, or insomnia. Patient should be watched closely for signs of mental depression.
- Effect of drug may last for 10 days after discontinuation.
- This drug can cause drowsiness.
- Female patient should report pregnancy.
- Orthostatic hypotension can be minimized by rising slowly and avoiding sudden position changes. Mouth dryness can be relieved with sugarless chewing gum, sour hard candy, or ice chips.
- Patient should contact doctor if relief is needed for nasal stuffiness.
- This drug should be taken with meals.
- Patient should weigh himself daily and report any weight gain.
- 1 mg of alseroxylon is approximately equal to 0.1 mg of reserpine.

Interactions:

INSULIN AND HYPOGLYCEMIC DRUGS (ORAL): can alter dosage requirements in previously stablilized diabetics. Observe patient carefully.

CARDIAC GLYCOSIDES: excessive bradycardia and increased depressant effect on myocardium. Use together cautiously.

Special considerations:

- Contraindicated in sinus bradycardia and greater than first degree conduction block, and cardiogenic shock.
- Use cautiously in patients with cardiac failure.
- Similar to metoprolol, atenolol is a cardioselective beta blocker. Although atenolol can be used in patients with bronchospastic diseases such as asthma and emphysema, the drug should still be used cautiously in such patients–especially when 100 mg are given.
- Dosage should be reduced if patient has renal insufficiency.
- Once-a-day dosage encourages patient compliance. Patient should take the drug at a regular time every day. Drug can be dispensed in a 28-day calendar pack.
- Patient's apical pulse should always be checked before giving this drug; apical pulse rate slower than 60 bpm should be reported and medication held.
- Blood pressure should be monitored frequently. If patient develops severe hypotension, a vasopressor may be prescribed.
- Abrupt discontinuation can exacerbate angina and MI.
- Patient should understand his disease and therapy. He should take this drug even when he's feeling well. Patient should not discontinue drug suddenly, but report unpleasant side effects.
- This drug masks common signs of shock and hypoglycemia.

NAMES, INDICATIONS AND DOSAGES	SIDE EFFECTS

captopril
Capoten

Treatment of severe hypertension:
ADULTS: 25 mg t.i.d. initially. If blood pressure isn't satisfactorily controlled in 1 to 2 weeks, dose may be increased to 50 mg t.i.d. If not satisfactorily controlled after another 1 to 2 weeks, a diuretic should be added to regimen. If further blood pressure reduction is necessary, dose may be raised to as high as 150 mg t.i.d. while continuing the diuretic. Maximum dose is 450 mg/day.

Blood: *leukopenia, agranulocytosis, pancytopenia.*
CNS: dizziness, fainting.
CV: *tachycardia,* hypotension, angina pectoris, congestive heart failure.
EENT: *loss of taste (dysgeusia).*
GU: *proteinuria, nephrotic syndrome, membranous glomerulopathy, renal failure,* urinary frequency.
GI: anorexia.
Skin: *urticarial rash, maculopapular rash,* pruritus.
Other: fever, angioedema of face and extremities, transient increases in liver enzymes.

---

clonidine hydrochloride
Catapres♦

Essential, renal, and malignant hypertension:
ADULTS: initially, 0.1 mg P.O. b.i.d. Then increase by 0.1 to 0.2 mg daily on a weekly basis. Usual dose range: 0.2 to 0.8 mg daily in divided doses. Infrequently, doses as high as 2.4 mg daily.
No dosing recommendations for children.

CNS: *drowsiness,* dizziness, fatigue, sedation, nervousness, headache.
CV: orthostatic hypotension, bradycardia.
EENT: *mouth dryness.*
GI: *constipation.*
GU: urinary retention.
Other: impotence.

---

cryptenamine acetate
Unitensen Aqueous
cryptenamine tannate
Unitensen, Unitensyl♦♦

Mild-to-moderate hypertension, toxemia:
ADULTS: initially, 2 mg P.O. b.i.d., increased at weekly intervals, depending on response. Total daily dose not to exceed 12 mg daily. I.V. (for hypertensive crises and convulsive toxemia)—0.5 ml (130 CSR units) diluted to 20 ml with 5% dextrose in water. Administer at infusion rate of 1 ml/minute. When giving this drug I.V., record blood pressure approximately every minute.

CNS: mental confusion.
CV: *orthostatic hypotension,* cardiac arrhythmias, *bradycardia.*
EENT: blurred vision, excessive salivation, unpleasant taste.
GI: *nausea, vomiting,* epigastric burning, hiccups.
Other: respiratory depression, bronchial constriction.

---

deserpidine
Harmonyl

Mild essential hypertension:
ADULTS: 0.25 mg P.O. t.i.d. to q.i.d. for up

CNS: mental confusion, *depression, drowsiness, nervousness,* anxiety, nightmares, sedation.
CV: bradycardia.
EENT: *mouth dryness, nasal stuffiness,* glaucoma.

♦ Available in U.S. and Canada. ♦♦ Available in Canada only.
All other products (no symbol) available in U.S. only. Italicized side effects are common or life-threatening.

INTERACTIONS AND SPECIAL CONSIDERATIONS

No significant interactions.

Special considerations:

- Use cautiously in patients with impaired renal function or serious autoimmune disease (particularly systemic lupus erythematosus), or those who have been exposed to other drugs known to affect white cell counts or immune response.
- Proteinuria and nephrotic syndrome may occur in patients who are on captopril therapy. Those who develop persistent proteinuria or proteinuria that exceeds 1 g/day should have their captopril therapy reevaluated.
- Patient's blood pressure and pulse rate should be monitored frequently.
- WBC and differential counts should be performed before starting treatment, every 2 weeks for the first 3 months of therapy, and periodically thereafter.
- Patients should report any sign of infection (sore throat, fever).
- Because captopril may cause serious side effects, it should be reserved for those patients who have developed undesirable side effects from or failed to respond to other antihypertensive drugs. Commonly used in patients who fail to respond to triple-drug therapy (a diuretic, a beta blocker, and a vasodilator).
- Although captopril can be used alone, its beneficial effects are increased when a thiazide diuretic is added.
- May cause dizziness or fainting; patients should avoid sudden postural changes.
- Impaired taste sensation is possible.
- Should be taken 1 hour before meals since food in the GI tract may reduce absorption.

Interactions:

TRICYCLIN ANTIDEPRESSANTS AND MAO INHIBITORS: may decrease antihypertensive effect. Use together cautiously.

PROPRANOLOL AND OTHER BETA BLOCKERS: paradoxical hypertensive response. Monitor carefully.

Special considerations:

- Use cautiously in patients with severe coronary insufficiency, myocardial infarction, cerebrovascular disease, chronic renal failure, history of depression, or those taking other antihypertensives.
- Blood pressure and pulse rate should be monitored frequently. Dosage is usually adjusted to patient's blood pressure and tolerance.
- Dose should be reduced gradually over 2 to 4 days. If discontinued abruptly, this drug may cause severe hypertension.
- Patient should understand his disease and therapy. He should take this drug exactly as prescribed, even when he's feeling well. Patient should not discontinue this drug suddenly, but report unpleasant side effects. This drug can cause drowsiness.
- Orthostatic hypotension can be minimized by rising slowly and avoiding sudden position changes. Mouth dryness can be relieved with sugarless chewing gum, sour hard candy, or ice chips.
- Last dose should be taken immediately before retiring.
- Has been used investigationally to decrease the subjective symptoms of opiate withdrawal, migraine headache prophylaxis, and dysmenorrhea.

Interactions:

ANESTHETIC AGENTS: may cause additive hypotensive effect. Observe patient carefully.

TRICYCLIC ANTIDEPRESSANTS: may diminish hypotensive response. Avoid if possible.

Special considerations:

- Contraindicated in patients with pheochromocytoma. Use cautiously in patients with angina, cerebrovascular disease, bronchial asthma, or renal insufficiency, or in those taking other antihypertensives.
- Blood pressure and pulse rate should be monitored closely. If severe hypotension develops, infusion should be stopped; phenylephrine or ephedrine may be ordered to counteract effect. Hypotension should dissipate in 60 to 90 minutes. If patient develops bradycardia, he may require atropine.
- The range between therapeutic and toxic doses of this drug is narrow. Side effects may develop.
- Patient should understand his disease and therapy. He should take this drug exactly as prescribed, even when he's feeling well. Patient should not discontinue this drug suddenly, but report unpleasant side effects. This drug can cause drowsiness.
- Orthostatic hypotension can be minimized by rising slowly and avoiding sudden position changes. Unpleasant taste can be relieved with sugarless chewing gum, sour hard candy, or ice chips.

Interactions:

MAO INHIBITORS: may cause excitability and hypertension. Avoid if possible.

Special considerations:

- Contraindicated in patients with mental depression. Use cautiously in patients with severe cardiac or cerebrovascular disease, peptic ulcer, ulcerative colitis, gallstones, or mental

(continued on following page)

NAMES, INDICATIONS AND DOSAGES	SIDE EFFECTS

deserpidine
(continued)

to 2 weeks, then maintenance dose of 0.25 mg once daily may be adequate.

No dosing recommendations for children.

GI: *hypersecretion of gastric acid, nausea, vomiting,* gastrointestinal bleeding.
Skin: pruritus, rash.
Other: *impotence, weight gain.*

---

diazoxide
Hyperstat♦ (I.V. only)

Hypertensive crisis:

ADULTS: 300 mg I.V. bolus push, administered in 30 seconds or less into peripheral vein. Repeat at intervals of 4 to 24 hours, p.r.n. Miniboluses of 1 to 3 mg/kg repeated at intervals of 5 to 15 minutes or infusions of 15 mg/minute are equally effective. Switch to therapy with oral antihypertensives as soon as possible.

CHILDREN: 5 mg/kg I.V. rapid bolus push.

CNS: *headaches,* dizziness, light-headedness, euphoria.
CV: *sodium and water retention, orthostatic hypotension,* sweating, flusing, warmth, angina, myocardial ischemia, arrhythmias, EKG changes.
GI: *nausea, vomiting,* abdominal discomfort.
Metabolic: *hyperglycemia,* hyperuricemia.
Local: inflammation and pain from extravasation.

---

guanethidine sulfate
Ismelin♦

For moderate-to-severe hypertension; usually used in combination with other antihypertensives:

ADULTS: initially, 10 mg P.O. daily. Increase by 10 mg at weekly to monthly intervals, p.r.n. Usual dose is 25 to 50 mg daily. Some patients may require up to 300 mg.

CHILDREN: initially, 200 mcg/kg P.O. daily. Increase gradually every 1 to 3 weeks to maximum of 8 times initial dose.

CNS: *dizziness, weakness, syncope.*
CV: *orthostatic hypotension, bradycardia,* congestive heart failure, arrhythmias.
EENT: *nasal stuffiness,* mouth dryness.
GI: *diarrhea.*
Other: *edema, weight gain, inhibition of ejaculation.*

---

hydralazine hydrochloride
Apresoline♦, Dralzine, Hydralyn, Nor-Pres 25, Rolazine

Essential hypertension (oral, alone or in combination with other antihypertensives); to reduce afterload in severe congestive heart failure (with nitrates); and severe essential hypertension (parenteral to lower blood pressure quickly):

CNS: peripheral neuritis, *headache,* dizziness.
CV: orthostatic hypotension, *tachycardia,* arrhythmias, *angina, palpitations, sodium retention.*
GI: *nausea, vomiting, diarrhea, anorexia.*
Skin: rash.
Other: *lupus erythematosus–like syndrome, weight gain.*

♦ Available in U.S. and Canada. ♦♦ Available in Canada only.
All other products (no symbol) available in U.S. only. Italicized side effects are common or life-threatening.

INTERACTIONS AND SPECIAL CONSIDERATIONS

depressive disorders; in patients undergoing surgery; and in patients taking other antihypertensives or anticonvulsants.
• Patient's blood pressure and pulse rate should be monitored frequently.
• Patient should understand his disease and therapy. He should take this drug exactly as prescribed, even when he's feeling well. Patient should not discontinue this drug suddenly, but report unpleasant side effects, such as mental depression, insomnia, or loss of appetite. Drug can cause drowsiness.
• Patient should be monitored closely for signs of mental depression; should report promptly having nightmares.
• Patient should avoid alcohol and follow prescribed diet.
• Mouth dryness can be relieved with sugarless chewing gum, sour hard candy, or ice chips. Patient should contact doctor if relief is needed for nasal stuffiness.
• To increase absorption, should be taken with meals.
• Patient should weigh himself daily and report any weight gain.
• The 0.1-mg dosage strength contains tartrazine dye, which may produce allergic reactions in susceptible patients.

Interactions:
HYDRALAZINE: may cause severe hypotension. Use together cautiously.
THIAZIDE DIURETICS: may increase the effects of diazoxide. Use together cautiously.

Special considerations:
• Use cautiously in patients with impaired cerebral or cardiac function, diabetes, uremia, or in those taking other antihypertensives.
• Monitor blood pressure frequently. Severe hypotension may develop. Levarterenol should be available.
• Patient's intake and output should be monitored carefully; furosemide may be ordered if fluid or sodium retention develops.
• Extravasation should be avoided.
• This drug may alter requirements for insulin, diet, or oral hypoglycemic drugs in previously controlled patients with diabetes.
• Patients should be weighed daily and any weight increase reported.
• Patients with diabetes should be watched closely for signs of severe hyperglycemia or hyperosmolar nonketotic coma. Insulin may be needed.
• Patient's uric acid levels should be checked frequently.
• Orthostatic hypotension can be minimized by rising slowly and avoiding sudden position changes. Patient should remain supine for 30 minutes after injection.
• Infusion of diazoxide has been shown to be as effective as a bolus in some patients.

Interactions:
LEVODOPA, ALCOHOL: may increase hypotensive effect of guanethidine. Use together cautiously.
MAO INHIBITORS, EPHEDRINE, LEVARTERENOL, METHYLPHENIDATE, TRICYCLIC ANTIDEPRESSANTS, AMPHETAMINES, PHENOTHIAZINES: may inhibit the antihypertensive effect of guanethidine. Adjust dose accordingly.

Special considerations:
• Contraindicated in patients with pheochromocytoma. Use cautiously in patients with severe cardiac disease, recent MI, cerebrovascular disease, peptic ulcer, impaired renal function, or bronchial asthma, or in those taking other antihypertensives.
• Drug should be discontinued 2 to 3 weeks before elective surgery to reduce the possibility of vascular collapse and cardiac arrest during anesthesia.
• Patient should understand his disease and therapy. He should take this drug exactly as prescribed, even when he's feeling well. Patient should not discontinue this drug suddenly, but report unpleasant side effects. This drug can cause drowsiness.
• Patient should avoid strenuous exercise.
• Orthostatic hypotension can be minimized by rising slowly and avoiding sudden position changes. Mouth dryness can be relieved with sugarless chewing gum, sour hard candy, or ice chips.
• This drug should be taken with meals to increase absorption.
• If patient develops diarrhea, atropine or paregoric may be ordered.

Interactions:
DIAZOXIDE: may cause severe hypotension. Use together cautiously.

Special considerations:
• Use cautiously in patients with cardiac disease or in those taking other antihypertensives.
• Patient's blood pressure and pulse rate should be monitored frequently.
• Development of sore throat, fever, muscle and joint aches, or skin rash (signs of lupus erthematosus–like syndrome) should be reported immediately.
• Patient should understand his disease and therapy. He should take this drug exactly as prescribed, even when he's feeling well. Patient should not discontinue this drug suddenly, but report unpleasant side effects.
• Orthostatic hypotension can be minimized by rising slowly and avoiding sudden position

(continued on following page)

NAMES, INDICATIONS AND DOSAGES	SIDE EFFECTS
hydralazine hydrochloride *(continued)* ADULTS: initially, 10 mg P.O. q.i.d.; gradually increased to 50 mg q.i.d. Maximum recommended dosage is 200 mg daily, but some patients may require 300 to 400 mg daily. I.V.—20 to 40 mg given slowly and repeated as necessary, generally q 4 to 6 hours. Switch to oral antihypertensives as soon as possible. I.M.—20 to 40 mg repeated as necessary, generally q 4 to 6 hours. Switch to oral antihypertensives as soon as possible. CHILDREN: initially, 0.75 mg/kg P.O. daily in 4 divided doses (25 mg/m^2 daily). May increase gradually to 10 times this dose, if necessary. I.V.—give slowly 1.7 to 3.5 mg/kg daily or 50 to 100 mg/m^2 daily in 4 to 6 divided doses. I.M.—1.7 to 3.5 mg/kg daily or 50 to 100 mg/m^2 daily in 4 to 6 divided doses.	
mecamylamine hydrochloride Inversine **For moderate-to-severe essential hypertension and uncomplicated malignant hypertension:** ADULTS: initially, 2.5 mg P.O. b.i.d. Increase by 2.5 mg daily every 2 days. Average daily dose 25 mg given in 3 divided doses. No dosing recommendations for children.	**CNS:** *paresthesias*, sedation, *fatigue*, *tremor*, *choreiform movements*, convulsions, psychic changes, dizziness, *weakness*, *headaches*. **CV:** *orthostatic hypotension*. **EENT:** *mouth dryness*, glossitis, dilated pupils, *blurred vision*. **GI:** *anorexia*, *nausea*, *vomiting*, *constipation*, *adynamic ileus*, *diarrhea*. **GU:** urinary retention. **Other:** decreased libido, impotence.
methyldopa Aldomet♦, Dopamet♦♦, Medimet-250♦♦, Novomedopa♦♦ **For sustained mild-to-severe hypertension; should not be used for acute treatment of hypertensive emergencies:** ADULTS: 250 mg P.O. b.i.d. to t.i.d. in first 48 hours. Then increase p.r.n. q 2 days. Dosages may need adjustment if other antihypertensive drugs are added to or deleted from therapy. Maintenance dosages—500 mg to 2 g daily in 2 to 4 divided doses. Maximum recommended daily dose is 3 g. I.V.—500 mg to 1 g q 6 hours, diluted in 5% dextrose in water, and administered over 30 to 60 minutes. Switch to oral antihypertensives as soon as possible. CHILDREN: initially, 10 mg/kg/day P.O. in 2 to 3 divided doses; or 20 to 40 mg/kg/day I.V. in 4 divided doses. Increase dose daily until desired response occurs. Maximum daily dose 65 mg/kg.	**Blood:** *hemolytic anemia*, reversible granulocytopenia, thrombocytopenia. **CNS:** *sedation*, headache, asthenia, weakness, dizziness, *decreased mental acuity*, involuntary choreoathetotic movements, psychic disturbances, depression. **CV:** bradycardia, *orthostatic hypotension*, aggravated angina, myocarditis, *edema and weight gain*. **EENT:** *dry mouth*, *nasal stuffiness*. **GI:** diarrhea. **Hepatic:** *hepatic necrosis*. **Other:** gynecomastia, lactation, skin rash, drug-induced fever, impotence.

INTERACTIONS AND SPECIAL CONSIDERATIONS

changes.
- This drug should be taken with meals to increase absorption.
- Compliance may be improved by administering this drug twice a day.

Interactions:
SODIUM BICARBONATE AND ACETAZOLAMIDE: may increase effect of mecamylamine. Use together cautiously. Watch for increased hypotensive effects and toxicity.

Special considerations:
- Contraindicated in patients with recent MI, uremia, or chronic pyelonephritis. Use cautiously in patients with lower urinary tract pathology, renal insufficiency, glaucoma, pyloric stenosis, coronary insufficiency, cerebrovascular insufficiency, or in those taking other antihypertensives.
- Effects of drug increased by high environmental temperature, fever, stress, severe illness.
- This drug should not be withdrawn suddenly; rebound hypertension may occur.
- Blood pressure should be monitored frequently while patient is standing.
- Should be taken with meals for better absorption. Sodium intake should not be restricted.
- If patient develops constipation from this drug, milk of magnesia may be ordered; patient should avoid bulk laxatives.
- Patient should understand his disease and therapy. He should take drug exactly as prescribed, even when feeling well.
- Orthostatic hypotension minimized by rising slowly and avoiding sudden position changes. Mouth dryness relieved with sugarless chewing gum, hard candy, ice chips.

Interactions:
NOREPINEPHRINE, PHENOTHIAZINES, TRICYCLIC ANTIDEPRESSANTS, AND AMPHETAMINES: may cause hypertensive effects. Monitor carefully.

Special considerations:
- Use cautiously in patients receiving other antihypertensives or MAO inhibitors. Blood pressure and pulse rate should be monitored frequently.
- Side effects, particularly unexplained fever, should be reported.
- Patient requiring blood transfusion should have direct and indirect Coombs' tests to avoid cross-matching problems.
- Blood studies (complete blood count) should be monitored before and during therapy.
- If patient has been on this drug for several months, positive reaction to direct Coombs' tests indicates hemolytic anemia.
- Patient should be weighed daily. Salt and water retention may occur but can be relieved with diuretics.
- Urine may turn dark in toilet bowls treated with bleach.
- Patient should understand his disease and therapy. He should take this drug exactly as prescribed, even when he's feeling well. Patient should not stop this drug suddenly, but report unpleasant side effects. Once-daily dosage given at bedtime will minimize drowsiness during daytime.
- Orthostatic hypotension can be minimized by rising slowly and avoiding position changes. Mouth dryness can be relieved with sugarless chewing gum, sour hard candy, or ice chips.

NAMES, INDICATIONS AND DOSAGES	SIDE EFFECTS
metoprolol tartrate Betaloc♦♦, Lopresor♦♦, Lopressor **For hypertension; may be used alone or in combination with other antihypertensives:** ADULTS: 50 mg b.i.d. P.O. initially. Up to 200 to 400 mg daily in 2 to 3 divided doses. No dosage recommendations for children.	**CNS:** *fatigue, lethargy,* vivid dreams, hallucinations. **CV:** *bradycardia, hypotension, congestive heart failure,* peripheral vascular disease. **GI:** nausea, vomiting, diarrhea. **Metabolic:** hypoglycemia without tachycardia. **Skin:** rash. **Other:** fever.
metyrosine Demser **Preoperative preparation of patients with pheochromocytoma; management of such patients when surgery is contraindicated; to control or prevent hypertension before or during pheochromocytomectomy:** ADULTS AND CHILDREN OVER 12 YEARS: 2,150 mg P.O. q.i.d. May be increased by 250 to 500 mg q day to a maximum of 4 g/day in divided doses. When used for preoperative preparation, optimally effective dosage should be given for at least 5 to 7 days.	**CNS:** *sedation,* extrapyramidal symptoms such as speech difficulty and tremors, disorientation. **GI:** *diarrhea,* nausea, vomiting, abdominal pain. **GU:** *crystalluria,* hematuria. **Other:** impotence, hypersensitivity.
minoxidil Loniten **Treatment of severe hypertension:** ADULTS: 5 mg P.O. initially as a single dose. Effective dosage range is usually 10 to 40 mg/day. Maximum dose 100 mg/day. CHILDREN UNDER 12 YEARS: 0.2 mg/kg as a single daily dose. Effective dosage range usually 0.25 to 1.0 mg/kg/day. Maximum dose is 50 mg.	**CV:** *edema, tachycardia, pericardial effusion and tamponade, congestive heart failure,* EKG changes. **Other:** *hypertrichosis* (elongation, thickening, and enhanced pigmentation of fine body hair), breast tenderness.
nadolol Corgard♦ **Treatment of hypertension:** ADULTS: 40 mg P.O. once daily. Dosage may be increased in 40- to 80-mg increments until optimum response. Usual maintenance dosage range: 80 to 320 mg once daily. Doses of 640 mg may be necessary in rare cases. **Long-term management of angina pectoris:** ADULTS: 40 mg P.O. once daily. initially. Dosage may be increased in 40- to 80-mg increments until optimum response. Usual maintenance dosage range: 80 to 240 mg once daily.	**CNS:** *fatigue, lethargy,* vivid dreams, hallucinations. **CV:** *bradycardia, hypotension, congestive heart failure,* peripheral vascular disease. **GI:** nausea, vomiting, diarrhea. **Metabolic:** hypoglycemia without tachycardia. **Skin:** rash. **Other:** *increased airway resistance,* fever.

♦ Available in U.S. and Canada. ♦♦ Available in Canada only.
All other products (no symbol) available in U.S. only. Italicized side effects are common or life-threatening.

INTERACTIONS AND SPECIAL CONSIDERATIONS

Interactions:
INSULIN AND HYPOGLYCEMIC DRUGS (ORAL): can alter dosage requirements in previously stabilized diabetics. Observe patient carefully.
CARDIOTONIC GLYCOSIDES: excessive bradycardia and increased depressant effect on myocardium. Use together cautiously.

Special considerations:
- Use cautiously in patients with heart block, congestive heart failure, diabetes, respiratory disease, or in those taking other antihypertensives. Patient's apical pulse rate should be checked before this drug is given. Pulse rate slower than 60 bpm requires withholding drug.
- Blood pressure should be monitored frequently. If patient develops severe hypotension, a vasopressor should be administered.
- Abrupt discontinuation can exacerbate angina and MI.
- Patient should understand his disease and therapy. He should take this drug, even when he's feeling well. Patient should not discontinue drug suddenly; abrupt discontinuation can exacerbate angina and MI.
- Food may increase the absorption of metoprolol. Should be taken consistently with meals.

Interactions:
PHENOTHIAZINES AND HALOPERIDOL: increased inhibition of catecholamine synthesis may result in extrapyramidal symptoms. Use cautiously.

Special considerations:
- During surgery, blood pressure and EKG should be monitored continuously. If a serious arrhythmia occurs during anesthesia and surgery, treatment with a beta-blocking drug or lidocaine may be necessary.
- Sedation almost always occurs in those treated with metyrosine. Sedation usually subsides after several days' treatment.
- Patient should increase daily fluid intake to prevent crystalluria. Daily urine volume should be 2,000 ml or more.
- Patient should report any of the listed side effects.
- Insomnia may occur when metyrosine is stopped.
- If patient's hypertension is not adequately controlled by metyrosine, an alpha-adrenergic–blocking agent, such as phenoxybenzamine, should be added to the regimen.
- Available as 250-mg capsules.

Interactions:
GUANETHIDINE: may cause severe orthostatic hypotension. Advise patient to stand up slowly.

Special considerations:
- Contraindicated in patients with pheochromocytoma.
- A potent vasodilator: Use only when other antihypertensives have failed.
- About 8 out of 10 patients will experience hypertrichosis within 3 to 6 weeks of beginning treatment. Unwanted hair can be controlled with a depilatory or shaving. Extra hair will disappear within 1 to 6 months of stopping minoxidil. However, patient should not discontinue drug without doctor's consent.
- Drug is usually prescribed with a beta-blocking drug to control tachycardia and a diuretic to counteract fluid retention. Patient should comply with total treatment regimen.
- A patient package insert has been prepared by the manufacturer of minoxidil, describing in layman's terms the drug and its side effects. Patient should receive this insert and read it thoroughly. Provide oral explanation also.
- Available as a 2.5-mg and 10-mg tablet.

Interactions:
INSULIN AND HYPOGLYCEMIC DRUGS (ORAL): can alter dosage requirements in previously stabilized diabetics. Observe patient carefully.
CARDIOTONIC GLYCOSIDES: excessive bradycardia and increased depressant effect on myocardium. Use together cautiously.
EPINEPHRINE: severe vasocontriction. Monitor blood pressure and observe patient carefully.

Special considerations:
- Contraindicated in patients with bronchial asthma, sinus bradycardia and greater than first-degree conduction block, and cardiogenic shock.
- Use cautiously in patients with heart failure, chronic bronchitis, and emphysema.
- Patient's apical pulse should always be checked before giving this drug. Report apical pulse rate slower than 60 bpm and hold medication.
- Blood pressure should be monitored frequently. If patient develops severe hypotension, a vasopressor may be prescribed.
- Patient should understand his disease and therapy. He should take this drug, even when he's feeling well. Outpatient should not discontinue drug suddenly, but report unpleasant side effects. Abrupt discontinuation can exacerbate angina and MI.
- This drug masks common signs of shock and hypoglycemia.
- May be taken with food.

NAMES, INDICATIONS AND DOSAGES	SIDE EFFECTS
nitroprusside sodium Nipride♦ **To lower blood pressure quickly in hypertensive emergencies; to control hypotension during anesthesia; to reduce preload and afterload in cardiac pump failure or cardiogenic shock; may be used with or without dopamine:** ADULTS: 50-mg vial diluted with 2 to 3 ml of 5% dextrose in water I.V. and then added to 250, 500, or 1,000 ml 5% dextrose in water. Infuse at 0.5 to 10 mcg/kg/minute. Average dose: 3 mcg/kg/minute. Maximum infusion rate: 10 mcg/kg/minute. Patients taking other antihypertensive drugs along with nitroprusside are very sensitive to this drug. Adjust dosage accordingly.	*The following effects generally indicate overdosage:* **CNS:** *headache, dizziness,* ataxia, loss of consciousness, coma, weak pulse, absent reflexes, widely dilated pupils, *restlessness, muscle twitching, diaphoresis.* **CV:** distant heart sounds, palpitations, dyspnea, shallow breathing. **GI:** *vomiting, nausea, abdominal pain.* **Metabolic:** acidosis. **Skin:** pink color. **Local:** *tissue sloughing and necrosis with extravasation.*
pargyline hydrochloride Eutonyl **For moderate-to-severe hypertension, usually given in combination with other drugs:** ADULTS: initially, 25 to 50 mg P.O. once daily, if not receiving any other antihypertensive drugs. Then increase dosage by 10 mg daily at weekly intervals. Maximum daily dosage 200 mg. Usual daily dose for patients over 65 years or those who've had sympathectomy: 10 to 25 mg. When used in combination with other drugs, total daily dose of pargyline should not exceed 25 mg. No dosage recommendations for children.	**CNS:** *tremors,* convulsions, choreiform movements, psychic changes, *nightmares, hyperexcitability, sweating,* dizziness, fainting, drowsiness. **CV:** palpitations, *orthostatic hypotension,* fluid retention. **EENT:** *mouth dryness,* optic damage. **GI:** *nausea, vomiting, increased appetite, constipation.* **Other:** impotence.
phenoxybenzamine hydrochloride Dibenzyline **To control hypertension and sweating secondary to pheochromocytoma; may be used in combination with propranolol to control excessive tachycardia:** ADULTS: initially, 10 mg P.O. daily. Increase by 10 mg daily every 4 days. Maintenance dose: 20 to 60 mg daily. CHILDREN: initially, 0.2 mg/kg or 6 mg/m^2 P.O. daily in a single dose. Maintenance dose: 12 to 36 mg/m^2 daily as a single dose or in divided doses.	**CNS:** lethargy, drowsiness. **CV:** *orthostatic hypotension, tachycardia,* shock. **EENT:** *nasal stuffiness, dry mouth, miosis.* **GI:** vomiting, abdominal distress. **Other:** *impotence.*

♦ Available in U.S. and Canada. ♦♦ Available in Canada only.
All other products (no symbol) available in U.S. only. Italicized side effects are common or life-threatening.

INTERACTIONS AND SPECIAL CONSIDERATIONS

No significant interactions.

Special considerations:
• Use cautiously in patients with hypothyroidism, hepatic or renal disease, or in those receiving other antihypertensives.
• Due to light sensitivity, I.V. solution should be wrapped in foil or black tape; not necessary to wrap the tubing in foil. Fresh solution should have faint brownish tint and be discarded after 4 hours.
• Baseline vital signs should be obtained before this drug is given, and parameters should be determined.
• Blood pressure should be monitored every 5 minutes at start of infusion and every 15 minutes thereafter. If severe hypotension occurs, I.V. nitroprusside should be turned off; effects of drug quickly reversed. If possible, an arterial pressure line should be started and drug flow regulated to specified level.
• Bacteriostatic water for injection or sterile saline should not be used for reconstitution.
• Should be infused with motorized infusion pump.
• This drug is best run piggyback through a peripheral line with no other medication. Rate of main I.V. line should not be regulated while this drug is running. Even small bolus of nitroprusside can cause severe hypotension.
• This drug can cause cyanide toxicity, so serum thiocyanate levels should be checked every 72 hours. Signs of thiocyanate toxicity: profound hypotension, metabolic acidosis, dyspnea, headache, loss of consciousness, ataxia, vomiting. If these occur, drug should be discontinued immediately.
• Extravasation can cause tissue irritation.

Interactions:
AMPHETAMINES, EPHEDRINE, LEVODOPA, METARAMINOL, METHOTRIMEPRAZINE, METHYLPHENIDATE, PHENYLEPHRINE, PHENYLPROPANOLAMINE, AND PSEUDOEPHEDRINE: enhanced pressor effects. Use together cautiously.
ALCOHOL, BARBITURATES, AND OTHER SEDATIVES; TRANQUILIZERS; NARCOTICS; DEXTROMETHORPHAN; AND TRICYCLIC ANTIDEPRESSANTS: unpredictable interactions. Should be used with caution and in reduced dosage.

Special considerations:
• Contraindicated in patients with advanced renal failure, pheochromocytoma, hyperthyroidism, or Parkinson's disease; in patients who are hyperactive and hyperexcitable. Use cautiously in patients receiving other antihypertensives, or who have hepatic disease.
• This drug should be discontinued at least 2 weeks before elective surgery.
• Hypotensive effects of this drug are increased by high temperatures, fever, stress, or severe illness. Ephedrine or phenylephrine counteracts severe hypotension.
• Blood pressure and pulse rate should be monitored frequently. Blood pressure should be taken while patient is standing.
• Patient should have periodic ophthalmic evaluations during therapy.
• If patient is scheduled for surgery and has been taking this drug, narcotic dosages should be reduced.
• This drug may require up to several weeks to reach optimal effect.
• Patient should not take any other medications, including over-the-counter cold remedies, without doctor approval.
• This drug is an MAO inhibitor. Patient should not eat foods with high tyramine content, for example, aged cheese, chianti wine, sour cream, canned figs, raisins, chicken livers, yeast extract, chocolate, pickled herring, caffeine, cyclamates, cola drinks.
• Patient should understand his disease and therapy. He should take this drug exactly as prescribed, even when he's feeling well. Patient should not discontinue this drug suddenly, but report unpleasant side effects.
• Orthostatic hypotension can be minimized by rising slowly and avoiding sudden position changes. Mouth dryness can be relieved with sugarless chewing gum, sour hard candy, or ice chips.

No significant interactions.

Special considerations:
• Use cautiously in patients with cerebrovascular or coronary insufficiency, advanced renal disease, respiratory disease.
• If severe hypotension develops, patient may require levarterenol to counteract effect.
• Nasal congestion, miosis, and impotence usually decrease with continued therapy.
• Patient with tachycardia may require concurrent propranolol therapy.
• Patient's heart rate and blood pressure should be monitored frequently.
• This drug may take several weeks to achieve optimal effect.
• Respiratory status should be monitored carefully: this drug may aggravate symptoms of pneumonia and asthma.
• Patient should understand his disease and therapy. He should take this drug exactly as prescribed, even when he's feeling well. Patient should not discontinue this drug suddenly, but report unpleasant side effects.
• Orthostatic hypotension can be minimized by rising slowly and avoiding sudden position changes. Mouth dryness relieved with sugarless chewing gum, hard candy, ice chips.

NAMES, INDICATIONS AND DOSAGES	SIDE EFFECTS
phentolamine hydrochloride Regitine **phentolamine methanesulfonate** Regitine, Rogitine♦♦ **To aid in diagnosis of pheochromocytoma; to control or prevent hypertension before or during pheochromocytomectomy:** ADULTS: P.O. therapeutic dose: 50 mg q.i.d. I.V. diagnostic dose: 5 mg, with close monitoring of blood pressure. Before surgical removal of tumor, give 2 to 5 mg I.M. or I.V. During surgery, patient may need small I.V. doses (1 mg) or small I.M. doses (3 mg). CHILDREN: P.O. therapeutic dose: 5 mg/kg daily or 150 mg/m^2 daily in 4 to 6 divided doses. I.V. diagnostic dose: 0.1 mg/kg or 3 mg/m^2 as single dose, with close monitoring of blood pressure. Before surgical removal of tumor give 1 mg I.V. or 3 mg I.M. During surgery, patient may need small I.V. doses (1 mg).	**CNS:** *dizziness, weakness, flushing.* **CV:** *hypotension,* shock, *arrhythmias,* palpitations, *tachycardia,* angina pectoris. **GI:** *diarrhea,* abdominal pain, *nausea, vomiting,* hyperperistalsis. **Other:** *nasal stuffiness,* hypoglycemia.
prazosin hydrochloride Minipress♦ **For mild-to-moderate hypertension; used alone or in combination with a diuretic or other antihypertensive drugs; also used to decrease afterload in severe chronic congestive heart failure:** ADULTS: P.O. test dose: 1 mg given before bedtime to prevent first-dose syncope. Initial dose: 1 mg t.i.d. Increase dosage slowly. Maximum daily dose 20 mg. Maintenance dose: 3 to 20 mg daily in 3 divided doses. A few patients have required dosages larger than this (up to 40 mg daily). If other antihypertensive drugs or diuretics are added to this drug, decrease prazosin dosage to 1 to 2 mg t.i.d. and retitrate.	**CNS:** *dizziness,* headache, drowsiness, weakness, *first-dose syncope,* depression. **CV:** orthostatic hypotension, *palpitations.* **EENT:** blurred vision, dry mouth. **GI:** vomiting, diarrhea, abdominal cramps, constipation, *nausea.* **GU:** priapism.
propranolol hydrochloride Inderal♦ **Hypertension (usually used with thiazide diuretics):** ADULTS: initial treatment of hypertension: 80 mg P.O. daily in 2 to 4 divided doses. Increase at 3- to 7-day intervals to maximum daily dose of 640 mg. Usual maintenance dose for hypertension: 160 to 480 mg daily. No dosing recommendations for children.	**CNS:** *fatigue, lethargy,* vivid dreams, hallucinations. **CV:** *bradycardia, hypotension, congestive heart failure,* peripheral vascular disease. **GI:** nausea, vomiting, diarrhea. **Metabolic:** hypoglycemia without tachycardia. **Skin:** rash. **Other:** *increased airway resistance,* fever.

INTERACTIONS AND SPECIAL CONSIDERATIONS

No significant interactions.

Special considerations:

- Contraindicated in patients with angina, coronary artery disease, and history of MI. Use cautiously in patients with gastritis or peptic ulcer and in those receiving other antihypertensives.
- When this drug is given for diagnostic test, patient's blood pressure should be checked first and frequently during administration.
- Diagnosis positive for pheochromocytoma if severe hypotension results from I.V. test dose.
- Levarterenol counteracts severe hypotensive effect of this drug. Epinephrine should not be administered to raise blood pressure, as this may cause further drop.
- Sedatives or narcotics should not be given 24 hours prior to diagnostic test.

Interactions:

PROPRANOLOL AND OTHER BETA BLOCKERS: syncope with loss of consciousness may occur more frequently. Advise patient to sit or lie down if he feels dizzy.

Special considerations:

- Use cautiously in patients receiving other antihypertensive drugs.
- Patient's blood pressure and pulse rate should be monitored frequently.
- If initial dose is greater than 1 mg, patient may develop severe syncope with loss of consciousness (first-dose syncope). Dosage should be increased slowly. Patient should sit or lie down if he experiences dizziness.
- Patient should understand his disease and therapy. He should take this drug exactly as prescribed, even when he's feeling well. Patient should not discontinue this drug suddenly, but report unpleasant side effects.
- Orthostatic hypotension can be minimized by rising slowly and avoiding sudden position changes. Mouth dryness can be relieved with sugarless chewing gum, hard candy, ice chips.
- Compliance *may* be improved by taking this drug on a once-daily basis.

Interactions:

INSULIN, HYPOGLYCEMIC DRUGS (ORAL): can alter requirements for these drugs in previously stabilized diabetics. Monitor for hypoglycemia.

CARDIOTONIC GLYCOSIDES: excessive bradycardia and increased depressant effect on myocardium. Use together cautiously.

AMINOPHYLLINE: antagonize beta-blocking effects of propranolol. Use together cautiously.

ISOPROTERENOL AND GLUCAGON: antagonize propranolol effect. May be used therapeutically and in emergencies.

CIMETIDINE: inhibits propranolol's metabolism. Monitor for greater beta-blocking effect.

EPINEPHRINE: severe vasoconstriction. Monitor blood pressure and observe patient carefully.

Special considerations:

- Contraindicated in diabetes mellitus, asthma, allergic rhinitis; during ethyl ether anesthesia; in sinus bradycardia and heart block greater than first degree; in cardiogenic shock; in right ventricular failure secondary to pulmonary hypertension. Use with caution in patients with congestive heart failure, respiratory disease, and in patients taking other antihypertensive drugs.
- Patient's apical pulse rate should always be checked before this drug is taken. Report extremes in pulse rates and hold medication.
- Monitor blood pressure frequently. Severe hypotension may require a vasopressor.
- Patient should understand his disease and therapy. He should take this drug exactly as prescribed, even when he's feeling well. Patient should not discontinue this drug suddenly; abrupt discontinuation can exacerbate angina and MI. Unpleasant side effects should be reported.
- Drug masks shock and hypoglycemia.
- Food may increase the absorption of propranolol. Should be taken consistently with meals.
- Compliance may be improved by administering this drug on a twice-daily basis.

NAMES, INDICATIONS AND DOSAGES	SIDE EFFECTS
rauwolfia serpentina HBP, Hiwolfia, Hyper-Rauw, Hywolfia, Rau, Raudixin♦, Rauja, Raumason, Rauneed, Raupoid, Rauserpin, Rausertina, Rauval, Rauwoldin, Rawfola, Ru-Hy-T, Serfia, Serfolia, T-Rau, Wolfina **Mild-to-moderate hypertension:** ADULTS: initially and for 1 to 3 weeks thereafter, 200 to 400 mg P.O. daily as a single dose or in 2 divided doses. Maintenance dose: 50 to 300 mg/day. No dosing recommendations for children.	**CNS:** mental confusion, *depression, drowsiness, nervousness,* anxiety, nightmares, sedation, headache. **CV:** *orthostatic hypotension, bradycardia, syncope.* **EENT:** *mouth dryness, nasal stuffiness,* glaucoma. **GI:** *hypersecretion of gastric acid, nausea, vomiting,* gastrointestinal bleeding. **Skin:** pruritus, rash. **Other:** *impotence, weight gain.*
rescinnamine Anaprel, Cinnasil, Moderil **For mild-to-moderate hypertension; may be used alone or in combination with other antihypertensives:** ADULTS: initially, 0.5 mg b.i.d. Maintenance dose: 0.25 to 0.5 mg daily. No dosing recommendations for children.	**CNS:** mental confusion, *depression, drowsiness, nervousness, anxiety, nightmares,* sedation, parkinsonism. **CV:** *orthostatic hypotension, bradycardia, syncope.* **EENT:** *mouth dryness, nasal stuffiness,* glaucoma. **GI:** *hypersecretion of gastric acid, nausea, vomiting,* gastrointestinal bleeding. **Skin:** pruritus, rash. **Other:** *impotence, weight gain.*
reserpine Alkarau, Arcum R-S, Bonapene, Broserpine, De Serpa, Elserpine, Hyperine, Lemiserp, Maso-Serpine, Neo-Serp♦♦, Rauloydin, Rau-Sed, Rauserpin, Releserp-5, Reserjen, Reserfia♦♦, Reserpanca♦♦, Reserpaneed, Reserpoid, Rolserp, Sandril, Serp, Serpalan, Serpena, Serpanray, Serpasil♦, Serpate, Sertabs, Sertina, Tensin, T-Serp, Zepine **Mild-to-moderate essential hypertension (oral); hypertensive emergencies (parenteral):** ADULTS: initially, 0.5 mg P.O. daily for 1 to 2 weeks. Maintenance dose: 0.1 to 0.5 mg daily. I.M—initially, 0.5 to 1 mg, followed by doses of 2 to 4 mg at 2-hour intervals. Maximum recommended dose 4 mg. CHILDREN: 0.07 mg/kg or 2 mg/m² with hydralazine I.M. every 12 to 24 hours.	**CNS:** mental confusion, *depression, drowsiness, nervousness, anxiety, nightmares,* sedation. **CV:** *orthostatic hypotension, bradycardia, syncope.* **EENT:** *mouth dryness, nasal stuffiness,* glaucoma. **GI:** *hyperacidity, nausea, vomiting,* gastrointestinal bleeding. **Skin:** pruritus, rash. **Other:** *impotence, weight gain.*
timolol maleate Blocadren **Hypertension:** ADULTS: Initial dosage is 10 mg P.O. b.i.d. Usual daily maintenance dosage is 20 to 40 mg.	**CNS:** *fatigue, lethargy,* vivid dreams, hallucinations, dizziness. **CV:** *bradycardia, hypotension, congestive heart failure (CHF)* peripheral vascular disease. **GI:** nausea, vomiting, diarrhea. **Metabolic:** hypoglycemia without tachycardia.

♦ Available in U.S. and Canada. ♦♦ Available in Canada only.
All other products (no symbol) available in U.S. only. Italicized side effects are common or life-threatening.

INTERACTIONS AND SPECIAL CONSIDERATIONS

Interactions:
MAO INHIBITORS: excitability and hypertension. Use together cautiously.

Special considerations:
• Contraindicated in patients with depression. Use cautiously in patients with severe cardiac or cerebrovascular disease, impaired renal function, peptic ulcer, ulcerative colitis, gallstones; in those undergoing surgery; and in those taking other antihypertensives or tricyclic antidepressants.
• Patient's blood pressure and pulse rate should be monitored frequently.
• Patient should understand his disease and therapy. He should take this drug exactly as prescribed, even when he's feeling well. Patient should not discontinue this drug suddenly, but report unpleasant side effects. This drug can cause drowsiness.
• Patient should be monitored closely for signs of mental depression; should report promptly having nightmares.
• Orthostatic hypotension can be minimized by rising slowly and avoiding sudden position changes. Mouth dryness can be relieved with sugarless chewing gum, sour hard candy, or ice chips. Patient should contact doctor if relief is needed for nasal stuffiness.
• This drug should be taken with meals.
• Patient should weigh himself daily and report any weight gain.
• Effects of this drug may last for 10 days after it's been discontinued.

Interactions:
MAO INHIBITORS: excitability and hypertension. Use together cautiously.

Special considerations:
• Contraindicated in patients with depression. Use cautiously in patients with severe cardiac or cerebrovascular disease, peptic ulcer, ulcerative colitis, gallstones, or in those undergoing surgery. Also use cautiously in patients taking other antihypertensives.
• Patient's blood pressure and pulse rate should be monitored frequently.
• Patient should understand his disease and therapy. He should take this drug exactly as prescribed, even when he's feeling well. Patient should not discontinue this drug suddenly, but report unpleasant side effects. This drug can cause drowsiness.
• Patient should be monitored closely for signs of mental depression. He should report promptly having nightmares.
• Orthostatic hypotension can be minimized by rising slowly and avoiding sudden position changes. Mouth dryness can be relieved with sugarless chewing gum, sour hard candy, or ice chips. Patient should contact doctor if relief is needed for nasal stuffiness.
• This drug should be taken with meals.
• Patient should weigh himself daily and report any weight gain.
• Effects of this drug may last for 10 days after it's been discontinued.

Interactions:
MAO INHIBITORS: excitability and hypertension. Use together cautiously.

Special considerations:
• Contraindicated in patients with depression. Use cautiously in patients with severe cardiac or cerebrovascular disease, peptic ulcer, ulcerative colitis, gallstones, mental depressive disorders; in those undergoing surgery; and in those taking other antihypertensive drugs.
• Patient's blood pressure and pulse rate should be monitored frequently.
• Patient should understand his disease and therapy. He should take this drug exactly as prescribed, even when he's feeling well. Patient should not discontinue this drug suddenly, but report unpleasant side effects. This drug can cause drowsiness.
• Female patient should report pregnancy.
• Patient should be monitored closely for signs of mental depression. He should report promptly having nightmares.
• Orthostatic hypotension can be minimized by rising slowly and avoiding sudden position changes. Mouth dryness can be relieved with sugarless chewing gum, sour hard candy, or ice chips. Patient should contact doctor if relief is needed for nasal stuffiness.
• This drug should be taken with meals.
• Patient should weigh himself daily and report any weight gain.
• Effects of this drug may last for 10 days after it's been discontinued.
• Parenteral form erratically absorbed; largely replaced by other antihypertensives for hypertensive emergencies.

Interactions:
INSULIN, AND HYPOGLYCEMIC DRUGS (ORAL): can alter requirements for these drugs in previously stablized diabetics. Monitor for hypoglycemia.
CARDIC GLYCOSIDES: excessive bradycardia and increased depressant effect on myocardium. Use together cautiously.

Special considerations:
• Contraindicated in diabetes mellitus, asthma, allergic rhinitis; during ethyl ether anesthesia;

(continued on following page)

NAMES, INDICATIONS AND DOSAGES	SIDE EFFECTS
timolol maleate *(continued)* Maximum daily dosage is 60 mg. Drug is used either alone or in combination with diuretics. **Myocardial infarction:** ADULTS: Recommend dosage for long-term prophylaxis in survivors of acute myocardial infarction (MI) is 10 mg P.O. b.i.d.	**Skin:** rash. **Other:** *increased airway resistance,* fever.
trimethaphan camsylate Arfonad♦ **To lower blood pressure quickly in hypertensive emergencies; for controlled hypotension during surgery:** ADULTS: 500 mg (10 ml) diluted in 500 ml dextrose 5% in water to yield concentration of 1 mg/ml I.V. Start I.V. drip at 1 to 2 mg/minute and titrate to achieve desired hypotensive response. Range: 0.3 mg to 6 mg/minute.	**CNS:** dilated pupils, *extreme weakness.* **CV:** *severe orthostatic hypotension, tachycardia.* **GI:** anorexia, *nausea, vomiting, dry mouth.* **GU:** *urinary retention.* **Other:** respiratory depression.

INTERACTIONS AND SPECIAL CONSIDERATIONS

in sinus bradycardia and heart block greater than first degree; in cardiogenic shock; in right ventricular failure secondary to pulmonary hypertension. Use with caution in CHF and respiratory disease, and in patients taking other antihypertensives.

• Patient's apical pulse rate should always be checked before giving this drug. Extremes in pulse rates should be reported and medication withheld.

• Blood pressure should be monitored frequently. If patient develops severe hypotension, a vasopressor may be prescribed.

• Patient should understand his disease and therapy. He should take drug exactly as prescribed, even when he's feeling well. Patient should not discontinue drug suddenly; abrupt discontinuation can exacerbate angina and MI. Patient should report unpleasant side effects.

• This drug masks common signs of shock and hypoglycemia.

• If patient is taking the drug for hypertension, he should not increase the dosage without first consulting his doctor. At least 7 days should intervene between increases in dosage.

• Timolol is the first beta blocker approved for use in post-MI patients. Like other beta blockers, it prolongs survival of MI patients.

No significant interactions.

Special considerations:

• Contraindicated in patients with anemia and respiratory insufficiency. Use cautiously in patients with arteriosclerosis; cardiac, hepatic, or renal disease; degenerative CNS disorders; Addison's disease; diabetes. Also use cautiously in patients receiving glucocorticoids and in those receiving other antihypertensives.

• Patient's blood pressure and vital signs should be monitored frequently.

• Extreme hypotension should be reported and drug discontinued. Phenylephrine or mephentermine counteracts hypotension.

• Respiratory distress possible, especially if large doses are used.

• Infusion pump should be used to administer this drug slowly.

• Drug should be discontinued before wound closure in surgery to allow blood pressure to return to normal.

• Patient should be positioned to avoid cerebral anoxia.

• Patient should receive oxygen therapy during use of this agent.

CHECKING FOR HYPERTENSION? FOLLOW THESE NEW RECOMMENDATIONS

You'll probably be performing more blood pressure checks and seeing more drug therapy for patients with mild hypertension.

Why? The 1980 recommendations of the National Institutes of Health (NIH) Joint National Committee on Detection, Evaluation, and Treatment of High Blood Pressure are being implemented. These recommendations update those issued in 1977. Since then, NIH received results of a massive clinical study showing that early detection and treatment of mild hypertension can reduce mortality and morbidity.

According to the 1977 recommendations, hypertension therapy was indicated only for patients with diastolic blood pressures of 105 mmHg or higher. *The new recommendations indicate that all adults with diastolic blood pressure of 95 mmHg or higher on first screening should have the elevation confirmed promptly.* (For outpatients, "promptly" means within 1 month, generally.)

A hospitalized patient with a diastolic blood pressure of 90 to 95 mmHg should be periodically checked until he's discharged. Within 3 months after discharge from the hospital, the patient's blood pressure should be checked again during an office visit.

According to NIH recommendations, *a diastolic reading of 115 mmHg or higher warrants immediate referral.* This contrasts with the 1977 reading of 120 mmHg.

The earlier recommendations didn't mention nondrug hypertension therapies. However, the update suggests that dietary management—weight control and sodium restriction—be used as an adjunct to drug therapy.

22

Vasodilators

amyl nitrite
cyclandelate
dipyridamole
erythrityl tetranitrate
ethaverine hydrochloride
isosorbide dinitrate
isoxsuprine hydrochloride
mannitol hexanitrate
nicotinyl alcohol
nitroglycerin
nylidrin hydrochloride
papaverine hydrochloride
pentaerythritol tetranitrate
tolazoline hydrochloride

Vasodilators can be grouped into two categories: peripheral vasodilators and coronary vasodilators.

Peripheral vasodilators include cyclandelate, ethaverine, isoxsuprine, nicotinyl alcohol, nylidrin, papaverine, and tolazoline. Although these drugs have limited clinical value in patients with obstructive vascular disease, they may be useful in patients with minimal organic involvement. Studies in healthy persons indicate that the peripheral vasodilators increase blood flow to vascular areas. Although we lack evidence of their vasodilating effect in diseased vascular areas, these drugs are still widely used.

The *coronary vasodilators,* or antianginal agents, include drugs that abort acute angina episodes (amyl nitrite, isosorbide dinitrate, and nitroglycerin) and long-term prophylactic drugs (erythrityl tetranitrate, isosorbide dinitrate, mannitol hexanitrate, nitroglycerin, and pentaerythritol tetranitrate).

Major uses

Peripheral vasodilators are used to treat symptoms of peripheral vascular and vasospastic conditions as well as cerebrovascular disease.

Coronary vasodilators combat acute episodes of angina or furnish long-term anginal prophylaxis.

- Dipyridamole (in combination with aspirin or warfarin) inhibits platelet aggregation to reduce risk of thrombus formation.
- Isosorbide dinitrate and nitroglycerin act as therapeutic adjuncts in chronic congestive heart failure.

Mechanism of action

- Some peripheral vasodilators directly relax smooth muscle. This effect may be due to the inhibition of phosphodiesterase, resulting in increased concentrations of cyclic adenosine monophosphate, which causes the vasodilation.
- Other peripheral vasodilators have a different mechanism of action. Tolazoline blocks alpha receptors; isoxsuprine and nylidrin stimulate beta receptors. Although isoxsuprine originally was thought only to stimulate beta receptors, newer evidence indicates that it may also be a direct-acting peripheral vasodilator.
- Coronary vasodilation occurs in normal but not in diseased arteries. Thus, the assumption that coronary vasodilators relieve angina by dilating coronary arteries is only partly correct. Coronary vasodilators cause a pooling of venous blood, which decreases the heart's work load by lowering ventricular diastolic pressure and reducing the stretching of myocardial fibers.
- Dipyridamole, originally classified as a coronary vasodilator, has no value in treating acute attacks of angina. In fact, we lack evidence that its long-term use is beneficial in preventing chronic angina. It does, however, inhibit platelet adhesion.
- Nitrates are effective in chronic congestive heart failure refractory to standard therapy.

THERAPEUTIC ACTIVITY

THERAPEUTIC ACTIVITY OF SELECTED VASODILATORS

DRUG	FORM	ONSET	DURATION
amyl nitrite	inhalant	instantaneous	4 to 8 min
erythrityl tetranitrate	chewable	5 min	2 hr
	oral	30 min	3 to 4 hr
	sublingual	5 to 10 min	3 to 4 hr
isosorbide dinitrate	chewable	2 to 5 min	1 to 2 hr
	oral	30 min	4 hr
	sublingual	2 min	1 to 2 hr
mannitol hexanitrate	oral	15 to 30 min	4 to 6 hr
nitroglycerin	oral (extended-release)	1 hr	4 to 6 hr
	sublingual	1 to 2 min	30 min
	topical	15 to 30 min	4 to 6 hr
pentaerythritol tetranitrate	oral	1 hr	4 to 5 hr

Dilating effect of nitrates on venous circulation promotes more efficient contraction.

Absorption, distribution, metabolism, and excretion
Vasodilators are well absorbed, widely distributed in body tissues, metabolized in the liver, and excreted mainly in the urine.

Onset and duration
Onset and duration of vasodilators depend on the drug used, form selected, and route of administration. The chart above shows onset and duration for these drugs.

PATIENT-TEACHING AID

HOW TO USE NITROGLYCERIN OINTMENT

Dear Patient:

The doctor has prescribed your nitroglycerin as an ointment. In this form, nitroglycerin is continuously absorbed through the skin into the circulation; it's effective for about 4 hours.

To get the most from your therapy, follow these instructions carefully:

1. Apply ointment to a hairless or shaved area of skin (chest, arm, thigh, abdomen, forehead, ankle, or back) to promote uniform absorption. Choose a new site each time you apply a new dose to prevent minor skin irritations. Remove any traces of ointment left from previous application.
2. Use the ruled applicator paper that comes with the ointment to measure your dose accurately.
3. Use the applicator paper to apply the ointment in a thin, uniform layer over an area of about 7.5 to 15 cm (3″ to 6″). Leave the applicator paper on the site.
4. Cover the applicator paper with plastic wrap and secure it with tape. This will protect your clothing and ensure maximum absorption.

Call your doctor immediately if you experience headache, feel dizzy or faint, or notice any redness or irritation at the application site. He may want to adjust your dosage or check the application site.

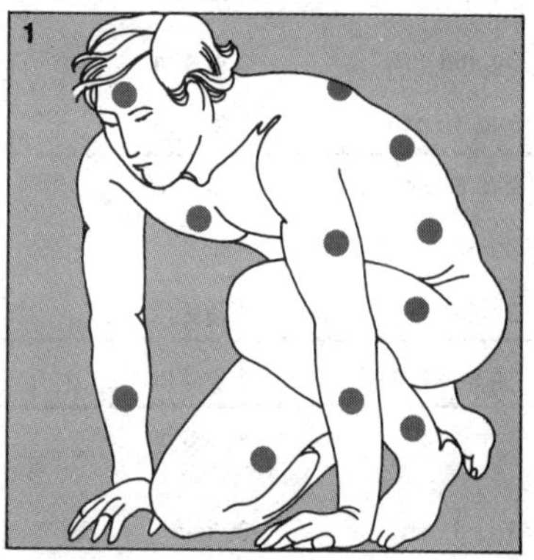

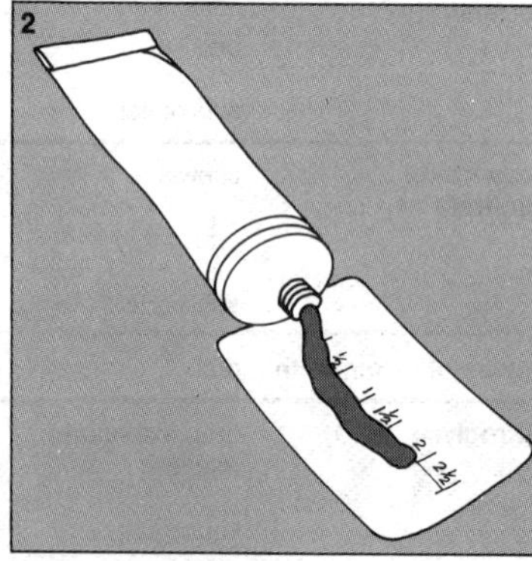

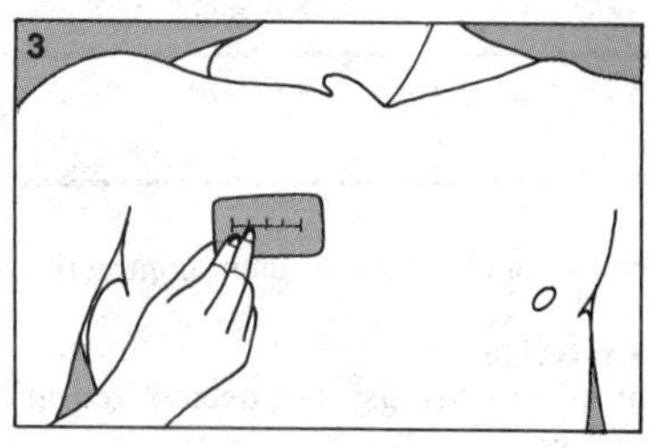

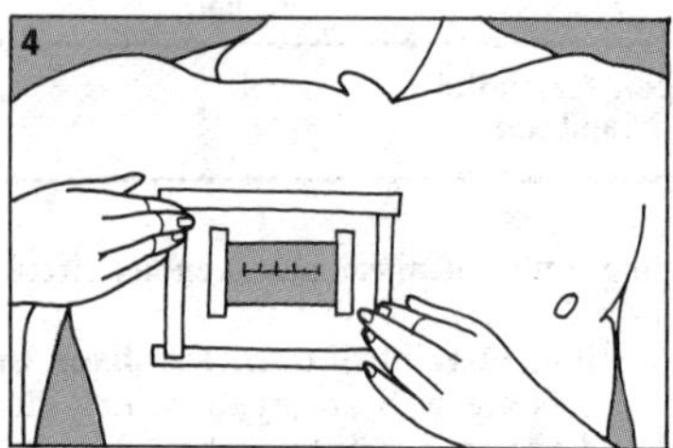

This patient-teaching aid may be reproduced by office copier for distribution to patients.

PATIENT-TEACHING AID

HOW TO TAKE SUBLINGUAL NITROGLYCERIN TABLETS

Dear Patient:

Nitroglycerin relieves anginal pain by temporarily dilating veins and arteries. This brings more blood and oxygen to the heart so it doesn't have to work as hard.

To get the most from your therapy, follow these instructions carefully:

- When you experience anginal pain, lie down and put a tablet under your tongue. Let it dissolve completely, and hold the saliva in your mouth for 1 or 2 minutes before swallowing. Don't stand up until you've swallowed the saliva or you may become dizzy. If you feel headachy or your face flushes after taking your tablet, don't worry. These effects are only temporary.
- Take up to three tablets—one every 4 to 5 minutes—if necessary. Record each dose. If the pain doesn't go away after 30 minutes, call the doctor at once or go to the hospital emergency department.
- Don't stop taking your tablets altogether without asking the doctor. But don't worry about taking them as often as you need; they aren't habit-forming.
- Keep your tablets in their original container, but remove the cotton. They will lose their strength if they're exposed to light, moisture, or heat, or if they're more than 3 months old. Fresh tablets produce a slight burning sensation under your tongue.

Call the doctor immediately if you notice unusually severe or prolonged pain, fainting, or dizziness.

Always have a supply of tablets with you when you go out. Keep a bottle in your car, at work, and at home if you can. Nitroglycerin is available in different strengths, so don't lend tablets or borrow them from anyone else taking this medication.

Combination products

CARDILATE-P: erythrityl tetranitrate 10 mg and phenobarbital 15 mg.
CARTRAX-10: pentaerythritol tetranitrate 10 mg and hydroxyzine HCl 10 mg.
CARTRAX-20: pentaerythritol tetranitrate 20 mg together with hydroxyzine HCl 10 mg.
COROVAS TYMCAPS: pentaerythritol tetranitrate 30 mg and secobarbital 50 mg.
DEAPRIL-ST: dihydroergocornine mesylate 0.167 mg, dihydroergocristine mesylate 0.167 mg, and dihydroergocryptine mesylate 0.167 mg.
EQUANITRATE 10: pentaerythritol tetranitrate 10 mg and meprobamate 200 mg.
EQUANITRATE 20: pentaerythritol tetranitrate 20 mg and meprobamate 200 mg.
HYDERGINE: dihydroergocornine mesylate 0.167 mg, dihydroergocristine mesylate 0.167 mg, and dihydroergocryptine mesylate 0.167 mg.
ISORIL WITH PHENOBARBITAL: isosorbide dinitrate 10 mg and phenobarbital 15 mg.
MILTRATE-10: pentaerythritol tetranitrate 10 mg and meprobamate 200 mg.
MILTRATE-20: pentaerythritol tetranitrate 20 mg and meprobamate 200 mg.
PAPAVATRAL L.A. CAPSULES: pentaerythritol tetranitrate 50 mg and ethaverine HCl 30 mg.
PERITRATE WITH PHENOBARBITAL: pentaerythritol tetranitrate 10 mg and phenobarbital 15 mg.
PERITRATE WITH PHENOBARBITAL: pentaerythritol tetranitrate 20 mg and phenobarbital 15 mg.

NAMES, INDICATIONS AND DOSAGES	SIDE EFFECTS
amyl nitrite **Antidote for cyanide poisoning:** 0.2 or 0.3 ml by inhalation for 30 to 60 seconds q 5 minutes until conscious. **Relief of angina pectoris, bronchospasm, biliary spasm:** ADULTS AND CHILDREN: 0.2 to 0.3 ml by inhalation (1 glass ampul inhaler), p.r.n.	**Blood:** methemoglobinemia. **CNS:** *headache, sometimes with throbbing;* dizziness; weakness. **CV:** *orthostatic hypotension, tachycardia,* flushing, palpitations, fainting. **GI:** nausea, vomiting. **Skin:** cutaneous vasodilation. **Other:** hypersensitivity reactions.
cyclandelate Cyclanfor, Cyclospasmol♦ **Adjunct in intermittent claudication, arteriosclerosis obliterans, vasospasm and muscular ischemia associated with thrombophlebitis, nocturnal leg cramps, Raynaud's phenomenon, selected cases of ischemic cerebral vascular disease:** ADULTS: initially, 200 mg P.O. q.i.d. (before meals and h.s.); maximum 400 mg P.O. q.i.d. When clinical response is noted, decrease dosage gradually until maintenance dosage is reached. Maintenance dose 400 to 800 mg daily in divided doses.	**CNS:** *headache, tingling of the extremities, dizziness.* **CV:** *mild flushing,* tachycardia. **GI:** pyrosis, eructation, nausea, heartburn. **Other:** *sweating.*
dipyridamole Persantine♦ **Long-term therapy for chronic angina pectoris, prevention of recurrent transient ischemic attack:** ADULTS: 50 mg P.O. t.i.d. at least 1 hour before meals, to maximum of 400 mg daily. **Inhibition of platelet adhesion in patients with prosthetic heart valves, in combination with warfarin:** ADULTS: 100 to 400 mg P.O. daily. **Transient ischemic attack:** ADULTS: 100 mg P.O. daily as a single dose.	**CNS:** *headache, dizziness,* weakness. **CV:** flushing, fainting, *hypotension.* **GI:** *nausea,* vomiting, diarrhea. **Skin:** rash.
erythrityl tetranitrate Anginar, Cardilate♦ **Prophylaxis and long-term management of frequent or recurrent anginal pain, reduced exercise tolerance associated with angina pectoris:** ADULTS: 5 mg sublingually or bucally t.i.d. or 10 mg P.O., a.c. chewed t.i.d., increasing in 2 to 3 days if needed.	**CNS:** *headache, sometimes with throbbing; dizziness;* weakness. **CV:** *orthostatic hypotension, tachycardia, flushing, palpitations,* fainting. **GI:** nausea, vomiting. **Local:** sublingual burning. **Skin:** cutaneous vasodilation. **Other:** hypersensitivity reactions.

♦ Available in U.S. and Canada. ♦♦ Available in Canada only.
All other products (no symbol) available in U.S. only. Italicized side effects are common or life-threatening.

INTERACTIONS AND SPECIAL CONSIDERATIONS

No significant interactions.

Special considerations:
• Contraindicated in hypersensitivity to nitrites. Use with caution in cerebral hemorrhage, hypotension, head injury, and glaucoma.
• Patient can minimize orthostatic hypotension by sitting down and avoiding rapid position changes while inhaling drug.
• Extinguish all cigarettes before using or ampule may ignite.
• Ampule should be wrapped in cloth, crushed, and held near patient's nose and mouth so vapor is inhaled.
• Effective within 30 seconds but has a short duration (4 to 8 minutes).
• Head-low position, deep breathing, and movement of extremities may help relieve dizziness, syncope, or weakness from postural hypotension.
• Drug is often abused. Claimed to have aphrodisiac benefits. Sometimes called Amy.

No significant interactions.

Special considerations:
• Use with extreme caution in severe obliterative coronary artery or cerebrovascular disease, since circulation to these diseased areas may be compromised by vasodilatory effects of the drug elsewhere (coronary steal syndrome). Use with caution in glaucoma and hypotension.
• Should be taken with food or antacids to lessen GI distress.
• Should be used in conjunction with, not as a substitute for, appropriate medical or surgical therapy of peripheral or cerebrovascular disease.
• Short-term therapy of little benefit. Patient should expect long-term treatment and continue to take medication.
• Side effects usually disappear after several weeks of therapy.

No significant interactions.

Special considerations:
• Use with caution in hypotension and anticoagulant therapy.
• Patient may develop side effects, especially with large doses. Blood pressure should be monitored.
• Should be administered 1 hour before meals.
• Signs of bleeding, prolonged bleeding time (large doses, long-term) should be watched for.
• Clinical response to antianginal therapy may not be evident before second or third month. Patient should continue drug despite lack of observable response.

No significant interactions.

Special considerations:
• Contraindicated in hypersensitivity to nitrites, idiosyncrasy, head trauma, cerebral hemorrhage, severe anemia. Use with caution in hypotension.
• Blood pressure and intensity and duration of response to drug should be monitored.
• May cause headaches, especially at first. Treat headache with aspirin or acetaminophen. Dosage may need to be reduced temporarily, but tolerance usually develops.
• Patient should take medication regularly, even long-term, if ordered, and keep it easily accessible at all times. Physiologically necessary but not habit-forming.
• Additional dose may be taken before anticipated stress or at bedtime if angina is nocturnal.
• Patient should avoid alcoholic beverages; they may produce unpleasant disulfiram-like side effects.
• May cause orthostatic hypotension. Patient should get out of bed, go up and down stairs, and change position slowly, and should lie down at first sign of dizziness.
• Patient should take sublingual tablet at first sign of attack. He should wet the tablet with saliva, place it under the tongue until completely absorbed, and sit down and rest. Burning sensation indicates potency. Dose may be repeated every 10 to 15 minutes for a maximum of 3 doses. If no relief, patient should call doctor or go to hospital emergency room. If patient complains of tingling, he may try holding tablet in buccal pouch.

(continued on following page)

NAMES, INDICATIONS AND DOSAGES	SIDE EFFECTS
erythrityl tetranitrate *(continued)*	
ethaverine hydrochloride Cebral, Circubid, Etalent, Ethaquin, Ethatab, Ethavex, Isovex, Laverin, Myoquin, Pavaspan, Rolidiol, Spasodil **Long-term treatment of peripheral and cerebrovascular insufficiency associated with arterial spasm; spastic conditions of gastrointestinal and genitourinary tracts:** ADULTS: 100 to 200 mg P.O. t.i.d. or 150 mg of sustained-release preparation P.O. q 12 hours.	**CNS:** *headache,* drowsiness. **CV:** *hypotension, flushing,* sweating, vertigo, cardiac depression, arrhythmias. **GI:** *nausea; anorexia; abdominal distress; dryness of throat;* constipation; diarrhea. **Hepatic:** jaundice, altered liver function studies. **Skin:** rash. **Other:** respiratory depression, malaise, lassitude.
isosorbide dinitrate Angidil, Coronex♦♦, Dilatrate-SR, Iso-Bid, Iso-D, Isosorb, Isordil♦, Isotrate, Onset, Sorate, Sorbitrate **Treatment of acute anginal attacks (sublingual and chewable only); prophylaxis in situations likely to cause attacks; treatment of chronic ischemic heart disease (by preload reduction); adjunct with other vasodilators, such as hydralazine and prazosin, in the treatment of severe chronic congestive heart failure:** ADULTS: *Sublingual form*—2.5 to 10 mg under the tongue for prompt relief of anginal pain, repeated q 2 to 3 hours during acute phase, or q 4 to 6 hours for prophylaxis. *Chewable form*—5 to 10 mg, p.r.n., for acute attack or q 2 to 3 hours for prophylaxis but only after initial test dose of 5 mg to determine risk of severe hypotension. *Oral form*—5 to 30 mg P.O. q.i.d. for prophylaxis only (use smallest effective dose); sustained-release forms 40 mg P.O. q 6 to 12 hours.	**CNS:** *headache, sometimes with throbbing; dizziness;* weakness. **CV:** *orthostatic hypotension, tachycardia, palpitations,* fainting. **GI:** nausea, vomiting. **Local:** sublingual burning. **Skin:** cutaneous vasodilation, *flushing.* **Other:** hypersensitivity reactions.
isoxsuprine hydrochloride Rolisox, Vasodilan♦, Vasoprine **Adjunct for relief of symptoms associated with cerebral vascular insufficiency, peripheral vascular diseases (such as arteriosclerosis obliterans, thromboangiitis obliterans, Raynaud's disease):** ADULTS: 10 to 20 mg P.O. t.i.d. or q.i.d.; initially, 5 to 10 mg I.M. b.i.d. or t.i.d. in severe or acute conditions, to maximum of 10 mg. Intramuscular doses greater than 10 mg may be associated with hypotension and tachycardia and are not recommended.	**CNS:** *dizziness,* nervousness, weakness, trembling, *light-headedness.* **CV:** *hypotension, tachycardia, transient palpitations.* **GI:** vomiting, abdominal distress, intestinal distention. **Skin:** severe rash.

♦ Available in U.S. and Canada. ♦♦ Available in Canada only.
All other products (no symbol) available in U.S. only. Italicized side effects are common or life-threatening.

INTERACTIONS AND SPECIAL CONSIDERATIONS

• Patient should take oral tablet on empty stomach, either ½ hour before or 1 to 2 hours after meals; swallow oral tablets whole; and chew chewable tablets thoroughly before swallowing.
• Drug should not be discontinued abruptly—coronary vasospasm may occur.
• Store medication in cool place, in tightly closed container, away from light. To assure freshness, replace supply every 3 months. Remove cotton from container, since it absorbs drug.

No significant interactions.

Special considerations:
• Contraindicated in complete AV dissociation and in severe hepatic disease. Use with caution in women who are pregnant or of childbearing age, and in patients with glaucoma or pulmonary embolus; may precipitate arrhythmias.
• Dose should be held if signs of hepatic hypersensitivity (GI symptoms, altered liver function studies, jaundice, eosinophilia) develop.
• Vital signs should be monitored throughout therapy.
• FDA has announced this drug may not be effective for disease states indicated.

No significant interactions.

Special considerations:
• Contraindicated in hypersensitivity to nitrites, head trauma, cerebral hemorrhage, severe anemia. Use with caution in hypotension.
• Blood pressure and intensity and duration of response to drug should be monitored.
• May cause headaches, especially at first. Treat headache with aspirin or acetaminophen. Dosage may need to be reduced temporarily, but tolerance usually develops.
• Patient should take medication regularly, even long-term, if ordered, and keep it easily accessible at all times. Physiologically necessary but not habit-forming.
• Additional dose may be taken before anticipated stress or at bedtime if angina is nocturnal.
• Patient should avoid alcoholic beverages; they may produce unpleasant disulfiram-like side effects.
• May cause orthostatic hypotension. Patient should get out of bed, go up and down stairs, and change position slowly, and should lie down at first sign of dizziness.
• Patient should take sublingual tablet at first sign of attack. He should wet the tablet with saliva, place it under the tongue until completely absorbed, and sit down and rest. Burning sensation indicates potency. Dose may be repeated every 10 to 15 minutes for a maximum of 3 doses. If no relief, patient should call doctor or go to hospital emergency room. If patient complains of tingling, he may try holding tablet in buccal pouch.
• Patient should not confuse sublingual with oral form.
• Patient should take oral tablet on empty stomach, either ½ hour before or 1 to 2 hours after meals; swallow oral tablets whole; and chew chewable tablets thoroughly before swallowing.
• Drug should not be discontinued abruptly; coronary vasospasm may occur.
• Store in cool place, in tightly closed container, away from light.
• Has been used investigationally in treatment of congestive heart failure.

No significant interactions.

Special considerations:
• Contraindicated in immediate postpartum period and arterial bleeding; I.M. contraindicated in hypotension or tachycardia.
• Safe use in pregnancy and lactation not established, although drug has been used to inhibit contractions in premature labor.
• Should not be given intravenously.
• Possible hypotension and tachycardia with parenteral use. Blood pressure and pulse rate should be monitored.
• Should be discontinued if rash develops.

NAMES, INDICATIONS AND DOSAGES	SIDE EFFECTS
mannitol hexanitrate Mannex, Vascunitol **Chronic prophylaxis against attacks of angina pectoris:** ADULTS: 15 to 60 mg P.O. q 4 to 6 hours.	**CNS:** *headache, sometimes with throbbing; dizziness;* weakness, increased intracranial pressure. **CV:** *orthostatic hypotension, tachycardia, flushing, palpitations,* fainting. **EENT:** rise in intraocular tension. **GI:** nausea, vomiting. **Local:** sublingual burning. **Skin:** cutaneous vasodilation. **Other:** hypersensitivity.
nicotinyl alcohol Roniacol♦ **Treatment of conditions of deficient circulation such as peripheral vascular disease, vascular spasm, varicose ulcers, decubital ulcers, Ménière's syndrome, vertigo:** ADULTS: 50 to 100 mg regular tablets P.O. b.i.d. or t.i.d. (may increase to 150 to 200 mg P.O. t.i.d. or q.i.d.); 150 to 300 mg sustained-release tablets P.O. b.i.d.; 5 to 10 ml of elixir P.O. t.i.d.	**CNS:** paresthesias. **CV:** *transient flushing.* **GI:** *gastric irritation.* **Skin:** minor rashes. **Other:** allergic reactions.
nitroglycerin Ang-O-Span, Cardabid, Corobid, Glyceryl Trinitrate, Gly-Trate, Nitrobid, Nitrocap, Nitrocels, Nitro-Dial, Nitroglyn, Nitrol♦, Nitro-Lyn, Nitrong♦, Nitrospan, Nitrostabilin♦♦, Nitrostat♦, Nitrotym, Nyglycon, Trates, Vasoglyn **Prophylaxis against chronic anginal attacks:** ADULTS: 1 sustained-release capsule q 8 to 12 hours; or 2% ointment: Start with ½" ointment, increasing with ½" increments until headache occurs, then decreasing to previous dose. Range of dosage with ointment 2" to 5". Usual dose 1" to 2". Alternatively, transdermal disc or pad may be applied to hairless site once daily. **Relief of acute angina pectoris, prophylaxis to prevent or minimize anginal attacks when taken immediately prior to stressful events:** ADULTS: 1 sublingual tablet (gr 1/400, 1/200, 1/150, 1/100) dissolved under the tongue or in the buccal pouch immediately upon indication of anginal attack. May repeat q 5 minutes for 15 minutes.	**CNS:** *headache, sometimes with throbbing; dizziness;* weakness. **CV:** *orthostatic hypotension, tachycardia, flushing, palpitations,* fainting. **GI:** nausea, vomiting. **Skin:** cutaneous vasodilation. **Local:** sublingual burning. **Other:** hypersensitivity reactions.
nylidrin hydrochloride Arlidin♦, Pervadil♦♦, Rolidrin **To increase blood supply in vasospastic disorders (arteriosclerosis obliterans, thromboangiitis obliterans, diabetic vascular disease, night leg cramps, Raynaud's phenomenon and disease, ischemic ulcer, frostbite,**	**CNS:** trembling, *nervousness,* weakness, *dizziness (not associated with labyrinth artery insufficiency).* **CV:** *palpitations, hypotension,* flushing. **GI:** *nausea, vomiting.*

♦ Available in U.S. and Canada. ♦♦ Available in Canada only.
All other products (no symbol) available in U.S. only. Italicized side effects are common or life-threatening.

INTERACTIONS AND SPECIAL CONSIDERATIONS

No significant interactions.

Special considerations:
• Contraindicated in head trauma, cerebral hemorrhage, severe anemia. Use with caution in hypotension.
• Blood pressure and intensity and duration of response to drug should be monitored.
• Medication may cause headaches, especially at first. Treat headache with aspirin or acetaminophen. Dosage may need to be reduced temporarily, but tolerance usually develops.
• Patient should take medication regularly, even long-term, if ordered. Physiologically necessary but not habit-forming.
• Additional doses may be taken before anticipated stress or at bedtime if angina is nocturnal.
• Alcoholic beverages should be avoided, since they may produce unpleasant disulfiram-like side effects.
• Medication may cause orthostatic hypotension. Patient should get out of bed, go up and down stairs, or change position slowly, and should lie down at first sign of dizziness.
• Store medication in cool dark place, in tightly covered container.
• Effective within 15 to 30 minutes; duration 4 to 6 hours.

Interactions:
CLONIDINE: may inhibit vasodilation. Observe for lack of response.

Special considerations:
• Contraindicated in active peptic ulcer or gastritis.
• Tolerance to side effects develops with continued therapy.

No significant interactions.

Special considerations:
• Contraindicated in hypersensitivity to nitrites, head trauma, cerebral hemorrhage, severe anemia. Use with caution in hypotension.
• Blood pressure and intensity and duration of response to drug should be monitored.
• May cause headaches, especially at first. Treat headaches with aspirin or acetaminophen. Dosage may need to be reduced temporarily, but tolerance usually develops.
• Patient should take medication regularly, even long-term, if ordered, and keep it easily accessible at all times. Physiologically necessary but not habit-forming.
• Additional dose may be taken before anticipated stress or at bedtime if angina is nocturnal.
• Patient should avoid alcoholic beverages; they may produce unpleasant disulfiram-like side effects.
• May cause orthostatic hypotension. Patient should get out of bed, go up and down stairs, and change position slowly, and should lie down at first sign of dizziness.
• Patient should take sublingual tablet at first sign of attack. He should wet the tablet with saliva, place it under the tongue until completely absorbed, and sit down and rest. Burning sensation indicates potency. Dose may be repeated every 10 to 15 minutes for a maximum of 3 doses. If no relief, patient should call doctor or go to hospital emergency room. If patient complains of tingling, he may try holding tablet in buccal pouch.
• Patient should take oral tablet on empty stomach, either ½ hour before or 1 to 2 hours after meals; swallow oral tablets whole; and chew chewable tablets thoroughly before swallowing.
• Store in cool dark place, in tightly closed container. To assure freshness, replace every 3 months. Cotton absorbs drug; remove from container.
• To apply ointment: spread in uniform thin layer on any nonhairy area; do not rub in; cover with plastic film to aid absorption and to protect clothing.
• Doctor may prescribe nitroglycerin by its chemical name, glyceryl trinitrate (GTN).

No significant interactions.

Special considerations:
• Contraindicated in acute myocardial infarction, paroxysmal tachycardia, angina pectoris, thyrotoxicosis. Use with caution in uncompensated heart disease or peptic ulcer.

(continued on following page)

NAMES, INDICATIONS AND DOSAGES	SIDE EFFECTS
nylidrin hydrochloride *(continued)* **acrocyanosis, acroparesthesia, sequelae of thrombophlebitis); and in circulatory disturbances of the middle ear (primary cochlear ischemia, cochlear striae, vascular ischemia, macular or ampullar ischemia); other disturbances due to labyrinth artery spasm or obstruction:** ADULTS: 3 to 12 mg P.O. t.i.d. or q.i.d.	
papaverine hydrochloride Blupav, BP-Papaverine, Cerebid, Cerespan, Cirbed, Delapav, DiPav, Kavrin, Lapav, Meta-Kaps, Myobid, Papacon, Papalease, PapKaps-150, P-A-V, Pavabid, Pavacap, Pavacen, Pavaclor, Pavacron, Pavadel, Pavadur, Pavadyl, Pavakey S.A., Pava-lyn, Pava-Par, Pava-Rx, Pavasule, Pavatime, Pava-Wol, Paverolan, Pavex, PT-300, Ro-Papav, S.M.R.-Kaps, Sustaverine, Vasal, Vasocap, Vasospan, Vazosan **Relief of cerebral and peripheral ischemia associated with arterial spasm and myocardial ischemia; treatment of smooth muscle spasm (coronary occlusion, angina pectoris, sequelae of peripheral and pulmonary embolism, certain cerebral angiospastic states); and visceral spasms (biliary, ureteral, or gastrointestinal colic):** ADULTS: 60 to 300 mg P.O. 1 to 5 times daily, or 150 to 300 mg sustained-release preparations q 8 to 12 hours; 30 to 120 mg I.M. or I.V. q 3 hours, as indicated.	**CNS:** *headache.* **CV:** *increased heart rate, increased blood pressure* (with parenteral use), depressed AV and intraventricular conduction, arrhythmias. **GI:** constipation, *nausea.* **Other:** *sweating, flushing,* malaise, increased depth of respiration.
pentaerythritol tetranitrate Angijen Green, Arcotrate Nos. 1 & 2, Baritrate, Blaintrate, Desatrate 30, Desatrate 50, Dilar, Dinate, Duotrate, Kaytrate, Maso-Trol, Nitrin, Penta-Cap-No. 1, Penta-E., Penta-E. S.A., Pentaforte-T, Penta-Tal No. 1 & 2, Pentestan-80, Pentetra, Pentraspan, Pentrate T.D., Pentritol, Pent-T-80, Pentylan, Peritrate♦, PETN, Petro-20 mg, P-T♦♦, P-T-T, Quintrate, Rate, Vasolate, Vasolate-80 **Prophylaxis against angina pectoris:** ADULTS: 10 to 20 mg P.O. q.i.d.; may be titrated upward to 40 mg P.O. q.i.d. ½ hour before or 1 hour after meals and h.s.; 80 mg sustained-release preparations P.O. b.i.d.	**CNS:** *headache, sometimes with throbbing; dizziness;* weakness. **CV:** *orthostatic hypotension, tachycardia, flushing, palpitations,* fainting. **GI:** nausea, vomiting. **Skin:** cutaneous vasodilation. **Other:** hypersensitivity reactions.
tolazoline hydrochloride Tazol, Toloxan, Tolzol **Spastic peripheral vascular disorders associated with acrocyanosis, acroparesthesia, arteriosclerosis obliterans, Buerger's disease, causalgia, diabetic arteriosclerosis, gangrene, endarteritis, sequelae of frostbite, postthrombotic conditions, Raynaud's dis-**	**CV:** *arrhythmias, anginal pain, hypertension, flushing,* transient postural vertigo, palpitations. **GI:** *nausea, vomiting, diarrhea, epigastric discomfort, exacerbation of peptic ulcer.* **Local:** burning at injection site. **Other:** weakness, paradoxical response in seriously damaged limbs, increased pilomotor activity, tingling, chilliness, apprehension.

INTERACTIONS AND SPECIAL CONSIDERATIONS

No significant interactions.

Special considerations:
• Contraindicated for I.V. use in complete AV block. Use with caution in glaucoma.
• Blood pressure, heart rate and rhythm should be monitored, especially in cardiac disease. If changes occur, dose should be withheld.
• Not often used parenterally, except when immediate effect is desired.
• I.V. should be given slowly (over 1 to 2 minutes) to avoid side effects.
• Most effective when given early in the course of a disorder.
• Patient should take medication regularly; long-term therapy is required.
• Should not add lactated Ringer's injection to the injectable form; will precipitate.
• FDA has announced this drug may not be effective for disease states indicated.

No significant interactions.

Special considerations:
• Contraindicated in head trauma, cerebral hemorrhage, severe anemia. Use with caution in hypotension and glaucoma.
• Blood pressure and intensity and duration of response to drug should be monitored.
• Medication may cause headaches, especially at first. Treat with aspirin or acetaminophen. Dosage may need to be reduced temporarily, but tolerance usually develops.
• Medication should be taken regularly, even long-term, if ordered. Physiologically necessary but not habit-forming.
• Additional doses may be taken before anticipated stress or at bedtime for nocturnal angina.
• Not to be used for relief of acute anginal attacks.
• Medication may cause orthostatic hypotension. Patient should get out of bed, go up and down stairs, or change position slowly, and should lie down at first sign of dizziness.
• Drug should not be discontinued abruptly; coronary vasospasm may occur.
• Store medication in cool place in tightly covered, light-resistant container.

Interactions:
ETHYL ALCOHOL: possible disulfiram reaction from accumulation of acetaldehyde. Use together cautiously.

Special considerations:
• Contraindicated in coronary artery disease, active peptic ulcer, or following cerebrovascular accident. Use with caution in patients with history of peptic ulcer disease, gastritis, or known or suspected mitral stenosis.
• Patient should be kept warm during parenteral administration to increase response.
• Appearance of flushing usually indicates maximum tolerable dose.
• Vital signs should be monitored, especially blood pressure changes and arrhythmias.
• Patient should avoid alcohol; chills and flush-

(continued on following page)

NAMES, INDICATIONS AND DOSAGES	SIDE EFFECTS
tolazoline hydrochloride *(continued)* **ease, scleroderma:** ADULTS: *Oral*—25 mg 4 to 6 times daily, gradually increasing to maximum of 50 mg 6 times daily. *Parenteral*—10 to 50 mg S.C., I.V., or I.M. q.i.d. Start with low dose, increasing gradually until optimal response (as determined by appearance of flushing) is reached. *Intra-arterial*—50 to 75 mg/injection, depending on response; 1 or 2 injections may be required initially, then dose of 2 or 3 injections weekly to maintain circulation, possibly coupled with oral tolazoline between injections.	

INTERACTIONS AND SPECIAL CONSIDERATIONS

ing may occur.

- Due to risks, technique, and precautions, intra-arterial injection should be done only by experienced personnel, in selected cases, and only after maximum benefit has been achieved with oral and parenteral therapy.
- Exposure to cold can aggravate tissue damage.
- Often used to distinguish between functional (vasospastic) and organic (obstructive) forms of peripheral vascular disease.

23

Antilipemics

cholestyramine
clofibrate
colestipol hydrochloride
dextrothyroxine sodium
niacin
probucol
sitosterols

Antilipemics can retard, and even arrest, atherosclerosis and its resultant complications. Atherosclerosis is associated with increased levels of certain blood lipids. Research thus far, however, has not been able to show a direct clinical relationship between lowered blood lipid levels and reduced incidence of atherosclerosis since other risk factors are reduced as well during the treatment period.

Dietary restriction and physical exercise are essential in treating all hyperlipidemias. If strict dietary therapy does not effectively lower lipid levels after 2 or 3 months, drug therapy may be started.

Hyperlipidemias may be primary or secondary to conditions such as hypothyroidism, hepatic disorders, renal failure, nephrosis, pancreatic insufficiency, malabsorption syndromes, and diabetes mellitus.

Major uses

Antilipemics counteract high concentrations of lipids in the blood. They do this by lowering levels of cholesterol or triglycerides or both, to different degrees.

Mechanism of action

The drug chosen to reduce blood lipid levels depends on which fraction or fractions of the blood lipids are elevated.

- Both cholestyramine and colestipol combine with bile acid to form an insoluble compound that is excreted.
- Clofibrate—used when triglycerides are high and cholesterol levels are only moderately elevated—seems to inhibit biosynthesis of cholesterol, but the exact mechanism is unknown.
- Dextrothyroxine accelerates hepatic catabolism of cholesterol and increases bile secretion to lower cholesterol levels. The drug's serious cardiovascular side effects restrict its use to young patients with no history of coronary artery disease.
- Niacin, by an unknown mechanism, decreases synthesis of low-density lipoproteins and inhibits lipolysis in adipose tissue.
- Probucol inhibits cholesterol transport from the intestine and may also decrease cholesterol synthesis. The drug appears to be more effective in patients with mild cholesterol elevations than in those with severe hypercholesterolemia.
- Sitosterols, structurally similar to cholesterol, compete with it to reduce absorption.

Absorption, distribution, metabolism, and excretion

- Cholestyramine, colestipol, and the sitosterols are not appreciably absorbed from the gastrointestinal (GI) tract. They are eliminated in the feces.
- Clofibrate and niacin are well absorbed from the GI tract.
- Dextrothyroxine is poorly absorbed from the GI tract.

TYPES OF HYPERLIPOPROTEINEMIA

TYPE AND NAME	FREQUENCY	POSSIBLE TREATMENTS
I—Fat-induced hyperlipemia	Rare	• Very low-fat diet
II—Familial hyper-cholesterolemia	Common	• If severe, possibly antiplatelet therapy • Fat-controlled diet • Colestipol or cholestyramine (first choice); clofibrate or nicotinic acid (second choice)
III—Broad beta disease	Rare	• Low-calorie diet if overweight • Fat-controlled diet • Clofibrate
IV—Endogenous hypertriglycer-idemia	Common	• Low-calorie diet if overweight • Fat-controlled diet • Exercise • Clofibrate • Avoidance of oral contraceptives and estrogens
V—Mixed hyper-lipemia	Uncommon	• Diet low in cholesterol, fat, and carbohydrates • Clofibrate

• Probucol is very poorly absorbed from the GI tract. It is passed into the bile for elimination in the feces.

Onset and duration

Response to antilipemic therapy varies with adherence to drug and dietary regimens. Drug treatment is effective only when combined with an adequate dietary plan. For maximum benefit, blood cholesterol and triglyceride levels should be tested several times during the first few months of therapy and periodically thereafter.

After administration of dietary or drug therapy, a new lipid steady-state level is reached in 4 weeks. Lipid levels should be rechecked at this time and the regimen changed, if necessary.

• Clofibrate and probucol take up to 2 months to achieve maximum effect.

• Niacin's effect is transient; therefore, free fatty acid levels rebound between meals and at night. The bedtime dose is especially important to counteract the striking rise of free fatty acid levels during the nocturnal fast.

NAMES, INDICATIONS AND DOSAGES	SIDE EFFECTS
cholestyramine Questran ♦ **Primary hyperlipidemia, pruritus, and diarrhea due to excess bile acid:** ADULTS: 4 g before meals and h.s., not to exceed 32 g daily. Each scoop or packet of Questran contains 4 g cholestyramine. CHILDREN: 240 mg/kg/day P.O. in 3 divided doses with beverage or food. Safe dosage not established for children under 6 years.	**GI:** *constipation,* fecal impaction, hemorrhoids, *abdominal discomfort,* flatulence, *nausea,* vomiting, steatorrhea. **Skin:** *rashes,* irritation of skin, tongue, and perianal area. **Other:** *vitamin A, D, and K deficiency from decreased absorption;* hyperchloremic acidosis with long-term use or very high dosage.
clofibrate Atromid-S ♦ **Hyperlipidemia and xanthoma tuberosum:** ADULTS: 2 g P.O. daily in 4 divided doses. Some patients may respond to lower doses as assessed by serum lipid monitoring. Should not be used in children.	**Blood:** leukopenia. **CNS:** fatigue, weakness. **GI:** *nausea, diarrhea, vomiting,* stomatitis, *dyspepsia,* flatulence. **GU:** decreased libido. **Hepatic:** gallstones, *transient and reversible elevations of liver function studies.* **Skin:** rashes, urticaria, pruritus, dry skin and hair. **Other:** *myalgias and arthralgias,* resembling a flulike syndrome; *weight gain; polyphagia;* fever.
colestipol hydrochloride Colestid **Primary hypercholesterolemia and xanthomas:** ADULTS: 15 to 30 g P.O. daily in 2 to 4 divided doses.	**GI:** *constipation (common, may require decreasing the dosage),* fecal impaction, hemorrhoids, abdominal discomfort, flatulence, nausea, vomiting, steatorrhea. **Skin:** rashes, irritation of skin, tongue, and perianal area. **Other:** vitamins A, D, and K deficiencies from decreased absorption; hyperchloremic acidosis with long-term use or very high dosage.
dextrothyroxine sodium Choloxin ♦ **Hyperlipidemia in euthyroid patients, especially when cholesterol and triglyceride levels are elevated:** ADULTS: initial dose 1 to 2 mg daily, increased by 1 to 2 mg daily at monthly intervals to a total of 4 to 8 mg daily. CHILDREN: initial dose 0.05 mg/kg daily, increased by 0.05 mg/kg daily at monthly intervals to a total of 4 mg daily.	**CV:** palpitations, angina pectoris, arrhythmias, ischemic myocardial changes on EKG, myocardial infarction. **EENT:** visual disturbances, ptosis. **GI:** nausea, vomiting, diarrhea, constipation, decreased appetite. **Metabolic:** *insomnia, weight loss, sweating,* flushing, hyperthermia, hair loss, menstrual irregularities.
niacin Diacin, Niac, Niacalex, Niacels, NICL, Nicobid, Nicocap, Nico-400, Nicolar, NiCord XL, Nico-Span, Nicotinex, Ni-Span, Tega-Span **Adjunctive treatment of hyperlipidemias, especially with hypercholesterolemia:** ADULTS: 1.5 to 3 g daily in 3 divided doses with or after meals, increased at intervals to 6 g daily.	**CV:** *flushing* (which usually subsides in a few weeks). **GI:** *nausea,* dyspepsia, vomiting, diarrhea, anorexia, flatulence, epigastric pain. **Hepatic:** abnormal liver function studies. **Metabolic:** *glucose intolerance resulting in hyperglycemia in previously well-controlled diabetics, hyperuricemia.* **Skin:** *pruritus,* sensation of burning or stinging.

♦ Available in U.S. and Canada. ♦♦ Available in Canada only.
All other products (no symbol) available in U.S. only. Italicized side effects are common or life-threatening.

INTERACTIONS AND SPECIAL CONSIDERATIONS

No significant interactions.

Special considerations:
• To mix, sprinkle powder on surface of preferred beverage or wet food. Let stand a few minutes, then stir to obtain uniform suspension.
• Mixing with carbonated beverages may result in excess foaming. To avoid, use large glass, mix slowly.
• All other medications should be administered at least 1 hour before or 4 to 6 hours after cholestyramine to avoid blocking their absorption.
• Bowel habits should be observed and constipation treated as needed. If severe constipation develops, dosage should be decreased, stool softener added, or drug stopped.
• Cardiotonic glycoside levels should be monitored in patients receiving both medications concurrently. Should cholestyramine therapy be discontinued, cardiotonic glycoside toxicity may result unless dosage is adjusted.
• Deficiencies of vitamins A, D, and K possible.
• May cause decreased absorption of many drugs due to binding. Drug interaction list of individual drugs should be checked.

Interactions:
ORAL CONTRACEPTIVES: may antagonize clofibrate's lipid-lowering effect. Monitor blood lipid level.

Special considerations:
• Contraindicated in patients with severe renal or hepatic disease.
• Patient should report flulike symptoms immediately.
• Kidney and hepatic function, blood counts, serum electrolyte, and blood sugar levels should be monitored. If liver function studies show steady rise, clofibrate should be discontinued.
• Should not be used indiscriminately. May pose increased risk of gallstones and cancer.
• If significant lipid lowering is not achieved within 3 months, drug should be discontinued.

Interactions:
ORAL HYPOGLYCEMICS: may antagonize response to colestipol. Monitor blood lipid level.

Special considerations:
• All other medications should be administered at least 1 hour before or 4 to 6 hours after colestipol to avoid blocking their absorption.
• Cardiotonic glycoside levels should be monitored in patients receiving both medications concurrently. Should colestipol therapy be discontinued, cardiotonic glycoside toxicity may result unless dosage is adjusted.
• Vitamins A, D, and K deficiencies possible.
• Lowering dosage or adding stool softener may relieve constipation.
• May cause decreased absorption of many drugs due to binding. Drug interaction list of individual drugs should be checked.

No significant interactions.

Special considerations:
• Contraindicated in patients with hepatic or renal disease, or iodism. Patients with history of cardiac disease, including arrhythmias, hypertension, or angina pectoris, should receive very small doses.
• May increase need for insulin, diet therapy, or oral hypoglycemics in patients with diabetes.
• Drug should be discontinued 2 weeks before surgery to avoid possible potentiation of anticoagulant effect.
• Patient should be observed for signs of hyperthyroidism, such as nervousness, insomnia, weight loss. If these occur, dosage should be decreased or drug discontinued.

No significant interactions.

Special considerations:
• Use cautiously in patients with gout, diabetes, gallbladder or hepatic disease, peptic ulcer.
• Pruritus and flushing noted in first few weeks of therapy usually lessen with continued use.
• Therapy should begin with small doses; then increased gradually.
• Should be taken with meals to minimize GI irritation. Cold water eases swallowing.
• Blood glucose and liver function studies should be performed routinely during early therapy.

NAMES, INDICATIONS AND DOSAGES	SIDE EFFECTS
probucol Lorelco♦ **Primary hypercholesterolemia:** ADULTS: 2 tablets (500 mg total) P.O. b.i.d. with morning and evening meals. Not recommended in children.	**GI:** *diarrhea, flatulence, abdominal pain, nausea, vomiting.* **Other:** *hyperhidrosis,* fetid sweat, angioneurotic edema.
sitosterols Cytellin **Adjunctive therapy for hypercholesterolemia or hyperbetalipoproteinemia:** ADULTS: 15 ml (3 g) P.O. before meals to a total of 45 ml (9 g) daily. May increase to 30 ml before large or high-fat meals; give fraction of usual dose before snacks.	**GI:** anorexia; *diarrhea;* abdominal cramps; *bulky, light-colored stools;* nausea.

♦ Available in U.S. and Canada. ♦♦ Available in Canada only.
All other products (no symbol) available in U.S. only. Italicized side effects are common or life-threatening.

LETHAL LIPIDS

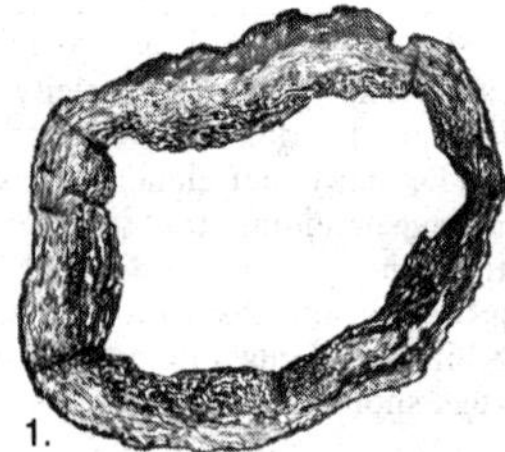

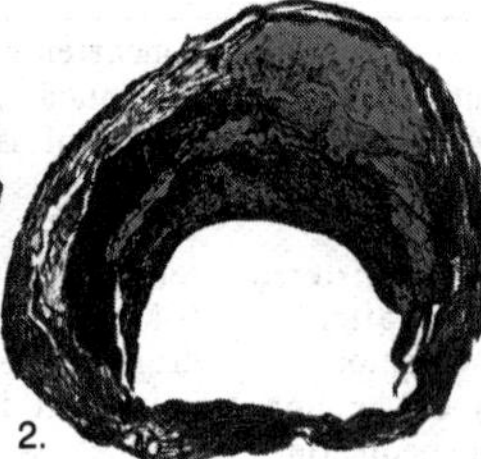

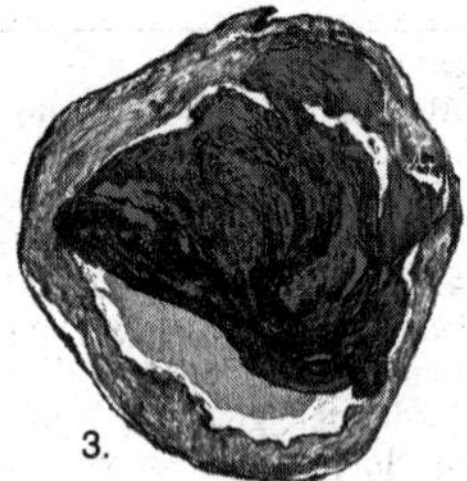

As atherosclerosis develops, a normal coronary artery (illustration 1) becomes roughened and narrowed by lipid deposits (illustration 2). This condition can be treated with antilipemic drugs and a fat-controlled diet. But if left untreated, a blood clot may develop and potentially clog the artery (illustration 3), depriving the heart of its blood supply and causing a heart attack.

INTERACTIONS AND SPECIAL CONSIDERATIONS

No significant interactions.

Special considerations:

- Contraindicated in patients with arrhythmias. Drug should be stopped in any patient whose EKG shows prolonged Q-T interval.
- Drug's effect is enhanced when taken with food.

No significant interactions.

Special considerations:

- Other medications should be administered 1 hour before or 4 hours after sitosterols.
- Sitosterols should be taken immediately before meals or snacks.
- Mix with milk, tea, coffee, or fruit juice for palatability.
- Maximum therapeutic effect during second and third month of therapy.

ANTILIPEMICS' EFFECTS ON BLOOD LIPIDS

DRUG	EFFECT ON CHOLESTEROL	EFFECT ON TRIGLYCERIDES
cholestyramine	⬇	O or ⇧
clofibrate	⇩	⬇
colestipol	⬇	O or ⇧
dextrothyroxine	⬇	⇩ or ⇧
niacin	⬇	⬇
probucol	⬇	O or ⇧
sitosterols	⇩	O

KEY: ⇩ = Mild decrease ⬇ = Moderate decrease ⬇ = Marked decrease

⇧ = Mild increase O = No change

24

Nonnarcotic analgesics and antipyretics

Morphine-like analgesics
butorphanol tartrate
nalbuphine hydrochloride

Salicylates
aspirin
choline magnesium trisalicylate
choline salicylate
magnesium salicylate
salicylamide
salsalate
sodium salicylate
sodium thiosalicylate

Urinary tract analgesics
ethoxazene hydrochloride
phenazopyridine hydrochloride

Miscellaneous
acetaminophen
ethoheptazine citrate
methotrimeprazine
phenacetin
zomepirac sodium

(All drugs are listed in alphabetical order in the tables that follow.)

Nonnarcotic analgesics and antipyretics are probably the most common drugs in medicine. Aspirin, of course, and most salicylate derivatives are available without a doctor's prescription. Acetaminophen, and to a lesser extent phenacetin, are also widely available without prescriptions. Salicylates, acetaminophen, and phenacetin are combined with one another in varying amounts in many proprietary preparations that are widely advertised in the mass media. Both the morphine-like and urinary tract analgesics necessitate a doctor's prescription.

Major uses

• Morphine-like analgesics relieve moderate-to-severe pain.

• Salicylates relieve mild-to-moderate pain; alleviate inflammation of rheumatoid arthritis, osteoarthritis, gout, and other conditions; and reduce fever. Aspirin also inhibits platelet aggregation, hindering coagulation.

• Urinary tract analgesics ease the pain of frequent urination (burning and urgency) associated with cystitis, prostatitis, and urethritis. Although once thought to have antiseptic properties, urinary tract analgesics are ineffective against microorganisms responsible for urinary tract infections.

• Among the miscellaneous drugs, acetaminophen, ethoheptazine, and phenacetin relieve mild-to-moderate pain and fever. Methotrimeprazine alleviates moderate-to-severe pain; zomepirac is effective against mild-to-moderately severe pain.

Mechanism of action

• Morphine-like analgesics bind to receptor sites in the central nervous system to alter the individual's perception of and response to pain.

• Salicylates produce analgesia by an ill-defined effect on the hypothalamus (central action) and by blocking generation of pain impulses (peripheral action). The peripheral action may involve inhibition of prostaglandin synthesis.

Salicylates probably exert an anti-inflammatory effect by inhibiting prostaglandin synthesis and may inhibit synthesis or action of other mediators of inflammation.

They relieve fever by acting on the hypothalamic heat-regulating center to produce peripheral vasodilation. This increases peripheral blood supply and promotes sweating, which leads to loss of heat and cooling by evaporation. Aspirin also appears to impede coagulation by blocking prostaglandin synthetase action, which prevents formation of platelet-aggregating substance thromboxane A_2.

• The exact mechanism of action of the urinary tract analgesics is unknown.

• Among the miscellaneous drugs, acetaminophen and phenacetin produce analgesia by blocking generation of pain impulses. This action is probably due to inhibition of prostaglandin synthesis; it may also be due to inhibition of the synthesis or action of other substances that sensitize pain receptors to mechanical or chemical stimulation. Both drugs relieve fever by central action in the hypothalamic heat-regulating center.

Ethoheptazine's mechanism of action is unknown.

Methotrimeprazine is thought to suppress sensory impulses by acting on sites in the thalamus, hypothalamus, and reticular activating and limbic systems.

Zomepirac's mechanism of action is unknown but is probably related to inhibition of prostaglandin synthesis.

Absorption, distribution, metabolism, and excretion

All oral and I.M. forms of the analgesics and antipyretics are well absorbed. The drugs are distributed in most body tissues and fluids, largely metabolized in the liver, and eliminated as inactive metabolites in urine and—through the bile—in feces. The urinary tract analgesics are eliminated as both inactive metabolites and unchanged drug.

Onset and duration

All the nonnarcotic analgesics and antipyretics begin to act 30 to 60 minutes after oral administration and 15 to 30 minutes after I.M. injection. Peak blood levels are reached in 2 to 3 hours. Duration of action of these drugs is generally 4 to 6 hours.

Combination products

ANACIN: aspirin 400 mg and caffeine 32 mg.
A.P.C.: aspirin 227 mg, phenacetin 162 mg, and caffeine 32 mg.
BUTAZOLIDIN ALKA: phenylbutazone 100 mg, dried aluminum hydroxide gel 100 mg, and magnesium trisilicate 150 mg.
DARVOCET-N 50: acetaminophen 325 mg and propoxyphene napsylate 50 mg.
DARVON COMPOUND-65: aspirin 227 mg, phenacetin 162 mg, caffeine 32.4 mg, and propoxyphene HCl 65 mg.
DOLENE AP-65: acetaminophen 650 mg and propoxyphene HCl 65 mg.
DOLENE COMPOUND-65: aspirin 227 mg, phenacetin 162 mg, propoxyphene HCl 65 mg, and caffeine 32.4 mg.
EQUAGESIC: aspirin 250 mg, ethoheptazine citrate 75 mg, and meprobamate 150 mg.
EXCEDRIN TABLETS: aspirin 194.4 mg, acetaminophen 97.2 mg, caffeine 64.8 mg, and salicylamide 129.6 mg.
FEMCAPS: aspirin 162 mg, phenacetin 65 mg, caffeine 32 mg, ephedrine sulfate 8 mg, and atropine sulfate 0.0325 mg.
FIORINAL: butalbital 50 mg, aspirin 200 mg, phenacetin 130 mg, caffeine 40 mg.
SYNALGOS: promethazine HCl 6.25 mg, aspirin 194.4 mg, phenacetin 162 mg, caffeine 30 mg.
TALWIN COMPOUND CAPLETS: aspirin 325 mg and pentazocine (as HCl) 12.5 mg.
TRILISATE: choline salicylate 293 mg and magnesium salicylate 362 mg.
VANQUISH: aspirin 227 mg, acetaminophen 194 mg, caffeine 33 mg, aluminum hydroxide 25 mg, and magnesium hydroxide 50 mg.
ZACTIRIN: aspirin 325 mg and ethoheptazine citrate 75 mg.

NAMES, INDICATIONS AND DOSAGES	SIDE EFFECTS
acetaminophen Acephen, Atasol♦♦, Campain♦♦, Datril, Dolanex, Liquiprin, Paralgin♦♦, Phendex, Robigesic♦♦, Rounox♦♦, SK-Apap, Tapar, Tempra♦, Tivrin♦♦, Tylenol♦, Valadol **Mild pain or fever:** ADULTS AND CHILDREN OVER 10 YEARS: 325 to 650 mg P.O. or rectally q 4 hours, p.r.n. Maximum 2.6 g daily. CHILDREN UNDER 1 YEAR: 15 to 60 mg/dose. 1 YEAR: 60 mg/dose. 2 YEARS: 120 mg/dose. 3 YEARS: 180 mg/dose. 4 YEARS: 240 mg/dose. 5 TO 10 YEARS: 325 mg/dose. May give P.O. or rectally q 4 to 6 hours. Maximum 1.2 g daily.	**Hepatic:** severe hepatotoxicity with large doses. **Skin:** rash, urticaria.
aspirin Acetal♦♦, Acetyl-Sal♦♦, Ancasal♦♦, A.S.A., Aspergum, Aspirjen Jr., Aspirin♦♦, Bayer Timed-Release, Buffinol, Ecotrin♦, Empirin, Entrophen♦♦, Measurin, Neopirine No. 25♦♦, Nova-Phase♦♦, Novasen♦♦, Rhonal♦♦, Sal-Adult♦♦, Sal-Infant♦♦, Supasa♦♦, Triaphen-10♦♦ ADULTS: **Arthritis:** 2.6 to 5.2 g P.O. daily in divided doses. **Mild pain or fever:** 325 to 650 mg P.O. or rectally q 4 hours, p.r.n. **Thromboembolic disorders:** 325 to 650 mg P.O. daily or b.i.d. **Transient ischemic attacks:** 650 mg P.O. b.i.d. or 325 mg q.i.d. CHILDREN: **Arthritis:** 90 to 130 mg/kg P.O. daily divided q 4 to 6 hours. **Fever:** 40 to 80 mg/kg P.O. or rectally daily divided q 6 hours, p.r.n. **Mild pain:** 65 to 100 mg/kg P.O. or rectally daily divided q 4 to 6 hours, p.r.n.	**Blood:** *prolonged bleeding time.* **EENT:** *tinnitus and hearing loss (first signs of toxicity).* **GI:** *nausea, vomiting, gastrointestinal distress, occult bleeding.* **Hepatic:** abnormal liver function studies. **Skin:** *rash.* **Other:** *hypersensitivity manifested by anaphylaxis.*
butorphanol tartrate Stadol **Moderate-to-severe pain:** ADULTS: 1 to 4 mg I.M. q 3 to 4 hours, p.r.n.; or 0.5 to 2 mg I.V. q 3 to 4 hours, p.r.n.	**CNS:** *sedation, headache, vertigo, floating sensation,* lethargy, confusion, nervousness, unusual dreams, agitation, euphoria, hallucinations, flushing. **CV:** palpitations, fluctuation in blood pressure. **EENT:** diplopia, blurred vision. **GI:** *nausea,* vomiting, dry mouth. **Skin:** rash, hives, *clamminess, excessive sweating.* **Other:** *respiratory depression.*
choline magnesium trisalicylate Trilisate **Arthritis, mild:** ADULTS: 1 to 2 tsp or tablets, each tablet or teaspoon equal to 500 mg salicylate, b.i.d.	**Blood:** *prolonged bleeding time.* **EENT:** *tinnitus and hearing loss (first signs of toxicity).* **GI:** *nausea, vomiting, gastrointestinal distress, occult bleeding.* **Hepatic:** abnormal liver function studies.

♦ Available in U.S. and Canada. ♦♦ Available in Canada only.
All other products (no symbol) available in U.S. only. Italicized side effects are common or life-threatening.

INTERACTIONS AND SPECIAL CONSIDERATIONS

No significant interactions.

Special considerations:
- Has no anti-inflammatory effect.
- High doses or unsupervised chronic use can cause hepatic damage. Excessive ingestion of alcoholic beverages may hasten hepatotoxicity.
- Has little or no effect on prothrombin time.
- For symptoms and treatment of acute toxicity, see APPENDIX.

Interactions:
AMMONIUM CHLORIDE (AND OTHER URINE ACIDIFIERS): increases blood levels of aspirin products. Monitor for aspirin toxicity.
ANTACIDS (AND OTHER URINE ALKALINIZERS): decrease levels of aspirin products. Monitor for decreased aspirin effect.
CARBONIC ANHYDRASE INHIBITORS: may elevate salicylate levels. Monitor for toxicity.
CORTICOSTEROIDS: enhance salicylate elimination. Monitor for decreased salicylate effect.
ORAL ANTICOAGULANTS: increase risk of bleeding. Avoid using together if possible.

Special considerations:
- Contraindicated in GI ulcer, GI bleeding, aspirin hypersensitivity. Use cautiously in hypoprothrombinemia, vitamin K deficiency, bleeding disorders, Hodgkin's disease (may cause profound hypothermia), and in those with asthma with nasal polyps (may cause severe bronchospasm).
- Febrile, dehydrated children can develop toxicity rapidly.
- Should be taken with food, milk, antacid, or large glass of water to reduce GI side effects.
- Patients should check with doctor or pharmacist before taking over-the-counter combinations containing aspirin.
- Therapeutic serum salicylate level in arthritis is 20 to 30 mg/100 ml.
- Alcohol may increase GI blood loss.
- May cause increase in serum levels of SGOT, SGPT, alkaline phosphatase, and bilirubin. May produce false-negative test results for urine glucose by glucose oxidase methods (Clinistix, Tes-Tape) and false-positive results using Clinitest.
- Keep out of reach of children—aspirin is one of the leading causes of poisoning in children.
- Patients taking large doses of aspirin for an extended period of time should maintain adequate fluid intake and watch for petechiae, bleeding gums, and signs of GI bleeding. Hemoglobin and prothrombin tests should be obtained periodically.
- For symptoms and treatment of acute toxicity, see APPENDIX.

No significant interactions.

Special considerations:
- Contraindicated in narcotic addiction; may precipitate narcotic abstinence syndrome. Use cautiously in head injury, increased intracranial pressure, acute MI, ventricular dysfunction, coronary insufficiency, respiratory diseases or depression, renal or hepatic dysfunction.
- Unlikely to cause dependence.
- Respiratory depression does not increase with increased dosage.
- Subcutaneous route not recommended.
- Also approved for use as a preoperative medication, as the analgesic component of balanced anesthesia, and for relief of postpartum pain.

Interactions:
AMMONIUM CHLORIDE (AND OTHER URINE ACIDIFIERS): increases blood levels of salicylates. Monitor for salicylate toxicity.
ANTACIDS (AND OTHER URINE ALKALINIZERS): decrease levels of salicylates. Monitor for decreased salicylate effect.
CARBONIC ANHYDRASE INHIBITORS: may elevate salicylate levels. Monitor for toxicity.
CORTICOSTEROIDS: enhance salicylate elimination. Monitor for decreased salicylate effect.
ORAL ANTICOAGULANTS: increase risk of bleed-

(continued on following page)

NAMES, INDICATIONS AND DOSAGES	SIDE EFFECTS
choline magnesium trisalicylate *(continued)* **Rheumatoid arthritis and osteoarthritis:** ADULTS: 2 to 3 teaspoonfuls or tablets b.i.d. Each tablet or teaspoonful equal in salicylate content to 650 mg aspirin.	**Skin:** *rash.* **Other:** *hypersensitivity manifested by anaphylaxis.*
choline salicylate Arthropan♦ **Arthritis:** ADULTS: 5 to 10 ml P.O. q.i.d. **Minor pain or fever:** ADULTS: 870 mg (5 ml) P.O. q 3 to 4 hours, p.r.n. CHILDREN 3 TO 6 YEARS: 105 to 210 mg P.O. q 4 hours, p.r.n. Each 870 mg (5 ml) equals 650 mg aspirin.	**Blood:** *prolonged bleeding time.* **EENT:** *tinnitus and hearing loss (first signs of toxicity).* **GI:** *nausea, vomiting, gastrointestinal distress, occult bleeding.* **Hepatic:** abnormal liver function studies. **Skin:** *rash.* **Other:** *hypersensitivity manifested by anaphylaxis.*
ethoheptazine citrate Zactane **Mild pain:** ADULTS: 75 to 150 mg P.O. t.i.d. or q.i.d.	**CNS:** dizziness, headache, syncope, nervousness. **EENT:** visual disturbances. **GI:** nausea, vomiting. **Skin:** pruritus.
ethoxazene hydrochloride Serenium **Pain with urinary tract irritation or infection:** ADULTS: 100 mg a.c. P.O. t.i.d.	**GI:** nausea, vomiting.
magnesium salicylate Analate, Arthrin, Lorisal, Magan, Mobidin, MSG-600, Triact ADULTS: **Arthritis:** up to 9.6 g daily in divided doses.	**Blood:** *prolonged bleeding time.* **EENT:** *tinnitus and hearing loss (first signs of toxicity).* **GI:** *nausea, vomiting, gastrointestinal distress, occult bleeding.* **Hepatic:** abnormal liver function studies.

INTERACTIONS AND SPECIAL CONSIDERATIONS

ing. Avoid using together if possible.

Special considerations:
• Contraindicated in GI ulcer, GI bleeding, aspirin hypersensitivity. Use cautiously in patients with hypoprothrombinemia, vitamin K deficiency, bleeding disorders, Hodgkin's disease (may cause profound hypothermia) and in those with asthma with nasal polyps (may cause severe bronchospasm).
• May cause less GI distress than aspirin. If needed, antacid should be taken 2 hours after meals and choline magnesium trisalicylate taken before meals.
• May mix drug with water, fruit juice, or carbonated drinks.
• Febrile, dehydrated children can develop toxicity rapidly.
• Patient should check with doctor before taking over-the-counter combinations containing aspirin.
• Therapeutic blood salicylate level in arthritis is 20 to 30 mg/100 ml.
• Alcohol may increase gastrointestinal blood loss.
• May cause an increase in serum levels of SGOT, SGPT, alkaline phosphatase, and bilirubin. May produce false-negative test results for urine glucose by glucose oxidase methods (Clinistix, Tes-Tape) and false-positive results using Clinitest.
• Hemoglobin and prothrombin tests should be obtained periodically in patients receiving large doses over an extended period of time.

Interactions:
AMMONIUM CHLORIDE (AND OTHER URINE ACIDIFIERS): increases blood levels of salicylates. Monitor for salicylate toxicity.
ANTACIDS (AND OTHER URINE ALKALINIZERS): decrease levels of salicylates. Monitor for decreased salicylate effect.
CARBONIC ANHYDRASE INHIBITORS: may elevate salicylate levels. Monitor for toxicity.
CORTICOSTEROIDS: enhance salicylate elimination. Monitor for decreased salicylate effect.
ORAL ANTICOAGULANTS: increase risk of bleeding. Avoid using together if possible.

Special considerations:
• Contraindicated in GI ulcer, GI bleeding, aspirin hypersensitivity. Use cautiously in patients with hypoprothrombinemia, vitamin K deficiency, bleeding disorders, Hodgkin's disease (may cause profound hypothermia), and in those with asthma with nasal polyps (may cause severe bronchospasm).
• May cause less GI distress than aspirin. If antacid needed, should be taken 2 hours after meals and choline salicylate taken before meals.
• May mix drug with water, fruit juice, or carbonated drinks.
• Febrile, dehydrated children can develop toxicity rapidly.
• Patient should check with doctor before taking over-the-counter combinations containing aspirin.
• Therapeutic serum salicylate level in arthritis is 20 to 30 mg/100 ml.
• Alcohol may increase GI blood loss.
• May cause an increase in serum levels of SGOT, SGPT, alkaline phosphatase, and bilirubin. May produce false-negative test results for urine glucose by glucose oxidase methods (Clinistix, Tes-Tape) and false-positive results using Clinitest.
• Hemoglobin and prothrombin tests should be obtained periodically in patients receiving large doses over an extended period of time.
• For symptoms and treatment of acute toxicity, see APPENDIX.

No significant interactions.

Special considerations:
• May be used with aspirin for arthritic pain.
• Doesn't lower fever; may be used alone when fever is valuable for diagnosis.
• Side effects other than GI distress and pruritus usually occur only when recommended dosage exceeded.

No significant interactions.

Special considerations:
• Contraindicated in hepatic and renal disease. Use cautiously in GI disorders.
• Colors urine reddish-orange. May stain fabrics.
• Use only as analgesic. Use with antibiotic to treat urinary tract infection.

Interactions:
AMMONIUM CHLORIDE (AND OTHER URINE ACIDIFIERS): increases blood levels of aspirin products. Monitor for aspirin toxicity.
ANTACIDS (AND OTHER URINE ALKALINIZERS): decrease levels of aspirin products. Monitor for decreased aspirin effect.
CARBONIC ANHYDRASE INHIBITORS: may elevate salicylate levels. Monitor for toxicity.
CORTICOSTEROIDS: enhance salicylate elimination. Monitor for decreased salicylate effect.
ORAL ANTICOAGULANTS: increase risk of bleed-

(continued on following page)

NAMES, INDICATIONS AND DOSAGES	SIDE EFFECTS
magnesium salicylate *(continued)* **Mild pain or fever:** 600 mg P.O. t.i.d. or q.i.d.	**Skin:** *rash.* **Other:** *hypersensitivity manifested by anaphylaxis.*
methotrimeprazine Levoprome, Nozinan♦♦ **Moderate-to-severe pain in nonambulatory patients:** ADULTS: 10 to 20 mg deep I.M. into large muscle mass, q 4 to 6 hours, p.r.n. Maximum dose 40 mg.	**Blood:** *agranulocytosis.* **CNS:** confusion, dizziness, *sedation,* weakness, amnesia, slurred speech. **CV:** *orthostatic hypotension.* **EENT:** nasal congestion. **GI:** dry mouth, nausea, vomiting. **GU:** difficulties in urination. **Local:** pain, inflammation at injection site. **Other:** chills.
nalbuphine hydrochloride Nubain **Moderate-to-severe pain:** S.C., I.M., or I.V. ADULTS: 10 to 20 mg q 3 to 6 hours p.r.n. Maximum daily dose 160 mg.	**CNS:** *sedation,* nervousness, depression, restlessness, crying, euphoria, hostility, unusual dreams, confusion, hallucinations, delusions. **GI:** cramps, dyspepsia, bitter taste. **GU:** urinary urgency. **Skin:** itching, burning, urticaria. **Other:** *respiratory depression,* physical and psychological dependence.
phenacetin **Mild pain or fever:** ADULTS: 300 mg P.O. q 3 to 4 hours, p.r.n. Maximum 2.4 g daily.	**Blood:** methemoglobinemia in toxic doses, hemolytic anemia in G-6-PD deficiency. **GI:** nausea, vomiting. **GU:** *papillary necrosis and chronic interstitial nephritis with long-term high doses.* **Skin:** rash.
phenazopyridine hydrochloride Azodine, Azogesic, Azo-Pyridon, Azo-Standard, Azo-Sulfizin, Baridium, Di-Azo, Diridone, Phenazo♦♦, Phen-Azo, Phenazodine, Pyridiate, Pyridium♦, Urodine **Pain with urinary tract irritation or infection:** ADULTS: 100 to 200 mg P.O. t.i.d. CHILDREN: 100 mg P.O. t.i.d.	**CNS:** headache. **GI:** nausea.

♦ Available in U.S. and Canada. ♦♦ Available in Canada only.
All other products (no symbol) available in U.S. only. Italicized side effects are common or life-threatening.

INTERACTIONS AND SPECIAL CONSIDERATIONS

ing. Avoid using together if possible.

Special considerations:

• Contraindicated in severe chronic renal insufficiency because of risk of magnesium toxicity; in GI ulcer, GI bleeding, aspirin hypersensitivity. Use cautiously in patients with hypoprothrombinemia, vitamin K deficiency, bleeding disorders, and Hodgkin's disease (may cause profound hypothermia).
• Febrile, dehydrated children can develop toxicity rapidly.
• Should be taken with food, milk, antacid, or large glass of water to reduce GI side effects.
• Patient should check with doctor before taking over-the-counter combinations containing aspirin.
• Therapeutic serum salicylate level in arthritis is 20 to 30 mg/100 ml.
• Alcohol may increase GI blood loss.
• May cause an increase in serum levels of SGOT, SGPT, alkaline phosphatase, and bilirubin. May produce false-negative test results for urine glucose by glucose oxidase methods (Clinistix, Tes-Tape) and false-positive results using Clinitest.
• Hemoglobin and prothrombin tests should be obtained periodically in patients receiving large doses over an extended period of time.
• For symptoms and treatment of acute toxicity, see APPENDIX.

Interactions:

ALL ANTIHYPERTENSIVE AGENTS AND MAO INHIBITORS: increased orthostatic hypotension. Select other analgesic.

Special considerations:

• Contraindicated in phenothiazine hypersensitivity; cardiac, renal or hepatic disease; hypotension; coma; convulsive disorders. Use with extreme caution in elderly or debilitated patients with cardiac disease or in any patients who may suffer severe consequences from a sudden drop in blood pressure.
• Used mainly in nonambulatory patients because of hypotension. Patient should be kept in bed or assisted when out of bed for at least 6 hours after initial dose. Tolerance to this effect usually develops, but patient should be watched closely after each dose.
• May be mixed with atropine or scopolamine but not with other drugs.

No significant interactions.

Special considerations:

• Contraindicated in emotional instability, drug abuse, head injury, increased intracranial pressure. Should be used cautiously in patients with hepatic and renal disease. These patients may overreact to customary doses.
• Causes respiratory depression which at 10 mg is equal to the respiratory depression produced by 10 mg of morphine.
• Psychological and physiologic dependence may occur, but it is less than that of pentazocine (Talwin).
• Respiratory depression can be reversed with naloxone.
• Also acts as a narcotic antagonist.
• Patient should avoid hazardous tasks until response to drug is determined.

No significant interactions.

Special considerations:

• Repeated use contraindicated in anemia; cardiac, pulmonary, hepatic, or renal disease.
• Contained in many analgesic combinations. Patient should check ingredients of combination over-the-counter products.

No significant interactions.

Special considerations:

• Contraindicated in renal and hepatic insufficiency.
• Colors urine red or orange. May stain fabrics.
• Should be used only as analgesic. Should be used with antibiotic to treat urinary tract infection.
• Drug may be stopped in 3 days if pain relieved.
• May alter Clinistix or Tes-Tape results. Clinitest should be used for accurate urinary glucose test results.
• Drug should be stopped if skin or sclera becomes yellow tinged. May indicate accumulation due to impaired renal excretion.

NAMES, INDICATIONS AND DOSAGES	SIDE EFFECTS
salicylamide Amid-Sal, Doldram, Salamide **Mild pain or fever:** ADULTS: 650 mg P.O. q.i.d., p.r.n. CHILDREN: 65 mg/kg/day divided into 6 doses.	**Blood:** *prolonged bleeding time.* **EENT:** *tinnitus and hearing loss (first signs of toxicity).* **GI:** *nausea, vomiting, gastrointestinal distress, occult bleeding.* **Hepatic:** abnormal liver function studies. **Skin:** *rash.* **Other:** *hypersensitivity manifested by anaphylaxis.*
salsalate Disalcid **Minor pain or fever, arthritis:** ADULTS: 1 g P.O. b.i.d., t.i.d., or q.i.d., p.r.n.	**Blood:** *prolonged bleeding time.* **EENT:** *tinnitus and hearing loss (first signs of toxicity).* **GI:** *nausea, vomiting, gastrointestinal distress, occult bleeding.* **Hepatic:** abnormal liver function studies. **Skin:** *rash.* **Other:** *hypersensitivity manifested by anaphylaxis.*
sodium salicylate Uracel **Minor pain or fever:** ADULTS: 325 to 650 mg P.O. q 4 to 6 hours, p.r.n., or 500 mg slow I.V. infusion over 4 to 8 hours. Maximum dose 1 g daily. CHILDREN: 40 to 100 mg/kg P.O. q 4 to 6 hours, p.r.n.	**Blood:** *prolonged bleeding time.* **EENT:** *tinnitus and hearing loss (first signs of toxicity).* **GI:** *nausea, vomiting, gastrointestinal distress, occult bleeding.* **Hepatic:** abnormal liver function studies. **Skin:** *rash.* **Other:** *hypersensitivity manifested by anaphylaxis.*

INTERACTIONS AND SPECIAL CONSIDERATIONS

Interactions:
AMMONIUM CHLORIDE (AND OTHER URINE ACIDIFIERS): increases blood levels of aspirin products. Monitor for aspirin toxicity.
ANTACIDS (AND OTHER URINE ALKALINIZERS): decrease levels of aspirin products. Monitor for decreased aspirin effect.
CARBONIC ANHYDRASE INHIBITORS: may elevate salicylate levels. Monitor for toxicity.
CORTICOSTEROIDS: enhance salicylate elimination. Monitor for decreased salicylate effect.
ORAL ANTICOAGULANTS: increase risk of bleeding. Avoid using together if possible.

Special considerations:
• Contraindicated in GI ulcer, GI bleeding, aspirin hypersensitivity. Use cautiously in hypoprothrombinemia, vitamin K deficiency, bleeding disorders, and Hodgkin's disease (may cause profound hypothermia).
• Should be taken with food, milk, antacid, or large glass of water to reduce GI side effects.
• Patient should check with doctor before taking over-the-counter combinations containing aspirin.
• Alcohol may increase GI blood loss.
• May increase serum alkaline phosphatase, bilirubin, SGOT, and SGPT levels. May produce false-negative test results for urine glucose using glucose oxidase methods (Clinistix, Tes-Tape) and false-positive results using Clinitest.
• Patients taking large doses for an extended period of time should maintain adequate fluid intake and watch for petechiae, bleeding gums, and signs of GI bleeding. Hemoglobin and prothrombin tests should be obtained periodically.
• For symptoms and treatment of acute toxicity, see APPENDIX.

Interactions:
AMMONIUM CHLORIDE (AND OTHER URINE ACIDIFIERS): increases blood levels of aspirin products. Monitor for aspirin toxicity.
ANTACIDS (AND OTHER URINE ALKALINIZERS): decrease levels of aspirin products. Monitor for decreased aspirin effect.
CARBONIC ANHYDRASE INHIBITORS: may elevate salicylate levels. Monitor for toxicity.
CORTICOSTEROIDS: enhance salicylate elimination. Monitor for decreased salicylate effect.
ORAL ANTICOAGULANTS: increase risk of bleeding. Avoid using together if possible.

Special considerations:
• Contraindicated in GI ulcer, GI bleeding, aspirin hypersensitivity. Use cautiously in patients with hypoprothrombinemia, vitamin K deficiency, bleeding disorders, and Hodgkin's disease (may cause profound hypothermia).
• Should be taken with food, milk, antacid, or large glass of water to reduce GI side effects.
• Patient should check with doctor before taking over-the-counter combinations containing aspirin.
• Therapeutic serum salicylate level in arthritis is 20 to 30 mg/100 ml.
• Alcohol may increase GI blood loss.
• May increase serum alkaline phosphatase, bilirubin, SGOT, and SGPT levels. May produce false-negative test results for urine glucose using glucose oxidase methods (Clinistix, Tes-Tape) and false-positive results using Clinitest.
• Patients receiving large doses for extended period of time should maintain adequate fluid intake and watch for petechiae, bleeding gums, and signs of GI bleeding. Hemoglobin and prothrombin tests should be obtained periodically.
• For symptoms and treatment of acute toxicity, see APPENDIX.

Interactions:
AMMONIUM CHLORIDE (AND OTHER URINE ACIDIFIERS): increases blood levels of aspirin products. Monitor for aspirin toxicity.
ANTACIDS (AND OTHER URINE ALKALINIZERS): decrease levels of aspirin products. Monitor for decreased aspirin effect.
CARBONIC ANHYDRASE INHIBITORS: may elevate salicylate levels. Monitor for toxicity.
CORTICOSTEROIDS: enhance salicylate elimination. Monitor for decreased salicylate effect.
ORAL ANTICOAGULANTS: increase risk of bleeding. Avoid using together if possible.

Special considerations:
• Contraindicated in GI ulcer, GI bleeding, aspirin hypersensitivity. Use cautiously in patients with hypoprothrombinemia, vitamin K deficiency, bleeding disorders, asthma with nasal polyps (may cause severe bronchospasm), and Hodgkin's disease (may cause profound hypothermia).
• Febrile, dehydrated children can develop toxicity rapidly.
• Should be taken with food, milk, antacid, or large glass of water to reduce GI side effects.
• Enteric-coated or timed-release preparations are absorbed erratically and are ineffective for long-term therapy.
• Patient should check with doctor before taking over-the-counter combinations containing aspirin.
• Therapeutic serum salicylate level in arthritis is 20 to 30 mg/100 ml.
• Tinnitus, headache, dizziness, confusion, fever, sweating, thirst, drowsiness, dim vision, hyperventilation, and increased pulse rate are signs of mild toxicity.
• Alcohol may increase GI blood loss.
• May increase serum alkaline phosphatase, bilirubin, SGOT, and SGPT levels. May produce false-negative results for urine glucose using

(continued on following page)

NAMES, INDICATIONS AND DOSAGES	SIDE EFFECTS
sodium salicylate *(continued)*	
sodium thiosalicylate Arthrolate, Nalate, Osteolate, Thiodyne, Thiolate, Thiosal, TH Sal **Mild pain:** ADULTS: 50 to 100 mg I.M. daily or every other day. **Arthritis:** ADULTS: 100 mg I.M. daily. **Rheumatic fever:** ADULTS:100 to 150 mg I.M. b.i.d. until asymptomatic. **Acute gout:** ADULTS: 100 mg I.M. q 3 to 4 hours for 2 days, then 100 mg I.M. daily until asymptomatic.	**Blood:** *prolonged bleeding time.* **EENT:** *tinnitus and hearing loss (first signs of toxicity).* **GI:** *nausea, vomiting, gastrointestinal distress, occult bleeding.* **Hepatic:** abnormal liver function studies. **Skin:** *rash.* **Other:** *hypersensitivity manifested by anaphylaxis.*
zomepirac sodium Zomax **Mild-to-moderately severe pain:** ADULTS: 100 mg P.O. q 4 to 6 hours as required p.r.n. In mild pain, 50 mg q 4 to 6 hours may be adequate. Don't exceed 600 mg/day. Not recommended for children.	**EENT:** tinnitus. **CNS:** *drowsiness, dizziness, insomnia,* paresthesia, nervousness. **CV:** *edema, hypertension,* cardiac irregularity, palpitations. **GI:** *nausea, vomiting, diarrhea, dyspepsia,* constipation, flatulence, anorexia. **GU:** urinary frequency, urinary tract infection, elevated BUN and creatinine, vaginitis. **Skin:** rash, pruritus. **Other:** chills, alterations in sense of taste.

♦ Available in U.S. and Canada. ♦♦ Available in Canada only.
All other products (no symbol) available in U.S. only. Italicized side effects are common or life-threatening.

ASPIRIN'S ROLE IN TRANSIENT ISCHEMIC ATTACKS AND REYE'S SYNDROME

Aspirin, if taken daily, can help prevent the recurrence of transient ischemic attacks (TIAs) in men. These temporary blackouts, which last from seconds to hours, are considered a warning signal of impending major cerebrovascular accident.

Studies show that a dose of two regular aspirin tablets twice a day, or one tablet four times a day, can reduce the risk of a TIA by 19% and the incidence of major stroke and death by 31%. Aspirin blocks production of a certain clot-promoting prostaglandin (called thromboxane A_2) in blood platelets, thus helping to prevent formation of stroke-producing clots in the brain. Since new platelets develop constantly, repeated doses of aspirin are necessary to halt synthesis of new prostaglandins. Too high a dose, however, inhibits the clot-*dissolving* prostaglandin prostacyclin and restores the danger of clotting.

Current test findings are definitive for men but not for women. Aspirin has reduced the number of minor strokes in women, but figures are insignificant.

INTERACTIONS AND SPECIAL CONSIDERATIONS

glucose oxidase methods (Clinistix, Tes-Tape) and false-positive results using Clinitest.
• Patients receiving large doses for extended period of time should maintain adequate fluid intake and watch for petechiae, bleeding gums, and signs of GI bleeding. Hemoglobin and prothrombin tests should be obtained periodically.
• For symptoms and treatment of acute toxicity, see APPENDIX.

Interactions:
AMMONIUM CHLORIDE (AND OTHER URINE ACIDIFIERS): increases blood levels of aspirin products. Monitor for aspirin toxicity.
ANTACIDS (AND OTHER URINE ALKALINIZERS): decrease levels of aspirin products. Monitor for decreased aspirin effect.
CARBONIC ANHYDRASE INHIBITORS: may elevate salicylate levels. Monitor for toxicity.
CORTICOSTEROIDS: enhance salicylate elimination. Monitor for decreased salicylate effect.
ORAL ANTICOAGULANTS: increase risk of bleeding. Avoid using together if possible.

Special considerations:
• Contraindicated in GI ulcer, GI bleeding, aspirin hypersensitivity. Use cautiously in patients with hypoprothrombinemia, vitamin K deficiency, bleeding disorders, asthma with nasal polyps (may cause severe bronchospasm), and Hodgkin's disease (may cause profound hypothermia).
• Tinnitus, headache, dizziness, confusion, fever, sweating, thirst, drowsiness, dim vision, hyperventilation, and increased pulse rate are signs of mild toxicity.
• Alcohol may increase GI blood loss.
• May increase serum alkaline phosphatase, bilirubin, SGOT, and SGPT levels. May produce false-negative results for urine glucose using glucose oxidase methods (Clinistix, Tes-Tape) and false-positive results using Clinitest.
• Patients receiving large doses for extended period of time should maintain adequate fluid intake and watch for petechiae, bleeding gums, and signs of GI bleeding. Hemoglobin and prothrombin tests should be obtained periodically.
• For symptoms and treatment of acute toxicity, see APPENDIX.

No significant interactions.

Special considerations:
• Contraindicated in patients in whom aspirin and nonsteroidal anti-inflammatory drugs induce bronchospasm, rhinitis, urticaria, or other hypersensitivity reactions. Should be given cautiously to patients with a history of GI bleeding, fluid retention, hypertension, and heart failure.
• A nonnarcotic analgesic with narcotic potency. In several studies has been shown to be as effective as morphine.
• No evidence of addiction with zomepirac.
• Should be taken with food or antacids if GI symptoms occur.

Testing is now underway to determine the efficacy of aspirin for healthy persons who have never had attacks.

Link to Reye's syndrome?
Studies done by several state health departments have shown an increased risk of Reye's syndrome in children given aspirin for fever accompanying influenza and varicella. The Center for Disease Control (C.D.C) in Atlanta asked a panel of experts to evaluate the study data. These experts concluded that the link between Reye's syndrome and salicylates probably couldn't be attributed solely to the limitations of the studies. Therefore, they advised that the use of salicylates be avoided during influenza and varicella in children up to age 18.

The C.D.C., however, has announced that until definitive statistical information either confirming or denying this association is available, it is advising parents and doctors of the possible increased risk of Reye's syndrome associated with such use of aspirin in children.

25

Nonsteroidal anti-inflammatory agents

fenoprofen calcium
ibuprofen
indomethacin
meclofenamate
mefenamic acid
naproxen
naproxen sodium
oxyphenbutazone
phenylbutazone
sulindac
tolmetin sodium

The nonsteroidal anti-inflammatory agents may be particularly useful when a patient cannot tolerate the gastrointestinal (GI) side effects of the salicylates. Tolmetin and the propionic acid derivatives (fenoprofen, ibuprofen, and naproxen) are new drugs that cause fewer GI side effects than the older, established alternatives to salicylates (indomethacin, oxyphenbutazone, and phenylbutazone).

Major uses
The nonsteroidal anti-inflammatory agents are used to reduce inflammation associated with osteoarthritis, rheumatoid arthritis, gout, and other conditions. Some are also used to treat symptoms of dysmenorrhea.

Mechanism of action
Although their exact mechanism of action is unknown, these drugs probably inhibit prostaglandin synthesis.

Absorption, distribution, metabolism, and excretion
Oral forms of the nonsteroidal anti-inflammatory agents are well absorbed from the GI tract. Distributed in most body tissues and fluids, these drugs are largely metabolized in the liver. The inactive metabolites are eliminated in urine and—through the bile—in feces.

Onset and duration
Onset after oral administration is within 30 to 60 minutes; after I.M. injection, within 15 to 30 minutes. Blood levels peak within 2 to 3 hours. Duration of action for most of the drugs is 4 to 6 hours. Optimal anti-inflammatory action develops only after 2 to 4 weeks of therapy.
• Naproxen and sulindac have a longer duration of action and are generally given twice daily.

Combination products
None.

DYSMENORRHEA: NEW INDICATION FOR PROSTAGLANDIN INHIBITORS

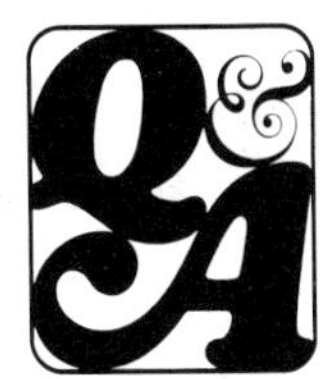

Mefenamic acid (Ponstel) and ibuprofen (Motrin) were the first prostaglandin inhibitors approved for use in dysmenorrhea, but others may be prescribed.

Studies now show that primary dysmenorrhea (of idiopathic origin) results when the endometrium overproduces prostaglandin hormones. The cause is still unknown, but the effect is strong uterine contractions and cramping pain. Increased prostaglandin production also stimulates synthesis of vasodilators bradykinin and histamine, which may cause menstrual headaches and nausea. Thus, drugs that inhibit prostaglandins are a logical choice to relieve dysmenorrhea.

Will any prostaglandin inhibitor work?

Theoretically, all should relieve dysmenorrhea, but some, like indomethacin (Indocin), may cause severe side effects. Mefenamic acid and ibuprofen will probably be prescribed most often. Four daily doses of 250 mg of mefenamic acid significantly decrease the frequency and severity of symptoms and reduce the patient's need for an additional analgesic. Ibuprofen's usual dosage is 400 mg four times a day. Reduced doses of either drug may also be effective.

What side effects might patients taking mefenamic acid or ibuprofen report?

Both drugs are relatively free of side effects when dosage is below recommended levels. However, at recommended dosage, some patients may report dizziness and gastrointestinal (GI) upsets, such as nausea, heartburn, and diarrhea. If taking the drugs with food or milk doesn't relieve these symptoms, the dose may be reduced. Agranulocytosis, a blood dyscrasia, rarely occurs with mefenamic acid, but periodic complete blood counts can help detect it. The patient should report all symptoms.

The patient's history should be checked for incidence of peptic ulcer or asthma. A patient with either of these conditions shouldn't take prostaglandin inhibitors since they produce GI side effects, and some patients with asthma develop allergies to them.

What other prostaglandin inhibitors might be prescribed to treat dysmenorrhea?

Possible alternatives are naproxen (Naprosyn), fenoprofen (Nalfon), sulindac (Clinoril), and tolmetin (Tolectin). Aspirin and acetaminophen inhibit prostaglandins but not enough to relieve symptoms. Oral contraceptives relieve dysmenorrhea by suppressing ovulation and thus lowering prostaglandin levels, but these drugs have many side effects.

Is there any special advice that should be given to the patient taking a prostaglandin inhibitor?

She should start the medication *after* her menstrual flow begins, unless ordered otherwise. Although starting the drug a few days before her period begins may help prevent dysmenorrhea, the patient could be pregnant—and pregnant women shouldn't take a prostaglandin inhibitor.

NAMES, INDICATIONS AND DOSAGES	SIDE EFFECTS
fenoprofen calcium Nalfon♦ **Rheumatoid arthritis and osteoarthritis:** ADULTS: 300 to 600 mg P.O. q.i.d. Maximum 3.2 g daily.	**Blood:** prolonged bleeding time, anemia. **CNS:** headache, drowsiness, dizziness. **GI:** *epigastric distress,* nausea, *occult blood loss.* **GU:** reversible renal failure. **Skin:** pruritus, rash, urticaria.
ibuprofen Motrin♦ Rufen **Arthritis, primary dysmenorrhea, postextraction dental pain:** ADULTS: 300 to 600 mg P.O. q.i.d.	**Blood:** prolonged bleeding time. **CNS:** headache, drowsiness, dizziness. **EENT:** visual disturbances, tinnitus. **GI:** *epigastric distress,* nausea, *occult blood loss.* **GU:** reversible renal failure. **Skin:** pruritus, rash, urticaria. **Other:** aseptic meningitis, bronchospasm, edema.
indomethacin Indocid♦♦, Indocin **Moderate-to-severe arthritis:** ADULTS: 25 mg P.O. b.i.d. or t.i.d. with food or antacids; may increase dose by 25 mg daily q 7 days up to 200 mg daily. *Acute gouty arthritis*—50 mg t.i.d. Reduce dose as soon as possible, then stop.	**Blood:** *hemolytic anemia, aplastic anemia, agranulocytosis,* leukopenia, *thrombocytopenic purpura,* iron deficiency anemia. **CNS:** *headache, dizziness,* depression, drowsiness, confusion, peripheral neuropathy, convulsions, psychic disturbances, syncope, *vertigo.* **CV:** hypertension, edema. **EENT:** blurred vision, corneal and retinal damage, hearing loss, tinnitus. **GI:** *nausea, vomiting,* anorexia, *diarrhea, severe GI bleeding.* **GU:** hematuria, hyperkalemia, acute renal failure. **Skin:** pruritus, urticaria. **Other:** hypersensitivity (shocklike symptoms, rash, respiratory distress, angioedema).
meclofenamate Meclomen **Rheumatoid arthritis and osteoarthritis:** ADULTS: 200 to 400 mg/day P.O. in 3 or 4 equally divided doses.	**Blood:** leukopenia, thrombocytopenia, *agranulocytosis, aplastic anemia.* **CNS:** drowsiness, dizziness, nervousness, headache. **EENT:** blurred vision, eye irritation. **GI:** nausea, vomiting, *diarrhea,* hemorrhage. **GU:** dysuria, hematuria, nephrotoxicity. **Hepatic:** hepatotoxicity. **Skin:** rash, urticaria.
mefenamic acid Ponstan♦♦, Ponstel **Mild-to-moderate pain, dysmenorrhea:** ADULTS AND CHILDREN OVER 14 YEARS: 500 mg P.O. initially, then 250 mg q 4 hours, p.r.n. Maximum therapy 1 week.	**Blood:** leukopenia, thrombocytopenia, *agranulocytosis, aplastic anemia.* **CNS:** drowsiness, dizziness, nervousness, headache. **EENT:** blurred vision, eye irritation. **GI:** nausea, vomiting, *diarrhea,* hemorrhage. **GU:** dysuria, hematuria, nephrotoxicity. **Hepatic:** hepatotoxicity. **Skin:** rash, urticaria.

INTERACTIONS AND SPECIAL CONSIDERATIONS

No significant interactions.

Special considerations:
• Contraindicated in patients with renal disease and in those with asthma with nasal polyps. Use cautiously in patients with GI disorders, cardiac disease, or allergy to other noncorticosteroid anti-inflammatory drugs.
• Therapeutic effect may be delayed for 2 to 4 weeks.
• Renal, hepatic, and auditory function should be checked periodically in long-term therapy and drug stopped if abnormalities occur.
• Dose should be taken either 30 minutes before or 2 hours after meals. If GI side effects occur, should be taken with milk or meals.
• Prothrombin time may be prolonged in patients receiving coumarin-type anticoagulants. Fenoprofen decreases platelet aggregation and may prolong bleeding time.

No significant interactions.

Special considerations:
• Contraindicated in patients with asthma with nasal polyps. Use cautiously in GI disorders, allergy to other noncorticosteroid anti-inflammatory drugs, hepatic or renal disease, cardiac decompensation, or known intrinsic coagulation defects.
• Therapeutic effect may be delayed for 2 to 4 weeks.
• Renal and hepatic function should be checked periodically in long-term therapy and drug stopped if abnormalities occur.
• Patient should report immediately any GI symptoms or signs of bleeding, visual disturbances, skin rashes, weight gain, or edema.
• Should be taken with meals or milk to reduce GI side effects.

Interactions:
PROBENECID: decreases indomethacin excretion; watch for increased incidence of indomethacin side effects.
FUROSEMIDE: impaired response to both drugs. Avoid if possible.

Special considerations:
• Contraindicated in aspirin allergy and GI disorders. Use cautiously in patients with epilepsy, parkinsonism, hepatic or renal disease, infection, history of mental illness, and in elderly patients.
• Severe headache may occur within 1 hour. Drug should be stopped if headache persists.
• Patient should report immediately any visual or hearing changes. Patients taking drug long-term should have regular eye examinations and hearing tests.
• Very irritating to GI tract. Should be taken with meals.
• CNS side effects are more common and serious in elderly patients.
• Patients receiving anticoagulants should be monitored for bleeding.
• Causes sodium retention; patients with hypertension should be monitored for increased blood pressure.
• Used investigationally as prophylaxis for gout when colchicine is not well tolerated.
• Patients taking drug long-term should receive periodic testing of CBC and renal function.

No significant interactions.

Special considerations:
• Contraindicated in GI ulceration or inflammation. Use cautiously in patients with hepatic or renal disease, blood dyscrasias, and diabetes mellitus, and in those with asthma with nasal polyps.
• Patient should avoid activities that require alertness until CNS response is determined.
• Drug should be discontinued if rash or diarrhea develops.
• Should not be administered for more than 1 week at a time.
• Should be taken with food to minimize GI side effects.
• Almost identical in chemical structure to mefenamic acid.
• Available as 50- and 100-mg capsules.
• False-positive reactions for urine bilirubin using the diazo tablet test have been reported.
• Patients taking drug long-term should receive periodic testing of CBC, and renal and hepatic function.

No significant interactions.

Special considerations:
• Contraindicated in GI ulceration or inflammation. Use cautiously with hepatic or renal disease, blood dyscrasias, and diabetes mellitus, and in those with asthma with nasal polyps.
• Patient should avoid activities requiring alertness until response to drug is determined.
• Severe hemolytic anemia may occur with prolonged use. Should not be administered for more than 1 week at a time. Drug should be stopped if rash or diarrhea develops.
• Should be administered with food to minimize GI side effects.
• Can be used to treat menstrual pain.
• False-positive reactions for urine bilirubin using the diazo tablet test have been reported.

NAMES, INDICATIONS AND DOSAGES	SIDE EFFECTS
naproxen Naprosyn♦ **naproxen sodium** Anaprox **Arthritis:** ADULTS: 250 to 500 mg P.O. b.i.d. Maximum 1,000 mg daily. **Mild-to-moderate pain and for treatment of primary dysmenorrhea (naproxen sodium only):** ADULTS: 2 tablets (275 mg each tablet) to start, followed by 275 mg q 6 to 8 hours as needed. Maximum daily dose should not exceed 1,375 mg.	**Blood:** prolonged bleeding time. **CNS:** headache, drowsiness, dizziness. **GI:** *epigastric distress, occult blood loss,* nausea. **GU:** reversible renal failure. **Skin:** pruritus, rash, urticaria.
oxyphenbutazone Oxalid, Tandearil **Pain, inflammation in arthritis, bursitis, superficial venous thrombosis:** ADULTS: 100 to 200 mg P.O. with food or milk t.i.d. or q.i.d. **Acute gouty arthritis:** ADULTS: 400 mg initially as single dose, then 100 mg q 4 hours for 4 days or until relief is obtained.	**Blood:** *bone marrow depression (fatal aplastic anemia, agranulocytosis, thrombocytopenia),* hemolytic anemia, leukopenia. **CNS:** restlessness, confusion, lethargy. **CV:** hypertension, *pericarditis, myocarditis, cardiac decompensation.* **EENT:** optic neuritis, blurred vision, retinal hemorrhage or detachment, hearing loss. **GI:** *nausea, vomiting, diarrhea,* ulceration, occult blood loss. **GU:** proteinuria, hematuria, glomerulonephritis, nephrotic syndrome, *renal failure.* **Hepatic:** *hepatitis.* **Metabolic:** toxic and nontoxic goiter, respiratory alkalosis, and metabolic acidosis. **Skin:** petechiae, pruritus, purpura, various dermatoses from rash to *toxic necrotizing epidermolysis.*
phenylbutazone Algoverine♦♦, Anevral♦♦, Azolid, Butagesic♦♦, Butazolidin♦, Intrabutazone♦♦, Malgesic♦♦, Nadozone♦♦, Neo-Zoline♦♦, Phen-butazone♦♦, Phenylbetazone♦♦ **Pain, inflammation in arthritis, bursitis, acute superficial thrombophlebitis:** ADULTS: initially, 100 to 200 mg P.O. t.i.d. or q.i.d. Maximum dose 600 mg/day. When improvement is obtained, decrease dose to 100 mg t.i.d. or q.i.d. **Acute, gouty arthritis:** ADULTS: 400 mg initially as single dose, then 100 mg q 4 hours for 4 days or until relief is obtained.	**Blood:** *bone marrow depression (fatal aplastic anemia, agranulocytosis,* thrombocytopenia), hemolytic anemia, leukopenia. **CNS:** agitation, confusion, lethargy. **CV:** hypertension, edema, *pericarditis, myocarditis, cardiac decompensation.* **EENT:** optic neuritis, blurred vision, retinal hemorrhage or detachment, hearing loss. **GI:** *nausea, vomiting, diarrhea,* ulceration, occult blood loss. **GU:** proteinuria, hematuria, glomerulonephritis, nephrotic syndrome, *renal failure.* **Hepatic:** *hepatitis.* **Metabolic:** hyperglycemia, toxic and nontoxic goiter, respiratory alkalosis, and metabolic acidosis. **Skin:** petechiae, pruritus, purpura, various dermatoses from rash to *toxic necrotizing epidermolysis.*
sulindac Clinoril **Osteoarthritis, rheumatoid arthritis, ankylosing spondylitis:** ADULTS: 150 mg P.O. b.i.d. initially; may	**Blood:** prolonged bleeding time, *aplastic anemia.* **CNS:** dizziness, headache, nervousness. **EENT:** tinnitus, transient visual disturbances. **GI:** *epigastric distress, occult blood loss,* nausea.

♦ Available in U.S. and Canada. ♦♦ Available in Canada only.
All other products (no symbol) available in U.S. only. Italicized side effects are common or life-threatening.

INTERACTIONS AND SPECIAL CONSIDERATIONS

No significant interactions.

Special considerations:
- Use cautiously in patients with renal disease, GI disorders, in those allergic to noncorticosteroid anti-inflammatory agents, and in those with asthma with nasal polyps.
- Therapeutic effect may be delayed 2 to 4 weeks in patient taking the naproxen "free base" (not the sodium salt).
- Full therapeutic benefit of naproxen sodium should be seen during the first day of treatment, and usually within the first several hours.
- Patient should not take both forms of naproxen at the same time because both circulate in the blood as the naproxen anion.
- Renal and hepatic function should be checked periodically in long-term therapy and drug stopped if abnormalities occur.
- Dose can be given once daily very effectively. May increase patient compliance.
- False-positive reactions for urine bilirubin using the diazo tablet test have been reported.

Interactions:
METHANDROSTENOLONE: may increase oxyphenbutazone levels. Give together cautiously.

Special considerations:
- Contraindicated in senile patients; GI ulcer; blood dyscrasias; renal, hepatic, cardiac, and thyroid disease; polymyalgia rheumatica and temporal arteritis. Should not be used in patients receiving long-term anticoagulant therapy.
- Patient should stop drug and report immediately if fever, sore throat, mouth ulcers, GI discomfort, black or tarry stools, bleeding, bruising, rash, or weight gain occurs.
- Should be taken with food, milk, or antacid.
- Complete physical examination and laboratory evaluation are recommended before therapy. Patient needs close medical supervision and regular follow-up.
- CBC should be monitored every 2 weeks or weekly in elderly patients. Any abnormality should be reported immediately.
- Patient's weight and intake and output should be recorded daily. May cause sodium retention and edema.
- Response should be seen in 2 or 3 days. Drug should be stopped if no response within 1 week.
- Patients over 60 years should not receive drug for longer than 1 week.

Interactions:
BARBITURATES, ANTIDEPRESSANTS: may impair phenylbutazone effect. Use together cautiously.
CHOLESTYRAMINE: may alter phenylbutazone absorption. Give 1 hour before cholestyramine.

Special considerations:
- Contraindicated in children under 14 years and in patients with senility; GI ulcer; blood dyscrasias; renal, hepatic, cardiac, and thyroid disease; polymyalgia rheumatica; temporal arteritis; and hypertension.
- Patient should stop drug and report immediately if fever, sore throat, mouth ulcers, GI discomfort, black or tarry stools, bleeding, bruising, rash, or weight gain occurs.
- Should be taken with food, milk, or antacids.
- Complete physical examination and laboratory evaluation are recommended before therapy. Patient should remain under close medical supervision and keep all doctor and laboratory appointments.
- CBC should be monitored every 2 weeks or weekly in elderly patients. Any abnormalities should be reported immediately.
- Patient's weight and intake and output should be monitored daily. May cause sodium retention and edema.
- Response should be seen in 3 to 4 days. Drug should be stopped if no response within 1 week.
- Patients over 60 years should not receive drug for longer than 1 week.

No significant interactions.

Special considerations:
- Contraindicated in patients with acute asthma whose condition is precipitated by aspirin or other nonsteroidal anti-inflammatory agents; in patients who have active ulcers and GI bleeding. Use cautiously in patients with a history of ulcers and GI bleeding, renal dysfunction, compromised cardiac function, hypertension; or in those receiving oral anticoagulants or oral hypoglycemic agents.

(continued on following page)

NAMES, INDICATIONS AND DOSAGES	SIDE EFFECTS
sulindac *(continued)* increase to 200 mg P.O. b.i.d. **Acute subacromial bursitis or supraspinatus tendinitis, acute gouty arthritis:** ADULTS: 200 mg P.O. b.i.d. for 7 to 14 days. Dose may be reduced as symptoms subside.	**Skin:** rash, pruritus. **Other:** edema.
tolmetin sodium Tolectin♦, Tolectin DS **Rheumatoid arthritis and osteoarthritis, juvenile rheumatoid arthritis:** ADULTS: 400 mg P.O. t.i.d. or q.i.d. Maximum 2 g daily. CHILDREN 2 YEARS OR OLDER: 15 to 30 mg/kg/day in divided doses.	**Blood:** prolonged bleeding time. **CNS:** headache, dizziness, drowsiness. **GI:** *epigastric distress, occult blood loss,* nausea. **GU:** reversible renal failure. **Skin:** rash, urticaria, pruritus. **Other:** sodium retention, edema.

♦ Available in U.S. and Canada. ♦♦ Available in Canada only.
All other products (no symbol) available in U.S. only. Italicized side effects are common or life-threatening.

HOW PROSTAGLANDIN INHIBITORS WORK

Nonsteroidal anti-inflammatory agents are prostaglandin inhibitors that relieve pain and inflammation by blocking an early step in the inflammatory reaction.

Prostaglandins form when cell injury or maybe even distortion of cell membranes triggers a chain reaction: First, enzymes produced by phagocytes at the injury site split the phospholipids present within all cell membranes, freeing arachidonic acid. This normally dormant fatty acid is then activated by the enzyme cyclo-oxygenase (prostaglandin synthetase) to create the G and H series prostaglandins called endoperoxides. These highly unstable intermediate prostaglandins convert to thromboxanes and prostacyclin, which respectively promote and prevent platelet aggregation, and to series E, F, and D prostaglandins. These final prostaglandins, particularly the E series, cause inflammation and pain.

Prostaglandin inhibitors check the action of the cyclo-oxygenase enzyme complex and prevent conversion of arachidonic acid to the endoperoxides or intermediate prostaglandins. Prostaglandin inhibitors mediate but do not arrest the inflammatory response or its consequences. For example, in the patient with rheumatoid arthritis, these drugs may reduce pain, redness, and swelling, but joint destruction continues.

INTERACTIONS AND SPECIAL CONSIDERATIONS	
• To reduce GI side effects, should be taken with food, milk, or antacids. • Patient should report any visual disturbances and have complete physical examination. • Patient should report immediately if prolonged bleeding occurs. • If liver function studies are abnormal, drug should be stopped.	
No significant interactions. *Special considerations:* • Contraindicated in patients with asthma with nasal polyps. Use cautiously in cardiac and renal disease, and GI bleeding disorders. • Should be taken with food, milk, or antacids to reduce GI side effects. • Therapeutic effect should begin within 1 week.	• Double-strength capsule (400 mg) is available. • Extended therapy should be accompanied by periodic eye examinations and kidney function studies.

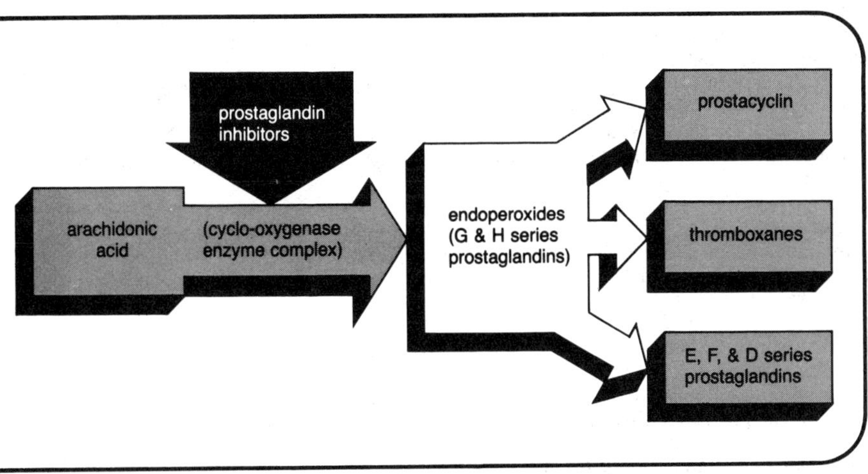

26

Narcotic analgesics

Brompton's cocktail
codeine phosphate
codeine sulfate
fentanyl citrate
hydromorphone hydrochloride
levorphanol tartrate
meperidine hydrochloride
methadone hydrochloride
morphine sulfate
oxycodone hydrochloride
oxymorphone hydrochloride
pentazocine hydrochloride
pentazocine lactate
propoxyphene hydrochloride
propoxyphene napsylate

Narcotic analgesics are defined by the Comprehensive Drug Abuse Prevention and Control Act of 1970 as controlled substances. They can change a patient's perception of pain so that it's qualitatively less disturbing, and use of these drugs may result in physical and psychological dependence. They should be reserved for treatment of severe pain unrelieved by nonnarcotic analgesics.

The concern about addiction is generally unwarranted when narcotic analgesics are used in terminally ill patients. For patients with intractable (particularly cancer-related) pain, these drugs should be administered around the clock—not p.r.n. When used in this manner, these drugs continually relieve pain and ease the patient's anxiety and anticipation of pain.

Major uses

Narcotic analgesics relieve moderate-to-severe pain and furnish preoperative sedation, alone or in combination with tranquilizers (such as chlorpromazine, diazepam, and hydroxyzine).

Mechanism of action

Narcotic analgesics bind with opiate receptors at many sites in the central nervous system (brain, brain stem, and spinal cord), altering both perception of and emotional response to pain. The precise mechanism of action, however, is unknown.

Absorption, distribution, metabolism, and excretion

Absorption of most narcotic analgesics is more effective after parenteral than after oral administration. However, Brompton's cocktail, oxycodone, and propoxyphene—available only in oral form—are well absorbed from the gastrointestinal tract.

All narcotic analgesics are well distributed in body tissues, metabolized in the liver, and excreted in the urine.

Onset and duration

The chart opposite lists the onset, peak, and duration time ranges for narcotic analgesics.

Combination products

EMPIRIN WITH CODEINE NO. 2: aspirin 325 mg and codeine phosphate 15 mg.
EMPIRIN WITH CODEINE NO. 3: aspirin 325 mg and codeine phosphate 30 mg.
EMPIRIN WITH CODEINE NO. 4: aspirin 325 mg and codeine phosphate 60 mg.
FIORINAL WITH CODEINE NO. 1: butalbital 50 mg, caffeine 40 mg, aspirin 200 mg, phenacetin 130 mg, and codeine phosphate 7.5 mg.
FIORINAL WITH CODEINE NO. 2♦: butalbital 50 mg, caffeine 40 mg, aspirin 200 mg,

THERAPEUTIC ACTIVITY OF NARCOTIC ANALGESICS

DRUG	ONSET	PEAK	DURATION
Brompton's cocktail*	10 to 15 min	2 to 3 hr	3 to 8 hr
codeine	15 to 30 min	60 to 90 min	4 to 6 hr
fentanyl	5 to 15 min	within 30 min	1 to 2 hr
hydromorphone	15 to 30 min	30 to 90 min	4 to 5 hr
levorphanol	within 1 hr	60 to 90 min	4 to 5 hr
meperidine	10 to 15 min	30 to 60 min	2 to 4 hr
methadone	10 to 15 min	1 to 2 hr	4 to 6 hr†
morphine	within 20 min	30 to 90 min	4 to 7 hr
oxycodone*	10 to 15 min	60 to 90 min	4 to 5 hr
oxymorphone	5 to 10 min	30 to 90 min	4 to 5 hr
pentazocine	10 to 15 min	30 to 60 min	2 to 3 hr
propoxyphene*	15 to 60 min	2 to 3 hr	4 to 6 hr

*Oral administration. (Other values in chart are for I.M. or S.Q. administration.)
†Increases with repeated use due to cumulative effects.

phenacetin 130 mg, and codeine phosphate 15 mg.
FIORINAL WITH CODEINE NO. 3♦: butalbital 50 mg, caffeine 40 mg, aspirin 200 mg, phenacetin 130 mg, and codeine 30 mg.
TYLENOL WITH CODEINE NO 1: acetaminophen 300 mg and codeine phosphate 7.5 mg.
TYLENOL WITH CODEINE NO. 2: acetaminophen 300 mg and codeine phosphate 15 mg.
TYLENOL WITH CODEINE NO. 3: acetaminophen 300 mg and codeine phosphate 30 mg.
TYLENOL WITH CODEINE NO. 4: acetaminophen 300 mg and codeine phosphate 60 mg.

NAMES, INDICATIONS AND DOSAGES	SIDE EFFECTS
Brompton's cocktail (Mixture containing varying amounts of the following ingredients: morphine or methadone, cocaine or amphetamine, syrup or honey, alcohol [90% to 98%] or gin, chloroform water) Controlled Substance Schedule II **Severe chronic pain of terminal cancer:** ADULTS: 10 to 20 ml of (standard pharmacy-prepared mixture) q 3 to 4 hours (if morphine is used) or q 6 to 8 hours (if methadone is used). Must be given around the clock. Dosage titrations can be made at 48- to 72-hour intervals. Maximum dose totally dependent on patient response.	**CNS:** *sedation, clouded sensorium, euphoria,* convulsions with large doses. **CV:** *hypotension,* bradycardia. **GI:** *nausea, vomiting, constipation,* ileus. **GU:** *urinary retention.* **Other:** *respiratory depression,* physical dependence.
codeine phosphate **codeine sulfate** Controlled Substance Schedule II **Mild-to-moderate pain:** ADULTS: 15 to 60 mg P.O. or 15 to 60 mg (phosphate) S.C. or I.M. q 4 hours, p.r.n. CHILDREN: 3 mg/kg daily P.O. divided q 4 hours, p.r.n.	**CNS:** *sedation, clouded sensorium, euphoria,* convulsions with large doses. **CV:** *hypotension,* bradycardia. **GI:** *nausea, vomiting, constipation,* ileus. **GU:** *urinary retention.* **Other:** *respiratory depression,* physical dependence.
fentanyl citrate Controlled Substance Schedule II Sublimaze♦ **Adjunct to general anesthetic:** ADULTS: 0.05 to 0.1 mg I.V. repeated q 2 to 3 minutes, p.r.n. Dose should be reduced in elderly and poor-risk patients. **Postoperatively:** ADULTS: 0.05 to 0.1 mg I.M. q 1 to 2 hours, p.r.n. CHILDREN 2 TO 12 YEARS: 0.02 to 0.03 mg/9 kg. **Preoperatively:** ADULTS: 0.05 to 0.1 mg I.M. 30 to 60 minutes before surgery.	**CNS:** *sedation, clouded sensorium, euphoria,* convulsions with large doses. **CV:** *hypotension,* bradycardia. **GI:** *nausea, vomiting, constipation,* ileus. **GU:** *urinary retention.* **Other:** *respiratory depression,* physical dependence.
hydromorphone hydrochloride Controlled Substance Schedule II Dilaudid♦ **Moderate-to-severe pain:** ADULTS: 2 to 4 mg P.O. q 4 to 6 hours, p.r.n.; or 2 to 4 mg I.M., S.C., or I.V. q 4 to 6 hours, p.r.n. (I.V. dose should be given over 3 to 5 minutes); or 3 mg rectal suppository at bedtime, p.r.n.	**CNS:** *sedation, clouded sensorium, euphoria,* convulsions with large doses. **CV:** *hypotension,* bradycardia. **GI:** *nausea, vomiting, constipation,* ileus. **GU:** *urinary retention.* **Local:** induration with repeated S.C. injection. **Other:** *respiratory depression,* physical dependence.

INTERACTIONS AND SPECIAL CONSIDERATIONS

No significant interactions.

Special considerations:
- Should be used with extreme caution in patients with head injury, increased intracranial pressure, shock, increased cerebrospinal fluid pressure, CNS depression, asthma, COPD, respiratory depression, seizures, hepatic or renal disease, hypothyroidism, Addison's disease, alcoholism, and in elderly or debilitated patients.
- Originated in Brompton Hospital in England to keep cancer patients in constant pain-free and euphoric state.
- Not commercially prepared—must be prepared by pharmacy.
- Has frequently proven to be effective when narcotic analgesics alone have failed to provide pain relief.
- Around-the-clock administration reduces patient's anticipation of pain and is major reason for effectiveness.
- If cocaine is ingredient in mixture—patient should swish mixture in mouth to aid absorption as cocaine is absorbed only through oral mucosa.
- Phenothiazines are occasionally added to increase analgesic effect and prevent nausea.
- Most formulations are stable for up to 4 weeks at room temperature; storage in refrigerator may increase stability to 8 weeks.

No significant interactions.

Special considerations:
- Use with extreme caution in patients with head injury, increased intracranial pressure, increased cerebrospinal fluid pressure, hepatic or renal disease, hypothyroidism, Addison's disease, acute alcoholism, seizures, severe CNS depression, bronchial asthma, COPD, respiratory depression, shock, and in elderly or debilitated patients.
- Ambulatory patient should avoid activities that require alertness.
- Respiratory and circulatory status and bowel function should be monitored.
- For full analgesic effect, should be given before patient has intense pain.
- Codeine and aspirin have additive effect and should be given together for maximum pain relief.
- Discolored injection solution should not be administered.
- If used with general anesthetics, other narcotic analgesics, tranquilizers, sedatives, hypnotics, alcohol, tricyclic antidepressants, or MAO inhibitors, CNS depression is increased. Should be used together with extreme caution and patient's response monitored.
- For symptoms and treatment of toxicity, see APPENDIX.

No significant interactions.

Special considerations:
- Contraindicated in patients who have received MAO inhibitors within 14 days and in those with myasthenia gravis. Use cautiously in patients with head injury, increased cerebrospinal fluid pressure, asthma, COPD, respiratory depression, seizures, hepatic or renal disease, hypothyroidism, Addison's disease, alcoholism, increased intracranial pressure, CNS depression, shock, and in elderly or debilitated patients.
- Narcotic antagonist (naloxone) and resuscitative equipment should be available when drug is given I.V.
- Respirations of newborn exposed to drug during labor need monitoring.
- As postoperative analgesic, should be used only in recovery room and another analgesic ordered for later use.
- Often used with droperidol (as Innovar) to produce neuroleptanalgesia.
- Circulatory and respiratory status should be monitored carefully.
- If used with other narcotic analgesics, general anesthetics, tranquilizers, alcohol, sedatives, hypnotics, tricyclic antidepressants, or MAO inhibitors, respiratory depression, hypotension, profound sedation, and coma may result. Fentanyl citrate dose should be reduced by ¼ to ⅓ and above drugs given in reduced dosages.
- For better analgesic effect, should be given before patient has intense pain.
- When used postoperatively, turning, coughing, and deep breathing should be encouraged to avoid atelectasis.
- For symptoms and treatment of toxicity, see APPENDIX.

No significant interactions.

Special considerations:
- Contraindicated in increased intracranial pressure and status asthmaticus. Use with extreme caution in patients with increased cerebrospinal fluid pressure, respiratory depression, hepatic or renal disease, hypothyroidism, shock, Addison's disease, acute alcoholism, seizures, head injury, severe CNS depression, brain tumor, bronchial asthma, COPD, and in elderly or debilitated patients.
- Ambulatory patient should avoid activities that require alertness.
- Respiratory and circulatory status and bowel function should be monitored.
- Narcotic antagonist (naloxone) should be kept available.
- Respiratory depression and hypotension can occur with I.V. administration. Should be given

(continued on following page)

NAMES, INDICATIONS AND DOSAGES	SIDE EFFECTS
hydromorphone hydrochloride *(continued)*	
levorphanol tartrate Controlled Substance Schedule II Levo-Dromoran♦ **Moderate-to-severe pain:** ADULTS: 2 to 3 mg P.O. or S.C. q 6 to 8 hours, p.r.n.	**CNS:** *sedation, clouded sensorium, euphoria,* convulsions with large doses. **CV:** *hypotension,* bradycardia. **GI:** *nausea, vomiting, constipation,* ileus. **GU:** *urinary retention.* **Other:** *respiratory depression,* physical dependence.
meperidine hydrochloride Controlled Substance Schedule II Demer-Idine♦♦, Demerol♦, Pethidine HCl B.P.♦♦ **Moderate-to-severe pain:** ADULTS: 50 to 150 mg P.O., I.M., or S.C. q 3 to 4 hours, p.r.n. CHILDREN: 1 mg/kg P.O., I.M., or S.C. q 4 to 6 hours. Maximum—100 mg q 4 hours, p.r.n. **Preoperatively:** ADULTS: 50 to 100 mg I.M. or S.C. 30 to 90 minutes before surgery. CHILDREN: 1 to 2.2 mg/kg I.M. or S.C. 30 to 90 minutes before surgery.	**CNS:** *sedation, clouded sensorium, euphoria,* convulsions with large doses. **CV:** *hypotension,* bradycardia. **GI:** *nausea, vomiting, constipation,* ileus. **GU:** *urinary retention.* **Local:** pain at injection site, local tissue irritation and induration after S.C. injection; phlebitis after I.V. injection. **Other:** *respiratory depression,* physical dependence.

INTERACTIONS AND SPECIAL CONSIDERATIONS

very slowly and monitored constantly.
• Injection sites should be rotated to avoid induration with subcutaneous injection.
• Commonly abused narcotic.
• If used with general anesthetics, other narcotic analgesics, tranquilizers, sedatives, hypnotics, alcohol, tricyclic antidepressants, or MAO inhibitors, CNS depression is increased. Hydromorphone dose should be reduced. Should be used together with caution and patient's response monitored.
• Oral dosage form is particularly convenient for patients with chronic pain because tablets are available in 1 mg, 2 mg, 3 mg, and 4 mg, which enables patients to titrate their own dose.
• For full analgesic effect, should be given before patient has intense pain.
• When used postoperatively, turning, coughing, and deep breathing should be encouraged to avoid atelectasis.
• For symptoms and treatment of toxicity, see APPENDIX.

No significant interactions.

Special considerations:
• Contraindicated in patients with acute alcoholism, bronchial asthma, increased intracranial pressure, respiratory and CNS depression, and anoxia. Use with extreme caution in patients with hepatic or renal disease, hypothyroidism, Addison's disease, seizures, head injury, severe CNS depression, brain tumor, COPD, shock, and in elderly or debilitated patients.
• Ambulatory patient should avoid activities that require alertness.
• Circulatory and respiratory status and bowel function should be monitored.
• Drug has bitter taste.
• Protect from light.
• Narcotic antagonist (naloxone) should be kept available.
• If used with general anesthetics, other narcotic analgesics, tranquilizers, sedatives, hypnotics, alcohol, tricyclic antidepressants, or MAO inhibitors, CNS depression is increased. Levorphanol dose should be reduced. Should be used together with extreme caution and patient's response monitored.
• For full analgesic effect, should be given before patient has intense pain.
• When used postoperatively, turning, coughing, and deep breathing should be encouraged to avoid atelectasis.
• For symptoms and treatment of toxicity, see APPENDIX.

Interactions:
MAO INHIBITORS, ISONIAZID: increase CNS excitation or depression, which can be severe or fatal. Don't use together.

Special considerations:
• Contraindicated if patient has used MAO inhibitors within 14 days. Use with extreme caution in patients with increased intracranial pressure, increased cerebrospinal fluid pressure, shock, CNS depression, head injury, asthma, COPD, respiratory depression, supraventricular tachycardias, seizures, acute abdominal conditions, hepatic or renal disease, hypothyroidism, Addison's disease, urethral stricture, prostatic hypertrophy, alcoholism, in children under age 12, and in elderly or debilitated patients.
• Meperidine and active metabolite normeperidine accumulate in renal failure. Patients with poor renal function should be monitored for increased toxic effect.
• Meperidine may be given slow I.V., preferably as a diluted solution. Subcutaneous injection very painful.
• Narcotic antagonist (naloxone) should be available when drug given I.V.
• Ambulatory patient should avoid activities that require alertness.
• Respirations of newborn exposed to drug during labor should be monitored and resuscitation equipment kept available.
• Oral dose less than half as effective as parenteral dose. Given I.M. if possible. When changing from parenteral to oral route, dose should be increased.
• Syrup has local anesthetic effect. Should be taken with full glass of water.
• Chemically incompatible with barbiturates. Should not be mixed.
• Respiratory and cardiovascular status should be monitored carefully. Should not be given if respirations below 12/minute or if change in pupils.
• Withdrawal symptoms possible if stopped abruptly after long-term use.
• If used with other narcotic analgesics, general anesthetics, phenothiazines, sedatives, hypnotics, tricyclic antidepressants, or alcohol, respiratory depression, hypotension, profound sedation, or coma may occur. Meperidine dose should be reduced. Should be used together with caution.
• For full analgesic effect, should be given before patient has intense pain.
• When used postoperatively, turning, coughing, and deep breathing should be encouraged to avoid atelectasis.
• For symptoms and treatment of toxicity, see APPENDIX.

NAMES, INDICATIONS AND DOSAGES	SIDE EFFECTS
methadone hydrochloride Controlled Substance Schedule II Dolophine, Methadone HCl Oral Solution **Severe pain:** ADULTS: 2.5 to 10 mg P.O., I.M., or S.C. q 3 to 4 hours, p.r.n. **Narcotic abstinence syndrome:** ADULTS: 15 to 40 mg P.O. daily (highly individualized). *Maintenance:* 20 to 120 mg P.O. daily. Adjust dose as needed. Daily doses greater than 120 mg require special state and federal approval.	**CNS:** *sedation, clouded sensorium, euphoria,* convulsions with large doses. **CV:** *hypotension,* bradycardia. **GI:** *nausea, vomiting, constipation,* ileus. **GU:** *urinary retention.* **Local:** pain at injection site, tissue irritation, induration following S.C. injection. **Other:** *respiratory depression,* physical dependence.
morphine sulfate♦ Controlled Substance Schedule II **Severe pain:** ADULTS: 5 to 15 mg S.C. or I.M., or 30 to 60 mg P.O. q 4 hours, p.r.n. or around the clock. May be injected slow I.V. (over 4 to 5 minutes) diluted in 4 to 5 ml water for injection. CHILDREN: 0.1 to 0.2 mg/kg dose S.C. Maximum 15 mg.	**CNS:** *sedation, clouded sensorium, euphoria,* convulsions with large doses. **CV:** *hypotension,* bradycardia. **GI:** *nausea, vomiting, constipation,* ileus. **GU:** *urinary retention.* **Other:** *respiratory depression, physical dependence.*
oxycodone hydrochloride Controlled Substance Schedule II Supeudol♦♦ *Combinations:* Percocet♦♦, Percocet 5, Percocet-Demi♦, Percodan♦, Percodan-Demi♦, Tylox **Moderate pain:** ADULTS: available in U.S. only in combination with other drugs, such as aspirin, phenacetin, and caffeine (Percodan, Percodan-Demi), or acetaminophen (Percocet 5, Tylox). 1 to 2 tablets P.O. q 6 hours, p.r.n. ADULTS: (Supeudol) 1 to 3 suppositories	**CNS:** *sedation, clouded sensorium, euphoria,* convulsions with large doses. **CV:** *hypotension,* bradycardia. **GI:** *nausea, vomiting, constipation,* ileus. **GU:** *urinary retention.* **Other:** *respiratory depression,* physical dependence.

♦ Available in U.S. and Canada. ♦♦ Available in Canada only.
All other products (no symbol) available in U.S. only. Italicized side effects are common or life-threatening.

INTERACTIONS AND SPECIAL CONSIDERATIONS

Interactions:

RIFAMPIN: withdrawal symptoms; reduced blood levels of methadone. Use together cautiously.

AMMONIUM CHLORIDE AND OTHER URINE ACIDIFIERS AND PHENYTOIN: may reduce methadone effect. Monitor for decreased pain control.

Special considerations:

• Contraindicated in obstetric analgesia. Give with extreme caution in patients with acute abdominal conditions, severe hepatic or renal impairment, hypothyroidism, Addison's disease, prostatic hypertrophy, urethral stricture, head injury, increased intracranial pressure, asthma, COPD, respiratory depression, CNS depression, and in elderly or debilitated patients.
• Safe use in adolescents as maintenance drug not established.
• Oral dose is half as potent as injected dose.
• Injection sites should be rotated.
• Has cumulative effect; marked sedation can occur after repeated doses.
• Circulatory and respiratory status and bowel function should be monitored.
• Ambulatory patient should avoid activities that require alertness.
• One daily dose adequate for maintenance. No advantage to divide doses.
• Oral form legally required in maintenance programs.
• Maintenance doses should be taken as oral liquid. Completely dissolve tablets in 120 ml of orange juice or powdered citrus drink.
• Constipation often severe with maintenance. Stool softener or other laxative should be ordered.
• Patient treated for narcotic abstinence syndrome will usually require an additional analgesic if pain control necessary.
• If used with general anesthetics, tranquilizers, sedatives, hypnotics, alcohol, tricyclic antidepressants, or MAO inhibitors, respiratory depression, hypotension, profound sedation, or coma may occur. Should be used together with extreme caution and patient's response monitored.
• Liquid form (1mg/ml) available for patients who are unable to swallow tablet.
• For symptoms and treatment of toxicity, see APPENDIX.

No significant interactions.

Special considerations:

• Use with extreme caution in patients with head injury, increased intracranial pressure, seizures, asthma, COPD, alcoholism, prostatic hypertrophy, severe hepatic or renal disease, acute abdominal conditions, hypothyroidism, Addison's disease, urethral stricture, cardiac arrhythmias, reduced blood volume, toxic psychosis, and in elderly or debilitated patients.
• Ambulatory patient should avoid activities that require alertness.
• Circulatory and respiratory status and bowel function should be monitored. Should not be given if respirations below 12/minute.
• Drug of choice in relieving pain of myocardial infarction. May cause transient decrease in blood pressure.
• Narcotic antagonist (naloxone) and resuscitative equipment should be kept available.
• If used with general anesthetics, tranquilizers, sedatives, hypnotics, alcohol, tricyclic antidepressants, or MAO inhibitors, respiratory depression, hypotension, profound sedation, or coma may occur. Morphine dose should be reduced. Should be used together with extreme caution and patient's response monitored.
• For full analgesic effect, should be given before patient has intense pain.
• When used postoperatively, turning, coughing, and deep breathing should be encouraged to avoid atelectasis.
• Patients with very severe pain may receive up to 150 mg of morphine sulfate every 3 hours.
• Newly available oral solution contains 10 mg/5 ml.
• For symptoms and treatment of toxicity, see APPENDIX.

Interactions:

ANTICOAGULANTS: oxycodone hydrochloride products containing aspirin may increase anticoagulant effect. Monitor clotting times. Use together cautiously.

Special considerations:

• Use with extreme caution in patients with head injury, increased intracranial pressure, increased cerebrospinal fluid pressure, seizures, asthma, alcoholism, prostatic hypertrophy, COPD, severe hepatic or renal disease, acute abdominal conditions, urethral stricture, hypothyroidism, Addison's disease, cardiac arrhythmias, reduced blood volume, toxic psychosis, and in elderly or debilitated patients.
• Should not be given to children, except for Percodan-Demi and Percocet-Demi.
• Ambulatory patient should avoid activities that require alertness.
• Circulatory and respiratory status and bowel function should be monitored. Should not be given if respirations below 12/minute.
• For full analgesic effect, should be given before patient has intense pain.
• High level of analgesia when given orally but poor choice due to high risk of addiction and presence of phenacetin in some combinations.

(continued on following page)

NAMES, INDICATIONS AND DOSAGES	SIDE EFFECTS
oxycodone hydrochloride *(continued)* rectally/day, p.r.n. CHILDREN: (Percodan-Demi) ¼ to ½ tablet P.O. q 6 hours, p.r.n.	
oxymorphone hydrochloride Controlled Substance Schedule II Numorphan♦ **Moderate-to-severe pain:** ADULTS: 1 to 1.5 mg I.M. or S.C. q 4 to 6 hours, p.r.n., or 0.5 mg I.V. q 4 to 6 hours, p.r.n., or 2.5 to 5 mg rectally q 4 to 6 hours, p.r.n.	**CNS:** *sedation, clouded sensorium, euphoria,* convulsions with large doses. **CV:** *hypotension,* bradycardia. **GI:** *nausea, vomiting, constipation,* ileus. **GU:** *urinary retention.* **Other:** *respiratory depression,* physical dependence.
pentazocine hydrochloride **pentazocine lactate** Controlled Substance Schedule IV Talwin♦ **Moderate-to-severe pain:** ADULTS: 50 to 100 mg P.O. q 3 to 4 hours, p.r.n. Maximum 600 mg daily or 30 mg I.M., I.V., or S.C. q 3 to 4 hours, p.r.n. Maximum 360 mg daily. Doses above 30 mg I.V. or 60 mg I.M. or S.C. not recommended.	**CNS:** *sedation,* visual disturbances, hallucinations, drowsiness, dizziness, light-headedness, confusion, euphoria, headache. **GI:** nausea, vomiting, dry mouth. **GU:** urinary retention. **Local:** induration, nodules, sloughing, and sclerosis of injection site. **Other:** *respiratory depression,* physical and psychological dependence.
propoxyphene hydrochloride Controlled Substance Schedule IV Darvon, Depronal♦♦, Dolene, Doraphen, Myospaz, Pargesic 65, Pro-65♦♦, Pro-Pox 65, Proxagesic, Ropoxy, Scrip-Dyne, SK-65, S-Pain-65, 642♦♦ **propoxyphene napsylate** Controlled Substance Schedule IV Darvocet-N, Darvon-N♦ **Mild-to-moderate pain:** ADULTS: 65 mg (hydrochloride) P.O. q 4 hours, p.r.n. **Mild-to-moderate pain:** ADULTS: 100 mg (napsylate) P.O. q 4 hours, p.r.n.	**CNS:** dizziness, headache, sedation, euphoria, paradoxical excitement, insomnia. **GI:** nausea, vomiting, constipation. **Other:** psychological and physical dependence.

INTERACTIONS AND SPECIAL CONSIDERATIONS

• Should be taken after meals or with milk.
• If used with general anesthetics, other narcotic analgesics, tranquilizers, sedatives, hypnotics, alcohol, tricyclic antidepressants, or MAO inhibitors, CNS depression is increased. Oxycodone dose should be reduced. Should be used together with extreme caution and patient's response monitored.
• For symptoms and treatment of toxicity, see APPENDIX.

No significant interactions.

Special considerations:
• Use with extreme caution in patients with head injury, increased intracranial pressure, seizures, asthma, COPD, alcoholism, increased cerebrospinal fluid pressure, acute abdominal conditions, prostatic hypertrophy, severe hepatic or renal disease, urethral stricture, CNS depression, respiratory depression, hypothyroidism, Addison's disease, cardiac arrhythmias, reduced blood volume, toxic psychosis, and in elderly or debilitated patients.
• Ambulatory patient should avoid activities that require alertness.
• Cardiovascular and respiratory status should be monitored. Should not be given if respirations below 12/minute.
• Well absorbed rectally. Alternative to narcotics with more limited dosage forms.
• Narcotic antagonist (naloxone) should be available.
• If used with general anesthetics, tranquilizers, sedatives, hypnotics, alcohol, tricyclic antidepressants, or MAO inhibitors, CNS depression is increased. Oxymorphone dose should be reduced. Should be used together with extreme caution and patient's response monitored.
• For full analgesic effect, should be given before patient has intense pain.
• When used postoperatively, turning, coughing, and deep breathing should be encouraged to avoid atelectasis.
• For symptoms and treatment of toxicity, see APPENDIX.

No significant interactions.

Special considerations:
• Contraindicated in emotional instability, drug abuse, head injury, increased intracranial pressure. Use cautiously in hepatic or renal disease, myocardial infarction with nausea, respiratory depression.
• Tablets not well absorbed.
• Possesses narcotic antgonist properties.
• Psychological and physiological dependence may occur.
• Respiratory depression can be reversed with naloxone.
• Should not be mixed in same syringe with soluble barbiturates.
• Ambulatory patient should avoid activities that require alertness.

No significant interactions.

Special considerations:
• Not to be prescribed in narcotic addiction.
• Ambulatory patient should avoid activities that require alertness until CNS response to drug has been established.
• Patient should not exceed recommended dosage.
• Caffeine or amphetamines should not be used to treat overdose; may cause fatal convulsions. Narcotic antagonist should be used instead.
• May cause false decreases in urinary steroid excretion tests.
• 65 mg propoxyphene HCl equals 100 mg propoxyphene napsylate.
• Can be considered a mild narcotic analgesic.
• Patients should limit their alcohol intake when taking this drug.
• For symptoms and treatment of acute toxicity, see APPENDIX.

27

Narcotic antagonists

levallorphan tartrate
naloxone

Because of their chemical similarity to narcotics, narcotic antagonists can compete with narcotics for receptor sites. They are antidotes for overdoses of narcotics, including pentazocine and propoxyphene. Narcotic antagonists are very potent and can reverse respiratory depression caused by a narcotic dose 10 to 100 times as great, as well as the narcotic's analgesic, cardiovascular, and gastrointestinal effects.

Levallorphan is ineffective against barbiturate- or anesthetic-induced respiratory depression. Indeed, levallorphan itself can induce respiratory depression and exacerbates such depression caused by nonnarcotic drugs. Naloxone, which does not worsen non-narcotic respiratory depression, is the antagonist of choice for respiratory depression of unknown cause.

Major uses

Narcotic antagonists are antidotes for narcotic-induced respiratory depression, including asphyxia neonatorum.

• Naloxone is used in diagnosis of suspected acute opiate overdosage.

Mechanism of action

Although the precise mechanism of action of narcotic antagonists is unknown, levallorphan and naloxone apparently displace previously administered narcotic analgesics from

QUESTIONS & ANSWERS

MORE BACKGROUND ON NALOXONE: AN EFFECTIVE ANTAGONIST WITH FEW SIDE EFFECTS

Why is naloxone chosen over other narcotic antagonists?

Naloxone is the most frequently used narcotic antagonist because it's the only one free of analgesic properties. And it doesn't produce unpleasant side effects, such as hallucinations, disorientation, tolerance or signs of physical dependence. It also has a high therapeutic index.

Does naloxone have any limitations?

Yes. Naloxone's duration of action is short compared with that of narcotic analgesics, so relapses are possible. When an opiate addict is being treated for an overdose, large doses of naloxone may cause severe withdrawal symptoms. These symptoms are much more severe and difficult to manage than those induced by narcotic abstinence alone.

When is naloxone used?

Naloxone is used to treat coma, respiratory depression, and convulsions whenever narcotic overdose is suspected.

How is naloxone administered?

Naloxone can be given I.V., I.M., or subcutaneously. However, in patients who have abused I.V. drugs, often no I.V. sites are available. I.M. and subcutaneous injections are inappropriate when the patient requires immediate antagonist therapy. In emergencies, sublingual or intra-arterial injections may be used.

NARCOTIC ANTAGONISTS: HOW THEY WORK

Narcotic antagonists can reverse the action of narcotic analgesics because they reach—and thus can affect—the same receptors in the body. This is possible because the chemical structure of these two types of drugs is similar.

The chemical structure of naloxone (a narcotic antagonist) and of oxymorphone (a narcotic analgesic) are illustrated below. As you can see, their basic structures are the same. But the groups highlighted in color are different, and these determine the drugs' effects on the patient. Naloxone has an allyl group, which makes it an antagonist; oxymorphone has a methyl group, which makes it an analgesic.

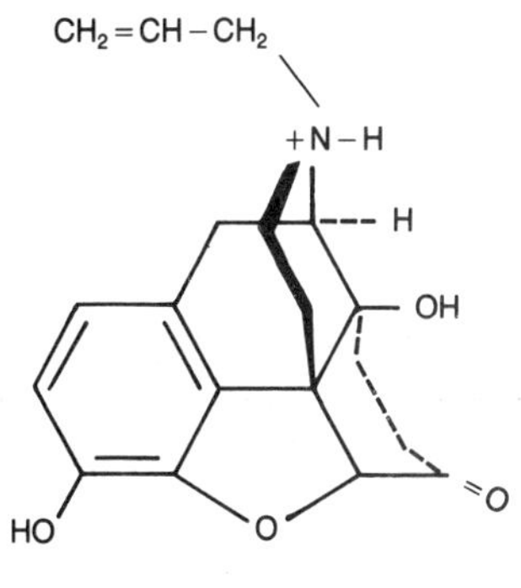

$CH_2=CH-CH_2$ +N−H H OH =O HO O

naloxone

CH_3 +N−H H OH =O HO O

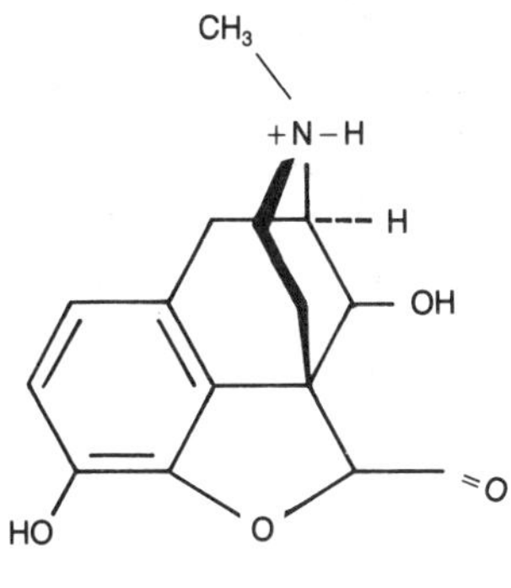

oxymorphone

their receptors (competitive antagonism).

- Levallorphan may have some narcotic *agonist* activity (narcotic analgesic effect), especially if administered alone, not as an antidote to narcotic analgesics.
- Naloxone—administered alone—has no pharmacologic activity.

Absorption, distribution, metabolism, and excretion

Narcotic antagonists are well absorbed after parenteral administration, rapidly metabolized in the liver, and excreted in the urine.

Onset and duration

- Levallorphan's onset of action is 1 to 2 minutes when given I.V.; 2 to 5 minutes when given I.M. or subcutaneously. The drug's duration of action by all parenteral routes of administration is 2 to 5 hours.
- Naloxone's onset of action is within 2 minutes after I.V. injection; approximately 2 to 5 minutes after I.M. or subcutaneous administration. Naloxone's duration of action when given I.V. is 45 minutes but longer when administered I.M. and subcutaneously.

NAMES, INDICATIONS AND DOSAGES	SIDE EFFECTS
levallorphan tartrate Lorfan **Severe narcotic-induced respiratory depression:** ADULTS: 1 mg I.V., then 1 to 2 doses of 0.5 mg at 10- to 15-minute intervals, p.r.n. Maximum total dose 3 mg. CHILDREN: 0.02 mg/kg I.V. May give 0.01 to 0.02 mg/kg in 10 to 15 minutes. NEONATES (ASPHYXIA NEONATORUM): 0.05 to 0.1 mg I.V. into umbilical vein immediately after delivery. May repeat in 5 to 10 minutes.	**CNS:** lethargy, dizziness, drowsiness, restlessness, sense of heaviness in limbs; with high doses: psychic disturbances (hallucinations, disorientation, vivid dreams); in neonates: irritability, increased crying. **CV:** pallor. **EENT:** miosis, pseudoptosis. **GI:** nausea. **Other:** sweating, respiratory depression.
naloxone Narcan♦ **Narcotic-induced respiratory depression, including pentazocine and propoxyphene:** ADULTS: 0.4 mg I.V., S.C., or I.M. May repeat q 2 to 3 minutes, p.r.n., for 3 doses. **Postoperative narcotic depression:** ADULTS: 0.1 to 0.2 mg I.V. q 2 to 3 minutes, p.r.n. Adult concentration is 0.4 mg/ml. CHILDREN: 0.01 mg/kg dose I.M., I.V., S.C. May repeat q 2 to 3 minutes for 3 doses. *Note:* If initial dose 0.01 mg/kg does not result in clinical improvement, up to 10 times this dose (0.1 mg/kg) may be needed to be effective. NEONATES (ASPHYXIA NEONATORUM): 0.01 mg/kg I.V. into umbilical vein. May repeat q 2 to 3 minutes for 3 doses. Neonatal concentration (for children also) is 0.02 mg/ml.	*With higher-than-recommended doses:* nausea, vomiting. *In narcotic addicts:* withdrawal symptoms.

INTERACTIONS AND SPECIAL CONSIDERATIONS

No significant interactions.

Special considerations:

• Contraindicated in mild respiratory depression and in narcotic addiction. (Violent withdrawal symptoms may occur.)

• Respiratory depth and rate should be monitored; should be prepared to give oxygen, ventilation, and other resuscitative measures.

• May increase mild respiratory depression or that caused by nonnarcotic agents. Repeated doses may produce tolerance and increased respiratory depression.

No significant interactions.

Special considerations:

• Use cautiously in patients with cardiac irritability and narcotic addiction.

• Safest drug to use when cause of respiratory depression uncertain.

• Respiratory depth and rate should be monitored; should be prepared to give oxygen, ventilation, and other resuscitative measures.

• Ineffective in respiratory depression caused by nonnarcotics.

• May dilute adult concentration (0.4 mg) by mixing 0.5 ml with 9.5 ml sterile water or saline for injection to make neonatal concentration (0.02 mg/ml).

28

Sedatives and hypnotics

amobarbital
amobarbital sodium
aprobarbital
barbital
butabarbital
butabarbital sodium
chloral hydrate
ethchlorvynol
ethinamate
flurazepam hydrochloride
glutethimide
hexobarbital
mephobarbital
methaqualone
methaqualone hydrochloride
methotrimeprazine hydrochloride
methyprylon
paraldehyde
pentobarbital
pentobarbital sodium
phenobarbital
phenobarbital sodium
propiomazine hydrochloride
secobarbital
secobarbital sodium
talbutal
temazepam
triclofos sodium

Most of the drugs in this chapter are barbiturates (amobarbital, aprobarbital, barbital, butabarbital, hexobarbital, mephobarbital, pentobarbital, phenobarbital, secobarbital, and talbutal). Until recently, these were used extensively as nighttime sedative-hypnotics to induce sleep. However, because of the high risk of barbiturate toxicity and dependence, most doctors no longer regard them as the drugs of choice for this indication.

The benzodiazepines, flurazepam and temazepam, are more desirable for nighttime sedation because they have a much greater therapeutic index (margin between toxic and therapeutic dose) than the barbiturates. Also, both are generally as therapeutically effective as the barbiturates. The other drugs in this chapter (except paraldehyde) more closely resemble the barbiturates in their potential to cause toxicity and drug dependence. Methaqualone has a particularly high potential for abuse.

Major uses

Sedatives and hypnotics are used to treat insomnia, induce sleep before operative or test procedures, and provide sedation and relief of anxiety.

- Mephobarbital and paraldehyde alleviate alcohol withdrawal syndrome.
- Phenobarbital controls acute psychotic agitation.

Mechanism of action

- Although their mechanism of action is not completely defined, barbiturates probably interfere with transmission of impulses from the thalamus to the cortex of the brain.
- Flurazepam and temazepam act on the limbic system, thalamus, and hypothalamus of the central nervous system to produce hypnotic effects.

Absorption, distribution, metabolism, and excretion

- The barbiturates are well absorbed from all administration routes; the sodium salts are more rapidly absorbed than the acids. They are distributed to all tissues and body fluids, with high concentrations in the brain and liver.

They are metabolized slowly in the liver. Both metabolites and unchanged drug are

SLEEP MEDICATIONS: ARE THEY ALWAYS NECESSARY?

Sleep problems are probably among patients' most common complaints. Approximately 40 million Americans have trouble sleeping, but researchers say sleep medications won't necessarily help such persons. Only a small percentage of the 2 million Americans who regularly take sleep medications may actually need them. Look at these facts:

- 85% of persons who claim they have insomnia really don't. Most persons tested for insomnia in sleep laboratories fall asleep in 20 minutes.
- Relief is only temporary. After a 2-week period, effectiveness usually wanes, and patients develop a false tolerance to the drug, requiring a higher dosage to get the same effect. (*Effective* dosage increases, but the *lethal* dosage remains the same.)
- 10% of all insomniacs seen at sleep disorder treatment centers—only a small number of the people taking drugs for insomnia—are victims of *drug-induced* insomnia.

Doubling and tripling the original dosage leads to *drug dependence.* Withdrawal symptoms occur mainly at night, in the form of nightmares and restless sleep. Unfortunately, these symptoms tend to reinforce the patient's perceived need for the drug; this is especially true of anxious patients and those with chronic illnesses.

A better judgment can be made about a patient's real need for sleep medications by remembering these facts and by closely observing a patient's condition. He may be experiencing *transient* sleep difficulties, caused by psychological or environmental influences. These sleep problems can be treated successfully with hypnotics, since only short-term therapy is necessary. Insomnia may also accompany use of certain drugs (amphetamines or caffeine, for example) or withdrawal of certain substances (alcoholic beverages or nicotine, for example).

Medical conditions characterized by pain, dyspnea, physical discomfort, fear, anxiety, and depression can also affect sleep habits. Remember:

- Patients with arthritis, neurogenic pain, and various kinds of headache may experience more pain or discomfort at night than during the day. (With *decreased* external stimulation, patients are more conscious of their body sensations.)
- Patients with nocturnal leg recumbency cramps (restless leg syndrome—tingling sensations and nighttime cramps) commonly complain of sleep problems and see sleep medication as the solution.
- Besides increased pain, patients with cancer may experience fear and anxiety while trying to fall asleep, and this inhibits restful sleep.
- Patients with angina pectoris and/or cardiac arrhythmias may fear attack at night and thus be afraid to sleep. This is common. Such patients who cannot readily fall asleep may become dependent on sleep medications to induce sleep.
- Some patients may actually have *sleep apnea.* This is a serious disorder in which they unknowingly stop breathing for as long as 2 minutes during the night, disturbing normal sleep patterns. They awake feeling tired and in need of more sleep, so may ask for something to help them sleep. Unusually explosive, intermittent snoring may be a key to this specific diagnosis.

Hypnotics may be useful in treating short-term sleep problems. But excessive or long-term use should be avoided. Insomnia is often only a symptom of other problems that need to be treated to overcome the sleeplessness.

excreted in urine. Trace amounts are also eliminated in feces and perspiration.

• Chloral hydrate is well absorbed from the gastrointestinal (GI) tract after oral or rectal administration. It is rapidly reduced and distributed to all tissues. Both the unchanged drug and active metabolites are detected in cerebrospinal fluid (CSF), umbilical cord blood, fetal blood, and amniotic fluid.

Chloral hydrate is metabolized in the liver and red cells. It is eliminated primarily in urine and partially in feces through the bile.

• Ethchlorvynol is rapidly absorbed from the GI tract after oral administration. Both the unchanged drug and metabolites are detected in the liver, kidneys, spleen, brain, bile, and CSF. The drug is metabolized primarily in the liver and excreted in urine.

• Ethinamate is well absorbed from the GI tract. Although it is rapidly destroyed in the tissues, its pattern of distribution is unknown. The liver is not significantly involved in the drug's metabolism. Small amounts are excreted in the urine.

• Flurazepam and temazepam are well absorbed from the GI tract after oral administration. Distributed to all tissues and metabolized in the liver, they are eliminated primarily in urine and partially in feces.

• Glutethimide is absorbed irregularly from the GI tract after oral administration. The unchanged drug and active metabolites are detected in the liver, kidneys, brain, and bile. The drug is metabolized in the liver and eliminated in both urine and feces.

• Methaqualone is absorbed rapidly from the GI tract after oral administration. The unchanged drug or its metabolites or both are detected in the liver, kidneys, heart, brain, spleen, skeletal muscles, and CSF. The drug is metabolized in the liver; some of the metabolites are excreted in urine, and the remainder passes through the bile for elimination in feces.

• Methotrimeprazine is rapidly absorbed after I.M. injection. It is well distributed to body tissues, including the CSF, metabolized in the liver, and eliminated slowly in urine and feces.

• Methyprylon's absorption and distribution are not well known. The drug is metabolized in the liver. Some of its metabolites are secreted in the bile and reabsorbed; the rest are excreted in urine.

• Paraldehyde is rapidly absorbed from either the GI tract or muscles, depending on the route of administration. Although its distribution is not well known, the drug is metabolized in the liver and excreted in urine and through the lungs. Significant quantities are exhaled unchanged, emitting a characteristic odor.

• Propiomazine is well absorbed from parenteral sites; distributed throughout the body; metabolized in the liver; and eliminated in urine and, through the bile, in feces.

• Triclofos is rapidly absorbed from the GI tract. Its distribution in body tissues is unclear. It is metabolized primarily in the liver and kidneys and slowly eliminated in urine and feces.

Onset and duration

The chart on the opposite page summarizes onset and duration.

Combination products

Barbiturates

BUTATRAX CAPSULES: amobarbital 20 mg and butabarbital 30 mg.

CARBRITAL KAPSEALS: pentobarbital sodium 97.5 mg and carbromal 260 mg.

ETHOBRAL CAPSULE: phenobarbital 50 mg, butabarbital sodium 30 mg, and secobarbital sodium 50 mg.

HYPTRAN TABLET: secobarbital 60 mg and phenyltoloxamine dihydrogen citrate 25 mg in outer layer (immediate release), phenyltoloxamine dihydrogen citrate 75 mg in core (delayed release).

THERAPEUTIC ACTIVITY OF SEDATIVES AND HYPNOTICS

ONSET AND DURATION	DRUGS P.O./I.M.	DRUGS I.V.
Ultra short-acting: few minutes' onset; short-term duration (less than 1 hour)	hexobarbital	amobarbital ethchlorvynol pentobarbital phenobarbital
Short-acting: 10 to 15 minutes' onset; 3 hours or less duration	paraldehyde pentobarbital secobarbital	
Intermediate-acting: 10 to 30 minutes' onset; 3 to 6 hours' duration	amobarbital aprobarbital butabarbital chloral hydrate ethchlorvynol ethinamate methotrimeprazine propiomazine talbutal tricloflos	
Long-acting: 30 to 60 minutes' onset; 6 or more hours' duration	barbital flurazepam glutethimide mephobarbital methaqualone methyprylon phenobarbital	

NIDAR TABLET: phenobarbital sodium 7.5 mg, butabarbital sodium 7.5 mg, secobarbital sodium 25 mg, and pentobarbital sodium 25 mg.
TRI-BARBS CAPSULE: phenobarbital 32 mg, butabarbital sodium 32 mg, and secobarbital sodium 32 mg.
TUINAL 50 MG PULVULES: amobarbital sodium 25 mg and secobarbital sodium 25 mg.
TUINAL 100 MG PULVULES♦: amobarbital sodium 50 mg and secobarbital sodium 50 mg.
TUINAL 200 MG PULVULES♦: amobarbital sodium 100 mg; secobarbital sodium 100 mg.

NAMES, INDICATIONS AND DOSAGES	SIDE EFFECTS
amobarbital Amytal♦, Isobec♦♦ **amobarbital sodium** Controlled Substance Schedule II Amytal Sodium♦ **Sedation:** ADULTS: usually 30 to 50 mg P.O. b.i.d. or t.i.d. but may range from 15 to 120 mg b.i.d. to q.i.d. CHILDREN: 3 to 6 mg/kg/day P.O. divided into 4 equal doses. **Insomnia:** ADULTS: 65 to 200 mg P.O. or deep I.M. at bedtime; I.M. injection not to exceed 5 ml in any one site. Maximum dose 500 mg. CHILDREN: 3 to 5 mg/kg deep I.M. at bedtime; I.M. injection not to exceed 5 ml in any one site. **Preanesthetic sedation:** ADULTS AND CHILDREN: 200 mg P.O. or I.M. 1 to 2 hours before surgery. **Manic reactions; anticonvulsant:** ADULTS AND CHILDREN OVER 6 YEARS: 65 to 500 mg slow I.V.; rate not to exceed 100 mg/minute. Maximum dose 1 g. CHILDREN UNDER 6 YEARS: 3 to 5 mg/kg slow I.V. or I.M.	**CNS:** *drowsiness, lethargy, hangover,* paradoxical excitement in elderly patients. **GI:** nausea, vomiting. **Skin:** rash, urticaria. **Local:** pain, irritation, sterile abscess at injection site. **Other:** *Stevens-Johnson syndrome,* angioedema.
aprobarbital Controlled Substance Schedule III **Sedation:** ADULTS: 15 to 40 mg P.O. t.i.d. or q.i.d.; usual dose 40 mg t.i.d. **Insomnia:** ADULTS: 40 to 160 mg P.O. at bedtime.	**CNS:** *drowsiness, lethargy, hangover,* paradoxical excitement in elderly patients. **GI:** nausea, vomiting. **Skin:** rash, urticaria. **Other:** *Stevens-Johnson syndrome,* angioedema.
barbital Controlled Substance Schedule IV Barbital Sodium **Insomnia:** ADULTS: 300 to 600 mg P.O. or I.M. 1 to 2 hours before bedtime.	**CNS:** *drowsiness, lethargy, hangover,* paradoxical excitement in elderly patients. **GI:** nausea, vomiting. **Skin:** rash, urticaria. **Local:** pain, swelling, thrombophlebitis. **Other:** *Stevens-Johnson syndrome,* angioedema.

♦ Available in U.S. and Canada. ♦♦ Available in Canada only.
All other products (no symbol) available in U.S. only. Italicized side effects are common or life-threatening.

INTERACTIONS AND SPECIAL CONSIDERATIONS

Interactions:
ALCOHOL OR OTHER CNS DEPRESSANTS, INCLUDING OTHER NARCOTIC ANALGESICS: excessive CNS and respiratory depression. Don't use together.
MAO INHIBITORS: inhibit metabolism of barbiturates; may cause prolonged CNS depression. Reduce barbiturate dosage.
RIFAMPIN: may decrease barbiturate levels. Monitor for decreased effect.

Special considerations:
- Contraindicated in patients with uncontrolled severe pain, respiratory disease with dyspnea or obstruction, hypersensitivity to barbiturates, previous addiction to sedatives, and porphyria. Use with caution in hepatic or renal impairment.
- Injection solution should be used within 30 minutes after opening container to minimize deterioration. Cloudy or precipitated solution should not be used. Should not shake solution; should be mixed with sterile water.
- I.V. injection should be reserved for emergency treatment under close supervision. Should be administered slow I.V.; not to exceed 100 mg/minute.
- I.M. injection should be administered deeply. Superficial injection may cause pain, sterile abscess, and sloughing.
- Barbiturates potentiate narcotics; dose should be reduced when given during labor. Excessive dose may cause respiratory depression in neonate.
- Cigarettes should be removed if patient receives hypnotic dose.
- Walking should be supervised and bed rails raised, especially for elderly patients.
- Long-term high dosage may cause drug dependence and severe withdrawal symptoms. Barbiturates should be withdrawn gradually.
- Patients who are depressed, suicidal, or drug-dependent, or who have a history of drug abuse should be prevented from hoarding or self-overdosing. Patient should be warned that alcohol increases effects of drug. Activities requiring alertness or skill should be avoided until CNS response is determined.
- Signs of barbiturate toxicity: coma, pupillary constriction, cyanosis, clammy skin, hypotension. Overdose can be fatal.
- Monitor prothrombin times when patient on amobarbital starts or ends anticoagulant therapy. Anticoagulant dose may need to be adjusted.
- For treatment of toxicity, see APPENDIX.

Interactions:
ALCOHOL OR OTHER CNS DEPRESSANTS, INCLUDING OTHER NARCOTIC ANALGESICS: excessive CNS and respiratory depression. Don't use together.
MAO INHIBITORS: inhibit metabolism of barbiturates; may cause prolonged CNS depression. Reduce barbiturate dosage.
RIFAMPIN: may decrease barbiturate levels. Monitor for decreased effect.

Special considerations:
- Contraindicated in patients with uncontrolled severe pain, respiratory disease with dyspnea or obstruction, hypersensitivity to barbiturates, previous addiction to sedatives, and porphyria. Use with caution in hepatic or renal impairment.
- Cigarettes should be removed if patient receives hypnotic dose.
- Walking should be supervised and bed rails raised, especially for elderly patients.
- Long-term high dosage may cause drug dependence and severe withdrawal symptoms. Barbiturates should be withdrawn gradually.
- Patients who are depressed, suicidal, or drug-dependent, or who have a history of drug abuse should be prevented from hoarding or self-overdosing. Patient should be warned that alcohol increases effects of drug. Activities requiring alertness or skill should be avoided until CNS response is determined.
- Available as elixir only, with alcohol 20%.
- Monitor prothrombin times when patient on aprobarbital starts or ends anticoagulant therapy. Anticoagulant dose may need to be adjusted.
- Signs of barbiturate toxicity: coma, pupillary constriction, cyanosis, clammy skin, hypotension. Overdose can be fatal.
- For treatment of toxicity, see APPENDIX.

Interactions:
ALCOHOL OR OTHER CNS DEPRESSANTS, INCLUDING OTHER NARCOTIC ANALGESICS: excessive CNS and respiratory depression. Don't use together.
MAO INHIBITORS: inhibit metabolism of barbiturates; may cause prolonged CNS depression. Reduce barbiturate dosage.
RIFAMPIN: may decrease barbiturate levels. Monitor for decreased effect.

Special considerations:
- Contraindicated in patients with uncontrolled severe pain, respiratory disease with dyspnea or obstruction, hypersensitivity to barbiturates, previous addiction to sedatives, and porphyria. Use with caution in hepatic, renal, cardiac, or respiratory impairment.

(continued on following page)

NAMES, INDICATIONS AND DOSAGES	SIDE EFFECTS

barbital
(continued)

Sedation:
ADULTS: 65 to 130 mg P.O. or I.M. b.i.d. or t.i.d.

---

butabarbital
Buta-Barb♦♦, Butisol, Day-Barb♦♦, Medarsed, Neo-Barb♦♦
butabarbital sodium
Controlled Substance Schedule III
Butal, Butisol Sodium♦

Sedation:
ADULTS: 15 to 30 mg P.O. t.i.d. or q.i.d.
CHILDREN: 6 mg/kg P.O. divided t.i.d. Dosage range 7.5 to 30 mg P.O. t.i.d.

Preoperatively:
ADULTS: 50 to 100 mg P.O. 60 to 90 minutes before surgery.

Insomnia:
ADULTS: 50 to 100 mg P.O. at bedtime.

CNS: *drowsiness, lethargy, hangover,* paradoxical excitement in elderly patients.
GI: nausea, vomiting.
Skin: rash, urticaria.
Other: *Stevens-Johnson syndrome,* angioedema.

---

chloral hydrate
Controlled Substance Schedule IV
Aquachloral Supprettes, Chloralvan♦♦, Cohidrate, Noctec♦, Novochlorhydrate♦♦, Oradrate, S K Chloral Hydrate

Sedation:
ADULTS: 250 mg P.O. or rectally t.i.d. after meals.
CHILDREN: 8 mg/kg P.O. t.i.d. Maximum 500 mg t.i.d.

Insomnia:
ADULTS: 500 mg to 1 g P.O. or rectally 15 to 30 minutes before bedtime.
CHILDREN: 50 mg/kg single dose. Maximum dose 1 g.

Premedication for EEG:
CHILDREN: 25 mg/kg single dose. Maximum dose 1 g.

CNS: *hangover, drowsiness,* nightmares, dizziness, ataxia.
GI: *nausea,* vomiting, diarrhea, flatulence.
Skin: hypersensitivity reactions.

♦ Available in U.S. and Canada. ♦♦ Available in Canada only.
All other products (no symbol) available in U.S. only. Italicized side effects are common or life-threatening.

INTERACTIONS AND SPECIAL CONSIDERATIONS

- Injection solution should be used within 30 minutes after opening container to minimize deterioration. Don't use cloudy solution.
- I.M. injection should be administered deeply. Superficial injection may cause pain, sterile abscess, and sloughing.
- Because barbiturates potentiate narcotics, dose should be reduced during labor. Overdose may cause respiratory depression in neonate.
- With hypnotic dose, remove patient's cigarettes.
- Walking should be supervised and bed rails raised, especially for elderly patients.
- Long-term high dosage may cause drug dependence and severe withdrawal symptoms. Barbiturates should be withdrawn gradually.
- Patients who are depressed, suicidal, or drug-dependent, or who have a history of drug abuse should be prevented from hoarding or self-overdosing. Patient should be warned that alcohol increases effects of drug. Activities requiring alertness or skill should be avoided until CNS response is determined.
- No analgesic action. May cause restlessness or delirium in presence of pain.
- Prothrombin times should be monitored when patient on barbital starts or ends anticoagulant therapy. Anticoagulant dose may need to be adjusted.
- Signs of barbiturate toxicity: coma, pupillary constriction, cyanosis, clammy skin, hypotension. Overdose can be fatal.
- For treatment of toxicity, see APPENDIX.

Interactions:

ALCOHOL OR OTHER CNS DEPRESSANTS, INCLUDING OTHER NARCOTIC ANALGESICS: excessive CNS and respiratory depression. Don't use together.

MAO INHIBITORS: inhibit the metabolism of barbiturates; may cause prolonged CNS depression. Reduce barbiturate dosage.

RIFAMPIN: may decrease barbiturate levels. Monitor for decreased effect.

Special considerations:

- Contraindicated in patients with uncontrolled severe pain, respiratory disease with dyspnea or obstruction, hypersensitivity to barbiturates, previous addiction to sedatives, and porphyria. Use with caution in hepatic or renal impairment.
- Cigarettes should be removed if patient receives hypnotic dose.
- Walking should be supervised and bed rails raised, especially for elderly patients.
- Long-term high dosage may cause drug dependence and severe withdrawal symptoms. Barbiturates should be withdrawn gradually.
- Patients who are depressed, suicidal, or drug-dependent, or who have a history of drug abuse should be prevented from hoarding or self-overdosing. Patient should be warned that alcohol increases effects of drug. Activities requiring alertness or skill should be avoided until CNS response is determined.
- Butisol Sodium Elixir is sugar free.
- Monitor prothrombin times carefully when patient on butabarbital starts or ends anticoagulant therapy. Anticoagulant dose may need to be adjusted.
- Signs of barbiturate toxicity: coma, pupillary constriction, cyanosis, clammy skin, hypotension. Overdose can be fatal.
- Prolonged administration not recommended: drug not effective after 14 days. A drug-free interval of at least 1 week is advised.
- For treatment of toxicity, see APPENDIX.

Interactions:

ALCOHOL OR OTHER CNS DEPRESSANTS, INCLUDING OTHER NARCOTIC ANALGESICS: excessive CNS depression or vasodilation reaction. Use together cautiously.

FUROSEMIDE I.V.: sweating, flushes, variable blood pressure, uneasiness. Use together cautiously. Use a different hypnotic drug.

Special considerations:

- Contraindicated in patients with marked hepatic or renal impairment, hypersensitivity to chloral hydrate or triclofos. Oral administration contraindicated in gastric disorders. Use with caution in severe cardiac disease, mental depression, suicidal tendencies.
- Dilute or take with liquid to minimize bad taste and stomach irritation. Take after meals.
- Patients who are depressed, suicidal, or drug-dependent, or who have a history of drug abuse should be prevented from hoarding or self-overdosing. Alcohol increases effects of drugs. Activities requiring alertness or skill should be avoided until CNS response is determined.
- Remove cigarettes if patient receives hypnotic dose. Supervise walking and raise bed rails, especially for elderly patients.
- May cause false-positive results in glycosuria tests using cupric sulfate as Benedict's solution. Clinitest, Clinistix, or Tes-Tape should be used.
- May interfere with fluorometric tests for urine catecholamines and Reddy, Jenkins, Thorn test for urinary 17-hydroxycorticosteroids. Don't give drug for 48 hours before fluorometric test. Large dosage may raise BUN level.
- Aqueous solutions incompatible with alkaline substances. Store in dark container. Store suppositories in refrigerator.
- If patient given anticoagulant, increased prothrombin times should be monitored during first few days of therapy. Anticoagulant dose may need to be adjusted.

NAMES, INDICATIONS AND DOSAGES	SIDE EFFECTS
ethchlorvynol Controlled Substance Schedule IV Placidyl♦ **Sedation:** ADULTS: 100 to 200 mg P.O. b.i.d. or t.i.d. **Insomnia:** ADULTS: 500 mg to 1 g P.O. at bedtime. May repeat 100 to 200 mg if awakened in early a.m.	**Blood:** thrombocytopenia. **CNS:** facial numbness, drowsiness, fatigue, nightmares, dizziness, residual sedation, muscular weakness, syncope, ataxia. **CV:** hypotension. **EENT:** unpleasant aftertaste, blurred vision. **GI:** distress, nausea, vomiting. **Skin:** rashes, urticaria.
ethinamate Controlled Substance Schedule IV Valmid **Insomnia:** ADULTS: 500 mg to 1 g P.O. 20 minutes before bedtime. Starting dose may be 250 mg for elderly or debilitated patients. **Preanesthetic:** ADULTS: 500 mg to 1 g P.O. 2½ hours preoperatively.	**Blood:** thrombocytopenia. **GI:** mild upset. **Skin:** rashes, purpura. **Other:** fever (allergic reaction).
flurazepam hydrochloride Controlled Substance Schedule IV Dalmane♦ **Insomnia:** ADULTS: 15 to 30 mg P.O. at bedtime.	**Blood:** leukopenia, granulocytopenia. **CNS:** *daytime sedation, dizziness, drowsiness, disturbed coordination,* lethargy, confusion, *headache.*
glutethimide Controlled Substance Schedule III Doriden♦, Rolathimide **Insomnia:** ADULTS: 250 to 500 mg P.O. at bedtime. May be repeated, but not less than 4 hours before intended awakening. Total daily dose should not	**CNS:** *residual sedation,* paradoxical excitation, headache, vertigo. **EENT:** dry mouth, blurred vision. **GI:** irritation, nausea, diarrhea. **GU:** bladder atony. **Skin:** rashes, urticaria.

♦ Available in U.S. and Canada. ♦♦ Available in Canada only.
All other products (no symbol) available in U.S. only. Italicized side effects are common or life-threatening.

INTERACTIONS AND SPECIAL CONSIDERATIONS

Interactions:
ALCOHOL OR OTHER CNS DEPRESSANTS, INCLUDING OTHER NARCOTIC ANALGESICS AND MAO INHIBITORS: excessive CNS depression. Use together cautiously.

Special considerations:
• Contraindicated in patients with uncontrolled pain and porphyria. Use cautiously in hepatic or renal impairment; in mental depression with suicidal tendencies; in elderly or debilitated patients; or in a patient who has previously overreacted to barbiturates or alcohol.
• Should be taken with milk or food to minimize transient dizziness or ataxia caused by rapid absorption.
• Prolonged use may cause dependence and severe withdrawal symptoms.
• Patients who are depressed, suicidal, or drug-dependent, or who have a history of drug abuse should be prevented from hoarding or self-overdosing. Overdosage very difficult to treat and has a high mortality rate. Patient should be warned that alcohol increases effects of drug. Activities requiring alertness or skill should be avoided until CNS response is determined.
• Toxicity signs: poor muscle coordination, confusion, hypothermia, speech or vision disturbances, tremors, or weakness.
• 750-mg strength contains tartrazine dye. May cause allergic reactions in susceptible patients.
• Cigarettes should be removed if patient receives hypnotic dose.
• Walking should be supervised and bed rails raised, especially for elderly patients.
• Slight darkening of liquid from exposure to air and light doesn't affect safety or potency, but store in tight, light-resistant container to avoid possible deterioration.
• Prothrombin times should be monitored carefully when patient on ethchlorvynol starts or ends anticoagulant therapy. Anticoagulant dose may need to be adjusted.
• Drug is effective for short-term use only; treatment period should not exceed 1 week.

No significant interactions.

Special considerations:
• Contraindicated for uncontrolled pain. Use cautiously in patients with mental depression, suicidal tendencies, or history of drug abuse.
• Not usually given for daytime sedation due to short duration of effect.
• Long-term use may cause dependence and severe withdrawal symptoms; should be withdrawn gradually.
• Patients who are depressed, suicidal, or drug dependent, or who have a history of drug abuse should be prevented from hoarding or self-overdosing. Patient should be warned that alcohol increases effects of drug. Activities requiring alertness or skill should be avoided until CNS response is determined.
• Abrupt withdrawal may cause blood pressure and pulse rate changes, sweating, and hallucinations.
• Patient's cigarettes should be removed after taking dose.
• Walking should be supervised and bed rails raised, especially for elderly patients.
• In overdosage, CNS and respiratory depression should be treated same as barbiturate intoxication; ethinamate is dialyzable.
• May cause falsely elevated urinary 17-ketosteroid (modified Zimmerman reaction) and 17-hydroxycorticosteroid levels (Porter-Silber test).
• Prolonged therapy not recommended; drug is not effective for more than 7 days.

Interactions:
CIMETIDINE: increased sedation. Monitor carefully.

Special considerations:
• Use cautiously in patients with impaired hepatic or renal function, mental depression, suicidal tendencies, or history of drug abuse. Use caution and low end of dosage range for elderly or debilitated patients.
• Patients who are depressed, suicidal, or drug-dependent, or who have a history of drug abuse should be prevented from hoarding or self-overdosing. Patient should be warned that alcohol increases effects of drug. Activities requiring alertness or skill should be avoided until CNS response is determined.
• Patient's cigarettes should be removed after taking dose.
• Walking should be supervised and bed rails raised, especially for elderly patients.

Interactions:
ALCOHOL OR OTHER CNS DEPRESSANTS, INCLUDING OTHER NARCOTIC ANALGESICS: excessive CNS depression. Use together cautiously.

Special considerations:
• Contraindicated in uncontrolled pain, severe renal impairment, and porphyria. Use cautiously in patients with mental depression, suicidal tendencies, history of drug abuse, prostatic hypertrophy, stenosing peptic ulcer, pyloroduodenal or bladder neck obstruction, narrow-angle glaucoma, cardiac arrhythmias.
• Drug is effective for short-term use only.
• Walking should be supervised and bed rails

(continued on following page)

NAMES, INDICATIONS AND DOSAGES	SIDE EFFECTS
glutethimide *(continued)* exceed 1 g. **Preoperatively:** ADULTS: 500 mg night before surgery; 500 mg to 1 g 1 hour before anesthestic. **First stage of labor:** 500 mg at onset of labor; repeat once if necessary. **Sedative:** ADULTS: 125 to 250 mg t.i.d. after meals.	**CNS:** *residual sedation,* paradoxical excitation, headache, vertigo. **EENT:** dry mouth, blurred vision. **GI:** irritation, nausea, diarrhea. **GU:** bladder atony. **Skin:** rashes, urticaria.
hexobarbital Controlled Substance Schedule III Sombulex **Sedation:** ADULTS: 250 mg P.O., repeated as needed, q 2 to 3 hours. **Insomnia:** ADULTS: 250 to 500 mg P.O. at bedtime.	**CNS:** *drowsiness, lethargy, hangover,* paradoxical excitement in elderly patients. **GI:** nausea, vomiting. **Skin:** rash, urticaria. **Other:** *Stevens-Johnson syndrome,* angioedema.
mephobarbital Controlled Substance Schedule IV Mebaral♦ **Sedation:** ADULTS: 32 to 100 mg P.O. t.i.d. to q.i.d. CHILDREN: 16 to 32 mg P.O. t.i.d. to q.i.d. *Incipient or active delirium tremens*—200 mg P.O. t.i.d.	**CNS:** drowsiness, vertigo, headache, depression, residual sedation after hypnotic dose, paradoxical excitement. **GI:** nausea, vomiting, diarrhea. **Skin:** hypersensitivity reactions, jaundice. **Other:** respiratory depression, apnea; discontinuance of hypnotic doses may induce nightmares or insomnia.

INTERACTIONS AND SPECIAL CONSIDERATIONS

raised, especially for elderly patients.
- Patient's cigarettes should be removed after taking dose.
- Patients who are depressed, suicidal, or drug-dependent, or who have a history of drug abuse should be prevented from hoarding or self-overdosing. Patient should be warned that alcohol increases effects of drug. Activities requiring alertness or skill should be avoided for 7 to 8 hours after receiving this drug.
- Abrupt withdrawal may produce nausea, vomiting, nervousness, tremors, chills, fever, nightmares, insomnia, tachycardia, delirium, numbness of extremities, hallucinations, dysphagia, convulsions. Should be withdrawn gradually.
- Prothrombin times should be monitored when patient on glutethimide starts or ends anticoagulant therapy. Anticoagulant dose may need to be adjusted.

Interactions:

ALCOHOL OR OTHER CNS DEPRESSANTS, INCLUDING OTHER NARCOTIC ANALGESICS: excessive CNS and respiratory depression. Do not use together.

MAO INHIBITORS: inhibit metabolism of barbiturates; may cause prolonged CNS depression. Reduce barbiturate dosage.

RIFAMPIN: may decrease barbiturate levels. Monitor for decreased effect.

Special considerations:

- Contraindicated in patients with uncontrolled severe pain, respiratory disease with dyspnea or obstruction, hypersensitivity to barbiturates, previous addiction to sedatives, and porphyria. Use with caution in hepatic or renal impairment.
- May be used preoperatively with atropine when morphine contraindicated.
- Because barbiturates potentiate narcotics, dose should be reduced when given during labor. Excessive dose may cause respiratory depression in neonate.
- Patient's cigarettes should be removed if he receives hypnotic dose.
- Walking should be supervised and bed rails raised, especially for elderly patients.
- Long-term high dosage may cause drug dependence and severe withdrawal symptoms. Barbiturates should be withdrawn gradually.
- Patients who are depressed, suicidal, or drug-dependent, or who have a history of drug abuse should be prevented from hoarding or self overdosing. Patient should be warned that alcohol increases effects of drug. Activities requiring alertness or skill should be avoided until CNS response is determined.
- Monitor prothrombin times when patient on hexobarbital starts or ends anticoagulant therapy. Anticoagulant dose may need to be adjusted.
- Signs of toxicity: coma, pupillary constriction (pupillary dilation with severe poisoning), clammy skin, hypotension. Overdose can be fatal.
- For treatment of toxicity, see APPENDIX.

Interactions:

ALCOHOL OR OTHER CNS DEPRESSANTS, INCLUDING OTHER NARCOTIC ANALGESICS: excessive CNS and respiratory depression. Do not use together.

MAO INHIBITORS: inhibit metabolism of barbiturates; may cause prolonged CNS depression. Reduce barbiturate dosage.

RIFAMPIN: may decrease barbiturate levels. Monitor for decreased effect.

Special considerations:

- Contraindicated in patients with uncontrolled severe pain, respiratory disease with dyspnea or obstruction, hypersensitivity to barbiturates, previous addiction to sedatives, and porphyria. Use with caution in hepatic or renal impairment, or impaired cardiac or respiratory function.
- Cigarettes should be removed if patient receives hypnotic dose.
- Walking should be supervised and bed rails raised, especially for elderly patients.
- Long-term high dosage may cause drug dependence and severe withdrawal symptoms. Barbiturates should be withdrawn gradually.
- Patients who are depressed, suicidal, or drug-dependent, or who have a history of drug abuse should be prevented from hoarding or self overdosing. Patient should be warned that alcohol increases effects of drug. Activities requiring alertness or skill should be avoided until CNS response is determined.
- Mephobarbital is metabolized to phenobarbital, the active agent.
- Prothrombin times should be monitored carefully when patient on mephobarbital starts or ends anticoagulant therapy. Anticoagulant dose may need adjustment.
- Toxicity possible.
- For treatment of toxicity, see APPENDIX.

NAMES, INDICATIONS AND DOSAGES	SIDE EFFECTS
methaqualone Mequin, Quaalude **methaqualone hydrochloride** Controlled Substance Schedule II Parest, Parest 400, Rouqualone♦♦, Sedalone♦♦, Somnafac, Somnafac Forte, Triador♦♦, Tualone♦♦, Vitalone♦♦ **Sedation (methaqualone):** ADULTS: 75 mg P.O. t.i.d. or q.i.d. **Insomnia (methaqualone):** ADULTS: 150 to 300 P.O. at bedtime. **Insomnia (methaqualone hydrochloride):** ADULTS: 200 to 400 mg P.O. at bedtime.	**CNS:** headache, dizziness, fatigue, residual sedation, *transient paresthesias of extremities,* restlessness, anxiety. **EENT:** dry mouth. **GI:** anorexia, *nausea, vomiting,* epigastric discomfort.
methotrimeprazine hydrochloride Levoprome, Nozinan♦♦ **Postoperative analgesia:** ADULTS AND CHILDREN OVER 12 YEARS: initially, 2.5 to 7.5 mg I.M. q 4 to 6 hours, then adjust dose. **Preanesthetic medication:** ADULTS AND CHILDREN OVER 12 YEARS: 2 to 20 mg I.M. 45 minutes to 3 hours before surgery. **Sedation, analgesia:** ADULTS AND CHILDREN OVER 12 YEARS: 10 to 20 mg deep I.M. q 4 to 6 hours as required. ELDERLY: 5 to 10 mg I.M. q 4 to 6 hours.	**Blood:** agranulocytosis and other dyscrasias after long-term high dosage. **CNS:** *orthostatic hypotension, fainting, weakness, dizziness,* drowsiness, excessive sedation, amnesia, disorientation, euphoria, headache, slurred speech. **CV:** *drop in blood pressure,* palpitations. **EENT:** dry mouth, nasal congestion. **GI:** nausea, vomiting, abdominal discomfort. **GU:** difficulty urinating. **Local:** *pain, inflammation, swelling at injection site.*
methyprylon Controlled Substance Schedule III Noludar♦ **Insomnia:** ADULTS: 200 to 400 mg P.O. 15 minutes before bedtime. CHILDREN OVER 3 MONTHS: 50 mg P.O. at bedtime, increased to 200 mg, if necessary. Maximum 400 mg/day.	**CNS:** morning drowsiness, dizziness, headache, paradoxical excitation. **GI:** nausea, vomiting, diarrhea, esophagitis. **Skin:** rash.
paraldehyde Controlled Substance Schedule IV Paral **Sedation:** ADULTS: 4 to 10 ml P.O. or rectally; or 5 ml deep I.M. in upper outer quadrant of buttock. 3 to 5 ml I.V. (in emergency only).	**CV:** *I.V. administration may cause pulmonary edema or hemorrhage,* dilation of right side of heart, circulatory collapse. **GI:** irritation, *foul breath odor.* **GU:** nephrosis with prolonged use. **Skin:** *erythematous rash.* **Local:** *pain,* sterile abscesses, sloughing of skin, fat necrosis, muscular irritation, nerve damage

♦ Available in U.S. and Canada. ♦♦ Available in Canada only.
All other products (no symbol) available in U.S. only. Italicized side effects are common or life-threatening.

INTERACTIONS AND SPECIAL CONSIDERATIONS

Interactions:
ALCOHOL OR OTHER CNS DEPRESSANTS, INCLUDING OTHER NARCOTIC ANALGESICS: excessive CNS depression. Use together cautiously.

Special considerations:
- Contraindicated in patients with history of drug abuse. Use cautiously in patients with hepatic impairment, mental depression, or suicidal tendencies.
- Cigarettes should be removed if patient receives hypnotic dose.
- Walking should be supervised and bed rails raised, especially for elderly patients.
- Patient should be warned that alcohol increases effects of drug. Activities requiring alertness or skill should be avoided until CNS response is determined.
- Switching from another hypnotic to methaqualone requires 5 to 7 consecutive nights of therapy to obtain satisfactory hypnotic effect.
- Prolonged administration of methaqualone is not recommended; drug not shown to be effective more than 14 days.
- One of major drugs of abuse on the street. Because of high abuse potential, methaqualone is rarely clinically indicated.
- For symptoms and treatment of toxicity, see APPENDIX.

Interactions:
ALL ANTIHYPERTENSIVE AGENTS: increase orthostatic hypotension. Don't use together.

Special considerations:
- Contraindicated in patients receiving concurrent antihypertensive drug therapy, including MAO inhibitors; also, in history of convulsive disorders; hypersensitivity to phenothiazines; severe cardiac, hepatic, or renal disease; previous overdose of CNS depressant; coma. Use with extreme caution in elderly or debilitated patient with heart disease or in any patient who may suffer serious consequences from a sudden drop in blood pressure.
- Low initial dose should be used in susceptible patient and increased gradually while frequently checking pulse rate, blood pressure, and circulation.
- Blood pressure drops 10 to 20 minutes after I.M. injection.
- Patient should be kept in bed or closely supervised for 6 to 12 hours after each of the first several injections because of orthostatic hypotension. Severe hypotension should be combated with phenylephrine, methoxamine, or levarterenol—not epinephrine.
- Should not be used for longer than 30 days except in terminal illness or when narcotics are contraindicated.
- In prolonged use, liver function and blood studies should be monitored periodically.
- I.M. should be injected into large muscle masses and sites rotated. Should not be administered subcutaneously, as local irritation results. I.V. injection not advised.
- May be mixed in same syringe with reduced dose of atropine and scopolamine. Should not be mixed with other drugs. Protect solution from light.

No significant interactions.

Special considerations:
- Contraindicated in intermittent porphyria. Use cautiously in patients with renal or hepatic impairment.
- Periodic blood counts are advisable during repeated or long-term use.
- Long-term high dosage may cause drug dependence and severe life-threatening withdrawal symptoms. Withdrawal should be gradual and closely monitored.
- Patients who are depressed, suicidal, or drug-dependent, or who have a history of drug abuse should be prevented from hoarding or self overdosing. Patient should be warned that alcohol increases effects of drug. Activities requiring alertness or skill should be avoided until CNS response determined.
- Patient's cigarettes should be removed after taking dose.
- Walking should be supervised and bed rails raised, especially for elderly patients.
- Value of this drug as a sedative has not been established.
- Overdosage symptoms include somnolence, confusion, constricted pupils, respiratory depression, hypotension, coma. Hemodialysis is useful in severe intoxication.
- For treatment of toxicity, see APPENDIX.

Interactions:
ALCOHOL: excessive CNS depression. Use with caution.
DISULFIRAM (ANTABUSE): increase in paraldehyde and acetaldehyde blood levels. Use together cautiously. May produce toxic disulfiram reaction.

Special considerations:
- Contraindicated in bronchopulmonary disease or gastroenteritis with ulceration. Use cautiously in patients with hepatic impairment.
- Rectal dose should be given in olive oil or cottonseed oil as retention enema: 1 part paraldehyde, 2 parts oil, and 200 ml 0.9% sodium chloride solution.

(continued on following page)

NAMES, INDICATIONS AND DOSAGES	SIDE EFFECTS
paraldehyde *(continued)* CHILDREN: 0.15 ml/kg P.O., rectally, or deep I.M. **Insomnia:** ADULTS: 10 to 30 ml P.O. or rectally; 10 ml I.M. or I.V. CHILDREN: 0.3 ml/kg P.O., rectally, deep I.M. **Alcohol withdrawal syndrome:** ADULTS: 5 to 10 ml P.O. or rectally; or 5 ml deep I.M. q 4 to 6 hours for the first 24 hours, not to exceed a total of 60 ml P.O. or 30 ml I.M.; then q 6 hours on following days, not to exceed 40 ml P.O. or 20 ml/24 hours I.M. **Tetanus:** ADULTS: 4 to 5 ml I.V. (well diluted) or 12 ml (diluted 1:10) by gastric tube q 4 hours, p.r.n.; 5 to 10 ml I.M., p.r.n. to control seizures.	at I.M. injection site (if injection is near nerve trunk). **Other:** *respiratory depression.*
pentobarbital Controlled Substance Schedule II Nebralin **pentobarbital sodium** Maso-Pent, Nembutal Sodium♦, Nova-Rectal♦♦, Penital, Pentogen♦♦ **Sedation:** ADULTS: 20 to 40 mg P.O. b.i.d., t.i.d., or q.i.d. CHILDREN: 6 mg/kg/day P.O. in divided doses. **Insomnia:** ADULTS: 100 to 200 mg P.O. at bedtime or 150 to 200 mg deep I.M.; 100 mg initially, I.V., then additional doses up to 500 mg; 120 to 200 mg rectally. CHILDREN: 3 to 5 mg/kg I.M. Maximum dose: 100 mg. Rectal dosages: 2 months to 1 year, 30 mg; 1 to 4 years, 30 to 60 mg; 5 to 12 years, 60 mg; 12 to 14 years, 60 to 120 mg. **Preanesthetic medication:** ADULTS: 150 to 200 mg I.M. or P.O. in 2 divided doses.	**CNS:** *drowsiness, lethargy, hangover,* paradoxical excitement in elderly patients. **GI:** nausea, vomiting. **Skin:** rash, urticaria. **Other:** *Stevens-Johnson syndrome,* angioedema.
phenobarbital Barbipil, Barbita, Eskabarb♦, Gardenal♦, Henomint, Luminal♦, Orprine, PBR 12, SK-Phenobarbital, Solfoton, Solu-barb, Stental	**CNS:** *drowsiness, lethargy, hangover,* paradoxical excitement in elderly patients. **GI:** nausea, vomiting. **Skin:** rash, urticaria. **Local:** pain, swelling, thrombophlebitis, necro-

INTERACTIONS AND SPECIAL CONSIDERATIONS

• Oral dose should be diluted with iced juice or milk to mask taste and odor and to reduce GI distress.
• Fresh supply should be used; bottles should be discarded if opened more than 24 hours. Should not be used if liquid has a brownish color, vinegary odor, or contains a precipitate.
• Drug reacts with plastic. Liquid should not be put in Styrofoam cup, and glass syringe should be used for parenteral dose.
• I.M. injection should be given deeply, away from nerve trunks, and injection site massaged. No more than 5 ml should be given per injection site.
• Respiratory depression possible, especially with repeated doses.
• Long-term high dosage may cause drug dependence and severe withdrawal symptoms. Should be withdrawn gradually, with close monitoring.
• Cigarettes should be removed if patient receives hypnotic dose.
• Walking should be supervised and bed rails raised, especially for elderly patients.
• Patient's room should be ventilated well to remove exhaled paraldehyde.
• No analgesic effect. May produce excitement or delirium in presence of pain.
• Oral or rectal administration of decomposed paraldehyde may cause severe corrosion of stomach or rectum.

Interactions:
ALCOHOL OR OTHER CNS DEPRESSANTS, INCLUDING OTHER NARCOTIC ANALGESICS: excessive CNS and respiratory depression. Do not use together.
MAO INHIBITORS: inhibit metabolism of barbiturates; may cause prolonged CNS depression. Reduce barbiturate dosage.
RIFAMPIN: may decrease barbiturate levels. Monitor for decreased effect.

Special considerations:
• Contraindicated in patients with uncontrolled severe pain, respiratory disease with dyspnea or obstruction, hypersensitivity to barbiturates, previous addiction to sedatives, and porphyria. Use with caution in hepatic or renal impairment.
• Injection solution should be used within 30 minutes after opening container to minimize deterioration. Cloudy solution should not be used.
• Parenteral solution alkaline. Extravasation may cause tissue necrosis.
• I.V. injection should be reserved for emergency treatment and given under close supervision. Should be prepared to give artificial respiration.
• I.M. injection should be administered deeply. Superficial injection may cause pain, sterile abscess, and sloughing.
• Should not be mixed with any other medication.
• Because barbiturates potentiate narcotics, dose should be reduced when given during labor. Excessive dose may cause respiratory depression in neonate.
• Cigarettes should be removed if patient receives hypnotic dose.
• Walking should be supervised and bed rails raised, especially for elderly patients.
• Long-term high dosage may cause drug dependence and severe withdrawal symptoms. Barbiturates should be withdrawn gradually.
• Patients who are depressed, suicidal, or drug-dependent, or who have a history of drug abuse should be prevented from hoarding or self-overdosing. Patient should be warned that alcohol increases effects of drug. Activities requiring alertness or skill should be avoided until CNS response is determined.
• No analgesic effect. May cause restlessness or delirium in presence of pain.
• Monitor prothrombin times when patient on pentobarbital starts or ends anticoagulant therapy. Anticoagulant dose may need to be adjusted.
• Signs of barbiturate toxicity: coma, pupillary constriction, cyanosis, clammy skin, hypotension. Overdose can be fatal.
• To ensure accurate dosage, rectal suppositories should not be divided.
• Nembutal sodium contains tartrazine dye; may cause allergic reactions in susceptible persons.
• For treatment of toxicity, see APPENDIX.

Interactions:
ALCOHOL OR OTHER CNS DEPRESSANTS, INCLUDING OTHER NARCOTIC ANALGESICS: excessive CNS and respiratory depression. Do not use together.
MAO INHIBITORS: inhibit metabolism of barbiturates; may cause prolonged CNS depression. Reduce barbiturate dosage.
RIFAMPIN: may decrease barbiturate levels. Monitor for decreased effect.

(continued on following page)

NAMES, INDICATIONS AND DOSAGES	SIDE EFFECTS

phenobarbital
(continued)

sis, nerve injury.
Other: *Stevens-Johnson syndrome*, angioedema.

phenobarbital sodium
Controlled Substance Schedule IV
Luminal Sodium♦

Sedation:
ADULTS: 30 to 120 mg P.O. daily in 2 or 3 divided doses.
CHILDREN: 6 mg/kg P.O. divided t.i.d.

Insomnia:
ADULTS: 100 to 320 mg P.O. or I.M.
CHILDREN: 3 to 6 mg/kg.

Preoperative sedation:
ADULTS: 100 to 200 mg I.M. 60 to 90 minutes before surgery.
CHILDREN: 16 to 100 mg I.M. 60 to 90 minutes before surgery.

Hyperbilirubinemia:
NEONATES: 7 mg/kg/day P.O. from first to fifth day of life, or 5 mg/kg/day I.M. on first day, repeated P.O. on second to seventh days.

Chronic cholestasis:
ADULTS: 90 to 180 mg P.O. daily in 2 or 3 divided doses.
CHILDREN UNDER 12 YEARS: 3 to 12 mg/kg/day P.O. in 2 or 3 divided doses.

---

propiomazine hydrochloride
Largon

Sedation:
ADULTS: 20 to 40 mg I.M. or I.V.

Preoperatively; during surgery; with local, nerve block, or spinal anesthetic:
ADULTS: 10 to 20 mg I.M. or I.V.

Obstetrics:
ADULTS: 20 to 40 mg I.M. or I.V. during early stages of labor, repeated q 3 hours, if necessary.

Sedation the night before surgery as a preanesthetic, or postoperatively:
CHILDREN UNDER 27 KG: 0.55 to 1.1 mg/kg I.M. or I.V.
CHILDREN 6 TO 12 YEARS: 25 mg I.M. or I.V. in a single dose.
CHILDREN 4 TO 6 YEARS: 15 mg I.M. or I.V. in a single dose.

CNS: dizziness, confusion, amnesia (primarily in the elderly), restlessness.
CV: tachycardia, rise in blood pressure, transient hypotension with rapid I.V. infusion.
EENT: dry mouth.
GI: distress.
Skin: rashes.
Local: vein irritation and thrombophlebitis after I.V. injection.
Other: respiratory depression.

---

secobarbital
Seconal
secobarbital sodium
Controlled Substance Schedule II
Secogen Sodium♦♦, Seconal Sodium♦, Seral♦♦

CNS: *drowsiness, lethargy, hangover*, paradoxical excitement in elderly patients.
GI: nausea, vomiting.
Skin: rash, urticaria.
Other: *Stevens-Johnson syndrome*, angioedema.

♦ Available in U.S. and Canada. ♦♦ Available in Canada only.
All other products (no symbol) available in U.S. only. Italicized side effects are common or life-threatening.

INTERACTIONS AND SPECIAL CONSIDERATIONS

PRIMIDONE: monitor for excessive phenobarbital blood levels.

Special considerations:

• Contraindicated in patients with uncontrolled severe pain, respiratory disease with dyspnea or obstruction, hypersensitivity to barbiturates, previous addiction to sedatives, and porphyria. Use with caution in patients with impaired hepatic, renal, cardiac, or respiratory function; hyperthyroidism; diabetes mellitus; anemia; and in elderly or debilitated patients.
• Injection solution should be used within 30 minutes after opening container to minimize deterioration. Cloudy solution should not be used.
• I.V. injection should be reserved for emergency treatment and given under close supervision. Should be prepared to give artificial respiration.
• When given I.V., should not be given more than 60 mg/minute.
• I.M. injection should be given deeply. Superficial injection may cause pain, sterile abscess, and sloughing.
• Because barbiturates potentiate narcotics, dose should be reduced when given during labor. Excessive dose may cause respiratory depression in neonate.
• Cigarettes should be removed if patient receives hypnotic dose.
• Walking should be supervised and bed rails raised, especially for elderly patients.
• Long-term high dosage may cause drug dependence and severe withdrawal symptoms. Barbiturates should be withdrawn gradually.
• Patients who are depressed, suicidal, or drug-dependent, or who have a history of drug abuse should be prevented from hoarding or self-overdosing. Patient should be warned that alcohol increases effects of drug. Activities requiring alertness or skill should be avoided until CNS response is determined.
• No analgesic action. May cause restlessness or delirium in presence of pain.
• Monitor prothrombin times when patient on phenobarbital starts or ends anticoagulant therapy. Anticoagulant dose may need to be adjusted.
• Signs of barbiturate toxicity: coma, pupillary constriction, cyanosis, clammy skin, hypotension. Overdose can be fatal.
• For treatment of toxicity, see APPENDIX.

No significant interactions.

Special considerations:

• Contraindicated if patients have received large doses of other CNS depressants or are comatose. Use extreme caution in patients with hypertensive crisis.
• I.V. injection should be given slowly to avoid transient fall in blood pressure.
• Should be injected in large, undamaged vein to minimize irritation. Extravasation should be avoided. Should not be injected into artery; irritation may cause severe arteriospasm, impaired circulation, and gangrene.
• Should not be given subcutaneously.
• Solution for injection should not be used if it is cloudy or contains a precipitate.
• Antiemetic effect may mask signs of drug overdose or other disorders.
• Patient should be warned about increased effects of alcohol, tranquilizers, antihistamines, and other CNS depressants and against performing hazardous activities requiring alertness or skill.
• Walking should be supervised and bed rails raised, especially in elderly patients.
• Propiomazine reverses vasopressor effect of epinephrine. Use norepinephrine when vasopressor effect needed.

Interactions:

ALCOHOL OR OTHER CNS DEPRESSANTS, INCLUDING OTHER NARCOTIC ANALGESICS: excessive CNS and respiratory depression. Do not use together.

MAO INHIBITORS: inhibit metabolism of barbiturates; may cause prolonged CNS depression. Reduce barbiturate dosage.

RIFAMPIN: may decrease barbiturate levels. Monitor for decreased effect.

(continued on following page)

NAMES, INDICATIONS AND DOSAGES	SIDE EFFECTS
secobarbital *(continued)* **Sedation, preoperatively:** ADULTS: 200 to 300 mg P.O. 1 to 2 hours before surgery. CHILDREN: 50 to 100 mg P.O. or 4 to 5 mg/kg rectally 1 to 2 hours before surgery. **Insomnia:** ADULTS: 100 to 200 mg P.O. or I.M. CHILDREN: 3 to 5 mg/kg I.M., not to exceed 100 mg, with no more than 5 ml injected in any one site. 4 to 5 mg/kg rectally. **Acute tetanus convulsion:** ADULTS AND CHILDREN: 5.5 mg/kg I.M. or slow I.V., repeated q 3 to 4 hours, if needed; I.V. injection rate not to exceed 50 mg/15 seconds. **Acute psychotic agitation:** ADULTS: 50 mg/minute I.V. up to 250 mg I.V. initially, additional doses given cautiously after 5 minutes if desired response is not obtained. Not to exceed 500 mg total. **Status epilepticus:** ADULTS AND CHILDREN: 250 to 350 mg I.M. or I.V.	
talbutal Controlled Substance Schedule III Lotusate **Insomnia:** ADULTS: 120 mg P.O. at bedtime.	**CNS:** *drowsiness, lethargy, hangover,* paradoxical excitement in elderly patients. **GI:** nausea, vomiting. **Skin:** rash, urticaria. **Other:** *Stevens-Johnson syndrome,* angioedema.
temazepam Controlled Substance Schedule IV Restoril **Insomnia:** ADULTS: 15 to 30 mg P.O. at bedtime.	**CNS:** *drowsiness, dizziness, lethargy,* disturbed coordination, daytime sedation, confusion. **GI:** anorexia, diarrhea.

♦ Available in U.S. and Canada. ♦♦ Available in Canada only.
All other products (no symbol) available in U.S. only. Italicized side effects are common or life-threatening.

INTERACTIONS AND SPECIAL CONSIDERATIONS

Special considerations:

• Contraindicated in patients with uncontrolled severe pain, respiratory disease with dyspnea or obstruction, hypersensitivity to barbiturates, previous addiction to sedatives, and porphyria. Use with caution in patients with hepatic or renal impairment; also, in pregnant women with toxemia or history of bleeding.

• Injection solution should be used within 30 minutes after opening container to minimize deterioration. Don't use cloudy solution.

• I.V. injection reserved for emergency treatment and given under close supervision. Be prepared to give artificial respiration.

• I.M. injection should be given deeply. Superficial injection may cause pain, sterile abscess, and sloughing.

• Because barbiturates potentiate narcotics, dose should be reduced when given during labor. Excessive dose may cause respiratory depression in neonate.

• Cigarettes should be removed if patient receives hypnotic dose.

• Walking should be supervised and bed rails raised, especially for elderly patients.

• Long-term high dosage may cause drug dependence and severe withdrawal symptoms. Barbiturates should be withdrawn gradually.

• Prevent patients who are depressed, suicidal, or drug-dependent, or who have a history of drug abuse from hoarding or self-overdosing. Warn patient that alcohol increases effects of drug. Activities requiring alertness should be avoided until CNS response determined.

• If patient has renal insufficiency, sterile drug reconstituted with sterile water for injection should be used. Commercial solution containing polyethylene glycol should be avoided; may irritate kidneys.

• Refrigerate secobarbital in polyethylene glycol. Secobarbital sodium injection not compatible with lactated Ringer's solution.

• Sterile secobarbital sodium compatible with Ringer's injection and normal saline solution. Don't mix with acidic solutions. To reconstitute, rotate ampule; don't shake.

• Prothrombin times should be monitored when patient on secobarbital starts or ends anticoagulant therapy. Anticoagulant dose may need to be adjusted.

• Signs of barbiturate toxicity: coma, pupillary constriction, cyanosis, clammy skin, hypotension. Overdose can be fatal.

• For treatment of toxicity, see APPENDIX.

Interactions:

ALCOHOL OR OTHER CNS DEPRESSANTS, INCLUDING OTHER NARCOTIC ANALGESICS: excessive CNS and respiratory depression. Don't use together.

MAO INHIBITORS: inhibit the metabolism of barbiturates; may cause prolonged CNS depression. Reduce barbiturate dosage.

RIFAMPIN: may decrease barbiturate levels. Monitor for decreased effect.

Special considerations:

• Contraindicated in patients with uncontrolled severe pain, respiratory disease with dyspnea or obstruction, hypersensitivity to barbiturates, previous addiction to sedatives, and porphyria. Use with caution in hepatic or renal impairment.

• With hypnotic dose, remove patient's cigarettes.

• Walking should be supervised and bed rails raised, especially for elderly patients.

• Long-term high dosage may cause drug dependence and severe withdrawal symptoms. Barbiturates should be withdrawn gradually.

• Prevent patients who are depressed, suicidal, or drug-dependent, or who have a history of drug abuse from hoarding or self-overdosing. Alcohol increases effects of drug. Activities requiring alertness or skill should be avoided until CNS response is determined.

• Prothrombin times should be monitored carefully when patient on talbutal starts or ends anticoagulant therapy. Anticoagulant dose may need to be adjusted.

• Signs of barbiturate toxicity: coma, pupillary constriction, cyanosis, clammy skin, hypotension. Overdose can be fatal.

• For treatment of toxicity, see APPENDIX.

No significant interactions.

Special considerations:

• Use cautiously in impaired hepatic or renal function; in patients with mental depression or suicidal tendencies; and in patients with history of drug abuse. Use caution and low end of dosage range for elderly or debilitated patients.

• Patients who are depressed, suicidal, or drug-dependent, or who have a history of drug abuse should be prevented from hoarding or self-overdosing. Patients should be warned about increased alcohol effects and against hazardous activity requiring alertness or skill.

• Remove cigarettes of patient receiving drug.

• Walking should be supervised and bed rails raised, especially for elderly patients.

• The newest benzodiazepine derivative.

• May have less residual sedative effects (hangover) the next day than flurazepam and diazepam. Relatively short acting.

NAMES, INDICATIONS AND DOSAGES	SIDE EFFECTS
triclofos sodium Triclos **Insomnia:** ADULTS: 1.5 g P.O. 15 to 20 minutes before bedtime. **To induce sleep in EEG:** CHILDREN UNDER 12 YEARS: 22 mg/kg P.O.	**CNS:** light-headedness, dizziness, hangover, *drowsiness*, headache, ataxia. **GI:** *nausea*, vomiting, flatulence, bad taste in mouth. **Skin:** hypersensitivity reactions.

♦ Available in U.S. and Canada. ♦♦ Available in Canada only.
All other products (no symbol) available in U.S. only. Italicized side effects are common or life-threatening.

INTERACTIONS AND SPECIAL CONSIDERATIONS

Interactions:
ALCOHOL OR OTHER CNS DEPRESSANTS, INCLUDING OTHER NARCOTIC ANALGESICS: excessive CNS depression or vasodilation. Use together cautiously.
FUROSEMIDE I.V.: possible sweating, flushes, variable blood pressure, uneasiness. Use together cautiously.

Special considerations:
- Contraindicated in patients with hepatic or renal impairment, hypersensitivity to triclofos sodium or chloral hydrate, and in women in labor. Use with caution in patients with cardiac arrhythmias, severe cardiac disease, mental depression, suicidal tendencies, or drug dependency.
- In prolonged use, blood and liver function should be monitored periodically.
- Should be withdrawn slowly after prolonged use to avoid delirium, tremors, hallucinations.
- Patients who are depressed, suicidal, or drug-dependent, or who have a history of drug abuse should be prevented from hoarding or self-overdosing. Patient should be warned that alcohol increases effects of drug. Activities requiring alertness or skill should be avoided until CNS response is determined.
- Walking should be supervised and bed rails raised, especially for elderly patients.
- May cause false-positive results in glycosuria tests using cupric sulfate as Benedict's or Fehling's solution. Clinitest, Clinistix, or Tes-Tape should be used.
- May interfere with fluorometric tests for urine catecholamines and Reddy, Jenkins, Thorn test for urinary 17-hydroxycorticosteroids. Drug should not be administered for 48 hours before fluorometric test.
- Prothrombin times should be monitored carefully when patient on triclofos starts or ends anticoagulant therapy. Anticoagulant dose may need to be adjusted.

WHAT YOU SHOULD KNOW ABOUT METHAQUALONE ABUSE

Since its introduction in 1965, methaqualone has become one of the ten most abused drugs in the United States, according to the Federal Bureau of Narcotics and Dangerous Drugs.

Abusers find methaqualone more enjoyable and satisfying than barbiturates because it:
- produces rapid, long-lasting effects
- reduces inhibitions in social situations
- promotes a perpetual state of sedation that eases life's pressures
- substitutes for narcotics when they're not available.

Several years after its introduction, methaqualone was classified as a controlled substance. Quaalude, the most publicized brand of methaqualone, had become notorious, so many doctors stopped prescribing it and many pharmacists avoided stocking it.

Now Quaalude's manufacturer—Lemmon Company—is marketing a new brand of methaqualone: Mequin. Mequin is an alternative for doctors and pharmacists who prefer not to handle the widely abused Quaalude. (*Note:* Mequin and Quaalude are chemically and therapeutically identical.)

Meanwhile, methaqualone abuse has increased. (In 1980, methaqualone abuse was up 1.3% from 1979.) Since methaqualone overdose can result in deep coma or even death, be alert for these symptoms:
- depressed respiratory and cardiovascular activity
- increased muscle tone (ranging from hypertonia and muscle spasms to tonic-clonic convulsions)
- increased salivation
- possible increased pupil reaction to light and rapid changes in pupil size
- vomiting
- lack of response to auditory stimulus or pain. High doses can increase a person's pain threshold, so that he is unaware of injury and its resulting pain. Some users may have a sense of indestructibility.

If a patient's coming out of a coma, he may experience excitation again. Complications may include:
- oliguria
- renal failure
- toxic polyneuropathy
- myocardial damage
- cutaneous, gastrointestinal, or retinal hemorrhage
- facial or pulmonary edema.

29

Anticonvulsants

acetazolamide
acetazolamide sodium
bromides
carbamazepine
clonazepam
diazepam
ethosuximide
ethotoin
magnesium sulfate
mephenytoin
mephobarbital
metharbital
methsuximide
paraldehyde
paramethadione
phenacemide
phenobarbital
phenobarbital sodium
phensuximide
phenytoin sodium (extended)
phenytoin sodium (prompt)
primidone
trimethadione
valproic acid
valproate sodium

Each anticonvulsant has indications for specific seizure disorders. Frequently, these drugs are used in combination for complex or mixed seizure disorders. Seizures may be of unknown origin (idiopathic) or secondary to some organic or acquired condition. When the etiology of seizures is known, therapy is often aimed at the underlying cause as well.

Major uses
Anticonvulsants prevent or reduce the frequency or severity of seizures of idiopathic epilepsy, or seizures secondary to drugs, hypoglycemia, hypomagnesemia, meningitis, eclampsia, encephalitis, alcohol withdrawal, or accident-related brain injury.

Mechanism of action
• Acetazolamide may inhibit carbonic anhydrase in the central nervous system (CNS) and decrease abnormal paroxysmal or excessive neuronal discharge.

HELPING A PATIENT DURING A GRAND MAL SEIZURE

To see the patient through the various stages of a grand mal seizure, follow these guidelines:

At onset:
• Place a stat stick or a padded tongue depressor between the patient's teeth *before* they're clenched, to keep him from biting his tongue. (After the patient has clenched his teeth, don't try to force anything between them.)
• Maintain an airway.
• Protect him from injury.
• Cushion his head, and turn it to the side.

During the *tonic phase,* the patient's teeth are clenched and his muscles are constantly tensed or contracted.

Next, the *clonic phase* appears; the patient experiences continuous and rapid spasms, with alternating relaxed and rigid states.

When the seizure is over:
• Place the patient in semiprone position or on his side, to keep his airway open.
• Watch him carefully until he's consciouo again.
• Allow him to rest: many patients are lethargic and sleepy after a seizure.

THERAPEUTIC ACTIVITY

THERAPEUTIC ACTIVITY OF COMMON ANTICONVULSANTS

DRUG	BLOOD LEVELS (mcg/ml)	HALF-LIFE	TIME TO REACH STEADY STATE*
carbamazepine	6 to 8	7 to 30 hr	2 to 4 days
clonazepam	0.013 to 0.072	20 to 30 hr	5 to 10 days
ethosuximide	40 to 80	2 to 3 days	5 to 8 days
methsuximide	0.1	2 to 4 hr	8 to 16 hr
phenobarbital	10 to 35	2 to 4 days	14 to 21 days
phenytoin	10 to 20	24 hr	5 to 10 days
primidone	6 to 12	3 to 12 hr	4 to 7 days
trimethadione	6 to 41	12 to 24 hr	2 to 5 days
valproic acid	50 to 100	5 to 20 hr	2 to 4 days

*Steady-state blood levels are achieved if the patient is initially given maintenance therapy rather than a loading dose.

• Barbiturate derivatives depress monosynaptic and polysynaptic transmission in the CNS and increase the threshold for seizure activity in the motor cortex.
• Benzodiazepine derivatives appear to act on the limbic system, thalamus, and hypothalamus to produce anticonvulsant effects.
• Bromides depress all nerve tissue, but their exact mechanism of CNS depression is unknown.
• Carbamazepine and paraldehyde's mechanisms of action are unknown.
• Hydantoin derivatives stabilize neuronal membranes and limit seizure activity by either increasing efflux or decreasing influx of sodium ions across cell membranes in the motor cortex during generation of nerve impulses.

USE OF ANTICONVULSANTS IN EPILEPTIC-TYPE SEIZURES

DRUG	GRAND MAL	PETIT MAL	MYOCLONIC	MIXED	PSYCHOMOTOR	STATUS EPILEPTICUS
Barbiturate derivatives						
mephobarbital	✓	✓				
metharbital	✓	✓	✓	✓		
phenobarbital	✓	✓	✓	✓	✓	
primidone	✓				✓	
Benzodiazepine derivatives						
clonazepam		✓	✓			
diazepam						✓
Hydantoin derivatives						
ethotoin	✓				✓	
mephenytoin	✓				✓	
phenacemide				✓	✓	
phenytoin	✓				✓	✓
Oxazolidone derivatives						
paramethadione		✓				
trimethadione		✓				
Succinimide derivatives						
ethosuximide		✓				
methsuximide		✓				
phensuximide		✓				
Miscellaneous						
acetazolamide		✓				
bromides*	✓	✓	✓	✓	✓	
carbamazepine	✓			✓	✓	
valproic acid		✓				

*Rarely used as drug of first or second choice

Note: Magnesium sulfate and paraldehyde are not included in this list since they are used to control nonepileptic seizures.

DRUG ALERT

KNOW ABOUT THE TWO FORMS OF PHENYTOIN

Oral phenytoin is often prescribed to prevent and control epileptic seizures. But phenytoin (Dilantin) is available in *two* forms; confusing one with the other may cause serious problems.

The FDA has determined that one of the phenytoins—Dilantin Kapseals—is absorbed more slowly and is longer-acting than other phenytoins. As a result, Dilantin Kapseals are designated extended-release and approved for once-a-day dosage. (All other phenytoins are designated prompt-release and labeled "not for once-a-day dosing.") Remember these points about administering phenytoins:

- Use of extended-release phenytoin may improve patient compliance. However, some patients can't be adequately controlled with a once-a-day dosage. These patients must take a prompt-release phenytoin two or three times a day.
- Prompt-release phenytoin attains higher blood levels sooner than the extended-release form. If a patient taking Dilantin Kapseals mistakenly takes a total daily dose of prompt-release phenytoin, he may experience phenytoin toxicity.

The patient should know the difference between the two forms of the drug. He should be warned not to allow generic phenytoin to be substituted for Dilantin Kapseals after he leaves the hospital.

- Magnesium sulfate may decrease acetylcholine released by nerve impulse, but its anticonvulsant mechanism is unknown.
- Oxazolidone derivatives raise the threshold for cortical seizure but do not modify seizure pattern. These drugs decrease projection of focal activity and reduce both repetitive spinal cord transmission and spike-and-wave patterns of absence (petit mal) seizures.
- Succinimide derivatives increase seizure threshold. They reduce the paroxysmal spike-and-wave pattern of absence seizures by depressing nerve transmisson in the motor cortex.
- Valproic acid may increase brain levels of gamma-aminobutyric acid, which transmits inhibitory nerve impulses in the CNS.

Absorption, distribution, metabolism, and excretion

Anticonvulsants are generally well absorbed from the gastrointestinal tract and widely distributed in the tissues, including the CNS. They're metabolized by the liver and excreted by the kidneys.

Because barbiturates induce microsomal enzymes in the liver, they may accelerate metabolism of other anticonvulsant drugs given concurrently.

Onset and duration

Onset and duration of action vary with each drug and from patient to patient. When parenteral preparations are used for acute episodes (status epilepticus or eclampsia, for example), onset is immediate.

Most anticonvulsants have half-lives of several hours to days, and they may require days or even weeks of therapy to achieve steady-state blood concentrations.

See chart on p. 303 for details on common anticonvulsants.

Combination products

DILANTIN WITH PHENOBARBITAL♦: phenytoin sodium 100 mg and phenobarbital 16 mg.
DILANTIN WITH PHENOBARBITAL♦: phenytoin sodium 100 mg and phenobarbital 32 mg.
PHELANTIN KAPSEALS♦: phenytoin 100 mg, phenobarbital 30 mg, and methamphetamine hydrochloride 2.5 mg.

NAMES, INDICATIONS AND DOSAGES	SIDE EFFECTS

acetazolamide
Acetazolam♦♦, Diamox♦, Hydrazol, Roxolamide
acetazolamide sodium
Diamox♦

Myoclonic seizures, refractory grand mal or petit mal, mixed seizures:
ADULTS: 375 mg P.O., I.M., or I.V. daily up to 250 mg q.i.d. Initial dose when used with other anticonvulsants usually 250 mg daily.
CHILDREN: 8 to 30 mg/kg daily, divided t.i.d. or q.i.d. Maximum dose 1.5 g daily, or 300 to 900 mg/m² daily.

Blood: leukopenia, *aplastic anemia.*
CNS: paresthesias, drowsiness.
EENT: transient myopia.
GI: anorexia, nausea, vomiting.
GU: crystalluria, renal calculi.
Metabolic: *hyperchloremic acidosis.*
Skin: rash.
Local: *pain at injection site,* sterile abscesses.

bromides
Bromide, Calcium Bromide, Lanabrom, Neurosine, Peacock's Bromides, Potassium Bromide, Sodium Bromide

Major motor and myoclonic seizures:
ADULTS: 1 to 2 g t.i.d.
CHILDREN: 50 to 100 mg/kg daily, divided equally t.i.d. Or, 1.5 to 3 g/m² daily in divided doses t.i.d.

CNS: *drowsiness,* mental dullness, toxic psychosis.
Skin: *rashes* (acneiform, morbilliform, granulomatous), Stevens-Johnson syndrome.

carbamazepine
Tegretol♦

Psychomotor, temporal lobe, grand mal, mixed seizure patterns:
ADULTS AND CHILDREN OVER 12 YEARS: 200 mg P.O. b.i.d. on day 1. May increase by 200 mg P.O./day, in divided doses at 6- to 8-hour intervals. Adjust to minimum effective level when control achieved. Usual maintenance 800 to 1,200 mg daily. Don't exceed 1 g total daily dose in 12- to 15-year-olds and 1,200 mg P.O. daily in patients over 15 years.
CHILDREN UNDER 12 YEARS: 10 to 20 mg/kg P.O daily in 2 to 4 divided doses.

Trigeminal neuralgia:
ADULTS: 100 mg P.O. b.i.d. with meals on day 1. Increase by 100 mg q 12 hours until pain relieved. Don't exceed 1.2 g daily. Maintenance dose 200 to 400 mg P.O. b.i.d.

Blood: *aplastic anemia, agranulocytosis,* eosinophilia, leukocytosis, *thrombocytopenia.*
CNS: dizziness, *vertigo, drowsiness,* fatigue, *ataxia.*
CV: congestive heart failure, hypertension, hypotension, aggravation of coronary artery disease.
EENT: conjunctivitis, dry mouth and pharynx, blurred vision, diplopia, nystagmus.
GI: *nausea,* vomiting, abdominal pain, diarrhea, anorexia, *stomatitis,* glossitis, *dry mouth.*
GU: urinary frequency or retention, impotence, albuminuria, glycosuria, elevated BUN.
Hepatic: abnormal liver function studies.
Metabolic: water intoxication.
Skin: rash, urticaria.
Other: diaphoresis, fever, chills.

clonazepam
Controlled Substance Schedule IV
Clonopin, Rivotril♦

Petit mal and petit mal variant (Lennox syndrome) seizures; akinetic and myoclonic seizures:
ADULTS: initial dose should not exceed 1.5 mg

Blood: leukopenia, thrombocytopenia, eosinophilia.
CNS: *drowsiness, ataxia, behavioral disturbances (especially in children),* slurred speech, tremor, confusion.
EENT: *increased salivation,* diplopia, nystagmus, abnormal eye movements.
GI: constipation, gastritis, change in appetite,

♦ Available in U.S. and Canada. ♦♦ Available in Canada only.
All other products (no symbol) available in U.S. only. Italicized side effects are common or life-threatening.

INTERACTIONS AND SPECIAL CONSIDERATIONS

Interactions:
METHENAMINE: antagonized methenamine effect. If used together, urine must be kept at pH 5.5 or lower.

Special considerations:
• Contraindicated in sulfonamide sensitivity, chronic pulmonary disease, renal or hepatic dysfunction, Addison's disease (adrenocortical insufficiency), hyponatremia, hypokalemia, hyperchloremic acidosis, chronic noncongestive angle-closure glaucoma. Use cautiously in hypercalciuria, diabetes mellitus, gout, and respiratory acidosis.
• CBC and serum electrolytes should be obtained every 3 months; serum calcium every 6 months.
• Drug should not be withdrawn suddenly, even if side effects develop.
• Patient should avoid activities that require alertness and good psychomotor coordination until CNS response to drug has been determined.
• This drug is also a diuretic. Diuretic precautions should be used.
• Chronic use results in tolerance to drug.
• 500-mg vial should be reconstituted with 5 ml sterile water for injection. Provides 100 mg/ml. Reconstituted solution should be refrigerated; discard in 24 hours.
• Oral liquid: soften 1 tablet in 2 teaspoonfuls of very warm water and add to 2 teaspoonfuls honey or syrup (chocolate, cherry), not fruit juice.
• May cause hyperglycemia in patients who are prediabetic or in those with diabetes on insulin or oral drugs. These patients should be monitored carefully.
• Hypokalemia or metabolic acidosis may occur.

No significant interactions.

Special considerations:
• Contraindicated in debilitated, dehydrated, or alcoholic patients, or in those with cerebral arteriosclerosis, organic brain damage, impaired renal function, severe depression, neurologic or psychologic disorders, tuberculosis or skin disorders (acne, dermatitis, herpetiformis). Especially in adults, use may lead to chronic toxicity (mental, psychic, GI, and neurologic disturbances; skin eruptions). May be mistaken for acute alcohol intoxication, tabes dorsalis, cerebral tumor, uremia, or multiple sclerosis.
• In adults, blood levels above 5 mEq/liter may cause toxicity.
• Therapeutic blood level in children is usually 20 to 25 mEq/liter (200 mg/100 ml), but range is 10 to 35 mEq/liter.
• Effect may not be seen for 2 to 3 weeks.
• Side effects are possible.

Interactions:
TROLEANDOMYCIN AND ERYTHROMYCIN: may increase carbamazepine blood levels. Use cautiously.
PROPOXYPHENE: may raise carbamazepine levels. Use another analgesic.

Special considerations:
• Contraindicated in patients with bone marrow depression or hypersensitivity to carbamazepine or tricyclic antidepressants. Use cautiously in cardiac, renal, or hepatic damage, or increased intraocular pressure.
• Patient should avoid activities that require alertness and good psychomotor coordination until response to drug has been determined.
• Don't withdraw drug suddenly when treating seizures or status epilepticus, even if side effects develop.
• CBC, platelet and reticulocyte counts, and serum iron should be obtained weekly for first 3 months, then monthly. If bone marrow depression develops, drug should be stopped. Urinalysis, BUN, and liver function studies should be obtained every 3 months. Periodic eye examinations recommended.
• Patient should report immediately fever, sore throat, mouth ulcers, or easy bruising.
• Therapeutic anticonvulsant serum level is 3 to 9 mcg/ml.
• When used for trigeminal neuralgia, every 3 months an attempt should be made to decrease dose or stop drug.

No significant interactions.

Special considerations:
• Contraindicated in hepatic disease; chlordiazepoxide, diazepam, or other benzodiazepine sensitivity; or acute narrow-angle glaucoma. Use with caution in chronic respiratory disease, impaired renal function, open-angle glaucoma.
• Patient should avoid activities that require alertness and good psychomotor coordination until CNS response to drug has been determined.
• Don't withdraw drug suddenly, even if side effects develop.
• Periodic CBC and liver function studies should be obtained.
• Patient should be monitored for oversedation.

(continued on following page)

NAMES, INDICATIONS AND DOSAGES	SIDE EFFECTS
clonazepam *(continued)* P.O./day, divided into 3 doses. May be increased by 0.5 to 1 mg q 3 days until seizures controlled. Maximum recommended daily dose is 20 mg. CHILDREN UP TO 10 YEARS OR 30 KG: 0.01 to 0.03 mg/kg P.O. daily (not to exceed 0.05 mg/kg daily), divided q 8 hours. Increase dosage by 0.25 to 0.5 mg q third day to a maximum maintenance dose of 0.1 mg to 0.2 mg/kg daily.	nausea, abnormal thirst, sore gums. **GU:** dysuria, enuresis, nocturia, urinary retention. **Skin:** rash. **Other:** respiratory depression.
diazepam Controlled Substance Schedule IV Valium♦ **Status epilepticus:** ADULTS: 5 to 10 mg slow I.V. push 5 mg/minute; may repeat q 10 minutes up to maximum total dose of 30 mg. Use 2 to 5 mg in elderly or debilitated patients. May repeat therapy in 2 to 4 hours with caution if seizures recur. CHILDREN: 0.1 to 0.3 mg/kg slow I.V. push (1 mg/minute over 3 minutes). May repeat q 15 minutes for 2 doses. Maximum single dose: children under 5 years—5 mg; children over 5 years—10 mg. **Adjunctive use in convulsive disorders:** ADULTS AND CHILDREN: 2 to 10 mg P.O. b.i.d., t.i.d., or q.i.d.	**Blood:** neutropenia. **CNS:** fatigue, *drowsiness, ataxia,* dizziness, headache, dysarthria, slurred speech, tremor. **CV:** hypotension, bradycardia, *cardiovascular collapse.* **EENT:** diplopia, blurred vision, nystagmus. **GI:** nausea, constipation, change in salivation. **GU:** incontinence, urinary retention. **Local:** *pain, phlebitis at injection site.* **Skin:** rash, urticaria.
ethosuximide Zarontin♦ **Petit mal seizures:** ADULTS AND CHILDREN OVER 6 YEARS: initially, 250 mg P.O. b.i.d. May increase by 250 mg q 4 to 7 days up to 1.5 g daily. CHILDREN 3 TO 6 YEARS: 250 mg P.O. daily or 125 mg P.O. b.i.d. May increase by 250 mg q 4 to 7 days up to 1.5 g daily.	**Blood:** leukopenia, eosinophilia, *agranulocytosis,* pancytopenia, *aplastic anemia.* **CNS:** *drowsiness,* headache, *fatigue, dizziness,* ataxia, irritability, hiccups, *euphoria, lethargy.* **EENT:** myopia. **GI:** *nausea, vomiting,* diarrhea, gum hypertrophy, weight loss, cramps, tongue swelling, *anorexia, epigastric and abdominal pain.* **GU:** vaginal bleeding. **Skin:** urticaria, pruritic and erythematous rashes, hirsutism.
ethotoin Peganone **Grand mal or psychomotor seizures:** ADULTS: initially, 250 mg P.O. q.i.d. after meals. May increase slowly over several days to 3 g daily divided q.i.d. CHILDREN: initially, 250 mg P.O. b.i.d. May increase up to 250 mg P.O. q.i.d.	**Blood:** thrombocytopenia, leukopenia, *agranulocytosis,* pancytopenia, megaloblastic anemia. **CNS:** fatigue, insomnia, dizziness, headache, numbness. **CV:** chest pain. **EENT:** diplopia, nystagmus. **GI:** nausea, vomiting, diarrhea, gingival hyperplasia (rare). **Skin:** rash. **Other:** fever, lymphadenopathy.

♦ Available in U.S. and Canada. ♦♦ Available in Canada only.
All other products (no symbol) available in U.S. only. Italicized side effects are common or life-threatening.

INTERACTIONS AND SPECIAL CONSIDERATIONS

- Withdrawal symptoms similar to barbiturates.

No significant interactions.

Special considerations:

- Contraindicated in shock, psychosis, coma, acute alcohol intoxication with depression of vital signs, acute narrow-angle glaucoma. Use cautiously in elderly or debilitated patients; those with limited pulmonary reserve, and those in whom blood pressure drop might cause cardiovascular complications; also in those with history of anxiety states with suicidal tendencies, blood dyscrasias, hepatic or renal damage, open-angle glaucoma, or alcoholism.
- Respirations should be monitored every 5 to 15 minutes and before each I.V. repeated dose. Emergency resuscitative equipment and oxygen should be at bedside.
- Should not be mixed with other drugs or I.V. fluids.
- Small veins such as those on dorsum of hand or wrist should not be used.
- Extravasation should be avoided.
- I.V. should be given slowly at a rate not exceeding 5 mg/minute. Phlebitis may occur at injection site.
- Should not be infused through plastic tubing or stored in plastic syringe.
- Drug should not be withdrawn abruptly.
- Heavy use of alcohol or other CNS depressants should be avoided.
- For symptoms and treatment of toxicity, see APPENDIX.

No significant interactions.

Special considerations:

- Contraindicated in hypersensitivity to succinimide derivatives. Use cautiously in hepatic or renal disease.
- Don't withdraw drug suddenly, even if side effects develop. Abrupt withdrawal may precipitate petit mal seizures.
- Patient should avoid activities that require alertness and good psychomotor coordination until CNS response to drug has been determined.
- CBC should be obtained every 3 months; urinalysis and liver function studies every 6 months.
- Therapeutic serum levels 40 to 80 mg/ml.
- May increase frequency of grand mal seizures when used alone in mixed epilepsy.
- May cause positive direct Coombs' test.

Interactions:

ALCOHOL, FOLIC ACID, AND LOXAPINE SUCCINATE: monitor for decreased ethotoin activity.
ORAL ANTICOAGULANTS, ANTIHISTAMINES, CHLORAMPHENICOL, DIAZEPAM, DIAZOXIDE, DISULFIRAM, ISONIAZID, PHENYLBUTAZONE, PHENYRAMIDOL, SALICYLATES, SULFAMETHIZOLE, AND VALPROATE: monitor for increased ethotoin activity and toxicity.

Special considerations:

- Contraindicated in patients with hydantoin hypersensitivity and in hepatic or hematologic disorders. Use cautiously in patients receiving other hydantoin derivatives.
- Don't withdraw drug suddenly, even if side effects develop.
- Patient should avoid activities that require alertness and good psychomotor coordination until response to drug has been determined.
- CBC and urinalysis should be obtained when therapy starts and monthly thereafter.
- Should be taken after meals. Doses should be scheduled as evenly as possible over 24 hours.
- Should be stopped at once if lymphadenopathy or lupuslike syndrome develops.
- Heavy use of alcohol may diminish benefits of drug.
- Hydantoin derivative of choice in young adults who are prone to gingival hyperplasia caused by phenytoin.

NAMES, INDICATIONS AND DOSAGES	SIDE EFFECTS
magnesium sulfate **Hypomagnesemic seizures:** ADULTS: 1 to 2 g (as 10% solution) I.V. over 15 minutes, then 1 g I.M. q 4 to 6 hours, based on the patient's response and magnesium blood levels. CHILDREN: seizures secondary to hypomagnesemia in acute nephritis—0.2 ml/kg of 50% solution I.M. q 4 to 6 hours, p.r.n. or 100 mg/kg of 10% solution I.V. very slowly. Titrate dosage according to magnesium blood levels and seizure response. **Prevention or control of seizures in preeclampsia or eclampsia:** WOMEN: initially, 4 g I.V. in 250 ml 5% dextrose in water and 4 g deep I.M. each buttock; then 4 g deep I.M. into alternate buttock q 4 hours, p.r.n. Subsequent doses based on magnesium blood levels and urinary magnesium excretion. Do not exceed 40 g daily.	**CNS:** sweating, drowsiness, depressed reflexes, flaccid paralysis, hypothermia. **CV:** hypotension, flushing, *circulatory collapse,* depressed cardiac function, heart block. **Other:** *respiratory paralysis,* hypocalcemia.
mephenytoin Mesantoin♦ **Refractory grand mal, focal, or psychomotor seizures:** ADULTS: 50 to 100 mg P.O. daily. May increase by 50 to 100 mg at weekly intervals up to 200 mg P.O. t.i.d. CHILDREN: initial dose 50 to 100 mg P.O. daily or 100 to 450 mg/m² P.O. daily in 3 divided doses. May increase slowly by 50 to 100 mg at weekly intervals up to 200 mg P.O. t.i.d., divided q 8 hours. Dosage must be adjusted individually.	**Blood:** *leukopenia,* neutropenia, *agranulocytosis,* thrombocytopenia, pancytopenia, eosinophilia. **CNS:** ataxia, *drowsiness,* fatigue, irritability, choreiform movements, depression, tremor, sleeplessness, dizziness (usually transient). **EENT:** photophobia, conjunctivitis, diplopia, nystagmus. **GI:** gingival hyperplasia, nausea and vomiting (with prolonged use). **Skin:** *rashes, exfoliative dermatitis.* **Other:** hypertrichosis, edema, dysarthria, lymphadenopathy, polyarthropathy, pulmonary fibrosis.
mephobarbital Controlled Substance Schedule IV Mebaral♦, Mentabal, Mephoral **Grand or petit mal seizures:** ADULTS: 400 to 600 mg P.O. daily or in divided doses. CHILDREN: 6 to 12 mg/kg P.O. daily, divided q 6 to 8 hours (smaller doses are given initially and increased over 4 to 5 days as needed).	**Blood:** megaloblastic anemia, agranulocytosis, thrombocytopenia. **CNS:** dizziness, headache, hangover, confusion, paradoxical excitation, exacerbation of existing pain, drowsiness. **CV:** hypotension. **GI:** nausea, vomiting, epigastric pain. **Skin:** urticaria, morbilliform rash, blisters, purpura, erythema multiforme. **Other:** allergic reactions (facial edema).

INTERACTIONS AND SPECIAL CONSIDERATIONS

Interactions:
NEUROMUSCULAR BLOCKING AGENTS: may cause increased neuromuscular blockade. Use cautiously.

Special considerations:
• Contraindicated in patients with impaired renal function, myocardial damage, heart block, and in women in labor.
• I.V. calcium gluconate should be kept available to reverse magnesium intoxication; however, should not be used in digitalized patient due to danger of arrhythmias.
• Vital signs should be monitored every 15 minutes when drug is given I.V.
• Respiratory depression and heart block possible. Respirations should be approximately 16/minute before each dose given.
• Intake and output should be monitored. Urinary output should be 100 ml or more in 4-hour period before each dose.
• Serum magnesium levels should be checked after repeated doses. Disappearance of knee jerk and patellar reflexes are signs of pending magnesium toxicity.
• Maximum infusion rate is 150 mg/minute. Rapid drip will induce uncomfortable feeling of heat.
• Side effects may occur.
• Especially when given I.V. to toxemic mothers within 24 hours before delivery, newborn should be observed for signs of magnesium toxicity, including neuromuscular or respiratory depression.

Interactions:
ALCOHOL, FOLIC ACID, AND LOXAPINE SUCCINATE: monitor for decreased mephenytoin activity.
ORAL ANTICOAGULANTS, ANTIHISTAMINES, CHLORAMPHENICOL, DIAZEPAM, DIAZOXIDE, DISULFIRAM, ISONIAZID, PHENYLBUTAZONE, PHENYRAMIDOL, SALICYLATES, SULFAMETHIZOLE, AND VALPROATE: monitor for increased mephenytoin activity and toxicity.

Special considerations:
• Contraindicated in hydantoin hypersensitivity. Use cautiously in patients receiving other hydantoin derivatives.
• Patient should report fever, sore throat, bleeding, or rash.
• CBC and platelet count should be checked initially and every 2 weeks thereafter, up to 2 weeks after full dose attained; then monthly for first year and every 3 months thereafter. Drug should be stopped if neutrophils less than 1,600/mm^3.
• Don't withdraw drug suddenly, even if side effects develop.
• Patient should avoid activities that require alertness and good psychomotor coordination until response to drug has been determined.
• Therapeutic serum level is 5 to 20 mcg/ml.
• Heavy use of alcohol may diminish benefit of drug.

Interactions:
ALCOHOL AND OTHER CNS DEPRESSANTS, INCLUDING NARCOTIC ANALGESICS: excessive CNS depression. Use cautiously.
MAO INHIBITORS: potentiated barbiturate effect. Monitor patient for increased CNS and respiratory depression.
RIFAMPIN: may decrease barbiturate levels. Monitor for decreased effect.

Special considerations:
• Contraindicated in barbiturate hypersensitivity, porphyria, and respiratory disease with dyspnea or obstruction. Use cautiously in hepatic, renal, cardiac, or respiratory function impairment, and in myasthenia gravis and myxedema.
• Don't withdraw drug suddenly, even if side effects develop.
• Patient should avoid activities that require alertness and good psychomotor coordination until CNS response to drug has been determined.
• Store in light-resistant container.
• In adults, total or largest dose should be taken at night if seizures occur then.
• Three quarters of drug metabolized to phenobarbital; therapeutic blood levels as phenobarbital are 15 to 40 mcg/ml.
• Prothrombin times should be monitored carefully when patient on mephobarbital starts or ends anticoagulant therapy. Anticoagulant dose may need to be adjusted.
• For symptoms and treatment of toxicity, see APPENDIX.

NAMES, INDICATIONS AND DOSAGES	SIDE EFFECTS
metharbital Controlled Substance Schedule III Gemonil **Grand or petit mal seizures; myoclonic or mixed seizures:** ADULTS: initially, 100 mg P.O. daily to t.i.d. May increase to 800 mg daily in divided doses. CHILDREN: 5 to 15 mg/kg P.O. daily, divided t.i.d. May increase to 50 to 100 mg P.O. daily, b.i.d., or t.i.d.	**Blood:** megaloblastic anemia, *agranulocytosis,* thrombocytopenia. **CNS:** dizziness, irritability, drowsiness, headache, confusion, excitation. **CV:** hypotension. **GI:** nausea, vomiting, discomfort. **Skin:** rash, urticaria, purpura, erythema multiforme.
methsuximide Celontin♦ **Refractory petit mal seizures:** ADULTS AND CHILDREN: initially, 300 mg P.O. daily. May increase by 300 mg weekly. Maximum daily dosage of 1.2 g in divided doses.	**Blood:** eosinophilia, leukopenia, monocytosis, pancytopenia. **CNS:** *drowsiness, ataxia, dizziness,* irritability, nervousness, headache, insomnia, confusion, depression, aggressiveness. **EENT:** blurred vision, photophobia, periorbital edema. **GI:** *nausea, vomiting, anorexia,* diarrhea, weight loss, abdominal or epigastric pain. **Skin:** urticaria, pruritic and erythematous rashes.
paraldehyde Controlled Substance Schedule IV Paral **Refractory grand mal seizures, status epilepticus:** ADULTS: 5 to 10 ml I.M. (divide 10 ml dose into 2 injections); 0.2 to 0.4 ml/kg in 0.9% saline injection I.V. CHILDREN: 0.15 ml/kg dose deep I.M. q 4 to 6 hours, p.r.n.; or 0.3 ml/kg rectally in olive oil q 4 to 6 hours; or 1 ml/year of age not to exceed 5 ml, repeated in 1 hour, p.r.n.; or dilute 5 ml in 95 ml 0.9% saline injection for I.V. infusion and titrate dose beginning at 5 ml/hour.	**CV:** *I.V. administration may cause pulmonary edema or hemorrhage,* dilatation of right side of heart, *circulatory collapse.* **GI:** irritation, *foul breath odor.* **GU:** nephrosis with prolonged use. **Skin:** *erythematous rash.* **Local:** *pain,* sterile abscesses, sloughing of skin, fat necrosis, muscular irritation, nerve damage (if injection is near nerve trunk) at I.M. injection site. **Other:** respiratory depression.
paramethadione Paradione♦ **Refractory petit mal seizures:** ADULTS: initially, 300 mg P.O. t.i.d. May increase by 300 mg weekly, up to 600 mg q.i.d., if needed. CHILDREN OVER 6 YEARS: 0.9 g P.O. daily in divided doses t.i.d. or q.i.d. CHILDREN 2 TO 6 YEARS: 0.6 g P.O. daily in divided doses t.i.d. or q.i.d. CHILDREN UNDER 2 YEARS: 0.3 g P.O. daily in divided doses b.i.d.	**Blood:** neutropenia, leukopenia, eosinophilia, thrombocytopenia, pancytopenia, *agranulocytosis, hypoplastic and aplastic anemia.* **CNS:** *drowsiness,* fatigue, vertigo, headache, paresthesias, irritability. **CV:** hypertension, hypotension. **EENT:** hemeralopia, photophobia, diplopia, epistaxis, retinal hemorrhage. **GI:** nausea, vomiting, abdominal pain, weight loss, bleeding gums. **GU:** albuminuria, vaginal bleeding. **Hepatic:** abnormal liver function studies. **Skin:** acneiform or morbilliform rash, *exfoliative dermatitis,* erythema multiforme, petechiae, alopecia. **Other:** lymphadenopathy, lupus erythematosus.

INTERACTIONS AND SPECIAL CONSIDERATIONS

Interactions:
ALCOHOL AND OTHER CNS DEPRESSANTS, INCLUDING NARCOTIC ANALGESICS: excessive CNS depression. Use cautiously.
MAO INHIBITORS: potentiated barbiturate effect. Monitor patient for increased CNS and respiratory depression.
RIFAMPIN: may decrease barbiturate levels. Monitor for decreased effect.

Special considerations:
• Contraindicated in barbiturate hypersensitivity, in manifest or latent porphyria, and in respiratory disease with dyspnea or obstruction. Use cautiously in hepatic, cardiac, or renal impairment.
• Drug should not be stopped abruptly, even if side effects develop.
• Patient should avoid activities that require alertness and good psychomotor coordination until CNS response to drug is determined.
• Prothrombin times should be monitored carefully when patient on metharbital starts or ends anticoagulant therapy. Anticoagulant dose may need to be adjusted.
• For symptoms and treatment of toxicity, see APPENDIX.

No significant interactions.

Special considerations:
• Contraindicated in hypersensitivity to succinimide derivatives. Use cautiously in hepatic or renal dysfunction.
• Don't withdraw drug suddenly, even if side effects develop. Abrupt withdrawal may precipitate petit mal seizures.
• Patient should avoid activities that require alertness and good psychomotor coordination until CNS response to drug has been determined.
• CBC should be obtained every 3 months; urinalysis and liver function studies every 6 months.
• May color urine pink or brown.
• Therapeutic serum levels 40 to 100 mcg/ml.

Interactions:
ALCOHOL: increased CNS depression. Use with caution.
DISULFIRAM: increased paraldehyde and acetaldehyde blood levels; possible toxic disulfiram reaction. Use together cautiously.

Special considerations:
• Contraindicated in gastroenteritis with ulceration. Use cautiously in impaired hepatic function, or in asthma or other pulmonary disease.
• Fresh supply should be used. Should not be used if exposed to air, if liquid is brown, has a vinegary odor, or container opened more than 24 hours.
• Respiratory depression possible, especially in repeated doses.
• Drug reacts with plastic. Glass syringe and bottle should be used for parenteral dose, and fresh I.V. solution should be prepared every 4 hours. I.V. administration hazardous.
• I.M. dose should be given deeply, away from nerve trunks, and injection site massaged.
• Paraldehyde should be diluted in olive oil or cottonseed oil 1:2 for rectal administration and given as retention enema. To prepare enema, 200 ml normal saline solution may also be used.
• Patient's room should be well-ventilated to remove exhaled paraldehyde.
• Long-term high dosage may cause drug dependence and severe withdrawal symptoms.
• Oral or rectal administration of decomposed paraldehyde may cause severe corrosion of stomach or rectum.

No significant interactions.

Special considerations:
• Contraindicated in renal and hepatic dysfunction, severe blood dyscrasias. Use cautiously in retinal or optic nerve diseases.
• Don't withdraw drug suddenly, even if side effects develop.
• Therapeutic serum levels 6 to 71 mcg/ml.
• Drug should be stopped if scotomata or signs of hepatitis, systemic lupus erythematosus, lymphadenopathy, skin rash, nephrosis, hair loss, or grand mal seizures appear.
• Patient should report sore throat, fever, malaise, bruises, petechiae, or epistaxis immediately. Patient should wear dark glasses if photophobia occurs and should not drive a car or operate machinery until CNS response to drug has been determined.
• Liver function studies and urinalysis should be obtained before therapy; then monthly.
• Oral solution should be diluted with water before given.
• CBC should be monitored. If neutrophil count falls below 2,500/mm^3, drug should be discontinued.
• 300-mg capsule contains tartrazine. May cause allergy in susceptible patients.

NAMES, INDICATIONS AND DOSAGES	SIDE EFFECTS
phenacemide Phenurone **Refractory, mixed psychomotor, grand mal, petit mal, and petit mal variant seizures:** ADULTS: 500 mg P.O. t.i.d. May increase by 500 mg weekly up to 5 g daily, p.r.n. CHILDREN 5 TO 10 YEARS: 250 mg P.O. t.i.d. May increase by 250 mg weekly, up to 1.5 g daily, p.r.n.	**Blood:** *aplastic anemia, agranulocytosis,* leukopenia. **CNS:** drowsiness, dizziness, insomnia, headaches, paresthesias, *depression, suicidal tendencies,* aggressiveness. **GI:** anorexia, weight loss. **GU:** nephritis with marked albuminuria. **Hepatic:** hepatitis, jaundice. **Skin:** rashes.
phenobarbital Bar, Barbipil, Barbita, Eskabarb♦, Floramine, Gardenal♦♦, Henomint, Luminal♦, Nova-Pheno♦♦, Orprine, PB, PBR, Solfoton, Solu-Barb, Stental **phenobarbital sodium** Controlled Substance Schedule IV Luminal Sodium♦ **All forms of epilepsy, febrile seizures in children:** ADULTS: 100 to 200 mg P.O. daily, divided t.i.d. or given as single dose at bedtime. CHILDREN: 4 to 6 mg/kg P.O. daily, divided q 12 hours. **Status epilepticus:** ADULTS: 90 to 120 mg I.V., followed by 30 to 60 mg q 10 to 15 minutes, as needed, up to 500 mg total. CHILDREN: 5 to 10 mg/kg I.V. May repeat q 10 to 15 minutes up to total of 20 mg/kg. I.V. injection rate should not exceed 60 mg/minute.	**CNS:** *drowsiness, lethargy, hangover,* paradoxical excitement in elderly patients. **GI:** nausea, vomiting. **Skin:** rash, Stevens-Johnson syndrome, urticaria. **Other:** angioedema.
phensuximide Milontin♦ **Petit mal seizures:** ADULTS AND CHILDREN: 500 mg to 1 g P.O. b.i.d. to t.i.d.	**Blood:** transient leukopenia, pancytopenia, *agranulocytosis.* **CNS:** muscular weakness, *drowsiness,* dizziness, ataxia, headache. **GI:** nausea, vomiting, anorexia. **GU:** urinary frequency, renal damage, hematuria. **Skin:** pruritus, eruptions, erythema.
phenytoin sodium (extended) Dilantin♦ **phenytoin sodium (prompt)** Di-Phen, Diphenylan, Ditan **Grand mal and psychomotor seizures, nonepileptic seizures (post–head trauma, Reye's syndrome):** ADULTS: loading dose 900 mg to 1.5 g I.V. at 50 mg/minute or P.O. divided t.i.d., then start maintenance dose of 300 mg P.O. daily (extended only) or divided t.i.d. (extended or prompt). CHILDREN: loading dose 15 mg/kg I.V. at	**Blood:** thrombocytopenia, leukopenia, *agranulocytosis,* pancytopenia, macrocytosis, megaloblastic anemia. **CNS:** *ataxia,* slurred speech, confusion, dizziness, insomnia, nervousness, twitching, headache. **CV:** hypotension, *ventricular fibrillation.* **EENT:** *nystagmus, diplopia,* blurred vision. **GI:** *nausea, vomiting, gingival hyperplasia (especially children).* **Hepatic:** *toxic hepatitis.* **Skin:** scarlatiniform or morbilliform rash; bullous, *exfoliative,* or purpuric *dermatitis;* Stevens-Johnson syndrome; lupus erythemato-

♦ Available in U.S. and Canada. ♦♦ Available in Canada only.
All other products (no symbol) available in U.S. only. Italicized side effects are common or life-threatening.

INTERACTIONS AND SPECIAL CONSIDERATIONS

No significant interactions.

Special considerations:
• Contraindicated in patients with preexisting personality disturbances. Use with caution in patients with hepatic dysfunction, history of allergy, and when a hydantoin is used concomitantly.
• Liver function studies, CBCs, and urinalyses should be obtained before and at monthly intervals during therapy.
• Patient should report sore throat or fever immediately.
• Patient should avoid activities that require alertness or good psychomotor coordination until CNS response to drug has been determined.
• Don't withdraw drug suddenly, even if side effects develop.
• Patient's family should report personality or psychological changes at once.
• Extremely toxic. Use only when other anticonvulsants are ineffective.
• Jaundice or other signs of hepatitis, abnormal urinary findings, or WBC below 4,000/mm³ may develop.

Interactions:
ALCOHOL AND OTHER CNS DEPRESSANTS, INCLUDING NARCOTIC ANALGESICS: excessive CNS depression. Use cautiously.
MAO INHIBITORS: potentiate barbiturate effect. Monitor for increased CNS and respiratory depression.
RIFAMPIN: may decrease barbiturate levels. Monitor for decreased effect.
PRIMIDONE: monitor for excessive phenobarbital blood levels.
VALPROIC ACID: increased phenobarbital levels. Monitor for toxicity.

Special considerations:
• Contraindicated in patients with barbiturate hypersensitivity, porphyria, hepatic dysfunction, respiratory disease with dyspnea or obstruction, nephritis, and in lactating women. Use cautiously in patients with hyperthyroidism, diabetes mellitus, anemia, and in elderly or debilitated patients.
• I.V. injection should be reserved for emergency treatment and should be given slowly under close supervision. Respirations should be monitored closely.
• Barbiturate toxicity signs: coma, asthmatic breathing, cyanosis, clammy skin, hypotension. Overdose can be fatal.
• Patient should avoid activities that require alertness and good psychomotor coordination until CNS response to drug is determined.
• Don't withdraw drug suddenly, even if side effects develop.
• Full therapeutic effects not seen for 2 to 3 weeks, except when loading dose is used.
• Injection solution should not be used if it contains a precipitate.
• Therapeutic serum levels are 15 to 40 mg/ml.
• Prothrombin times should be monitored carefully when patient on phenobarbital starts or ends anticoagulant therapy. Anticoagulant dose may need to be adjusted.
• Parenteral form should not be mixed with acidic solutions: precipitation may result.
• For symptoms and treatment of toxicity, see APPENDIX.

No significant interactions.

Special considerations:
• Contraindicated in hypersensitivity to succinimide derivatives. Use cautiously in patients with hepatic or renal disease.
• Don't withdraw drug suddenly, even if side effects develop. Abrupt withdrawal may precipitate petit mal seizures.
• CBCs should be obtained every 3 months; urinalyses and liver function studies every 6 months.
• May color urine pink or red to reddish brown.
• Therapeutic serum level 40 to 80 mcg/ml.
• May increase incidence of grand mal seizures if used alone to treat patients with mixed epilepsy.

Interactions:
ALCOHOL, FOLIC ACID, AND LOXAPINE: monitor for decreased phenytoin activity.
ORAL ANTICOAGULANTS, ANTIHISTAMINES, CHLORAMPHENICOL, DIAZEPAM, DIAZOXIDE, DISULFIRAM, ISONIAZID, PHENYLBUTAZONE, PHENYRAMIDOL, SALICYLATES, SULFAMETHIZOLE, THIORIDAZINE, AND VALPROATE: monitor for increased phenytoin activity and toxicity.

Special considerations:
• Contraindicated in phenacemide or hydantoin hypersensitivity, bradycardia, SA and AV block, Stokes-Adams syndrome. Use cautiously in patients with hepatic or renal dysfunction, hypotension, myocardial insufficiency, respiratory depression, in patients receiving other hydantoin derivatives, and in elderly or debilitated patients.
• Don't withdraw drug suddenly, even if side effects develop.
• Patient should avoid activities that require alertness and good psychomotor coordination until CNS response to drug is determined.
• Drug should not be mixed with 5% dextrose in water because it will precipitate. I.V. tubing should be cleared first with normal saline solution. Cloudy solution should never be used. Drug may be mixed with normal saline solution

(continued on following page)

NAMES, INDICATIONS AND DOSAGES	SIDE EFFECTS

phenytoin sodium
(continued)

50 mg/minute or P.O. divided q 8 to 12 hours, then start maintenance dose of 5 to 7 mg/kg P.O. or I.V. daily, divided q 12 hours.

A loading dose is given if patient has not taken phenytoin in the past. If patient has not received phenytoin previously or has no detectable blood level, use loading dose:
ADULTS: 900 mg to 1.5 g I.V. divided into t.i.d. at 50 mg/minute. Do not exceed 500 mg each dose.
CHILDREN: 15 mg/kg I.V. at 50 mg/minute.

If patient has been receiving phenytoin but has missed one or more doses and has subtherapeutic levels:
ADULTS: 100 to 300 mg I.V. at 50 mg/minute.
CHILDREN: 5 to 7 mg/kg I.V. at 50 mg/minute. May repeat lower dose in 30 minutes if needed.

Neuritic pain (migraine, trigeminal neuralgia, Bell's palsy):
ADULTS: 200 to 400 mg P.O. daily.

sus; hirsutism; toxic epidermal necrolysis.
Local: pain, necrosis, and inflammation at injection site.
Other: periarteritis nodosa, lymphadenopathy, hyperglycemia, osteomalacia, hypertrichosis.

---

primidone
Mysoline♦, Sertan♦♦

Grand mal, psychomotor, and focal seizures:
ADULTS AND CHILDREN OVER 8 YEARS: 250 mg P.O. daily. Increase by 250 mg weekly, up to maximum 2 g daily, divided q.i.d.
CHILDREN UNDER 8 YEARS: 125 mg P.O. daily. Increase by 125 mg weekly, up to maximum 1 g daily, divided q.i.d.

Blood: leukopenia, eosinophilia.
CNS: *drowsiness, ataxia,* emotional disturbances, vertigo, hyperirritability, fatigue.
EENT: *diplopia,* nystagmus, edema of the eyelids.
GI: anorexia, *nausea, vomiting.*
GU: impotence, polyuria.
Skin: morbilliform rash, alopecia.
Other: edema, thirst.

---

trimethadione
Tridione, Trimedone♦♦

Refractory petit mal seizures:
ADULTS: initially, 300 mg P.O. t.i.d. May increase by 300 mg weekly up to 600 mg P.O. q.i.d.
CHILDREN: 20 to 50 mg/kg P.O. daily, divided q 6 to 8 hours. May increase by 150 to 300 mg. Usual maintenance 40 mg/kg or 1 g/m^2 P.O. daily in divided doses t.i.d. or q.i.d.

Blood: neutropenia, leukopenia, eosinophilia, thrombocytopenia, pancytopenia, *agranulocytosis, hypoplastic and aplastic anemia.*
CNS: *drowsiness,* fatigue, *malaise,* insomnia, dizziness, headache, paresthesias, irritability.
CV: hypertension, hypotension.
EENT: *hemeralopia,* diplopia, photophobia, epistaxis, retinal hemorrhage.
GI: nausea, vomiting, anorexia, abdominal pain, bleeding gums.
GU: nephrosis, albuminuria, vaginal bleeding.
Hepatic: abnormal liver function studies.
Skin: acneiform and morbilliform rash, *exfoliative dermatitis,* erythema multiforme, petechiae, alopecia.
Other: lymphadenopathy.

♦ Available in U.S. and Canada. ♦♦ Available in Canada only.
All other products (no symbol) available in U.S. only. Italicized side effects are common or life-threatening.

INTERACTIONS AND SPECIAL CONSIDERATIONS

at a concentration of 100 mg/50 ml if necessary.
• Should not be given I.M. unless dosage adjustments are made. Drug may precipitate at injection site, cause pain, and give erratic blood levels.
• CBC and serum calcium should be obtained every 6 months. Folic acid and vitamin B_{12} may be ordered if megaloblastic anemia is evident.
• Drug may color urine pink or red to reddish brown.
• Patient should carry identification stating that he's taking phenytoin.
• Good oral hygiene and regular dental examinations important. Gingivectomy may be necessary periodically.
• Drug should be stopped if rash appears. If rash is scarlet or measleslike, drug may be resumed after rash clears. If rash reappears, therapy should be stopped. If rash is exfoliative, purpuric, or bullous, drug should not be resumed.
• Only clear solution should be used for injection. Slight yellow color acceptable. Should not be refrigerated.
• Divided doses given with or after meals may decrease GI side effects.
• Available as suspension. Should be shaken well before each dose. Solid form should be used (chewable tablets or capsules) if possible.
• Therapeutic serum level is 10 to 20 mcg/ml.
• Heavy use of alcohol may diminish benefits of drug.
• Phenytoin levels may be decreased in mononucleosis. Patient should be monitored for increased seizure activity.
• Dilantin brand is the only oral form that can be given on a once-daily basis. Toxic levels may result if any other brand is given once daily.
• Patient should not change brands once stabilized on therapy.
• The drug was formerly known as diphenylhydantoin.

Interactions:
PHENYTOIN: stimulated conversion of primidone to phenobarbital. Observe for increased phenobarbital effect.

Special considerations:
• Contraindicated in phenobarbital hypersensitivity and porphyria.
• Don't withdraw drug suddenly, even if side effects develop.
• Patient should avoid activities that require alertness and good psychomotor coordination until CNS response to drug has been determined.
• Therapeutic serum levels of primidone 7 to 15 mg/ml. Therapeutic serum levels of phenobarbital 15 to 40 mcg/ml.
• CBC and routine blood chemistry should be done every 6 months.
• Partially converted to phenobarbital; should be used cautiously with phenobarbital.
• Liquid suspension should be well shaken.
• For symptoms and treatment of toxicity, see APPENDIX.

No significant interactions.

Special considerations:
• Contraindicated in paramethadione and trimethadione hypersensitivity, severe blood dyscrasias, severe hepatic dysfunction. Use with extreme caution in retinal and optic nerve diseases.
• Don't withdraw drug suddenly, even if side effects develop. Abrupt withdrawal may precipitate petit mal seizures.
• CBC, hepatic function, and urinalysis should be checked before starting therapy and monthly thereafter. Drug should be stopped if neutrophil count falls below 2,500/mm^3.
• Impending toxicity may precipitate grand mal seizure.
• Patient should report skin rash, alopecia, sore throat, fever, bruises, or epistaxis immediately.
• Patient should avoid activities that require alertness and good psychomotor coordination until CNS response to drug has been determined.
• Blurred vision in bright light should be reported. Sunglasses should be suggested.
• If scotomata or rash occurs, drug should be stopped.
• Therapeutic serum levels 20 to 40 mcg/ml.
• May increase incidence of grand mal seizures if used alone to treat patients who have mixed types of seizures.

NAMES, INDICATIONS AND DOSAGES	SIDE EFFECTS
valproic acid Depakene **valproate sodium** Depakene Syrup **Simple and complex absence seizures (including petit mal), mixed seizure types (including absence seizures), investigationally in major motor (grand mal, tonic clonic) seizures:** ADULTS AND CHILDREN: initially, 15 mg/kg P.O. daily divided b.i.d. or t.i.d.; then may increase by 5 to 10 mg/kg daily at weekly intervals up to maximum of 30 mg/kg daily, divided b.i.d. or t.i.d.	Because drug usually used in combination with other anticonvulsants, side effects reported may not be caused by valproic acid alone. **Blood:** inhibited platelet aggregation, thrombocytopenia, increased bleeding time. **CNS:** *sedation,* emotional upset, depression, psychosis, aggression, hyperactivity, behavioral deterioration, muscle weakness, tremors. **GI:** *nausea, vomiting,* indigestion, diarrhea, abdominal cramps, constipation, increased appetite and weight gain, *anorexia,* pancreatitis. **Hepatic:** *enzyme elevations, toxic hepatitis.* **Other:** alopecia.

♦ Available in U.S. and Canada. ♦♦ Available in Canada only.
All other products (no symbol) available in U.S. only. Italicized side effects are common or life-threatening.

INTERACTIONS AND SPECIAL CONSIDERATIONS

No significant interactions.

Special considerations:
- Use cautiously in hepatic dysfunction.
- Don't withdraw drug suddenly, even if side effects develop.
- Liver function studies, platelet counts, and prothrombin time should be obtained before starting drug and every 2 months thereafter.
- Patient should avoid activities that require alertness and good psychomotor coordination until CNS response to drug is determined.
- Drug may be taken with food or milk to reduce GI side effects. Chewing capsules should not be encouraged; causes irritation of mouth and throat.
- Tremors may indicate the need for dosage reduction.
- Patient should take with meals; will produce more uniform blood levels.
- May produce false-positive test for ketones in urine.
- Available as tasty red syrup. Keep out of reach of children.
- Syrup is more rapidly absorbed. Peak effect within 15 minutes.
- Syrup shouldn't be mixed with carbonated beverages; may be irritating to mouth and throat.

QUESTIONS & ANSWERS

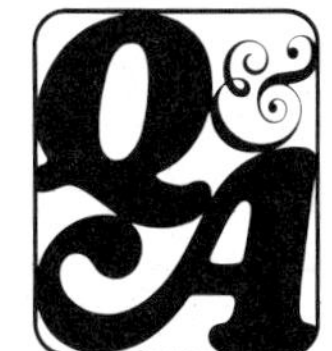

DRUG OR DISEASE: WHICH BRINGS ON ATAXIA?

Is ataxia caused by the grand mal convulsion or too much phenytoin?

Grand mal epileptic seizures can cause cerebellar dysfunction—staggered gait, ataxia, slurred speech, and tensed muscles. Unfortunately, too much phenytoin—a drug that's commonly used to *treat* grand mal seizures—can also produce ataxia. In fact, this is one of the major warning signs of phenytoin toxicity.

To help determine whether the ataxia is caused by the drug or the disease, the patient should be observed closely. Clinical signs can be the first indication that phenytoin blood levels are too high.

If the patient becomes ataxic, it should be reported immediately. Phenytoin dosage may be reduced or stopped until drug levels have been determined.

If ataxia persists even though phenytoin blood levels are normal (10 to 20 mcg/ml), the patient's ataxia is probably due to epilepsy, not drug therapy.

Antidepressants

Monoamine oxidase inhibitors
isocarboxazid
phenelzine sulfate
tranylcypromine sulfate

Tetracyclic antidepressants
maprotiline hydrochloride

Tricyclic antidepressants
amitriptyline hydrochloride
amoxapine
desipramine hydrochloride
doxepin hydrochloride
imipramine hydrochloride
nortriptyline hydrochloride
protriptyline hydrochloride
trimipramine maleate

(All drugs are listed in alphabetical order in the tables that follow.)

Tricyclic antidepressants (TCAs) are the drugs of choice for most types of depression. Since their introduction in the late 1950s, they have totally supplanted amphetamines and other psychomotor stimulants for this indication. This change has occurred because of the TCAs' effectiveness and relative lack of side effects.

Monoamine oxidase inhibitors (MAO inhibitors, or MAOIs) are another class of antidepressants. These can cause more serious side effects than the TCAs; thus they are generally reserved until two TCAs have been tried unsuccessfully. Despite the official warning against the combined use of a TCA and an MAO inhibitor, reports have documented the success of combination therapy.

Tetracyclic antidepressants are the most recent class of drugs to come on the market.

With all classes of antidepressants, the biggest problem in the past has been underdosage, that is, reluctance or failure to prescribe maximum recommended dose. The latest trend in psychotropic drug therapy is higher dosage for greater therapeutic effectiveness.

Major uses

All antidepressants are used to treat psychotic and neurotic endogenous depression and to prevent recurrent depression.

- Imipramine is used to treat enuresis in children and adolescents.
- MAO inhibitors may be effective in closely supervised patients who are unresponsive to other antidepressant therapy for severe reactive or endogenous depression.

Mechanism of action

- Tricyclic and tetracyclic antidepressants are thought to increase the amount of norepinephrine or serotonin, or both, in the central nervous system by blocking their reuptake by the presynaptic neurons. This action allows these neurotransmitters to accumulate.
- MAO inhibitors block MAO (which helps metabolize neurotransmitters at synapse), causing buildup of certain neurotransmitters and probably resulting in antidepressant action.

Absorption, distribution, metabolism, and excretion

- Tricyclic and tetracyclic antidepressants have rapid and uniformly good absorption after oral administration.
- All antidepressants are widely distributed to body tissues.
- Tricyclic and tetracyclic antidepressants are metabolized in the liver and excreted by the kidneys as inactive metabolites. Most of the drugs and metabolites are excreted within 72 hours.

PATIENT-TEACHING AID

FOODS TO AVOID WHEN TAKING MAO INHIBITORS

Dear Patient:

When your doctor prescribes an antidepressant, ask him if the medication is an MAO inhibitor. If it is, you should avoid foods with high-tyramine content. These include:

- most cheeses, but especially blue, Boursault, brick, Brie, Camembert, cheddar, Emmentaler, Gruyère, mozzarella, Parmesan, Romano, Roquefort, and Stilton
- caviar
- herring
- sausage meats, especially bologna, pepperoni, salami, and summer sausage
- yeast extracts, that is, those foods containing live yeast, such as compressed yeast cakes. (Cooking kills yeast cells, so baked goods won't cause adverse reactions.)
- chocolate
- Chianti wine and imported beers. (Feel free to drink white wines because they're made without the grape pulp and seeds, the possible source of the amino acid tyramine present in red wines.)

- MAO inhibitors are rapidly and uniformly absorbed after oral administration, metabolized by the liver, and excreted by the kidneys, usually within 24 hours. Although their half-lives are short, the pharmacologic effects of these drugs are long lasting because they permanently inactivate enzymes.

Onset and duration

- Tricyclic and tetracyclic antidepressants produce sedative effects within a few hours after oral administration. Also, anticholinergic side effects occur soon after therapy begins. Antidepressant effects occur 7 to 14 days after onset of therapy due to slow effect on the brain's neurotransmitter metabolism.

  The claim that some of the newer TCAs (amoxapine and trimipramine) supply a more rapid onset of action is not well substantiated.
- Of the MAO inhibitors, isocarboxazid and phenelzine have a very slow onset that may not occur for several weeks or months. Effects may persist for up to 3 weeks after therapy is stopped.

  Tranylcypromine has a more rapid onset of action (usually several days), and MAO activity is restored 3 to 5 days after the drug's discontinued.

Combination products

ETRAFON 2-10♦: perphenazine 2 mg and amitriptyline HCl 10 mg.
ETRAFON: perphenazine 2 mg and amitriptyline HCl 25 mg.
ETRAFON-A: perphenazine 4 mg and amitriptyline 10 mg.
ETRAFON-FORTE: perphenazine 4 mg and amitriptyline 25 mg.
LIMBITROL 10-25: chlordiazepoxide 10 mg and amitriptyline (as HCl) 25 mg.
TRIAVIL-2-10, TRIAVIL-4-10, TRIAVIL-2-25, TRIAVIL-4-25 are products identical to the Etrafon products listed above. Triavil is also available as TRIAVIL-4-50 (perphenazine 4 mg and amitriptyline HCl 50 mg).

NAMES, INDICATIONS AND DOSAGES	SIDE EFFECTS
amitriptyline hydrochloride Amiline♦♦, Amitid, Amitril, Deprex♦♦, Elavil♦, Endep, Levate♦♦, Meravil♦♦, Novotriptyn♦♦, Rolavil **Endogenous and other depression:** ADULTS: 50 to 100 mg P.O. h.s., increasing to 200 mg daily; maximum 300 mg daily if needed; or 20 to 30 mg I.M. q.i.d. Alternatively, the entire dosage can be given at bedtime. ELDERLY AND ADOLESCENTS: 30 mg P.O. daily in divided doses. May be increased to 150 mg.	**Blood:** *agranulocytosis.* **CNS:** *drowsiness,* excitation, seizures, tremors, weakness, confusion, headache. **CV:** *orthostatic hypotension, tachycardia, EKG changes,* hypertension. **EENT:** *blurred vision,* tinnitus, mydriasis. **GI:** *dry mouth, constipation,* nausea, vomiting, anorexia, paralytic ileus. **GU:** *urinary retention.* **Skin:** rash, urticaria. **Other:** *sweating, weight gain and craving for sweets,* allergy. **Abrupt cessation after long-term therapy:** nausea, headache, malaise. (Does not indicate addiction.)
amoxapine Asendin **Endogenous and other depression:** ADULTS: initial dose 50 mg P.O. t.i.d. May increase to 100 mg t.i.d. on third day of treatment. Increases above 300 mg daily should be made only if 300 mg daily has been ineffective during a trial period of at least 2 weeks. When effective dosage is established, entire dosage (not exceeding 300 mg) may be given at bedtime.	**Blood:** *agranulocytosis.* **CNS:** *drowsiness,* excitation, seizures, tremors, weakness, confusion, headache. **CV:** *orthostatic hypotension, tachycardia, EKG changes,* hypertension. **EENT:** *blurred vision,* tinnitus, mydriasis. **GI:** *dry mouth, constipation,* nausea, vomiting, anorexia, paralytic ileus. **GU:** *urinary retention.* **Skin:** rash, urticaria. **Other:** *sweating, weight gain and craving for sweets,* allergy. **Abrupt cessation after long-term therapy:** nausea, headache, malaise. (Does not indicate addiction.)
desipramine hydrochloride Norpramin♦, Pertofrane♦ **Endogenous and other depression:** ADULTS: 75 to 150 mdivided doses, increasing to maximum 200 mg dailyAlternatively, the entire dosage can be given at bedtime. ELDERLY AND ADOLESCENTS: 25 to 50 mg P.O. daily, increasing gradually to maximum 100 mg daily.	**Blood:** *agranulocytosis.* **CNS:** *drowsiness,* excitation, seizures, tremors, weakness, confusion, headache. **CV:** *orthostatic hypotension, tachycardia, EKG changes,* hypertension. **EENT:** *blurred vision,* tinnitus, mydriasis. **GI:** *dry mouth, constipation,* nausea, vomiting, anorexia, paralytic ileus. **GU:** *urinary retention.* **Skin:** rash, urticaria. **Other:** *sweating, weight gain and craving for sweets,* allergy.

INTERACTIONS AND SPECIAL CONSIDERATIONS

Interactions:
MAO INHIBITORS: may cause severe excitation, hyperpyrexia, convulsions, usually with high dose. Use together cautiously.
EPINEPHRINE, LEVARTERENOL: increase hypertensive effect. Use with caution.
BARBITURATES: decrease TCA blood levels. Monitor for decreased antidepressant effect.
METHYLPHENIDATE: increases TCA blood levels. Monitor for enhanced antidepressant effect.

Special considerations:
- Contraindicated during acute recovery phase of myocardial infarction and in patients with prostatic hypertrophy. Use with caution in those who are suicide risks or who have a history of seizures; in patients with urinary retention, narrow-angle glaucoma, increased intraocular pressure, cardiovascular disease, impaired hepatic function, hyperthyroidism; and in patients receiving thyroid medications, electroshock therapy, or elective surgery.
- Dose should be reduced in elderly or debilitated persons and in adolescents.
- Drug should not be withdrawn abruptly.
- If psychotic signs (mood changes, suicidal tendencies) increase, dose should be reduced; to lessen suicide risk, only minimum supply of tablets should be allowed.
- Urinary retention and constipation are possible, intake and output should be monitored. Fluids should be increased to lessen constipation and a stool softener suggested, if needed.
- Patient should avoid activities that require alertness and good psychomotor coordination until CNS response to drug is determined. Drowsiness and dizziness usually subside after first few weeks.
- Has strong anticholinergic effects; one of the most sedating tricyclic antidepressants. Should not be combined with alcohol or other depressants.
- Patient should expect time lag of up to 10 to 14 days before effect is noticeable. Full effect usually appears in 30 days.
- Dry mouth may be relieved with sugarless hard candy or gum.
- Patient should not take any other drugs (prescription or over-the-counter) without first consulting the doctor.

Interactions:
MAO INHIBITORS: may cause severe excitation, hyperpyrexia, convulsions, usually with high dose. Use together cautiously.
EPINEPHRINE, LEVARTERENOL: increase hypertensive effect. Use with caution.
BARBITURATES: decrease TCA blood levels. Monitor for decreased antidepressant effect.
METHYLPHENIDATE: increases TCA blood levels. Monitor for enhanced antidepressant effect.

Special considerations:
- Contraindicated in acute recovery phase of myocardial infarction, and in prostatic hypertrophy. Use with caution in patients who are suicide risks or who have a history of seizures; in patients with urinary retention, narrow-angle glaucoma, increased intraocular pressure, cardiovascular disease, impaired hepatic function, hyperthyroidism; and in patients receiving thyroid medications, electroshock therapy, or elective surgery.
- Dose should be reduced in elderly or debilitated persons and adolescents.
- Drug should not be withdrawn abruptly.
- If psychotic signs (mood changes, suicidal tendencies) increase, dose should be reduced. To lessen suicide risk, only minimum supply of tablets should be allowed.
- Urinary retention and constipation are possible; intake and output should be monitored. Fluids should be increased to lessen constipation and a stool softener suggested, if needed.
- Patient should avoid activities that require alertness and good psychomotor coordination until CNS response to drug is determined. Drowsiness and dizziness usually subside after first few weeks.
- Dry mouth may be relieved with sugarless hard candy or gum.
- Beneficial response may occur within 4 to 7 days.
- Whenever possible, patient should take full dose at bedtime.

Interactions:
MAO INHIBITORS: may cause severe excitation, hyperpyrexia, convulsions, usually with high dose. Use together cautiously.
EPINEPHRINE, LEVARTERENOL: increase hypertensive effect. Use with caution.
BARBITURATES: decrease TCA blood levels. Monitor for decreased antidepressant effect.
METHYLPHENIDATE: increases TCA blood levels. Monitor for enhanced antidepressant effect.

Special considerations:
- Contraindicated during acute recovery phase of myocardial infarction and in patients with prostatic hypertrophy. Use with caution in cardiovascular disease, urinary retention, narrow-angle glaucoma, thyroid disease, seizure disorders, blood dyscrasias, impaired hepatic function; in patients who are suicide risks; and in those receiving electroshock therapy, thyroid medication, or elective surgery.
- Dose should be reduced in elderly or debilitated persons and in adolescents.
- Drug should not be withdrawn abruptly.
- Orthostatic hypotension not as severe with this drug compared to that with other tricyclics.
- If psychotic signs (mood changes, suicidal tendencies) increase, dose should be reduced;

(continued on following page)

NAMES, INDICATIONS AND DOSAGES	SIDE EFFECTS
desipramine hydrochloride *(continued)*	**Abrupt cessation after long-term therapy:** nausea, headache, malaise. (Does not indicate addiction.)
doxepin hydrochloride Adapin, Sinequan♦ **Endogenous and other depression:** ADULTS: initially, 50 to 75 mg P.O. daily in divided doses, to maximum 300 mg daily. Alternatively, entire dosage may be given at bedtime.	**Blood:** *agranulocytosis.* **CNS:** *drowsiness,* excitation, seizures, tremors, weakness, confusion, headache. **CV:** *orthostatic hypotension, tachycardia, EKG changes,* hypertension. **EENT:** *blurred vision,* tinnitus, glossitis, mydriasis. **GI:** *dry mouth, constipation,* nausea, vomiting, anorexia, paralytic ileus. **GU:** *urinary retention.* **Skin:** rash, urticaria. **Other:** *sweating, weight gain and craving for sweets,* allergy. **Abrupt cessation after long-term therapy:** nausea, headache, malaise. (Does not indicate addiction.)
imipramine hydrochloride Antipress, Impril♦♦, Janimine, Novopramine♦♦, Praminil♦♦, Presamine, Ropramine, SK-Pramine, Tofranil♦ **Endogenous and other depression:** ADULTS: 75 to 100 mg P.O. or I.M. daily in divided doses, with 25- to 50-mg increments up to 200 mg. Maximum 300 mg daily. Alternatively, the entire dosage may be given at bedtime. (I.M. route rarely used.) **Childhood enuresis:** 25 to 75 mg P.O. daily.	**Blood:** *agranulocytosis.* **CNS:** *drowsiness,* excitation, seizures, tremors, weakness, confusion, headache. **CV:** *orthostatic hypotension, tachycardia, EKG changes,* hypertension. **EENT:** *blurred vision,* tinnitus, mydriasis. **GI:** *dry mouth, constipation,* nausea, vomiting, anorexia, paralytic ileus. **GU:** *urinary retention.* **Skin:** rash, urticaria. **Other:** *sweating, weight gain and craving for sweets,* allergy. **Abrupt cessation after long-term therapy:** nausea, headache, malaise. (Does not indicate addiction.)

♦ Available in U.S. and Canada. ♦♦ Available in Canada only.
All other products (no symbol) available in U.S. only. Italicized side effects are common or life-threatening.

INTERACTIONS AND SPECIAL CONSIDERATIONS

to lessen suicide risk, only minimum supply of tablets should be allowed.
• Urinary retention and constipation are possible; intake and output should be monitored. Fluids should be increased to lessen constipation and stool softener suggested, if needed.
• Patient should avoid activities that require alertness and good psychomotor coordination until CNS response to drug is determined. Drowsiness and dizziness usually subside after a few weeks.
• Dry mouth may be relieved with sugarless hard candy or gum.
• Drug has anticholinergic effect, is a metabolite of imipramine, and produces less sedation than amitriptyline or doxepin. Alcohol may antagonize effects of desipramine.
• Because it produces less tachycardia and other anticholinergic effects compared with other tricyclics, desipramine is often prescribed for cardiac patients.
• Patient should expect lag time of 10 to 14 days before noticeable effects. Full effect usually appears in 30 days.
• Patient should not take any other drugs (prescription or over-the-counter) without first consulting the doctor.

Interactions:
MAO INHIBITORS: may cause severe excitation, hyperpyrexia, convulsions, usually with high dose. Use together cautiously.
BARBITURATES: decrease TCA blood levels. Monitor for decreased antidepressant effect.
METHYLPHENIDATE: increases TCA blood levels. Monitor for enhanced antidepressant effect.

Special considerations:
• Contraindicated in patients with urinary retention, narrow-angle glaucoma, or prostatic hypertrophy. Use with caution in suicide risks.
• Reduce dose in elderly or debilitated persons, adolescents, and in those receiving other medications (especially anticholinergics).
• Dilute oral concentrate with 120 ml water, milk, or juice (orange, grapefruit, tomato, prune, or pineapple); avoid carbonated beverages.
• Patient should take most of daily dose at bedtime.
• If psychotic signs (mood changes, suicidal tendencies) increase, dose should be reduced.
• Urinary retention and constipation are possible; intake and output should be monitored. Fluids should be increased to lessen constipation and stool softener suggested, if needed.
• Patient should avoid activities that require alertness and good psychomotor coordination until CNS response to drug is determined. Drowsiness and dizziness usually subside after a few weeks.
• Patient should expect time lag of 10 to 14 days before effect is noticeable. Full effect usually appears within 30 days.
• Dry mouth may be relieved with sugarless hard candy or gum.
• Has strong anticholinergic effects; one of the most sedating tricyclic antidepressants. Should not be combined with alcohol or other depressants.
• Patient should not take any other drugs (over-the-counter or prescription) without first consulting the doctor.

Interactions:
MAO INHIBITORS: may cause severe excitation, hyperpyrexia, convulsions, usually with high dose. Use together cautiously.
EPINEPHRINE, LEVARTERENOL: increase hypertensive effect. Use with caution.
BARBITURATES: decrease TCA blood levels. Monitor for decreased antidepressant effect.
METHYLPHENIDATE: increases TCA blood levels. Monitor for enhanced antidepressant effect.

Special considerations:
• Contraindicated during acute recovery phase of myocardial infarction and in prostatic hypertrophy. Use with extreme caution in cardiovascular disease, urinary retention, narrow-angle glaucoma or increased intraocular pressure, thyroid disease, seizure disorders, blood dyscrasias, impaired hepatic function; in suicide risks; and in those receiving electroshock therapy, thyroid medication, or elective surgery.
• Dose should be reduced in elderly or debilitated persons, adolescents, and patients with aggravated psychotic symptoms.
• Drug should not be withdrawn abruptly.
• If psychotic signs (mood changes, suicidal tendencies) increase, dose should be reduced; to lessen suicide risk, only minimum supply of tablets should be allowed.
• Urinary retention and constipation are possible; intake and output should be monitored. Fluids should be increased to lessen constipation and stool softener suggested, if necessary.
• Patient should avoid activities that require alertness and good psychomotor coordination until CNS response to drug is determined. Drowsiness and dizziness usually subside after a few weeks.
• Should not be combined with alcohol or other depressants.
• Patient should expect time lag of 10 to 14 days before effect is noticeable. Full effect usually appears in 30 days.
• Dry mouth may be relieved with sugarless hard candy or gum.
• Patient should not take any other drugs (prescription or over-the-counter) without first consulting the doctor.

NAMES, INDICATIONS AND DOSAGES	SIDE EFFECTS
isocarboxazid Marplan♦ **Depression:** ADULTS: 30 mg P.O. daily in divided doses. Reduce to 10 to 20 mg daily when condition improves. Not recommended for children under 16 years.	**CNS:** dizziness, vertigo, weakness, headache, overactivity, hyperreflexia, tremors, muscle twitching, mania, *insomnia,* confusion, memory impairment, fatigue. **CV:** *orthostatic hypotension,* arrhythmias, paradoxical hypertension. **EENT:** blurred vision. **GI:** dry mouth, *anorexia,* nausea, diarrhea, constipation. **GU:** altered libido. **Skin:** rash. **Other:** peripheral edema, sweating, weight changes.
maprotiline hydrochloride Ludiomil **Treatment of depression associated with depressive neurosis and manic-depressive illness:** ADULTS: initial dose of 75 mg daily for patients with mild-to-moderate depression. The dosage may be increased as required to a dose of 150 mg daily. Maximum dose is 225 mg in patients who are not hospitalized. More severely depressed, hospitalized patients may receive up to 300 mg daily.	**Blood:** *agranulocytosis.* **CNS:** *drowsiness,* excitation, seizures, tremors, weakness, confusion, headache. **CV:** *orthostatic hypotension, tachycardia, EKG changes,* hypertension. **EENT:** *blurred vision,* tinnitus, mydriasis. **GI:** *dry mouth, constipation,* nausea, vomiting, anorexia, paralytic ileus. **GU:** *urinary retention.* **Skin:** rash, urticaria. **Other:** *sweating, weight gain and craving for sweets,* allergy. **Abrupt cessation after long-term therapy:** nausea, headache, malaise. (Does not indicate addiction.)

♦ Available in U.S. and Canada. ♦♦ Available in Canada only.
All other products (no symbol) available in U.S. only. Italicized side effects are common or life-threatening.

INTERACTIONS AND SPECIAL CONSIDERATIONS

Interactions:
AMPHETAMINES, EPHEDRINE, LEVODOPA, MEPERIDINE, METARAMINOL, METHOTRIMEPRAZINE, METHYLPHENIDATE, PHENYLEPHRINE, PHENYLPROPANOLAMINE: pressor effects of these drugs are enhanced by isocarboxazid. Use together very cautiously.
ALCOHOL, BARBITURATES, AND OTHER SEDATIVES; TRANQUILIZERS; NARCOTICS; DEXTROMETHORPHAN; TRICYCLIC ANTIDEPRESSANTS: unpredictable interaction. Use with caution and in reduced dosage.

Special considerations:
• Contraindicated in elderly or debilitated patients, and in patients with severe hepatic or renal impairment; congestive heart failure; pheochromocytoma; hypertensive, cardiovascular, or cerebrovascular disease; severe or frequent headaches. Also contraindicated with foods containing tryptophan or tyramine and excess caffeine. Also during therapy with other MAO inhibitor (including pargyline HCl, phenelzine sulfate, tranylcypromine sulfate) or within 10 days of such therapy; within 10 days of elective surgery requiring general anesthetic, cocaine, or local anesthetic containing sympathomimetic vasoconstrictors. Use cautiously with other psychotropic drugs or with spinal anesthetic; in hyperactive, agitated, or schizophrenic patients; in suicide risks; and in patients with diabetes or epilepsy.
• Used only when TCA or electroshock is ineffective or contraindicated.
• If symptoms of overdosage (palpitations or frequent headaches, jaundice or other hepatic symptoms, or severe orthostatic hypotension) occur, dose should be held and therapy reevaluated.
• Patient should be watched for suicidal tendencies.
• Dose is usually reduced to maintenance level as soon as possible.
• Drug should not be withdrawn abruptly.
• Patient should be weighed biweekly and checked for edema and urinary retention.
• Patient should avoid foods high in tyramine or tryptophan; large amounts of caffeine; and over-the-counter cold, hay fever, or diet preparations.
• Incidence of orthostatic hypotension is high. Walking should be supervised and patient told to get out of bed slowly, sitting up first for 1 minute. Wearing elastic stockings may help minimize orthostatic hypotension.
• Phentolamine (Regitine) should be available to counteract severe hypertension.
• Precautions should be continued 10 days after drug is stopped; long-lasting effects.
• Patient should expect time lag of 1 to 4 weeks before effect is noticeable.
• Drug is MAO inhibitor and is generally less effective than tricyclic antidepressant. Should not be combined with alcohol or other depressants.
• Baseline blood pressure readings, CBCs, and liver function studies should be obtained before beginning therapy and monitored throughout treatment.

Interactions:
MAO INHIBITORS: may cause severe excitation, hyperpyrexia, convulsions, usually with high dose. Use together cautiously.
EPINEPHRINE, LEVARTERENOL: increase hypertensive effect. Use with caution.
BARBITURATES: decrease maprotiline blood levels. Monitor for decreased antidepressant effect.
METHYLPHENIDATE: increases maprotiline blood levels. Monitor for enhanced antidepressant effect.

Special considerations:
• Contraindicated during acute recovery phase of myocardial infarction and in patients with prostatic hypertrophy. Use with caution in cardiovascular disease, urinary retention, narrow-angle glaucoma, thyroid disease or medication, seizure disorders, blood dyscrasias, impaired hepatic functon; in patients who are suicide risks; and in those receiving electroshock therapy or elective surgery.
• Dose should be reduced in elderly or debilitated persons and in adolescents.
• Drug should not be withdrawn abruptly.
• If psychotic signs (mood changes, suicidal tendencies) increase, dose should be reduced; to lessen suicide risk, only minimum supply of tablets should be allowed.
• Urinary retention and constipation are possible; intake and output should be monitored. Fluids should be increased to lessen constipation and stool softener suggested, if needed.
• Patient should avoid activities that require alertness and good psychomotor coordination until CNS response to drug is determined. Drowsiness and dizziness usually subside after a few weeks.
• Dry mouth may be relieved with sugarless hard candy or gum.
• Beneficial response may occur within 4 to 7 days.
• Whenever possible, patient should take full dose at bedtime.
• The first "tetracyclic" antidepressant.

NAMES, INDICATIONS AND DOSAGES	SIDE EFFECTS
nortriptyline hydrochloride Aventyl♦, Pamelor **Endogenous and other depression:** ADULTS: 25 mg P.O. t.i.d. or q.i.d., gradually increasing to maximum 100 mg daily. Alternatively, entire dose may be given at bedtime.	**Blood:** *agranulocytosis.* **CNS:** *drowsiness,* excitation, seizures, tremors, weakness, confusion, headache. **CV:** *orthostatic hypotension, tachycardia, EKG changes,* hypertension. **EENT:** *blurred vision,* tinnitus, mydriasis. **GI:** *dry mouth, constipation,* nausea, vomiting, anorexia, paralytic ileus. **GU:** *urinary retention.* **Skin:** rash, urticaria. **Other:** *sweating, weight gain and craving for sweets,* allergy. **Abrupt cessation after long-term therapy:** nausea, headache, malaise. (Does not indicate addiction.)
phenelzine sulfate Nardil♦ **Endogenous and other depression:** ADULTS: 45 mg P.O. daily in divided doses, increasing rapidly to 60 mg daily. Maximum 90 mg daily. Not recommended for children under 16 years.	**CNS:** dizziness, vertigo, headache, overactivity, hyperreflexia, tremors, muscle twitching, mania, jitters, *insomnia,* confusion, memory impairment, drowsiness, weakness, fatigue. **CV:** paradoxical hypertension, *orthostatic hypotension,* arrhythmias. **GI:** dry mouth, *anorexia,* nausea, constipation. **Other:** peripheral edema, sweating, weight changes.

INTERACTIONS AND SPECIAL CONSIDERATIONS

Interactions:
MAO INHIBITORS: may cause severe excitation, hyperpyrexia, convulsions, usually with high dose. Use together cautiously.
EPINEPHRINE, LEVARTERENOL: increase hypertensive effect. Use with caution.
BARBITURATES: decrease TCA blood levels. Monitor for decreased antidepressant effect.
METHYLPHENIDATE: increases TCA blood levels. Monitor for enhanced antidepressant effect.

Special considerations:
- Contraindicated during acute recovery phase of myocardial infarction and in patients with prostatic hypertrophy. Use with caution in patients with cardiovascular disease, urinary retention, glaucoma, thyroid disease, seizure disorders, impaired hepatic function, blood dyscrasias; in patients who are suicide risks; or in those receiving electroshock therapy, thyroid medication, or elective surgery.
- Dose should be reduced in elderly or debilitated persons and in adolescents.
- Drug should not be withdrawn abruptly.
- If psychotic signs (mood changes, suicidal tendencies) increase, dose should be reduced; to lessen suicide risk, only minimum supply of tablets should be allowed.
- Urinary retention and constipation are possible; intake and output should be monitored. Fluids should be increased to lessen constipation and stool softener suggested, if necessary.
- Patient should avoid activities that require alertness and good psychomotor coordination until CNS response to drug is determined. Drowsiness and dizziness usually subside after a few weeks.
- Patient should expect time lag of 10 to 14 days before effect is noticable. Full effect usually appears in 30 days.
- Dry mouth may be relieved by sugarless hard candy or gum.
- Drug is tricyclic antidepressant, similar in anticholinergic effects to other tricyclics. Should not be combined with alcohol or other depressants.
- Patient should not use other drugs (prescription or over-the-counter) without first consulting the doctor.

Interactions:
AMPHETAMINES, EPHEDRINE, LEVODOPA, MEPERIDINE, METARAMINOL, METHOTRIMEPRAZINE, METHYLPHENIDATE, PHENYLEPHRINE, PHENYLPROPANOLAMINE: enhance pressor effects. Use together cautiously.
ALCOHOL, BARBITURATES, AND OTHER SEDATIVES; TRANQUILIZERS; NARCOTICS; DEXTROMETHORPHAN; TRICYCLIC ANTIDEPRESSANTS: unpredictable interaction. Use with caution and in reduced dosage.

Special considerations:
- Contraindicated in elderly or debilitated patients, and in patients with hepatic impairment, congestive heart failure, pheochromocytoma, hypertension, cardiovascular or cerebrovascular disease, severe or frequent headaches; also contraindicated with foods containing tryptophan (broad beans) or tyramine and excess caffeine or chocolate. Also contraindicated during therapy with other MAO inhibitor, including pargyline HCl, isocarboxazid, tranylcypromine sulfate, or within 10 days of such therapy; within 10 days of elective surgery requiring general anesthetic, cocaine, or local anesthetic containing sympathomimetic vasoconstrictors; in hyperactive, agitated, or schizophrenic patients. Use cautiously with antihypertensive drugs containing thiazide diuretics or with spinal anesthetic; in suicide risk, diabetes, epilepsy.
- Should be used only when TCA or electroshock therapy is ineffective or contraindicated.
- If symptoms of overdose (jaundice or other hepatic symptoms, severe hypotension, palpitations, or frequent headaches) occur, dose should be held and therapy reevaluated.
- Suicidal tendencies should be watched for.
- Dose is usually reduced to maintenance level as soon as possible.
- Store drug in tight container, away from heat and light.
- Phentolamine (Regitine) counteracts severe hypertension.
- Patient should avoid foods high in tyramine or tryptophan; large amounts of caffeine; and self-medication with over-the-counter cold, hay fever, or diet preparations.
- Incidence of orthostatic hypotension is high. Walking should be supervised and patient told to get out of bed slowly, sitting up first for 1 minute.
- Precautions should be continued 10 days after stopping drug; long-lasting effects. Wearing elastic stockings may help minimize orthostatic hypotension.
- Patient should expect time lag of 1 to 4 weeks before effect is noticeable.
- Drug is MAO inhibitor and is generally less effective than tricyclic antidepressant. Should not be combined with alcohol or other depressants.
- Baseline blood pressure readings, CBCs, and liver function studies should be obtained before beginning therapy and monitored throughout treatment.

NAMES, INDICATIONS AND DOSAGES	SIDE EFFECTS
protriptyline hydrochloride Triptil♦♦, Vivactil **Endogenous and other depression:** ADULTS: 15 to 40 mg P.O. daily in divided doses, increasing gradually to maximum 60 mg daily.	**Blood:** *agranulocytosis.* **CNS:** excitation, seizures, tremors, weakness, confusion, headache. **CV:** *orthostatic hypotension, tachycardia, EKG changes,* hypertension. **EENT:** *blurred vision,* tinnitus, mydriasis. **GI:** *dry mouth, constipation,* nausea, vomiting, anorexia, paralytic ileus. **GU:** *urinary retention.* **Skin:** rash, urticaria. **Other:** *sweating, weight gain and craving for sweets,* allergy. **Abrupt cessation after long-term therapy:** nausea, headache, malaise. (Does not indicate addiction.)
tranylcypromine sulfate Parnate♦ **Endogenous or other depression:** ADULTS: 10 mg P.O. b.i.d. Increase to maximum 30 mg daily, if necessary, after 2 weeks. Not recommended for children under 16 years.	**CNS:** dizziness, vertigo, headache, overactivity, hyperreflexia, tremors, muscle twitching, mania, jitters, confusion, memory impairment, fatigue. **CV:** *orthostatic hypotension,* arrhythmias, paradoxical hypertension. **EENT:** blurred vision. **GI:** dry mouth, *anorexia,* nausea, diarrhea, constipation, abdominal pain. **GU:** changed libido, impotence. **Skin:** rash. **Other:** peripheral edema, sweating, weight changes, chills.

♦ Available in U.S. and Canada. ♦♦ Available in Canada only.
All other products (no symbol) available in U.S. only. Italicized side effects are common or life-threatening.

INTERACTIONS AND SPECIAL CONSIDERATIONS

Interactions:

MAO INHIBITORS: may cause severe excitation, hyperpyrexia, convulsions, and death, usually with high dose. Use together cautiously.

EPINEPHRINE, LEVARTERENOL: increase hypertensive effect. Use with caution.

BARBITURATES: decrease TCA blood levels. Monitor for decreased antidepressant effect.

METHYLPHENIDATE: increases TCA blood levels. Monitor for enhanced antidepressant effect.

Special considerations:

- Contraindicated during acute recovery phase of myocardial infarction and in prostatic hypertrophy. Use with caution in the elderly and in patients with cardiovascular disease, urinary retention, increased intraocular tension, thyroid disease, seizure disorders, blood dyscrasias; in suicide risks; and in those receiving electroshock therapy, thyroid medication, or elective surgery.
- Dose should be reduced in elderly or debilitated persons and in adolescents.
- Drug should not be withdrawn abruptly.
- If psychotic signs (mood changes, suicidal tendencies, anxiety, agitation, or cardiovascular reactions) increase, dose should be reduced; to lessen suicide risk, only minimum supply of tablets should be allowed.
- Urinary retention and constipation are possible; intake and output should be monitored. Fluids should be increased to lessen constipation and stool softener suggested, if necessary.
- Patient should avoid activities that require alertness and good psychomotor coordination until CNS response to drug is determined. Drowsiness and dizziness usually subside after a few weeks.
- Dry mouth may be relieved with sugarless hard candy or gum.
- Patient should expect time lag of 7 to 14 days before effect is noticeable.
- Drug is possibly the most rapid-acting but least sedating tricyclic antidepressant. Should not be combined with alcohol or other depressants.
- Entire dose should not be given at bedtime as patient may develop insomnia.
- Patient should not use other drugs (prescription or over-the-counter) without first consulting the doctor.

Interactions:

AMPHETAMINES, EPHEDRINE, LEVODOPA, MEPERIDINE, METARAMINOL, METHOTRIMEPRAZINE, METHYLPHENIDATE, PHENYLEPHRINE, PHENYLPROPANOLAMINE: pressor effects of these drugs are enhanced by tranylcypromine. Use together cautiously.

ALCOHOL, BARBITURATES, AND OTHER SEDATIVES; TRANQUILIZERS; NARCOTICS; DEXTROMETHORPHAN; TRICYCLIC ANTIDEPRESSANTS: use with caution and in reduced dosage.

Special considerations:

- Contraindicated in patients with severe hepatic or renal impairment; congestive heart failure; pheochromocytoma, hypertension, or cardiovascular or cerebrovascular disease; severe or frequent headaches; in patients taking antihypertensive drugs or diuretics; in elderly or debilitated patients; in patients for whom close supervision is not possible; and in hyperactive, agitated, or schizophrenic patients. Also contraindicated with foods containing tryptophan or tyramine and with excess caffeine. Also contraindicted during therapy with other MAO inhibitor (including pargyline HCl, phenelzine sulfate, isocarboxazid) or within 7 days of such therapy; within 7 days of elective surgery requiring general anesthetic, cocaine, or local anesthetic containing sympathomimetic vasoconstrictors. Use cautiously with anti-Parkinson drugs, spinal anesthetic; in renal disease, diabetes, epilepsy, hyperthyroidism; and in suicide risks.
- Should be used only when TCA or electroshock therapy is ineffective or contraindicated.
- If symptoms of overdose (palpitations, severe orthostatic hypotension) occur, dose should be held and therapy reevaluated.
- Suicidal tendencies should be watched for.
- Dose is usually reduced to maintenance level as soon as possible.
- Drug should not be withdrawn abruptly.
- Phentolamine (Regitine) counteracts severe hypertension.
- Patient should avoid foods high in tyramine or tryptophan; large amounts of caffeine; and self-medication with over-the-counter cold, hay fever, or diet preparations.
- Patient should get out of bed slowly, sitting up for 1 minute. Wearing elastic stockings may help minimize orthostatic hypotension.
- Precautions should be continued for 7 days after drug is stopped; effects last that long.
- Patient should expect time lag of 1 to 3 weeks before effect is noticeable.
- More rapid onset of action than isocarboxazid or phenelzine sulfate.
- MAO inhibitor most likely to cause hypertensive crisis in presence of high-tyramine ingestion. Generally less effective than tricyclic antidepressant. Should not be combined with alcohol or other depressants.
- Baseline blood pressure readings, CBCs, and liver function studies, should be obtained before beginning therapy and monitored throughout treatment.

NAMES, INDICATIONS AND DOSAGES	SIDE EFFECTS
trimipramine maleate Surmontil **Endogenous and other depression:** ADULTS: 75 mg daily in divided doses, increased to 200 mg/day. Dosages over 300 mg/day not recommended. **Enuresis:** CHILDREN OVER 6 YEARS: initial dose 25 mg P.O. 1 hour before bedtime; if no response, increase dose to 50 mg in children under 12 years, and to 75 mg in children over 12 years.	**Blood:** *agranulocytosis.* **CNS:** *drowsiness,* excitation, seizures, tremors, weakness, confusion, headache. **CV:** *orthostatic hypotension, tachycardia, EKG changes,* hypertension. **EENT:** *blurred vision,* tinnitus, mydriasis. **GI:** *dry mouth, constipation,* nausea, vomiting, anorexia, paralytic ileus. **GU:** *urinary retention.* **Skin:** rash, urticaria. **Other:** *sweating, weight gain and craving for sweets,* allergy. **Abrupt cessation after long-term therapy:** nausea, headache, malaise. (Does not indicate addiction.)

INTERACTIONS AND SPECIAL CONSIDERATIONS

Interactions:

MAO INHIBITORS: may cause severe excitation, hyperpyrexia, convulsions, usually with high dose. Use together cautiously.

EPINEPHRINE, LEVARTERENOL: increase hypertensive effect. Use with caution.

BARBITURATES: decrease TCA blood levels. Monitor for decreased antidepressant effect.

METHYLPHENIDATE: increases TCA blood levels. Monitor for enhanced antidepressant effects.

Special considerations:

- Contraindicated during acute recovery phase of myocardial infarction and in patients with prostatic hypertrophy. Use with extreme caution in patients with cardiovascular disease, urinary retention, narrow-angle glaucoma or increased intraocular pressure, thyroid disease, seizure disorders, blood dyscrasias, impaired hepatic function. Also contraindicated in patients who are suicide risks and in those receiving electroshock therapy, thyroid medication, or elective surgery.
- Dose should be reduced in elderly or debilitated persons and adolescents.
- Drug should not be withdrawn abruptly.
- If psychotic signs (mood changes, suicidal tendencies) increase, dose should be reduced; to lessen suicide risk, only minimum supply of tablets should be allowed.
- Urinary retention and constipation are possible; intake and output should be monitored. Fluids should be increased to lessen constipation and stool softener suggested, if needed.
- Patient should avoid activities that require alertness and good psychomotor coordination until CNS response to drug has been determined. Drowsiness and dizziness usually subside after a few weeks.
- Patient should expect time lag of 10 to 14 days before effect is noticeable. Full effect usually appears in 30 days.
- Dry mouth may be relieved with sugarless hard candy or gum.
- Most common tricyclic used for enuresis, but effectiveness may decrease over time. Similar in anticholinergic effects to other tricyclics.
- Patient should not use other drugs (prescription or over-the-counter) without first consulting the doctor.

31

Tranquilizers

alprazolam
chlordiazepoxide hydrochloride
chlormezanone
clorazepate dipotassium
diazepam
halazepam
hydroxyzine hydrochloride
hydroxyzine pamoate
lorazepam
meprobamate
oxazepam
prazepam
tybamate

Tranquilizers reduce anxiety without inducing sleep; they're indicated for patients suffering from various neuroses or mild depression. Most tranquilizers have muscle relaxant and anticonvulsant properties. They produce a dose-dependent, nonspecific depression of the central nervous system (CNS) and closely resemble sedative-hypnotic drugs (barbiturates) in pharmacologic properties.

Major uses

Tranquilizers are used to:

- treat anxiety
- relax skeletal muscle
- prevent and treat alcohol withdrawal symptoms (especially chlordiazepoxide, diazepam, and lorazepam) and convulsions
- treat status epilepticus (especially I.V. diazepam)
- supply premedication for I.V. general anesthetic for short procedures (especially diazepam and lorazepam).

Mechanism of action

- Benzodiazepines (alprazolam, chlordiazepoxide, clorazepate, diazepam, halazepam, lorazepam, oxazepam, and prazepam) appear to depress the CNS at the limbic and subcortical levels of the brain, with sedative, skeletal muscle relaxant, and anticonvulsant effects. They can produce dependence.
- The mechanisms of the other tranquilizers are still unclear.

Absorption, distribution, metabolism, and excretion

- Benzodiazepines are very well absorbed when given orally. Well distributed to body tissues and fluids, they're all metabolized in the gastrointestinal tract and the liver to either active or inactive metabolites. These metabolites are then excreted by the kidneys.

  Chlordiazepoxide and diazepam absorption, after I.M. injection, is variable, painful, and unpredictable.

  Lorazepam absorption, after I.M. injection, is much more dependable and less painful than that of diazepam and chlordiazepoxide.
- Chlormezanone, hydroxyzine, meprobamate, and tybamate are well absorbed orally, distributed to most body tissues, metabolized in the liver, and eliminated in both the urine and feces.

Onset and duration

- All benzodiazepines have a fairly prompt onset of action (1 to 2 hours); diazepam has the fastest (about 1 hour). Generally, those agents that are changed into active (long-acting) metabolites have longer duration of action (up to 24 hours) than those that are not changed. The long therapeutic half-lives of the active metabolites permit once-daily

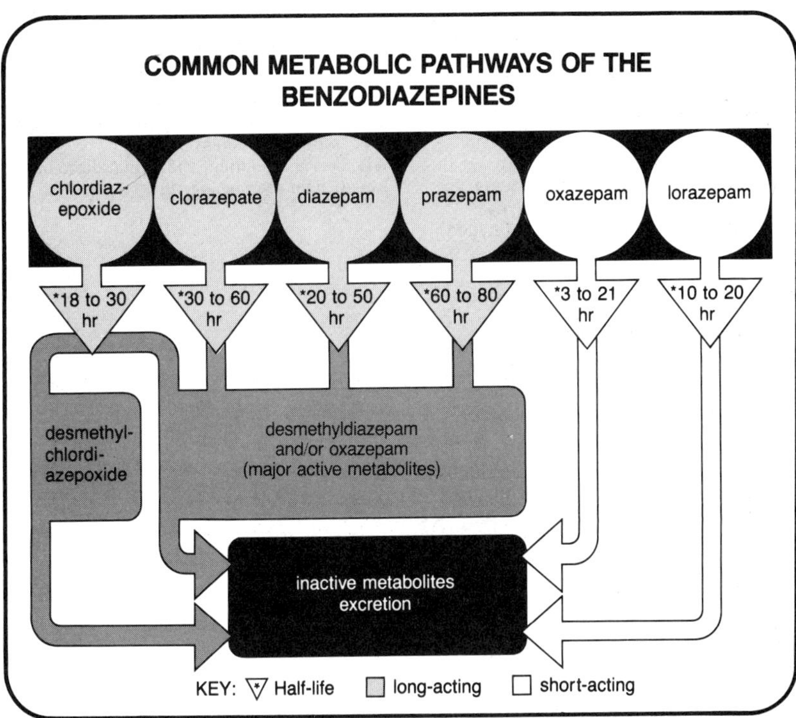

dosing when steady-state levels are reached.

Lorazepam and oxazepam, with shorter half-lives, must be given two to four times daily (see chart above).

- Chlormezanone acts within 15 to 30 minutes, and its effect lasts 6 hours.
- Hydroxyzine acts within 15 to 20 minutes, and its effect lasts 4 to 6 hours.
- Meprobamate begins its therapeutic action in 1 hour, peaks in 2 to 3 hours, and has a half-life of about 10 hours.
- Tybamate has an onset and peak similar to meprobamate but a shorter half-life (3 hours).

Combination products

EQUAGESIC: meprobamate 150 mg, ethoheptazine citrate 75 mg, and aspirin 250 mg.
LIBRAX CAPSULES: chlordiazepoxide hydrochloride 5 mg and clidinium bromide 2.5 mg.
LIMBITROL 5-12.5: chlordiazepoxide 5 mg and amitriptyline (as HCl) 12.5 mg.
LIMBITROL 10-25: chlordiazepoxide 10 mg and amitriptyline (as HCl) 25 mg.
MENRIUM 5-2: chlordiazepoxide 5 mg and esterified estrogens 0.2 mg.
MILPATH-400: meprobamate 400 mg and tridihexethyl chloride 25 mg.

NAMES, INDICATIONS AND DOSAGES	SIDE EFFECTS
alprazolam Xanax Controlled Substance Schedule IV **Anxiety and tension:** ADULTS: Usual starting dose is 0.25 to 0.5 mg t.i.d. Maximum total daily dosage is 4 mg in divided doses. In elderly or debilitated patients, usual starting dose is 0.25 mg b.i.d. or t.i.d.	**CNS:** *drowsiness, lightheadedness,* headache, confusion. **CV:** transient hypotension. **EENT:** dry mouth. **GI:** nausea, vomiting, discomfort.
chlordiazepoxide hydrochloride Controlled Substance Schedule IV A-poxide, Chlordiazachel, Corax♦♦, C-Tran♦♦, J-Liberty, Libritabs, Librium♦, Medilium♦♦, Nack♦♦, Novopoxide♦♦, Protensin♦♦, Relaxil♦♦, Sereen, SK-Lygen, Solium♦♦, Tenax, Trilium♦♦, Zetran **Mild-to-moderate anxiety and tension:** ADULTS: 5 to 10 mg t.i.d. or q.i.d. CHILDREN OVER 6 YEARS: 5 mg P.O. b.i.d. to q.i.d. Maximum 10 mg P.O. b.i.d. to t.i.d. **Severe anxiety and tension:** ADULTS: 20 to 25 mg t.i.d. or q.i.d. **Withdrawal symptoms of acute alcoholism:** ADULTS: 50 to 100 mg P.O., I.M., or I.V. Maximum 300 mg daily. **Preoperative apprehension and anxiety:** ADULTS: 5 to 10 mg P.O. t.i.d. or q.i.d. on day preceding surgery; or 50 to 100 mg I.M. 1 hour before surgery. *Note:* Parenteral form not recommended in children under 12 years.	**CNS:** *drowsiness, lethargy, hangover,* fainting. **CV:** transient hypotension. **GI:** nausea, vomiting, abdominal discomfort. **Local:** *pain at injection site.*
chlormezanone Fenarol, Trancopal♦ **Mild anxiety and tension, muscle relaxation:** ADULTS: 100 to 200 mg P.O. t.i.d. or q.i.d. CHILDREN 5 TO 12 YEARS: 50 to 100 mg P.O. t.i.d. or q.i.d.	**CNS:** *drowsiness,* mental depression, headache, dizziness, ataxia, lethargy, muscular weakness. **CV:** edema. **GI:** nausea, anorexia, dry mouth. **GU:** urinary retention. **Skin:** rash.
clorazepate dipotassium Controlled Substance Schedule IV Tranxene♦ **Acute alcohol withdrawal:** ADULTS: Day 1—30 mg P.O. initially, followed by 30 to 60 mg P.O. in divided doses; Day 2—45 to 90 mg P.O. in divided doses;	**CNS:** *drowsiness, lethargy, hangover,* fainting. **CV:** transient hypotension. **GI:** nausea, vomiting, abdominal discomfort.

♦ Available in U.S. and Canada. ♦♦ Available in Canada only.
All other products (no symbol) available in U.S. only. Italicized side effects are common or life-threatening.

INTERACTIONS AND SPECIAL CONSIDERATIONS

Interactions:
CIMETIDINE: possible increased sedation. Monitor patient carefully if used together.

Special considerations:
• Contraindicated in acute narrow-angle glaucoma, psychosis, and anxiety-free psychiatric disorders.
• Dosage should be reduced in elderly or debilitated patients.
• Drug should not be withdrawn abruptly. Abuse or addiction is possible. Withdrawal symptoms may occur.
• Patient should not combine drug with alcohol or other depressants, and should avoid activities that require alertness and psychomotor coordination until CNS response to drug is determined.
• Patient should not give medication to others.
• Drug should not be prescribed for everyday stress.
• Drug is not for long-term use (more than 4 months).
• Patient should not continue drug without doctors's approval.
• Alprazolam is the first of a new type of benzodiazepine, known as a triazolo-benzodiazepine. It's more rapidly metabolized and excreted than most of the other drugs in the benzodiazepine class and has a lower incidence of lethargy than other drugs of this class.

Interactions:
CIMETIDINE: increased sedation. Monitor carefully.

Special considerations:
• Use with caution in patients with mental depression, blood dyscrasias, hepatic or renal disease, or in those undergoing anticoagulant therapy.
• Dosage should be reduced in elderly or debilitated patients.
• Possibility of abuse and addiction. Drug should not be withdrawn abruptly; withdrawal symptoms may occur.
• Patient should avoid activities that require alertness and good psychomotor coordination until CNS response to drug is determined.
• Patient should not combine drug with alcohol or other depressants.
• Although package recommends I.M. use only, drug may be given I.V.
• Injectable form (as hydrochloride) comes as two ampules— diluent and powdered drug. For I.M., 2 ml of diluent should be added to powder and agitated gently until clear. Should be used immediately. I.M. form may be erratically absorbed.
• For I.V., 5 ml of saline injection or sterile water for injection should be used as diluent and given slowly over 1 minute. Packaged diluent should not be given I.V.
• Powder should be kept away from light, mixed just before use, and the remainder discarded.
• Injectable form should not be mixed with any other parenteral drug.
• Patient should not give medication to others.
• For symptoms and treatment of toxicity, see APPENDIX.

No significant interactions.

Special considerations:
• Use with caution in hepatic or renal disease.
• Dosage should be reduced in elderly or debilitated patients.
• Possibility of abuse and addiction exists. Drug should not be withdrawn abruptly; withdrawal symptoms may occur.
• Patient should avoid activities that require alertness and good psychomotor coordination until CNS response to drug is determined.
• Patient should not combine drug with alcohol or other depressants.
• Rapid onset of action (15 to 30 minutes), with effects lasting 4 to 6 hours.
• Chemically unrelated to other antianxiety agents.
• Chewing gum or sugarless hard candy suggested to relieve dry mouth.

Interactions:
CIMETIDINE: increased sedation. Monitor carefully.

Special considerations:
• Contraindicated in patients with acute narrow-angle glaucoma, depressive neuroses, psychotic reactions, and in children under 18 years. Use with caution when hepatic or renal damage is present.
• Dosage should be reduced in elderly or debilitated patients.
• Possibility of abuse and addiction exists. Drug should not be withdrawn abruptly; withdrawal symptoms may occur.
• Patient should avoid activities that require

(continued on following page)

NAMES, INDICATIONS AND DOSAGES	SIDE EFFECTS

clorazepate dipotassium
(continued)

Day 3—22.5 to 45 mg P.O. in divided doses; Day 4—15 to 30 mg P.O. in divided doses; gradually reduce daily dose to 7.5 to 15 mg.

Anxiety:
ADULTS: 15 to 60 mg P.O. daily.

As an adjunct in epilepsy:
ADULTS AND CHILDREN OVER 12 YEARS: Maximum recommended initial dosage is 7.5 mg P.O. t.i.d. Dosage increases should be no greater than 7.5 mg/week. Maximum daily dosage should not exceed 90 mg/day.
CHILDREN BETWEEN 9 AND 12 YEARS: Maximum recommended initial dosage is 7.5 mg P.O. b.i.d. Dosage increases should be no greater than 7.5 mg/week. Maximum daily dosage should not exceed 60 mg/day.

diazepam
Controlled Substance Schedule IV
D-Tran♦♦, E-Pam♦♦, Erital♦♦, Meval♦♦, NeoCalme♦♦, Novodipam♦♦, Paxel♦♦, Serenack♦♦, Stress-Pam♦♦, Valium♦, Vivol♦♦

Tension, anxiety, adjunct in convulsive disorders or skeletal muscle spasm:
ADULTS: 2 to 10 mg P.O. t.i.d. or q.i.d.
CHILDREN OVER 6 MONTHS: 1 to 2.5 mg P.O. t.i.d. or q.i.d.

Tension, anxiety, muscle spasm, endoscopic procedures, seizures:
ADULTS: 5 to 10 mg I.V. initially, up to 30 mg in 1 hour or possibly more for cardioversion or status epilepticus, depending on response.
CHILDREN 5 YEARS AND OVER: 1 mg I.V. or I.M. slowly q 2 to 5 minutes to maximum 10 mg. Repeat q 2 to 4 hours.
CHILDREN 30 DAYS TO 5 YEARS: 0.2 to 0.5 mg I.V. or I.M. slowly q 2 to 5 minutes to maximum 5 mg. Repeat q 2 to 4 hours.

Tetanic muscle spasms:
CHILDREN OVER 5 YEARS: 5 to 10 mg I.M. or I.V. q 3 to 4 hours, p.r.n.
INFANTS OVER 30 DAYS: 1 to 2 mg I.M. or I.V. q 3 to 4 hours, p.r.n.

Side effects:
CNS: *drowsiness, lethargy, hangover,* fainting.
CV: transient hypotension.
GI: nausea, vomiting, abdominal discomfort.
Local: desquamation, pain, phlebitis at injection site.

halazepam
Paxipam
Controlled Substance Schedule IV

Relief of anxiety and tension:
ADULTS: Usual dose is 20 to 40 mg P.O. t.i.d. or q.i.d.
Optimal daily dosage is generally 80 to 160 mg. Daily doses up to 600 mg have been given. In elderly or debilitated patients, initial dosage is

Side effects:
CNS: *drowsiness, lethargy, hangover,* fainting.
CV: transient hypotension.
EENT: dry mouth.
GI: nausea and vomiting, discomfort.

♦ Available in U.S. and Canada. ♦♦ Available in Canada only.
All other products (no symbol) available in U.S. only. Italicized side effects are common or life-threatening.

INTERACTIONS AND SPECIAL CONSIDERATIONS

alertness and good psychomotor coordination until CNS response to drug is determined.
• Patient should not combine drug with alcohol or other depressants.
• Sugarless chewing gum or hard candy suggested to relieve dry mouth.
• Patient should not give medication to others.
• Drug should not be prescribed regularly for everyday stress.

Interactions:
CIMETIDINE: increased sedation. Monitor carefully.

Special considerations:
• Contraindicated in shock, coma, acute alcohol intoxication, acute narrow-angle glaucoma, psychosis; in oral form for children under 6 months. Use with caution in patients with blood dyscrasias, hepatic or renal damage, depression, open-angle glaucoma; in elderly and debilitated patients; and in those with limited pulmonary reserve.
• Dosage should be reduced in elderly or debilitated patients.
• Possibility of abuse and addiction exists. Drug should not be withdrawn abruptly; withdrawal symptoms may occur.
• Patient should avoid activities that require alertness and good psychomotor coordination until CNS response to drug is determined.
• Patient should not combine drug with alcohol or other depressants.
• Should not be diluted with solutions or mixed with other drugs: incompatible.
• Extravasation should be avoided. Should not be injected into small veins.
• Phlebitis possible at injection site.
• Should be given I.V. slowly, at rate not exceeding 5 mg/minute.
• I.V. route more reliable; I.M. absorption variable, to be discouraged.
• Drug of choice (I.V. form) for status epilepticus.
• Diazepam should not be stored in plastic syringes.
• Patient should not give medication to others.
• Drug should not be prescribed regularly for everyday stress.
• For symptoms and treatment of toxicity, see APPENDIX.

Interactions:
CIMETIDINE: possible increased sedation. Monitor carefully.

Special considerations:
• Contraindicated in acute narrow-angle glaucoma, psychosis, and anxiety-free psychiatric disorders. Use with caution in hepatorenal impairment.
• Dosage should be reduced in elderly or debilitated patients.
• Abuse and addiction are possible. Drug should not be withdrawn abruptly; withdrawal symptoms may occur.
• Patient should not combine drug with alcohol or other depressant, and also avoid activities that require alertness and psychomotor coordination until CNS response to drug is determined.
• Patient should not give medication to others.
• Patient should not continue the drug without

(continued on following page)

NAMES, INDICATIONS AND DOSAGES	SIDE EFFECTS
halazepam *(continued)* 20 mg once or twice daily.	
hydroxyzine hydrochloride Atarax♦, Hyzine-50, Orgatrax, Quiess, Vistaril (parenteral) **hydroxyzine pamoate** Vistaril (oral) **Anxiety and tension:** ADULTS: 25 to 100 mg P.O. t.i.d. or q.i.d. **Anxiety, tension, hyperkinesia:** CHILDREN OVER 6 YEARS: 50 to 100 mg P.O. daily in divided doses. CHILDREN UNDER 6 YEARS: 50 mg P.O. daily in divided doses. **Preoperative and postoperative adjunctive therapy:** ADULTS: 25 to 100 mg I.M. q 4 to 6 hours. CHILDREN: 1.1 mg/kg I.M. q 4 to 6 hours.	**CNS:** *drowsiness,* involuntary motor activity. **GI:** *dry mouth.* **Local:** marked discomfort at site of I.M. injection.
lorazepam Controlled Substance Schedule IV Ativan♦ **Anxiety, tension, agitation, irritability, especially in anxiety neuroses or organic (especially GI or CV) disorders:** ADULTS: 2 to 6 mg P.O. daily in divided doses. Maximum 10 mg daily. **Insomnia:** ADULTS: 2 to 4 mg P.O. h.s. **Sedation, anxiety, and as a premedication before operative procedure:** ADULTS: 2 to 4 mg I.M. or I.V.	**CNS:** *drowsiness, lethargy, hangover,* fainting. **CV:** transient hypotension. **GI:** abdominal discomfort.
meprobamate Controlled Substance Schedule IV Arcoban, Bamate, Equanil, Kalmm, Lan-Dol♦♦, Maso-Bamate, Meditran, Mep-E, Mepriam, Meprocon, Meprotabs, Meribam, Miltown♦, Neo-Tran♦♦, Novomepro♦♦, Pax-400, Quietal♦♦, Saronil, Sedabamate, SK-Bamate, Tranmep **Anxiety and tension:** ADULTS: 1.2 to 1.6 g P.O. in 3 or 4 equally divided doses. Maximum 2.4 g daily. CHILDREN 6 TO 12 YEARS: 100 to 200 mg P.O. b.i.d. or t.i.d. Not recommended for children under 6 years.	**Blood:** *thrombocytopenia, leukopenia,* eosinophilia. **CNS:** *drowsiness,* ataxia, dizziness, slurred speech, headache, vertigo. **CV:** palpitation, tachycardia, hypotension. **GI:** anorexia, nausea, vomiting, diarrhea, stomatitis. **Skin:** pruritus, urticaria, erythematous maculopapular rash.

♦ Available in U.S. and Canada. ♦♦ Available in Canada only.
All other products (no symbol) available in U.S. only. Italicized side effects are common or life-threatening.

INTERACTIONS AND SPECIAL CONSIDERATIONS

the doctor's approval.
• Drug should not be prescribed for everyday stress.
• Halazepam is not for long-term use (more than 4 months).

No significant interactions.

Special considerations:
• Contraindicated in patients in shock or comatose states.
• Dosage should be reduced in elderly or debilitated patients.
• Possibility of abuse and addiction exists. Drug should not be withdrawn abruptly; withdrawal symptoms may occur.
• Patient should avoid activities that require alertness and good psychomotor coordination until CNS response to drug is determined.
• Patient should not combine drug with alcohol or other depressants.
• Excessive sedation possible due to potentiation with other CNS drugs.
• Used as an antiemetic and antianxiety drug.
• Used in psychogenically induced allergic conditions, such as chronic urticaria and pruritus.
• Parenteral form (hydroxyzine HCl) for I.M. use only; never I.V.
• Injection should be aspirated carefully to prevent inadvertent intravascular injection. Should be injected deeply into a large muscle.
• Sugarless gum or hard candy should be suggested to relieve dry mouth.

Interactions:
CIMETIDINE: increased sedation. Monitor carefully.

Special considerations:
• Contraindicated in myasthenia gravis, acute narrow-angle glaucoma, psychosis, mental depression. Use with caution in organic brain syndrome, renal or hepatic impairment.
• Dosage should be reduced in elderly or debilitated patients.
• Possibility of abuse and addiction exists. Drug should not be withdrawn abruptly; withdrawal symptoms may occur.
• When administering I.M., should be injected deeply into muscle mass. Should not be diluted.
• When administering I.V., should be diluted with an equal volume of sterile water for injection, sodium chloride injection, or 5% dextrose injection.
• Patient should avoid activities that require alertness or good psychomotor coordination until CNS response to drug is determined.
• Patient should not combine drug with alcohol or other depressants.
• Patient should not give medication to others.
• Drug should not be prescribed regularly for everyday stress.
• For symptoms and treatment of toxicity, see APPENDIX.

No significant interactions.

Special considerations:
• Contraindicated in patients with hypersensitivity to meprobamate, carisoprodol, mebutamate, tybamate, carbromal; and in those with renal insufficiency or porphyria. Use with caution in patients with impaired hepatic or renal function, in lactating women, and in patients with suicidal tendencies.
• Dosage should be reduced in elderly or debilitated patients.
• Possibility of abuse and addiction exists. Drug should be withdrawn gradually (over 2 weeks) or withdrawal symptoms may occur.
• Patient should avoid activities that require alertness or good psychomotor coordination until CNS response to drug is determined.
• Patient should not combine drug with alcohol or other depressants.
• Should be given deep I.M. into muscle.
• Should be taken P.O. with meals to reduce gastric distress.
• Therapeutic blood levels 0.5 to 2 mg/100 ml; levels above 20 mg/100 ml may cause coma and death.
• Periodic evaluation of CBC and liver function studies are indicated in patients receiving high doses.

NAMES, INDICATIONS AND DOSAGES	SIDE EFFECTS
oxazepam Controlled Substance Schedule IV Serax♦ **Alcohol withdrawal:** ADULTS: 15 to 30 mg P.O. t.i.d. or q.i.d. **Severe anxiety:** ADULTS: 15 to 30 mg P.O. t.i.d. or q.i.d. **Tension, mild-to-moderate anxiety:** ADULTS: 10 to 15 mg P.O. t.i.d. or q.i.d.	**CNS:** *drowsiness, lethargy, hangover,* fainting. **CV:** transient hypotension. **GI:** nausea, vomiting, abdominal discomfort.
prazepam Controlled Substance Schedule IV Verstran, Centrax **Anxiety:** ADULTS: 30 mg P.O. in divided doses. Range 20 to 60 mg daily. May be administered as single daily dose at bedtime. Start with 20 mg.	**CNS:** *drowsiness, lethargy, hangover,* fainting. **CV:** transient hypotension. **GI:** nausea, vomiting, abdominal discomfort.
tybamate Controlled Substance Schedule IV Tybatran **Anxiety and tension:** ADULTS: 750 mg to 2 g P.O. daily in divided doses; maximum 3 g daily. CHILDREN 6 TO 12 YEARS: 20 to 25 mg/kg daily, divided into 3 or 4 doses.	**Blood:** dyscrasias. **CNS:** *drowsiness,* dizziness, fatigue, weakness, ataxia, depressive or panic reactions, paradoxical irritability, excitement, confusion, euphoria, insomnia, headache, paresthesias. **CV:** flushing, light-headedness, hypotension, palpitation, tachycardia, fainting. **GI:** nausea, anorexia, dry mouth, glossitis. **Skin:** urticaria, pruritus, pruritus ani, rash.

♦ Available in U.S. and Canada. ♦♦ Available in Canada only.
All other products (no symbol) available in U.S. only. Italicized side effects are common or life-threatening.

INTERACTIONS AND SPECIAL CONSIDERATIONS

Interactions:
CIMETIDINE: increased sedation. Monitor carefully.

Special considerations:
- Contraindicated in psychoses. Use cautiously in patients with history of convulsive disorders, drug allergies, blood dyscrasias, renal disease, depression.
- Dose should be reduced in elderly or debilitated patients.
- Possibility of abuse and addiction exists. Drug should not be withdrawn abruptly; withdrawal symptoms may occur.
- Patient should avoid activities that require alertness or good psychomotor coordination until CNS response to drug is determined.
- Patient should not combine drug with alcohol or other depressants.
- Fewer cumulative effects than most other benzodiazepines due to short half-life.
- Patient should not give medication to others.
- Drug should not be prescribed for everyday stress.
- For symptoms and treatment of toxicity, see APPENDIX.

Interactions:
CIMETIDINE: increased sedation. Monitor carefully.

Special considerations:
- Contraindicated in patients with acute narrow-angle glaucoma, psychosis, and psychiatric disorders not showing anxiety. Use with caution in renal or hepatic impairment.
- Dosage should be reduced in elderly or debilitated patients.
- Possibility of abuse and addiction exists. Drug should not be withdrawn abruptly; withdrawal symptoms may occur.
- Patient should avoid activities that require alertness and good psychomotor coordination until CNS response to drug is determined.
- Patient should not combine drug with alcohol or other depressants.
- Patient should not give medication to others.
- Drug should not be prescribed for everyday stress.
- For symptoms and treatment of toxicity, see APPENDIX.

No significant interactions.

Special considerations:
- Contraindicated in patients with history of hypersensitivity to tybamate or related compounds, such as meprobamate, carisoprodol, or mebutamate; in patients with convulsive disorders, drug allergies, blood dyscrasias, or porphyria; and in lactating women. Use with caution in hepatic or renal dysfunction.
- Dosage should be reduced in elderly or debilitated patients.
- Possibility of abuse and addiction exists. Drug should not be withdrawn abruptly; withdrawal symptoms may occur.
- Patient should avoid activities that require alertness and good psychomotor coordination until CNS response to drug is determined.
- Patient should not combine drug with alcohol or other depressants.
- Shorter acting than meprobamate.
- Periodic evaluation of CBC and liver and kidney function studies are advised in patients receiving high doses or prolonged therapy.
- Sugarless gum or hard candy may relieve dry mouth.

32

Antipsychotics

acetophenazine maleate
carphenazine maleate
chlorpromazine hydrochloride
chlorprothixene
droperidol
fluphenazine decanoate
fluphenazine enanthate
fluphenazine hydrochloride
haloperidol
loxapine succinate
mesoridazine besylate
molindone hydrochloride
perphenazine
piperacetazine
prochlorperazine edisylate
prochlorperazine maleate
promazine hydrochloride
thioridazine hydrochloride
thiothixene
thiothixene hydrochloride
trifluoperazine hydrochloride
triflupromazine hydrochloride

Antipsychotic (neuroleptic) drugs may help control symptoms but not causes of organic psychoses. They modify thought disorders, blunted affect (deadened emotions and apathy), and behaviors associated with psychomotor and mental retardation. They lessen symptoms of paranoia, agitation, hallucinations, delusions, and autistic behavior. Some are used as antiemetics, antihistamines, or antipruritics. Antipyschotics may help patients be more receptive to psychotherapy. Introduced in the early 1950s, they have reduced the number of persons requiring institutionalization for psychotic disorders.

Antipsychotics can be classified on the basis of chemical structure into five groups. Many clinicians believe that one of these groups, the phenothiazines, should be treated as three distinct drug classes because of their differences in side effects (sedative properties, cardiovascular effects, and potential for inducing neuromuscular or extrapyramidal reactions). The three classes include aliphatics (which may cause sedation and anticholinergic effects), piperidines (which may cause sedation), and piperazines (which may cause extrapyramidal reactions). The other groups are butyrophenones, dibenzoxazepine, dihydroindole, and thioxanthines.

Because antipsychotics cause many side effects, they should be reserved for severe mental illnesses. For lesser disturbances, antianxiety drugs (benzodiazepines) are safer and probably more efficient. Patients undergoing antipsychotic drug therapy, however, should take their medications exactly as ordered. Symptoms of psychoses may return if these patients stop taking the medications.

Major uses

Antipsychotics may be used to treat symptoms of acute and chronic psychoses, especially those attended by increased psychomotor activity (including manic phase of manic-depressive illness, or bipolar disorders, and schizophrenia).

- Chlorpromazine and prochlorperazine may control nausea and vomiting.
- Haloperidol and thioridazine are more commonly used than other antipsychotics to control agitation in organic brain syndrome.

Mechanism of action

• As antipsychotics, these drugs block postsynaptic dopamine receptors in the brain. They also produce alpha-adrenergic blocking and depress release of hypothalamic and some pituitary hormones.
• As antiemetics, the drugs inhibit the medullary chemoreceptor trigger zone.
• As antiagitative drugs, they cause indirect reduction of stimuli to the brain stem reticular system.

Absorption, distribution, metabolism, and excretion

Although absorption after oral administration of these agents is efficient (faster with liquid concentrate than with tablets), it varies markedly from patient to patient. Absorption after I.M. administration is generally more complete (about one half the oral dose produces equal effect).

The agents are well distributed to body tissues, and highest concentrations of unchanged drug occur in the brain. Metabolites predominate in the lungs, liver, kidneys, and spleen.

All antipsychotics are metabolized in the liver; the metabolites are eliminated in the urine and—through the bile—in feces.

Onset and duration

• Onset of action is 2 to 6 hours for most drugs given orally and I.M., although haloperidol's onset (administered I.M.) is much shorter (20 to 30 minutes).
• Although symptoms may diminish with the first few doses, maximal effects may require weeks to months to develop.
• Long half-lives generally permit once-daily dosing (usually at bedtime).
• Divided doses are sometimes necessary for drugs causing significant hypotension (thioridazine and chlorpromazine, for example).

Administering large doses of the prescribed antipsychotic at the beginning of drug therapy (rapid neuroleptization) is becoming more popular. Drugs such as haloperidol and thiothixene are given hourly until symptoms abate.

Combination products

COMBID: prochlorperazine maleate 10 mg and isopropamide iodide 5 mg.
ESKATROL: prochlorperazine maleate 7.5 mg and dextroamphetamine sulfate 15 mg.
ETRAFON 2-10: perphenazine 2 mg and amitriptyline HCl 10 mg.
ETRAFON A: perphenazine 2 mg and amitriptyline HCl 25 mg.
ETRAFON-FORTE: perphenazine 4 mg and amitriptyline HCl 25 mg.
LIMBITROL 10-25: chlordiazepoxide 10 mg and amitriptyline (as HCl) 25 mg.
LIMBITROL 5-12.5: chlordiazepoxide 5 mg and amitriptyline (as HCl) 12.5 mg.
TRIAVIL 2-10, TRIAVIL 4-10, TRIAVIL 2-25 are identical to Etrafon products listed above; TRIAVIL 4-50: perphenazine 4 mg and amitriptyline HCl 50 mg.

NAMES, INDICATIONS AND DOSAGES	SIDE EFFECTS
acetophenazine maleate Tindal **Psychotic disorders:** ADULTS: initially, 20 mg P.O. t.i.d. or q.i.d. Daily dosage ranges from 40 to 80 mg in outpatients, or 80 to 120 mg in hospitalized patients, but in severe psychotic states up to 600 mg daily has been safely administered. Smallest effective dose should be used at all times.	**Blood:** *transient leukopenia, agranulocytosis.* **CNS:** *extrapyramidal reactions (high incidence),* sedation (low incidence), pseudoparkinsonism, EEG changes, dizziness. **CV:** *orthostatic hypotension,* tachycardia, EKG changes. **EENT:** *ocular changes, blurred vision.* **GI:** *dry mouth, constipation.* **GU:** *urinary retention,* dark urine, menstrual irregularities, gynecomastia, inhibited ejaculation. **Hepatic:** *cholestatic jaundice, abnormal liver function studies.* **Metabolic:** hyperprolactinemia. **Skin:** *mild photosensitivity,* dermal allergic reactions, *exfoliative dermatitis.* **Other:** weight gain, increased appetite. **After abrupt withdrawal:** gastritis, nausea, vomiting, dizziness, tremors, feeling of warmth or cold, sweating, tachycardia, headache, insomnia.
carphenazine maleate Proketazine **Psychotic disorders:** ADULTS: initially, 12.5 to 50 mg P.O., b.i.d. or t.i.d. Increase gradually to maximum 100 mg daily.	**Blood:** *transient leukopenia, agranulocytosis.* **CNS:** *extrapyramidal reactions (high incidence),* sedation (low incidence), pseudoparkinsonism, EEG changes, dizziness. **CV:** *orthostatic hypotension,* tachycardia, EKG changes. **EENT:** *ocular changes, blurred vision.* **GI:** *dry mouth, constipation.* **GU:** *urinary retention,* dark urine, menstrual irregularities, gynecomastia, inhibited ejaculation. **Hepatic:** *cholestatic jaundice, abnormal liver function studies.* **Metabolic:** hyperprolactinemia. **Skin:** *mild photosensitivity,* dermal allergic reactions, *exfoliative dermatitis.* **Other:** weight gain, increased appetite. **After abrupt withdrawal:** gastritis, nausea, vomiting, dizziness, tremors, feeling of warmth or cold, sweating, tachycardia, headache, insomnia.

INTERACTIONS AND SPECIAL CONSIDERATIONS

Interactions:
ANTACIDS: inhibit absorption of oral phenothiazines. Separate antacid and phenothiazine doses by at least 2 hours.
BARBITURATES: may decrease phenothiazine effect. Observe patient.

Special considerations:
• Contraindicated in CNS depression, bone marrow depression, subcortical damage, and coma; also with use of spinal or epidural anesthetic, or adrenergic blocking agents. Use cautiously with other CNS depressants and anticholinergics; in elderly or debilitated patients; and in patients with hepatic disease, arteriosclerosis or cardiovascular disease (may cause sudden drop in blood pressure), exposure to extreme heat or cold (including antipyretic therapy), respiratory disorders, hypocalcemia, convulsive disorders (may lower seizure threshold), severe reactions to insulin or electroshock therapy, suspected brain tumor or intestinal obstruction, glaucoma, or prostatic hypertrophy.
• If symptoms of blood dyscrasias (fever, sore throat, infection, cellulitis, weakness) or persistent (longer than a few hours) extrapyramidal reactions develop, or especially if such reactions develop during pregnancy, dose should be held and therapy reevaluated.
• Dose of 20 mg is therapeutic equivalent of 100 mg chlorpromazine.
• Therapy should be monitored by weekly bilirubin tests during first month; periodic blood tests (CBC, liver function); and ophthalmic tests (long-term use).
• Urinary retention or constipation may occur; intake and output should be monitored.
• Patient should use sunscreening agents and protective clothing to avoid photosensitivity reactions.
• Patient should avoid activities that require alertness or good psychomotor coordination until CNS response to drug is determined.
• Baseline measures of blood pressure should be obtained before starting therapy and monitored routinely. Orthostatic hypotension possible. Patient should get up slowly.
• Dry mouth may be relieved with sugarless gum, sour hard candy, or rinsing with mouthwash.
• Should not be combined with alcohol or other depressants.
• Should not be withdrawn abruptly unless required by severe side effects.
• Patient on maintenance may take medication at bedtime to facilitate sleep and decrease sedation during daytime.
• For symptoms and treatment of toxicity, see APPENDIX.

Interactions:
ANTACIDS: inhibit absorption of oral phenothiazines. Separate antacid and phenothiazine doses by at least 2 hours.
BARBITURATES: may decrease phenothiazine effect. Observe patient.

Special considerations:
• Contraindicated in CNS depression, bone marrow depression, subcortical damage, and coma; also contraindicated with use of spinal or epidural anesthetic, or adrenergic blocking agents. Use cautiously with other CNS depressants and anticholinergics; in elderly or debilitated patients; in patients with hepatic disease, arteriosclerosis or cardiovascular disease (may cause sudden drop in blood pressure), exposure to extreme heat or cold (including antipyretic therapy), respiratory disorders, hypocalcemia, convulsive disorders (may lower seizure threshold), severe reactions to insulin or electroshock therapy, suspected brain tumor or intestinal obstruction, glaucoma, or prostatic hypertrophy; and in acutely ill or dehydrated children.
• If symptoms of jaundice, blood dyscrasias (fever, sore throat, infection, cellulitis, weakness), or persistent (longer than a few hours) extrapyramidal reactions develop, dose should be held and therapy reevaluated.
• Therapy should be monitored by weekly bilirubin tests during first month; periodic blood tests (CBC, liver function); and ophthalmic tests (long-term use).
• Urinary retention or constipation are possible; intake and output should be monitored.
• Patient should use sunscreening agents and protective clothing to avoid photosensitivity reactions.
• Patient should avoid activities that require alertness or good psychomotor coordination until CNS response to drug is determined. Drowsiness and dizziness usually subside after a few weeks.
• Baseline measures of blood pressure should be obtained before starting therapy and monitored regularly. Orthostatic hypotension possible. Patient should get up slowly.
• Should not be combined with alcohol or other depressants.
• Should not be withdrawn abruptly unless required by severe side effects.
• Dry mouth may be relieved by sugarless gum, sour hard candy, or rinsing with mouthwash.
• Dose of 25 mg is therapeutic equivalent of 100 mg chlorpromazine.
• For symptoms and treatment of toxicity, see APPENDIX.

NAMES, INDICATIONS AND DOSAGES	SIDE EFFECTS

chlorpromazine hydrochloride
Chlorprom♦♦, Chlor-Promanyl♦♦, Chlorzine, Klorazine, Largactil♦♦, Ormazine, Promachlor, Promapar, Promaz, Sonazine, Terpium, Thoradex, Thorazine

Intractable hiccups:
ADULTS: 25 to 50 mg P.O. or I.M. t.i.d. or q.i.d.

Mild alcohol withdrawal, acute intermittent porphyria, and tetanus:
ADULTS: 25 to 50 mg I.M. t.i.d. or q.i.d.

Nausea and vomiting:
ADULTS: 10 to 25 mg P.O. or I.M. q 4 to 6 hours, p.r.n.; or 50 to 100 mg rectally q 6 to 8 hours, p.r.n.
CHILDREN: 0.25 mg/kg P.O. q 4 to 6 hours; or 0.25 mg/kg I.M. q 6 to 8 hours; or 0.5 mg/kg rectally q 6 to 8 hours.

Psychosis:
ADULTS: 500 mg P.O. daily in divided doses, increasing gradually to 2 g; or 25 to 50 mg I.M. q 1 to 4 hours, p.r.n.
CHILDREN: 0.25 mg/kg P.O. q 4 to 6 hours; or 0.25 mg/kg I.M. q 6 to 8 hours; or 0.5 mg/kg rectally q 6 to 8 hours. Maximum dose is 40 mg in children under 5 years, and 75 mg in children 5 to 12 years.

Blood: *transient leukopenia, agranulocytosis.*
CNS: *extrapyramidal reactions (moderate incidence), sedation (high incidence),* pseudoparkinsonism, EEG changes, dizziness.
CV: *orthostatic hypotension,* tachycardia, EKG changes.
EENT: *ocular changes, blurred vision.*
GI: *dry mouth, constipation.*
GU: *urinary retention,* dark urine, menstrual irregularities, gynecomastia, inhibited ejaculation.
Hepatic: *cholestatic jaundice, abnormal liver function studies.*
Metabolic: hyperprolactinemia.
Skin: *mild photosensitivity,* dermal allergic reactions, *exfoliative dermatitis.*
Local: pain on I.M. injection, sterile abscess.
Other: weight gain, increased appetite.
After abrupt withdrawal: gastritis, nausea, vomiting, dizziness, tremors, feeling of warmth or cold, sweating, tachycardia, headache, insomnia.

---

chlorprothixene
Taractan, Tarasan♦♦

Psychotic disorders:
ADULTS: initially, 10 mg P.O. t.i.d. or q.i.d. Increase gradually to maximum 600 mg daily.
CHILDREN OVER 6 YEARS: 10 to 25 mg P.O. t.i.d. or q.i.d.

Agitation of severe neurosis, depression, schizophrenia:
ADULTS: 25 to 50 mg P.O. or I.M. t.i.d. or q.i.d. Increase as needed up to maximum 600 mg.

Blood: *transient leukopenia, agranulocytosis.*
CNS: *extrapyramidal reactions (high incidence),* sedation (low incidence), pseudoparkinsonism, EEG changes, dizziness.
CV: *orthostatic hypotension,* tachycardia, EKG changes.
EENT: *ocular changes, blurred vision.*
GI: *dry mouth, constipation.*
GU: *urinary retention,* dark urine, menstrual irregularities, gynecomastia, inhibited ejaculation.
Hepatic: *cholestatic jaundice, abnormal liver function studies.*
Metabolic: hyperprolactinemia.
Skin: *mild photosensitivity,* dermal allergic reactions, *exfoliative dermatitis.*
Local: pain on I.M. injection, sterile abscess.
Other: weight gain, increased appetite.
After abrupt withdrawal: gastritis, nausea, vomiting, dizziness, tremors, feeling of warmth

INTERACTIONS AND SPECIAL CONSIDERATIONS

Interactions:
ANTACIDS: inhibit absorption of oral phenothiazines. Separate antacid and phenothiazine doses by at least 2 hours.
ANTICHOLINERGICS (INCLUDING ANTIDEPRESSANT AND ANTI-PARKINSON AGENTS): increased anticholinergic activity, aggravated Parkinson-like symptoms. Use with caution.
BARBITURATES: may decrease phenothiazine effect. Observe patient.
LITHIUM: possible decreased response to chlorpromazine. Observe patient.

Special considerations:
• Contraindicated in CNS depression, bone marrow depression, subcortical damage, Reye's syndrome, and coma; also contraindicated with use of spinal or epidural anesthetic, or adrenergic blocking agents. Use cautiously with other CNS depressants and anticholinergics; in elderly or debilitated patients; in patients with hepatic disease, arteriosclerosis or cardiovascular disease (may cause sudden drop in blood pressure), exposure to extreme heat or cold (including antipyretic therapy), respiratory disorders, hypocalcemia, convulsive disorders (may lower seizure threshold), severe reactions to insulin or electroshock therapy, suspected brain tumor or intestinal obstruction, glaucoma, or prostatic hypertrophy; and in acutely ill or dehydrated children.
• If jaundice, symptoms of blood dyscrasias (fever, sore throat, infection, cellulitis, weakness) or persistent (longer than a few hours) extrapyramidal reactions develop, or especially if such reactions develop during pregnancy or in children, dose should be held and therapy reevaluated.
• Therapy should be monitored by weekly bilirubin tests during first month; periodic blood tests (CBC, liver function); and ophthalmic tests (long-term use).
• Urinary retention or constipation are possible; intake and output should be monitored.
• Patient should use sunscreening agents and protective clothing to avoid photosensitivity reactions.
• Patient should avoid activities that require alertness or good psychomotor coordination until CNS response to drug is determined. Drowsiness and dizziness usually subside after first few weeks.
• Baseline measures of blood pressure should be obtained before starting therapy and monitored regularly. Orthostatic hypotension possible, especially with parenteral administration. Blood pressure should be monitored before and after I.M. administration and patient kept supine for 1 hour afterward; then patient should get up slowly.
• Should not be combined with alcohol or other depressants.
• I.M. should be given deeply only in upper outer quadrant of buttocks and skin massaged slowly afterward to prevent sterile abscess. Injection may sting.
• Keeping drug off patient's skin and clothes prevents contact dermatitis.
• Liquid concentrate should be protected from light and diluted with fruit juice, milk, or semisolid food just before administration.
• Slight yellowing of injection or concentrate is common; does not affect potency. Markedly discolored solutions should be discarded.
• Should not be withdrawn abruptly unless required by severe side effects.
• Dry mouth may be relieved by sugarless gum, sour hard candy, or rinsing with mouthwash.
• An aliphatic; has greater tendency to cause anticholinergic side effects.
• For symptoms and treatment of toxicity, see APPENDIX.

No significant interactions.

Special considerations:
• Contraindicated in coma, CNS depression, bone marrow depression, circulatory collapse, congestive failure, cardiac decompensation, coronary artery or cerebral vascular disorders, subcortical damage, with use of spinal or epidural anesthetic or adrenergic blocking agents. Use cautiously with other CNS depressants and anticholinergics; in elderly or debilitated patients; in patients with hepatic or renal disease, arteriosclerosis or cardiovascular disease (may cause sudden drop in blood pressure), exposure to extreme heat or cold (including antipyretic therapy), respiratory disorders, hypocalcemia, convulsive disorders (may lower seizure threshold), severe reactions to insulin or electroshock therapy, suspected brain tumor or intestinal obstruction, glaucoma, or prostatic hypertrophy; and acutely ill or dehydrated children.
• If symptoms of blood dyscrasias (fever, sore throat, infection, cellulitis, weakness), jaundice, or persistent (longer than a few hours) extrapyramidal reactions develop, or especially if such reactions develop in children, dose should be held and therapy reevaluated.
• Therapy should be monitored by weekly bilirubin tests during first month; periodic blood tests (CBC, liver function) before and during therapy; and ophthalmic tests (long-term therapy).
• Urinary retention and constipation are possible; intake and output should be monitored.
• Patient should use sunscreening agents and protective clothing to avoid photosensitivity reactions.
• Patient should avoid activities that require alertness or good psychomotor coordination until CNS response to drug is determined. Drows-

(continued on following page)

NAMES, INDICATIONS AND DOSAGES	SIDE EFFECTS
chlorprothixene *(continued)*	or cold, sweating, tachycardia, headache, insomnia.
droperidol Inapsine♦ **Premedication:** ADULTS: 2.5 to 10 mg (1 to 4 ml) I.M. 30 to 60 minutes preoperatively. CHILDREN 2 TO 12 YEARS: 1 to 1.5 mg (0.4 to 0.6 ml)/20 to 25 lb of body weight I.M.. **As induction agent:** ADULTS: 2.5 mg (1 ml)/20 to 25 lb I.V. with analgesic and/or general anesthetic. CHILDREN 2 TO 12 YEARS: 1 to 1.5 mg (0.4 to 0.6 ml)/20 to 25 lb I.V. Dose should be titrated. ELDERLY OR DEBILITATED PATIENTS: initial dose should be decreased. **Maintenance dose in general anesthesia:** 1.25 to 2.5 mg (0.5 to 1 ml) I.V.	**CNS:** extrapyramidal reactions (dystonia, akathisia), upward rotation of eyes and oculogyric crises, extended neck, flexed arms, fine tremor of limbs, dizziness, chills or shivering, facial sweating, restlessness. **CV:** hypotension, tachycardia.
fluphenazine decanoate Modecate Decanoate♦♦, Prolixin Decanoate **fluphenazine enanthate** Moditen Enanthate♦♦, Prolixin Enanthate **fluphenazine hydrochloride** Moditen Hydrochloride♦♦, Permitil Hydrochloride, Prolixin Hydrochloride **Psychotic disorders:** ADULTS: initially, 0.5 to 10 mg fluphenazine HCl P.O. daily in divided doses q 6 to 8 hours; may increase cautiously to 20 mg. Higher doses (50 to 100 mg) have been given. Maintenance: 1 to 5 mg P.O. daily. I.M. doses are ⅓ to ½ oral doses. Lower doses for geriatric patients (1 to 2.5 mg daily). CHILDREN: 0.25 to 3.5 mg fluphenazine HCl P.O. daily in divided doses q 4 to 6 hours; or ⅓ to ½ of oral dose I.M.; maximum 10 mg daily. ADULTS AND CHILDREN OVER 12 YEARS: 12.5 to 25 mg of long-acting esters (fluphenazine decanoate and enanthate) I.M. or S.C. q 1 to 6 weeks. Maintenance: 25 to 100 mg, p.r.n.	**Blood:** *transient leukopenia, agranulocytosis.* **CNS:** *extrapyramidal reactions (high incidence),* sedation (low incidence), pseudoparkinsonism, EEG changes, dizziness. **CV:** *orthostatic hypotension,* tachycardia, EKG changes. **EENT:** *ocular changes, blurred vision.* **GI:** *dry mouth, constipation.* **GU:** *urinary retention,* dark urine, menstrual irregularities, gynecomastia, inhibited ejaculation. **Hepatic:** *cholestatic jaundice, abnormal liver function studies.* **Metabolic:** hyperprolactinemia. **Skin:** *mild photosensitivity,* dermal allergic reactions, *exfoliative dermatitis.* **Other:** weight gain, increased appetite. **After abrupt withdrawal:** gastritis, nausea, vomiting, dizziness, tremors, feeling of warmth or cold, sweating, tachycardia, headache, insomnia.

♦ Available in U.S. and Canada. ♦♦ Available in Canada only.
All other products (no symbol) available in U.S. only. Italicized side effects are common or life-threatening.

INTERACTIONS AND SPECIAL CONSIDERATIONS

iness and dizziness usually subside after first few weeks.
• Baseline measures of blood pressure should be obtained before starting therapy and monitored regularly. Orthostatic hypotension possible, especially with parenteral administration, since adrenergic blockage is high. Patient should remain supine for 1 hour afterward and change positions slowly.
• Should not be combined with alcohol or other depressants.
• I.M. should be given deeply only in upper outer quadrant of buttocks or midlateral thigh, and skin massaged slowly afterward to prevent sterile abscess. Injection may sting.
• Liquid concentrate should be diluted with fruit juice, milk, or semisolid food just before administration.
• Medication should be protected from light. Slight yellowing of injection or concentrate is common; does not affect potency. Markedly discolored solutions should be discarded.
• Drug should not be withdrawn abruptly unless required by severe side effects.
• Keeping drug off patient's skin and clothes prevents contact dermatitis.
• Dry mouth may be relieved by sugarless gum, sour hard candy, or rinsing with mouthwash.
• Dose of 100 mg is therapeutic equivalent of 100 mg chlorpromazine.

No significant interactions.

Special considerations:
• Use cautiously in elderly or debilitated patients; and in patients with hypotension or other cardiovascular disease, impaired hepatic or renal function, and Parkinson's disease.
• Extrapyramidal reactions may develop.
• Approved by FDA *only* for use preoperatively and during induction and maintenance of anesthesia.
• A butyrophenone compound, related to haloperidol; has greater tendency to cause extrapyramidal reactions than other antipyschotics.
• Keep intravenous fluids and vasopressors handy for hypotension.
• If used with a narcotic analgesic such as fentanyl (Sublimaze), the special properties of each drug should be known, particularly the widely differing durations of action. Respiratory depression, apnea, and muscular rigidity possible, which could lead to respiratory arrest if untreated. Narcotic antagonist and CPR equipment should be on hand.
• Vital signs should be monitored frequently.
• Intravenous injections should be given slowly.
• Patient should not be placed in Trendelenburg position (shock position); severe hypotension, deeper anesthesia may result, causing respiratory arrest.
• Drug has been used to prevent cisplatinum–associated nausea and vomiting.

Interactions:
ANTACIDS: inhibit absorption of oral phenothiazines. Separate antacid and phenothiazine doses by at least 2 hours.
BARBITURATES: may decrease phenothiazine effect. Observe patient.

Special considerations:
• Contraindicated in coma, CNS depression, bone marrow depression or other blood dyscrasia, subcortical damage, hepatic damage, renal insufficiency; and with use of spinal or epidural anesthetic, or adrenergic blocking agents. Use cautiously with other CNS depressants and anticholinergics; in elderly or debilitated patients; in acutely ill or dehydrated children; and in patients with hepatic disease, pheochromocytoma, arteriosclerotic, cerebrovascular, or cardiovascular disease (may cause sudden drop in blood pressure), peptic ulcer, exposure to extreme heat or cold (including antipyretic therapy), respiratory disorders, hypocalcemia, convulsive disorders, (may lower seizure threshold), severe reactions to insulin or electroshock therapy, suspected brain tumor or intestinal obstruction, glaucoma, or prostatic hypertrophy.
• If symptoms of blood dyscrasias (fever, sore throat, infection, cellulitis, weakness) or persistent (longer than a few hours) extrapyramidal reactions develop, or especially if such reactions develop during pregnancy or in children, dose should be held and therapy reevaluated.
• Therapy should be monitored by weekly bilirubin tests during first month; periodic blood tests (CBC, liver function); periodic kidney function tests; and ophthalmic tests (long-term use).
• Urinary retention and constipation are possible; intake and output should be monitored.
• Patient should use sunscreening agents and protective clothing to avoid photosensitivity reactions.
• Patient should avoid activities that require alertness and good psychomotor coordination until CNS response to drug is determined. Drowsiness and dizziness usually subside after first few weeks.
• Should not be combined with alcohol or other depressants.
• Baseline measures of blood pressure should be obtained before starting therapy and monitored regularly. Orthostatic hypotension possible, especially with parenteral administration. Blood pressure should be monitored before and

(continued on following page)

NAMES, INDICATIONS AND DOSAGES	SIDE EFFECTS
fluphenazine *(continued)*	
haloperidol Haldol♦ **Psychotic disorders:** ADULTS: dosage varies for each patient. Initial range is 0.5 to 5 mg P.O. b.i.d. or t.i.d.; or 2 to 5 mg I.M. q 4 to 8 hours, increasing rapidly if necessary for prompt control. Maximum 100 mg P.O. daily. Doses over 100 mg have been used for patients with severely resistant conditions. **Control of tics, vocal utterances in Gilles de la Tourette's syndrome:** ADULTS: 0.5 to 5 mg P.O. b.i.d. or t.i.d., increasing p.r.n.	**Blood:** transient leukopenia and leukocytosis. **CNS:** *high incidence of severe extrapyramidal reactions,* low incidence of sedation. **CV:** low incidence of cardiovascular effects with therapeutic dosages. **EENT:** blurred vision, dry mouth. **GU:** urinary retention, menstrual irregularities, gynecomastia. **Skin:** rash.
loxapine succinate Loxapac♦♦, Loxitane, Loxitane-C **Psychotic disorders:** ADULTS: 10 mg P.O. or I.M. b.i.d. to q.i.d., rapidly increasing to 60 to 100 mg P.O. daily for most patients; dose varies from patient to patient.	**Blood:** *transient leukopenia.* **CNS:** *extrapyramidal reactions (moderate incidence), sedation (moderate incidence),* pseudoparkinsonism, EEG changes, dizziness. **CV:** *orthostatic hypotension,* tachycardia, EKG changes. **EENT:** *blurred vision.* **GI:** *dry mouth, constipation.* **GU:** *urinary retention,* dark urine, menstrual irregularities, gynecomastia. **Skin:** *mild photosensitivity,* dermal allergic reactions, *exfoliative dermatitis.* **Other:** weight gain, increased appetite.
mesoridazine besylate Serentil♦ **Alcoholism:** ADULTS AND CHILDREN OVER 12 YEARS: 25 mg P.O. b.i.d. up to maximum 200 mg daily. **Behavioral problems associated with chronic brain syndrome:** ADULTS AND CHILDREN OVER 12 YEARS: 25 mg P.O. t.i.d. up to maximum of 300 mg daily.	**Blood:** *transient leukopenia, agranulocytosis.* **CNS:** extrapyramidal reactions (low incidence), *sedation (high incidence),* EEG changes, dizziness. **CV:** *orthostatic hypotension,* tachycardia, EKG changes. **EENT:** *ocular changes, blurred vision,* pigmentary retinopathy. **GI:** *dry mouth, constipation.* **GU:** *urinary retention,* dark urine, menstrual irregularities, gynecomastia, inhibited ejaculation. **Hepatic:** *cholestatic jaundice, abnormal liver*

♦ Available in U.S. and Canada. ♦♦ Available in Canada only.
All other products (no symbol) available in U.S. only. Italicized side effects are common or life-threatening.

INTERACTIONS AND SPECIAL CONSIDERATIONS

after I.M. administration. Patient should remain supine for 1 hour afterward and change positions slowly.
• Dacanoate and enanthate may be given subcutaneously.
• For long-acting forms (decanoate and enanthate), which are oil preparations, a dry needle of at least 21G should be used and 24 to 96 hours allowed for onset of action. Adverse side effects in patients taking the long-acting drug forms should be reported.
• Keeping drug off patient's skin and clothes prevents contact dermatitis.
• Liquid concentrate should be diluted with water, fruit juice, milk, or semisolid food just before administration.
• Medication should be protected from light. Slight yellowing of injection or concentrate is common; does not affect potency. Markedly discolored solutions should be discarded.
• Dry mouth may be relieved by sugarless gum, sour hard candy, or rinsing with mouthwash.
• Drug should not be withdrawn abruptly unless required by severe side effects.
• Dose of 2 mg is therapeutic equivalent of 100 mg chlorpromazine.
• For symptoms and treatment of toxicity, see APPENDIX.

Interactions:
LITHIUM: lethargy and confusion with high doses. Observe patient.
METHYLDOPA: possible symptoms of dementia. Observe patient.

Special considerations:
• Contraindicated in parkinsonism, coma, or CNS depression. Use with caution in elderly and debilitated patients; in severe cardiovascular disorders, allergies, glaucoma, urinary retention; and in conjunction with anticonvulsant, anticoagulant, anti-Parkinson, or lithium medications.
• Patient should avoid activities that require alertness and good psychomotor coordination until CNS response to drug is determined. Drowsiness and dizziness usually subside after a few weeks.
• Should not be combined with alcohol or other depressants.
• Medication should be protected from light. Slight yellowing of injection or concentrate is common; does not affect potency. Markedly discolored solutions should be discarded.
• Drug should not be withdrawn abruptly unless required by severe side effects.
• Dry mouth may be relieved by sugarless gum, sour hard candy, and rinsing with mouthwash.
• Dose of 2 mg is therapeutic equivalent of 100 mg chlorpromazine.
• Only butyrophenone compound used as an antipsychotic in the United States.

No significant interactions.

Special considerations:
• Contraindicated in coma, severe CNS depression, drug-induced depressed states. Use with caution in epilepsy, cardiovascular disorders, glaucoma, urinary retention, suspected intestinal obstruction or brain tumor, and renal damage.
• Patient should avoid activities that require alertness and good psychomotor coordination until CNS response to drug is determined. Drowsiness and dizziness usually subside after first few weeks.
• Should not be combined with alcohol or other depressants.
• Baseline measures of blood should be obtained before starting therapy and monitored regularly. Patient should get up slowly to avoid orthostatic hypotension.
• Liquid concentrate should be diluted with orange or grapefruit juice just before administration.
• Dry mouth may be relieved by sugarless gum, sour hard candy, or rinsing with mouthwash.
• Periodic ophthalmic tests recommended.
• Tricyclic dibenzoxazepine; the only dibenzoxazepine derivative.
• Dose of 10 mg is therapeutic equivalent of 100 mg chlorpromazine.

Interactions:
ANTACIDS: inhibit absorption of oral phenothiazines. Separate antacid and phenothiazine doses by at least 2 hours.
BARBITURATES: may decrease phenothiazine effect. Observe patient.

Special considerations:
• Contraindicated in coma, CNS depression, bone marrow depression, subcortical damage, and with use of spinal or epidural anesthetic or adrenergic blocking agents. Use cautiously with other CNS depressants and anticholinergics; in elderly or debilitated patients; in acutely ill or dehydrated children; and in patients with hepatic disease, arteriosclerosis or cardiovascular disease (may cause sudden drop in blood pressure), exposure to extreme heat or cold (including antipyretic therapy), respiratory disorders, hypocalcemia, convulsive disorders, severe reactions to insulin or electroshock therapy, suspected brain tumor or intestinal obstruction, glaucoma, or prostatic hypertrophy.
• If jaundice, symptoms of blood dyscrasias (fever, sore throat, infection, cellulitis, weakness) or persistent (longer than a few hours)

(continued on following page)

NAMES, INDICATIONS AND DOSAGES	SIDE EFFECTS
mesoridazine besylate *(continued)* **Psychoneurotic manifestations (anxiety):** ADULTS AND CHILDREN OVER 12 YEARS: 10 mg P.O. t.i.d. up to maximum 150 mg daily. **Schizophrenia:** ADULTS AND CHILDREN OVER 12 YEARS: initially, 50 mg P.O. t.i.d. or 25 mg I.M. repeated in 30 to 60 minutes, p.r.n.	*function studies.* **Metabolic:** hyperprolactinemia. **Skin:** *mild photosensitivity,* dermal allergic reactions, *exfoliative dermatitis.* **Local:** pain at I.M. injection site, sterile abscess. **Other:** weight gain, increased appetite. **After abrupt withdrawal:** gastritis, nausea, vomiting, dizziness, tremors, feeling of warmth or cold, sweating, tachycardia, headache, insomnia.
molindone hydrochloride Lidone, Moban **Psychotic disorders:** ADULTS: 50 to 75 mg P.O. daily, increasing to maximum 225 mg daily. Doses up to 400 mg may be required.	**Blood:** *transient leukopenia.* **CNS:** *extrapyramidal reactions (moderate incidence), sedation (moderate incidence),* pseudoparkinsonism, EEG changes, dizziness. **CV:** *orthostatic hypotension,* tachycardia, EKG changes. **EENT:** *blurred vision.* **GI:** *dry mouth, constipation.* **GU:** *urinary retention,* dark urine, menstrual irregularities, gynecomastia, inhibited ejaculation. **Hepatic:** *cholestatic jaundice, abnormal liver function studies.* **Metabolic:** hyperprolactinemia. **Skin:** *mild photosensitivity,* dermal allergic reactions, *exfoliative dermatitis.* **Other:** weight gain, increased appetite.
perphenazine Phenazine♦♦, Trilafon♦ **Hospitalized psychiatric patients:** ADULTS: initially, 8 to 16 mg P.O. b.i.d., t.i.d., or q.i.d., increasing to 64 mg daily. CHILDREN OVER 12 YEARS: 6 to 12 mg P.O. daily in divided doses. **Mental disturbances, acute alcoholism, nausea, vomiting, hiccups:** ADULTS AND CHILDREN OVER 12 YEARS: 5 to 10 mg I.M., p.r.n. Maximum 15 mg daily in ambulatory patients, 30 mg daily in hospitalized patients.	**Blood:** *transient leukopenia, agranulocytosis.* **CNS:** *extrapyramidal reactions (high incidence),* sedation (low incidence), pseudoparkinsonism, EEG changes, dizziness. **CV:** *orthostatic hypotension,* tachycardia, EKG changes. **EENT:** *ocular changes, blurred vision.* **GI:** *dry mouth, constipation.* **GU:** *urinary retention,* dark urine, menstrual irregularities, gynecomastia, inhibited ejaculation. **Hepatic:** *cholestatic jaundice, abnormal liver function studies.* **Metabolic:** hyperprolactinemia. **Skin:** *mild photosensitivity,* dermal allergic reactions, *exfoliative dermatitis.* **Local:** pain at I.M. injection site, sterile abscess. **Other:** weight gain, increased appetite. **After abrupt withdrawal:** gastritis, nausea,

INTERACTIONS AND SPECIAL CONSIDERATIONS

extrapyramidal reactions develop, or especially if such reactions develop during pregnancy or in children over 12 years, dose should be held and therapy reevaluated.
• Therapy should be monitored by weekly bilirubin tests during first month; periodic blood tests (CBC, liver function); and ophthalmic tests (long-term use).
• Urinary retention and constipation are possible; intake and output should be monitored.
• Patient should use sunscreening agents and protective clothing to avoid photosensitivity reactions.
• Patient should avoid activities that require alertness and good psychomotor coordination until CNS response to drug is determined. Drowsiness and dizziness usually subside after a few weeks.
• Should not be combined with alcohol or other depressants.
• Baseline measures of blood pressure should be obtained before starting therapy and monitored regularly. Orthostatic hypotension possible, especially with parenteral administration. Patient should change positions slowly.
• I.M. should be given deeply only in upper outer quadrant of buttocks, and skin massaged slowly afterward to prevent sterile abscess. Injection may sting.
• Medication should be protected from light. Slight yellowing of injection or concentrate is common; does not affect potency. Markedly discolored solutions should be discarded.
• Keeping drug off patient's skin and clothes prevents contact dermatitis.
• Dry mouth relieved with sugarless gum, sour hard candy, or mouthwash.
• Drug should not be withdrawn abruptly unless required by severe side effects.
• Drug is a piperidine phenothiazine (a metabolite of thioridazine).
• Dose of 50 mg is therapeutic equivalent of 100 mg chlorpromazine.
• For symptoms and treatment of toxicity, see APPENDIX.

No significant interactions.

Special considerations:
• Contraindicated in coma or severe CNS depression. Use with caution when increased physical activity would be harmful, as this agent increases activity; in seizures, suicide risk, suspected brain tumor, or intestinal obstruction.
• Patient should avoid activities that require alertness or good psychomotor coordination until CNS response to drug is determined. Drowsiness and dizziness usually subside after first few weeks.
• Should not be combined with alcohol or other depressants.
• Dry mouth may be relieved with sugarless gum, sour hard candy, or rinsing with mouthwash.
• Drug is the only dihydroindolone derivative.
• Dose of 20 mg is therapeutic equivalent of 100 mg chlorpromazine.
• No injection available.
• Liquid oral concentrate is available.
• Lidone capsules contain tartrazine dye. May cause allergy in susceptible patients.
• May be administered in a single daily dose.

Interactions:
ANTACIDS: inhibit absorption of oral phenothiazines. Separate antacid and phenothiazine doses by at least 2 hours.
BARBITURATES: may decrease phenothiazine effect. Observe patient.

Special considerations:
• Contraindicated in coma, CNS depression, bone marrow depression, subcortical damage, use of spinal or epidural anesthetic or adrenergic blocking agents. Use cautiously with other CNS depressants and anticholinergics; in elderly or debilitated patients, in acutely ill or dehydrated children; and in patients with hepatic disease, arteriosclerosis or cardiovascular disease (may cause sudden drop in blood pressure), exposure to extreme heat or cold (including antipyretic therapy), respiratory disorders, hypocalcemia, convulsive disorders (may lower seizure threshold), severe reactions to insulin or electroshock therapy, suspected brain tumor or intestinal obstruction, glaucoma, prostatic hypertrophy.
• If jaundice, symptoms of blood dyscrasias (fever, sore throat, infection, cellulitis, weakness), or persistent (longer than a few hours) extrapyramidal reactions develop, or especially if such reactions develop during pregnancy or in children, dose should be held and therapy reevaluated.
• Therapy should be monitored by weekly bilirubin tests during first month; periodic blood tests (CBC, liver function); and ophthalmic tests (long-term use).
• Urinary retention and constipation are possible; intake and output should be monitored.
• Patient should use sunscreening agents and protective clothing to avoid photosensitivity reactions.
• Patient should avoid activities that require

(continued on following page)

NAMES, INDICATIONS AND DOSAGES	SIDE EFFECTS
perphenazine *(continued)*	vomiting, dizziness, tremors, feeling of warmth or cold, sweating, tachycardia, headache, insomnia.
piperacetazine Quide♦ **Psychotic disorders:** ADULTS: initially, 10 mg P.O. b.i.d. to q.i.d. Dosage may be gradually increased to 160 mg daily if necessary.	**Blood:** *transient leukopenia, agranulocytosis.* **CNS:** extrapyramidal reactions (low incidence), *sedation (high incidence),* EEG changes, dizziness. **CV:** *orthostatic hypotension,* tachycardia, EKG changes. **EENT:** *ocular changes, blurred vision,* pigmentary retinopathy. **GI:** *dry mouth, constipation.* **GU:** *urinary retention,* dark urine, menstrual irregularities, gynecomastia, inhibited ejaculation. **Hepatic:** *cholestatic jaundice, abnormal liver function studies.* **Metabolic:** hyperprolactinemia. **Skin:** *mild photosensitivity,* dermal allergic reactions, *exfoliative dermatitis.* **Other:** weight gain, increased appetite. **After abrupt withdrawal:** gastritis, nausea, vomiting, dizziness, tremors, feeling of warmth or cold, sweating, tachycardia, headache, insomnia.
prochlorperazine edisylate **prochlorperazine maleate** Compazine, Stemetil♦♦ **Mild-to-moderate emotional disturbances:** ADULTS: 5 to 10 mg P.O. t.i.d. or q.i.d.; extended-release 15 mg P.O. in a.m. or 10 mg q 12 hours; 25 mg rectally b.i.d.; 5 to 10 mg I.M. q 3 to 4 hours. CHILDREN 18 TO 38.5 KG: 5 mg P.O. or rectally b.i.d., to maximum of 15 mg daily.	**Blood:** *transient leukopenia, agranulocytosis.* **CNS:** *extrapyramidal reactions (high incidence),* sedation (low incidence), pseudoparkinsonism, EEG changes, dizziness. **CV:** *orthostatic hypotension,* tachycardia, EKG changes. **EENT:** *ocular changes, blurred vision.* **GI:** *dry mouth, constipation.* **GU:** *urinary retention,* dark urine, menstrual irregularities, gynecomastia, inhibited ejaculation.

♦ Available in U.S. and Canada. ♦♦ Available in Canada only.
All other products (no symbol) available in U.S. only. Italicized side effects are common or life-threatening.

INTERACTIONS AND SPECIAL CONSIDERATIONS

alertness or good psychomotor coordination until CNS response to drug is determined. Drowsiness and dizziness usually subside after a few weeks.

- Should not be combined with alcohol or other depressants.
- Baseline measures of blood pressure should be obtained before starting therapy and monitored regularly. Orthostatic hypotension possible, especially with parenteral administration. Patient should remain supine for 1 hour afterward and change positions slowly.
- Should be given deep I.M. only in upper outer quadrant of buttocks, and skin massaged slowly afterward to prevent sterile abscess. Injection may sting.
- Drug should not be withdrawn abruptly unless required by severe side effects.
- Medication should be protected from light. Slight yellowing of injection or concentrate is common; does not affect potency. Discard markedly discolored solutions.
- Keeping drug off patient's skin and clothes prevents contact dermatitis.
- Liquid concentrate should be diluted with fruit juice, milk, carbonated beverage, or semisolid food just before administration. Exceptions: oral concentrate causes turbidity or precipitation in colas, black coffee, grape or apple juice, or tea. Should not be mixed with these liquids.
- Dry mouth may be relieved with sugarless gum, sour hard candy, or rinsing with mouthwash.
- Dose of 8 mg is therapeutic equivalent of 100 mg chlorpromazine.
- For symptoms and treatment of toxicity, see APPENDIX.

Interactions:

ANTACIDS: inhibit absorption of oral phenothiazines. Separate antacid and phenothiazine doses by at least 2 hours.

BARBITURATES: may decrease phenothiazine effect. Observe patient.

Special considerations:

- Contraindicated in coma, CNS depression, bone marrow depression, thrombocytopenia and other blood dyscrasias, subcortical damage, and with use of spinal or epidural anesthetic or adrenergic blocking agents. Use cautiously with other CNS depressants and anticholinergics; in elderly or debilitated patients; in patients with hepatic disease, arteriosclerosis or cardiovascular disease (may cause sudden drop in blood pressure), exposure to extreme heat or cold (including antipyretic therapy), respiratory disorders, hypocalcemia, convulsive disorders (may lower seizure threshold), severe reactions to insulin or electroshock therapy, suspected brain tumor or intestinal obstruction, glaucoma, or prostatic hypertrophy.
- If jaundice, symptoms of blood dyscrasias (fever, sore throat, infection, cellulitis, weakness), or persistent (longer than a few hours) extrapyramidal reactions develop, or especially if such reactions develop during pregnancy, dose should be held and therapy reevaluated.
- Therapy should be monitored by weekly bilirubin tests during first month; periodic blood tests (CBC, liver function); and ophthalmic tests (long-term use).
- Urinary retention and constipation are possible; intake and output should be monitored.
- Patient should use sunscreening agents and protective clothing to avoid photosensitivity reactions.
- Patient should avoid activities that require alertness or good psychomotor coordination until CNS response to drug is determined. Drowsiness and dizziness usually subside after a few weeks.
- Should not be combined with alcohol or other depressants.
- Blood pressure should be monitored. Baseline measures of blood pressure should be obtained before starting therapy. Orthostatic hypotension possible.
- Protect tablets from light.
- Drug should not be withdrawn abruptly unless required by severe side effects.
- Dry mouth may be relieved with sugarless gum, sour hard candy, or rinsing with mouthwash.
- Drug is a piperidine phenothiazine.
- Dose of 10 mg is therapeutic equivalent of 100 mg chlorpromazine.
- For symptoms and treatment of toxicity, see APPENDIX.

Interactions:

ANTACIDS: inhibit absorption of oral phenothiazines. Separate antacid and phenothiazine doses by at least 2 hours.

BARBITURATES: may decrease phenothiazine effect. Observe patient.

Special considerations:

- Contraindicated in coma, depression, CNS depression, bone marrow depression, subcortical damage, pediatric surgery, and with use of spinal or epidural anesthetic, adrenergic blocking agents, or alcohol. Use cautiously with other CNS depressants and anticholinergics; in elderly or debilitated patients; in patients with hepatic disease, arteriosclerosis or cardiovascular disease (may cause sudden drop in blood pressure), exposure to extreme heat or cold (including antipyretic therapy), respiratory disorders, hypocalcemia, vomiting in children, convulsive disorders (may lower seizure threshold) or severe reactions to insulin or electroshock therapy, sus-

(continued on following page)

NAMES, INDICATIONS AND DOSAGES

prochlorperazine
(continued)

CHILDREN 13.5 TO 17.5 KG: 2.5 mg P.O. or rectally b.i.d. or t.i.d., up to maximum 10 mg daily.

CHILDREN 9 TO 13 KG: 2.5 mg P.O. or rectally daily or b.i.d. to maximum 7.5 mg daily. I.M. dose 0.13 mg/kg; repeat if necessary. Not recommended in children under 9 kg.

Psychomotor agitation in schizophrenia; manic phase of manic-depressive psychosis; involutional toxic and senile psychoses:

ADULTS: initially, 10 mg P.O. t.i.d. to q.i.d., increasing up to 50 to 150 mg daily; or 10 to 20 mg I.M. q 1 to 4 hours, p.r.n., up to 100 mg daily, until symptoms are controlled. Prolonged I.M. dosage 10 to 20 mg q 4 to 6 hours.

SIDE EFFECTS

Hepatic: *cholestatic jaundice, abnormal liver function studies.*
Metabolic: hyperprolactinemia.
Skin: *mild photosensitivity,* dermal allergic reactions, *exfoliative dermatitis.*
Local: pain at I.M. injection site, sterile abscess.
Other: weight gain, increased appetite.
After abrupt withdrawal: gastritis, nausea, vomiting, dizziness, tremors, feeling of warmth or cold, sweating, tachycardia, headache, insomnia.

promazine hydrochloride
Promabec♦♦, Promanyl♦♦, Promazettes♦♦, Sparine♦

Psychosis:

ADULTS: 25 to 200 mg P.O. or I.M. q 4 to 6 hours, up to 1 g daily. I.V. dose in concentrations no greater than 25 mg/ml for acutely agitated patients. Initial dose 50 to 150 mg; repeat within 5 to 10 minutes if necessary.

CHILDREN OVER 12 YEARS: 10 to 25 mg P.O. or I.M. q 4 to 6 hours.

Blood: *transient leukopenia, agranulocytosis.*
CNS: *extrapyramidal reactions (moderate incidence), sedation (high incidence),* pseudoparkinsonism, EEG changes, dizziness.
CV: *orthostatic hypotension,* tachycardia, EKG changes.
EENT: *ocular changes, blurred vision.*
GI: *dry mouth, constipation.*
GU: *urinary retention,* dark urine, menstrual irregularities, gynecomastia, inhibited ejaculation.
Hepatic: *cholestatic jaundice, abnormal liver function studies.*
Metabolic: hyperprolactinemia.
Skin: *mild photosensitivity,* dermal allergic reactions, *exfoliative dermatitis.*
Local: pain at I.M. injection site, sterile abscess.
Other: weight gain, increased appetite.
After abrupt withdrawal: gastritis, nausea, vomiting, dizziness, tremors, feeling of warmth or cold, sweating, tachycardia, headache, insomnia.

♦ Available in U.S. and Canada. ♦♦ Available in Canada only.
All other products (no symbol) available in U.S. only. Italicized side effects are common or life-threatening.

INTERACTIONS AND SPECIAL CONSIDERATIONS

pected brain tumor or intestinal obstruction, glaucoma, or prostatic hypertrophy; and in acutely ill or dehydrated children.
• If jaundice, symptoms of blood dyscrasias (fever, sore throat, infection, cellulitis, weakness), or persistent (longer than a few hours) extrapyramidal reactions develop, or especially if such reactions develop during pregnancy or in children, dose should be held and therapy reevaluated.
• Therapy should be monitored by weekly bilirubin tests during first month; periodic blood tests (CBC, liver function); and ophthalmic tests (long-term use).
• Urinary retention and constipation are possible; intake and output should be monitored.
• Patient should use sunscreening agents and protective clothing to avoid photosensitivity reactions.
• Patient should avoid activities that require alertness or good psychomotor coordination until CNS response to drug is determined. Drowsiness and dizziness usually subside after a few weeks.
• Should not be combined with alcohol or other depressants.
• Baseline measures of blood pressure should be obtained. Blood pressure and heart rate should be monitored regularly. Orthostatic hypotension possible, especially with parenteral administration. Patient should change positions slowly.
• Should be given deep I.M. only in upper outer quadrant of buttocks, and skin massaged slowly afterward to prevent sterile abscess. Injection may sting.
• Should not be mixed in same syringe with another drug.
• Medication should not be given subcutaneously.
• Should be protected from light. Slight yellowing of injection or concentrate is common; does not affect potency. Markedly discolored solutions should be discarded.
• Keeping drug off patient's skin and clothes prevents contact dermatitis.
• Liquid concentrate should be diluted with fruit juice, milk, coffee, tea, carbonated beverages, or semisolid food just before administration.
• Drug should not be withdrawn abruptly unless required by severe side effects.
• Dry mouth may be relieved with sugarless gum, sour hard candy, or rinsing with mouthwash.
• Piperidine phenothiazine; most commonly used as an antiemetic.
• If more than 4 doses needed in 24-hour period, medical supervision required.
• Injectable form may be mixed with solutions of 5% dextrose, 10% dextrose, 10% fructose, 5% invert sugar, 10% invert sugar, normal saline, Ringer's injection, lactated Ringer's I.V. infusion, and dextrose-saline combinations.
• For symptoms and treatment of toxicity, see APPENDIX.

Interactions:
ANTACIDS: inhibit absorption of oral phenothiazines. Separate antacid and phenothiazine doses by at least 2 hours.
ANTICHOLINERGICS (INCLUDING ANTIDEPRESSANT AND ANTI-PARKINSON AGENTS): increased anticholinergic activity, aggravated Parkinson-like symptoms. Use with caution.
BARBITURATES: may decrease phenothiazine effect. Observe patient.

Special considerations:
• Contraindicated in coma, CNS depression, bone marrow depression, subcortical damage, and with use of spinal or epidural anesthesia or adrenergic blocking agents. Use cautiously with other CNS depressants and anticholinergics; in elderly or debilitated patients; in patients with hepatic disease, arteriosclerosis or cardiovascular disease (may cause sudden drop in blood pressure), exposure to extreme heat or cold (including antipyretic therapy), respiratory disorders, hypocalcemia, convulsive disorders (may lower seizure threshold), severe reactions to insulin or electroshock therapy, suspected brain tumor or intestinal obstruction, glaucoma, prostatic hypertrophy; and in acutely ill or dehydrated children.
• If jaundice, symptoms of blood dyscrasias (fever, sore throat, infection, cellulitis, weakness), or persistent (longer than a few hours) extrapyramidal reactions develop, or especially if such reactions develop during pregnancy or in children, dose should be held and therapy reevaluated.
• Therapy should be monitored by weekly bilirubin tests during first month; periodic blood tests (CBC, liver function); and ophthalmic tests (long-term use).
• Urinary retention and constipation are possible; intake and output should be monitored.
• Patient should use sunscreening agents and protective clothing to avoid photosensitivity reactions.
• Patient should avoid activities that require alertness or good psychomotor coordination until CNS response to drug is determined. Drowsiness and dizziness usually subside after a few weeks.
• Should not be combined with alcohol or other depressants.
• Blood pressure should be monitored lying and standing before starting therapy, and routinely throughout course of treatment.
• Orthostatic hypotension possible, especially with parenteral administration. Patient should remain supine for 1 hour afterward and change positions slowly.

(continued on following page)

NAMES, INDICATIONS AND DOSAGES	SIDE EFFECTS

promazine hydrochloride
(continued)

thioridazine hydrochloride
Mellaril♦, Novoridazine♦♦

Psychosis:
ADULTS: initially, 50 to 100 mg P.O. t.i.d., with gradual increments up to 800 mg daily in divided doses, if needed. Dosage varies. Dose above 800 mg may be associated with ocular toxicity (pigmentary retinopathy).

Depressive neurosis, alcohol withdrawal, dementia in geriatric patients, behavioral problems in children:
ADULTS: initially, 25 mg P.O. t.i.d. Maintenance dose is 20 to 200 mg daily.
CHILDREN OVER 2 YEARS: 0.5 to 3 mg/kg daily in divided doses.

Blood: *transient leukopenias, agranulocytosis.*
CNS: extrapyramidal reactions (low incidence), *sedation (high incidence),* EEG changes, dizziness.
CV: *orthostatic hypotension,* tachycardia, EKG changes.
EENT: *ocular changes, blurred vision,* pigmentary retinopathy.
GI: *dry mouth, constipation.*
GU: *urinary retention,* dark urine, menstrual irregularities, gynecomastia, inhibited ejaculation.
Hepatic: *cholestatic jaundice.*
Metabolic: hyperprolactinemia.
Skin: *mild photosensitivity,* dermal allergic reactions, *exfoliative dermatitis.*
Other: weight gain, increased appetite.
After abrupt withdrawal: gastritis, nausea, vomiting, dizziness, tremors, feeling of warmth or cold, sweating, tachycardia, headache, insomnia.

thiothixene
thiothixene hydrochloride
Navane♦

Acute agitation:
ADULTS: 4 mg I.M. b.i.d. to q.i.d. Maximum 30 mg daily I.M. Change to P.O. as soon as possible.

Mild-to-moderate psychosis:
ADULTS: initially, 2 mg P.O. t.i.d. May increase gradually to 15 mg daily.

Blood: *transient leukopenia, agranulocytosis.*
CNS: *extrapyramidal reactions (high incidence),* sedation (low incidence), pseudoparkinsonism, EEG changes, dizziness.
CV: *orthostatic hypotension,* tachycardia, EKG changes.
EENT: *ocular changes, blurred vision.*
GI: *dry mouth, constipation.*
GU: *urinary retention,* dark urine, menstrual irregularities, gynecomastia, inhibited ejaculation.
Hepatic: *cholestatic jaundice.*
Metabolic: hyperprolactinemia.
Skin: *mild photosensitivity,* dermal allergic re-

INTERACTIONS AND SPECIAL CONSIDERATIONS

• Should be given deep I.M. only in upper outer quadrant of buttocks, and skin massaged slowly afterward to prevent sterile abscess. Injection may sting.
• Should be protected from light. Slight yellowing of injection or concentrate is common; does not affect potency. Markedly discolored solutions should be discarded.
• Keeping drug off patient's skin and clothes prevents contact dermatitis.
• Liquid concentrate should be diluted with fruit juice, milk, semisolid food, or chocolate-flavored drinks just before administration. For best taste, at least 10 ml diluent per 25 mg drug should be used.
• Drug should not be withdrawn abruptly unless required by severe side effects.
• Dry mouth may be relieved with sugarless gum, sour hard candy, or rinsing with mouthwash.
• Drug is an aliphatic phenothiazine; rarely used for psychiatric treatment.
• For symptoms and treatment of toxicity, see APPENDIX.

Interactions:
ANTACIDS: inhibit absorption of oral phenothiazines. Separate antacid and phenothiazine doses by at least 2 hours.
BARBITURATES: may decrease phenothiazine effect. Observe patient.

Special considerations:
• Contraindicated in coma, CNS depression, bone marrow depression, hypertensive or hypotensive cardiac disease, subcortical damage, and with use of spinal or epidural anesthetic or adrenergic blocking agents. Use cautiously with other CNS depressants and anticholinergics; in elderly or debilitated patients; in patients with hepatic disease, arteriosclerosis or cardiovascular disease (may cause sudden drop in blood pressure), exposure to extreme heat or cold (including antipyretic therapy), respiratory disorders, hypocalcemia, convulsive disorders, severe reactions to insulin or electroshock therapy, suspected brain tumor or intestinal obstruction, glaucoma, or prostatic hypertrophy; and in acutely ill or dehydrated children.
• If jaundice, symptoms of blood dyscrasias (fever, sore throat, infection, cellulitis, weakness), or persistent (longer than a few hours) extrapyramidal reactions develop, or especially if such reactions develop during pregnancy or in children, dose should be held and therapy reevaluated.
• Therapy should be monitored by weekly bilirubin tests during first month; periodic blood tests (CBC, liver function); and ophthalmic tests (long-term therapy).
• Urinary retention and constipation are possible; intake and output should be monitored.
• Blurred vision and dry mouth should be watched for; high incidence of anticholinergic effects.
• Patient should use sunscreening agents and protective clothing to avoid photosensitivity reactions.
• Blood pressure should be monitored.
• Patient should avoid activities that require alertness or good psychomotor coordination until CNS response to drug is determined. Drowsiness and dizziness usually subside after a few weeks.
• Should not be combined with alcohol or other depressants.
• Orthostatic hypotension possible, especially with parenteral administration. Patient should change positions slowly.
• Keeping drug off patient's skin and clothes prevents contact dermatitis.
• Liquid concentrate should be diluted with water or fruit juice just before administration.
• Drug should not be withdrawn abruptly unless required by severe side effects.
• Dry mouth may be relieved with sugarless gum, sour hard candy, or rinsing with mouthwash.
• Piperidine phenothiazine; used to continue antipsychotic therapy when parkinsonian effects require withdrawal of other phenothiazines.
• Dose of 100 mg is therapeutic equivalent of 100 mg chlorpromazine.
• For symptoms and treatment of toxicity, see APPENDIX.

No significant interactions.

Special considerations:
• Contraindicated in convulsive seizures, circulatory collapse, coma, CNS depression, blood dyscrasias, bone marrow depression, alcohol withdrawal, akathisia or restlessness, subcortical damage, and with use of spinal or epidural anesthetic or adrenergic blocking agents. Use cautiously with other CNS depressants and anticholinergics; in elderly or debilitated patients; and in patients with hepatic disease, arteriosclerosis or cardiovascular disease (may cause sudden drop in blood pressure), exposure to extreme heat or cold (including antipyretic therapy) or undue sunlight, respiratory disorders, hypocalcemia, severe reactions to insulin or electroshock therapy, suspected brain tumor or intestinal obstruction, glaucoma, or prostatic hypertrophy.
• If jaundice, symptoms of blood dyscrasias (fever, sore throat, infection, cellulitis, weakness), or persistent (longer than a few hours) extrapyramidal reactions develop, or especially if such reactions develop during pregnancy, dose should be held and therapy reevaluated.
• Therapy should be monitored by weekly bilirubin tests during first month; periodic blood

(continued on following page)

NAMES, INDICATIONS AND DOSAGES	SIDE EFFECTS
thiothixene *(continued)* **Severe psychosis:** ADULTS: initially, 5 mg P.O. b.i.d. May increase gradually to 15 to 30 mg daily. Maximum recommended daily dose 60 mg. Not recommended in children under 12 years.	actions, *exfoliative dermatitis.* **Local:** pain at I.M. injection site, sterile abscess. **Other:** weight gain, increased appetite. **After abrupt withdrawal:** gastritis, nausea, vomiting, dizziness, tremors, feeling of warmth or cold, sweating, tachycardia, headache, insomnia.
trifluoperazine hydrochloride Clinazine♦♦, Novoflurazine♦♦, Pentazine♦♦, Solazine♦♦, Stelazine♦, Terfluzine♦♦, Triflurin♦♦, Tripazine♦♦ **Anxiety states:** ADULTS: 1 to 2 mg P.O. b.i.d. **Schizophrenia and other psychotic disorders:** ADULTS: outpatients—1 to 2 mg P.O. b.i.d., up to 4 mg daily; hospitalized—2 to 5 mg P.O. b.i.d.; may gradually increase to 40 mg daily. 1 to 2 mg I.M. q 4 to 6 hours, p.r.n. More than 6 mg daily is rarely needed. CHILDREN 6 TO 12 YEARS (HOSPITALIZED OR UNDER CLOSE SUPERVISION): 1 mg P.O. daily or b.i.d.; may increase gradually to 15 mg daily.	**Blood:** *transient leukopenia, agranulocytosis.* **CNS:** *extrapyramidal reactions (high incidence),* sedation (low incidence), pseudoparkinsonism, EEG changes, dizziness. **CV:** *orthostatic hypotension,* tachycardia, EKG changes. **EENT:** *ocular changes, blurred vision.* **GI:** *dry mouth, constipation.* **GU:** *urinary retention,* dark urine, menstrual irregularities, gynecomastia, inhibited ejaculation. **Hepatic:** *cholestatic jaundice.* **Metabolic:** hyperprolactinemia. **Skin:** *mild photosensitivity,* dermal allergic reactions, *exfoliative dermatitis.* **Local:** pain at I.M. injection site, sterile abscess. **Other:** weight gain, increased appetite. **After abrupt withdrawal:** gastritis, nausea, vomiting, dizziness, tremors, feeling of warmth or cold, sweating, tachycardia, headache, insomnia.

INTERACTIONS AND SPECIAL CONSIDERATIONS

tests (CBC, liver function); and ophthalmic tests (long-term therapy).
• Urinary retention and constipation are possible; intake and output should be monitored.
• Patient should use sunscreening agents and protective clothing to avoid photosensitivity reactions.
• Patient should avoid activities that require alertness or good psychomotor coordination until CNS response to drug is determined. Drowsiness and dizziness usually subside after a few weeks.
• Should not be combined with alcohol or other depressants.
• Orthostatic hypotension possible, especially with parenteral administration. Patient should remain supine for 1 hour afterward and change positions slowly.
• Should be given I.M. only in upper outer quadrant of buttocks, or midlateral thigh, and skin massaged slowly afterward to prevent sterile abscess. Injection may sting.
• I.M. form must be stored in refrigerator.
• Slight yellowing of injection or concentrate is common; does not affect potency. Markedly discolored solutions should be discarded.
• Keeping drug off patient's skin and clothes prevents contact dermatitis.
• Liquid concentrate should be diluted with fruit juice, milk, or semisolid food just before administration.
• Drug should not be withdrawn abruptly unless required by severe side effects.
• Dry mouth may be relieved with sugarless gum, sour hard candy, or rinsing with mouthwash.
• Drug is a thioxanthene derivative but produces responses similar to phenothiazine and butyrophenones.
• Dose of 4 mg is therapeutic equivalent of 100 mg chlorpromazine.

Interactions:
ANTACIDS: inhibit absorption of oral phenothiazines. Separate antacid and phenothiazine doses by at least 2 hours.
BARBITURATES: may decrease phenothiazine effect. Observe patient.

Special considerations:
• Contraindicated in coma, CNS depression, bone marrow depression, subcortical damage, and with use of spinal or epidural anesthetic or adrenergic blocking agents. Use cautiously with other CNS depressants, anticholinergics; in elderly or debilitated patients; in patients with hepatic disease, arteriosclerosis or cardiovascular disease (may cause drop in blood pressure), exposure to extreme heat or cold (including antipyretic therapy), respiratory disorders, hypocalcemia, convulsive disorders, severe reactions to insulin or electroshock therapy, suspected brain tumor or intestinal obstruction, glaucoma, or prostatic hypertrophy; and in acutely ill or dehydrated children.
• If jaundice, symptoms of blood dyscrasias (fever, sore throat, infection, cellulitis, weakness), or persistent (longer than a few hours) extrapyramidal reactions develop, or especially if such reactions develop during pregnancy or in children, dose should be held and therapy reevaluated.
• Therapy should be monitored by weekly bilirubin tests during first month; periodic blood tests (CBC, liver function); and ophthalmic tests (long-term therapy).
• Urinary retention and constipation are possible; intake and output should be monitored.
• Patient should use sunscreening agents and protective clothing to avoid photosensitivity reactions.
• Patient should avoid activities that require alertness or good psychomotor coordination until CNS response to drug is determined. Drowsiness and dizziness usually subside after a few weeks.
• Drug should not be combined with alcohol or other depressants.
• Orthostatic hypotension possible, especially with parenteral administration. Patient should remain supine for 1 hour afterward and change positions slowly.
• Should be given deep I.M. only in upper outer quadrant of buttocks, and skin massaged slowly afterward to prevent sterile abscess. Injection may sting.
• Should be protected from light. Slight yellowing of injection or concentrate is common; does not affect potency. Markedly discolored solutions should be discarded.
• Keeping drug off patient's skin and clothes prevents contact dermatitis.
• Liquid concentrate should be diluted with 60 ml tomato or fruit juice, carbonated beverages, coffee, tea, milk, water, or semisolid food just before administration.
• Should not be withdrawn abruptly unless required by severe side effects.
• Dry mouth may be relieved with sugarless gum, sour hard candy, or rinsing with mouthwash.
• Drug is a prototype piperazine phenothiazine.
• Dose of 5 mg is therapeutic equivalent of 100 mg chlorpromazine.
• For symptoms and treatment of toxicity, see APPENDIX.

NAMES, INDICATIONS AND DOSAGES	SIDE EFFECTS

trifluopromazine hydrochloride

Vesprin

Acute, severe agitation:

ADULTS: 60 to 150 mg I.M. in 2 or 3 divided doses.

CHILDREN OVER 2½ YEARS: 0.2 to 0.25 mg/kg in divided doses. Maximum dose 10 mg daily.

Nausea and vomiting:

ADULTS: 20 to 30 mg P.O. daily; or 1 to 3 mg I.V. daily; or 5 to 15 mg I.M. daily up to maximum 60 mg daily.

CHILDREN: 0.2 mg/kg P.O. or I.M. up to maximum 10 mg daily.

Psychotic disorders (mild to moderate symptoms):

ADULTS: 10 to 25 mg P.O. b.i.d.

CHILDREN OVER 2½ YEARS: 10 mg P.O. t.i.d.

ELDERLY OR DEBILITATED PATIENTS: 10 mg b.i.d. or t.i.d.; increase gradually to desired effect.

Severe symptoms:

ADULTS: 50 mg P.O. b.i.d. or t.i.d.

CHILDREN OVER 2½ YEARS: 2 mg/kg P.O. in 3 divided doses; may increase gradually to 150 mg daily.

Blood: *transient leukopenia, agranulocytosis.*
CNS: *extrapyramidal reactions (moderate incidence), sedation (high incidence),* pseudoparkinsonism, EEG changes, dizziness.
CV: *orthostatic hypotension,* tachycardia, EKG changes.
EENT: *ocular changes, blurred vision.*
GI: *dry mouth, constipation.*
GU: *urinary retention,* dark urine, menstrual irregularities, gynecomastia, inhibited ejaculation.
Hepatic: *cholestatic jaundice.*
Metabolic: hyperprolactinemia.
Skin: *mild photosensitivity,* dermal allergic reactions, *exfoliative dermatitis.*
Local: pain at I.M. injection site, sterile abscess.
Other: weight gain, increased appetite.
After abrupt withdrawal: gastritis, nausea, vomiting, dizziness, tremors, feeling of warmth or cold, sweating, tachycardia, headache, insomnia.

INTERACTIONS AND SPECIAL CONSIDERATIONS

Interactions:

ANTACIDS: inhibit absorption of oral phenothiazines. Separate antacid and phenothiazine doses by at least 2 hours.

ANTICHOLINERGICS (INCLUDING ANTIDEPRESSANT AND ANTI-PARKINSON AGENTS): increased anticholinergic activity, aggravated Parkinson-like symptoms. Use with caution.

BARBITURATES: may decrease phenothiazine effect. Observe patient.

Special considerations:

• Contraindicated in coma, CNS depression, blood dyscrasias, bone marrow depression, subcortical brain damage, and with use of spinal or epidural anesthetic or adrenergic blocking agents. Use cautiously with other CNS depressants and anticholinergics; in elderly or debilitated patients; in patients with hepatic disease, arteriosclerosis or cardiovascular disease (may cause sudden drop in blood pressure), exposure to extreme heat or cold (including antipyretic therapy), respiratory disorders, pheochromocytoma, hypocalcemia, convulsive disorders, severe reactions to insulin or electroshock therapy, suspected brain tumor or intestinal obstruction, glaucoma, prostatic hypertrophy; and in acutely ill or dehydrated children.
• If jaundice, symptoms of blood dyscrasias (fever, sore throat, infection, cellulitis, weakness), or persistent (longer than a few hours) extrapyramidal reactions develop, or especially if such reactions develop during pregnancy or in children, dose should be held and therapy reevaluated.
• Therapy should be monitored by weekly bilirubin tests during first month; periodic blood tests (CBC, liver function); and ophthalmic tests in long-term therapy.
• Urinary retention and constipation are possible; intake and output should be monitored.
• Hypothermia reactions should be watched for.
• Patient should use sunscreening agents and protective clothing to avoid photosensitivity reactions.
• Patient should avoid activities that require alertness or good psychomotor coordination until CNS response to drug is determined. Drowsiness and dizziness usually subside after a few weeks.
• Should not be combined with alcohol or other depressants.
• Orthostatic hypotension possible, especially with parenteral administration. Patient should remain supine for 1 hour afterward and change positions slowly.
• Should be given I.M. only in upper outer quadrant of buttocks, and skin massaged slowly afterward to prevent sterile abscess. Injection may sting.
• Should be protected from light. Slight yellowing of injection or concentrate is common; does not affect potency. Markedly discolored solutions should be discarded.
• Liquid suspension should be kept tightly closed.
• Keeping drug off patient's skin and clothes prevents contact dermatitis.
• Drug should not be withdrawn abruptly unless required by severe side effects.
• Dry mouth may be relieved with sugarless gum, sour hard candy, or rinsing with mouthwash.
• Drug is an aliphatic phenothiazine.
• Dose of 25 mg is therapeutic equivalent of 10 mg chlorpromazine.

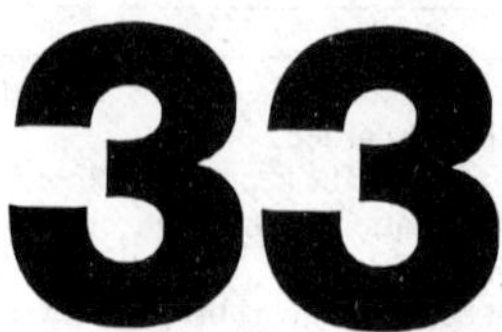

Miscellaneous psychotherapeutics

lithium carbonate
lithium citrate

Lithium salts have been used throughout the world for more than 20 years to combat manic-depressive illness (bipolar disorders). In the United States, however, lithium has been used only since 1970. (Many deaths had occurred during the 1940s when lithium was improperly used as a salt substitute.)

Under proper supervision, lithium may prevent up to 80% of manic and depressive episodes. Episodes that occur during lithium therapy are usually less severe and shorter than those that might occur without such therapy. Close monitoring to maintain therapeutic lithium blood levels allows safe use of this drug. However, lithium's toxic level is very close to its therapeutic level.

Consistent dietary sodium and fluid intake are necessary every day to help prevent toxicity. Conditions that may cause excess sodium and water loss (such as sweating or diarrhea) may require supplemental fluid or salt administration.

Major uses

Lithium salts are used to treat acute manic or hypomanic episodes of manic-depressive

PATIENT-TEACHING AID

WHAT YOU SHOULD KNOW ABOUT LITHIUM

Dear Patient:

To get the most from your drug therapy, follow these instructions carefully:
• If you experience diarrhea, vomiting, drowsiness, muscle weakness and coordination failure, tremors, restlessness, or confusion, call the doctor immediately. But don't abruptly stop taking your drug.
• Expect transient nausea, frequent urination, and thirst during the first few days of therapy.
• Expect a time lag of 1 to 3 weeks before you notice the drug's beneficial effects.
• Avoid activities that require complete mental alertness, such as operating machinery or driving, until your response to the drug is determined.
• Don't switch brands of lithium without asking the doctor first.
• Drink a full glass of water when you take your medication. Also, taking your medication after meals helps minimize nausea.
• Carry an identification card that gives instructions and toxicity and emergency information (available from your pharmacy).

LITHIUM MAY REDUCE INFECTION RISK DURING CANCER CHEMOTHERAPY

Studies indicate that lithium carbonate may prevent infectious complications in patients undergoing cancer chemotherapy.

In a landmark study reported in the *New England Journal of Medicine* (January 31, 1980), 20 patients were given 300 mg of lithium three times daily, from 24 hours before chemotherapy until 48 hours before the next chemotherapy cycle. Here's how their reactions to chemotherapy differed from 25 patients who hadn't received lithium.

They experienced:

- fewer days with severe neutropenia
- fewer days hospitalized with neutropenia and fever
- no neutropenic febrile episodes, in contrast with six cases in the control group
- no infection-related deaths, in contrast with five in the control group
- significantly longer infection-free survival
- fewer antineoplastic dose reductions
- shorter and less frequent delays in treatment.

Patients given lithium had higher leukocyte and neutrophil counts throughout their chemotherapy treatment than those who were not given lithium.

Thus, this study concludes that administration of lithium between chemotherapy cycles reduces the risk of infection-related mortality, which is due to the leukocyte and neutrophil depression that commonly develops between treatment cycles. However, further study is needed to check the safety and efficacy of this regimen.

disorders and to prevent their recurrence.

They're also used investigationally to stimulate white cell production in patients receiving antineoplastic drugs.

Mechanism of action

Lithium alters chemical transmitters in the central nervous system, possibly by interfering with ionic pump mechanisms in brain cells. Its exact mechanism of action in mania, however, is unknown.

Absorption, distribution, metabolism, and excretion

Lithium is readily absorbed orally. It is distributed to body tissues, with highest concentrations in the kidneys and lowest concentrations in brain tissue. The drug is almost entirely excreted through the kidneys as unchanged lithium ions.

Onset and duration

Blood levels of lithium peak within 2 to 4 hours. The antimanic action is delayed for 5 to 10 days.

Combination products

None.

NAMES, INDICATIONS AND DOSAGES	SIDE EFFECTS

lithium carbonate
Carbolith♦♦, Eskalith, Lithane♦, Lithizine♦♦, Lithobid, Lithonate, Lithotabs
lithium citrate
Cibalith-S

Prevention or control of mania:
ADULTS: 300 to 600 mg P.O. up to 4 times daily, increasing on the basis of blood levels to achieve optimal dosage. Recommended therapeutic lithium blood levels: 1 to 1.5 mEq/liter for acute mania; 0.6 to 1.2 mEq/liter for maintenance therapy; and 2 mEq/liter as maximum.
ADULTS: 5 ml lithium citrate (liquid) contains 8 mEq lithium equal to 300 mg lithium carbonate.

Blood: *leukocytosis of 14,000 to 18,000 (reversible).*
CNS: tremors, drowsiness, headache, confusion, restlessness, dizziness, psychomotor retardation, stupor, lethargy, coma, blackouts, epileptiform seizures, EEG changes, worsened organic brain syndrome, impaired speech, ataxia, muscle weakness, incoordination, hyperexcitability.
CV: *reversible EKG changes,* arrhythmia, hypotension, peripheral circulatory collapse, allergic vasculitis, ankle and wrist edema.
EENT: tinnitus, impaired vision.
GI: nausea, vomiting, anorexia, diarrhea, fecal incontinence, dry mouth, thirst, metallic taste.
GU: *polyuria,* glycosuria, incontinence, renal toxicity.
Metabolic: transient hyperglycemia, goiter, hypothyroidism (lowered T_3, T_4, and PBI, but elevated ^{131}I uptake), hyponatremia.
Skin: pruritus, rash, diminished or lost sensation, drying and thinning of hair.

♦ Available in U.S. and Canada. ♦♦ Available in Canada only.
All other products (no symbol) available in U.S. only. Italicized side effects are common or life-threatening.

INTERACTIONS AND SPECIAL CONSIDERATIONS

Interactions:
DIURETICS: increased reabsorption of lithium by kidneys, with possible toxic effect. Use with extreme caution, and monitor lithium and electrolyte levels (especially sodium).
HALOPERIDOL: encephalopathic syndrome (lethargy, tremors, extrapyramidal symptoms). Watch for syndrome, and stop drug if it occurs.
APHYLLINE, SODIUM BICARBONATE, SODIUM CHLORIDE: ingestion of these salts increases lithium excretion. Avoid salt loads and monitor lithium levels.
PROBENECID, INDOMETHACIN, METHYLDOPA: increased effect of lithium. Monitor for lithium toxicity.

Special considerations:
- Contraindicated if therapy cannot be closely monitored. Use with caution with haloperidol, other antipsychotics, neuromuscular blocking agents, and diuretics; in elderly or debilitated persons; and in thyroid disease, epilepsy, renal or cardiovascular disease, brain damage, severe debilitation or dehydration, and sodium depletion.
- Baseline EKG, thyroid and renal studies, and electrolyte levels should be monitored. Serum lithium levels should be monitored 8 to 12 hours after first dose, usually before a.m. dose, 2 to 3 times weekly first month, then weekly to monthly on maintenance.
- When blood levels of lithium are below 1.5 mEq/liter, side effects generally remain mild.
- Fluid intake and output should be checked, especially when surgery is scheduled.
- Patient and family should watch for signs of toxicity (diarrhea, vomiting, drowsiness, muscular weakness, ataxia) and expect transient nausea, polyuria, thirst, and discomfort during first few days. Patient should withhold one dose and call doctor if toxic symptoms appear, but not stop drug abruptly.
- Patient should expect lag of 1 to 3 weeks before drug's beneficial effects are noticed.
- Patient should be weighed daily; edema or sudden weight gain possible.
- Fluid and salt ingestion should be adjusted to compensate if excessive loss occurs through protracted sweating or diarrhea. Under normal conditions, patients should have fluid intake of 2,500 to 3,000 ml/day and a balanced diet with adequate salt intake.
- Patient should have outpatient follow-up of thyroid and renal functions every 6 to 12 months. Thyroid should be palpated to check for enlargement.
- Identification/instruction card (available from pharmacy) with toxicity and emergency information should be carried.
- Ambulatory patient should avoid activities that require alertness and good psychomotor coordination until CNS response to drug is determined.
- Should be administered with plenty of water, and after meals to minimize GI upset.
- Urine should be checked for specific gravity, and level below 1.015, which may indicate diabetes insipidus syndrome, should be reported.
- Has been used to treat syndrome of inappropriate antidiuretic hormone.
- Patient should not switch brands of lithium or take other drugs (prescription or over-the-counter) without doctor's guidance.
- Investigationally used to increase white cells in patients undergoing cancer chemotherapy.
- Also used investigationally for treatment of cluster headaches, aggression, organic brain syndrome, and tardive dyskinesia.
- For symptoms and treatment of toxicity, see APPENDIX.

34

Cerebral stimulants

amphetamine hydrochloride
amphetamine phosphate
amphetamine sulfate
benzphetamine hydrochloride
caffeine
caffeine, citrated
caffeine sodium benzoate injection
chlorphentermine hydrochloride
clortermine hydrochloride
deanol acetamidobenzoate
dextroamphetamine phosphate
dextroamphetamine sulfate
diethylpropion hydrochloride
fenfluramine hydrochloride
mazindol
methamphetamine hydrochloride
methylphenidate hydrochloride
pemoline
phendimetrazine tartrate
phenmetrazine hydrochloride
phentermine hydrochloride

Amphetamines are the prototypes for central nervous system (CNS) stimulants. They're the first agents to have been used as appetite suppressants (anorexigenics). Recently, however, the Food and Drug Administration proposed that weight reduction in obesity be deleted as an approved indication for these drugs. Their use as anorexigenics should be limited to short-term weight control only as prescribed by a doctor.

Amphetamines, or "uppers" in street language, are common drugs of abuse (many are pictured in the special color section on pp. 36 to 57).

Also included in this class are isomers of amphetamines (amphetamine-like drugs). These have less potential for abuse because their euphoric effects aren't as great.

All the agents discussed in this chapter, except caffeine and deanol, are officially listed by the Drug Enforcement Agency as controlled substances.

Major uses

- The amphetamines and amphetamine-like drugs may suppress appetite, promote weight reduction in exogenous obesity, and supply short-term adjunctive therapy for weight control and dieting.
- Deanol, dextroamphetamine, methamphetamine, methylphenidate, and pemoline are used as therapeutic adjuncts in minimal brain dysfunction in children, such as hyperkinesia.
- Dextroamphetamine and methylphenidate are used to treat narcolepsy.

Mechanism of action

- Amphetamines and amphetamine-like drugs, caffeine, methylphenidate, and pemoline are sympathomimetics whose main sites of activity appear to be the cerebral cortex and the reticular activating system. They probably promote nerve impulse transmission by releasing stored noreinephrine from nerve terminals in the brain.
- In children with hyperkinesia, amphetamines have a paradoxical calming effect that is probably related to the actions of the drug on CNS neurotransmitters. The mechanism by which amphetamines produce mental and behavioral effects in children, however, has not been established.
- Deanol probably elicits a CNS-stimulating effect by increasing brain levels of choline—a precursor of acetylcholine.

Absorption, distribution, metabolism, and excretion

Cerebral stimulants are readily absorbed from the GI tract. They are well distributed to most body tissues, with high concentrations in the brain and cerebrospinal fluid.

DEALING WITH AMPHETAMINE ADDICTION

Prevention

- The patient should be educated concerning the misuse of caffeine and amphetamines.
- Monitor amphetamine-induced side effects by:

—teaching the obese patient who is taking amphetamines to report such symptoms as nervousness, insomnia, and cardiac palpitations.

—observing the depressed patient who is being treated with amphetamines for insomnia, loss of appetite, restlessness, and agitation.

—watching the patient on powerful central nervous system stimulants such as dextroamphetamine, which is twice as potent as amphetamine. Dextroamphetamine, in large doses, is more likely to cause fatigue, mental depression, increased blood pressure, cyanosis, respiratory failure, disorientation, hallucinations, convulsions, and coma.

- Observation of drug-induced symptoms may require discontinuation of medication.

Patient care

- The health-care professional should be aware of his own attitude toward drug addiction and abuse. If he respects the amphetamine addict as a human being, the patient's motivation will be increased. He should be straightforward with the patient and firm in setting limits without irritating or humiliating the patient unnecessarily when enforcing them.
- A special effort should be made to establish a supportive relationship with the addicted patient during his withdrawal from amphetamines. This critical stage of rehabilitation can have a favorable effect on the patient's final recovery.

- Amphetamines and amphetamine-like drugs are excreted by the kidneys, largely unchanged, in about 3 hours. They and fenfluramine hydrochloride are excreted more readily in acidic urine than they are in alkaline urine.
- Caffeine, deanol, and methylphenidate are partially metabolized by the liver and excreted by the kidneys.
- Pemoline probably undergoes the greatest metabolic change of these drugs, with more than 50% being metabolized to pemoline dione, an active metabolite, before being excreted by the kidneys.

Onset and duration

Onset is usually within 1 to 2 hours. Duration is from 4 to 10 hours, with most drugs requiring multiple doses for continued anorexigenic effect. Some are longer-acting (6 to 12 hours).

Combination products

AMPHAPLEX-10/OBETROL-10: dextroamphetamine saccharate 2.5 mg, amphetamine aspartate 2.5 mg, amphetamine sulfate 2.5 mg, and dextroamphetamine sulfate 2.5 mg.
AMPHAPLEX-20/OBETROL-20: dextroamphetamine saccharate 5 mg, amphetamine aspartate 5 mg, amphetamine sulfate 5 mg, and dextroamphetamine sulfate 5 mg.
BIPHETAMINE 12½: dextroamphetamine 6.25 mg and amphetamine 6.25 mg.
BIPHETAMINE 20: dextroamphetamine 10 mg and amphetamine 10 mg.
ESKATROL: dextroamphetamine sulfate 15 mg and prochlorperazine maleate 7.5 mg.

NAMES, INDICATIONS AND DOSAGES	SIDE EFFECTS
amphetamine hydrochloride **amphetamine phosphate** **amphetamine sulfate** Controlled Substance Schedule II Benzedrine♦ **Minimal brain dysfunction:** CHILDREN 6 YEARS AND OLDER: 5 mg P.O. daily, with 5-mg increments weekly, p.r.n. CHILDREN 3 TO 5 YEARS: 2.5 mg P.O. daily, with 2.5-mg increments weekly, p.r.n. **Narcolepsy:** ADULTS: 5 to 60 mg P.O. daily in divided doses. CHILDREN OVER 12 YEARS: 10 mg P.O. daily, with 10-mg increments weekly, p.r.n. CHILDREN 6 TO 12 YEARS: 5 mg P.O. daily, with 5-mg increments weekly, p.r.n. **Short-term adjunct in exogenous obesity:** ADULTS: single 10- or 15-mg long-acting capsule daily, or 2 if needed, up to 30 mg daily; or 5 to 30 mg daily in divided doses 30 to 60 minutes before meals. Not recommended for children under 12 years.	**CNS:** *restlessness,* tremor, *hyperactivity, talkativeness, insomnia,* irritability, dizziness, headache, chills, overstimulation, dysphoria. **CV:** *tachycardia, palpitations,* hypertension, hypotension. **GI:** nausea, vomiting, cramps, dry mouth, diarrhea, constipation, metallic taste, anorexia, weight loss. **Other:** urticaria, impotence, changes in libido.
benzphetamine hydrochloride Controlled Substance Schedule III Didrex **Short-term adjunct in exogenous obesity:** ADULTS: 25 to 50 mg P.O. daily, b.i.d., or t.i.d.	**CNS:** *restlessness,* tremor, *hyperactivity, talkativeness, insomnia,* irritability, dizziness, headache, chills, overstimulation, dysphoria. **CV:** *tachycardia, palpitations,* hypertension, hypotension. **GI:** nausea, vomiting, cramps, dry mouth, diarrhea, constipation, metallic taste, anorexia, weight loss. **Skin:** urticaria. **Other:** impotence, changes in libido.

INTERACTIONS AND SPECIAL CONSIDERATIONS

Interactions:
MAO INHIBITORS: severe hypertension; possible hypertensive crisis. Don't use together.
SODIUM BICARBONATE, ACETAZOLAMIDE: increased renal reabsorption. Monitor for enhanced effect.
AMMONIUM CHLORIDE, ASCORBIC ACID: observe for decreased amphetamine effect.
PHENOTHIAZINES, HALOPERIDOL: observe for decreased amphetamine effect.

Special considerations:
• Contraindicated in symptomatic cardiovascular diseases, hyperthyroidism, nephritis, angina pectoris, moderate-to-severe hypertension, parkinsonism due to arteriosclerosis, certain types of glaucoma, advanced arteriosclerosis, agitated states, or history of drug abuse. Use with caution in patients with diabetes mellitus and in elderly, debilitated, or hyperexcitable patients.
• Psychic dependence or habituation may occur, especially in patients with history of drug addiction. Prolonged use should be avoided. When used long-term, lower dosage gradually to prevent acute rebound depression.
• When used for obesity, patient should also follow a weight-reduction program. Drug should be taken 30 to 60 minutes before meals.
• Fatigue may result as drug effects wear off. Patient will need more rest.
• Patient should avoid caffeinic drinks, which increase the effects of amphetamines and related amines.
• Vital signs should be checked regularly and patient observed for signs of excessive stimulation.
• Urinary acidification enhances renal excretion; urinary alkalinization enhances renal reabsorption and recycling.
• When tolerance to anorexigenic effect develops, dosage should not be increased, but drug discontinued.
• Use to combat fatigue should be discouraged.
• Patient should avoid activities that require alertness or good psychomotor coordination until CNS response to drug is determined.
• May alter insulin needs in patients with diabetes. Blood and urine sugars should be monitored.
• Use as analeptic is usually discouraged, since CNS stimulation superimposed on CNS depression can lead to neuronal instability and seizures.
• May reverse beneficial effect of antihypertensives. Blood pressure should be monitored.

Interactions:
MAO INHIBITORS: severe hypertension; possible hypertensive crisis. Don't use together.
SODIUM BICARBONATE, ACETAZOLAMIDE: increased renal reabsorption. Monitor for enhanced effects.
AMMONIUM CHLORIDE, ASCORBIC ACID: observe for decreased benzphetamine effects.
PHENOTHIAZINES, HALOPERIDOL: observe for decreased benzphetamine effects.

Special considerations:
• Contraindicated in symptomatic cardiovascular diseases, hyperthyroidism, nephritis, angina pectoris, moderate-to-severe hypertension, parkinsonism due to arteriosclerosis, certain types of glaucoma, advanced arteriosclerosis, agitated states, or in patients with history of drug abuse. Use with caution in patients with diabetes mellitus and in elderly, debilitated, or hyperexcitable patients.
• Psychic dependence or habituation may occur, especially in patients with history of drug addiction. Prolonged use should be avoided. When used long-term, lower dosage gradually to prevent acute rebound depression.
• Should be used with weight-reduction program. Should be taken 30 to 60 minutes before meals.
• Fatigue may result as drug effects wear off. Patient will need more rest.
• Patient should avoid caffeinic drinks, which increase the effect of amphetamines and related amines.
• Vital signs should be checked regularly and patient observed for signs of excessive stimulation.
• Urinary acidification enhances renal excretion; urinary alkalinization enhances renal reabsorption and recycling.
• When tolerance to anorexigenic effect develops, dosage should not be increased but drug discontinued.
• Patient should avoid activities that require alertness or good psychomotor coordination until CNS response to drug is determined.
• May alter insulin needs in patients with diabetes. Blood and urine sugars should be monitored.

NAMES, INDICATIONS AND DOSAGES	SIDE EFFECTS
caffeine Ban-Drowz, Kirkaffeine, Nodoz, Tirend, Vivarin **caffeine, citrated** **caffeine sodium benzoate injection** **Respiratory and central nervous system stimulant:** ADULTS: 100 to 200 mg anhydrous caffeine P.O.; 500 mg to 1 g caffeine sodium benzoate I.M. or I.V. in emergency only.	**CNS:** *stimulation, insomnia,* restlessness, nervousness, mild delirium, headache, excitement, agitation, muscle tremors, twitches. **CV:** *tachycardia.* **GI:** nausea, vomiting. **GU:** *diuresis.* **Skin:** hyperesthesia.
chlorphentermine hydrochloride Controlled Substance Schedule III Chlorophen, Pre-Sate♦ **Short-term adjunct in exogenous obesity:** ADULTS: 65 mg P.O. taken after breakfast.	**CNS:** *insomnia,* overstimulation, nervousness, dizziness, paradoxical sedation, headache. **CV:** *tachycardia, palpitations,* increased blood pressure. **GI:** nausea, dry mouth, constipation. **Skin:** urticaria.
clortermine hydrochloride Controlled Substance Schedule III Voranil **Short-term adjunct in exogenous obesity:** ADULTS: 50 mg P.O. taken at midmorning.	**CNS:** *restlessness,* dizziness, *insomnia,* euphoria, tremor, headache. **CV:** *tachycardia, palpitations,* arrhythmias, increased blood pressure. **GI:** dry mouth, diarrhea, constipation. **Skin:** urticaria. **Other:** impotence, libido changes.
deanol acetamidobenzoate Deaner, Deaner-100♦♦, Deaner-250 **Minimal brain dysfunction:** CHILDREN OVER 6 YEARS: initially, 500 mg P.O. daily after breakfast; may reduce to maintenance 250 to 500 mg daily. Dose adjusted to patient's needs and response. **Dyskinesia, blepharospasm:** ADULTS: 600 mg to 1.6 g P.O. daily.	**CNS:** insomnia, mild overstimulation, irritability, headache, muscle twitching, tenseness. **CV:** postural hypotension. **EENT:** increased nasal and oral secretions. **GI:** constipation. **Skin:** transient rash. **Other:** dyspnea.

♦ Available in U.S. and Canada. ♦♦ Available in Canada only.
All other products (no symbol) available in U.S. only. Italicized side effects are common or life-threatening.

INTERACTIONS AND SPECIAL CONSIDERATIONS

No significant interactions.

Special considerations:
- Contraindicated in patients with gastric or duodenal ulcer.
- Tolerance or psychological dependence may develop.
- Signs of overdose: GI pain, mild delirium, insomnia, diuresis, dehydration, and fever. Should be treated with short-acting barbiturates, gastric emesis, or lavage.
- Single dose should not exceed 1 g.
- Caffeine content in cola beverages, 17 to 55 mg/180 ml; tea, 40 to 100 mg/180 ml; instant coffee, 60 to 180 mg/180 ml; brewed coffee, 100 to 150 mg/180 ml.
- Caffeine does not reverse alcohol intoxication or depressant effects of alcohol. Overvigorous therapy with caffeine may aggravate depression in an already depressed patient.
- Use as analeptic is discouraged.

Interactions:
MAO INHIBITORS: severe hypertension; possible hypertensive crisis. Don't use together.
SODIUM BICARBONATE, ACETAZOLAMIDE: increased renal reabsorption. Monitor for enhanced effects.
AMMONIUM CHLORIDE, ASCORBIC ACID: observe for decreased chlorphentermine effects.

Special considerations:
- Contraindicated in hyperexcitability states, hyperthyroidism, hypertension, angina pectoris, severe cardiovascular disease, glaucoma, or in patients with history of drug abuse.
- Psychic dependence and habituation may occur. When tolerance to anorexigenic effect develops, dose should not be increased but drug discontinued.
- May alter insulin needs in patients with diabetes. Blood and urine sugars should be monitored.
- Patient should follow a good dietary plan and exercise program.
- Drug should be withdrawn gradually.
- Fatigue may result as drug effects wear off. Patient will need more rest.
- Patient should avoid caffeinic drinks, which increase the effects of amphetamines and related amines.
- Vital signs should be checked regularly and patient observed for signs of excessive stimulation.
- Urinary acidification enhances renal excretion; urinary alkalinization enhances renal reabsorption and recycling.

Interactions:
MAO INHIBITORS: severe hypertension; possible hypertensive crisis. Don't use together.
SODIUM BICARBONATE, ACETAZOLAMIDE: increased renal reabsorption. Monitor for enhanced effects.
AMMONIUM CHLORIDE, ASCORBIC ACID: observe for decreased clortermine effects.

Special considerations:
- Contraindicated in hyperthyroidism, glaucoma, severe hypertension, cardiovascular diseases, agitated states, and in patients with history of drug abuse. Use with caution in diabetes mellitus. Insulin requirements may be altered. Blood and urine sugars should be monitored.
- Patient should avoid activities that require alertness or good psychomotor coordination until CNS response to drug is determined.
- Patient should follow a sensible dietary regimen.
- Drug should be discontinued when tolerance develops.
- Fatigue may result as drug effects wear off. Patient will need more rest.
- Patient should avoid caffeinic drinks, which increase the effects of amphetamines and related amines.
- Vital signs should be checked regularly and patient observed for signs of excessive stimulation.
- Urinary acidification enhances renal excretion; urinary alkalinization enhances renal reabsorption and recycling.

No significant interactions.

Special considerations:
- Contraindicated for patients with grand mal epilepsy.
- In long-term use, child should be monitored closely for signs of growth suppression.
- Beneficial effects may not appear until after several weeks of therapy.
- Used with some success in treatment of tardive dyskinesia.

NAMES, INDICATIONS AND DOSAGES	SIDE EFFECTS
dextroamphetamine phosphate **dextroamphetamine sulfate** Controlled Substance Schedule II Dexampex, Dexedrine♦, Ferndex, Robese, Spancap #1 and #4, Tidex **Narcolepsy:** ADULTS: 5 to 60 mg P.O. daily in divided doses. CHILDREN OVER 12 YEARS: 10 mg P.O. daily, with 10-mg increments weekly, p.r.n. CHILDREN 6 TO 12 YEARS: 5 mg P.O. daily, with 5-mg increments weekly, p.r.n. **Short-term adjunct in exogenous obesity:** ADULTS: single 10- to 15-mg long-acting capsule, up to 30 mg daily; or in divided doses, 5 to 10 mg ½ hour before meals. **Minimal brain dysfunction:** CHILDREN 6 YEARS AND OVER: 5 mg once daily or b.i.d., with 5-mg increments weekly, p.r.n. CHILDREN 3 TO 5 YEARS: 2.5 mg P.O. daily, with 2.5-mg increments weekly, p.r.n.	**CNS:** *restlessness*, tremor, *hyperactivity, talkativeness, insomnia*, irritability, dizziness, headache, chills, overstimulation, dysphoria. **CV:** *tachycardia, palpitations*, hypertension, hypotension. **GI:** nausea, vomiting, cramps, dry mouth, diarrhea, constipation, metallic taste, anorexia, weight loss. **Skin:** urticaria. **Other:** impotence, changes in libido.
diethylpropion hydrochloride Controlled Substance Schedule IV Dietec♦♦, D.I.P.♦♦, Nobesine♦♦, Nu-Dispoz, Regibon♦♦, Ro-Diet, Tenuate♦, Tepanil **Short-term adjunct in exogenous obesity:** ADULTS: 25 mg P.O. before meals, t.i.d.; or 75 mg controlled-release tablet P.O. in midmorning.	**CNS:** headache, *nervousness*, dizziness. **CV:** *tachycardia, palpitations*, rise in blood pressure. **EENT:** blurred vision. **GI:** nausea, abdominal cramps, dry mouth, diarrhea, constipation. **Skin:** urticaria. **Other:** impotence, libido changes, menstrual upset.
fenfluramine hydrochloride Controlled Substance Schedule IV Pondimin♦ **Short-term adjunct in exogenous obesity:** ADULTS: initially, 20 mg P.O. t.i.d. before meals. Maximum 40 mg t.i.d. Adjust dosage according to patient's response.	**CNS:** dizziness, incoordination, headache, euphoria or depression, anxiety, *insomnia*, weakness or fatigue, agitation. **CV:** *palpitations*, hypotension, hypertension, chest pain. **EENT:** eye irritation, blurred vision. **GI:** diarrhea, dry mouth, nausea, vomiting, abdominal pain, constipation. **GU:** dysuria, increased urinary frequency, impotence, increased libido. **Skin:** rashes, urticaria, burning sensation. **Other:** sweating, chills, fever.

♦ Available in U.S. and Canada. ♦♦ Available in Canada only.
All other products (no symbol) available in U.S. only. Italicized side effects are common or life-threatening.

INTERACTIONS AND SPECIAL CONSIDERATIONS

Interactions:
MAO INHIBITORS: severe hypertension; possible hypertensive crisis. Don't use together.
SODIUM BICARBONATE, ACETAZOLAMIDE: increased renal reabsorption. Monitor for enhanced amphetamine effects.
AMMONIUM CHLORIDE, ASCORBIC ACID: observe for decreased amphetamine effects.
PHENOTHIAZINES, HALOPERIDOL: observe for decreased amphetamine effects.

Special considerations:
- Contraindicated in patients with hyperthyroidism, nephritis, severe hypertension, angina pectoris or other severe cardiovascular disease, some types of glaucoma, or history of drug abuse. Use with caution in patients with diabetes mellitus and in elderly, debilitated, or hyperexcitable patients.
- Psychic dependence or habituation may occur, especially in patients with history of drug addiction. Prolonged use should be avoided. When used long-term, lower dosage gradually to prevent acute rebound depression.
- When used for obesity, patient should also follow a weight-reduction program. Should be taken 30 to 60 minutes before meals. Should not be taken within 6 hours of bedtime.
- Fatigue may result as drug effects wear off. Patient will need more rest.
- Patient should avoid caffeinic drinks, which increase the effects of amphetamines and related amines.
- Vital signs should be checked regularly and patient observed for signs of excessive stimulation.
- Urinary acidification enhances renal excretion; urinary alkalinization enhances renal reabsorption and recycling.
- When tolerance to anorexigenic effect develops, dosage should not be increased but drug discontinued.
- Use to combat fatigue should be discouraged.
- Patient should avoid activities that require alertness or good psychomotor coordination until CNS response to drug is determined.
- May alter daily insulin needs in patients with diabetes. Blood and urine sugars should be monitored.
- Use as analeptic is usually discouraged, since CNS stimulation superimposed on CNS depression can lead to neuronal instability and seizures.

Interactions:
MAO INHIBITORS: hypertension; possible hypertensive crisis. Don't use together.

Special considerations:
- Contraindicated in patients with hyperthyroidism, hypertension, angina pectoris, severe cardiovascular disease, glaucoma, or history of drug abuse. Use with caution in epilepsy, diabetes mellitus, or hyperexcitability states. May alter insulin requirements. Blood and urine sugars should be monitored.
- When tolerance to anorexigenic effect develops, dosage should not be increased but drug discontinued.
- Habituation or psychic dependence may occur.
- Patient should also follow a weight-reduction program.
- Can be used to stop nighttime eating. Rarely causes insomnia.
- Fatigue may result as drug effects wear off. Patient will need more rest.
- Patient should avoid caffeinic drinks, which increase the effects of amphetamines and related amines.
- Vital signs should be checked regularly and patient observed for signs of excessive stimulation.
- Urinary acidification enhances renal excretion; urinary alkalinization enhances renal reabsorption and recycling.
- Use as analeptic is usually discouraged, since CNS stimulation superimposed on CNS depression can lead to neuronal instability and seizures.

Interactions:
MAO INHIBITORS: severe hypertension; possible hypertensive crisis. Don't use together.

Special considerations:
- Contraindicated in glaucoma, hypersensitivity to sympathomimetic amines, symptomatic cardiovascular disease, alcoholism, or history of drug abuse. Use with caution in hypertension, history of mental depression, diabetes mellitus.
- Because of possible hypoglycemia, patients with diabetes may have altered insulin or sulfonylurea requirements. Blood and urine sugars should be monitored.
- Vital signs should be checked regularly and patient observed for signs of excessive sedation, depression, or excessive stimulation. Blood pressure should be closely monitored.
- Patient should follow a weight-reduction program.
- Tolerance or dependence may occur. Prolonged administration should be avoided.
- Fatigue may result as drug effects wear off. Patient will need more rest.
- Patient should avoid caffeinic drinks, which increase the effects of amphetamines and related amines.

NAMES, INDICATIONS AND DOSAGES	SIDE EFFECTS
mazindol Controlled Substance Schedule IV Sanorex♦ **Short-term adjunct in exogenous obesity:** ADULTS: 1 mg t.i.d. 1 hour before meals, or 2 mg daily 1 hour before lunch. Use lowest effective dose.	**CNS:** *nervousness,* restlessness, dizziness, *insomnia,* dysphoria, headache, depression, drowsiness, weakness, tremors. **CV:** *palpitations, tachycardia.* **GI:** dry mouth, nausea, constipation, diarrhea, unpleasant taste. **GU:** difficulty initiating micturition, impotence, libido changes. **Skin:** rash, clamminess, pallor. **Other:** shivering, excessive sweating.
methamphetamine hydrochloride Controlled Substance Schedule II Desoxyn, Methampex **Minimal brain dysfunction:** CHILDREN 6 YEARS AND OVER: 2.5 to 5 mg P.O. once daily or b.i.d., with 5-mg increments weekly, p.r.n. Usual effective dosage is 20 to 25 mg daily. **Short-term adjunct in exogenous obesity:** ADULTS: 2.5 to 5 mg P.O. once to t.i.d. 30 minutes before meals; or 1 long-acting 5- to 15-mg tablet daily before breakfast.	**CNS:** *nervousness, insomnia,* irritability, *talkativeness,* dizziness, headache, hyperexcitability, tremor. **CV:** hypertension or hypotension, *tachycardia, palpitations,* cardiac arrhythmias. **EENT:** blurred vision, mydriasis. **GI:** nausea, vomiting, abdominal cramps, diarrhea or constipation, dry mouth, anorexia, metallic taste. **Skin:** urticaria. **Other:** impotence, libido changes.
methylphenidate hydrochloride Controlled Substance Schedule II Methidate♦♦, Ritalin♦ **Minimal brain dysfunction (hyperkinetic behavior disorders):** CHILDREN 6 YEARS AND OVER: initial dose 5 to 10 mg P.O. daily before breakfast and lunch, with 5- to 10-mg increments weekly as needed, up to 60 mg daily. **Narcolepsy:** ADULTS: 10 mg P.O. b.i.d. or t.i.d. ½ hour before meals. Dosage varies with patient needs. Dosage range is 5 to 50 mg daily.	**CNS:** *nervousness, insomnia,* dizziness, headache, akathisia, dyskinesia. **CV:** *palpitations,* angina, *tachycardia,* changes in blood pressure and pulse rate. **EENT:** difficulty with accommodation and blurring of vision. **GI:** nausea, dry throat, abdominal pain, anorexia, weight loss. **Skin:** rash, urticaria, *exfoliative dermatitis,* erythema multiforme.

♦ Available in U.S. and Canada. ♦♦ Available in Canada only.
All other products (no symbol) available in U.S. only. Italicized side effects are common or life-threatening.

INTERACTIONS AND SPECIAL CONSIDERATIONS

Interactions:
MAO INHIBITORS: severe hypertension; possible hypertensive crisis. Don't use together.

Special considerations:
• Contraindicated in patients with glaucoma, cardiovascular disease including arrhythmias, agitated states, history of drug abuse. Use with caution in diabetes mellitus, hypertension, hyperexcitability states.
• Patient should avoid activities that require alertness or good psychomotor coordination until CNS response has been determined.
• Fatigue may result as drug effects wear off. Patient will need more rest.
• Patient should avoid caffeinic drinks, which increase the effects of amphetamines and related amines.
• Check vital signs regularly. Observe for signs of excessive stimulation.
• Tolerance or dependence may develop. Prolonged use should be avoided.
• Patient should also follow a weight-reduction program.
• May alter insulin needs in patients with diabetes. Blood and urine sugars should be monitored.

Interactions:
MAO INHIBITORS: severe hypertension; possible hypertensive crisis. Don't use together.
SODIUM BICARBONATE, ACETAZOLAMIDE: increased renal reabsorption. Monitor for enhanced effects.
AMMONIUM CHLORIDE, ASCORBIC ACID: observe for decreased amphetamine effects.
PHENOTHIAZINES, HALOPERIDOL: observe for decreased amphetamine effects.

Special considerations:
• Contraindicated in patients with hypertension, hyperthyroidism, nephritis, angina pectoris or other severe cardiovascular disease, glaucoma, parkinsonism due to arteriosclerosis, agitated states, or history of drug abuse. Use with caution in patients with diabetes mellitus and in patients who are elderly, debilitated, asthenic, psychopathic, or who have a history of suicidal or homicidal tendencies.
• High potential for abuse. Use to combat fatigue should be discouraged.
• May alter insulin needs in patients with diabetes. Blood and urine sugars should be monitored.
• When used for obesity, patient should be on a weight-reduction program.
• Patient should avoid caffeinic drinks, which increase the effects of amphetamines and related amines.
• Vital signs should be checked regularly and patient observed for signs of excessive stimulation.
• Urinary acidification enhances renal excretion; urinary alkalinization enhances renal reabsorption and recycling.
• When tolerance to anorexigenic effect develops, dosage should not be increased but drug discontinued.
• Patient should avoid activities that require alertness or good psychomotor coordination until CNS response to drug is determined.

Interactions:
MAO INHIBITORS: severe hypertension; possible hypertensive crisis. Don't use together.

Special considerations:
• Contraindicated in patients with symptomatic cardiac disease; hyperthyroidism; moderate-to-severe hypertension; angina pectoris; advanced arteriosclerosis; severe depression of either endogenous or exogenous forms; glaucoma; parkinsonism; history of drug abuse or dependency; history of marked anxiety, tension, or agitation. Use with caution in elderly, debilitated, or hyperexcitable patients and in those with history of cardiovascular disease, diabetes, or seizures.
• Blood pressure should be closely monitored and patient observed for signs of excessive stimulation.
• Use to combat fatigue should be discouraged.
• Patient should be observed for interactions, as treatment of other disease states may be affected. May alter daily insulin needs in patients with diabetes. Blood and urine sugars should be monitored. May decrease seizure threshold in patients with seizure disorders.
• Drug of choice for minimal brain dysfunction. Usually stopped postpuberty.
• Used in treatment for nocturnal enuresis in children.
• Periodic CBC, differential, and platelet counts advised with long-term use.
• Tolerance, psychic dependence, or habituation may occur, especially in patients with history of drug addiction. High abuse potential. Prolonged administration should be avoided. When used long-term, dosage should be lowered gradually to prevent acute rebound depression.
• Fatigue may result as drug effects wear off. Patient will need more rest.
• Patient should avoid caffeinic drinks, which increase the effects of amphetamines and related amines.
• Patient should avoid activities that require alertness or good psychomotor coordination until CNS response to drug is determined.

NAMES, INDICATIONS AND DOSAGES	SIDE EFFECTS
pemoline Controlled Substance Schedule IV Cylert **Minimal brain dysfunction:** CHILDREN 6 YEARS AND OVER: initially, 37.5 mg P.O. given in the morning. Daily dose can be raised by 18.75 mg weekly. Effective dosage range 56.25 to 75 mg daily; maximum is 112.5 mg daily.	**CNS:** *insomnia,* malaise, irritability, fatigue, mild depression, dizziness, headache, drowsiness, hallucinations, nervousness (large doses), seizures. **CV:** tachycardia (large doses). **GI:** anorexia, abdominal pain, nausea, diarrhea. **Hepatic:** liver enzyme elevations. **Skin:** rash.
phendimetrazine tartrate Controlled Substance Schedule IV Anorex, Bacarate, Bontril PDM, Delcozine, Di-Ap-Trol, Ex-Obese, Limit, Metra, Obalan, Obepar, Obeval, Obezine, Phenazine♦, Phenzine, Plegine, Sprx 1,2,3, Sprx-105, Statobex, Trimstat, Trimtabs **Short-term adjunct in exogenous obesity:** ADULTS: 35 mg P.O. 2 to 3 times daily 1 hour before meals. Maximum dosage is 70 mg t.i.d. Use lowest effective dosage. Adjust dose to individual response.	**CNS:** *nervousness,* dizziness, *insomnia,* tremor, headache. **CV:** *tachycardia, palpitations,* rise in blood pressure. **EENT:** blurred vision. **GI:** dry mouth, nausea, abdominal cramps, diarrhea or constipation. **GU:** dysuria.
phenmetrazine hydrochloride Controlled Substance Schedule II Preludin **Short-term adjunct in exogenous obesity:** ADULTS: 25 mg P.O. b.i.d. or t.i.d. 1 hour before meals, up to 75 mg daily; or single 50- to 75-mg extended-release tablet daily in midmorning.	**CNS:** *nervousness,* dizziness, *insomnia,* headache. **CV:** *tachycardia, palpitations,* increased blood pressure. **EENT:** blurred vision. **GI:** dry mouth, nausea, abdominal cramps, constipation. **Skin:** urticaria. **Other:** libido changes, impotence.
phentermine hydrochloride Controlled Substance Schedule IV Adipex, Anoxine, Fastin, Ionamin♦, Parmine, Phentrol, Rolaphent, Wilpowr **Short-term adjunct in exogenous obesity:** ADULTS: 8 mg P.O. t.i.d. ½ hour before meals; or 15 to 30 mg daily before breakfast (resin complex).	**CNS:** *nervousness,* dizziness, *insomnia.* **CV:** *palpitations, tachycardia,* increased blood pressure. **GI:** dry mouth, unpleasant taste, nausea, constipation, diarrhea. **Skin:** urticaria. **Other:** libido changes, impotence.

INTERACTIONS AND SPECIAL CONSIDERATIONS

No significant interactions.

Special considerations:

• Use with caution in patients with impaired renal function. Drug may accumulate.
• Safety and efficacy for more than 2 years of administration has not been established. Patients on long-term therapy should be closely monitored for possible hepatic function abnormalities and for growth suppression.
• Structurally dissimilar to amphetamines or methylphenidate.
• Therapeutic effects may not be evident for 2 to 3 weeks.

Interactions:

MAO INHIBITORS: severe hypertension; possible hypertensive crisis. Don't use together.
SODIUM BICARBONATE, ACETAZOLAMIDE: increased renal reabsorption. Monitor for enhanced effects.
AMMONIUM CHLORIDE, ASCORBIC ACID: observe for decreased phendimetrazine effects.
PHENOTHIAZINES, HALOPERIDOL: observe for decreased effect.

Special considerations:

• Contraindicated in hyperthyroidism, hypertension, angina pectoris or other severe cardiovascular disease, glaucoma. Use with caution in hyperexcitability states or in patients with history of addiction.
• Patient should avoid activities that require alertness or good psychomotor coordination until CNS response to drug has been determined.
• Encourage weight-reduction program.
• Tolerance or dependence can develop. Not advised for prolonged use.
• Fatigue may result as drug effects wear off.
• Patient should avoid caffeinic drinks, which increase the effects of amphetamines and related amines.
• Check vital signs regularly and observe patient for signs of excessive stimulation.
• Urinary acidification enhances renal excretion; urinary alkalinization enhances renal reabsorption and recycling.
• May alter daily insulin needs in patients with diabetes. Blood and urine sugars should be monitored.

Interactions:

MAO INHIBITORS: severe hypertension; possible hypertensive crisis. Don't use together.
SODIUM BICARBONATE, ACETAZOLAMIDE: increased renal reabsorption. Monitor for enhanced effects.
AMMONIUM CHLORIDE, ASCORBIC ACID: observe for decreased phenmetrazine effects.
PHENOTHIAZINES, HALOPERIDOL: observe for decreased effect.

Special considerations:

• Contraindicated in patients with hyperthyroidism, hypertension, angina pectoris or other cardiovascular disease, glaucoma, or history of drug abuse. Use with caution in hyperexcitability states.
• Tolerance or dependence may develop. High abuse potential. Not advised for prolonged use.
• Encourage weight-reduction program.
• Fatigue may result as drug effects wear off.
• Avoid caffeinic drinks, which increase the effects of amphetamine and related amines.
• Check vital signs regularly and observe patient for signs of excessive stimulation.
• Urinary acidification enhances renal excretion; urinary alkalinization enhances renal reabsorption and recycling.

Interactions:

MAO INHIBITORS: severe hypertension; possible hypertensive crisis. Don't use together.
SODIUM BICARBONATE, ACETAZOLAMIDE: increased renal reabsorption. Monitor for enhanced effects.
AMMONIUM CHLORIDE, ASCORBIC ACID: observe for decreased phentermine effects.
PHENOTHIAZINES, HALOPERIDOL: observe for decreased effect.

Special considerations:

• Contraindicated in hyperthyroidism, hypertension, angina pectoris or other severe cardiovascular disease, glaucoma. Use with caution in hyperexcitability states or in patients with history of drug addiction.
• Tolerance or dependence may develop. Prolonged administration should be avoided.
• Should be used with weight-reduction program and taken 30 minutes before meals.
• Fatigue may result as drug effects wear off.
• Patient should avoid caffeinic drinks, which increase the effects of amphetamine and related amines.
• Check vital signs regularly and observe patient for signs of excessive stimulation.
• Urinary acidification enhances renal excretion; urinary alkalinization enhances renal reabsorption and recycling.

35

Respiratory stimulants

ammonia, aromatic spirits
doxapram hydrochloride
nikethamide
pentylenetetrazol

Respiratory stimulants, or analeptics, have limited usefulness in treating respiratory depression in patients with postanesthetic apnea caused by drugs other than muscle relaxants.

Doxapram is the most common respiratory stimulant. Aromatic spirits of ammonia are essentially smelling salts and are still commonly used. Pentylenetetrazol and nikethamide are seldom used today.

All these drugs except ammonia are dangerous because they're epileptogenic, or able to precipitate seizures.

Major uses

The respiratory stimulants combat effects of central nervous system depressants.

- Ammonia stimulates respiration through peripheral irritation. It is also sometimes used as an antacid and a carminative.
- Pentylenetetrazol enhances physical and mental activity in elderly patients.

Mechanism of action

Respiratory stimulants act either directly on the central respiratory centers in the medulla or indirectly on the chemoreceptors.

- Ammonia causes irritation of the sensory receptors in the nasal membranes, producing reflex stimulation of the respiratory centers.

Absorption, distribution, metabolism, and excretion

Generally, respiratory stimulants are quickly absorbed after oral (pentylenetetrazol) or I.V. administration and well distributed to the body tissues.

- Doxapram is rapidly metabolized in the liver and eliminated in both urine and feces.
- Nikethamide is partly metabolized in the liver to niacinamide, which is excreted in the urine as N-methylniacinamide.
- Pentylenetetrazol is metabolized in the liver to at least five inactive metabolites, which are largely excreted in the urine.

Onset and duration

Onset of respiratory stimulants is quick, usually within 1 to 2 minutes; duration of

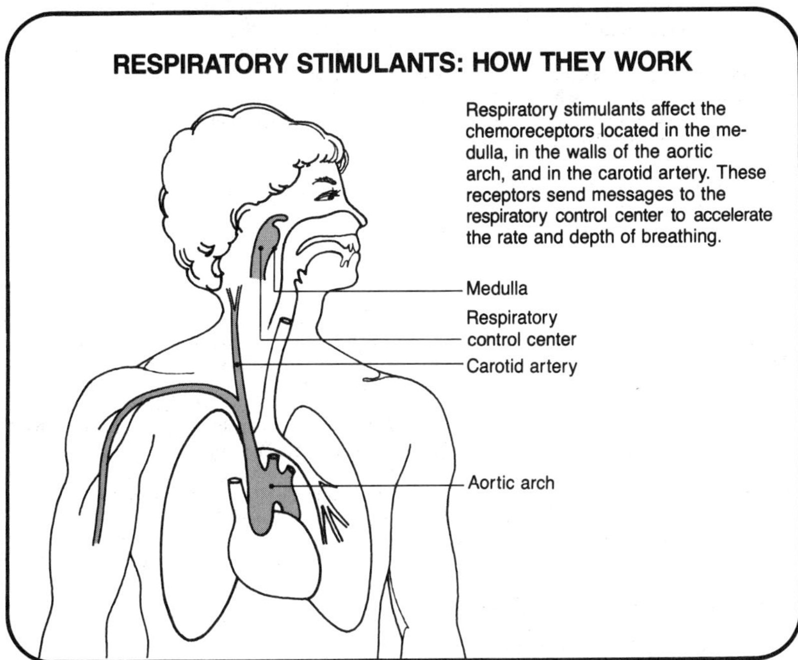

respiratory stimulants varies (usually 2 to 15 minutes).

RESPIRATORY STIMULANTS: HOW THEY WORK
Respiratory stimulants affect the chemoreceptors located in the medulla, in the walls of the aortic arch, and in the carotid artery. These receptors send messages to the respiratory control center to accelerate the rate and depth of breathing.
Medulla
Respiratory control center
Carotid artery
Aortic arch

- Pentylenetetrazol (the only orally administered drug in this group) has an onset of 1 to 2 hours and a duration of 4 to 6 hours.

Combination products

GERONIAZOL: pentylenetetrazol 200 mg and niacin 100 mg.
NICO-METRAZOL: pentylenetetrazol 100 mg and niacin 50 mg.

NAMES, INDICATIONS AND DOSAGES	SIDE EFFECTS
ammonia, aromatic spirits **Fainting:** ADULTS AND CHILDREN: inhale as needed.	None reported.
doxapram hydrochloride Dopram♦ **Postanesthesia respiratory stimulant, drug-induced central nervous system depression, and chronic pulmonary disease associated with acute hypercapnia:** ADULTS: 0.5 to 1 mg/kg of body weight (up to 2 mg/kg in CNS depression), I.V. injection or infusion. Maximum 4 mg/kg, up to 3 g in 1 day. Infusion rate 1 to 3 mg/minute (initial: 5 mg/minute for postanesthesia). **Chronic obstructive pulmonary disease:** ADULTS: infusion, 1 to 2 mg/minute. Maximum 3 mg/minute for a maximum duration of 2 hours.	**CNS:** seizures, headache, dizziness, apprehension, disorientation, pupillary dilation, bilateral Babinski's signs, flushing, sweating, paresthesias. **CV:** chest pain and tightness, variations in heart rate, hypertension, lowered T waves. **GI:** nausea, vomiting, diarrhea. **GU:** urinary retention, or stimulation of the bladder with incontinence. **Other:** sneezing, coughing, laryngospasm, bronchospasm, hiccups, rebound hypoventilation, pruritus.
nikethamide Coramine♦, Kardonyl♦♦ **Acute alcoholism:** ADULTS: 1.25 to 5 g I.V.; repeat as necessary. **Carbon monoxide poisoning:** ADULTS: 1.25 to 2.5 g I.V. initially, then 1.25 g q 5 minutes for first hour, depending on response. **Cardiac arrest associated with anesthetic overdose:** ADULTS: 125 to 250 mg intracardially. **Combat respiratory paralysis:** ADULTS: 3.75 g I.V.; repeat as required. **Overcome respiratory depression:** ADULTS: 1.25 to 2.5 g I.V. **Shock:** ADULTS: 2.5 to 3.75 g I.V. or I.M. initially; repeat as indicated. **Shorten narcosis:** ADULTS: 1 g I.V. or I.M. **Adjunct in neonatal asphyxia:** NEONATES: 375 mg injected into umbilical vein. **Oral maintenance:** ADULTS AND CHILDREN: 3 to 5 ml oral solution q 4 to 6 hours.	**CNS:** seizure, restlessness, muscle twitching or fasciculations, fear. **CV:** increased heart rate and blood pressure. **EENT:** unpleasant burning or itching at back of nose, sneezing, coughing. **GI:** nausea, vomiting. **Other:** increased respiratory rate, flushing, feeling of warmth, sweating.

INTERACTIONS AND SPECIAL CONSIDERATIONS

No significant interactions.

Special considerations:
- Stimulates mucous membranes of upper respiratory tract.

Interactions:
MAO INHIBITORS: potentiate adverse cardiovascular effects. Use together cautiously.

Special considerations:
- Contraindicated in convulsive disorders; head injury; cardiovascular disorders; frank uncompensated heart failure; severe hypertension; cerebrovascular accidents; respiratory failure or incompetence secondary to neuromuscular disorders, muscle paresis, flail chest, obstructed airway, pulmonary embolism, pneumothorax, restrictive respiratory disease, acute bronchial asthma, extreme dyspnea; hypoxia not associated with hypercapnia. Use with caution in bronchial asthma, severe tachycardia or cardiac arrhythmias, cerebral edema or increased cerebrospinal fluid pressure, hyperthyroidism, pheochromocytoma, or profound metabolic disorders.
- Adequate airway should be established before drug is administered, and patient should be prevented from aspirating vomitus.
- Blood pressure, heart rate, deep tendon reflexes, and arterial blood gases should be monitored before drug is given and every 30 minutes afterward.
- Signs of overdosage: hypertension, tachycardia, arrhythmias, skeletal muscle hyperactivity, dyspnea. Should be discontinued if patient shows signs of increased arterial carbon dioxide or oxygen tension, or if mechanical ventilation is started. I.V. injection of anticonvulsant may be given for convulsions.
- Should be used only in surgical or emergency room situations such as thiopental sodium; doxapran is acidic.
- Should not be combined with alkaline solutions such as thiopental sodium; doxapram is acidic.

No significant interactions.

Special considerations:
- Patient's respiratory rate and volume should be monitored.
- Mechanical support of breathing is often preferred over nikethamide.
- Should not be injected intra-arterially; arterial spasm and thrombosis may result.
- Signs of overdosage: muscle tremors or spasm, retching, tachycardia, arrhythmias, hyperpnea, hyperpyrexia, convulsions, psychotic reactions, postictal depression. I.V. injection of diazepam or barbiturate such as thiopental sodium may be given for convulsions. Induced emesis and gastric lavage aren't effective.

NAMES, INDICATIONS AND DOSAGES	SIDE EFFECTS
pentylenetetrazol Metrazol, Nelex-100, Nioric, Petrazole **Overdose of CNS depressants:** ADULTS: 100 to 500 mg I.V. Repeat, if necessary, followed by 100 to 200 mg I.M., p.r.n. **In depression from barbiturates:** 5 ml of 10% solution I.V. within 3 to 5 seconds. If necessary, may be repeated until patient awakens. **To improve mental and physical activity in elderly patients:** ADULTS: 100 to 200 mg P.O. t.i.d.	Few side effects with oral administration; narrow margin of safety with parenteral administration. *Signs of overdose:* **CNS:** fasciculations, clonic convulsions. **CV:** slight increases in blood pressure, bradycardia. **GI:** nausea, vomiting. **Other:** hypersalivation, coughing, hyperthermia.

♦ Available in U.S. and Canada. ♦♦ Available in Canada only.
All other products (no symbol) available in U.S. only. Italicized side effects are common or life-threatening.

INTERACTIONS AND SPECIAL CONSIDERATIONS

No significant interactions.

Special considerations:

- Should be used with caution in patients with history of seizures or focal brain lesion. If dosage is high, use with caution in patients with cardiac disease.
- Analeptic use is not recommended.
- False-positive response to hCG pregnancy test.

CLEARING A PATIENT'S AIRWAY

When an unconscious patient lies in supine position, his relaxed muscles allow his lower jaw to drop backward and permit the back of his tongue to block his airway (illustration 1). To relieve this obstruction easily and quickly, use the head-tilt maneuver (illustration 2). This raises the tongue from the back of the throat and, in some cases, may be enough to start the patient breathing.

If tilting the patient's head doesn't open his airway, try the jaw thrust. Place your fingers behind the angles of the patient's jaw and push forward. Exert enough pressure to maintain the head tilt.

Caution: If you suspect a neck injury, don't use the head-tilt maneuver. Try opening the airway with a modified jaw thrust. Push the jaw forward, but don't hyperextend the neck or move the head to either side.

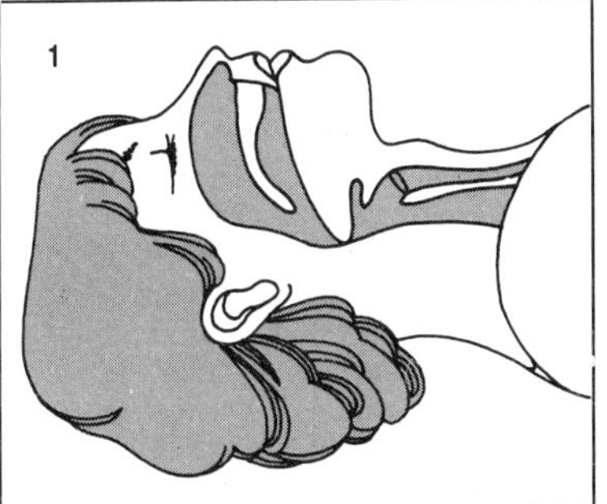

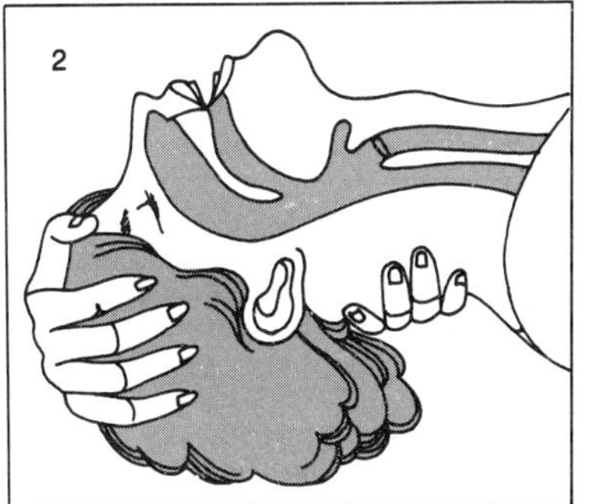

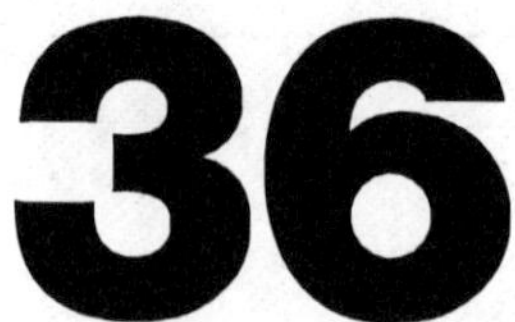

Cholinergics (parasympathomimetics)

ambenonium chloride
bethanechol chloride
edrophonium chloride
neostigmine bromide
neostigmine methylsulfate
physostigmine salicylate
pyridostigmine bromide

Cholinergics mimic the action of acetylcholine in that they produce parasympathetic responses. They are not organ-specific. When bethanechol, for example, is administered to treat postoperative urinary retention, it is distributed through the body, and other organs innervated by the parasympathetic system are activated. Thus, these drugs can produce a therapeutic effect at one location (such as preventing urinary retention in the bladder) and annoying side effects at another (such as causing excess production of saliva by the salivary glands).

The parasympathetic division of the autonomic nervous system innervates various body organs and systems and acts on the heart, gastrointestinal (GI) tract, urinary bladder, and respiratory tract. The parasympathetic division works in concert with its sympathetic counterpart to provide continuous control of those functions which occur without conscious thought (for example, digestion, respiration, and maintenance of blood pressure).

When stimulated, parasympathetic nerves release acetylcholine from their nerve endings. This chemical binds to specific sites (muscarinic receptors) in the tissue innervated by the parasympathetic nerve. This interaction starts the mechanisms that result in a typical parasympathetic response.

Nerves that innervate skeletal muscle also release acetylcholine when stimulated. The released acetylcholine binds to specific sites in skeletal muscle, triggering contraction. Disordered release of acetylcholine from these nerves or impaired binding with skeletal muscle leads to profound muscle weakness (myasthenia gravis). Drugs that promote the accumulation of acetylcholine at skeletal muscle sites (for example, neostigmine) improve muscular performance in patients with this disease.

Major uses

- Ambenonium, neostigmine, and pyridostigmine are used to treat symptoms of myasthenia gravis.
- Bethanechol is used to prevent and treat postoperative urinary retention, postoperative gastric atony and retention, abdominal distention, and megacolon.
- Edrophonium aids differential diagnosis of myasthenia gravis.
- Neostigmine is used to prevent and treat postoperative urinary retention.
- Neostigmine and pyridostigmine reverse the effect of neuromuscular blocking agents used in surgery.

• Physostigmine is an antidote in anticholinergic poisoning, particularly poisoning caused by tricyclic antidepressants.

Mechanism of action
• Ambenonium, edrophonium, neostigmine, physostigmine, and pyridostigmine inhibit the destruction of acetylcholine released from the parasympathetic nerves. Acetylcholine accumulates, promoting increased stimulation of the receptor.
• Bethanechol and neostigmine directly bind to muscarinic receptors, mimicking the action of acetylcholine.

Absorption, distribution, metabolism, and excretion
All cholinergics except physostigmine are poorly absorbed orally. They are widely distributed to organs innervated by the parasympathetic nervous system, metabolized by the liver, and excreted by the kidneys as water-soluble metabolites.
• Physostigmine is the only cholinergic drug that effectively crosses the blood-brain barrier, which makes physostigmine useful for tricyclic antidepressant and anticholinergic poisoning.

Onset and duration
• Ambenonium's onset and duration are variable. The drug's effects on skeletal muscle usually lasts 4 to 8 hours.
• Bethanechol has an onset between 60 and 90 minutes (occasionally as soon as 30 minutes) after oral administration. Therapeutic effects persist for about 1 hour. After subcutaneous injection, onset occurs within 5 to 15 minutes, and action peaks in 15 to 30 minutes. Therapeutic effects wane thereafter and disappear after 2 hours.
• Edrophonium's onset, after I.V. infusion, occurs within 30 to 60 seconds; therapeutic activity lasts 5 to 10 minutes. When the drug is given I.M., onset occurs in 2 to 10 minutes, and its duration of action is 5 to 30 minutes.
• Neostigmine has an onset of action on the GI tract 2 to 4 hours after oral administration, 10 to 30 minutes after I.M. injection. Duration of action on skeletal muscle, after I.M. injection, is 2½ to 4 hours.
• Physostigmine's onset occurs in 3 to 8 minutes after parenteral administration; its duration of action is 30 minutes to 5 hours.
• Pyridostigmine's action on skeletal muscle begins within 30 to 45 minutes when the drug is given orally. Its action persists 3 to 6 hours. After I.M. injection, onset occurs within 15 minutes. After I.V. infusion, onset occurs in 2 to 5 minutes; its duration of action is 2 to 3 hours.

NAMES, INDICATIONS AND DOSAGES	SIDE EFFECTS

ambenonium chloride
Mytelase♦

Symptomatic treatment of myasthenia gravis in patients who cannot take neostigmine bromide and pyridostigmine bromide:
ADULTS: dose must be individualized for each patient, but usually ranges from 5 to 25 mg P.O. q 3 to 4 hours while awake. Starting dose usually 5 mg P.O. q 3 to 4 hours. Increase gradually and adjust at 1- to 2-day intervals to avoid drug accumulation and overdosage. May range from 5 mg to as much as 75 mg/dose.

CNS: headache, dizziness, muscle weakness, convulsions, mental confusion, jitters, sweating, respiratory depression.
CV: bradycardia, hypotension.
EENT: miosis.
GI: *nausea, vomiting, diarrhea, abdominal cramps,* increased salivation.
GU: urinary frequency, incontinence.
Other: bronchospasm, *muscle cramps,* bronchoconstriction.

bethanechol chloride
Duvoid, Mictrol-10, Mictrol-25, Myotonachol, Urecholine♦, Vesicholine

Acute postoperative and postpartum nonobstructive (functional) urinary retention, neurogenic atony of urinary bladder with retention, abdominal distention, megacolon:
ADULTS: 10 to 30 mg P.O. t.i.d. to q.i.d. Never give I.M. or I.V. When used for urinary retention, some patients may require 50 to 100 mg P.O. per dose. Use such doses with extreme caution.
Test dose: 2.5 mg S.C. repeated at 15- to 30-minute intervals to total of 4 doses to determine the minimal effective dose; then use minimal effective dose q 6 to 8 hours. All doses must be adjusted individually.

Dose-related:
CNS: headache, malaise.
CV: bradycardia, hypotension, *cardiac arrest,* tachycardia.
EENT: lacrimation, miosis.
GI: *abdominal cramps, diarrhea,* salivation, nausea, vomiting, belching, borborygmus.
GU: urinary urgency.
Skin: flushing, sweating.
Other: bronchoconstriction.

INTERACTIONS AND SPECIAL CONSIDERATIONS

Interactions:
PROCAINAMIDE, QUINIDINE: may reverse cholinergic effect on muscle. Observe for lack of drug effect.

Special considerations:
• Contraindicated in patients with mechanical obstruction of intestine or urinary tract, bradycardia, hypotension.
• Use with extreme caution in patients with bronchial asthma.
• Use cautiously in patients with epilepsy, recent coronary occlusion, vagotonia, hyperthyroidism, cardiac arrhythmias, peptic ulcer.
• Large dose should be avoided in patients with decreased gastrointestinal motility or megacolon.
• All other cholinergics should be discontinued before this drug is given.
• Patient should be watched very closely for side effects, particularly if total dose is greater than 200 mg daily. Side effects may indicate drug toxicity and should be reported immediately.
• Vital signs should be monitored frequently, especially respirations. For possible respiratory distress: always have atropine injection readily available; be prepared to give atropine 0.5 mg subcutaneously or slow I.V. push; and provide respiratory support as needed.
• Each dose should be administered exactly as ordered, on time. Amount and frequency of dosage should vary with patient's activity level. Larger doses may be prescribed when patient is fatigued, for example, in the afternoon and at mealtime.
• If muscle weakness is severe, determination should be made if drug-induced toxicity or exacerbation of myasthenia gravis. A test dose of edrophonium I.V. will aggravate drug-induced weakness but will temporarily relieve weakness that results from the disease.
• Patient should know how to observe and record variations in muscle strength.
• When given for myasthenia gravis, this drug relieves symptoms of ptosis, double vision, difficulty in chewing and swallowing, trunk and limb weakness. This drug should be taken exactly as ordered. Patient should know the drug's effect on myasthenia gravis and know that he must take the drug for life.
• Intake and output should be monitored.
• Patient may develop resistance to drug.
• When indicated, hospitalized patient may have bedside supply of tablets to take himself. Patients with long-standing disease often insist on this.
• Drug taken with milk or food produces fewer muscarinic side effects.
• Patient should wear identification tag indicating he has myasthenia gravis.

Interactions:
PROCAINAMIDE, QUINIDINE: may reverse cholinergic effects on muscle. Observe for lack of drug effect.

Special considerations:
• Contraindicated in patients with uncertain strength or integrity of bladder wall; when increased muscular activity of GI or urinary tract is harmful; in mechanical obstructions of GI or urinary tract; in hyperthyroidism, peptic ulcer, latent or active bronchial asthma, cardiac or coronary artery disease, vagotonia, epilepsy, Parkinson's disease, bradycardia, chronic obstructive pulmonary disease, hypotension. Use cautiously in hypertension, vasomotor instability, peritonitis, or other acute inflammatory conditions of GI tract.
• Should *never* be given I.M. or I.V.; could cause circulatory collapse, hypotension, severe abdominal cramping, bloody diarrhea, shock, cardiac arrest.
• All other cholinergics should be stopped before this drug is given.
• Side effects may indicate drug toxicity, especially with subcutaneous administration.
• Vital signs should be monitored frequently, especially respirations. For possible respiratory distress: always have atropine injection readily available; be prepared to give atropine 0.5 mg subcutaneously or slow I.V. push; and provide respiratory support as needed.
• If used to treat urinary retention, bedpan should be handy, and intake and output monitored.
• When used to prevent abdominal distention and GI distress, a rectal tube inserted to help passage of gas may also be ordered.
• Poor and variable oral absorption requires larger oral doses. Oral and subcutaneous doses are *not* interchangeable.
• Drug usually effective 5 to 15 minutes after injection and 30 to 90 minutes after oral use.
• Should be taken on empty stomach; if taken after meals, may cause nausea and vomiting.
• For symptoms and treatment of toxicity, see APPENDIX.

NAMES, INDICATIONS AND DOSAGES

edrophonium chloride
Tensilon♦

As a curare antagonist (to reverse neuromuscular blocking action):
ADULTS: 10 mg I.V. given over 30 to 45 seconds. Dose may be repeated as necessary to 40 mg maximum dose. Larger doses may potentiate rather than antagonize effect of curare.

Diagnostic aid in myasthenia gravis (the Tensilon test):
ADULTS: 1 to 2 mg I.V. within 15 to 30 seconds, then 8 mg if no response (increase in muscular strength).
CHILDREN OVER 34 KG: 2 mg I.V. If no response within 45 seconds, give 1 mg q 45 seconds to maximum of 10 mg.
CHILDREN UP TO 34 KG: 1 mg I.V. If no response within 45 seconds, give 1 mg q 45 seconds to maximum of 5 mg.
INFANTS: 0.5 mg I.V.

To differentiate myasthenic crisis from cholinergic crisis:
ADULTS: 1 mg I.V. If no response in 1 minute, repeat dose once. Increased muscular strength confirms myasthenic crisis; no increase or exaggerated weakness confirms cholinergic crisis.

Paroxysmal supraventricular tachycardia:
ADULTS: 10 mg I.V. given over 1 minute or less.

SIDE EFFECTS

CNS: weakness, respiratory paralysis, sweating.
CV: hypotension, bradycardia.
EENT: miosis.
GI: nausea, vomiting, *diarrhea, abdominal cramps,* excessive salivation.
Other: increased bronchial secretions, bronchospasm, muscle cramps, muscle fasciculation.

---

neostigmine bromide
Prostigmin Bromide♦
neostigmine methylsulfate
Prostigmin♦

Antidote for tubocurarine:
ADULTS: 0.5 to 2 mg I.V. slowly. Repeat p.r.n. Give 0.6 to 1.2 mg atropine sulfate I.V. before antidote dose.

Functional amenorrhea: 1 mg I.M. or S.C. daily for 3 days.

Postoperative abdominal distention and bladder atony:
ADULTS: 0.5 to 1 mg I.M. or S.C. q 4 to 6 hours.

Postoperative ileus:
ADULTS: 0.25 to 1 mg I.M. or S.C. q 4 to 6 hours.

Treatment of myasthenia gravis:
ADULTS: 15 to 30 mg t.i.d. (range 15 to 375 mg/day); or 0.5 to 2 mg I.M. or I.V. q 1 to 3 hours. Dose must be individualized, depending on response and tolerance of side effects. Therapy may be required day and night.

CNS: dizziness, muscle weakness, mental confusion, jitters, sweating, respiratory depression.
CV: bradycardia, hypotension.
EENT: miosis.
GI: *nausea, vomiting, diarrhea, abdominal cramps,* excessive salivation.
Skin: rash (bromide).
Other: bronchospasm, *muscle cramps,* bronchoconstriction.

♦ Available in U.S. and Canada. ♦♦ Available in Canada only.
All other products (no symbol) available in U.S. only. Italicized side effects are common or life-threatening.

INTERACTIONS AND SPECIAL CONSIDERATIONS

Interactions:
PROCAINAMIDE, QUINIDINE: may reverse cholinergic effects on muscle. Observe for lack of drug effect.

Special considerations:
- Contraindicated in mechanical obstruction of intestine or urinary tract, bradycardia, hypotension. Use cautiously in hyperthyroidism, cardiac disease, peptic ulcer, bronchial asthma.
- All other cholingerics should be stopped before this drug is given.
- Side effects may indicate toxicity.
- Vital signs should be monitored frequently, especially respirations. For possible respiratory distress: always have atropine injection readily available; be prepared to give atropine 0.5 mg subcutaneously or slow I.V. push; and provide respiratory support as needed.
- When drug is given to differentiate myasthenic crisis from cholinergic crisis, patient's muscle strength should be observed closely.
- Edrophonium not effective against muscle relaxation induced by decamethonium bromide and succinylcholine chloride.
- This cholinergic has the most rapid onset but shortest duration; therefore not used for treatment of myasthenia gravis.
- For easier parenteral administration, a tuberculin syringe with an I.V. needle should be used.
- I.M. route may be used in children due to difficulty with the I.V. route: for children under 34 kg, inject 2 mg I.M.; children over 34 kg, 5 mg I.M. Same reactions expected as with I.V. test, but these appear after 2- to 10-minute delay.
- When used as antidote for curariform drugs, each dose given should be recorded.
- For symptoms and treatment of toxicity, see APPENDIX.

Interactions:
PROCAINAMIDE, QUINIDINE: may reverse cholinergic effect on muscle. Observe for lack of drug effect.

Special considerations:
- Contraindicated in hypersensitivity to cholinergics or to bromide, mechanical obstruction of the intestine or urinary tract, bradycardia, hypotension. Use with extreme caution in bronchial asthma. Use cautiously in epilepsy, recent coronary occlusion, peritonitis, vagotonia, hyperthyroidism, cardiac arrhythmias, or peptic ulcer.
- All other cholinergics should be stopped before this drug is given.
- Side effects may indicate toxicity.
- Vital signs should be monitored frequently, especially respirations. For possible respiratory distress: always have atropine injection readily available; be prepared to give atropine 0.5 mg subcutaneously or slow I.V. push; and provide respiratory support as needed.
- Patient's response after each dose helps determine optimum dose. Patient should know how to observe and record variations in muscle strength.
- For myasthenia gravis, this drug will relieve ptosis, double vision, difficulty in chewing and swallowing, and trunk and limb weakness. Patient should take drug exactly as ordered. Drug must be taken for life. The drug's effect on myasthenic symptoms should be explained.
- If patient has dysphagia, dose should be scheduled 30 minutes before each meal.
- When used to prevent abdominal distention and GI distress, a rectal tube inserted to help passage of gas may be ordered.
- Patients sometimes develop a resistance to neostigmine.
- When used for functional amenorrhea, vaginal bleeding should be checked for and patient should report any vaginal bleeding. If no bleeding in 72 hours after third injection, the patient has nonfunctional amenorrhea.
- If muscle weakness is severe, determination should be made if it is caused by drug-induced toxicity or exacerbation of myasthenia gravis. Test dose of edrophonium I.V. will aggravate drug-induced weakness but will temporarily relieve weakness caused by disease.
- Medical regimen of hospitalized patients with long-standing myasthenia who request bedside supply of tablets should be supervised.
- GI side effects may be reduced by taking drug with milk or food.
- Patient should wear an identification tag indicating that he has myasthenia gravis.

(continued on following page)

NAMES, INDICATIONS AND DOSAGES	SIDE EFFECTS

neostigmine
(continued)

CHILDREN: 7.5 to 15 mg P.O. t.i.d. to q.i.d.
Note: 1:1,000 solution of injectable solution contains 1 mg/1 ml; 1:2,000 solution contains 0.5 mg/ml.

---

physostigmine salicylate
Antilirium♦

Anticholinergic poisoning:
ADULTS: 0.5 to 4 mg P.O., I.M., or I.V. q 2 hours.

Tricyclic antidepressant poisoning:
ADULTS: 0.5 to 3 mg P.O., I.M., or I.V. (1 mg/minute I.V.) repeated as necessary if life-threatening signs recur (coma, convulsions, arrhythmias).

CNS: hallucinations, muscular twitching, muscle weakness, ataxia, *restlessness, excitability, sweating.*
CV: irregular pulse, palpitations.
EENT: miosis.
GI: nausea, vomiting, epigastric pain, *diarrhea, excessive salivation.*
Other: bronchospasm, bronchial constriction, dyspnea.

---

pyridostigmine bromide
Mestinon♦, Regonol♦

Curariform antagonist:
ADULTS: 10 to 30 mg I.V. preceded by atropine sulfate 0.6 to 1.2 mg I.V.

Myasthenia gravis:
ADULTS: 60 to 180 mg P.O. b.i.d. or q.i.d. Usual dose 600 mg daily but higher doses may be needed (up to 1,500 mg/day). Give 1/30 of oral dose I.M. or I.V. Dose must be adjusted for each patient, depending on response and tolerance of side effects.

CNS: headache (with high doses), weakness, sweating, convulsions.
CV: bradycardia, hypotension.
EENT: miosis.
GI: abdominal cramps, nausea, vomiting, diarrhea, excessive salivation.
Skin: rash.
Local: thrombophlebitis.
Other: bronchospasm, bronchoconstriction, increased bronchial secretions, muscle cramps.

♦ Available in U.S. and Canada. ♦♦ Available in Canada only.
All other products (no symbol) available in U.S. only. Italicized side effects are common or life-threatening.

INTERACTIONS AND SPECIAL CONSIDERATIONS

• For symptoms and treatment of toxicity, see APPENDIX.

Interactions:
PROCAINAMIDE, QUINIDINE: may reverse cholinergic effects on muscle. Observe for lack of drug effect.

Special considerations:
• Use cautiously in preexisting conditions: mechanical obstruction of intestine or urogenital tract, bronchial asthma, gangrene, diabetes, cardiovascular disease, vagotonia, bradycardia, hypotension, epilepsy, Parkinson's disease, hyperthyroidism, peptic ulcer.
• Side effects, particularly CNS disturbances, may indicate drug toxicity. Side rails should be used if patient becomes restless or hallucinates.
• Vital signs should be monitored frequently, especially respirations. For possible respiratory distress: always have atropine injection readily available; be prepared to give atropine 0.5 mg subcutaneously or slow I.V. push; and provide respiratory support as needed.
• Only clear solution should be used; darkening may indicate loss of potency.
• Should be given I.V. at controlled rate: use slow, direct injection at no more than 1 mg/minute.
• Only cholinergic that crosses blood/brain barrier; therefore the only one useful for treating CNS effects of anticholinergic or tricyclic antidepressant therapy.
• Effectiveness often immediate and dramatic but may be transient and may require repeat dose.
• For symptoms and treatment of toxicity, see APPENDIX.

Interactions:
PROCAINAMIDE, QUINIDINE: may reverse cholinergic effects on muscle. Observe for lack of drug effect.

Special considerations:
• Contraindicated in mechanical obstruction of intestine or urinary tract, bradycardia, hypotension. Use with extreme caution in bronchial asthma. Use cautiously in epilepsy, recent coronary occlusion, vagotonia, hyperthyroidism, cardiac arrhythmias, peptic ulcer. Large doses should be avoided in decreased GI motility or megacolon.
• Patient's response after each dose helps determine optimum dosage.
• All other cholinergics should be stopped before this drug is given.
• Side effects may indicate toxicity.
• Vital signs should be monitored frequently, especially respirations. For possible respiratory distress: always have atropine injection readily available; be prepared to give atropine 0.5 mg subcutaneously or slow I.V. push; and provide respiratory support as needed.
• If muscle weakness is severe, determination should be made if it is caused by drug-induced toxicity or exacerbation of myasthenia gravis. Test dose of edrophonium I.V. will aggravate drug-induced weakness but will temporarily relieve weakness caused by disease.
• For myasthenia gravis, drug should be taken exactly as ordered, on time, in evenly spaced doses. Patient must take extended-release tablets at the same time each day, at least 6 hours apart. Patient should know the drug's effect on myasthenia symptoms and know that he must take the drug for life.
• Has longest duration of the cholinergics used for myasthenia gravis.
• Available in 60-mg tablets, sustained-release (180 mg) tablets, injection, and syrup.
• For symptoms and treatment of toxicity, see APPENDIX.

37

Cholinergic blockers (parasympatholytics)

atropine sulfate
benztropine mesylate
biperiden hydrochloride
biperiden lactate
chlorphenoxamine hydrochloride
cycrimine hydrochloride
glycopyrrolate
procyclidine hydrochloride
scopolamine hydrobromide
trihexyphenidyl hydrochloride

Cholinergic blockers inhibit action of acetylcholine released by parasympathetic and some sympathetic nerves. Because parasympathetic nerves innervate many organs, parasympatholytic action can be widespread. Effects of parasympatholytics are typically opposite those of parasympathetic stimulation. Parasympathetic (vagal) stimulation of the heart decreases heart rate, but atropine, a parasympatholytic drug, increases heart rate.

Several of these drugs (for example, benztropine and trihexyphenidyl) can enter the brain, where they antagonize the actions of cerebral acetylcholine. The cholinergic blockers help to control the clinical effects of parkinsonism (a disease partly attributable to overactivity of certain cholinergic pathways in the brain) and dyskinesias associated with the use of major tranquilizers.

Parasympatholytic drugs are not organ-specific. The administration of atropine to reverse severe bradycardia, for example, can dry oral and respiratory secretions. Likewise, the use of benztropine for parkinsonism can produce urinary retention, especially in men with prostatic hypertrophy. (For cholinergic blockers used specifically for gastrointestinal disorders, see Chapter 49, GASTROINTESTINAL ANTICHOLINERGICS.)

Major uses

- Atropine may be used for poisoning due to organic phosphate insecticides and certain mushrooms.
- Atropine and scopolamine, as preanesthetic medications, are used to reduce salivary and respiratory secretions.
- Benztropine, biperiden, cycrimine, procyclidine, and trihexyphenidyl are used to treat parkinsonism and extrapyramidal reactions associated with the use of neuroleptics.

Mechanism of action

Cholinergic blockers inhibit the effect of acetylcholine—as the neurotransmitter for impulses in the parasympathetic nervous system—at the junction between postganglionic nerve endings and effector organs.

Absorption, distribution, metabolism, and excretion

Cholinergic blockers generally are well absorbed from GI tract, distributed to body organs innervated by parasympathetic nervous system, and excreted unchanged in urine.

- Atropine, benztropine, biperiden, scopolamine, and trihexyphenidyl are more likely to penetrate the central nervous system than the other cholinergic blockers.

Onset and duration

All cholinergic blockers take effect within 30 minutes when injected I.M. or subcuta-

WHAT CHOLINERGIC BLOCKERS DO

INNERVATED ORGAN	When body naturally releases neurohormone acetylcholine:	When cholinergic blockers are given:
Heart	▼	▲
Bronchioles	▲	▼
GI tract	▲	▼
Bladder	▲	▼
Bladder sphincter	▼	▲
Blood vessels	▼	▲
Sweat and salivary glands	▲	▼

KEY: ▼ = relaxes or dilates ▲ = constricts or stimulates

neously, and within 30 to 60 minutes when given orally.

The duration of these agents (except benztropine) is from 2 to 6 hours when given I.M. or subcutaneously, and from 4 to 6 hours when given orally. Effects of large doses can last as long as 24 hours.

• Benztropine's duration of action is 24 hours after I.M., subcutaneous, or oral administration.

Combination products

Cholinergic blocking agents are available in tablets and capsules, combined with varying amounts of sedatives.

NAMES, INDICATIONS AND DOSAGES	SIDE EFFECTS
atropine sulfate **Antidote for anticholinesterase insecticide poisoning:** ADULTS AND CHILDREN: 2 mg I.M. or I.V. repeated at hourly intervals until muscarinic symptoms disappear. Severe cases may require up to 6 mg I.M. or I.V. q 1 hour. **Preoperatively for diminishing secretions and blocking cardiac vagal reflexes:** ADULTS: 0.4 to 0.6 mg I.M. 45 to 60 minutes before anesthetic. CHILDREN: 0.01 mg/kg I.M. up to a maximum dose of 0.4 mg 45 to 60 minutes before anesthetic.	With usual doses of 0.4 to 0.6 mg, there are few side effects other than dry mouth. However, individual tolerance varies greatly. **CNS:** disorientation, restlessness, irritability, incoherence, hallucinations, headache. **CV:** palpitations, tachycardia, paradoxical bradycardia with doses less than 0.4 mg. **EENT:** *dilated pupils, blurred vision,* photophobia, increased intraocular pressure, eye pain, dysphagia. **GI:** *constipation, mouth dryness,* nausea, vomiting. **GU:** *urinary hesitancy or retention.* **Skin:** flushing, dryness. **Other:** bronchial plugging, fever. Side effects above may be due to pending atropine toxicity and are dose-related.
benztropine mesylate Cogentin♦ **Acute dystonic reaction:** ADULTS: 2 mg I.V. or I.M. followed by 1 to 2 mg P.O. b.i.d. to prevent recurrence. **Parkinsonism:** ADULTS: 0.5 to 6 mg P.O. daily. Initial dose 0.5 mg to 1 mg. Increase 0.5 mg every 5 to 6 days. Adjust dosage to meet individual requirements.	**CNS:** disorientation, restlessness, irritability, incoherence, hallucinations, headache, sedation, depression, muscular weakness. **CV:** palpitations, tachycardia, paradoxical bradycardia. **EENT:** dilated pupils, blurred vision, photophobia, difficulty swallowing. **GI:** *constipation, mouth dryness,* nausea, vomiting, epigastric distress. **GU:** urinary hesitancy or retention. Some side effects may be due to pending atropine-like toxicity and are dose related.
biperiden hydrochloride Akineton♦ **biperiden lactate** Akineton Lactate♦ **Extrapyramidal disorders:** ADULTS: 2 to 6 mg P.O. daily, b.i.d., or t.i.d., depending on severity. Usual dose is 2 mg daily, or 2 mg I.M. or I.V. q ½ hour, not to exceed 4 doses or 8 mg total daily. **Parkinsonism:** ADULTS: 2 mg P.O. t.i.d. to q.i.d.	**CNS:** disorientation, euphoria, restlessness, irritability, incoherence, dizziness, increased tremor. **CV:** transient postural hypotension. **EENT:** blurred vision. **GI:** *constipation, mouth dryness,* nausea, vomiting, epigastric distress. **GU:** urinary hesitancy or retention. Side effects are dose-related and may resemble atropine toxicity.
chlorphenoxamine hydrochloride Phenoxene♦ **Parkinsonism:** ADULTS: 50 mg P.O. t.i.d.; in severe cases, 300 to 400 mg daily, 100 mg t.i.d. to q.i.d.	**CNS:** drowsiness, sedation, increased tremors. **EENT:** blurred vision. **GI:** *constipation, dry mouth,* nausea, vomiting, epigastric distress.

INTERACTIONS AND SPECIAL CONSIDERATIONS

No significant interactions.

Special considerations:

• Contraindicated in narrow-angle glaucoma, obstructive uropathy, obstructive disease of GI tract, myasthenia gravis, paralytic ileus, intestinal atony, unstable cardiovascular status in acute hemorrhage, and toxic megacolon. Use with caution in autonomic neuropathy, hyperthyroidism, coronary artery disease, cardiac arrhythmias, congestive heart failure, hypertension, hiatal hernia associated with reflux esophagitis, hepatic or renal disease, ulcerative colitis, in patients over 40 years because of the increased incidence of glaucoma, and in children under 6 years. Use with caution in hot or humid environments. Drug-induced heat stroke possible.

• All dosages should be checked carefully. Even slight overdose could lead to toxicity.

• Vital signs should be monitored carefully. Side effects possible, especially in elderly or debilitated patients.

• When given I.V., may cause paradoxical initial bradycardia. Usually disappears within 2 minutes.

• Intake and output should be monitored. Drug causes urinary retention and hesitancy; patient should void before drug is administered.

• Many of the side effects (such as dry mouth and constipation) are an extension of the drug's pharmacologic activity and may be expected.

• For symptoms and treatment of toxicity, see APPENDIX.

Interactions:

AMANTADINE: anticholinergic side effects, such as confusion and hallucinations. Reduce dosage before administering amantadine.

Special considerations:

• Contraindicated in narrow-angle glaucoma. Use cautiously in patients with prostatic hypertrophy, tendency to tachycardia, and in elderly or debilitated patients; produces atropine-like side effects.

• Vital signs should be monitored carefully. Side effects possible, especially in elderly or debilitated patients.

• This drug should never be discontinued abruptly. Dosages must be reduced gradually.

• Patient should avoid activities that require alertness until CNS response to drug is known. If patient receives single daily dose, should be given at bedtime.

• Drug may take 2 to 3 days to exert full effect.

• Intake and output should be monitored; urinary hesitancy and retention may develop.

• Intermittent constipation, distention, and abdominal pain may be onset of paralytic ileus.

• Dry mouth relieved with cool drinks, ice chips, sugarless gum, or hard candy.

• Administration after meals helps prevent gastric irritation.

• For symptoms and treatment of toxicity, see APPENDIX.

No significant interactions.

Special considerations:

• Use with caution in narrow-angle glaucoma, prostatism, cardiac arrhythmias.

• Vital signs should be monitored carefully. Side effects possible, especially in elderly or debilitated patients.

• Oral doses given with or after meals decrease GI side effects.

• When given parenterally, patient should remain supine. Parenteral use may cause transient postural hypotension and coordination disturbances.

• I.V. injections should be made very slowly.

• Because of possible dizziness, patient may need help getting out of bed.

• Tolerance may develop and may require increased dosage.

• In severe parkinsonism, tremors may increase as spasticity is relieved.

• Patient should avoid activities that require alertness until CNS response to drug is determined.

• Intake and output should be monitored; urinary hesitancy and retention may develop.

• Dry mouth relieved with cool drinks, ice chips, sugarless gum, or hard candy.

• For symptoms and treatment of toxicity, see APPENDIX.

No significant interactions.

Special considerations:

• Use cautiously in narrow-angle glaucoma, tachycardia, or prostatic hypertrophy.

• Vital signs should be monitored carefully. Side effects possible, especially in elderly or debilitated patients.

• Patient should avoid activities that require alertness until CNS reaction determined.

• Doses should be administered with milk after meals to decrease GI side effects.

• In severe parkinsonism, tremors may increase as spasticity is relieved.

• Tolerance may develop and may require increased dosage.

• Dry mouth relieved with cool drinks, ice chips, sugarless gum, or hard candy.

• For symptoms and treatment of toxicity, see APPENDIX.

NAMES, INDICATIONS AND DOSAGES	SIDE EFFECTS
cycrimine hydrochloride Pagitane Hydrochloride **Idiopathic and arteriosclerotic parkinsonism:** ADULTS: initially, 1.25 to 2.5 mg P.O. t.i.d.; gradually increase dosage to 5 mg q.i.d. **Postencephalitic parkinsonism:** ADULTS: 5 mg t.i.d. or up to 5 mg q 2 hours while awake.	**CNS:** disorientation, incoherence, weakness, drowsiness, dizziness. **EENT:** blurred vision. **GI:** epigastric distress, sore mouth and tongue, *constipation, mouth dryness.* Also transient nausea and anorexia 30 minutes to 1 hour after administration. **Skin:** flushing, dryness, rash. **Other:** fever.
glycopyrrolate Robinul **To reverse neuromuscular blockade:** ADULTS: 0.2 mg I.V. for each 1 mg neostigmine or equivalent dose of pyridostigmine. May be given intravenously without dilution or may be added to dextrose injection and given by infusion. **Preoperatively to diminish secretions and block cardiac vagal reflexes:** ADULTS: 0.002 mg/lb of body weight I.M. 30 to 60 minutes before anesthetic.	**CNS:** disorientation, irritability, incoherence, weakness, nervousness, drowsiness, dizziness, headache. **CV:** palpitations, tachycardia, paradoxical bradycardia. **EENT:** *dilated pupils, blurred vision,* photophobia, increased intraocular pressure, difficulty swallowing. **GI:** *constipation, mouth dryness,* nausea, vomiting, epigastric distress. **GU:** urinary hesitancy or retention. **Skin:** flushing, dryness, rash. **Local:** burning at injection site. **Other:** bronchial plugging, fever.
procyclidine hydrochloride Kemadrin♦, Procyclid♦♦ **Parkinsonism, muscle rigidity:** ADULTS: initially, 2 to 2.5 mg P.O. t.i.d., after meals. Increase as needed to maximum 60 mg daily. Also used to relieve extrapyramidal dysfunction that accompanies treatment with phenothiazines and rauwolfia derivatives. Also controls sialorrhea from neuroleptic medications.	**CNS:** light-headedness, giddiness. **EENT:** blurred vision, mydriasis. **GI:** *constipation, mouth dryness,* nausea, vomiting, epigastric distress. **Skin:** rash.
scopolamine hydrobromide **Postencephalitic parkinsonism and other spastic states:** ADULTS: 0.5 to 1 mg P.O. t.i.d. to q.i.d.; 0.3 to 0.6 mg S.C., I.M., or I.V. (with suitable dilution) t.i.d. to q.i.d. CHILDREN: 0.006 mg/kg P.O. or S.C. t.i.d. to q.i.d.; or 0.2 mg/m^2.	**CNS:** disorientation, restlessness, irritability, incoherence, headache. **CV:** palpitations, tachycardia, paradoxical bradycardia. **EENT:** dilated pupils, blurred vision, photophobia, increased intraocular pressure, difficulty swallowing. **GI:** *constipation, mouth dryness, nausea, vomiting, epigastric distress.* **GU:** urinary hesitancy or retention. **Skin:** flushing, dryness. **Other:** bronchial plugging, fever, depressed respirations. Side effects may be due to pending atropine-like toxicity and are dose related. Individual tolerance varies greatly.

♦ Available in U.S. and Canada. ♦♦ Available in Canada only.
All other products (no symbol) available in U.S. only. Italicized side effects are common or life-threatening.

INTERACTIONS AND SPECIAL CONSIDERATIONS

No significant interactions.

Special considerations:

• Use with caution in narrow-angle glaucoma; in the elderly with arteriosclerotic changes; and in tachycardia or tendency toward urinary retention.
• Vital signs should be monitored carefully.
• Side effects, especially vertigo, disorientation, and weakness, may require dosage to be reduced or stopped.
• Mild side effects, such as dry mouth, blurred vision, epigastric distress, disappear with continued administration.
• Doses should be administered with milk or after meals to decrease GI side effects.
• Dry mouth relieved with cool drinks, ice chips, sugarless gum, or hard candy.
• For symptoms and treatment of toxicity, see APPENDIX.

No significant interactions.

Special considerations:

• Contraindicated in narrow-angle glaucoma, obstructive uropathy, obstructive disease of the GI tract, myasthenia gravis, paralytic ileus, intestinal atony, unstable cardiovascular status in acute hemorrhage, toxic megacolon. Use with caution in patients with autonomic neuropathy, hyperthyroidism, coronary artery disease, cardiac arrhythmias, congestive heart failure, hypertension, hiatal hernia associated with reflux esophagitis, hepatic or renal disease, ulcerative colitis, and in patients over 40 years because of increased incidence of glaucoma. Use with caution in hot or humid environments. Drug-induced heat stroke possible.
• Dosages should be checked carefully. Slight overdose could be toxic.
• Should not be mixed with I.V. solution of sodium chloride or bicarbonate.
• Vital signs should be monitored carefully. Side effects possible, especially in elderly or debilitated patients.
• Intake and output should be monitored. Causes urinary retention or hesitancy.
• Patient should avoid activities that require alertness until CNS response to drug is determined.
• Side effects less likely than with other parasympatholytics, unless dosages are excessive.
• For symptoms and treatment of toxicity, see APPENDIX.

No significant interactions.

Special considerations:

• Contraindicated in narrow-angle glaucoma. Use cautiously in tachycardia, hypotension, urinary retention, or prostatic hypertrophy.
• Mental confusion, disorientation, agitation, hallucinations, and psychotic symptoms possible, especially in the elderly.
• In severe parkinsonism, tremors may increase as spasticity is relieved.
• Should be taken after meals to minimize GI distress.
• Patient should avoid activities that require alertness until CNS response to drug is determined.
• Dry mouth relieved with cool drinks, ice chips, sugarless gum, or hard candy.
• For symptoms and treatment of toxicity, see APPENDIX.

No significant interactions.

Special considerations:

• Contraindicated in narrow-angle glaucoma, obstructive uropathy, obstructive disease of the GI tract, asthma, chronic pulmonary disease, myasthenia gravis, paralytic ileus, intestinal atony, unstable cardiovascular status in acute hemorrhage, or toxic megacolon. Use with caution in patients with autonomic neuropathy, hyperthyroidism, coronary artery disease, cardiac arrhythmias, congestive heart failure, hypertension, hiatal hernia associated with reflux esophagitis, hepatic or renal disease, ulcerative colitis, in patients over 40 years because of the increased incidence of glaucoma, and in children under 6 years. Use with caution in hot or humid environments. Drug-induced heat stroke possible.
• Some patients become temporarily excited or disoriented. Symptoms disappear when sedative effect is complete. Bed rails should be used as precaution.
• Patients should avoid activities requiring alertness until CNS response to drug is determined.
• Intake and output should be monitored; urinary hesitancy or retention may develop.
• Tolerance may develop when administered over a long period of time.
• Many of the side effects (such as dry mouth, constipation) are extensions of the drug's pharmacologic activity and may be expected.
• For symptoms and treatment of toxicity, see APPENDIX.

NAMES, INDICATIONS AND DOSAGES	SIDE EFFECTS
trihexyphenidyl hydrochloride Aparkane♦♦, Artane♦, Hexaphen, Novohexidyl♦♦, T.H.P., Tremin, Trihexane, Trihexidyl, Trihexy♦♦, Trixyl♦♦ **Drug-induced parkinsonism:** ADULTS: 1 mg P.O. 1st day, 2 mg 2nd day, then increase 2 mg every 3 to 5 days until total of 6 to 10 mg given daily. Usually given t.i.d. with meals and, if needed, q.i.d. (last dose should be before bedtime). Postencephalitic parkinsonism may require 12 to 15 mg total daily dose.	**CNS:** nervousness, dizziness, headache, restlessness, agitation, hallucinations, euphoria, delusion, amnesia. **CV:** tachycardia. **EENT:** blurred vision, mydriasis, increased intraocular pressure. **GI:** constipation, *dry mouth, nausea.* **GU:** urinary hesitancy or retention. Side effects are dose related.

INTERACTIONS AND SPECIAL CONSIDERATIONS

Interactions:

AMANTADINE: anticholinergic side effects, such as confusion and hallucinations. Reduce dosage before administering amantadine.

Special considerations:

- Use cautiously in patients with narrow-angle glaucoma; cardiac, hepatic, or renal disorders; hypertension; obstructive disease of the GI and the genitourinary tracts; possible prostatic hypertrophy; in patients over 60 years; and in those with arteriosclerosis or history of drug hypersensitivities.
- Patient should avoid activities that require alertness until CNS response to drug is determined.
- Causes nausea if taken before meals.
- Dry mouth relieved with cool drinks, ice chips, sugarless gum, or hard candy.
- Patient may develop a tolerance to this drug.
- Intake and output should be monitored; urinary hesistancy or retention may develop.
- Gonioscopic evaluation and close monitoring of intraocular pressures advised, especially in patients over 40 years.
- For symptoms and treatment of toxicity, see APPENDIX.

NEW TREATMENT FOR DRY MOUTH

Moi-stir is a new nonprescription mouth moistener produced by Kingswood Laboratories. It relieves dry mouth (depressed salivary function), a common side effect of anticholinergic drugs.

Moi-stir contains sorbitol, sodium carboxymethylcellulose, potassium chloride, dibasic sodium phosphate, calcium chloride, sodium chloride, and magnesium chloride. Use Moi-stir cautiously in patients on sodium- or potassium-restricted diets. It's supplied in 120-ml bottles; a manual spray pump delivers about 0.5 ml of the moistener per stroke. Advise patients to spray Moi-stir once or twice into the mouth, as needed.

38

Adrenergics (sympathomimetics)

albuterol
dobutamine hydrochloride
dopamine hydrochloride
ephedrine sulfate
epinephrine
epinephrine bitartrate
epinephrine hydrochloride
ethylnorepinephrine hydrochloride
isoetharine hydrochloride 1%
isoetharine mesylate
isoproterenol hydrochloride
isoproterenol sulfate
mephentermine sulfate
metaproterenol sulfate
metaraminol bitartrate
methoxamine hydrochloride
norepinephrine injection (formerly levarterenol bitartrate)
pseudoephedrine hydrochloride
pseudoephedrine sulfate
terbutaline sulfate

Adrenergics produce their effect by either mimicking the actions of epinephrine or norepinephrine at receptor sites in the sympathetic nervous system or by displacing natural norepinephrine from neural storage sites. Because these drugs do not simulate all classes of adrenergic receptors equally, their effects and indications for use differ.

As with most drugs, the actions of adrenergics are not organ- or site-specific: they may occur at other than the desired sites.

The sympathetic nervous system innervates numerous organs (for example, the heart, blood vessels, respiratory tract, liver, urinary bladder, and intestines) and significantly affects the regulation of many body functions. When stimulated, sympathetic nerves release norepinephrine (except for sympathetic nerves that innervate sweat glands, which release acetylcholine). Norepinephrine combines with receptor sites on the innervated organ to elicit a response.

The three major types of receptors within the sympathetic system are alpha, beta, and dopaminergic. Stimulation of alpha receptors causes vasoconstriction and uterine and sphincter contraction. Beta receptors are divided into two subgroups, $beta_1$ and $beta_2$. $Beta_1$ receptors are largely in the heart; when stimulated, they increase the rate and force of myocardial contraction and the rate of atrioventricular node conduction. $Beta_2$ receptors are primarily in the bronchi, blood vessels, and uterus; stimulation produces bronchodilation, vasodilation, and uterine relaxation, respectively. Dopaminergic receptors are primarily in splanchnic blood vessels; stimulation dilates these vessels.

The adrenal medulla is a major part of the sympathetic nervous system. During times of danger or acute stress, it releases large amounts of epinephrine into the systemic circulation. Epinephrine activates alpha and beta receptors, ultimately producing physiologic and metabolic effects that prepare the person to cope with the stress (as in the fight-or-flight response).

Major uses

- Dobutamine, dopamine, mephentermine, metaraminol, methoxamine, and norepinephrine raise blood pressure and cardiac output in severely decompensated states, such as cardiogenic shock and heart failure.
- Albuterol, ephedrine, ethylnorepinephrine, isoetharine, isoproterenol, metaproterenol, and terbutaline relieve bronchoconstriction.
- Epinephrine and isoproterenol are used to treat heart block, certain arrhythmias such as paroxysmal atrial tachycardia, and cardiac arrest.
- Epinephrine and pseudoephedrine are used to treat anaphylaxis and other allergic

reactions (common in asthmatic attacks) and to relieve congestion.

Mechanism of action
Adrenergics simulate or increase the effect of epinephrine and norepinephrine on alpha- and beta-adrenergic receptors within the sympathetic nervous system. Effects vary and include bronchodilation, release of glucose from the liver, increase in heart rate and ventricular contractility, central nervous system excitation, dilation (beta effect) of blood vessels in skeletal muscles, and constriction (alpha effect) of blood vessels in cutaneous areas.

Absorption, distribution, metabolism, and excretion
- Albuterol is slowly absorbed following inhalation. It is partially metabolized in the liver and excreted in the urine both as metabolite and unchanged drug.
- Dobutamine and dopamine are not absorbed from the gastrointestinal (GI) tract and must be given parenterally. They're metabolized by the liver to inactive compounds and excreted in urine.
- Ephedrine is rapidly absorbed after oral, I.M., or subcutaneous administration. Some of the drug is metabolized by the liver; both unchanged compound and metabolites are excreted in the urine.
- Epinephrine and ethylnorepinephrine are not well absorbed from the GI tract after oral administration. Absorption is efficient, however, after I.M. or subcutaneous injection. The drugs are extensively metabolized in the liver and excreted in the urine.
- Isoetharine is rapidly absorbed from the respiratory tract after inhalation. It is partly metabolized by enzymes in the lungs and other tissues. Both the parent compound and metabolite are excreted in the urine.
- Isoproterenol is irregularly absorbed after oral or sublingual administration, but is well absorbed following parenteral administration or oral inhalation. It is metabolized in the liver and other tissues and excreted in the urine.
- Mephentermine is not absorbed from the GI tract and must be given parenterally. It is metabolized in the liver and excreted in the urine; excretion is increased in an acidic urine.
- Metaproterenol, well absorbed after oral administration, is subject to the first-pass effect. Conjugates of the parent compound are excreted in the urine.
- Metaraminol is erratically absorbed from the GI tract after being given orally, so must be given parenterally. Distribution, metabolism, and route of excretion are not completely known. Its pharmacologic effects are stopped by its uptake into body tissues.
- Methoxamine is not absorbed from the GI tract, so must be given parenterally. Its metabolism and excretion patterns are unclear.
- Norepinephrine is not absorbed after oral administration and is poorly absorbed after subcutaneous injection. The drug is taken up by nerve endings where it is metabolized; norepinephrine is also metabolized by the liver and other tissues. Metabolites are excreted in urine.
- Pseudoephedrine, effective when administered orally, is metabolized by the liver. The metabolites are excreted in the urine. Excretion increases in an acidic urine.
- Terbutaline is partially absorbed after oral administration but is well absorbed subcutaneously. It is eliminated in the urine and feces in both metabolized and unchanged form.

THERAPEUTIC ACTIVITY

THERAPEUTIC ACTIVITY OF ADRENERGICS

DRUG	ROUTE	ONSET	DURATION
albuterol	inhalation	within 15 min	1 to 4 hr
dobutamine	I.V.	within 2 min	until shortly after infusion is stopped
dopamine	I.V.	within 5 min	less than 10 min, or as long as infusion is continued
ephedrine	P.O.	less than 1 hr	4 to 12 hr, depending on form of P.O. dosage
epinephrine	I.M. S.C.	3 to 5 min	20 to 30 min
ethylnor-epinephrine	I.M. S.C.	3 to 5 min	20 to 30 min
isoetharine	inhalation	rapid; peaks in 5 to 15 min	1 to 4 hr
isoproterenol	I.V. P.O.	immediate 20 min	as long as infusion is continued 1 hr
mephentermine	I.M. I.V.	5 to 15 min immediate	1 to 4 hr 15 to 30 min after injection
metaproterenol	inhalation P.O.	1 min; peaks in 1 hr 15 min; peaks in 1 hr	up to 4 hr up to 4 hr
metaraminol	I.M. I.V. S.C.	within 10 min 1 to 2 min 5 to 20 min	1 hr 5 to 15 min 1 hr
methoxamine	I.M. I.V.	15 to 20 min immediate	60 to 90 min 5 to 15 min
norepinephrine	I.V.	immediate	until shortly after infusion is stopped
pseudo-ephedrine	P.O.	30 min	4 to 6 hr
terbutaline	P.O. S.C.	20 to 30 min 10 to 20 min	6 hr 4 to 6 hr

Onset and duration

The chart on the opposite page summarizes the onset and duration of the adrenergics.

Combination products

Only a few of the many combinations are included here as examples of this group.

Inhalants

DUO-MEDIHALER: isoproterenol hydrochloride 0.16 mg and phenylephrine bitartrate 0.24 mg/dose.

Oral bronchodilators

AMESEC♦: aminophylline 130 mg, ephedrine HCl 25 mg, and amobarbital 25 mg.
BRONCHOBID DURACAPS: theophylline 260 mg and ephedrine HCl 35 mg.
MARAX♦: theophylline 130 mg, ephedrine sulfate 25 mg, and hydroxyzine HCl 10 mg.
QUADRINAL♦: theophylline calcium salicylate 65 mg, ephedrine hydrochloride 24 mg, potassium iodide 320 mg, and phenobarbital 24 mg.
QUIBRON PLUS: theophylline 150 mg, ephedrine hydrochloride 25 mg, guaifenesin 100 mg, and butabarbital 20 mg.
TEDRAL SA♦: theophylline 180 mg, ephedrine hydrochloride 48 mg, and phenobarbital 25 mg.
(OTC) ASMA-LIEF: theophylline 130 mg, ephedrine hydrochloride 24 mg, and phenobarbital 8 mg.
(OTC) TEDRAL: theophylline 130 mg, ephedrine hydrochloride 24 mg, and phenobarbital 8 mg.
(OTC) THALFED: theophylline 120 mg, ephedrine hydrochloride 25 mg, and phenobarbital 8 mg.

Decongestants

ACTIFED: pseudoephedrine hydrochloride 60 mg and triprolidine hydrochloride 2.5 mg.
CONGESPRIN: phenylephrine hydrochloride 1.25 mg and aspirin 81 mg.
DRISTAN: phenylephrine hydrochloride 5 mg, chlorpheniramine maleate 2 mg, aspirin 325 mg, and caffeine 16.2 mg.
HISTASPAN-PLUS: phenylephrine hydrochloride 20 mg and chlorpheniramine maleate 8 mg.
NALDECON: phenylpropanolamine hydrochloride 40 mg, phenylephrine hydrochloride 10 mg, chlorpheniramine maleate 5 mg, and phenyltoloxamine citrate 15 mg.
ORNEX: phenylpropanolamine hydrochloride 18 mg and acetaminophen 325 mg.
PHENERGAN-D: pseudoephedrine hydrochloride 60 mg and promethazine hydrochloride 6.25 mg.
SINUTAB-II: phenylpropanolamine hydrochloride 25 mg and acetaminophen 325 mg.
TRIAMINIC: phenylpropanolamine hydrochloride 50 mg, pyrilamine maleate 25 mg, and pheniramine maleate 25 mg.

NAMES, INDICATIONS AND DOSAGES	SIDE EFFECTS
albuterol Proventil, Ventolin **Relief of bronchospasm in patients with reversible obstructive airway disease:** ADULTS AND CHILDREN 12 YEARS OR OLDER: 1 to 2 inhalations q 4 to 6 hours. More frequent administration or a greater number of inhalations is not recommended. Not recommended in children under 12 years.	**CNS:** *tremor, nervousness,* dizziness, insomnia. **CV:** tachycardia, palpitations, hypertension. **EENT:** drying and irritation of nose and throat. **GI:** heartburn, nausea, vomiting.
dobutamine hydrochloride Dobutrex **Refractory heart failure and as adjunct in cardiac surgery:** ADULTS: 2.5 to 10 mcg/kg/minute as an I.V. infusion. Rarely, infusion rates up to 40 mcg/kg/minute have been required. May be reconstituted with 5% dextrose in water, normal saline solution, or lactated Ringer's solution.	**CNS:** headache. **CV:** *increased heart rate, hypertension, premature ventricular beats,* angina, nonspecific chest pain. **GI:** nausea, vomiting. **Other:** shortness of breath.
dopamine hydrochloride Intropin♦ **To treat shock and correct hemodynamic imbalances; to improve perfusion to vital organs, increase cardiac output; to correct hypotension:** ADULTS: 2 to 5 mcg/kg/minute I.V. infusion, up to 50 mcg/kg/minute. Titrate the dosage to the desired hemodynamic and/or renal response.	**CNS:** headache. **CV:** ectopic beats, tachycardia, anginal pain, palpitations, *hypotension.* Less frequently, bradycardia, widening of QRS complex, conduction disturbances, vasoconstriction. **GI:** nausea, vomiting. **Local:** necrosis and tissue sloughing with extravasation. **Other:** piloerection, dyspnea.

♦ Available in U.S. and Canada. ♦♦ Available in Canada only.
All other products (no symbol) available in U.S. only. Italicized side effects are common or life-threatening.

INTERACTIONS AND SPECIAL CONSIDERATIONS

Interactions:
PROPRANOLOL AND OTHER BETA BLOCKERS: blocked effect of albuterol and vice versa. Monitor patient carefully if used together.

Special considerations:
• Use cautiously in patients with cardiovascular disorders, including coronary insufficiency and hypertension; in patients with hyperthyroidism or diabetes mellitus; and in patients who are unusually responsive to adrenergics.
• Patient should be warned about the possibility of paradoxical bronchospasm. If this occurs, the drug should be discontinued immediately.
• Albuterol reportedly produces less cardiac stimulation than other sympathomimetics, especially isoproterenol.
• Albuterol is also known by the generic name of salbutamol.
• Patient should know how to administer metered dose correctly: shake container; exhale through nose; administer aerosol while inhaling deeply on mouthpiece of inhaler; hold breath for a few seconds, then exhale slowly. Two minutes should be allowed between inhalations.
• Store drug in light-resistant container.

Interactions:
PROPRANOLOL, METOPROLOL: These beta blockers may make dobutamine ineffective. Do not use together.

Special considerations:
• Contraindicated in idiopathic hypertrophic subaortic stenosis.
• A unique agent. Increases contractility of failing heart without inducing marked tachycardia, except at high doses.
• Dobutamine is a chemical modification of isoproterenol.
• Often used with nitroprusside for additive effects.
• EKG, blood pressure, pulmonary wedge pressure, and cardiac output should be monitored continuously. Urinary output should be monitored also.
• Incompatible with alkaline solutions. Should not be mixed with sodium bicarbonate injection.
• Infusions of up to 72 hours produce no more adverse effects than shorter infusions.
• Oxidation of drug may slightly discolor admixtures containing dobutamine. This does not indicate a significant loss of potency.
• Intravenous solutions remain stable for 24 hours.

Interactions:
ERGOT ALKALOIDS: extreme elevations in blood pressure. Don't use together.
PHENYTOIN: may lower blood pressure of dopamine-stabilized patients. Monitor carefully.

Special considerations:
• Contraindicated in uncorrected tachyarrhythmias, pheochromocytoma, ventricular fibrillation. Use cautiously in patients with occlusive vascular disease, cold injuries, diabetic endarteritis, arterial embolism; also, in pregnant patients and in those taking MAO inhibitors.
• Not a substitute for blood or fluid volume deficits. If volume deficits exist, these should be replaced before vasopressors are given.
• Don't mix with alkaline solutions. 5% dextrose in water, normal saline, or combination of 5% dextrose in water and saline should be used. Mix before use.
• Dopamine solutions deteriorate after 24 hours. Should be discarded at that time or earlier if solution is discolored.
• Large vein should be used, as in antecubital fossa, to minimize risk of extravasation. Site should be watched carefully for signs of extravasation. Infusion should be stopped immediately if extravasation occurs. Effect may be counteracted by infiltrating the area with 5 to 10 mg phentolamine and 10 to 15 ml normal saline.
• Blood pressure, pulse rate, urinary output, and extremity color and temperature should be checked often during infusion; infusion rate titrated according to findings. Use microdrip or infusion pump to regulate flow rate.
• If adverse effects develop, dosage may need to be adjusted or stopped.
• If a disproportionate rise in the diastolic pressure (a marked decrease in pulse pressure) is observed in patients receiving dopamine, infusion rate should be decreased and patient observed carefully for further evidence of predominant vasoconstrictor activity, unless such an effect is desired.
• Most patients satisfactorily maintained on less than 20 mcg/kg/minute.
• If doses exceed 50 mcg/kg/minute, urinary output should be checked often. If urine flow decreases without hypotension, reducing dose should be considered.
• If drug is stopped, sudden drop in blood pressure possible.
• Should not be mixed with alkaline solutions. Should be prepared with 5% dextrose in water, normal saline solution, or combination of 5% dextrose in water and saline solution and mixed just before use.
• Other drugs should not be mixed in bottle containing dopamine.
• Alkaline drugs (sodium bicarbonate, phenytoin sodium) should not be given through I.V. line containing dopamine.

NAMES, INDICATIONS AND DOSAGES	SIDE EFFECTS
ephedrine sulfate **To correct hypotensive states; to support ventricular rate in Adams-Stokes syndrome:** ADULTS: 25 to 50 mg I.M. or S.C., or 10 to 25 mg I.V. p.r.n. to maximum 150 mg/24 hours. CHILDREN: 3 mg/kg S.C. or I.V. daily, divided into 4 to 6 doses. **Bronchodilator or nasal decongestant:** ADULTS: 12.5 to 50 mg P.O. b.i.d., t.i.d., or q.i.d. Maximum 400 mg/day in 6 to 8 divided doses. CHILDREN: 2 to 3 mg/kg P.O. daily in 4 to 6 divided doses.	**CNS:** *insomnia, nervousness,* dizziness, headache, muscle weakness, sweating, euphoria, confusion, delirium. **CV:** *palpitations,* tachycardia, hypertension. **EENT:** dryness of nose and throat. **GI:** nausea, vomiting, anorexia. **GU:** urinary retention, painful urination due to visceral sphincter spasm.
epinephrine Inhalants: Bronkaid Mist♦, Primatene Mist **epinephrine bitartrate** Inhalants: AsthmaHaler, Medihaler-Epi♦ **epinephrine hydrochloride** Adrenalin Chloride, Asmolin, Sus-Phrine♦ **Bronchospasm, hypersensitivity reactions, and anaphylaxis:** ADULTS: 0.1 to 0.5 ml of 1:1,000 S.C. or I.M. Repeat q 10 to 15 minutes, p.r.n. Or 0.1 to 0.25 ml 1:1,000 I.V. CHILDREN: 0.01 ml (10 mcg) of 1:1,000/kg S.C. Repeat q 20 minutes to 4 hours, p.r.n.; 0.005 ml/kg of 1:200 (Sus-Phrine). Repeat q 8 to 12 hours, p.r.n. **Hemostatic:** ADULTS: 1:50,000 to 1:1,000, applied topically. **Acute asthmatic attacks (inhalation):** ADULTS AND CHILDREN: 1 or 2 inhalations of 1:100 or 2.25% racemic, p.r.n.; 0.2 mg/dose usual content. **To prolong local anesthetic effect:** ADULTS AND CHILDREN: 0.2 to 0.4 ml of 1:1,000 intraspinal; 1:500,000 to 1:50,000 local mixed with local anesthetic. **To restore cardiac rhythm in cardiac arrest:** ADULTS: 0.5 to 1 mg I.V. or into endotracheal tube. May be given intracardiac if no I.V. route or intratracheal route available. CHILDREN: 10 mcg/kg I.V. or 5 to 10 mcg (0.05 to 0.1 ml of 1:10,000)/kg intracardiac. *Note:* 1 mg = 1 ml of 1:1,000 or 10 ml of 1:10,000.	**CNS:** *nervousness,* tremor, euphoria, anxiety, coldness of extremities, vertigo, *headache,* sweating, cerebral hemorrhage, disorientation, agitation. In patients with Parkinson's disease, the drug increases rigidity and tremor. **CV:** *palpitations;* widened pulse pressure; hypertension; *tachycardia; ventricular fibrillation; CVA;* anginal pain; EKG changes, including a decrease in the T-wave amplitude. **Metabolic:** *hyperglycemia,* glycosuria. **Other:** pulmonary edema, dyspnea, *pallor.*

♦ Available in U.S. and Canada. ♦♦ Available in Canada only.
All other products (no symbol) available in U.S. only. Italicized side effects are common or life-threatening.

INTERACTIONS AND SPECIAL CONSIDERATIONS

Interactions:
MAO INHIBITORS AND TRICYCLIC ANTIDEPRESSANTS: when given with sympathomimetics, may cause severe hypertension (hypertensive crisis). Don't use together.
METHYLDOPA: may inhibit effect of ephedrine. Give together cautiously.

Special considerations:
- Contraindicated in porphyria, severe coronary artery disease, cardiac arrhythmias, narrow-angle glaucoma, psychoneurosis, and in patients on MAO inhibitor therapy. Use with caution in elderly patients, and in those with hypertension, hyperthyroidism, nervous or excitable states, cardiovascular disease, and prostatic hypertrophy.
- Not a substitute for blood or fluid volume deficit. Volume deficit should be replaced before vasopressors are administered.
- I.V. injection should be given slowly.
- Hypoxia, hypercapnia, and acidosis, which may reduce effectiveness or increase the incidence of adverse effects, must be identified and corrected before or during ephedrine administration.
- Effectiveness decreases after 2 to 3 weeks, then increased dosage may be needed. Tolerance develops, but not known to cause addiction.
- To prevent insomnia, should not be given within 2 hours of bedtime.
- Patient should not take over-the-counter drugs containing ephedrine without informing doctor.

Interactions:
TRICYCLIC ANTIDEPRESSANTS: when given with sympathomimetics, may cause severe hypertension (hypertensive crisis). Don't give together.
PROPRANOLOL: vasoconstriction and reflex bradycardia. Monitor patient carefully.

Special considerations:
- Contraindicated in narrow-angle glaucoma, shock (other than anaphylactic shock), organic brain damage, cardiac dilatation and coronary insufficiency. Also during general anesthesia with halogenated hydrocarbons or cyclopropane and in labor (may delay second stage). Use with extreme caution in patients with long-standing bronchial asthma and emphysema who have developed degenerative heart disease. Use with caution in elderly patients, and in those with hyperthyroidism, angina, hypertension, psychoneurosis, diabetes.
- Should not be mixed with alkaline solutions. 5% dextrose in water, normal saline, or a combination of 5% dextrose in water and saline should be used. Should be mixed just before use.
- Epinephrine is rapidly destroyed by oxidizing agents, such as iodine, chromates, nitrates, nitrites, oxygen, and salts of easily reducible metals such as iron.
- Epinephrine solutions deteriorate after 24 hours. Should be discarded after that time or before if solution is discolored or contains precipitate. Solution should be kept in light-resistant container and not removed before use.
- Massaging site after injection counteracts possible vasoconstriction. Repeated local injection can cause necrosis at site due to vasoconstriction.
- Intramuscular administration of oil injection into buttocks should be avoided. Gas gangrene may occur because epinephrine reduces oxygen tension of the tissues, encouraging the growth of contaminating organisms.
- This drug may widen patient's pulse pressure.
- In the event of a sharp blood pressure rise, rapid-acting vasodilators, such as the nitrites or alpha-adrenergic–blocking agents, can be given to counteract the marked pressor effect of large doses of epinephrine.
- If adverse effects develop, dosage may need to be adjusted or stopped.
- If patient has acute hypersensitivity reactions, it may be necessary to instruct him to self-inject epinephrine at home.
- Drug of choice in emergency treatment of severe acute anaphylactic reactions, including anaphylactic shock.

NAMES, INDICATIONS AND DOSAGES	SIDE EFFECTS
ethylnorepinephrine hydrochloride Bronkephrine **To relieve bronchospasm due to asthma:** ADULTS: 0.5 to 1 ml S.C. or I.M. CHILDREN: 0.1 to 0.5 ml S.C. or I.M.	**CNS:** *headache,* dizziness. **CV:** changes in blood pressure, *elevation in pulse rate,* palpitations. **GI:** nausea.
isoetharine hydrochloride 1% Beta-Z Solution, Bronkosol **isoetharine mesylate** Bronkometer **Bronchial asthma and reversible bronchospasm that may occur with bronchitis and emphysema:** ADULTS: (hydrochloride): administered by hand nebulizer, oxygen aerosolization, or IPPB. **Method** — **Dose** — **Dilution** Hand — 3 to 7 inhalations — undiluted Oxygen aerosolization — 0.5 ml — 1:3 with saline IPPB — 0.5 ml — 1:3 with saline ADULTS: (mesylate) 1 to 2 inhalations. Occasionally, more may be required.	**CNS:** *tremor, headache,* dizziness, excitement. **CV:** *palpitations,* increased heart rate. **GI:** nausea, vomiting.
isoproterenol hydrochloride Isuprel♦, Proternol (tabs) Inhalants: Norisodrine, Vapo-Iso **isoproterenol sulfate** Iso-Autohaler, Luf-Iso Inhalation, Medihaler-Iso♦, Norisodrine **Bronchial asthma and reversible bronchospasm (hydrochloride):** ADULTS: 10 to 20 mg S.L. q 6 to 8 hours. CHILDREN: 5 to 10 mg S.L. q 6 to 8 hours. Not recommended for children under 6 years. **Bronchospasm (sulfate):** ADULTS AND CHILDREN: acute dyspneic episodes—1 inhalation initially. May repeat if needed after 2 to 5 minutes. Maintenance—1 to 2 inhalations q.i.d. to 6 times daily. May repeat once more 10 minutes after second dose. Not more than 3 doses should be administered for each attack. **Heart block and ventricular arrhythmias (sulfate):** ADULTS: initially, 0.02 to 0.06 mg I.V. Subsequent doses 0.01 to 0.2 mg I.V. or 5 mcg/minute I.V.; or 0.2 mg I.M. initially, then 0.02 to 1 mg, p.r.n. CHILDREN: may give ½ of initial adult dose. **Maintenance for Stokes-Adams disease or AV block (sulfate):**	**CNS:** *headache,* mild tremor, weakness, dizziness, nervousness, insomnia. **CV:** *palpitations,* tachycardia, anginal pain; blood pressure may be elevated and then fall. **GI:** nausea, vomiting. **Metabolic:** hyperglycemia. **Other:** sweating, flushing of face, bronchial edema and inflammation.

INTERACTIONS AND SPECIAL CONSIDERATIONS

No significant interactions.

Special considerations:

• Use with caution in patients with cardiovascular disease or history of stroke.
• Safer than epinephrine for use in hypertensive or severely ill patients in whom significant pressor effects are undesirable.
• Valuable when used in children due to low incidence of adverse effects; may be useful in patients who are diabetic with asthma due to low glycogenolytic activity.
• Anatomic injection site should be chosen carefully to avoid inadvertent intraneural or intravascular injection.

No significant interactions.

Special considerations:

• Use cautiously in patients with hyperthyroidism, hypertension, coronary disease, or in those with sensitivity to sympathomimetics.
• Excessive use can lead to decreased effectiveness.
• Patients should be monitored for severe paradoxical bronchoconstriction after excessive use. Drug should be discontinued immediately if bronchoconstriction occurs.
• Although isoetharine has minimal effects on the heart, should be used cautiously in patients receiving general anesthetics that sensitize the myocardium to sympathomimetic drugs.
• Patient should know how to use aerosol and mouthpiece.

Interactions:

PROPRANOLOL AND OTHER BETA BLOCKERS: blocked effect of isoproterenol and vice versa. Monitor patient carefully if used together.

Special considerations:

• Contraindicated in tachycardia caused by digitalis intoxication and in patients with preexisting arrhythmias, especially tachycardia, because chronotropic effect on the heart may aggravate such disorders. Contraindicated in recent myocardial infarction. Use cautiously in coronary insufficiency, diabetes, hyperthyroidism.
• Not a substitute for blood or fluid volume deficit. If deficit exists, it should be replaced before vasopressors are administered.
• If heart rate exceeds 110 bpm, may be advisable to decrease infusion rate or temporarily stop infusion. Doses sufficient to increase heart rate to more than 130 bpm may induce ventricular arrhythmias.
• If precordial distress or anginal pain occurs, drug should be stopped immediately.
• When I.V. isoproterenol is administered for shock, blood pressure, CVP, EKG, arterial blood gas measurements, and urinary output should be monitored closely and infusion rate carefully adjusted according to these measurements.
• Oral and sublingual tablets are poorly and erratically absorbed.
• Patient should hold tablet under tongue until it dissolves and is absorbed and not swallow saliva until that time. Prolonged use of sublingual tablets can cause tooth decay. Patient should rinse mouth with water between doses. This will also help prevent dryness of oropharynx.
• If possible, should not be taken at bedtime; it interrupts sleep patterns.
• Oral tablets not for sublingual use must be swallowed whole, not broken. Store in cool, dry place in airtight, light-resistant container. Keep bottle tightly capped after opening.
• This drug may cause a slight rise in systolic blood pressure and a slight to marked drop in diastolic blood pressure.
• A microdrip or infusion pump should be used to regulate infusion flow rate.
• If adverse effects develop, dosage may need to be adjusted or stopped.
• Patient should understand how to use oral inhalation correctly with a metered-dose nebulizer:
  —Clear nasal passages and throat.
  —Breathe out, expelling as much air from lungs as possible.
  —Place mouthpiece well into mouth as dose is released; inhale deeply.
  —Hold breath for several seconds, remove mouthpiece, and exhale slowly.
• Instructions for metered powder nebulizer are the same, except that deep inhalation is not necessary.
• Patient may develop a tolerance to this drug and should be warned against overuse.
• Oral inhalant form of drug may turn sputum and saliva pink.

(continued on following page)

NAMES, INDICATIONS AND DOSAGES	SIDE EFFECTS
isoproterenol *(continued)* ADULTS: 30 to 180 mg timed-release tablets P.O. daily swallowed whole. **Shock (sulfate):** ADULTS AND CHILDREN: 0.5 to 5 mcg/ minute by continuous I.V. infusion. Usual concentration: 1 mg (5 ml) in 500 ml 5% dextrose in water. Adjust rate according to heart rate, central venous pressure, blood pressure, and urine flow.	
mephentermine sulfate Wyamine♦ **Hypotension following spinal anesthetic:** ADULTS: 30 to 45 mg I.V. in a single injection, then 30 mg I.V. repeated p.r.n. Maintenance of blood pressure: continuous I.V. infusion of 0.1% solution of mephentermine in 5% dextrose in water. **Hypotension following spinal anesthetic during obstetric procedures:** ADULTS: initially, 15 mg I.V., p.r.n. **Prevention of hypotension during spinal anesthetic:** ADULTS: 30 to 40 mg I.M. 10 to 20 minutes prior to anesthetic. **Treatment of shock and hypotension:** ADULTS: 0.5 mg/kg I.V. CHILDREN: 0.4 mg/kg I.V.	**CNS:** euphoria, nervousness, anxiety, tremor, incoherence, drowsiness, convulsions. **CV:** arrhythmias, marked elevation of blood pressure (with large doses).
metaproterenol sulfate Alupent♦, Metaprel **Acute episodes of bronchial asthma:** ADULTS AND CHILDREN: 2 to 3 inhalations. Should not repeat inhalations more often than q 3 to 4 hours. Should not exceed 12 inhalations daily. **Bronchial asthma and reversible bronchospasm:** ADULTS: 20 mg P.O. q 6 to 8 hours. CHILDREN OVER 9 YEARS OR OVER 27 KG: 20 mg P.O. q 6 to 8 hours. (0.4 mg to 0.9 mg/kg/dose t.i.d.) CHILDREN 6 TO 9 YEARS OR LESS THAN 27 KG: 10 mg P.O. q 6 to 8 hours. (0.4 mg to 0.9 mg/kg/dose t.i.d.) Not recommended for children under 6 years.	**CNS:** nervousness, weakness, drowsiness, tremor. **CV:** tachycardia, hypertension, palpitations; *with excessive use, cardiac arrest.* **GI:** vomiting, nausea, bad taste in mouth. **Other:** paradoxical bronchiolar constriction with excessive use.
metaraminol bitartrate Aramine♦ **Prevention of hypotension:** ADULTS: 2 to 10 mg I.M. or S.C.	**CNS:** apprehension, restlessness, dizziness, headache, tremor, weakness; with excessive use, convulsions. **CV:** hypertension; hypotension; precordial pain; palpitations; arrhythmias, including sinus or ventricular tachycardia; bradycardia; premature

INTERACTIONS AND SPECIAL CONSIDERATIONS

• May aggravate ventilation perfusion abnormalities; even while ease of breathing is improved, arterial oxygen tension may fall paradoxically.
• Inhalation solution should be discarded if it is discolored or contains precipitate.

No significant interactions.

Special considerations:
• Contraindicated in concealed hemorrhage or hypotension from hemorrhage, except in emergencies; also in patients receiving phenothiazines, or in those who have received MAO inhibitors within 2 weeks. Use cautiously with arteriosclerosis, cardiovascular disease, hyperthyroidism, hypertension, and chronic illness.
• Not a substitute for blood or fluid volume deficits. If deficits exist, these should be replaced before vasopressors are administered.
• During infusion, blood pressure should be checked every 5 minutes until stabilized; then every 15 minutes.
• If adverse effects develop, dosage may need to be adjusted or discontinued.
• Blood pressure should be monitored even after drug is stopped.
• I.M. route may be used since drug is not irritating to tissue.
• I.V. drug is not irritating to tissue, and extravasation is not dangerous. To prepare 0.1% I.V. solution: 16.6 ml mephentermine (30 mg/ml) should be added to 500 ml 5% dextrose in water.
• Can be given I.V. undiluted.
• May increase uterine contractions during third trimester of pregnancy.
• Hypercapnia, hypoxia, and acidosis may reduce effectiveness or increase adverse effects. Should be identified and corrected before and during administration.

No significant interactions.

Special considerations:
• Contraindicated in tachycardia and in arrhythmias associated with tachycardia. Use with caution in hypertension, coronary artery disease, hyperthyroidism, diabetes.
• Safe use of inhalant in children under 12 years not established.
• Patient should know how to administer metered dose correctly: shake container; exhale through nose; administer aerosol while inhaling deeply on mouthpiece of inhaler; hold breath for a few seconds, then exhale slowly. Allow 2 minutes between inhalations. Store drug in light-resistant container.
• Inhalant solution can be administered by IPPB diluted in saline solution or by a hand nebulizer at full strength.
• Patient should notify doctor if no response to dosage. Patient should not change dose without medical supervision.

Interactions:
MAO INHIBITORS: may cause severe hypertension (hypertensive crisis). Don't use together.

Special considerations:
• Contraindicated in peripheral or mesenteric thrombosis, pulmonary edema, hypercapnia and acidosis; also during anesthesia with cyclopropane or halogenated hydrocarbon anesthetics. Use cautiously in patients with hypertension, thyroid disease, diabetes, cirrhosis, or malaria, and in those receiving digitalis.

(continued on following page)

NAMES, INDICATIONS AND DOSAGES	SIDE EFFECTS
metaraminol bitartrate *(continued)* **Severe shock:** ADULTS: 0.5 to 5 mg direct I.V. followed by I.V. infusion. **Treatment of hypotension due to shock:** ADULTS: 15 to 100 mg in 500 ml normal saline solution or 5% dextrose in water I.V. infusion. Adjust rate to maintain blood pressure. **All indications:** CHILDREN: 0.01 mg/kg as single I.V. injection; 1 mg/25 ml 5% dextrose in water as I.V. infusion. Adjust rate to maintain blood pressure in normal range. 0.1 mg/kg I.M. as single dose, p.r.n. Allow at least 10 minutes to elapse before increasing dose because maximum effect is not immediately apparent.	supraventricular beats; atrioventricular dissociation. **GI:** nausea, vomiting. **GU:** decreased urinary output. **Metabolic:** hyperglycemia. **Skin:** flushing, pallor, sweating. **Local:** irritation upon extravasation. **Other:** *metabolic acidosis in hypovolemia, increased body temperature, respiratory distress.*
methoxamine hydrochloride **Moderate fall in blood pressure:** ADULTS: 5 to 10 mg I.M. **Paroxysmal supraventricular tachycardia:** ADULTS: 5 to 15 mg I.V. injected slowly. 10 to 20 mg I.M. Allow 15 minutes before additional increased doses to evaluate effects of initial dose and prevent a cumulative effect. **Prevention of hypotension during spinal anesthetic:** ADULTS: 10 to 15 mg I.M. before or with spinal anesthetic. **Support and restoration of blood pressure during anesthesia (including cyclopropane); termination of paroxysmal supraventricular tachycardia; emergency situations; systolic falls below 60 mmHg:** ADULTS: initially, 3 to 5 mg slow I.V. injection, followed by 10 to 15 mg I.M. to prolong effect. CHILDREN: direct I.V. dose is 80 mcg/kg of body weight or 2.5 mg/m^2 of body surface area, injected slowly.	**CNS:** paresthesias, chills, severe headache, restlessness, tremors, dizziness, anxiety, nervousness. **CV:** hypertension, bradycardia, cardiac depression, precordial pain, heart failure in diseased myocardium. **GI:** projectile vomiting. **GU:** urinary urgency, decreased urinary output. **Skin:** gooseflesh, pallor. **Other:** respiratory distress, *metabolic acidosis.*
norepinephrine injection (formerly levarterenol bitartrate) Levophed♦ **To restore blood pressure in acute hypotensive states:** ADULTS: initially, 8 to 12 mcg/minute I.V.	**CNS:** *headache,* anxiety, weakness, dizziness, tremor, restlessness, insomnia. **CV:** bradycardia, severe hypertension, marked increase in peripheral resistance, decreased cardiac output, arrhythmias, *ventricular tachycardia, fibrillation,* bigeminal rhythm, atrioventricular dissociation, precordial pain.

INTERACTIONS AND SPECIAL CONSIDERATIONS

• Not a substitute for blood or fluid volume deficits. Fluid deficit should be replaced before vasopressors are administered.
• Keep solution in light-resistant container, away from heat.
• Large veins should be used as in antecubital fossa, to minimize risk of extravasation, and infusion site watched carefully for signs of extravasation. If it occurs, infusion should be stopped immediately.
• During infusion, blood pressure should be checked every 5 minutes until stabilized; then every 15 minutes; also pulse rates, urinary output, and color and temperature of extremities. Infusion rate should be titrated according to findings.
• A microdrip or infusion pump should be used to regulate infusion flow rate.
• If adverse effects develop, dosage may need to be adjusted or stopped.
• For I.V. therapy, 2-bottle setup should be used so I.V. can run if this drug is stopped.
• Blood pressure should be raised to slightly less than the patient's normal level, avoiding excessive blood pressure response. Rapidly induced hypertensive response can cause acute pulmonary edema, arrhythmias, and cardiac arrest.
• Because of prolonged action, cumulative effect possible. With an excessive vasopressor response, elevated blood pressure may persist after drug is stopped.
• Urinary output may decrease initially, then increase as blood pressure reaches normal. Persistent decreased urinary output should be monitored.
• When discontinuing therapy with this drug, infusion rate should be slowed gradually; vital signs monitored, watching for possible severe drop in blood pressure; and equipment kept nearby to start drug again, if necessary. Pressor therapy should not be reinstated until the systolic blood pressure falls below 70 to 80 mmHg.
• These emergency drugs reverse effects of metaraminol: atropine for reflex bradycardia, phentolamine to decrease vasopressor effects, and propranolol for arrhythmias.
• Patients with diabetes should be monitored; insulin dose may need adjustment.
• Metaraminol should not be mixed with other drugs.

No significant interactions.

Special considerations:
• Contraindicated in patients with severe cardiac disease or in those taking MAO inhibitors; in shock due to myocardial infarction, or peripheral or mesenteric vascular thrombosis; and in elderly or pregnant patients. Use cautiously in hyperthyroidism or hypertension and after use of ergot alkaloids.
• Should not be used with local anesthetics to prolong their effect.
• Not a substitute for blood volume or fluid volume deficit. If deficit exists, should be replaced before vasopressors are given. Hypoxia and acidosis should also be corrected before or during therapy.
• Methoxamine solutions deteriorate after 24 hours. Should be discarded after that time or before if discolored or contain precipitate.
• Has potent, prolonged pressor action. Does not increase cardiac rate or irritability of cyclopropane-sensitized heart.
• Does not stimulate the CNS.
• Response should be monitored by checking blood pressure and adjusting dose accordingly. Blood pressure should be raised to slightly less than normal level. In previously normotensive patients, systolic blood pressure should be maintained at 80 to 100 mmHg; in previously hypertensive patients, systolic blood pressure should be maintained at 30 to 40 mmHg below usual level.
• Side effects may require adjusted or discontinued dosage.
• These emergency drugs reverse effects of methoxamine: atropine for reflex bradycardia and propranolol for arrhythmias.
• Sudden changes in blood pressure and pulse rate should be monitored even after stopping drug.

Interactions:
TRICYCLIC ANTIDEPRESSANTS: when given with sympathomimetics, may cause severe hypertension (hypertensive crisis). Don't give together.

Special considerations:
• Contraindicated in mesenteric or peripheral vascular thrombosis, pregnancy, profound hypoxia, hypercapnia, hypotension from blood volume deficits, or during cyclopropane or halothane anesthesia. Use cautiously in hypertension, hyperthyroidism, severe cardiac disease. Use with extreme caution in patients receiving MAO inhibitors or tricyclic antidepressants.
• Not a substitute for blood or fluid volume deficit. If deficit exists, these should be replaced

(continued on following page)

NAMES, INDICATIONS AND DOSAGES	SIDE EFFECTS
norepinephrine injection *(continued)* infusion, then adjust to maintain normal blood pressure. Average maintenance dose 2 to 4 mcg/minute.	**GU:** *decreased urinary output.* **Metabolic:** *metabolic acidosis,* hyperglycemia, increased glycogenolysis. **Local:** irritation with extravasation. **Other:** fever, respiratory difficulty.
pseudoephedrine hydrochloride Besan, Cenafed, D-Feda, Eltor♦♦, First Sign, Gyrocaps, Novafed, Robidrine♦♦, Ro-Fedrin, Sudabid, Sudafed♦, Sudafed SA **pseudoephedrine sulfate** Afrinol Repetabs **Nasal and eustachian tube decongestant:** ADULTS: 60 mg P.O. q 4 hours. CHILDREN 6 TO 12 YEARS: 30 mg P.O. q 4 hours. Maximum 120 mg/day. CHILDREN 2 TO 6 YEARS: 15 mg P.O. q 4 hours. Maximum 60 mg/day. Extended-relief tablets: ADULTS AND CHILDREN OVER 12 YEARS: 60 to 120 mg P.O. q 12 hours. This form contraindicated for children under 12 years. **Relief of nasal congestion:** ADULTS: 120 mg every 12 hours.	**CNS:** *anxiety,* transient stimulation, tremors, dizziness, headache, insomnia, *nervousness.* **CV:** arrhythmias, *palpitations,* tachycardia. **GI:** anorexia, nausea, vomiting, dry mouth. **GU:** difficulty in urination. **Skin:** pallor.
terbutaline sulfate Brethine, Bricanyl ♦ **Bronchodilator:** ADULTS: 2.5 to 5 mg P.O. q 8 hours; or 0.25 mg S.C. If no improvement in 15 to 30 minutes, repeat dose. Do not exceed 0.5 mg in 4 hours. CHILDREN 12 TO 15 YEARS: 2.5 mg P.O. t.i.d. Not recommended for children under 12 years.	**CNS:** *nervousness, tremors, headache,* drowsiness, sweating. **CV:** palpitations, increased heart rate. **GI:** vomiting, nausea.

INTERACTIONS AND SPECIAL CONSIDERATIONS

before vasopressors are administered.
• Norepinephrine solutions deteriorate after 24 hours. Should be discarded after that time.
• Large vein should be used as in antecubital fossa, to minimize risk of extravasation. Site should be checked frequently for signs of extravasation. Infusion should be stopped immediately if extravasation occurs. Effect may be counteracted by infiltrating area with 5 to 10 mg phentolamine and 10 to 15 ml normal saline solution. Also, blanching along course of infused vein should be checked; may progress to superficial slough. During infusion, blood pressure should be checked every 2 minutes until stabilized; then every 5 minutes. Also, pulse rates, urinary output, and color and temperature of extremities should be monitored and infusion rate titrated according to findings. In previously hypertensive patients, blood pressure should be raised no more than 40 mmHg below preexisting systolic pressure.
• Patient should never be left unattended.
• Use a microdrip or infusion pump to regulate infusion flow rate.
• For I.V. therapy, two-bottle setup with Y-port should be used so I.V. can continue if norepinephrine is stopped.
• If prolonged I.V. therapy needed, injection site should be changed frequently.
• When stopping drug, infusion rate should be slowed gradually and vital signs monitored, even after stopping. Possible severe drop in blood pressure.
• These emergency drugs reverse effects of norepinephrine: atropine for reflex bradycardia; propranolol for arrhythmias; phentolamine for increased vasopressor effects.
• Should be given in dextrose and saline solution; saline alone is not recommended.

Interactions:
MAO INHIBITORS: may cause severe hypertension (hypertensive crisis). Don't use together.

Special considerations:
• Contraindicated in patients with severe hypertension or severe coronary artery disease; in those receiving MAO inhibitors; and in breast-feeding mothers. Use cautiously in hypertension, cardiac disease, glaucoma, hyperthyroidism, or prostatic hypertrophy.
• Patient should stop drug if he becomes unusually restless, and report symptoms promptly.
• Patient should not use over-the-counter products containing ephedrine or other sympathomimetic amines.
• Patient should not take drug within 2 hours of bedtime because it can cause insomnia.
• Dry mouth relieved with sugarless gum or sour hard candy.

Interactions:
MAO INHIBITORS: when given with sympathomimetics, may cause severe hypertension (hypertensive crisis). Don't use together.
PROPRANOLOL AND OTHER BETA BLOCKERS: blocked effects of terbutaline. Monitor patient carefully if used together.

Special considerations:
• Use cautiously in patients with diabetes, hypertension, hyperthyroidism, severe cardiac disease, or cardiac arrhythmias.
• Injection should be protected from light; should not be used if discolored.
• Patient's family should understand why patient is taking drug.
• Subcutaneous injections should be given in lateral deltoid area.
• Tolerance may develop with prolonged use.

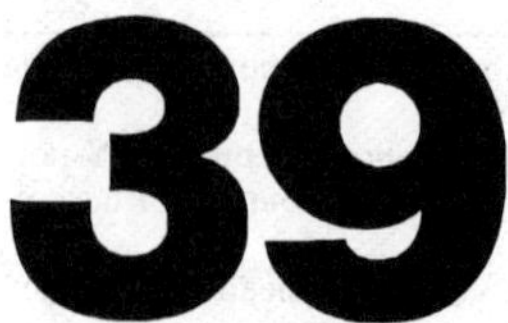

Adrenergic blockers (sympatholytics)

dihydroergotamine mesylate
ergotamine tartrate
methysergide maleate
phenoxybenzamine hydrochloride
phentolamine hydrochloride
phentolamine mesylate
propranolol hydrochloride

Adrenergic blockers inhibit the effects of epinephrine and norepinephrine released from sympathetic nerve endings, as well as the effects of other sympathomimetic amines.

The sympathetic nervous system has two types of receptors: alpha and beta. Stimulation of alpha receptors—located in smooth muscle—causes smooth muscle contraction, such as vasoconstriction and sphincteric and uterine contraction. The alpha blockers are dihydroergotamine, ergotamine, methysergide, phenoxybenzamine, and phentolamine.

Beta receptors are classified as $beta_1$ and $beta_2$. $Beta_1$ receptors—located mainly in the heart—increase heart rate, cardiac contraction, and atrioventricular conduction. $Beta_2$ receptors—in bronchi, blood vessels, and uterus—are responsible for smooth muscle relaxation, such as vasodilation, bronchodilation, and uterine relaxation. Propranolol, a prophylactic in migraine headache, is the only beta blocker discussed in this chapter. For more information on propranolol and the other beta blockers, see Chapter 20, ANTIARRHYTHMICS, and Chapter 21, ANTIHYPERTENSIVES.

Major uses

- Dihydroergotamine, ergotamine, methysergide, and propranolol are effective in prophylaxis and treatment of vascular headaches.
- Phenoxybenzamine is used to treat symptoms of spastic peripheral vascular disease. Both phentolamine and phenoxybenzamine furnish temporary relief of hypertension caused by pheochromocytoma.

Mechanism of action

- Alpha blockers inhibit the effects of epinephrine, norepinephrine, and other sympathomimetic amines on both smooth muscle and exocrine glands, preventing sympathetic stimulation.
- Methysergide specifically blocks serotonin (a neurotransmitter); other alpha blockers may also have some antiserotonin effects.
- Propranolol's beta-blocking action prevents vasodilation of the cerebral arteries.

Absorption, distribution, metabolism, and excretion

Although absorption varies with the specific drug, all adrenergic blockers are widely distributed to organs innervated by the sympathetic nervous system.

- Dihydroergotamine and ergotamine are well absorbed after parenteral administration. Ergotamine is also well absorbed orally, and rapidly and well absorbed sublingually. Distribution, metabolism, and excretion of ergot alkaloids are not completely defined.
- Methysergide and propranolol are well absorbed orally, metabolized in the liver, and excreted in the urine.
- Phenoxybenzamine is variably absorbed when given orally; it is excreted by the kidneys as both the parent compound and inactive metabolites.
- Little is known about phentolamine absorption, distribution, metabolism, and excretion.

DRUG ADVANCES

ANOTHER USE FOR PROPRANOLOL

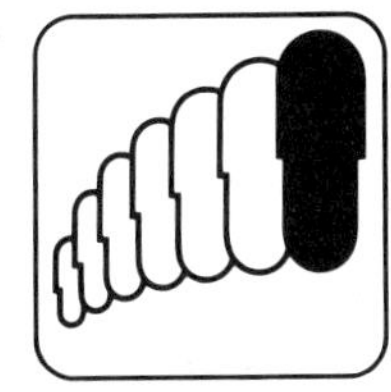

The Food and Drug Administration has approved a new use for propranolol: prevention of migraine headaches.

The benefits of propranolol in migraine therapy were discovered by chance. Migraine sufferers taking propranolol for angina pectoris mentioned to their doctors that they weren't having as many migraine headaches. Therefore doctors theorized that the propranolol lessened migraine attacks.

Subsequent studies showed that two-thirds of all patients with chronic migraine headaches reported good-to-excellent responses when treated with propranolol; for some, the number of headaches was cut in half.

How does propranolol prevent migraine headaches? The most likely cause of migraine headaches is the dilation of cerebral blood vessels. Propranolol's beta-blocking action prevents this vasodilation.

Onset and duration

• Onset of the adrenergic blockers after oral administration varies from 30 minutes for ergot alkaloids to several hours for phenoxybenzamine. Duration of action varies from 3 to 4 hours for the ergot alkaloids, methysergide, and propranolol to 3 to 4 days for phenoxybenzamine and phentolamine.

• Onset after I.M. or subcutaneous injection of ergot alkaloids is 15 to 30 minutes. Onset after I.V. administration (recommended for acute symptomatic episodes) is immediate.

Combination products

ALLYGESIC W/ERGOTAMINE: ergotamine tartrate 1 mg, allobarbital 15 mg, aspirin 150 mg, acetaminophen 100 mg, and aluminum aspirin 100 mg.
CAFERGOT: ergotamine tartrate 1 mg and caffeine 100 mg.
CAFERGOT SUPPOSITORIES: ergotamine tartrate 2 mg and caffeine 100 mg.
CAFERGOT P-B (SUPPOSITORIES): ergotamine tartrate 2 mg, caffeine 100 mg, pentobarbital 30 mg, and levorotatory belladonna alkaloids 0.125 mg.
ERGOCAF: ergotamine tartrate 1 mg and caffeine 100 mg.
MIGRAL: ergotamine tartrate 1 mg, caffeine 50 mg, and cyclizine HCl 25 mg.
WIGRAINE♦: ergotamine tartrate 1 mg, caffeine 100 mg, levorotatory belladonna alkaloids 0.1 mg, and phenacetin 130 mg.
WIGRAINE SUPPOSITORIES: ergotamine tartrate 1 mg, caffeine 100 mg, levorotatory belladonna alkaloids 0.1 mg, and phenacetin 130 mg.

NAMES, INDICATIONS AND DOSAGES	SIDE EFFECTS
dihydroergotamine mesylate D.H.E. 45 **Vascular or migraine headache:** ADULTS: 1 mg I.M. or I.V. May repeat q 1 to 2 hours, p.r.n., up to total of 3 mg. Maximum weekly dose is 6 mg.	**CV:** numbness and tingling in fingers and toes, transient tachycardia or bradycardia, precordial distress and pain, increased arterial pressure. **GI:** nausea, vomiting. **Skin:** itching. **Other:** weakness in legs, muscle pains in extremities, localized edema.
ergotamine tartrate Ergomar♦, Ergostat, Gynergen♦, Medihaler-Ergotamine♦ **Vascular or migraine headache:** ADULTS: initially, 2 mg P.O. S.L., then 1 to 2 mg P.O. q hour or S.L. q ½ hour, to maximum 6 mg daily and 10 mg weekly; or initially, 0.25 mg I.M. or S.C.; repeat in 40 minutes if needed. Maximum dose 0.5 mg/24 hours and 1 mg/week; or 1 inhalation initially, if not relieved in 5 minutes, use another inhalation. May repeat inhalations at least 5 minutes apart up to maximum of 6/24 hours.	**CV:** numbness and tingling in fingers and toes, transient tachycardia or bradycardia, precordial distress and pain, increased arterial pressure, angina pectoris. **GI:** nausea, vomiting, diarrhea, abdominal cramps. **Skin:** itching. **Other:** weakness in legs, muscle pains in extremities, localized edema.
methysergide maleate Sansert♦ **Prevention of frequent, severe, uncontrollable, or disabling migraine or vascular headache:** ADULTS: 2 to 4 mg P.O. b.i.d. with meals.	**Blood:** neutropenia, eosinophilia. **CNS:** insomnia, drowsiness, *euphoria, vertigo,* ataxia, *light-headedness,* hyperesthesia, weakness, *hallucinations or feelings of dissociation.* **CV:** *fibrotic thickening of cardiac valves and aorta, inferior vena cava, and common iliac branches;* vasoconstriction, causing chest pain, abdominal pain, vascular insufficiency of lower limbs; cold, numb, painful extremities with or without paresthesias and diminished or absent pulses; postural hypotension; tachycardia; peripheral edema; murmurs; bruits. **EENT:** nasal stuffiness. **GI:** nausea, vomiting, diarrhea, constipation, epigastric pain. **Skin:** hair loss, dermatitis, sweating, flushing, rash. **Other:** *retroperitoneal fibrosis,* causing general malaise, fatigue, weight gain, backache, low-grade fever, urinary obstruction; *pulmonary fibrosis,* causing dyspnea, tightness and pain in chest, pleural friction rubs and effusion, arthralgia, myalgia.

♦ Available in U.S. and Canada. ♦♦ Available in Canada only.
All other products (no symbol) available in U.S. only. Italicized side effects are common or life-threatening.

INTERACTIONS AND SPECIAL CONSIDERATIONS

Interactions:
PROPRANOLOL AND OTHER BETA BLOCKERS: blocked natural pathway for vasodilation in patients receiving ergot alkaloids and thus could result in excessive vasoconstriction. Watch closely if drugs are used together.

Special considerations:
• Contraindicated in patients with peripheral and occlusive vascular disease, coronary artery disease, hypertension, hepatic or renal dysfunction, sepsis.
• Prolonged administration should be avoided; recommended dosage should not be exceeded.
• Patient should report any feeling of coldness in extremities or tingling of fingers and toes due to vasoconstriction. Severe vasoconstriction may result in tissue damage.
• Most effective when used to prevent migraine or as soon after onset as possible. A quiet, low-light environment should be provided to help patient relax.
• Patient should be helped to evaluate underlying causes of physical or emotional stress, which may precipitate attacks.
• Ampuls should be protected from heat and light. Solution should be discarded if discolored.
• Best results are obtained by adjusting the dose in order to determine the most effective, minimal dose.

Interactions:
PROPRANOLOL AND OTHER BETA BLOCKERS: blocked natural pathway for vasodilation in patients receiving ergot alkaloids and thus could result in excessive vasoconstriction. Watch closely if drugs are used together.

Special considerations:
• Contraindicated in patients with peripheral and occlusive vascular diseases, coronary artery disease, hypertension, hepatic or renal dysfunction, sepsis.
• Prolonged administration should be avoided; recommended dosage should not be exceeded.
• Most effective when used to prevent migraine or as soon after onset as possible.
• A quiet, low-light environment should be provided to help patient relax.
• Patient should be helped to evaluate underlying causes of physical or emotional stress, which may precipitate attacks.
• Patient on long-term therapy should check for and report any feeling of coldness in extremities or tingling of fingers and toes due to vasoconstriction. Severe vasoconstriction may result in tissue damage.
• Store drug in light-resistant container.
• Sublingual tablet is preferred during early stage of attack because of its rapid absorption.
• Patient should not increase dosage without first consulting the doctor.
• An accurate dietary history should be obtained from patient to determine if a relationship exists between certain foods and onset of headache.

No significant interactions.

Special considerations:
• Contraindicated in patients with severe hypertension, arteriosclerosis, peripheral vascular insufficiency, renal or hepatic disease, severe coronary artery diseases, thromboembolic disorders, phlebitis or cellulitis of lower limbs, fibrotic processes, valvular heart disease, and in debilitated patients. Use cautiously in patients with peptic ulcers or suspected coronary artery disease. EKG and cardiac status evaluation advisable before drug is given to patients over 40 years.
• GI effects may be prevented by gradual introduction of medication and by taking with meals.
• Laboratory studies of cardiac and renal function, blood count, and sedimentation rate should be obtained before and during therapy.
• Stop drug every 6 months; then restart after at least 3 or 4 weeks.
• Patient should not stop drug abruptly; may cause rebound headaches. Should be stopped gradually over 2 to 3 weeks.
• Patient should keep daily weight record and report unusually rapid weight gain. He should check for peripheral edema and follow low-salt diet if necessary.
• Drug should be taken for 3 weeks before evaluating effectiveness.
• Patient should report to doctor promptly if he experiences cold, numb, or painful hands and feet; leg cramps when walking; pelvic, chest, or flank pain.
• Not for treatment of migraine or vascular headache in progress, or for treatment of tension (muscle contraction) headaches.
• Indicated only for patients who are unresponsive to other drugs and who can be kept under close medical supervision.

NAMES, INDICATIONS AND DOSAGES	SIDE EFFECTS
phenoxybenzamine hydrochloride Dibenzyline **To control or prevent hypertension and sweating associated with pheochromocytoma; Raynaud's syndrome; frostbite; acrocyanosis:** ADULTS: initially, 10 mg P.O., then increase by 10 mg q 4 days to a maximum of 60 mg daily.	**CNS:** sedation, fatigue, lassitude. **CV:** tachycardia, *postural hypotension with dizziness.* **EENT:** miosis, nasal congestion. **GI:** irritation. **GU:** inhibition of ejaculation.
phentolamine hydrochloride Regitine, Rogitine♦♦ **phentolamine mesylate** **To control or prevent hypertension before or during pheochromocytomectomy:** ADULTS: 50 to 100 mg P.O. 4 to 6 times daily; or 5 mg I.M. or I.V. 1 to 2 hours preoperatively. May repeat if needed. During surgery, 5 mg I.V. may be given as needed. CHILDREN: 25 mg P.O. daily, divided q 4 to 6 hours; or 1 mg I.M. or I.V. 1 to 2 hours preoperatively. May repeat if needed. During surgery, 1 mg I.V. may be given as needed. *To treat extravasation*—infiltrate area with 5 to 10 mg phentolamine in 10 ml normal saline solution. Must be done within 12 hours.	**CV:** acute and prolonged hypotension, tachycardia, cardiac arrhythmia, angina, orthostatic hypotension, flushing. **EENT:** nasal congestion. **GI:** nausea, vomiting, diarrhea, exacerbation of peptic ulcer.
propranolol hydrochloride Inderal♦ **Prevention of frequent, severe, uncontrollable, or disabling migraine or vascular headache:** ADULTS: initially, 80 mg daily in divided doses. Usual maintenance dose: 160 to 240 mg daily, divided t.i.d. or q.i.d.	**CNS:** *fatigue, lethargy,* vivid dreams, hallucinations. **CV:** *bradycardia, hypotension, congestive heart failure,* peripheral vascular disease. **GI:** nausea, vomiting, diarrhea. **Metabolic:** hypoglycemia without symptoms. **Skin:** rash. **Other:** *increased airway resistance,* fever.

INTERACTIONS AND SPECIAL CONSIDERATIONS

No significant interactions.

Special considerations:

- Contraindicated whenever a fall in blood pressure is undesirable. Use cautiously in cerebral or coronary arteriosclerosis, renal damage, or respiratory disease.
- May aggravate symptoms of respiratory infections.
- Safe use in pregnancy has not been established, but drug has been used during the third trimester to treat hypertension caused by pheochromocytoma without apparent harm to mother or fetus.
- Gastric irritation may be reduced by taking with milk or in divided doses.
- Patient should change position slowly to prevent possible hypotension. Patient should dangle his legs for a few minutes before standing if he has been lying down.
- Overdosed patient should be placed in Trendelenburg position. Hypotension should be treated with I.V. infusion of norepinephrine.
- Full therapeutic effect may not be seen for several weeks.
- Store drug in airtight containers, protected from light.

No significant interactions.

Special considerations:

- Contraindicated in angina, coronary artery disease, or in history of myocardial infarction. Use with caution in gastritis or peptic ulcer.
- If cardiac arrhythmias occur, digitalis glycosides should not be given until cardiac rhythm returns to normal.
- Overdosed patient should be placed in Trendelenburg position. Hypotension should be treated with I.V. infusion of norepinephrine.
- Blood pressure should be monitored closely, especially after parenteral administration. Patient should be in supine position when receiving drug parenterally.
- To reconstitute injection, 1 ml sterile water for injection should be added to 5-mg vial of drug. Should be used immediately after reconstitution.

Interactions:

INSULIN, HYPOGLYCEMIC DRUGS (ORAL): can alter requirements for these drugs in previously stabilized diabetics. Monitor for hypoglycemia.
CARDIOTONIC GLYCOSIDES: excessive bradycardia and increased depressant effect on myocardium. Monitor pulse rate.
AMINOPHYLLINE: antagonized beta-blocking effects of propranolol. Use together cautiously.
ISOPROTERENOL, GLUCAGON: antagonized propranolol effect. May be used therapeutically and in emergencies.
CIMETIDINE: inhibits propranolol's metabolism. Monitor for greater beta-blocking effect.
EPINEPHRINE: severe vasoconstriction. Monitor blood pressure and observe patient carefully.

Special considerations:

- Contraindicated in diabetes mellitus, asthma, or allergic rhinitis; during ethyl ether anesthesia; in sinus bradycardia and in heart block greater than first degree; in cardiogenic shock; in right ventricular failure secondary to pulmonary hypertension. Use with caution in congestive heart failure or respiratory disease.
- Withdraw drug slowly in patients with coronary artery disease. Abrupt withdrawal might precipitate myocardial infarction or aggravate angina or pheochromocytoma. Abrupt withdrawal in thyrotoxicosis may exacerbate hyperthyroidism or precipitate thyroid storm. In thyrotoxicosis, propranolol may mask signs of hyperthyroidism.
- Should not be stopped before surgery for pheochromocytoma. Before any surgical procedure, anesthesiologist should be notified patient is on propranolol.
- Blood pressure should be monitored frequently. Patient should notify doctor if he develops excessive hypotension. Orthostatic hypotension can be minimized by rising slowly and avoiding sudden position changes.
- This drug masks common signs of shock and hypoglycemia.

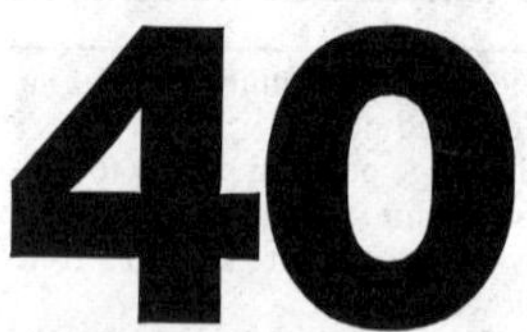

Skeletal muscle relaxants

baclofen
carisoprodol
chlorphenesin carbamate
chlorzoxazone
cyclobenzaprine
dantrolene sodium
metaxalone
methocarbamol
orphenadrine citrate

Skeletal muscle relaxants can be divided into two categories: those routinely used to treat painful muscle spasms associated with acute, self-limiting conditions, such as lower back pain, and those used to treat more serious skeletal muscle spasticity associated with disease, such as multiple sclerosis, or spasticity secondary to spinal cord transection. The first category includes all the above drugs except baclofen and dantrolene, the more powerful drugs of the second category. These drugs must not be used in trivial situations, but only for their appropriate indications. None of the skeletal muscle relaxants is effective in treating rigidity due to parkinsonism.

Major uses

- Baclofen treats spasticity of multiple sclerosis. It is not recommended for spasticity secondary to stroke or cerebral palsy.
- Carisoprodol, chlorphenesin, chlorzoxazone, cyclobenzaprine, metaxalone, methocarbamol, and orphenadrine are used as adjuncts in the treatment of painful musculoskeletal disorders.
- Oral dantrolene is used to treat spasticity in paraplegia and hemiplegia; the I.V. form controls malignant hyperthermia.

Mechanism of action

- Baclofen's mechanism of action is unclear.
- Carisoprodol, chlorphenesin, chlorzoxazone, cyclobenzaprine, metaxalone, methocarbamol, and orphenadrine reduce transmission of impulses from the spinal cord to skeletal muscle.
- Dantrolene acts directly on skeletal muscle to interfere with intracellular calcium movement.

Absorption, distribution, metabolism, and excretion

All skeletal muscle relaxants are well absorbed after oral administration; all the parenteral forms except dantrolene are well absorbed after I.M. administration. (The parenteral form of dantrolene should be given only by I.V. infusion.) These drugs are widely distributed in body tissues, with high concentrations in the brain. Metabolized in the liver, they are excreted by the kidneys as both unchanged parent compound and metabolites.

Onset and duration

Onset is generally between 30 and 60 minutes, and blood levels peak in 2 to 3 hours. Duration is 4 to 6 hours.

Combination products

NORGESIC: orphenadrine citrate 25 mg, aspirin 225 mg, phenacetin 160 mg, caffeine 30 mg.
NORGESIC FORTE: orphenadrine citrate 50 mg, aspirin 450 mg, phenacetin 320 mg, and caffeine 60 mg.

DANTROLENE CONTROLS MALIGNANT HYPERTHERMIA

Malignant hyperthermia—also known as malignant hyperpyrexia—occurs when a genetically susceptible patient is exposed to inhalation anesthetics. Standard presurgery screening (taking the patient's history, for example) may not detect patients predisposed to this condition. Since 1962, when malignant hyperthermia was first recognized, researchers have concentrated on finding the treatment for this rare but deadly condition. Both procainamide and dantrolene sodium have been studied for their usefulness in controlling malignant hyperthermia, but only dantrolene (I.V.) has proved successful enough to be approved for this use.

How does dantrolene work during a malignant hyperthermia crisis? The crisis begins when an inhalation anesthetic, such as halothane, is administered to a susceptible patient. This patient apparently has a defect in his muscle cell membranes that allows the anesthetic to trigger a sudden rise of calcium within muscle cells.

The increased amount of calcium sets off a series of biochemical reactions that increase the metabolic rate, eventually liberating heat. Muscle contractions also increase, liberating more heat.

The most consistent early symptom of malignant hyperthermia is sudden, unexplained tachycardia. The patient's temperature rises, ranging from 39° to 42° C. (102.2° to 107.6° F.). Rapid breathing, cyanotic mottling of the skin, hypotension, acidosis, muscle rigidity, and cardiac arrhythmias usually follow, causing even more calcium to flow into the muscle cells. If this cycle continues uninterrupted, the patient dies.

Dantrolene presumably breaks the cycle by interfering with the release of calcium ions within the muscle fiber. If this drug is administered before bradycardia or cardiac arrest develops, the patient will probably recover.

During and after a malignant hyperthermia crisis, patient care should focus on three major problems: elevated temperature, anoxia, and tachycardia. Here's a summary:

For elevated temperature:
- Monitor temperature.
- Initiate cooling measures with a light cover, sponging, or hypothermia blanket, depending on your orders.
- Keep the patient clean and dry. Provide good mouth care.
- Increase fluids.
- Observe seizure precautions.
- Assess neurologic function.

For anoxia:
- Monitor respirations.
- Administer oxygen.
- Limit the patient's activity.

For tachycardia:
- Monitor apical pulse rate.
- Assess the patient's cardiovascular system.
- Limit the patient's activity.

Before discharge, the patient should understand what happened. He should be advised to wear a medical identification bracelet or necklace that will inform others of his susceptibility to malignant hyperthermia in case of an emergency.

PARAFON FORTE♦: chlorzoxazone 250 mg and acetaminophen 300 mg.
ROBAXISAL♦: methocarbamol 400 mg and aspirin 325 mg.
SOMA COMPOUND♦: carisoprodol 200 mg, phenacetin 160 mg, and caffeine 32 mg.
SOMA COMPOUND WITH CODEINE: carisoprodol 200 mg, phenacetin 160 mg, caffeine 32 mg, and codeine phosphate 16 mg.

NAMES, INDICATIONS AND DOSAGES	SIDE EFFECTS
baclofen Lioresal **Spasticity in multiple sclerosis, spinal cord injury:** ADULTS: initially, 5 mg t.i.d. for 3 days, 10 mg t.i.d. for 3 days, 15 mg t.i.d. for 3 days, 20 mg t.i.d. for 3 days. Increase according to response up to maximum 80 mg daily.	**CNS:** *drowsiness, dizziness,* headache, *weakness, fatigue,* confusion, insomnia. **CV:** hypotension. **EENT:** nasal congestion. **GI:** *nausea,* constipation. **GU:** urinary frequency. **Hepatic:** increased SGOT, alkaline phosphatase. **Metabolic:** hyperglycemia. **Skin:** rash, pruritus. **Other:** ankle edema, excessive perspiration, weight gain.
carisoprodol Rela♦, Soma♦ **As an adjunct in acute, painful musculoskeletal conditions:** ADULTS AND CHILDREN OVER 12 YEARS: 350 mg P.O. t.i.d. and at bedtime. Not recommended for children under 12 years.	**CNS:** *drowsiness, dizziness,* vertigo, ataxia, tremor, agitation, irritability, headache, depressive reactions, insomnia. **CV:** orthostatic hypotension, tachycardia, facial flushing. **GI:** nausea, vomiting, hiccups, increased bowel activity, epigastric distress. **Skin:** rash, *erythema multiforme,* pruritus. **Other:** asthmatic episodes, fever, angioneurotic edema, *anaphylaxis.*
chlorphenesin carbamate Maolate **As an adjunct in short-term, acute, painful musculoskeletal conditions:** ADULTS: initial dose 800 mg P.O. t.i.d. Maintenance 400 mg P.O. q.i.d. for maximum of 8 weeks.	**Blood:** blood dyscrasia. **CNS:** *drowsiness, dizziness,* confusion, headache, weakness. Dose-related side effects include paradoxical stimulation, agitation, insomnia, nervousness, headache. **GI:** *nausea, epigastric distress.* **Other:** *anaphylaxis.*
chlorzoxazone Paraflex **As an adjunct in acute, painful musculoskeletal conditions:** ADULTS: 250 to 750 mg t.i.d. or q.i.d. CHILDREN: 20 mg/kg daily divided t.i.d. or q.i.d.	**CNS:** *drowsiness, dizziness, light-headedness,* malaise, headache, overstimulation. **GI:** anorexia, nausea, vomiting, heartburn, abdominal distress, constipation, diarrhea. **GU:** urine discoloration (orange or purple-red). **Hepatic:** liver dysfunction. **Skin:** urticaria, redness, itching, petechiae, bruising.
cyclobenzaprine Flexeril♦ **Short-term treatment of muscle spasm:** ADULTS: 10 mg P.O. t.i.d. for 7 days. Maximum: 60 mg/day for 2 to 3 weeks.	**CNS:** *drowsiness,* euphoria, weakness, headache, insomnia, nightmares, paresthesias, dizziness. **CV:** tachycardia. **EENT:** blurred vision. **GI:** abdominal pain, dyspepsia, peculiar taste, constipation, dry mouth. **GU:** urinary retention.

♦ Available in U.S. and Canada. ♦♦ Available in Canada only.
All other products (no symbol) available in U.S. only. Italicized side effects are common or life-threatening.

INTERACTIONS AND SPECIAL CONSIDERATIONS

No significant interactions.

Special considerations:
- Use cautiously in patients with impaired renal function, stroke (minimal benefit, poor tolerance), epilepsy, and when spasticity is used to maintain motor functions.
- Should be taken with meals or milk to prevent gastric distress.
- Amount of relief determines if dosage (and drowsiness) can be reduced.
- Patient should avoid activities that require alertness until CNS response to drug is determined. Drowsiness is usually transient.
- Increased seizures in epileptics possible.
- Sensitivity reactions such as fever, skin eruptions, and respiratory distress are possible.
- Patient should follow doctor's orders regarding rest and physical therapy.
- Drug should not be withdrawn abruptly unless required by severe side effects. May precipitate hallucinations or rebound spasticity.
- Overdosage treatment supportive only; emesis should not be induced or respiratory stimulant used in obtunded patients.
- Used investigationally for treatment of unstable bladder.

No significant interactions.

Special considerations:
- Contraindicated in hypersensitivity to related compounds (including meprobamate or tybamate); or intermittent porphyria. Use with caution in impaired hepatic or renal function.
- Possible idiosyncratic reactions after first to fourth dose (weakness, ataxia, visual and speech difficulties, fever, skin eruptions, mental changes) or severe reactions, including bronchospasm, hypotension, anaphylactic shock. Immediate discontinuation and reevaluation of therapy required.
- Amount of relief determines whether dosage can be reduced.
- Patient should avoid activities that require alertness until CNS response to drug is determined. Drowsiness is transient.
- Should not be combined with alcohol or other depressants.
- Patient should follow doctor's orders regarding rest and physical therapy.
- Mild withdrawal symptoms (such as insomnia, headache, nausea, abdominal cramps) may occur if drug is stopped abruptly.
- For treatment of anaphylaxis, see APPENDIX.

No significant interactions.

Special considerations:
- Use cautiously in hepatic disease or impaired renal function.
- Safe use for periods exceeding 8 weeks not established.
- Should be taken with meals or milk to prevent gastric distress.
- Amount of relief determines if dosage (and drowsiness) can be reduced.
- Possible sensitivity reactions such as fever, skin eruptions, and respiratory distress. Patient should hold dose and report any unusual reactions.
- Blood studies should be monitored.
- Unusual bleeding and infectious problems may indicate blood dyscrasia.
- For treatment of anaphylaxis, see APPENDIX.

No significant interactions.

Special considerations:
- Contraindicated in impaired hepatic function. Use cautiously in patients with history of drug allergies.
- Amount of relief determines whether dosage can be reduced.
- Signs of hepatic dysfunction require immediate discontinuation and reevaluation of therapy.
- Patient should avoid activities that require alertness until CNS response to drug is determined. Drowsiness is transient.
- Should not be combined with alcohol or other depressants.
- Patient should expect urine color to change.
- Patient should follow doctor's orders regarding rest and physical therapy.
- Should be taken with meals or milk to prevent gastric distress.

No significant interactions.

Special considerations:
- Contraindicated in patients who have received MAO inhibitors within 14 days; during acute recovery phase of myocardial infarction; and in heart block, arrhythmias, conduction disturbances, or congestive heart failure. Use cautiously in patients with urinary retention, narrow-angle glaucoma, increased intraocular pressure, cardiovascular disease, impaired hepatic function, seizures; and in elderly or debilitated patients.
- Withdrawal symptoms (nausea, headache, malaise) may occur if drug stopped abruptly after long-term therapy.
- Symptoms of overdose, including possible cardiotoxicity, should be reported. Physostig-

(continued on following page)

NAMES, INDICATIONS AND DOSAGES	SIDE EFFECTS
cyclobenzaprine *(continued)*	**Skin:** rash, urticaria, pruritus. **Other:** in high doses, watch for side effects like those of other tricyclic drugs (amitriptyline, imipramine).
dantrolene sodium Dantrium♦, Dantrium I.V. **Spasticity and sequelae secondary to severe chronic disorders (multiple sclerosis, cerebral palsy, spinal cord injury, stroke):** ADULTS: 25 mg P.O. daily. Increase gradually in increments of 25 mg, up to 100 mg b.i.d. to q.i.d. to maximum of 400 mg/day for 4 to 7 days. CHILDREN: 1 mg/kg/day P.O. b.i.d. to q.i.d. Increase gradually as needed by 1 mg/kg/day to maximum of 100 mg q.i.d. **Management of malignant hyperthermia:** ADULTS AND CHILDREN: 1 mg/kg I.V. initially; may repeat dose up to cumulative dose of 10 mg/kg.	**Blood:** eosinophilia. **CNS:** *muscle weakness, drowsiness,* dizziness, light-headedness, malaise, headache, confusion, nervousness, insomnia. **CV:** tachycardia, blood pressure changes. **EENT:** excessive tearing, visual disturbances. **GI:** anorexia, constipation, cramping, dysphagia, *severe diarrhea.* **GU:** urinary frequency, incontinence, nocturia, dysuria, crystalluria, difficulty achieving erection. **Hepatic:** *hepatitis.* **Skin:** eczematoid eruption, pruritus, urticaria, photosensitivity. **Other:** abnormal hair growth, drooling, sweating, pleural effusion, myalgia, chills, fever.
metaxalone Skelaxin♦ **As an adjunct in acute, painful musculoskeletal conditions:** ADULTS AND CHILDREN OVER 12 YEARS: 800 mg P.O. t.i.d. or q.i.d.	**Blood:** leukopenia, hemolytic anemia. **CNS:** *drowsiness,* dizziness, headache, nervousness, irritability, exacerbation of grand mal epilepsy. **GI:** *nausea, vomiting.* **Hepatic:** jaundice. **Skin:** light rash with or without pruritus.
methocarbamol Delaxin, Forbaxin, Metho-500, Robamol, Robaxin♦, Romethocarb, SK-Methocarbamol, Spenaxin **As an adjunct in acute, painful musculoskeletal conditions:** ADULTS: 1.5 g P.O. for 2 to 3 days, then 1 g P.O. q.i.d., or not more than 500 mg (5 ml) I.M. into each gluteal region. May repeat q 8 hours. Or 1 to 3 g/day (10 to 30 ml) I.V. directly into vein at 3 ml/minute, or 10 ml may be added to no more than 250 ml of 5% dextrose in water or normal saline solution. Maximum dose 3 g/day.	**Blood:** hemolysis, increased hemoglobin (I.V. only). **CNS:** drowsiness, dizziness, light-headedness, headache, vertigo, mild muscular incoordination (I.M. or I.V. only), convulsions (I.V. only). **CV:** hypotension, bradycardia (I.M. or I.V. only). **GI:** *nausea, anorexia, GI upset.* **GU:** red blood cells in urine (I.V. only), discoloration of urine. **Skin:** urticaria, pruritus, rash. **Local:** thrombophlebitis, extravasation (I.V. only). **Other:** fever, metallic taste, flushing, *anaphylactic reactions (I.M. or I.V. only).*

INTERACTIONS AND SPECIAL CONSIDERATIONS

mine should be available.
• Intake and output should be checked; urinary retention possible. Constipation may be treated with increased fluid intake and a stool softener.
• Patient should avoid activities that require alertness until CNS response to drug is known. Drowsiness and dizziness usually subside after 2 weeks.
• Alcohol or other depressants should not be combined with cyclobenzaprine.
• Dry mouth relieved with sugarless candy or gum.

No significant interactions.

Special considerations:
The following are considerations for the oral form only:
• Contraindicated when spasticity is used to maintain motor function; in spasms in rheumatic disorders; lactation. Use with caution in patients with severely impaired cardiac or pulmonary function or preexisting hepatic disease; and in females and all patients over 35 years.
• Safety and efficacy in long-term use not established; value may be determined by therapeutic trial. Should not be given more than 45 days if no benefits observed.
• Should be taken with meals or milk to prevent gastric distress.
• Oral suspension prepared for single dose by dissolving capsule contents in juice or other suitable liquid. For multiple dose, acid vehicle used, such as citric acid in USP Syrup; should be refrigerated and used within several days.
• Amount of relief determines whether dosage can be reduced.
• Hepatitis (fever, jaundice), severe diarrhea or weakness, or sensitivity reactions (fever, skin eruptions) require immediate discontinuation and reevaluation of therapy.
• Patient should avoid activities that require alertness until CNS response to drug is determined. Side effects should subside after 4 days.
• Patient should avoid combining with alcohol or other depressants; avoid photosensitivity reactions by using sunscreening agents and protective clothing; report abdominal discomfort or GI problems immediately; and follow doctor's orders regarding rest and physical therapy.

The following are considerations for the I.V. form only:
• Should be administered as soon as malignant hyperthermia reaction is recognized.
• Each vial should be reconstituted by adding 60 ml of sterile water for injection and shaking vial until clear.
• Contents should be protected from light and used within 6 hours.

No significant interactions.

Special considerations:
• Contraindicated in patients with impaired hepatic or renal function and in those with a history of drug-induced hemolytic or other anemias.
• Hepatic function should be tested periodically. May cause abnormalities in liver function studies; tests should be repeated after drug discontinued.
• Amount of relief determines if dosage can be reduced.
• Sensitivity reactions, such as rash with pruritus, possible.
• Patient should avoid combining with alcohol or other depressants.
• Patient should follow doctor's orders regarding rest and physical therapy.
• Should be taken with meals or milk to prevent gastric distress.
• False-positive results in glucose tests if cupric sulfate is used. Glucose oxidase should be used instead.

No significant interactions.

Special considerations:
• Contraindicated in patients with impaired renal function (injectable form), epilepsy (injection form); in children under 12 years (except in tetanus); and in patients receiving anticholinesterase agents.
• I.V. irritates veins, may cause phlebitis, aggravates seizures, may cause fainting if injected rapidly.
• In tetanus management, methocarbamol should be used with tetanus antitoxin, penicillin, tracheotomy, and aggressive supportive care. Long course of I.V. methocarbamol required.
• Possible sensitivity reactions such as fever and skin eruptions.
• Patient should avoid activities that require alertness until CNS response to drug is determined. Drowsiness subsides.
• Should not be combined with alcohol or other depressants.
• Patient should follow doctor's orders regarding rest and physical therapy.
• Urine may turn green, black, or brown.
• Should be given with meals or milk to prevent gastric distress.
• Orthostatic hypotension possible, especially with parenteral administration. Patient should remain supine for 15 minutes afterward and get up slowly.
• Should be given slow I.V. Maximum rate 300 mg (3 ml)/minute; should be given deep I.M., only in upper outer quadrant of buttocks,

(continued on following page)

NAMES, INDICATIONS AND DOSAGES	SIDE EFFECTS
methocarbamol *(continued)* **Supportive therapy in tetanus management:** ADULTS: 1 to 2 g into tubing of running I.V. or 1 to 3 g in infusion bottle q 6 hours. CHILDREN: 15 mg/kg I.V. q 6 hours.	
orphenadrine citrate Banflex, Flexon, Myolin, Norflex♦, Ro-Orphena, Tega-Flex, X-Otag **Adjunctive treatment in painful, acute musculoskeletal conditions:** ADULTS: 100 mg P.O. b.i.d., or 60 mg I.V. or I.M. q 12 hours, p.r.n.	**CNS:** disorientation, restlessness, irritability, weakness, *drowsiness*, headache. **CV:** palpitations, tachycardia. **EENT:** dilated pupils, blurred vision, difficulty swallowing. **GI:** constipation, *dry mouth*, nausea, vomiting, paralytic ileus, epigastric distress. **GU:** urinary hesitancy or retention.

♦ Available in U.S. and Canada. ♦♦ Available in Canada only.
All other products (no symbol) available in U.S. only. Italicized side effects are common or life-threatening.

INTERACTIONS AND SPECIAL CONSIDERATIONS

with maximum of 5 ml in each buttock, and injected slowly; should not be given subcutaneously.
• Epinephrine, antihistamines, and corticosteroids should be available.
• Liquid prepared by crushing tablets into water or saline solution and given through nasogastric tube.
• WBC count should be obtained periodically during prolonged therapy.
• For treatment of anaphylaxis, see APPENDIX.

No significant interactions.

Special considerations:
• Contraindicated in patients with narrow-angle glaucoma; prostatic hypertrophy; pyloric, duodenal, or bladder-neck obstruction; myasthenia gravis; tachycardia; severe hepatic or renal disease; ulcerative colitis. Use cautiously in elderly or debilitated patients with cardiac disease or arrhythmias; and in those exposed to high temperatures.
• All dosages should be checked carefully. Even a slight overdose can lead to toxicity. Early signs are excessive dry mouth, dilated pupils, blurred vision, skin flushing, fever.
• Vital signs should be monitored carefully.
• When given I.V., may cause paradoxical initial bradycardia. Usually disappears in 2 minutes.
• Intake and output should be monitored. Causes urinary retention and hesitancy; patient should void before drug is administered.
• Dry mouth relieved with cool drinks, ice chips, sugarless gum, or hard candy.
• Patient may develop a tolerance to this drug.

41

Neuromuscular blockers

decamethonium bromide
gallamine triethiodide
hexafluorenium bromide
metocurine iodide
pancuronium bromide
succinylcholine chloride
tubocurarine chloride

Neuromuscular blockers are sometimes called peripherally acting skeletal muscle relaxants. They must be used parenterally (unlike the centrally acting skeletal muscle relaxants in Chapter 40 that are commonly given orally).

Potentially dangerous drugs, neuromuscular blockers should be administered either by a doctor or under his direct supervision. They effectively paralyze skeletal muscle, thereby reducing anesthetic requirements and facilitating manipulation during surgery. However, because they also paralyze muscles essential for respiration (diaphragm and intercostals), mechanical ventilatory support must be available whenever they're administered.

Major uses

Neuromuscular blockers potentiate surgical anesthetics, allowing use of a lighter level of anesthesia. They facilitate intubation, abdominal surgical procedures, correction of dislocations, and setting of fractures.

They're also used to control respirations of patients on mechanical ventilators, muscle contraction in electroconvulsive therapy, and muscle spasms in convulsive states (tetanus, status epilepticus, drug intoxication, and black widow spider bites).

- Hexafluorenium enhances the action of succinylcholine.
- Tubocurarine aids differential diagnosis of myasthenia gravis.

Mechanism of action

These agents block transmission of nerve impulses at the skeletal neuromuscular junction by one of two mechanisms:

- Decamethonium and succinylcholine (depolarizing agents) prolong depolarization of the muscle end-plate. (Hexafluorenium inhibits the enzymatic breakdown of succinylcholine, prolonging its duration.)
- Gallamine, metocurine, pancuronium, and tubocurarine (nondepolarizing agents) prevent acetylcholine from binding to the receptors on the muscle end-plate, thus blocking depolarization.

Absorption, distribution, metabolism, and excretion

Neuromuscular blockers are ineffective orally because they're poorly absorbed from the gastrointestinal tract; they're slowly and unpredictably absorbed from I.M. injection sites. Rapidly distributed from I.V. sites, these drugs (except succinylcholine) are poorly metabolized and remain effective in the body until they're eliminated in urine and—through the bile—in feces as unchanged drug.

- Succinylcholine is hydrolyzed by pseudocholinesterase in the blood and liver.

Onset and duration

- Decamethonium has an onset of 1 to 3 minutes after I.V. administration and a duration of 4 to 8 minutes. Recovery occurs 15 to 20 minutes after injection.

WHERE NEUROMUSCULAR BLOCKING AGENTS ACT

Neuromuscular blocking agents block acetylcholine at the neuromuscular synapse. Here's how they work:

The basic unit of the nervous system is the nerve cell or neuron. It consists of a central cell body and threadlike projections of cytoplasm known as nerve fibers. These are of two types: the axon, which conducts impulses away from the cell body, and the dendrite, which conducts impulses to the cell body. Most neurons have multiple dendrites and a single axon.

Axons are surrounded by a white fatty substance called myelin, which insulates and protects the delicate inner fiber.

Neurons receive and transmit impulses at junctions called synapses, where one structure almost touches another. When information flows, one of the structures releases acetylcholine, a transmitting chemical that crosses the narrow cleft between them and activates the receiving cell. This is where the synapse is blocked.

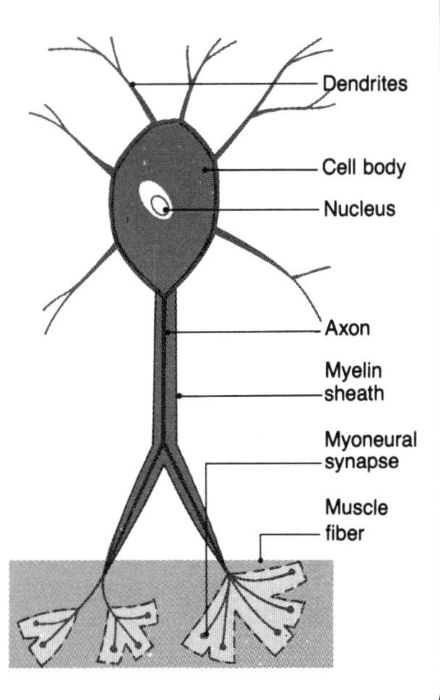

- Gallamine begins to work within 1 to 3 minutes after I.V. administration; its peak effect occurs in about 3 minutes. Duration of action depends on total dosage and number of doses administered.
- Hexafluorenium takes effect rapidly after I.V. administration; its action lasts 15 to 30 minutes.
- Metocurine and tubocurarine take effect within 1 to 3 minutes after I.V. administration; duration is 25 to 90 minutes. The drugs accumulate after repeated doses.
- Pancuronium's onset occurs within a few minutes after I.V. administration. Its duration is 25 to 60 minutes, or more prolonged when large doses are given.
- Succinylcholine, administered I.V., takes effect in 1 to 3 minutes; its duration is only 5 minutes but can be prolonged when used with hexafluorenium.

Combination products
None.

NAMES, INDICATIONS AND DOSAGES	SIDE EFFECTS
decamethonium bromide Syncurine♦ **Adjunct to anesthetic to induce skeletal muscle relaxation; facilitate intubation, lessen muscle contractions in pharmacologically or electrically induced convulsions; assist with mechanical ventilation:** Dose depends on anesthetic used, individual needs, and response. Doses are representative and must be adjusted. ADULTS: initially, 0.5 to 3 mg I.V., at a rate of 0.5 mg to 1 mg/minute, then 0.5 to 1 mg q 10 to 30 minutes for sustained relaxation. CHILDREN AND INFANTS: initially, 0.05 to 0.08 mg/kg I.V., then 0.02 to 0.03 mg/kg at 10- to 30-minute intervals.	**CV:** bradycardia, tachycardia, hypotension and hypertension. **Other:** *dose-related prolonged apnea,* residual muscle weakness, increased oropharyngeal secretions, allergic or idiosyncratic hypersensitivity reactions, *postoperative muscle pain.*
gallamine triethiodide Flaxedil♦ **Adjunct to anesthetic to induce skeletal muscle relaxation; facilitate intubation; reduction of fractures and dislocations; lessen muscle contractions in pharmacologically or electrically induced convulsions; assist with mechanical ventilation:** Dose depends on anesthetic used, individual needs, and response. Doses are representative and must be adjusted. ADULTS AND CHILDREN OVER 1 MONTH: initially, 1 mg/kg I.V. to maximum of 100 mg, regardless of patient's weight; then 0.5 mg to 1 mg/kg q 30 to 40 minutes. CHILDREN UNDER 1 MONTH BUT OVER 5 KG (11 LB): initially, 0.25 to 0.75 mg/kg I.V., then 0.01 to 0.05 mg/kg q 30 to 40 minutes.	**CV:** tachycardia. **Other:** *respiratory paralysis, dose-related prolonged apnea,* residual muscle weakness, increased oropharyngeal secretions, allergic or idiosyncratic hypersensitivity reactions.
hexafluorenium bromide Mylaxen **Adjunct for use with succinylcholine to prolong neuromuscular blockade and reduce muscular fasciculations:**	**CNS:** *prolonged neuromuscular blockade.* **CV:** hypotension, hypertension, tachycardia, bradycardia. **EENT:** increased intraocular pressure. **Other:** increased bronchial tone, *bronchospasm.*

INTERACTIONS AND SPECIAL CONSIDERATIONS

Interactions:
AMINOGLYCOSIDE ANTIBIOTICS (INCLUDING AMIKACIN, GENTAMICIN, KANAMYCIN, NEOMYCIN, STREPTOMYCIN); POLYMYXIN ANTIBIOTICS (POLYMYXIN B SULFATE, COLISTIN); CLINDAMYCIN, QUINIDINE: potentiated neuromuscular blockade, leading to increased skeletal muscle relaxation and possible respiratory paralysis. Use cautiously during surgical and postoperative periods.
NARCOTIC ANALGESICS: potentiated neuromuscular blockade, leading to increased skeletal muscle relaxation and possible respiratory paralysis. Use with extreme caution.

Special considerations:
• Contraindicated in hypersensitivity to bromides, impaired renal function, shock, myasthenia gravis, surgical procedures lasting longer than 20 minutes. Use cautiously in patients undergoing surgery in Trendelenburg or lithotomy positions; in patients recently digitalized; elderly or debilitated patients; and in hepatic or pulmonary impairment, respiratory depression, myasthenic syndrome of lung cancer, dehydration, thyroid disorders, collagen disease, porphyria, electrolyte disturbances, fractures, muscle spasms, and (in large doses) cesarean section.
• Seldom used due to uncertain effects and lack of suitable antidote.
• Multiple doses not often recommended; may cause reduced response and prolonged apnea.
• Baseline electrolyte determinations (electrolyte imbalance, especially potassium, calcium, and magnesium, can potentiate neuromuscular effects) and vital signs, especially respiration, should be monitored.
• Intake and output should be measured; renal dysfunction prolongs duration of action, since drug is unchanged before excretion.
• Clear airway should be maintained and emergency respiratory support (endotracheal equipment, respirator, oxygen, atropine, neostigmine, or edrophonium) kept available.
• Postoperative stiffness is normal and will soon subside.
• Only fresh solutions should be used.
• Should be given slow I.V. (not more than 1 mg/minute).
• Should not be given without direct supervision of doctor or experienced clinician.

Interactions:
AMINOGLYCOSIDE ANTIBIOTICS (INCLUDING AMIKACIN, GENTAMICIN, KANAMYCIN, NEOMYCIN, STREPTOMYCIN); POLYMYXIN ANTIBIOTICS (POLYMYXIN B SULFATE, COLISTIN); CLINDAMYCIN, QUINIDINE: potentiated neuromuscular blockade, leading to increased skeletal muscle relaxation and possible respiratory paralysis. Use cautiously during surgical and postoperative periods.
NARCOTIC ANALGESICS: potentiated neuromuscular blockade, leading to increased skeletal muscle relaxation and possible respiratory paralysis. Use with extreme caution, and reduce dose of gallamine.

Special considerations:
• Contraindicated in patients with hypersensitivity to iodides, impaired renal function, myasthenia gravis; patients in shock; and patients in whom tachycardia may be hazardous. Use cautiously in elderly or debilitated patients; in those with hepatic or pulmonary impairment, respiratory depression, myasthenic syndrome of lung cancer, dehydration, thyroid disorders, collagen diseases, porphyria, electrolyte disturbances, fractures, muscle spasms, and in patients undergoing cesarean section.
• Baseline electrolyte determinations (electrolyte imbalance can potentiate neuromuscular effects) should be monitored.
• Respiration should be watched for early symptoms of paralysis: inability to keep eyelids open and eyes focused, difficulty in swallowing and speaking.
• Vital signs should be monitored every 15 minutes, especially for developing tachycardia.
• Intake and output should be measured; renal dysfunction prolongs duration of action, since drug is unchanged before excretion.
• Clear airway should be maintained and emergency respiratory support (endotracheal equipment, respirator, oxygen, atropine, neostigmine) kept available.
• Postoperative stiffness is normal and will soon subside.
• Should be determined whether patient has iodide allergy.
• Drug should be protected from light or excessive heat and only fresh solutions used.
• Do not mix solution with meperidine HCl or barbiturate solutions.
• Should be given slow I.V. (over 30 to 90 seconds).
• Should not be given without direct supervision of doctor.

Interactions:
None reported for this drug alone; always used with succinylcholine. See succinylcholine chloride.

Special considerations:
• Contraindicated in hypersensitivity to bromides and in bronchial asthma. Use cautiously in elderly or debilitated patients; in renal, hepatic, or pulmonary impairment, respiratory depression, myasthenia gravis, myasthenic syndrome of lung cancer, dehydration, thyroid disorders, collagen diseases, porphyria, electrolyte disturbances, and glaucoma; and during ocular

(continued on following page)

NAMES, INDICATIONS AND DOSAGES	SIDE EFFECTS

hexafluorenium bromide
(continued)

Dose depends on individual needs and response. Doses are representative and must be adjusted.

ADULTS AND CHILDREN: use in ratio of 2 mg/1 mg succinylcholine. Maximum hexafluorenium bromide 10 to 36 mg; should not be administered more frequently than q 15 to 30 minutes.

metocurine iodide
Metubine

Adjunct to anesthetic to induce skeletal muscle relaxation; facilitate intubation, reduction of fractures and dislocations:

Dose depends on anesthetic used, individual needs, and response. Doses are representative and must be adjusted. Administer as sustained injection over 30 to 60 seconds.

ADULTS: given cyclopropane—2 to 4 mg I.V. (2.68 mg average); given ether—1.5 to 3 mg I.V. (2.1 mg average); given nitrous oxide—4 to 7 mg I.V. (4.79 mg average). Supplemental injections of 0.5 to 1 mg in 25 to 90 minutes, repeated p.r.n.

Lessen muscle contractions in pharmacologically or electrically induced convulsions:

ADULTS: 1.75 to 5.5 mg I.V.

CV: hypotension secondary to histamine release, ganglionic blockade in rapid dose or overdose.

Other: *dose-related prolonged apnea,* residual muscle weakness, increased oropharyngeal secretions, allergic or idiosyncratic hypersensitivity reactions, *bronchospasm.*

pancuronium bromide
Pavulon♦

Adjunct to anesthetic to induce skeletal muscle relaxation; facilitate intubation, lessen muscle contractions in pharmacologically or electrically induced convulsions; assist with mechanical ventilation:

Dose depends on anesthetic used, individual needs, and response. Doses are representative and must be adjusted.

ADULTS: initially, 0.04 to 0.1 mg/kg I.V.; then 0.01 mg/kg q 30 to 60 minutes.

CHILDREN OVER 10 YEARS: initially, 0.04 to 0.1 mg/kg I.V., then ⅕ initial dose q 30 to 60 minutes.

CV: tachycardia, increased blood pressure.

Local: burning sensation.

Skin: transient rashes.

Other: excessive sweating and salivation, *prolonged dose-related apnea,* residual muscle weakness, allergic or idiosyncratic hypersensitivity reactions.

INTERACTIONS AND SPECIAL CONSIDERATIONS

surgery and (in large doses) cesarean section.
• Not used extensively in clinical practice.
• Baseline electrolyte determinations (electrolyte imbalance potentiates neuromuscular effects) and vital signs (especially respirations) should be monitored.
• Airway should be kept clear and emergency respiratory support (endotracheal equipment, respirator, oxygen, atropine, neostigmine) on hand.
• Postoperative stiffness is normal and will soon subside.
• Should be determined whether patient has bromide allergy.
• Only fresh solutions usable; not given without medical supervision.

Interactions:

AMINOGLYCOSIDE ANTIBIOTICS (INCLUDING AMIKACIN, GENTAMICIN, KANAMYCIN, NEOMYCIN, STREPTOMYCIN); POLYMYXIN ANTIBIOTICS (POLYMYXIN B SULFATE, COLISTIN); CLINDAMYCIN, QUINIDINE: potentiated neuromuscular blockade, leading to increased skeletal muscle relaxation and possible respiratory paralysis. Use cautiously during surgical and postoperative periods.

NARCOTIC ANALGESICS: potentiated neuromuscular blockade, leading to increased skeletal muscle relaxation and possible respiratory paralysis. Use with extreme caution, and reduce dose of metocurine iodide.

Special considerations:

• Contraindicated in patients with hypersensitivity to iodides and in those for whom histamine release is a hazard (asthmatic or atopic patients). Use cautiously in elderly or debilitated patients; and in renal, hepatic, or pulmonary impairment, respiratory depression, myasthenia gravis, myasthenic syndrome of lung cancer, dehydration, thyroid disorders, collagen diseases, porphyria, electrolyte disturbances, hyperthermia, and (in large doses) cesarean section.
• Neostigmine, edrophonium, and epinephrine may be used to reverse effects of metocurine because of their anticurare effects.
• Doses of 1 mg therapeutic equivalent of 3 mg *d*-tubocurarine chloride.
• Baseline electrolyte determinations (electrolyte imbalance, especially potassium, calcium, and magnesium, can potentiate neuromuscular effects) and vital signs, especially respiration, should be monitored.
• Intake and output should be measured; renal dysfunction prolongs duration of action, since drug is mainly unchanged before excretion.
• Clear airway should be maintained and emergency respiratory support (endotracheal equipment, respirator, oxygen, atropine, edrophonium, epinephrine, and neostigmine) kept available.
• Postoperative stiffness is normal and will soon subside.
• Should be determined whether patient has iodide allergy.
• Solution should be stored away from heat, sunlight; should not be mixed with barbiturates, methohexital, or thiopental (precipitate will form); and only fresh solutions should be used.
• Should not be given without direct supervision of doctor.

Interactions:

AMINOGLYCOSIDE ANTIBIOTICS (INCLUDING AMIKACIN, GENTAMICIN, KANAMYCIN, NEOMYCIN, STREPTOMYCIN); POLYMYXIN ANTIBIOTICS (POLYMYXIN B SULFATE, COLISTIN); CLINDAMYCIN, QUINIDINE: potentiated neuromuscular blockade, leading to increased skeletal muscle relaxation and possible respiratory paralysis. Use cautiously during surgical and postoperative periods.

LITHIUM, NARCOTIC ANALGESICS: potentiated neuromuscular blockade, leading to increased skeletal muscle relaxation and possible respiratory paralysis. Use with extreme caution, and reduce dose of pancuronium.

Special considerations:

• Contraindicated in hypersensitivity to bromides; preexisting tachycardia; and in patients for whom even a minor increase in heart rate is undesirable. Use cautiously in elderly or debilitated patients; renal, hepatic, or pulmonary impairment; respiratory depression, myasthenia gravis, myasthenic syndrome of lung cancer, dehydration, thyroid disorders, collagen diseases, porphyria, electrolyte disturbances, hyperthermia, toxemic states, and (in large doses) cesarean section.
• Causes no histamine release or hypotension.
• Dose of 1 mg is the approximate therapeutic equivalent of 5 mg *d*-tubocurarine chloride.
• Baseline electrolyte determinations (electrolyte imbalance can potentiate neuromuscular effects) and vital signs (especially respiration and heart rate) should be monitored.
• Intake and output should be measured; renal dysfunction may prolong duration of action, since 25% of the drug is unchanged before excretion.
• Emergency respiratory support (endotracheal equipment, respirator, oxygen, atropine, neostigmine) should be available.
• Effects of succinylcholine should be allowed to subside before pancuronium is given.

(continued on following page)

NAMES, INDICATIONS AND DOSAGES	SIDE EFFECTS
pancuronium bromide *(continued)*	
succinylcholine chloride Anectine♦, Anectine Flo-Pack Powder, Sux-Cert **Adjunct to anesthetic to induce skeletal muscle relaxation; facilitate intubation and assist with mechanical ventilation or orthopedic manipulations (drug of choice); lessen muscle contractions in pharmacologically or electrically induced convulsions:** Dose depends on anesthetic used, individual needs, and response. Doses are representative and must be adjusted. ADULTS: 25 to 75 mg I.V., then 2.5 mg/minute, p.r.n., or 2.5 mg/kg I.M. up to maximum 150 mg I.M. in deltoid muscle. CHILDREN: 1 to 2 mg/kg I.M. or I.V. Maximum I.M. dose 150 mg. (Children may be less sensitive to succinylcholine than adults.)	**CV:** bradycardia, tachycardia, hypertension, hypotension, arrhythmias. **EENT:** increased intraocular pressure. **Other:** *prolonged respiratory depression, apnea, malignant hyperthermia,* muscle fasciculation, *postoperative muscle pain,* myoglobinemia, excessive salivation, allergic or idiosyncratic hypersensitivity reactions.
tubocurarine chloride Tubarine♦♦ **Adjunct to anesthetic to induce skeletal muscle relaxation; facilitate intubation, orthopedic manipulations:** Dose depends on anesthetic used, individual needs, and response. Doses listed are representative and must be adjusted. ADULTS: 1 unit/kg or 0.15 mg/kg I.V. slowly over 60 to 90 seconds. Average, initially, 40 to 60 units I.V. May give 20 to 30 units in 3 to 5 minutes. For longer procedures, give 20 units, p.r.n. CHILDREN: 1 unit/kg or 0.15 mg/kg.	**CV:** hypotension, circulatory depression. **Other:** profound and prolonged muscle relaxation, *respiratory depression to the point of apnea,* hypersensitivity, idiosyncrasy, residual muscle weakness, *bronchospasm.*

♦ Available in U.S. and Canada. ♦♦ Available in Canada only.
All other products (no symbol) available in U.S. only. Italicized side effects are common or life-threatening.

INTERACTIONS AND SPECIAL CONSIDERATIONS

• Should be stored in refrigerator but not in plastic containers or syringes, although plastic syringes may be used for administration.
• Should not be mixed with barbiturate solutions and only fresh solutions used.
• Should not be given without direct supervision of doctor.

Interactions:
AMINOGLYCOSIDE ANTIBIOTICS (INCLUDING AMIKACIN, GENTAMICIN, KANAMYCIN, NEOMYCIN, PAROMOMYCIN, STREPTOMYCIN); POLYMYXIN ANTIBIOTICS (POLYMYXIN B SULFATE, COLISTIN); ECHOTHIOPHATE: potentiated neuromuscular blockade, leading to increased skeletal muscle relaxation and possible respiratory paralysis. Use cautiously during surgical and postoperative periods.
NARCOTIC ANALGESICS, LIDOCAINE, PROCAINE, METHOTRIMEPRAZINE: potentiated neuromuscular blockade, leading to increased skeletal muscle relaxation and possible respiratory paralysis. Use with extreme caution.
MAO INHIBITORS, LITHIUM, CYCLOPHOSPHAMIDE: prolonged apnea. Use with caution.
MAGNESIUM SULFATE (PARENTERALLY): potentiated neuromuscular blockade, increased skeletal muscle relaxation, and possible respiratory paralysis. Use with caution, preferably with reduced doses.
CARDIOTONIC GLYCOSIDES: possible cardiac arrhythmias. Use together cautiously.

Special considerations:
• Contraindicated in abnormally low plasma pseudocholinesterase levels. Use with caution in patients with personal or family history of malignant hypertension or hyperthermia; elderly or debilitated patients; and in hepatic, renal, or pulmonary impairment, respiratory depression, severe burns or trauma, electrolyte imbalances, quinidine or digitalis therapy, hyperkalemia, paraplegia, spinal neuraxis injury, degenerative or dystrophic neuromuscular disease, myasthenia gravis, myasthenic syndrome of lung cancer, dehydration, thyroid disorders, collagen diseases, porphyria, fractures, muscle spasms, glaucoma, eye surgery or penetrating eye wounds, pheochromocytoma, and (in large doses) cesarean section.
• Drug of choice for short procedures (less than 3 minutes) and for orthopedic manipulations; caution should be used in fractures or dislocations.
• Duration of action prolonged to 20 minutes by continuous I.V. infusion or single-dose administration, along with hexafluorenium bromide.
• Repeated or continuous infusions of succinylcholine alone not advised; may cause reduced response or prolonged apnea.
• Baseline electrolyte determinations and vital signs should be monitored; respiration should be checked every 5 to 10 minutes during infusion.
• Clear airway should be maintained and emergency respiratory support (endotracheal equipment, respirator, oxygen, atropine, neostigmine) kept available.
• Postoperative stiffness is normal and will soon subside.
• Injectable form should be stored in refrigerator; powder form at room temperature, tightly closed. Should be used immediately after reconstitution. Should not be mixed with alkaline solutions (thiopental, sodium bicarbonate, barbiturates).
• Test dose (10 mg I.M. or I.V.) should be given after patient has been anesthetized. Normal response (no respiratory depression, or transient depression lasting less than 5 minutes) indicates drug may be given. Should not be given if patient develops respiratory paralysis sufficient to permit endotracheal intubation. (Recovery within 30 to 60 minutes.)
• Should not be given without direct supervision of doctor.
• Should be given deep I.M., preferably high into deltoid muscle.

Interactions:
AMINOGLYCOSIDE ANTIBIOTICS (INCLUDING AMIKACIN, GENTAMICIN, KANAMYCIN, NEOMYCIN, PAROMOMYCIN, STREPTOMYCIN); POLYMYXIN ANTIBIOTICS (POLYMYXIN B SULFATE, COLISTIN): potentiated neuromuscular blockade, leading to increased skeletal muscle relaxation and possible respiratory paralysis. Use cautiously during surgical and postoperative periods.
QUINIDINE: prolonged neuromuscular blockade. Use together with caution. Monitor closely.
THIAZIDE DIURETICS, FUROSEMIDE, ETHACRYNIC ACID, AMPHOTERICIN B, PROPRANOLOL, METHOTRIMEPRAZINE, NARCOTIC ANALGESICS: potentiated neuromuscular blockade, leading to increased respiratory paralysis. Use with extreme caution during surgical and postoperative periods.

Special considerations:
• Contraindicated in patients for whom histamine release is a hazard (those with asthma). Use cautiously in elderly or debilitated patients; in hepatic or pulmonary impairment, respiratory depression, myasthenia gravis, myasthenic syndrome of lung cancer, dehydration, thyroid disorders, collagen diseases, porphyria, electrolyte disturbances, fractures, muscle spasms, and (in large doses) cesarean section.

(continued on following page)

NAMES, INDICATIONS AND DOSAGES	SIDE EFFECTS

tubocurarine chloride
(continued)

Assist with mechanical ventilation:
ADULTS AND CHILDREN: initially, 0.0165 mg/kg I.V. (average 1 mg or 7 units), then adjust subsequent doses to patient's response.

Diagnose myasthenia gravis:
ADULTS AND CHILDREN: 0.0041 to 0.033 mg/kg I.V. or 1/15 to 1/5 normal adult dose for electroshock. Positive result: profound exaggeration of myasthenic symptoms. Dose may also be given I.M. when necessary.

Lessen muscle contractions in pharmacologically or electrically induced convulsions:
ADULTS AND CHILDREN: 1 unit/kg or 0.15 mg/kg slowly over 60 to 90 seconds. Initial dose 20 units (3 mg) less than calculated dose.

INTERACTIONS AND SPECIAL CONSIDERATIONS

- Small margin of safety between therapeutic dose and dose causing respiratory paralysis.
- Used to diagnose myasthenia gravis, but procedure is hazardous.
- Succinylcholine effects should be allowed to subside before tubocurarine is given.
- Baseline electrolyte determinations should be monitored; electrolyte imbalance can potentiate neuromuscular effects.
- Respiration should be watched closely for early symptoms of paralysis: inability to keep eyelids open and eyes focused or difficulty in swallowing and speaking.
- Vital signs should be checked every 15 minutes for changes.
- Intake and output should be measured; renal dysfunction prolongs duration of action, since much of drug is unchanged before excretion.
- Clear airway should be maintained and emergency respiratory support (endotracheal equipment, respirator, oxygen, atropine, edrophonium, epinephrine, and neostigmine) kept available.
- Postoperative stiffness is normal and will soon subside.
- Inhalation anesthetics require decreased dose.
- Should not be mixed with barbiturates. Only fresh solutions should be used; if discolored, should be discarded.
- Should be given slow I.V. (60 to 90 seconds); should be given deep I.M. into deltoid muscle.
- Should not be given without direct supervision of doctor.

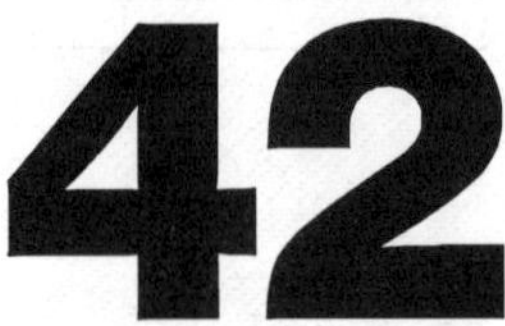

Antihistamines

azatadine maleate
brompheniramine maleate
carbinoxamine maleate
chlorpheniramine maleate
clemastine fumarate
cyproheptadine hydrochloride
dexchlorpheniramine maleate
dimethindene maleate
diphenhydramine hydrochloride
diphenylpyraline hydrochloride
doxylamine succinate
methdilazine hydrochloride
promethazine hydrochloride
trimeprazine tartrate
tripelennamine hydrochloride
triprolidine hydrochloride

Antihistamines are thought to block the physiologic action of histamine, the humoral compound that causes symptoms associated with allergic reactions. They compete with histamine for receptor sites (by the process of competitive inhibition: see Chapter 2, PHARMACOLOGY, for a detailed discussion of this concept).

Many compounds from different chemical classes are called antihistamines. All antihistamines have *qualitatively* similar pharmacologic effects. *Quantitatively,* however, they may differ in potency and range of effect. Drowsiness, a side effect common to all antihistamines, may vary in intensity from drug to drug—and sometimes from patient to patient.

Major uses

- Antihistamines (except cyproheptadine, methdilazine, and trimeprazine) are used to relieve symptoms of allergy-related rhinitis and conjunctivitis.
- Cyproheptadine, methdilazine, and trimeprazine are used to treat mild, uncomplicated urticaria or pruritus resulting from allergic dermatoses.
- Diphenhydramine is used as a nighttime sedative.
- Diphenhydramine is a therapeutic adjunct for anaphylaxis or less severe allergic reactions caused by drugs, blood, or plasma. It is also used as a local anesthetic in dental procedures.
- Promethazine is used to prevent motion sickness.

Mechanism of action

- Antihistamines compete with histamine for H_1-receptor sites on effector cells. They can prevent but they can't reverse histamine-mediated responses, particularly histamine's effects on the smooth muscle of the bronchial tubes, gastrointestinal tract, uterus, and blood vessels.
- Anticholinergic actions of antihistamines dry the nasal mucosa and also relieve vertigo and motion sickness.
- Diphenhydramine, structurally related to local anesthetics, provides anesthesia by preventing initiation and transmission of nerve impulses.

Absorption, distribution, metabolism, and excretion

Antihistamines are well absorbed after oral or parenteral administration. They are distributed to most body tissues, extensively metabolized in the liver, and excreted in the urine as inactive metabolites within 24 hours.

Onset and duration

Antihistamines begin to act within 15 to 30 minutes; blood levels peak in about 1 hour.

Duration of action varies, but symptoms are usually relieved for 4 to 6 hours. Action of the sustained-release forms may last 8 to 12 hours.

Combination products

ACTIFED: pseudoephedrine hydrochloride 60 mg and triprolidine hydrochloride 2.5 mg.

ALLEREST: phenylpropanolamine hydrochloride 18.7 mg; chlorpheniramine maleate 2 mg.

ALLERGY RELIEF MEDICINE: phenylpropanolamine hydrochloride 37.5 mg and chlorpheniramine maleate 4 mg.

BENDECTIN: doxylamine succinate 10 mg and pyridoxine hydrochloride 10 mg.

CHLOR-TRIMETON DECONGESTANT: chlorpheniramine maleate 4 mg and pseudoephedrine sulfate 60 mg.

CODIMAL DH: hydrocodone bitartrate 1.66 mg, phenylephrine hydrochloride 5 mg, pyrilamine maleate 8.33 mg, potassium guaiacolsulfonate 83.3 mg, sodium citrate 216 mg, and citric acid 50 mg.

CO-PYRONIL PULVULES: cyclopentamine hydrochloride 12.5 mg and pyrrobutamine phosphate 15 mg.

DEMAZIN SYRUP: phenylephrine hydrochloride 2.5 mg, chlorpheniramine maleate 1 mg, and alcohol 7.5%.

DIMETANE DECONGESTANT: phenylephrine hydrochloride 10 mg and brompheniramine maleate 4 mg.

DIMETAPP EXTENTABS: brompheniramine maleate 12 mg, phenylephrine hydrochloride 15 mg, and phenylpropanolamine hydrochloride 15 mg.

DISOPHROL CHRONOTAB: dexbrompheniramine maleate 6 mg and pseudoephedrine sulfate 120 mg.

DRIXORAL♦: dexbrompheniramine maleate 6 mg and pseudoephedrine sulfate 120 mg.

HISTALET FORTE: phenylpropanolamine hydrochloride 50 mg, phenylephrine hydrochloride 10 mg, chlorpheniramine maleate 4 mg, and pyrilamine maleate 25 mg.

HISTALET SYRUP: pseudoephedrine hydrochloride 45 mg, chlorpheniramine maleate 3 mg, and alcohol 0.45%.

HISTASPAN-D: chlorpheniramine maleate 8 mg, phenylephrine hydrochloride 20 mg, and methscopolamine nitrate 2.5 mg.

NALDECON: phenylephrine hydrochloride 10 mg, phenylpropanolamine hydrochloride 40 mg, phenyltoloxamine citrate 15 mg, and chlorpheniramine maleate 5 mg.

NALDECON SYRUP: phenylpropanolamine hydrochloride 20 mg, phenylephrine hydrochloride 5 mg, chlorpheniramine maleate 2.5 mg, and phenyltoloxamine citrate 7.5 mg.

NOVAFED A: pseudoephedrine hydrochloride 120 mg and chlorpheniramine maleate 8 mg.

NOVAHISTINE ELIXIR: phenylpropanolamine hydrochloride 18.7 mg, chlorpheniramine maleate 2 mg, and alcohol 5%/5 ml.

ORNADE: isopropamide iodide 2.5 mg, phenylpropanolamine hydrochloride 50 mg, and chlorpheniramine maleate 8 mg.

PHENERGAN-D: pseudoephedrine hydrochloride 60 mg, promethazine hydrochloride 6.25 mg.

RONDEC: carbinoxamine maleate 4 mg and pseudoephedrine hydrochloride 60 mg.

RONDEC TABLETS: pseudoephedrine hydrochloride 60 mg and carbinoxamine maleate 4 mg.

TRIAMINIC TABLETS: phenylpropanolamine hydrochloride 50 mg, pheniramine maleate 25 mg, and pyrilamine maleate 25 mg.

NAMES, INDICATIONS AND DOSAGES	SIDE EFFECTS
azatadine maleate Optimine♦ **Rhinitis, allergy symptoms, chronic urticaria:** ADULTS: 1 to 2 mg P.O. b.i.d. Maximum 4 mg daily.	**Blood:** thrombocytopenia. **CNS (especially in the elderly):** *drowsiness, dizziness,* vertigo, disturbed coordination. **CV:** hypotension, palpitations. **GI:** anorexia, *nausea,* vomiting, *dry mouth and throat.* **GU:** urinary retention. **Skin:** urticaria, rash. **Other:** thickening of bronchial secretions.
brompheniramine maleate Dimetane♦, Dimetane-Ten, Rolabromophen, Spentane, Veltane **Rhinitis, allergy symptoms:** ADULTS: 4 to 8 mg P.O. t.i.d. or q.i.d.; or (timed-release) 8 to 12 mg P.O. b.i.d. or t.i.d.; or 5 to 20 mg q 6 to 12 hours I.M., I.V., or S.C. Maximum 40 mg daily. CHILDREN OVER 6 YEARS: 2 to 4 mg t.i.d. or q.i.d.; or (timed-release) 8 to 12 mg q 12 hours; or 0.5 mg/kg daily I.M., I.V., or S.C. divided t.i.d. or q.i.d. CHILDREN UNDER 6 YEARS: 0.5 mg/kg daily P.O., I.M., I.V., or S.C. divided t.i.d. or q.i.d.	**Blood:** thrombocytopenia, *agranulocytosis.* **CNS (especially in the elderly):** dizziness, tremors, irritability, insomnia, *drowsiness.* **CV:** hypotension, palpitations. **GI:** anorexia, nausea, vomiting, *dry mouth and throat.* **GU:** urinary retention. **Skin:** urticaria, rash. **After parenteral administration:** local reaction, sweating, syncope.
carbinoxamine maleate Clistin, Clistin RA **Rhinitis, allergy symptoms:** ADULTS: 4 to 8 mg P.O. t.i.d. to q.i.d., or (timed-release) 8 to 12 mg q 8 to 12 hours. CHILDREN OVER 6 YEARS: 4 mg P.O. t.i.d. to q.i.d. CHILDREN 3 TO 6 YEARS: 2 to 4 mg P.O. t.i.d. to q.i.d. CHILDREN 1 TO 3 YEARS: 2 mg P.O. t.i.d. to q.i.d.	**CNS (especially in the elderly):** *drowsiness, dizziness.* **GI:** anorexia, nausea, vomiting, *dry mouth.*
chlorpheniramine maleate Allerid-O.D., AL-R, Chloramate, Chlormene, Chlortab, Chlor-Trimeton, Chlor-Tripolon♦♦, Histalon♦♦, Histaspan, Histex, Histrey, Novopheniram♦♦, Pyranistan, Teldrin **Rhinitis, allergy symptoms:** ADULTS: 2 to 4 mg P.O. t.i.d. or q.i.d.; or (timed-release) 8 to 12 mg P.O. b.i.d. or t.i.d.; or 5 to 40 mg I.M., I.V., or S.C. Give I.V. injection over 1 minute. CHILDREN 6 TO 12 YEARS: 2 mg P.O. t.i.d. or q.i.d.; or (timed-release) 8 mg P.O. daily or b.i.d. CHILDREN 2 TO 6 YEARS: 1 mg P.O. t.i.d. or q.i.d.	**CNS (especially in the elderly):** sedation, *drowsiness.* **CV:** hypotension, palpitations. **GI:** epigastric distress, *dry mouth.* **GU:** urinary retention. **Other:** thickening of bronchial secretions. **After parenteral administration:** local stinging, burning sensation, pallor, weak pulse, transient hypotension.

INTERACTIONS AND SPECIAL CONSIDERATIONS

No significant interactions.

Special considerations:

• Contraindicated in acute asthmatic attack. Use cautiously in elderly patients, and in patients with increased intraocular pressure, hyperthyroidism, cardiovascular or renal disease, hypertension, bronchial asthma, narrow-angle glaucoma, urinary retention, prostatic hypertrophy, bladder-neck obstruction.
• Patient should avoid alcoholic beverages during therapy and driving or other activities that require alertness until CNS response to drug is determined.
• Taking with food or milk reduces GI distress.
• Coffee or tea may reduce drowsiness. Sugarless gum, sour hard candy, or ice chips may relieve dry mouth.
• Each patient's dose should be titrated; response to drug varies.
• If tolerance develops, another antihistamine may be substituted.
• Patient should stop taking drug 4 days before allergy skin tests; otherwise, accuracy of tests may be affected.
• Blood counts should be monitored during long-term therapy; blood dyscrasias possible.

No significant interactions.

Special considerations:

• Contraindicated in acute asthmatic attack. Use cautiously in elderly patients, and in patients with increased intraocular pressure, hyperthyroidism, cardiovascular or renal disease, hypertension, bronchial asthma, narrow-angle glaucoma, urinary retention, prostatic hypertrophy, bladder-neck obstruction.
• Patient should avoid alcoholic beverages during therapy and driving or other activities that require alertness until CNS response to drug is determined.
• Taking drug with food or milk reduces GI distress.
• Coffee or tea may reduce drowsiness. Sugarless gum, sour hard candy, or ice chips may relieve dry mouth.
• Each patient's dose should be titrated; response to drug varies.
• If tolerance develops, another antihistamine may be substituted.
• Patient should stop taking drug 4 days before allergy skin tests; otherwise, accuracy of tests may be affected.
• Injectable form containing 10 mg/ml can be given diluted or undiluted very slow I.V. The 100 mg/ml injection should not be given I.V.
• Blood counts should be monitored during long-term therapy; blood dyscrasias possible.

No significant interactions.

Special considerations:

• Contraindicated in acute asthmatic attack. Use cautiously in elderly patients, and in patients with increased intraocular pressure, hyperthyroidism, cardiovascular or renal disease, hypertension, bronchial asthma, narrow-angle glaucoma, urinary retention, prostatic hypertrophy, bladder-neck obstruction.
• Patient should avoid alcoholic beverages during therapy and driving or other activities that require alertness until CNS response to drug is determined.
• Taking drug with food or milk reduces GI distress.
• Coffee or tea may reduce drowsiness. Sugarless gum, sour hard candy, or ice chips may relieve dry mouth.
• Each patient's dose should be titrated; response to drug varies.
• If tolerance develops, another antihistamine may be substituted.
• Patient should stop taking drug 4 days before allergy skin tests; otherwise, accuracy of tests may be affected.

No significant interactions.

Special considerations:

• Contraindicated in acute asthmatic attack. Use cautiously in elderly patients, and in patients with increased intraocular pressure, hyperthyroidism, cardiovascular or renal disease, hypertension, bronchial asthma, narrow-angle glaucoma, urinary retention, prostatic hypertrophy, bladder-neck obstruction.
• Patient should avoid alcoholic beverages and other CNS depressants during therapy and driving or other activities that require alertness until CNS response to drug is determined.
• Coffee or tea may reduce drowsiness.
• Each patient's dose should be titrated; response to drug varies.
• If tolerance develops, another antihistamine may be substituted.
• Patient should stop taking drug 4 days before allergy skin tests; otherwise, accuracy of tests may be affected.
• Only injectable forms *without* preservatives can be given I.V. Give *slowly*.
• If symptoms occur after parenteral dose, drug should be stopped.

NAMES, INDICATIONS AND DOSAGES	SIDE EFFECTS
clemastine fumarate Tavist, Tavist-1 **Rhinitis, allergy symptoms:** ADULTS: 1.34 to 2.68 mg once daily. Maximum recommended daily dosage is 8.04 mg; or (timed-release) 1.34 mg (long-acting tablet) b.i.d., not to exceed 8.04 mg (6 long-acting tablets) per day. **Allergic skin manifestation of urticaria and angioedema:** ADULTS: 2.68 mg up to t.i.d. maximum.	**Blood:** hemolytic anemia, thrombocytopenia, *agranulocytosis.* **CNS (especially in the elderly):** *sedation, drowsiness.* **CV:** hypotension, palpitations, tachycardia. **GI:** epigastric distress, anorexia, nausea, vomiting, constipation, *dry mouth.* **GU:** urinary retention. **Skin:** rash, urticaria. **Other:** thickening of bronchial secretions.
cyproheptadine hydrochloride Periactin♦, Vimicon♦♦ **Allergy symptoms, pruritus:** ADULTS: 4 mg P.O. t.i.d. or q.i.d. Maximum 0.5 mg/kg daily. CHILDREN 7 TO 14 YEARS: 4 mg P.O. b.i.d. or t.i.d. CHILDREN 2 TO 6 YEARS: 2 mg P.O. b.i.d. or t.i.d.	**CNS (especially in the elderly):** *drowsiness,* dizziness, headache, fatigue. **GI:** anorexia, nausea, vomiting, *dry mouth.* **Skin:** rash. **Other:** weight gain.
dexchlorpheniramine maleate Polaramine♦ **Rhinitis, allergy symptoms, contact dermatitis, pruritus:** ADULTS: 1 to 2 mg P.O. t.i.d. or q.i.d.; or (timed-release) 4 to 6 mg b.i.d. or t.i.d. CHILDREN UNDER 12 YEARS: 0.15 mg/kg P.O. daily divided into 4 doses. Do not use timed-release tablets for children younger than 6 years.	**CNS (especially in the elderly):** *drowsiness,* dizziness. **GI:** nausea, *dry mouth.* **GU:** polyuria, dysuria.
dimethindene maleate Forhistal, Triten **Allergy symptoms:** ADULTS AND CHILDREN OVER 6 YEARS: (timed-release) 2.5 mg P.O. daily b.i.d.	**CNS (especially in the elderly):** *drowsiness,* dizziness, insomnia, irritability, headache. **GI:** anorexia, nausea, vomiting, *dry mouth,* diarrhea. **GU:** urinary frequency.
diphenhydramine hydrochloride Allerdryl, Baramine, Bax, Benachlor, Benadryl♦, Benahist, Ben-Allergin, Bendylate, Bentrac, Bonyl, Eldadryl, Fenylhist, Nordryl, Phen-Amin 50, Phenamine, Rodryl, Rohydra,	**CNS (especially in the elderly):** *drowsiness,* confusion, insomnia, headache, vertigo. **CV:** palpitations. **EENT:** photosensitivity, diplopia, nasal stuffiness.

INTERACTIONS AND SPECIAL CONSIDERATIONS

No significant interactions.

Special considerations:
• Contraindicated in acute asthmatic attack. Use cautiously in elderly patients, and in patients with increased intraocular pressure, hyperthyroidism, cardiovascular or renal disease, hypertension, bronchial asthma, narrow-angle glaucoma, urinary retention, prostatic hypertrophy, bladder-neck obstruction.
• Patient should avoid alcoholic beverages during therapy and driving or other activities that require alertness until CNS response to drug is determined.
• Coffee or tea may reduce drowsiness. Sugarless gum, sour hard candy, or ice chips may relieve dry mouth.
• Each patient's dose should be titrated; response to drug varies.
• If tolerance develops, another antihistamine may be substituted.
• Patient should stop taking drug 4 days before allergy skin tests; otherwise, accuracy of tests may be affected.
• Tablets are available as 1.34 and 2.68 mg. Long-acting tablets are 1.34 mg.
• Blood counts should be monitored during long-term therapy; blood dyscrasias possible.

No significant interactions.

Special considerations:
• Contraindicated in acute asthmatic attack. Use cautiously in elderly patients, and in patients with increased intraocular pressure, hyperthyroidism, cardiovascular or renal disease, hypertension, bronchial asthma, narrow-angle glaucoma, urinary retention, prostatic hypertrophy, bladder-neck obstruction.
• Patient should avoid alcoholic beverages during therapy and driving or other activities that require alertness until CNS response to drug is determined.
• Taking drug with food or milk reduces GI distress.
• Coffee or tea may reduce drowsiness. Sugarless gum, sour hard candy, or ice chips may relieve dry mouth.
• Each patient's dose should be titrated; response to drug varies.
• If tolerance develops, another antihistamine may be substituted.
• Patient should stop taking drug 4 days before allergy skin tests; otherwise, accuracy of tests may be affected.
• Used experimentally to stimulate appetite and increase weight gain in children.

No significant interactions.

Special considerations:
• Contraindicated in acute asthmatic attack. Use cautiously in elderly patients, and in patients with increased intraocular pressure, hyperthyroidism, cardiovascular or renal disease, hypertension, bronchial asthma, narrow-angle glaucoma, urinary retention, prostatic hypertrophy, bladder-neck obstruction.
• Patient should avoid alcoholic beverages during therapy and driving or other activities that require alertness until CNS response to drug is determined.
• Coffee or tea may reduce drowsiness.
• Each patient's dose should be titrated; response to drug varies.
• If tolerance develops, another antihistamine may be substituted.
• Patient should stop taking drug 4 days before allergy skin tests; otherwise, accuracy of tests may be affected.

No significant interactions.

Special considerations:
• Contraindicated in acute asthmatic attack. Use cautiously in elderly patients, and in patients with increased intraocular pressure, hyperthyroidism, cardiovascular or renal disease, hypertension, bronchial asthma, narrow-angle glaucoma, urinary retention, prostatic hypertrophy, bladder-neck obstruction.
• Patient should avoid alcoholic beverages during therapy and driving or other activities that require alertness until CNS response to drug is determined.
• Taking drug with food or milk reduces GI distress.
• Coffee or tea may reduce drowsiness. Sugarless gum, sour hard candy, or ice chips may relieve dry mouth.
• Each patient's dose should be titrated; response to drug varies.
• If tolerance develops, another antihistamine may be substituted.
• Patient should stop taking drug 4 days before allergy skin tests; otherwise, accuracy of tests may be affected.

No significant interactions.

Special considerations:
• Contraindicated in acute asthmatic attack. Use cautiously in prostatic hypertrophy, peptic ulcer, pyloroduodenal and bladder-neck obstruction; in newborns, and in asthmatic, hypertensive, or cardiac patients.
• Injection sites should be alternated to prevent irritation. Should be administered deep I.M. into large muscle.
• Patient should avoid alcoholic beverages dur-

(continued on following page)

NAMES, INDICATIONS AND DOSAGES	SIDE EFFECTS
diphenhydramine hydrochloride *(continued)* SK-Diphenhydramine, Span-Lanin, Valdrene, Wehdryl **Rhinitis, allergy symptoms, motion sickness, antiparkinsonism:** ADULTS: 25 to 50 mg P.O. t.i.d. to q.i.d.; or 10 to 50 mg deep I.M. or I.V. Maximum 400 mg daily. CHILDREN UNDER 12 YEARS: 5 mg/kg daily P.O., deep I.M., or I.V. divided q.i.d. Maximum 300 mg daily. **Sedation:** ADULTS: 25 to 50 mg P.O., deep I.M., p.r.n.	**GU:** dysuria. **Skin:** urticaria.
diphenylpyraline hydrochloride Diafen, Hispril **Rhinitis, allergy symptoms:** ADULTS: 2 mg P.O. q 4 hours, p.r.n.; or (timed-release) 5 mg P.O. q 12 hours. CHILDREN OVER 6 YEARS: 2 mg P.O. q 6 hours, p.r.n.; or (timed-release) 5 mg P.O. daily. CHILDREN 2 TO 6 YEARS: 1 to 2 mg P.O. q 8 hours, p.r.n.	**CNS (especially in the elderly):** *drowsiness,* dizziness, headache. **EENT:** nasal congestion. **GI:** *dry mouth and throat,* epigastric distress. **Skin:** flushing.
doxylamine succinate Bendectin, Decapryn, Unisom **Rhinitis, allergy symptoms:** ADULTS: 12.5 to 25 mg P.O. q 4 to 6 hours, p.r.n. CHILDREN 6 TO 12 YEARS: 6.25 to 12.5 mg P.O. q 4 to 6 hours, p.r.n. **Nausea and vomiting of pregnancy:** ADULTS: 2 Bendectin tablets at bedtime. Maximum 4 tablets daily.	**CNS (especially in the elderly):** *drowsiness,* dizziness, insomnia, disorientation, confusion, tremor, irritability, vertigo. **CV:** palpitations. **GI:** *dry mouth and throat.*
methdilazine hydrochloride Dilosyn♦♦, Tacaryl **Pruritus:** ADULTS: 8 mg P.O. b.i.d. to q.i.d. or (chewable tablets) 7.2 mg P.O. b.i.d. to q.i.d. CHILDREN OVER 3 YEARS: 4 mg P.O. b.i.d. to q.i.d. or (chewable tablets) 3.6 mg P.O. b.i.d. to q.i.d.	**CNS (especially in the elderly):** *drowsiness,* dizziness, headache. **GI:** nausea, *dry mouth and throat.* **Hepatic:** cholestatic jaundice. **Skin:** rash.

♦ Available in U.S. and Canada. ♦♦ Available in Canada only.
All other products (no symbol) available in U.S. only. Italicized side effects are common or life-threatening.

INTERACTIONS AND SPECIAL CONSIDERATIONS

ing therapy and driving or other activities that require alertness until CNS response to drug is determined.
• Taking drug with food or milk reduces GI distress.
• Coffee or tea may reduce drowsiness. Sugarless gum, sour hard candy, or ice chips may relieve dry mouth.
• Each patient's dose should be titrated; response to drug varies.
• If tolerance develops, another antihistamine may be substituted.
• Patient should stop taking drug 4 days before allergy skin tests; otherwise, accuracy of tests may be affected.
• Used with epinephrine in anaphylaxis.
• One of most sedating antihistamines; often used as a nighttime sedative.

No significant interactions.

Special considerations:
• Contraindicated in acute asthmatic attack. Use cautiously in elderly patients, and in patients with increased intraocular pressure, hyperthyroidism, cardiovascular or renal disease, hypertension, bronchial asthma, narrow-angle glaucoma, urinary retention, prostatic hypertrophy, bladder-neck obstruction.
• Patient should avoid alcoholic beverages during therapy and driving or other activities that require alertness until CNS response to drug is determined.
• Taking drug with food or milk reduces GI distress.
• Coffee or tea may reduce drowsiness. Sugarless gum, sour hard candy, or ice chips may relieve dry mouth.
• Each patient's dose should be titrated; response to drug varies.
• If tolerance develops, another antihistamine may be substituted.
• Patient should stop taking drug 4 days before allergy skin tests; otherwise, accuracy of tests may be affected.

No significant interactions.

Special considerations:
• Contraindicated in acute asthmatic attack. Use cautiously in elderly patients, and in patients with increased intraocular pressure, hyperthyroidism, cardiovascular or renal disease, hypertension, bronchial asthma, narrow-angle glaucoma, urinary retention, prostatic hypertrophy, bladder-neck obstruction.
• Patient should avoid alcoholic beverages during therapy and driving or other activities that require alertness until CNS response to drug is determined.
• Coffee or tea may reduce drowsiness. Sugarless gum, sour hard candy, or ice chips may relieve dry mouth.
• Each patient's dose should be titrated; response to drug varies.
• If tolerance develops, another antihistamine may be substituted.
• Patient should stop taking drug 4 days before allergy skin tests; otherwise, accuracy of tests may be affected.
• Although Bendectin is indicated in the treatment of nausea and vomiting of pregnancy, it should only be used in extreme cases. Advise your patient to request Bendectin only if other measures, such as eating crackers or toast or drinking hot or cold liquids, have proven unsuccessful.

Interactions:
PHENOTHIAZINES: increased effects. Don't use together.

Special considerations:
• Contraindicated in acute asthmatic attack. Use cautiously in elderly or debilitated patients; acutely ill or dehydrated children; and in patients with pulmonary, hepatic, or cardiovascular disease, asthma, hypertension, narrow-angle glaucoma, peptic ulcer, prostatic hypertrophy, bladder-neck obstruction, CNS depression.
• Patient should avoid alcoholic beverages during therapy and driving or other activities that require alertness until CNS response to drug is determined.
• Taking drug with food or milk reduces GI distress.
• Coffee or tea may reduce drowsiness. Sugarless gum, sour hard candy, or ice chips may relieve dry mouth.
• Each patient's dose should be titrated; response to drug varies.
• If tolerance develops, another antihistamine may be substituted.
• Available as chewable tablet for children.

(continued on following page)

NAMES, INDICATIONS AND DOSAGES	SIDE EFFECTS
methdilazine hydrochloride *(continued)*	
promethazine hydrochloride Ganphen, Histantil♦♦, K-Phen, Methazine, Pentazine♦, Phencen-50, Phenergan♦, Promethamead, Promethazine, Prorex, Provigan, Remsed, Rolamethazine, Sigazine **Motion sickness:** ADULTS: 25 mg P.O. b.i.d. CHILDREN: 12.5 to 25 mg P.O., I.M., or rectally b.i.d. **Nausea:** ADULTS: 12.5 to 25 mg P.O., I.M., or rectally q 4 to 6 hours, p.r.n. CHILDREN: 0.25 to 0.5 mg/kg I.M. or rectally q 4 to 6 hours, p.r.n. **Rhinitis, allergy symptoms:** ADULTS: 12.5 mg P.O. q.i.d.; or 25 mg P.O. at bedtime. CHILDREN: 6.25 to 12.5 mg P.O. t.i.d. or 25 mg P.O. at bedtime. **Sedation:** ADULTS: 25 to 50 mg P.O., I.M. at bedtime or p.r.n. CHILDREN: 12.5 to 25 mg P.O., I.M., or rectally at bedtime.	**CNS (especially in the elderly):** *sedation,* confusion, restlessness, tremors, *drowsiness.* **CV:** hypotension. **EENT:** transient myopia, nasal congestion. **GI:** anorexia, nausea, vomiting, constipation, *dry mouth.* **Other:** *photosensitivity.*
trimeprazine tartrate Panectyl♦♦, Temaril **Pruritus:** ADULTS: 2.5 mg P.O. q.i.d.; or (timed-release) 5 mg P.O. b.i.d. CHILDREN 3 TO 12 YEARS: 2.5 mg P.O. h.s. or t.i.d., p.r.n. CHILDREN 6 MONTHS TO 3 YEARS: 1.25 mg P.O. h.s. or t.i.d., p.r.n.	**Blood:** *agranulocytosis,* leukopenia. **CNS (especially in the elderly):** *drowsiness,* dizziness, confusion, headache, restlessness, tremors, irritability, insomnia. **CV:** hypotension, palpitations, tachycardia. **GI:** anorexia, nausea, vomiting, *dry mouth and throat.* **GU:** urinary frequency or retention. **Skin:** urticaria, rash.
tripelennamine hydrochloride PBZ-SR, Pyribenzamine♦, Ro-Hist **Rhinitis, allergy symptoms:** ADULTS: 25 to 50 mg P.O. q 4 to 6 hours; or (timed-release) 100 mg b.i.d. to t.i.d. Maximum 600 mg daily. CHILDREN OVER 5 YEARS: 50 mg P.O. q 8 to 12 hours (timed-release).	**CNS (especially in the elderly):** *drowsiness,* dizziness, confusion, restlessness, tremors, irritability, insomnia. **CV:** palpitations. **GI:** anorexia, diarrhea or constipation, *nausea, vomiting, dry mouth.* **GU:** urinary frequency or retention. **Skin:** urticaria, rash. **Other:** thickening of bronchial secretions.

♦ Available in U.S. and Canada. ♦♦ Available in Canada only.
All other products (no symbol) available in U.S. only. Italicized side effects are common or life-threatening.

INTERACTIONS AND SPECIAL CONSIDERATIONS

Child should chew completely and swallow promptly; may cause local anesthetic effect in mouth.
• Patient should stop taking drug 4 days before allergy skin tests; otherwise, accuracy of tests may be affected.

Interactions:
PHENOTHIAZINES: increased effects. Don't give together.

Special considerations:
• Contraindicated in narrow-angle glaucoma, peptic ulcer, intestinal obstruction, prostatic hypertrophy, bladder-neck obstruction, epilepsy, bone marrow depression, coma, CNS depression, pregnancy (except during labor), lactation, and in newborns and acutely ill or dehydrated children. Use cautiously in pulmonary, hepatic, or cardiovascular disease; asthma; hypertension, and in elderly or debilitated patients.
• Patient should avoid alcoholic beverages during therapy and driving or other activities that require alertness until CNS response to drug is determined.
• Taking drug with food or milk reduces GI distress.
• Coffee or tea may reduce drowsiness. Sugarless gum, sour hard candy, or ice chips may relieve dry mouth.
• Each patient's dose should be titrated; response to drug varies.
• If tolerance develops, another antihistamine may be substituted.
• Patient should stop taking drug 4 days before allergy skin tests; otherwise, accuracy of tests may be affected.
• Pronounced sedative effect limits use in many ambulatory patients.
• May cause false-positive immunologic urinary pregnancy test (Gravindex). Also may interfere with blood grouping in ABO system.
• When treating motion sickness, patient should take first dose 30 to 60 minutes before travel. On succeeding days of travel, he should take dose upon arising and with evening meal.
• I.M. injection should be deep into large muscle mass.
• Patient should be warned about possible photosensitivity reaction and informed of the precautions he should take to avoid it.

Interactions:
PHENOTHIAZINES: increased effects. Don't use together.

Special considerations:
• Contraindicated in acute asthmatic attack. Use cautiously in pulmonary, hepatic, or cardiovascular disease; asthma, hypertension, narrow-angle glaucoma, peptic ulcer, intestinal obstruction, prostatic hypertrophy, bladder-neck obstruction, epilepsy, bone marrow depression, coma, CNS depression; in elderly or debilitated patients, and acutely ill or dehydrated children.
• Patient should avoid alcoholic beverages during therapy and driving or other activities that require alertness until CNS response to drug is determined.
• Taking drug with food or milk reduces GI distress.
• Coffee or tea may reduce drowsiness. Sugarless gum, sour hard candy, or ice chips may relieve dry mouth.
• Each patient's dose should be titrated; response to drug varies.
• If tolerance develops, another antihistamine may be substituted.
• Patient should stop taking drug 4 days before allergy skin tests; otherwise, accuracy of tests may be affected.
• Blood counts should be monitored during long-term therapy.

No significant interactions.

Special considerations:
• Contraindicated in acute asthmatic attack. Use cautiously in elderly patients, and in patients with increased intraocular pressure, hyperthyroidism, cardiovascular or renal disease, hypertension, bronchial asthma, narrow-angle glaucoma, urinary retention, prostatic hypertrophy, bladder-neck obstruction.
• Patient should avoid alcoholic beverages during therapy and driving or other activities that require alertness until CNS response to drug is determined.
• Taking drug with food or milk reduces GI distress.
• Coffee or tea may reduce drowsiness. Sugarless gum, sour hard candy, or ice chips may

(continued on following page)

NAMES, INDICATIONS AND DOSAGES	SIDE EFFECTS
tripelennamine hydrochloride *(continued)* CHILDREN UNDER 5 YEARS: 5 mg/kg daily P.O. in 4 to 6 divided doses. Maximum 300 mg daily.	
triprolidine hydrochloride Actidil ♦ **Colds and allergy symptoms:** ADULTS: 2.5 mg P.O. t.i.d. or q.i.d. CHILDREN OVER 6 YEARS: 1.25 mg t.i.d. or q.i.d. CHILDREN UNDER 6 YEARS: 0.3 to 0.6 mg t.i.d. or q.i.d.	**CNS (especially in the elderly):** *drowsiness,* dizziness, confusion, restlessness, insomnia. **GI:** anorexia, diarrhea or constipation, nausea, vomiting, *dry mouth*. **GU:** urinary frequency or retention. **Skin:** urticaria, rash.

INTERACTIONS AND SPECIAL CONSIDERATIONS

relieve dry mouth.
- Each patient's dose should be titrated; response to drug varies.
- If tolerance develops, another antihistamine may be substituted.
- Patient should stop taking drug 4 days before allergy skin tests; otherwise, accuracy of tests may be affected.

No significant interactions.

Special considerations:
- Contraindicated in acute asthmatic attack. Use cautiously in elderly patients, and in patients with increased intraocular pressure, hyperthyroidism, cardiovascular or renal disease, hypertension, diabetes mellitus, bronchial asthma, narrow-angle glaucoma, urinary retention, prostatic hypertrophy, bladder-neck obstruction.
- Patient should avoid alcoholic beverages during therapy and driving or other activities that require alertness until CNS response to drug is determined.
- Taking drug with food or milk reduces GI distress.
- Coffee or tea may reduce drowsiness. Sugarless gum, sour hard candy, or ice chips may relieve dry mouth.
- Each patient's dose should be titrated; response to drug varies.
- Patient should stop taking drug 4 days before allergy skin tests; otherwise, accuracy of tests may be affected.

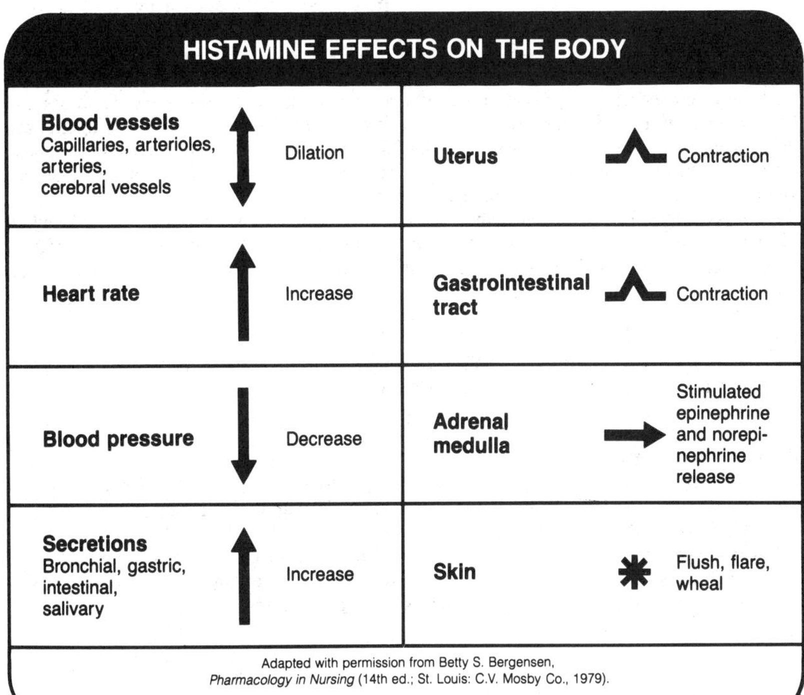

Adapted with permission from Betty S. Bergensen, *Pharmacology in Nursing* (14th ed.; St. Louis: C.V. Mosby Co., 1979).

43

Expectorants and antitussives

Expectorants
acetylcysteine
ammonium chloride
guaifenesin (formerly glyceryl guaiacolate)
hydriodic acid
iodinated glycerol
potassium iodide (SSKI)
terpin hydrate
tyloxapol

Antitussives
benzonatate
chlophedianol hydrochloride
codeine
codeine phosphate
codeine sulfate
dextromethorphan hydrobromide
diphenhydramine hydrochloride
hydrocodone bitartrate
hydromorphone hydrochloride
levopropoxyphene napsylate
noscapine hydrochloride

(All drugs are listed in alphabetical order in the tables that follow.)

Expectorants may decrease sputum viscosity and ease expectoration. Although they are used to loosen secretions (provide mucolytic action) in chronic pulmonary disorders and the common cold, their therapeutic efficacy is doubtful. Nevertheless, these agents are included in many prescription and over-the-counter cough and cold preparations. These agents should probably be used only in conjunction with a total care plan that includes adequate fluid intake and a cool mist or steam vaporizer.

Antitussives, or cough suppressants, reduce the frequency of a cough, especially when it is dry and nonproductive. Cough suppression is desirable when a chronic cough produces extreme fatigue (as in lung cancer). Most patients with a common cold don't need antitussives; cough drops will do.

Major uses

- Expectorants may facilitate expectoration in pneumonia, bronchitis, cystic fibrosis, tuberculosis, emphysema, atelectasis, and bronchial asthma.
- Antitussives suppress nonproductive coughs.

Mechanism of action

- Expectorants may increase production of respiratory tract fluids to help liquefy and reduce the viscosity of thick, tenacious secretions. Tyloxapol also lowers surface tension of sputum to facilitate expectoration.
- Antitussives suppress the cough reflex by direct action on the cough center in the medulla (brain) or by peripheral action on sensory nerve endings. Benzonatate, chlophedianol, and diphenhydramine also act as local anesthetics.

DO EXPECTORANTS REALLY HELP?

You're probably familiar with traditional expectorants, such as guaifenesin, potassium iodide and other iodides, terpin hydrate, and syrup of ipecac. But did you know that all these drugs have been the subjects of studies to determine the actual effectiveness of expectorants?

Guaifenesin (Robitussin), the most popular expectorant, has come under especially close scrutiny. It's been found:

- no better than the placebo in controlled studies.
- ineffective as an expectorant in patients with chronic bronchitis.
- effective in some studies but only when extremely high doses of this drug are administered.

Fortunately, new and effective trends have developed in expectorant therapy. These include the use of:

- *mucolytic agents*, which lower sputum viscosity and aid expectoration
- *corticosteroids*, which reduce mucus volume and lower sputum viscosity, and are effective in severe conditions such as bronchial asthma
- *oral, parenteral, mist, or steam hydration*, which helps to loosen thick secretions. (Hydration should be administered only when ordered. Since water increases mucus volume, further airway obstruction can result. Use hydration with a bronchodilator, a heated ultrasonic nebulizer, or a similar device if ordered.)

Absorption, distribution, metabolism, and excretion

All expectorants and antitussives are well absorbed after oral administration, metabolized in the liver, and excreted in the urine.

- Acetylcysteine and tyloxapol are also well absorbed after inhalation.
- Potassium iodide is also excreted through the respiratory tract.

Onset and duration

Expectorants and antitussives begin to act within 30 minutes. Their effects generally last 4 to 6 hours; benzonatate, however, may act as long as 8 hours.

Combination products

Preparations are available in the following combinations: expectorants with decongestants or antihistamines, or both; antitussives with decongestants or antihistamines, or both; expectorants and antitussives; expectorants and antitussives with decongestants or antihistamines, or both.

NAMES, INDICATIONS AND DOSAGES	SIDE EFFECTS
acetylcysteine Airbron♦♦, Mucomyst♦, NAC♦♦ **Pneumonia, bronchitis, tuberculosis, cystic fibrosis, emphysema, atelectasis (adjunct), complications of thoracic surgery and CV surgery:** ADULTS AND CHILDREN: 1 to 2 ml 10% to 20% solution by direct instillation into trachea as often as every hour; or 3 to 5 ml 20% solution, or 6 to 10 ml 10% solution, by mouthpiece t.i.d. or q.i.d. **Acetaminophen toxicity:** 140 mg/kg initially P.O., followed by 70 mg/kg q 4 hours for 17 doses (a total of 1,330 mg/kg).	**EENT:** *rhinorrhea, hemoptysis.* **GI:** *stomatitis, nausea.* **Other:** *bronchospasm (especially in patients with asthma).*
ammonium chloride **As expectorant:** ADULTS: 250 to 500 mg P.O. q 2 to 4 hours.	**CNS:** headache, drowsiness, confusion, excitation alternating with coma, twitching, hyperreflexia, EEG abnormalities. **CV:** bradycardia. **GI:** *anorexia, nausea, vomiting.* **GU:** renal impairment, glycosuria. **Metabolic:** acidosis, decreased potassium, hypocalcemic tetany, hyperglycemia. **Skin:** rash. **Other:** thirst.
benzonatate Tessalon♦ **Nonproductive cough:** ADULTS AND CHILDREN OVER 10 YEARS: 100 mg P.O. t.i.d.; up to 600 mg daily. CHILDREN UNDER 10 YEARS: 8 mg/kg P.O. in 3 to 6 divided doses.	**CNS:** dizziness, drowsiness. **EENT:** nasal congestion, sensation of burning in eyes. **GI:** nausea, constipation. **Skin:** rash.
chlophedianol hydrochloride Ulo, Ulone♦♦ **Nonproductive cough:** ADULTS AND CHILDREN OVER 12 YEARS: 25 mg P.O. t.i.d. or q.i.d. CHILDREN 6 TO 12 YEARS: 12.5 to 25 mg P.O. t.i.d. or q.i.d. CHILDREN 2 TO 6 YEARS: 12.5 mg P.O. t.i.d. or q.i.d.	**CNS:** *drowsiness,* dizziness, excitation, irritability, nightmares, hallucinations. **GI:** *nausea,* vomiting.
codeine **codeine phosphate** **codeine sulfate** Controlled Substance Schedule II **Nonproductive cough:** ADULTS: 8 to 20 mg P.O. q 4 to 6 hours. Maximum 120 mg/24 hours. CHILDREN: 1 to 1.5 mg/kg P.O. daily in 4 divided doses. Maximum 60 mg/24 hours.	**CNS:** *dizziness, sedation.* **CV:** palpitations. **GI:** *nausea,* vomiting; with repeated doses, *constipation.* **Skin:** pruritus. **Other:** tolerance and physical dependence.

INTERACTIONS AND SPECIAL CONSIDERATIONS

No significant interactions.

Special considerations:
- Use cautiously in patients with asthma or severe respiratory insufficiency, and in elderly or debilitated patients.
- Classified as a mucolytic.
- Plastic, glass, stainless steel, or another nonreactive metal should be used when administered by nebulization. Handbulb nebulizers not recommended because output too small and particle size too large.
- After opening, should be stored in refrigerator and used within 96 hours.
- Incompatible with oxytetracycline, tetracycline, and erythromycin lactobionate.
- Cough type and frequency should be monitored. For maximum effect, patient should clear his airway by coughing before aerosol administration.
- Available in combination with isoproterenol in a 4-ml vial.
- Large doses are used orally to treat acetaminophen overdose. For dose in acetaminophen toxicity, see APPENDIX.

Interactions:
SPIRONOLACTONE: systemic acidosis. Use cautiously.

Special considerations:
- Contraindicated in hepatic or renal impairment. Use cautiously in pulmonary insufficiency and congestive heart failure.
- Should be taken with full glass of water.
- Cough type and frequency should be monitored.
- Deep-breathing exercises should be encouraged.
- Possible potentiated diuresis when used with diuretics.
- Also used to acidify urine.

No significant interactions.

Special considerations:
- Patient should not chew tablets or leave in mouth to dissolve; local anesthesia will result.
- A cough suppressant; should not be used when cough is valuable diagnostic sign or is beneficial (as after thoracic surgery).
- Cough type and frequency should be monitored.
- Should be used with percussion and chest vibration.
- Fluid intake should be maintained to help liquify sputum.

No significant interactions.

Special considerations:
- An antitussive; should not be used when cough is valuable diagnostic sign or is beneficial (as after thoracic surgery).
- Cough type and frequency should be monitored.
- Should be used with percussion and chest vibration.
- CNS side effects disappear when drug is stopped.

No significant interactions.

Special considerations:
- Contraindicated in increased intracranial or CSF pressure. Use cautiously in debilitated patients, in dehydrated postoperative patients; in those with asthma, emphysema, head injury, history of drug abuse, hepatic or renal disease, hypothyroidism, Addison's disease, acute alcoholism, seizures, severe CNS depression, chronic obstructive pulmonary disease, psychosis; after thoracotomies or laparotomies; and when other CNS depressants are given. Patient should be monitored carefully.
- Should be used with percussion and chest vibration.
- Patient should avoid driving or other activities that require alertness until CNS response to drug is determined.
- An antitussive; should not be used when cough is valuable diagnostic sign or is beneficial (as after thoracic surgery).
- Cough type and frequency should be monitored.

NAMES, INDICATIONS AND DOSAGES	SIDE EFFECTS
dextromethorphan hydrobromide Balminil DM♦♦, Broncho-Grippol-DM♦♦, Contratuss♦♦, Pertussin 8-hour, Romilar Chewable Tablets for Children, St. Joseph Cough Syrup for Children, Sedatuss♦♦, Silence Is Golden. More commonly available in combination products such as Benylin-DM, Coryban-D Cough Syrup, Dimacol, Naldetuss, Novahistine DMX, Ornacol, Phenergan Expectorant with Dextromethorphan, Robitussin DM, Romilar CF, Rondec-DM, Triaminicol, Trind-DM, Tussi-Organidin-DM, 2G-DM **Nonproductive cough:** ADULTS: 10 to 20 mg q 4 hours, or 30 mg q 6 to 8 hours. Maximum 120 mg/day. CHILDREN 6 TO 12 YEARS: 5 to 10 mg q 4 hours, or 15 mg q 6 to 8 hours. Maximum 60 mg/day. CHILDREN 2 TO 6 YEARS: 2.5 mg q 4 hours, or 7.5 mg q 6 to 8 hours. Maximum 30 mg/day.	**CNS:** drowsiness. **GI:** nausea.
diphenhydramine hydrochloride Allerdryl, Baramine, Bax, Benachlor, Benadryl♦, Benahist, Ben-Allergin, Bendylate, Bentrac, Benylin Cough Syrup♦♦, Eldadryl, Fenylhist, Hyrexin, Nordryl, Phen-Amin 50, Phenamine, Rodryl, Rohydra, Valdrene, Wehdryl **Nonproductive cough:** ADULTS: 25 mg P.O. q 4 hours (not to exceed 100 mg/day). CHILDREN 6 TO 12 YEARS: 12.5 mg P.O. q 4 hours (not to exceed 50 mg/day). CHILDREN 2 TO 6 YEARS: 6.25 mg P.O. q 4 hours (not to exceed 25 mg/day).	**CNS:** *sedation,* confusion, restlessness, insomnia, headache. **CV:** palpitations. **EENT:** diplopia, blurred vision, nasal congestion. **GI:** *dry mouth and throat,* nausea, vomiting, diarrhea, constipation. **GU:** dysuria. **Skin:** urticaria.
guaifenesin (formerly glyceryl guaiacolate) Anti-Tuss, Balminil♦♦, Bowtussin, Breonesin, Colrex, Cosin-GG, Demo-Cineol♦♦, Dilyn, 2/G, G-100, G-200, GG-CEN, Glycotuss, Gly-O-Tussin, Glytuss, G-Tussin, Guaiatussin, Hytuss, Malotuss, Motussin♦♦, Nortussin, Proco, Recsei-Tuss, Resyl♦♦, Robitussin♦, Sedatuss♦♦, Tursen, Tussanca♦♦, Wal-Tussin DM **Productive and nonproductive cough:** ADULTS: 100 to 200 mg P.O. q 2 to 4 hours. Maximum 800 mg/day. CHILDREN: 12 mg/kg P.O. daily in 6 divided doses.	**CNS:** drowsiness. **GI:** vomiting and nausea occur with large doses.

♦ Available in U.S. and Canada. ♦♦ Available in Canada only.
All other products (no symbol) available in U.S. only. Italicized side effects are common or life-threatening.

INTERACTIONS AND SPECIAL CONSIDERATIONS

Interactions:
MAO INHIBITORS: hypotension, coma, hyperpyrexia, and death have occurred. Do not use together.

Special considerations:
• Contraindicated in patients currently taking or within 2 weeks of stopping MAO inhibitors.
• Produces no analgesia or addiction and little or no CNS depression.
• An antitussive; should not be used when cough is valuable diagnostic sign or is beneficial (as after thoracic surgery).
• Patient should not take fluids immediately after taking drug.
• Should be used with percussion and chest vibration.
• Cough type and frequency should be monitored.
• Available in most over-the-counter cough medicines.

No significant interactions.

Special considerations:
• Contraindicated in acute asthma, narrow-angle glaucoma, prostatic hypertrophy, peptic ulcer, pyloroduodenal and bladder neck obstruction. Use cautiously in asthma, hypertensive, or cardiac patients.
• Patient should avoid alcoholic beverages during therapy and driving or other activities that require alertness until CNS response to drug is determined.
• Liquid preparations are recommended for antitussive effect.
• Patient should not take fluids immediately after taking drug.
• Coffee and tea may reduce drowsiness. Sugarless gum, sour hard candy, or ice chips may relieve dry mouth.
• If tolerance develops, another antihistamine may be substituted.
• Patient should stop taking drug 4 days before allergy skin tests; otherwise, accuracy of tests may be affected.

No significant interactions.

Special considerations:
• May interfere with certain laboratory tests for 5-hydroxyindoleacetic acid and vanillylmandelic acid.
• Possible bleeding gums, hematuria, and bruising if given to patients on heparin. Should such symptoms appear, guaifenesin should be discontinued.
• Liquefies thick, tenacious sputum; fluid intake should be maintained; patient should take with a glass of water whenever possible.
• Cough type and frequency should be monitored.
• An expectorant.
• Deep-breathing exercises should be encouraged.
• Although a very popular expectorant, many medical authorities doubt its efficacy.

NAMES, INDICATIONS AND DOSAGES	SIDE EFFECTS
hydriodic acid **Chronic bronchitis, bronchial asthma:** ADULTS: 1.25 to 5 ml syrup well diluted in water P.O. b.i.d. or t.i.d.	**EENT:** tooth damage.
hydrocodone bitartrate Controlled Substance Schedule II Coditrate, Codone, Corutol DH♦♦, Dicodethal, Dicodid, Hycodan♦, Robidone♦♦ **Nonproductive cough:** ADULTS: 5 to 10 mg P.O. t.i.d. or q.i.d., p.r.n. Maximum single dose 15 mg. CHILDREN: 0.6 mg/kg P.O. daily in 3 or 4 divided doses.	**CNS:** *drowsiness, dizziness.* **EENT:** dryness of throat. **GI:** *nausea, constipation.* **Other:** tolerance and physical dependence after long-term use.
hydromorphone hydrochloride Controlled Substance Schedule II Dilaudid Cough Syrup♦ **Cough:** ADULTS: 1 mg P.O. q 3 to 4 hours, p.r.n. CHILDREN 6 TO 12 YEARS: 0.5 mg P.O. q 3 to 4 hours, p.r.n.	**CNS:** *dizziness, somnolence,* respiratory depression. **CV:** hypotension. **GI:** *nausea,* vomiting, anorexia, constipation.
iodinated glycerol Organidin♦ **Bronchial asthma, bronchitis, emphysema (adjunct):** ADULTS: 60 mg P.O. q.i.d. (tablets), or 20 drops (solution) P.O. q.i.d. with fluids, or 1 teaspoonful (elixir) P.O. q.i.d. CHILDREN: up to ½ adult dose based on child's weight.	**After long-term use:** **GI:** *nausea,* gastrointestinal distress. **Skin:** *eruptions.* **Other:** acute parotitis, thyroid enlargement.
levopropoxyphene napsylate Novrad **Nonproductive cough:** ADULTS: 50 to 100 mg q 4 hours. CHILDREN 23 TO 45 KG: 50 mg q 4 hours. CHILDREN UP TO 23 KG: 25 mg q 4 hours.	**CNS:** *drowsiness,* jitters, *dizziness,* headache. **EENT:** visual disturbances, dry mouth. **GI:** *nausea,* vomiting, diarrhea, *epigastric burning.* **GU:** urinary frequency or urgency. **Skin:** rash, urticaria.

♦ Available in U.S. and Canada. ♦♦ Available in Canada only.
All other products (no symbol) available in U.S. only. Italicized side effects are common or life-threatening.

INTERACTIONS AND SPECIAL CONSIDERATIONS

No significant interactions.

Special considerations:
• Should be diluted well and straw used to avoid injuring teeth; syrup is very acidic.
• Liquefies thick, tenacious sputum; fluid intake should be maintained; patient should take with a glass of water whenever possible.
• Should not be used if syrup is deep brown color.
• Cough type and frequency should be monitored.
• Deep-breathing exercises should be encouraged.
• An expectorant.

Interactions:
CNS DEPRESSANTS: increased sedation. Use together cautiously.

Special considerations:
• Contraindicated in glaucoma. Use cautiously in asthma, emphysema, drug dependence; after thoracotomy or laparotomy; and in debilitated or dehydrated patients.
• Patient should avoid driving or other activities that require alertness until CNS response to drug is determined.
• Patient's need for drug, which is addictive, should be evaluated.
• An antitussive; should not be used when cough is valuable diagnostic sign or is beneficial (as after thoracic surgery).
• Should be used with percussion and chest vibration.
• Cough type and frequency should be monitored.

Interactions:
CNS DEPRESSANTS: increased sedation. Use together cautiously.

Special considerations:
• Contraindicated in increased intracranial pressure and status asthmaticus. Use cautiously in hepatic or renal disease, hypothyroidism, Addison's disease, acute alcoholism, seizures, head injury, severe CNS depression, brain tumor, bronchial asthma, chronic obstructive pulmonary disease, or psychosis.
• Patient should avoid driving and other activities that require alertness until CNS response to drug is determined.
• Respiration, pupil size, and bowel function should be monitored.
• An antitussive; should not be used when cough is a valuable diagnostic sign or is beneficial (as after thoracic surgery).
• Should be used with percussion and chest vibration.
• Cough type and frequency should be monitored.
• Smoking should be discouraged and hard candy offered.
• Addictive.
• CNS depressants cause potentiation. Should be used together cautiously.

No significant interactions.

Special considerations:
• Contraindicated in hypothyroidism and iodine sensitivity.
• Skin rash or other hypersensitivity reaction may require stopping drug.
• May liquefy thick, tenacious sputum; fluid intake should be maintained.
• Cough type and frequency should be monitored.
• Deep-breathing exercises should be encouraged.
• An expectorant.

No significant interactions.

Special considerations:
• Contraindicated in first trimester of pregnancy.
• An antitussive; should not be used when cough is valuable diagnostic sign or is beneficial (as after thoracic surgery).
• Patient should not take fluids just after liquid preparation.
• Should be used with percussion and chest vibration.
• Cough type and frequency should be monitored.
• Patient should avoid driving or other activities that require alertness until CNS response to drug is determined.

NAMES, INDICATIONS AND DOSAGES	SIDE EFFECTS
noscapine hydrochloride Noscatuss♦♦, Tusscapine **Nonproductive cough:** ADULTS: 15 to 30 mg P.O. q 4 to 6 hours as chewable tablet. CHILDREN 6 TO 12 YEARS: 7.5 to 15 mg P.O. t.i.d. or q.i.d. as syrup. CHILDREN 2 TO 6 YEARS: 5 to 10 mg P.O. t.i.d. or q.i.d. as syrup.	**CNS:** slight drowsiness. **EENT:** acute vasomotor rhinitis, conjunctivitis. **GI:** nausea.
potassium iodide (SSKI) **Chronic bronchitis, bronchial asthma:** ADULTS: 300 to 600 mg P.O. q 2 hours until desired response obtained. CHILDREN: 0.25 to 1 ml of saturated solution (1 g/ml) b.i.d., t.i.d., or q.i.d. **Nuclear radiation protection:** ADULTS AND CHILDREN: 0.13 ml P.O. of SSKI immediately before or after initial exposure will block 90% of radioactive iodine. Same dose given 3 to 4 hours after exposure will provide 50% block. Should be administered for up to 10 days under medical supervision. INFANTS UNDER 1 YEAR: ½ adult dose.	**GI:** nonspecific small bowel lesions, *nausea,* vomiting, *epigastric pain,* metallic taste. **Metabolic:** goiter, hyperthyroid adenoma, hypothyroidism (with excessive use), collagen disease-like syndrome. **Skin:** rash. **Prolonged use:** chronic iodine poisoning, soreness of mouth, coryza, sneezing, swelling of eyelids.
terpin hydrate Creoterp, Terp **Excessive bronchial secretions:** ADULTS: 5 to 10 ml P.O. of elixir.	None.
tyloxapol Alevaire **Bronchitis, emphysema, pulmonary abscess, bronchiectasis, atelectasis (by inhalation only):** ADULTS: up to 500 ml 0.125% solution q 12 to 24 hours by continuous aerosol inhalation, adjusting rate of flow, p.r.n.; or 10 to 20 ml 0.125% solution by intermittent inhalation for 30 to 90 minutes t.i.d. or q.i.d.	**GI:** *nausea.* **Local:** irritation.

♦ Available in U.S. and Canada. ♦♦ Available in Canada only.
All other products (no symbol) available in U.S. only. Italicized side effects are common or life-threatening.

INTERACTIONS AND SPECIAL CONSIDERATIONS

No significant interactions.

Special considerations:
• An antitussive; should not be used when cough is valuable diagnostic sign or is beneficial (as after thoracic surgery).
• Patient should not take fluids just after liquid preparation.
• Should be used with percussion and chest vibration.
• Cough type and frequency should be monitored.

Interactions:
LITHIUM CARBONATE: may cause hypothyroidism. Don't use together.

Special considerations:
• Contraindicated in iodine hypersensitivity, tuberculosis, hyperkalemia, acute bronchitis, hyperthyroidism.
• Fluid intake should be maintained to help liquefy sputum.
• Has strong, salty, metallic taste. Should be diluted with milk or fruit juice to reduce GI distress and disguise taste.
• If given over long period, sudden withdrawal may precipitate thyroid storm.
• Cough type and frequency should be monitored.
• Deep-breathing exercises should be encouraged.
• If skin rash appears, use should be discontinued.
• An expectorant.
• Patient should not use any over-the-counter drugs without first consulting doctor.

No significant interactions.

Special considerations:
• Contraindicated on empty stomach, in peptic ulcer, or severe diabetes mellitus. Use cautiously in patients with history of alcohol or drug abuse.
• Should not be given in large doses: high alcoholic content of elixir (86 proof).
• Cough type and frequency should be monitored.

No significant interactions.

Special considerations:
• Aerosols may induce bronchial spasm in some patients with asthma.
• A surfactant with detergent properties.
• Lowers surface tension and reduces viscosity of thick, tenacious sputum to facilitate expectoration; fluid intake should be maintained. Most benefit results from humidification of inspired air.
• Cough type and frequency should be monitored.
• Deep-breathing exercises should be encouraged.
• If used as a vehicle, phenylephrine or isoproterenol should be added just before use.

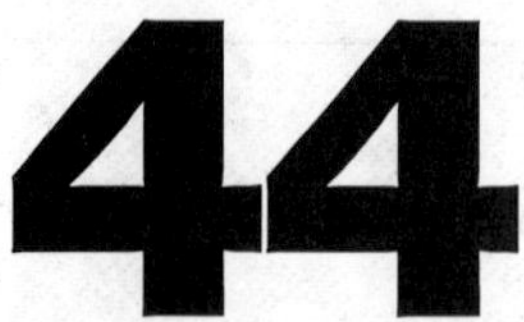

Antacids, adsorbents, and antiflatulents

activated charcoal
aluminum carbonate
aluminum hydroxide
aluminum phosphate
calcium carbonate
dihydroxyaluminum aminoacetate
dihydroxyaluminum sodium carbonate
magaldrate
magnesia magma (MOM)
magnesium carbonate
magnesium oxide
magnesium trisilicate
oxethazaine
simethicone
sodium bicarbonate

Antacids are used to treat peptic ulcers (localized lesions of the gastric and duodenal mucosa). They may consist of various combinations of aluminum, calcium, and magnesium salts; magaldrate; and oxethazaine. But most of them are combinations of aluminum and magnesium salts. Although the antacidic properties of inorganic salts cited have been known for more than 2,000 years, until the modern era their use was mainly empirical and subjective. Today, however, use and action of antacids are well known and medically respected.

The products vary in their ability to neutralize acid. Adequate doses and proper timing of administration promote healing of duodenal ulcers.

Many patients on salt-restricted diets may not realize that the antacids they're taking contain sodium in the form of the salt sodium chloride. Sometimes the salt content is high enough to aggravate conditions such as congestive heart failure and hypertension.

Adsorbents (specifically, activated charcoal) effectively inhibit gastrointestinal (GI) absorption of various drugs, chemicals, and toxins. However, activated charcoal doesn't adsorb cyanide, ethanol, methanol, iron, sodium chloride, alkalis, mineral acids, or organic solvents.

Antiflatulents, such as simethicone, have a defoaming action. They're usually combined with antacids to relieve hyperacidity and gas.

Major uses

- Antacids neutralize gastric acidity and help control ulcer pain. They're also used to treat the retrosternal burning sensation (heartburn) due to reflux esophagitis.
- Adsorbents are general-purpose antidotes in acute episodes of certain oral poisonings (phenol ingestion and acetaminophen overdose, for example).
- Antiflatulents relieve painful symptoms of excess gas in the digestive tract.

Mechanism of action

- Antacids reduce total acid load in the GI tract and elevate gastric pH to reduce pepsin activity. They also strengthen the gastric mucosal barrier and increase esophageal sphincter tone. They don't seem to have a coating effect on ulcers.

  Oxethazaine is a potent local anesthetic that may adhere to receptor sites, producing a prolonged topical anesthetic effect on the gastric mucosa.
- Adsorbents adhere to many drugs and chemicals, inhibiting their absorption from the GI tract.
- Antiflatulents, by the defoaming action of simethicone, disperse or prevent formation of mucus-surrounded gas pockets in the GI tract. These preparations form a film in the GI tract that causes gas bubbles to collapse.

Absorption, distribution, metabolism, and excretion

• Absorption of antacids varies. Prolonged use of antacids that contain magnesium or calcium may cause systemic absorption of magnesium or calcium ions in toxic quantities. Excessive aluminum antacid therapy can lead to hypophosphatemia. Antacids are distributed throughout the GI tract and are eliminated primarily in feces.

• Adsorbents are neither absorbed in the GI tract nor metabolized. They are eliminated unchanged in the feces.

• Because antiflatulents are physiologically inactive, they're not absorbed in the GI tract and don't interfere with gastric secretion or nutrient absorption. They're eliminated unchanged in the feces.

Onset and duration

• Antacids' onset of action is generally immediate. Duration of action is usually only 1 hour when taken on an empty stomach but as long as 3 hours if taken after meals.

• Adsorbents' onset of action is immediate. Duration varies, depending on amount of poison swallowed and absorbed, as well as amount of activated charcoal given.

• Antiflatulents' onset of action is immediate; duration of effect is as long as 3 hours.

Combination products

CAMALOX♦: aluminum hydroxide 225 mg, magnesium hydroxide 200 mg, and calcium carbonate 250 mg.

DELCID SUSPENSION: aluminum hydroxide 600 mg, magnesium hydroxide 665 mg, and sodium < 15 mg/5 ml.

DI-GEL: aluminum hydroxide and magnesium carbonate 282 mg, magnesium hydroxide 85 mg, simethicone 25 mg, and sodium 10.6 mg.

GAVISCON♦: aluminum hydroxide 80 mg, magnesium trisilicate 20 mg, sodium bicarbonate 70 mg, alginic acid 200 mg, and approximately 0.8 mEq sodium.

GELUSIL♦: aluminum hydroxide 200 mg, magnesium hydroxide 200 mg, simethicone 25 mg, and sodium 1.4 mg.

GELUSIL-II: aluminum hydroxide 400 mg, magnesium hydroxide 400 mg, simethicone 30 mg, and sodium 2.7 mg.

GELUSIL-M: aluminum hydroxide 300 mg, magnesium hydroxide 200 mg, simethicone 25 mg, and sodium 3 mg.

KOLANTYLWAFERS♦: aluminum hydroxide 180 mg and magnesium hydroxide 170 mg.

MAALOX NO. 1: aluminum hydroxide 200 mg and magnesium hydroxide 200 mg.

MAALOX NO. 2: aluminum hydroxide 400 mg and magnesium hydroxide 400 mg.

MAALOX PLUS♦: aluminum hydroxide 200 mg, magnesium hydroxide 200 mg, simethicone 25 mg, and sodium 1.6 mg.

MAALOX THERAPEUTIC CONCENTRATE: aluminum hydroxide 600 mg, magnesium hydroxide 300 mg, and sodium 1.25 mg.

MYLANTA♦: aluminum hydroxide 200 mg, magnesium hydroxide 200 mg, simethicone 20 mg, and sodium 0.5 mg.

MYLANTA-II♦: aluminum hydroxide 400 mg, magnesium hydroxide 400 mg, simethicone 30 mg, and sodium 1 mg.

RIOPAN PLUS SUSPENSION: magaldrate 400 mg, simethicone 20 mg, and sodium < 0.65 mg/5 ml.

NAMES, INDICATIONS AND DOSAGES	SIDE EFFECTS
activated charcoal Charcocaps, Charcodote, Charcotabs, Digestalin **Flatulence or dyspepsia:** ADULTS: 600 mg to 5 g P.O. **Poisoning:** ADULTS AND CHILDREN: 5 to 10 times estimated weight of drug or chemical ingested. Minimum dose 30 g in 250 ml water to make a slurry. Give orally, preferably within 30 minutes of poisoning. Larger doses are necessary if food is in the stomach. For treatment of poisoning or overdosage with acetaminophen, amphetamines, aspirin, antimony, atropine, arsenic, barbiturates, camphor, cocaine, cardiotonic glycosides, glutethimide, ipecac, malathion, morphine, poisonous mushrooms, opium, oxalic acid, parathion, phenol, phenothiazines, potassium permanganate, propoxyphene, quinine, strychnine, sulfonamides, tricyclic antidepressants.	**GI:** black stools.
aluminum carbonate Basaljel♦ **As antacid:** ADULTS: suspension: 5 to 10 ml, p.r.n. Extra-strength suspension: 2.5 to 5 ml, p.r.n. Tablets: 1 to 2, p.r.n. Capsules: 1 to 2, p.r.n. **To prevent formation of urinary phosphate stones (with low-phosphate diet):** ADULTS: suspension: 15 to 30 ml suspension in water or juice 1 hour after meals and h.s.; 5 to 15 ml extra-strength in water or juice 1 hour after meals and h.s.; 2 to 6 tablets or capsules 1 hour after meals and h.s.	**GI:** anorexia, *constipation,* intestinal obstruction. **Metabolic:** hypophosphatemia.
aluminum hydroxide ALternaGel, Alu-Cap, Al-U-Creme, Aluminett, Amphojel♦, Basaljel♦♦, Dialume, Hydroxal, No-Co-Gel, Nutrajel **Antacid:** ADULTS: 600 mg P.O. (5 to 10 ml of most products) 1 hour after meals and h.s.; 300- or 600-mg tablet, chewed before swallowing, taken with milk or water 5 to 6 times daily after meals and h.s. **Hyperphosphatemia in renal failure:** ADULTS: 500 mg to 2 g b.i.d. to q.i.d.	**GI:** anorexia, *constipation,* intestinal obstruction. **Metabolic:** hypophosphatemia.

♦ Available in U.S. and Canada. ♦♦ Available in Canada only.
All other products (no symbol) available in U.S. only. Italicized side effects are common or life-threatening.

INTERACTIONS AND SPECIAL CONSIDERATIONS

No significant interactions.

Special considerations:

- Because activated charcoal absorbs and inactivates syrup of ipecac, should be given after emesis.
- Should not be given in ice cream, which decreases absorptive capacity.
- Powder form most effective. Should be mixed with tap water to form consistency of thick syrup. Small amount of fruit juice may be added to make more palatable.
- Doses should be spaced at least 1 hour apart from other drugs if activated charcoal is being used for any indication other than poisoning.
- Patient should be warned that feces will be black.

No significant interactions.

Special considerations:

- Use cautiously in elderly patients, especially in those with decreased bowel motility (those receiving antidiarrheals, antispasmodics, or anticholinergics), dehydration, fluid restriction, chronic renal disease, and suspected intestinal obstruction.
- Amount and consistency of stools should be monitored. Constipation should be managed with laxatives or stool softeners. Should be alternated with magnesium-containing antacids (if not renal disease patient).
- Shake suspension well. Should be taken with milk or water to assure passage to stomach. For nasogastric instillation: check tube position and patency; flush tube with water after instillation to facilitate passage.
- Long-term, high-dose use in patient on restricted sodium intake should be monitored.
- Patient should not take aluminum carbonate indiscriminately and should not switch antacids without doctor's advice.
- Because it contains aluminum, it is used in patients with renal failure to help control hyperphosphatemia. Binds phosphate in GI tract.
- Serum phosphate levels should be monitored.
- Possible hypophosphatemia with prolonged use (anorexia, malaise, muscle weakness); can also lead to resorption of calcium and bone demineralization.
- If patient is able, he should be responsible for taking antacid while hospitalized.
- May cause enteric-coated drugs to be released prematurely in stomach. Doses should be separated by 1 hour.

No significant interactions.

Special considerations:

- Use cautiously in elderly, especially those with decreased bowel motility (those taking antidiarrheals, antispasmodics, or anticholinergics), dehydration, fluid restriction, chronic renal disease, suspected intestinal obstruction.
- Monitor amount and consistency of stools. Manage constipation with laxatives or stool softeners. Alternate with magnesium-containing antacids (if not renal disease patient).
- Shake suspension well; should be taken with milk or water to assure passage to stomach. For nasogastric instillation: check tube position and patency; flush tube with water after instillation.
- Long-term, high-dose use in patient on restricted sodium intake should be monitored.
- Patient should not take aluminum hydroxide indiscriminately and should not switch antacids without doctor's advice.
- Because it contains aluminum, it is used in renal failure patients to help control hyperphosphatemia. Binds phosphate in the GI tract.
- Serum phosphate levels should be monitored.
- Possible hypophosphatemia with prolonged use (anorexia, malaise, muscle weakness); can also lead to resorption of calcium and bone demineralization.
- If patient is able, he should be responsible for taking antacid while hospitalized.
- May cause enteric-coated drugs to be released prematurely in stomach. Doses should be separated by 1 hour.

NAMES, INDICATIONS AND DOSAGES	SIDE EFFECTS
aluminum phosphate Phosphaljel **Antacid:** ADULTS: 15 to 30 ml undiluted q 2 hours between meals and h.s.	**GI:** *constipation,* intestinal obstruction.
calcium carbonate Alka-2, Amitone, Calcilac, Calglycine, Dicarbosil, El-Da-Mint, Equilet, Gustalac, Mallamint, P.H. Tablets, Spentacid, Titracid, Titralac, Trialea, Tums **Antacid:** ADULTS: 1-g tablet, 4 to 6 times daily, chewed well and taken with water; or 1 g of suspension (5 ml of most products) 1 hour after meals and h.s.	**GI:** *constipation,* gastric distention, flatulence, acid-rebound, *nausea.* **Metabolic:** *hypercalcemia;* if taken with milk—milk-alkali syndrome.
dihydroxyaluminum aminoacetate Alkam, Hyperacid, Robalate♦ **Antacid:** ADULTS: 0.5 to 1 g (1 to 2 tablets) after meals and h.s., chewed before swallowing and taken with milk or water.	**GI:** anorexia, *constipation,* intestinal obstruction. **Metabolic:** hypophosphatemia.
dihydroxyaluminum sodium carbonate Rolaids **Antacid:** ADULTS: chew 1 to 2 tablets (334 mg to 668 mg), p.r.n.	**GI:** anorexia, *constipation,* intestinal obstruction.

♦ Available in U.S. and Canada. ♦♦ Available in Canada only.
All other products (no symbol) available in U.S. only. Italicized side effects are common or life-threatening.

INTERACTIONS AND SPECIAL CONSIDERATIONS

No significant interactions.

Special considerations:
• Use cautiously in elderly patients, especially in those with decreased bowel motility (those receiving antidiarrheals, antispasmodics, or anticholinergics), dehydration, fluid restriction, chronic renal disease, and suspected intestinal obstruction.
• Amount and consistency of stools should be monitored. Constipation should be managed with laxatives or stool softeners. Should be alternated with magnesium-containing antacids (if patient does not have renal disease).
• Shake well; should be taken alone or with milk or water. For nasogastric instillation: check tube position and patency; flush tube with water after instillation.
• Long-term, high-dose use in patient on restricted sodium intake should be monitored.
• Patient should not take aluminum phosphate indiscriminately and should not switch antacids without doctor's advice.
• This drug is a very weak antacid.
• Can reverse hypophosphatemia induced by aluminum hydroxide.
• If patient is able, he should be responsible for taking antacid while hospitalized.
• May cause enteric-coated drugs to be released prematurely in stomach. Doses should be separated by 1 hour.

No significant interactions.

Special considerations:
• Contraindicated in severe renal disease. Use cautiously in the elderly, especially those with decreased bowel motility (receiving antidiarrheals, antispasmodics, anticholinergics), dehydration, fluid restriction, chronic renal disease, and suspected intestinal obstruction.
• Should not be administered with milk or other foods high in vitamin D. Can cause milk-alkali syndrome (headache, confusion, distaste for food, nausea, vomiting, hypercalcemia, hypercalciuria, calcinosis, hyperphosphatemia).
• Amount and consistency of stools should be monitored. Constipation should be managed with laxatives or stool softeners.
• Hypercalcemia (nausea, vomiting, headache, mental confusion, anorexia) possible.
• Serum calcium levels, especially in mild renal impairment, should be monitored.
• Patient should not take calcium carbonate indiscriminately and should not switch antacids without doctor's advice. It is *not* candy.
• If patient is able, he should be responsible for taking antacid while hospitalized.
• Has been known to cause rebound hyperacidity.
• May cause enteric-coated tablets to be released prematurely in stomach. Doses should be separated by 1 hour.

No significant interactions.

Special considerations:
• Use cautiously in elderly patients, especially in those with decreased bowel motility (those receiving antidiarrheals, antispasmodics, or anticholinergics), dehydration, fluid restriction, chronic renal disease, and suspected intestinal obstruction.
• Amount and consistency of stools should be monitored. Less constipating than aluminum hydroxide. Constipation should be managed with laxatives or stool softeners. Should be alternated with magnesium-containing antacids (if not patient with renal disease).
• Possible hypophosphatemia with prolonged use (anorexia, malaise, muscle weakness); can also lead to resorption of calcium and bone demineralization.
• Serum phosphate levels should be monitored.
• Long-term, high-dose use in patient on restricted sodium intake should be monitored.
• Patient should not take dihydroxyaluminum aminoacetate indiscriminately and should not switch antacids without doctor's advice.
• If patient is able, he should be responsible for taking antacid while hospitalized.
• May cause enteric-coated drugs to be released prematurely in stomach. Doses should be separated by 1 hour.

No significant interactions.

Special considerations:
• Use cautiously in elderly patients, especially in those with decreased bowel motility (those receiving antidiarrheals, antispasmodics, or anticholinergics), dehydration, fluid restriction, chronic renal disease, and suspected intestinal obstruction.
• Has high sodium content and may increase sodium and water retention.
• Monitor amount and consistency of stools. Manage constipation with laxatives or stool softeners. Alternate with magnesium-containing antacids (if patient does not have renal disease).
• Long-term, high-dose use in patient on restricted sodium intake should be monitored.
• Patient should not take drug indiscriminately. It is *not* candy.
• If patient is able, he should be responsible for taking antacid while hospitalized.
• May cause enteric-coated drugs to be released prematurely in stomach. Doses should be separated by 1 hour.

NAMES, INDICATIONS AND DOSAGES	SIDE EFFECTS
magaldrate (aluminum-magnesium complex) Riopan♦ **Antacid:** ADULTS: suspension: 400 to 800 mg (5 to 10 ml) between meals and h.s. with water. Tablet: 400 to 800 mg (1 to 2 tablets) P.O. with water between meals and h.s. Chewable tablet: 400 to 800 mg (1 to 2 tablets) chewed before swallowing, between meals and h.s.	**GI:** mild constipation or diarrhea.
magnesia magma (MOM) (magnesium hydroxide) Milk of Magnesia, Mint-O-Mag **Antacid:** ADULTS: 5 to 10 ml or 1 to 2 tablets chewed before swallowing q.i.d., usually after meals and h.s. **Oral replacement therapy in mild hypomagnesemia:** ADULTS: 5 to 10 ml q.i.d., usually after meals and h.s. Monitor serum magnesium response.	**GI:** *diarrhea,* abdominal pain, nausea. **Metabolic:** hypermagnesemia.
magnesium carbonate **Antacid:** ADULTS: 0.5 to 2 g of powder product or chewable tablets between meals with ½ glass of water. **Laxative:** ADULTS: 8 g of powder product or chewable tablets with water h.s.	**GI:** *diarrhea,* gastric distention, flatulence, abdominal pain, nausea. **Metabolic:** hypermagnesemia.
magnesium oxide Mag-Ox, Maox, Niko-Mag, Oxabid, Par-Mag, Uro-Mag **Antacid:** ADULTS: 250 mg to 1 g with water or milk after meals and h.s. **Laxative:** ADULTS: 4 g with water or milk, usually h.s.	**GI:** *diarrhea,* nausea, abdominal pain. **Metabolic:** hypermagnesemia.

INTERACTIONS AND SPECIAL CONSIDERATIONS

No significant interactions.

Special considerations:
- Contraindicated in severe renal disease. Use cautiously in elderly patients, especially in those with decreased bowel motility (those receiving antidiarrheals, antispasmodics, or anticholinergics), dehydration, fluid restriction, and mild renal impairment.
- Amount and consistency of stools should be monitored.
- Shake suspension well; should be taken with small amount of water to assure passage to stomach. For nasogastric instillation: check tube position and patency; flush tube with water after instillation to assure passage to stomach and to maintain tube patency.
- Serum magnesium should be monitored in mild renal impairment. Symptomatic hypermagnesemia usually occurs only in severe renal failure.
- Not usually used in patients with renal failure (although it contains aluminum) to help control hypophosphatemia, since it contains magnesium, which may accumulate in renal failure.
- Good for patient on restricted sodium intake; very low sodium content.
- Patient should not take magaldrate indiscriminately and should not switch antacids without doctor's advice.
- If patient is able, he should be responsible for taking antacid while hospitalized.
- May cause enteric-coated drugs to be released prematurely in stomach. Doses should be separated by 1 hour.

No significant interactions.

Special considerations:
- Contraindicated in severe renal disease. Use cautiously in elderly patients and in those with mild renal impairment.
- Usually not used as antacid, even though it is very effective and potent, due to increased frequency of stools. Usually used as laxative.
- Amount and consistency of stools should be monitored.
- Shake suspension well; should be taken with small amount of water when used as antacid. For nasogastric instillation: check tube position and patency; flush tube with water after instillation to assure passage to stomach and to maintain tube patency.
- Possible hypermagnesemia with prolonged use and some degree of renal impairment (hypotension, nausea, vomiting, depressed reflexes, respiratory depression, coma). Serum magnesium levels should be monitored.
- May cause enteric-coated drugs to be released prematurely in stomach. Doses should be separated by 1 hour.
- If diarrhea occurs with antacid doses, alternative preparation should be suggested.
- Subcathartic doses also used as oral magnesium replacement therapy in hypomagnesemia.
- Patient should not take magnesia magma indiscriminately and should not switch antacids without doctor's advice.
- If able, patient should be responsible for taking antacid while hospitalized.

No significant interactions.

Special considerations:
- Contraindicated in severe renal disease. Use cautiously in elderly patients and in those with mild renal impairment.
- Possible hypermagnesemia with prolonged use and some degree of renal impairment (hypotension, nausea, vomiting, depressed reflexes, respiratory depression, coma). Serum magnesium levels should be monitored.
- When used as laxative, other oral drugs should not be taken 1 to 2 hours before or after.
- Amount and consistency of stools should be monitored.
- Patient should not take magnesium carbonate indiscriminately and should not switch antacids without doctor's advice.
- If patient is able, he should be responsible for taking antacid while hospitalized.
- May cause enteric-coated drugs to be released prematurely in stomach. Doses should be separated by 1 hour.

No significant interactions.

Special considerations:
- Contraindicated in severe renal disease. Use cautiously in elderly patients and in those with mild renal impairment.
- Possible hypermagnesemia with prolonged use and some degree of renal impairment (hypotension, nausea, vomiting, depressed reflexes, respiratory depression, coma). Serum magnesium levels should be monitored.
- When used as laxative, other oral drugs should not be taken 1 to 2 hours before or after.
- If diarrhea occurs on antacid doses, alternate preparation should be suggested.
- Patient should not take magnesium oxide indiscriminately and should not switch antacids without doctor's advice.
- If patient is able, he should be responsible for taking antacid while hospitalized.
- May cause enteric-coated drugs to be released prematurely in stomach. Doses should be separated by 1 hour.

(continued on following page)

NAMES, INDICATIONS AND DOSAGES	SIDE EFFECTS
magnesium oxide *(continued)* **Oral replacement therapy in mild hypomagnesemia:** ADULTS: 650-mg to 1.3-g tablet or capsule daily. Monitor serum magnesium response.	
magnesium trisilicate Trisomin **Antacid:** ADULTS: 1- to 4-g tablet t.i.d. chewed well and taken with ½ glass of water.	**GI:** *diarrhea,* gastric distention, flatulence, nausea, abdominal pain. **GU:** possible formation of silica renal calculi with prolonged use. **Metabolic:** hypermagnesemia.
oxethazaine Oxaine (oxethazaine in aluminum hydroxide gel) **Adjunctive therapy for hyperacidity:** ADULTS: 10 to 20 mg suspended in 5 to 10 ml aluminum hydroxide gel (equivalent to 5 to 10 ml of commercial product) q.i.d. 15 minutes before meals and h.s.	**CNS:** with high doses (120 mg oxethazaine daily): dizziness, faintness, drowsiness. **GI:** anorexia, *constipation,* intestinal obstruction.
simethicone Mylicon, Silain **Flatulence, functional gastric bloating:** ADULTS AND CHILDREN OVER 12 YEARS: 40 to 100 mg after each meal and h.s.	**GI:** expulsion of excessive liberated gas as belching, rectal flatus.
sodium bicarbonate Bell-ans, Soda Mint **Antacid:** ADULTS: 300 mg to 2 g tablets chewed well and taken with full glass of water, p.r.n.	**GI:** *gastric distention, belching, flatulence.* **GU:** renal calculi or crystals. **Metabolic:** systemic alkalosis (prolonged use), sodium and water retention; if taken with milk—milk-alkali syndrome.

INTERACTIONS AND SPECIAL CONSIDERATIONS

No significant interactions.

Special considerations:
• Contraindicated in severe renal disease. Use cautiously in elderly patients and in those with mild renal impairment.
• Possible hypermagnesemia with prolonged use and some degree of renal impairment (hypotension, nausea, vomiting, depressed reflexes, respiratory depression, coma). Serum magnesium levels should be monitored.
• If diarrhea occurs on antacid doses, alternate preparation should be suggested.
• Patient should not take magnesium trisilicate indiscriminately and should not switch antacids without doctor's advice.
• If patient is able, he should be responsible for taking antacid while hospitalized.
• May cause enteric-coated drugs to be released prematurely in stomach. Doses should be separated by 1 hour.

No significant interactions.

Special considerations:
• Use cautiously in elderly patients, especially in those with decreased bowel motility (those receiving antidiarrheals, antispasmodics, or anticholinergics), dehydration, fluid restriction, chronic renal disease, suspected intestinal obstructions.
• Amount and consistency of stools should be monitored and constipation managed with laxatives or stool softeners.
• Shake suspension well; should be taken with small amount of water to assure passage to stomach. For nasogastric instillation: check tube position and patency; flush tube with water after instillation to assure passage to stomach and maintain tube patency.
• *Caution:* Local anesthetic can affect gastric mucosa for up to 6 hours. Prolonged use may mask extension of ulcerative disease and may lead to perforation. Also may mask symptoms of gastric neoplasm.
• Patient should not take oxethazaine indiscriminately and should not switch antacids without doctor's advice.
• If patient is able, he should be responsible for taking antacid while hospitalized.
• May cause enteric-coated drugs to be released prematurely in stomach. Doses should be separated by 1 hour.

No significant interactions.

Special considerations:
• Patient should be observed for effectiveness.
• Patient should not take simethicone indiscriminately.
• Tablets should be chewed, not swallowed whole.

No significant interactions.

Special considerations:
• Contraindicated in congestive heart failure, hypertension, advanced renal disease, sodium restriction, tendency toward edema; in patients losing chloride from continuous GI suction; and in those receiving diuretics that cause hypochloremic alkalosis. Also contraindicated for long-term use. Use cautiously in elderly patients and in those with mild renal impairment.
• Use as antacid should be discouraged; nonabsorbable alternative antacid should be offered if it is to be used repeatedly.
• If patient is able, he should be responsible for taking antacid while hospitalized.
• Should not be administered with milk; can cause milk-alkali syndrome (headache, confusion, distaste for food, nausea, vomiting, hypercalcemia, hypercalciuria, calcinosis, hyperphosphatemia).
• May be used with caution to treat chronic metabolic acidosis.

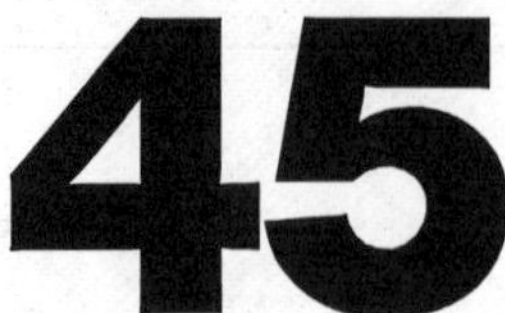

Digestants

bile salts
dehydrocholic acid
glutamic acid hydrochloride
hydrochloric acid, diluted
ketocholanic acids
pancreatin
pancrelipase

Digestants promote digestion in the gastrointestinal tract. Used in patients lacking such digestive substances as bile salts, gastric acid, or pancreatic enzymes, they can provide replacement therapy in specific deficiencies. The most widely used digestants are bile salts, hydrochloric acid, and pancreatic enzymes (pancreatin and pancrelipase).

Major uses

- Bile salts are used to treat uncomplicated constipation and to help maintain normal cholesterol solubility in the bile.
- Dehydrocholic and ketocholanic acids (synthetic bile salts) increase the solubility of cholesterol, preventing its buildup in recurring biliary calculi or strictures, recurring noncalculous cholangitis, biliary dyskinesia and chronic partial obstruction of the common bile duct, prolonged drainage from biliary fistulas or drainage of infected bile duct through a T tube, and sclerosing choledochitis. They may also prevent bacterial accumulation after biliary tract surgery.
- Glutamic acid hydrochloride and dilute hydrochloric acid (gastric acidifiers) are used to treat hypochlorhydria and achlorhydria.
- Pancreatin and pancrelipase (enzymes) supplement or replace exocrine pancreatic secretions, which are lacking in such disorders as cystic fibrosis.

Mechanism of action

- Bile salts, dehydrocholic acid, and ketocholanic acid stimulate bile flow from the liver, promoting normal digestion and absorption of fats, fat-soluble vitamins, and cholesterol.
- Glutamic and hydrochloric acids replace gastric acid.
- Pancreatin and pancrelipase replace endogenous exocrine pancreatic enzymes and aid intestinal digestion of starches, fats, and proteins.

Absorption, distribution, metabolism, and excretion

About 80% to 90% of bile salts are reabsorbed primarily in the ileum. They return to the liver and reenter the bile acid pool. As natural body substances, the rest of these digestants assume the normal physiology of the body.

Onset and duration

Onset and duration of digestants are unknown.

Combination products

ACCELERASE-PB CAPSULES: lipase 4,000 units, amylase 15,000 units, protease 15,000 units, cellulase 2 mg, mixed conjugated bile salts 65 mg, calcium carbonate 20 mg, l-alkaloids of belladonna 0.2 mg, and phenobarbital 16 mg.
BILOGEN TABLETS: pancreatin 250 mg, ox bile extract 120 mg, oxidized mixed ox bile acids 75 mg, and desoxycholic acid 30 mg.
BILRON♦: bile salts and iron.

SOME BACKGROUND ON ENZYMES

Enzymes are complex protein catalysts that increase chemical reaction rates without being changed in the process. They consist of a pure protein portion (apoenzyme) and a nonprotein portion (coenzyme), which, when combined, form the activated enzyme.

Enzymes are selective. Each enzyme works on only one compound or type of substance, which is called its substrate.

Enzymes are efficient. One key enzyme in the nervous system may produce a reaction up to a million times faster than any inorganic catalyst could. A relatively small amount of an enzyme can transform large quantities of its substrate; invertase, for example, can convert one million times its weight of sucrose into invert sugar.

The earliest names for enzymes ended in *-in* to indicate protein composition, such as pepsin and trypsin. Some enzymes were named for their source or method of separation.

Today, an enzyme is usually named by adding *-ase* to the root of its substrate (urease breaks down urea) or to the process it catalyzes (peptidases break peptide bonds).

BUTIBEL-ZYME TABLETS: proteolytic enzyme 10 mg, amylolytic enzyme 20 mg, lipolytic enzyme 100 mg, cellulolytic enzyme 5 mg, iron ox bile 30 mg, belladonna extract 15 mg, and sodium butabarbital 15 mg.
CHOLAN-HMB TABLETS: dehydrocholic acid 250 mg, homatropine methylbromide 2.5 mg, and phenobarbital 8 mg.
COTAZYM-B TABLETS: lipase 4,000 units, amylase 15,000 units, protease 15,000 units, cellulase 2 mg, and mixed conjugated bile salts 65 mg.
DONNAZYME TABLETS: pancreatin 300 mg, pepsin 150 mg, bile salts 150 mg, hyoscyamine sulfate 0.0518 mg, atropine sulfate 0.0097 mg, hyoscine hydrobromide 0.0033 mg, and phenobarbital 8.1 mg.
ENTOZYME TABLETS♦: pancreatin 300 mg, pepsin 250 mg, and bile salts 150 mg.
ENZYPAN TABLETS: pancreatin (in sufficient quantity to digest 19 g protein, 43 g starch, 10 g fat), pepsin 9 mg, and desiccated ox bile 56 mg.
FESTAL ENTERIC-COATED TABLETS: protease 17 units, amylase 10 units, lipase 10 units, bile constituents 25 mg, and hemicellulase 50 mg.
FESTALAN TABLETS: protease 17 units, amylase 10 units, lipase 10 units, lipase 10 units, bile constituents 25 mg, hemicellulase 50 mg, and atropine methylnitrate 1 mg.
KANULASE TABLETS: pancreatin 500 mg, pepsin 150 mg, ox bile extract 100 mg, cellulase 9 mg, and glutamic acid hydrochloride 200 mg.
MURIPSIN TABLETS: glutamic acid hydrochloride 500 mg and pepsin 35 mg.
PHAZYME TABLETS (enteric-coated): pancreatin 240 mg and simethicone 60 mg.
PHAZYME-95 TABLETS (enteric-coated): pancreatin 240 mg and simethicone 95 mg.
PHAZYME PB TABLETS (enteric-coated): pancreatin 240 mg, phenobarbital 15 mg, and simethicone 60 mg.
PROBILAGOL LIQUID: d-sorbitol 4.5 g and homatropine methylbromide 1 mg/5 ml.
RO-BILE TABLETS (enteric-coated): enzyme concentrate 75 mg (lipase equivalent to 750 mg pancreatin, amylase and protease equivalent to 300 mg pancreatin), ox bile extract 100 mg, dehydrocholic acid 30 mg, belladonna extract 8 mg, and pepsin 260 mg.

NAMES, INDICATIONS AND DOSAGES	SIDE EFFECTS
bile salts Biso, Chobile, Ox-Bile Extract Enseals **Uncomplicated constipation:** ADULTS AND CHILDREN: 300 to 500 mg (enteric-coated tablets) b.i.d. or t.i.d. after meals; or 150 to 450 mg capsules with or after meals.	**GI:** loose stools and mild cramping (with large doses).
dehydrocholic acid Bio-Cholin♦♦, Cholan-DH, Cholyphyl♦♦, Decholin♦, Dycholium♦♦, Hepahydrin, Idrocrine♦♦, Neocholan **Constipation, biliary tract conditions:** ADULTS: 250 to 500 mg P.O. b.i.d. to t.i.d. after meals for 4 to 6 weeks.	None reported.
glutamic acid hydrochloride Acidulin♦ **Hypoacidity:** ADULTS: 1 to 3 capsules P.O. t.i.d. before meals.	**Metabolic:** systemic acidosis in massive overdose.
hydrochloric acid, diluted **Hypoacidity:** ADULTS: 2 to 8 ml P.O. well diluted in 25 to 50 ml water.	**Metabolic:** systemic acidosis in massive overdose. **Other:** *tooth enamel damage.*
ketocholanic acids Ketochol **Constipation, biliary tract conditions:** ADULTS: 250 mg to 500 mg P.O. t.i.d. with meals.	None reported.
pancreatin Elzyme, Panteric Double Strength, Viokase **Exocrine pancreatic secretion insufficiency, digestive aid in cystic fibrosis:** ADULTS AND CHILDREN: 325 mg to 1 g P.O. with meals.	**GI:** nausea, diarrhea with high doses.

♦ Available in U.S. and Canada. ♦♦ Available in Canada only.
All other products (no symbol) available in U.S. only. Italicized side effects are common or life-threatening.

INTERACTIONS AND SPECIAL CONSIDERATIONS	
No significant interactions. *Special considerations:* • Contraindicated in marked hepatic dysfunction, except in malnutrition with steatorrhea and vitamin K deficiency with hypoprothrombinemia. • Ox-Bile Extract should be used cautiously in obstructive jaundice.	• Ox-Bile Extract should not be used if other preparations are available, since it doesn't provide an adequate amount of conjugated bile salts.
No significant interactions. *Special considerations:* • Contraindicated in complete mechanical biliary obstruction. Use cautiously in prostatic hypertrophy, acute hepatitis, asthmatic bronchitis, partial GI or GU tract obstruction, and in elderly patients. • Should not be used when patient is nauseated, vomiting, or has abdominal pain. • Simultaneous administration of bile salts may be needed in biliary fistula.	• Used to prevent bacterial accumulation after biliary tract surgery. • Probably much less effective than natural bile salts in lowering surface tension and promoting absorption. • Dehydrocholic acid should not be used to accelerate healing in patients with jaundice. • Frequent use may result in dependence on laxatives.
No significant interactions. *Special considerations:* • Contraindicated in gastric hyperacidity or peptic ulcer. • Use instead of hydrochloric acid so tooth enamel won't be damaged; however, glutamic acid HCl is not as effective in increasing gastric pH. • Gastric acidifier.	
No significant interactions. *Special considerations:* • Contraindicated in gastric hyperacidity or peptic ulcer. • Tooth enamel protected by sipping through glass straw during meal. • Alleviates primary functional hypoacidity or hypoacidity caused by organic disease such as pernicious anemia, certain allergies, chronic gastritis, other chronic debilitating diseases, or gastric resection. • Gastric acidifier; usual dose not sufficient to release free acid in stomach; no evidence that even larger doses are beneficial for this.	
No significant interactions. *Special considerations:* • Use cautiously in prostatic hypertrophy, acute hepatitis, asthmatic bronchitis, partial GI or GU tract obstruction, and in elderly patients. • Bile salt; derived from beef bile.	• Approximately equivalent to 250 mg dehydrocholic acid. • Should not be used when patient is nauseated, vomiting, or has abdominal pain. • Frequent use may result in dependence on laxatives.
No significant interactions. *Special considerations:* • Use cautiously in patients who are hypersensitive to pork. Bovine preparations are available for these patients, but are less effective. • Fat, protein, and starch intake should be balanced to avoid indigestion. Dosage varies according to degree of maldigestion and malabsorption, amount of fat in diet, and enzyme activity of individual preparations. • Pancreatin therapy shouldn't delay or replace treatment of primary disorder. • Adequate replacement decreases number of bowel movements and improves stool consistency. • Should be used only after confirmed diagnosis of exocrine pancreatic insufficiency. Not effective in GI disorders unrelated to pancreatic enzyme deficiency. • For infants, powder should be mixed with applesauce and given with meals. Older children may swallow capsules with food. • Enteric coating on some products may reduce availability of enzyme in upper portion of jejunum where it is primarily required. • Should be stored in tight containers at room temperature.	

NAMES, INDICATIONS AND DOSAGES	SIDE EFFECTS
pancrelipase Cotazym♦, Ilozyme, Ku-Zyme HP, Pancrease **Dose must be titrated to patient's response. Exocrine pancreatic secretion insufficiency, cystic fibrosis in adults and children, steatorrhea and other disorders of fat metabolism secondary to insufficient pancreatic enzymes:** ADULTS AND CHILDREN: dosage range 1 to 3 capsules or tablets P.O. before or with meals and 1 capsule or tablet with snack; or 1 to 2 powder packets before meals or snacks.	**GI:** *nausea*, diarrhea with high doses.

♦ Available in U.S. and Canada. ♦♦ Available in Canada only.
All other products (no symbol) available in U.S. only. Italicized side effects are common or life-threatening.

COMPARISON OF SOME POPULAR PANCREATIC ENZYME PRODUCTS

DIGESTANT	TRADE NAME	ENZYME CONTENT (UNITS)			FAT DIGESTION INDEX*
		Lipase	Amylase	Protease	
pancreatin	Beef Viokase				
	Tablet (1)	1,950	4,000	16,250	0.5
	Powder (1 tsp)	13,500	28,125	112,500	3.2
	Viokase				
	Tablet (1)	6,500	48,000	32,000	1.4
	Powder (1 tsp)	45,000	337,500	225,000	9.2
pancrelipase	Cotazym				
	Capsule (1)	8,000	30,000	30,000	1
	Packet (1)	16,000	60,000	60,000	2
	Cherry-flavored packet (1)	40,000	150,000	150,000	5
	Ilozyme				
	Tablet (1)	9,600	40,000	40,000	1.6

*Relative fat digestion activity. For example, the activity of a Beef Viokase tablet is half that of a Cotazyme capsule (0.5 vs. 1).

Adapted with permission from W.W. Waring, "Current Management of Cystic Fibrosis," in L.A. Barness et al., eds., *Advances in Pediatrics*, Vol. 23 (Chicago: Yearbook Medical Publishers, 1976).

INTERACTIONS AND SPECIAL CONSIDERATIONS

No significant interactions.

Special considerations:

- Contraindicated in patients with severe pork hypersensitivity.
- Pancrelipase therapy shouldn't delay or replace treatment of primary disorder.
- Should be used only after confirmed diagnosis of exocrine pancreatic insufficiency. Not effective in GI disorders unrelated to enzyme deficiency.
- Lipase activity greater than with other pancreatic enzymes.
- For infants, powder should be mixed with applesauce and given at mealtime. Avoid inhalation of powder. Older children may swallow capsules with food.
- Dosage varies with degree of maldigestion and malabsorption, amount of fat in diet, and enzyme activity of individual preparations.
- Adequate replacement decreases number of bowel movements and improves stool consistency.
- Enteric coating on some products may reduce availability of enzyme in upper portion of jejunum where it is primarily required.
- Crushing or chewing of capsule interferes with the enteric coating.

PARENT-TEACHING AID

WHAT YOU SHOULD KNOW ABOUT YOUR CHILD'S PANCREATIC ENZYME REPLACEMENT THERAPY

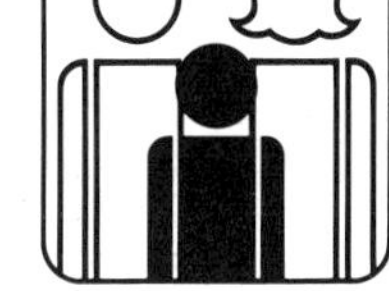

Dear Parent:

Your doctor has prescribed pancreatic enzyme replacement therapy to improve your child's digestion and absorption of fat and protein. To help your child benefit from his therapy, follow these instructions:

- Give your child pancreatic enzymes with snacks as well as with regular meals. After he starts pancreatic enzyme replacement therapy, his appetite will be dramatically decreased.
- If your child can't tolerate or is allergic to pork, be sure to tell the doctor. (Many enzyme preparations are made with pork.)
- If the pancreatic enzyme is in powder form, mix it with applesauce or other fruit to make it more palatable.
- Don't mix enzymes with foods containing protein. The enzymes would immediately break down the proteins and turn the food into a watery substance.
- To facilitate the absorption of fats and proteins, give enzymes at the beginning of a meal.
- Don't let the enzymes remain on your child's lips and skin; they may cause his skin to break down.
- If you know your child will be eating a greasy meal, call the doctor; he'll probably increase the amount of enzymes your child should take with this meal.
- If your child has diarrhea, call the doctor; he'll probably decrease the amount of enzymes your child is taking.

Symptoms of inadequate pancreatic replacement and excessive intake of fat include abdominal cramps and distention, light-colored mushy stools, foul-smelling gas, rectal seepage of oil, rectal prolapse, and failure to thrive despite a voracious appetite. Call the doctor if any of these occur so he can adjust your child's replacement regimen accordingly.

46

Antidiarrheals

bismuth subcarbonate
bismuth subgallate
bismuth subsalicylate
calcium polycarbophil
diphenoxylate hydrochloride (with atropine sulfate)
kaolin and pectin mixtures
lactobacillus
loperamide
opium tincture
opium tincture, camphorated

Antidiarrheals reduce the fluidity of the stool and the frequency of defecation.

Diarrhea is the abnormally frequent passage of watery stools with an average daily weight of more than 300 g. (Healthy adults have an average daily fecal weight of 100 to 150 g.)

In the absence of other symptoms, diarrhea usually reflects a minor and transient gastrointestinal (GI) disorder. In more serious conditions, however, it is usually one of several symptoms. Diarrhea may be caused by foods or drugs, laxative abuse, allergies, endocrine dysfunction, malabsorption, neurologic or inflammatory diseases, mechanical obstruction, parasitic infection, gastric resection, or radiation poisoning.

Major uses

- All antidiarrheals are used in the treatment of the acute, mild, or chronic stages of nonspecific diarrhea.
- Bismuth subgallate also neutralizes or absorbs fecal odors in patients with a colostomy or ileostomy.
- Loperamide also reduces the volume of ileostomy discharge and decreases daily fecal volume and fluid and electrolyte loss.

Mechanism of action

- Bismuth subcarbonate, subgallate, and subsalicylate have a mild water-binding capacity; they also may adsorb toxins and provide protective coating for intestinal mucosa.
- Calcium polycarbophil absorbs excess fecal water, forming a gel that gives form to the stool. This slows the stool's passage through the colon.
- Diphenoxylate hydrochloride and opium tinctures increase smooth muscle tone in the GI tract, inhibit motility and propulsion, and diminish digestive secretions.
- Kaolin and pectin decrease the stool's fluid content, although *total* water loss seems to remain the same.
- Lactobacillus cultures may suppress the growth of pathogenic microorganisms to help reestablish normal intestinal flora.
- Loperamide inhibits peristaltic activity, prolonging transit of intestinal contents.

Absorption, distribution, metabolism, and excretion

Adsorbent antidiarrheals (bismuth salts, calcium polycarbophil, kaolin, pectin, and lactobacillus) are not systemically absorbed.

- Diphenoxylate hydrochloride is well absorbed from the GI tract, metabolized in the liver, and eliminated in both urine and feces.
- Loperamide is poorly absorbed orally, metabolized in the liver, and eliminated primarily in feces.
- Opium tinctures are absorbed moderately from the GI tract as morphine, metabolized in the liver, and excreted in urine.

QUESTIONS & ANSWERS

TREATING DIARRHEA

What's best for diarrhea? Lomotil, Imodium ... or codeine?

Since the actions of Lomotil and Imodium are practically identical, both drugs are fine choices. Either 5 mg (2 tablets) of Lomotil or 2 to 4 mg (1 to 2 capsules) of Imodium will probably be prescribed until the patient's diarrhea subsides.

Although codeine phosphate may be preferred over Lomotil and Imodium—especially in the treatment of chronic diarrhea—codeine is not specific for diarrhea treatment. And remember, compared with Lomotil and Imodium, codeine is more habit-forming; it's a more controlled substance. Codeine is classified as a Schedule II substance whereas Lomotil and Imodium are classified as Schedule V drugs.

Onset and duration

- Bismuth salts, calcium polycarbophil, kaolin, pectin, and lactobacillus begin to act within 30 minutes; their therapeutic effects can last 4 to 6 hours.
- Diphenoxylate hydrochloride begins to act within 45 to 60 minutes. Its effect lasts as long as 4 hours.
- Loperamide's peak levels occur in 4 hours; half-life is about 40 hours.
- Opium tinctures begin to act rapidly. Duration of action varies.

Combination products

CORRECTIVE MIXTURE: zinc sulfocarbolate 10 mg, phenyl salicylate 22 mg, bismuth subsalicylate 85 mg, pepsin 45 mg, and alcohol 1.5% in 5-ml suspension.
CORRECTIVE MIXTURE WITH PAREGORIC: paregoric 0.6 ml, zinc sulfocarbolate 10 mg, phenyl salicylate 22 mg, bismuth subsalicylate 85 mg, pepsin 45 mg, and alcohol 2% in 5-ml suspension.
DONNAGEL SUSPENSION♦: kaolin 6 g, pectin 142.8 mg, hyoscyamine sulfate 0.1037 mg, atropine sulfate 0.0194 mg, hyoscine hydrobromide 0.0065 mg, and alcohol 3.8% in 30-ml suspension.
DONNAGEL-MB♦♦: kaolin 6 g, pectin 142.8 mg, and alcohol 3.8% in 30-ml suspension.
DONNAGEL-PG: powdered opium 24 mg, kaolin 6 g, pectin 142.8 mg, hyoscyamine sulfate 0.1037 mg, atropine sulfate 0.0194 mg, hyoscine hydrobromide 0.0065 mg, and alcohol 5% in 30-ml suspension.
KENPECTIN-P: opium 16.27 mg (equivalent to 3.7 ml paregoric), kaolin 5.85 g, pectin 195 mg, alcohol 6%, and aluminum hydroxide 650 mg in 30-ml suspension.
PAREPECTOLIN: opium 15 mg (equivalent to paregoric 3.7 ml), kaolin 5.85 g, pectin 162 mg, and alcohol 0.69% in 30-ml suspension.
PECTOCEL: kaolin 5.85 g, pectin 292.5 mg, and zinc phenolsulfonate 73.13 mg in 30-ml suspension.
PEKTAMALT: kaolin 6.5 g, pectin 600 mg, potassium gluconate 1.1 g, and sodium citrate 318 mg in 30-ml suspension.
POLYMAGMA PLAIN: activated attapulgite 500 mg, pectin 45 mg, and hydrated alumina powder 50 mg.

NAMES, INDICATIONS AND DOSAGES	SIDE EFFECTS
bismuth subcarbonate **bismuth subgallate** Devrom **Deodorize fecal odors in colostomy and ileostomy (subcarbonate):** ADULTS: 600 mg P.O. t.i.d. after each meal. **Mild, nonspecific diarrhea (subgallate):** ADULTS: 1 to 2 tablets chewed or swallowed whole t.i.d.	**CNS:** personality changes. Prolonged use (especially in colostomy and ileostomy patients) may lead to reversible deterioration of mental ability, confusion, tremors, and impaired coordination. **GI:** *transient darkened tongue and stool* (both with subgallate); fecal impaction or ulceration (in infants, elderly, or debilitated patients) after chronic use; *constipation*.
bismuth subsalicylate Pepto-Bismol **Mild, nonspecific diarrhea:** ADULTS: 30 ml or 2 tablets q ½ to 1 hour up to a maximum of 8 doses and for no longer than 2 days. CHILDREN 10 TO 14 YEARS: 20 ml. CHILDREN 6 TO 10 YEARS: 10 ml. CHILDREN 3 TO 6 YEARS: 5 ml.	**GI:** temporary darkening of tongue and stools. **Other:** salicylism (high doses).
calcium polycarbophil Mitrolan **Diarrhea associated with irritable bowel syndrome, as well as acute nonspecific diarrhea (tablets must be chewed before swallowing):** ADULTS: 1 g P.O. q.i.d. as required. Maximum 6 g in 24-hour period. CHILDREN 6 TO 12 YEARS: 500 mg P.O. t.i.d. as required. Maximum 3 g in 24-hour period. CHILDREN 3 TO 6 YEARS: 500 mg P.O. b.i.d. as required. Maximum 1.5 g in 24-hour period.	**GI:** abdominal fullness and increased flatus, intestinal obstruction.
diphenoxylate hydrochloride (with atropine sulfate) Controlled Substance Schedule V Colonaid, Diaction, Lofene, Loflo, Lomo-Plus, Lomotil♦, Lonox, Lotrol, Ro-Diphen-Atro, SK-Diphenoxylate **Acute, nonspecific diarrhea:** ADULTS: initially, 5 mg P.O. q.i.d., then adjust dose to individual response. CHILDREN 2 TO 12 YEARS: 0.3 to 0.4 mg/kg P.O. daily in divided doses, using liquid form only. Not recommended for children under 2 years.	**CNS:** *sedation, dizziness,* headache, drowsiness, lethargy, restlessness, depression, euphoria. **CV:** tachycardia. **EENT:** mydriasis. **GI:** *dry mouth,* nausea, vomiting, abdominal discomfort or distention, *paralytic ileus,* anorexia, fluid retention in bowel (may mask depletion of extracellular fluid and electrolytes, especially in young children treated for acute gastroenteritis). **GU:** urinary retention. **Skin:** pruritus, giant urticaria, rash. **Other:** possibly physical dependence in long-term use, angioedema, respiratory depression.
kaolin and pectin mixtures Baropectin, Kaoparin, Kaopectate♦, Kapectin, Keotin, Pectokay **Mild, nonspecific diarrhea:** ADULTS: 60 to 120 ml after each bowel movement; CHILDREN OVER 12: 60 ml after each bowel movement; CHILDREN 6 TO 12: 30 to 60 ml after each bowel movement; CHILDREN 3 TO 6: 15 to 30 ml after each bowel movement.	**GI:** drug absorbs nutrients and enzymes; fecal impaction or ulceration in infants, elderly, debilitated patients after chronic use; constipation.

♦ Available in U.S. and Canada. ♦♦ Available in Canada only.
All other products (no symbol) available in U.S. only. Italicized side effects are common or life-threatening.

INTERACTIONS AND SPECIAL CONSIDERATIONS

No significant interactions.

Special considerations:
- GI adsorbent.
- Should not replace specific therapy for underlying cause.
- May reduce absorption of other oral drugs, requiring dosage adjustment.
- Should be stored in tight, light-resistant containers.

No significant interactions.

Special considerations:
- Has been used successfully to treat turista (traveler's diarrhea).
- Patient should be warned that this drug contains a large amount of salicylate. Should be used cautiously in patients already taking aspirin products.

No significant interactions.

Special considerations:
- Contraindicated in patients with signs of GI obstruction.
- Should not be used for more than 2 days.
- Should not replace specific therapy for underlying cause of the diarrhea.
- Patient should chew tablets thoroughly before swallowing. When used as an antidiarrheal, patient should *not* drink a glass of water afterward.
- For episodes of severe diarrhea, the dose may be repeated every half hour, but maximum daily dosage should not be exceeded.
- Also used as a bulk laxative.

No significant interactions.

Special considerations:
- Contraindicated in acute diarrhea resulting from poison until toxic material is eliminated from GI tract; in acute diarrhea caused by organisms that penetrate intestinal mucosa; in diarrhea resulting from antibiotic-induced pseudomembranous enterocolitis; and in patients with jaundice. Use cautiously in children, and in hepatic disease, narcotic dependence, pregnancy. Use cautiously in acute ulcerative colitis. Stop therapy immediately if abdominal distention or other signs of toxic megacolon develop.
- Risk of physical dependence increases with high dose and long-term use. Long-term or unsupervised use should be discouraged. Atropine sulfate is included to discourage abuse.
- Patient should not exceed recommended dosage.
- Dehydration, especially in young children, may increase risk of delayed toxicity. Fluid and electrolyte disturbances should be corrected before starting drug.
- Dose of 2.5 mg as effective as 5 ml camphorated tincture of opium.
- Not indicated in treatment of antibiotic-induced diarrhea.
- For symptoms and treatment of toxicity, see APPENDIX.

No significant interactions.

Special considerations:
- Contraindicated in suspected obstructive bowel lesions.
- Should not be used for more than 2 days.
- Should not replace specific therapy for underlying cause.
- May reduce absorption of other oral drugs, requiring dosage adjustments.
- GI absorbent.

NAMES, INDICATIONS AND DOSAGES	SIDE EFFECTS
lactobacillus Bacid♦, DoFUS, Lactinex♦ **Diarrhea, especially that caused by antibiotics:** ADULTS: 2 capsules (Bacid) P.O. b.i.d., t.i.d., or q.i.d., preferably with milk; or 4 tablets or 1 packet (Lactinex) P.O. t.i.d. or q.i.d., preferably with food, milk, or juice; or 1 tablet (DoFUS) P.O. daily before meals.	**GI:** (with Bacid and DoFUS) increased intestinal flatus at beginning of therapy; subsides with continued therapy.
loperamide Controlled Substance Schedule V Imodium♦ **Acute, nonspecific diarrhea:** ADULTS: initially, 4 mg P.O., then 2 mg after each unformed stool. Maximum 16 mg daily. **Chronic diarrhea:** ADULTS: initially, 4 mg P.O., then 2 mg after each unformed stool until diarrhea subsides. Adjust dose to individual response.	**CNS:** drowsiness, fatigue, dizziness. **GI:** dry mouth; abdominal pain, distention, or discomfort; *constipation;* nausea; vomiting. **Skin:** rash.
opium tincture **opium tincture, camphorated** Controlled Substance Schedule III Paregoric♦ **Acute, nonspecific diarrhea:** ADULTS: 0.6 ml opium tincture (range 0.3 to 1 ml) P.O. q.i.d. Maximum dose 6 ml daily; or 5 to 10 ml camphorated opium tincture daily b.i.d., t.i.d., or q.i.d. until diarrhea subsides. CHILDREN: 0.25 to 0.5 ml/kg camphorated opium tincture daily, b.i.d., t.i.d., or q.i.d. until diarrhea subsides.	**GI:** nausea, vomiting. **Other:** physical dependence after long-term use.

♦ Available in U.S. and Canada. ♦♦ Available in Canada only.
All other products (no symbol) available in U.S. only. Italicized side effects are common or life-threatening.

ADVISING PATIENTS ABOUT TRAVELER'S DIARRHEA

Traveler's diarrhea, or *turista,* is a self-limiting but acute form of diarrhea caused by ingesting food or water contaminated with bacteria (usually enterotoxigenic *Escherichia coli*). When on vacation, a patient can prevent it by:

- drinking only boiled or carbonated water.
- not eating ice, salads, or unpeeled fruit.

Prophylactic drug therapy may be the best way to prevent traveler's diarrhea, and may include:

- doxycycline—an extremely effective →

INTERACTIONS AND SPECIAL CONSIDERATIONS

No significant interactions.

Special considerations:
- Bacid and DoFUS contraindicated in fever.
- Bacid should not be used for more than 2 days.
- Store in refrigerator.
- Diet containing large amounts of carbohydrate (up to 400 g), such as lactose, lactulose, and dextrin, may be more effective than lactobacillus in reestablishing normal flora after antibiotic therapy.
- Controversial form of diarrhea treatment.
- May be used prophylactically in history of antibiotic-induced diarrhea.

No significant interactions.

Special considerations:
- Contraindicated in acute diarrhea resulting from poison until toxic material is removed from GI tract, when constipation must be avoided, and in acute diarrhea caused by organisms that penetrate intestinal mucosa. Use cautiously in patients with severe prostatic hypertrophy, hepatic disease, and history of narcotic dependence.
- Drug should be stopped immediately if abdominal distention or other symptoms develop in patients with acute ulcerative colitis.
- In acute diarrhea, drug should be stopped if no improvement within 48 hours; in chronic diarrhea, drug should be stopped if no improvement after taking 16 mg daily for at least 10 days.
- Appears to have low potential for abuse.
- Patient should not exceed recommended dosage.
- Produces antidiarrheal action similar to diphenoxylate HCl but without as many CNS side effects; three times more potent than diphenoxylate HCl.

No significant interactions.

Special considerations:
- Contraindicated in acute diarrhea resulting from poisons until toxic material is removed from GI tract, and in acute diarrhea caused by organisms that penetrate intestinal mucosa. Use cautiously in asthma, severe prostatic hypertrophy, hepatic disease, narcotic dependence.
- Risk of physical dependence increases with long-term use. Long-term or unsupervised use should be discouraged.
- An effective and prompt-acting antidiarrheal.
- Opium content of opium tincture 25 times greater than camphorated tincture of opium. Camphorated opium tincture is more dilute, and teaspoonful doses easier to measure than dropper quantities of opium tincture.
- Not used as widely today as in past, but unique because dose can be adjusted precisely to patient's needs.
- Milky fluid forms when camphorated opium tincture is added to water.
- Camphorated opium tincture 0.06 to 0.5 ml daily has been used to treat infants with mild narcotic physical dependence.

---

agent against enterotoxigenic *E. coli* and thus far the most effective preventive treatment. However, it's ineffective against *Salmonella* or *Shigella* organisms. Since doxycycline is a tetracycline, its adverse effects may include photosensitivity and increased skin pigmentation.

- neomycin, iodochlorhydroxyquin (Entero-vioform*), or a variety of sulfonamides.
- a bismuth subsalicylate suspension such as Pepto-Bismol. This may be effective only when large doses are taken.

If the patient loses a lot of fluid, he'll need to replenish the loss with an oral hydration formula containing glucose and salts. A pharmacist can mix and pack these ingredients before the patient leaves.

Antimotility agents (such as Paregoric or tincture of opium) can relieve the abdominal cramps associated with traveler's diarrhea. But the patient shouldn't be fooled by kaolin-pectin preparations; they may alter stool consistency, but they don't relieve any other symptoms of the disease.

*Not available in the United States

47

Laxatives

barley-malt extract
bisacodyl
calcium polycarbophil
cascara sagrada
castor oil
danthron
docusate calcium (formerly dioctyl calcium sulfosuccinate)
docusate potassium (formerly dioctyl potassium sulfosuccinate)
docusate sodium (formerly dioctyl sodium sulfosuccinate)
glycerin
lactulose
magnesium salts
methylcellulose
mineral oil
phenolphthalein
psyllium
senna
sodium biphosphate
sodium phosphate

Laxatives (also historically known as cathartics, drastics, and purgatives) ease the passage of feces from the colon and rectum. The accumulation of feces in the lower bowel results from constipation, which is defined as a decrease in the frequency of fecal elimination, characterized by the passage of hard, dry stools. In an effort to alleviate constipation, many people overuse laxatives.

Laxatives can be classified according to the way they work: hyperosmolar, bulk-forming, lubricant, emollient or stool softener, or stimulant.

Major uses

Laxatives may relieve or prevent constipation. They are used to evacuate the bowel before rectal or bowel examination, exposure of abdominal X-ray films, barium enema, or various surgical procedures.

- The docusate salts are commonly used to soften stools and prevent straining during defecation.
- Lactulose is also used to treat hepatic encephalopathy.

Mechanism of action

- Bulk-forming laxatives absorb water and expand to increase bulk and moisture content of the stool. The increased bulk encourages peristalsis and bowel movement.
- Emollient laxatives, or stool softeners, reduce surface tension of interfacing liquid contents of the bowel. This mechanism, or detergent activity, promotes incorporation of additional liquid into the stool, forming a softer mass.
- Among the hyperosmolar laxatives, glycerin draws water from the tissues into the feces and thus stimulates reflex evacuation.

Lactulose produces an osmotic effect in the colon and is biodegraded by the intestinal flora into lactic, formic, and acetic acids. Distention of the bowel from fluid accumulation promotes peristalsis and bowel movement.

The saline agents (magnesium salts, sodium diphosphate, and sodium phosphate) produce an osmotic effect in the small intestine by drawing water into the intestinal lumen. Fluid accumulation produces distention, which then encourages peristalsis and bowel movement. Saline laxatives also promote cholecystokinin secretion, stimulating intestinal motility and inhibiting fluid and electrolyte absorption from the jejunum and ileum.

- Lubricant laxatives increase water retention in the stool by creating a barrier between colon wall and feces that prevents colonic reabsorption of fecal water.

- Stimulant laxatives may increase peristalsis by direct effect on the smooth muscle of the intestine. Although the precise mechanism is unknown, stimulant laxatives are thought either to irritate the musculature or to stimulate the colonic intramural plexus. These drugs also promote fluid accumulation in the colon and small intestine, increasing the laxative effect.

Absorption, distribution, metabolism, and excretion

- Bulk-forming laxatives are not absorbed systemically.
- Emollient laxatives are systemically absorbed and eliminated in the bile.
- Among the hyperosmolar laxatives, glycerin suppositories and lactulose are not absorbed systemically.

  About 20% of the magnesium in magnesium salts is systemically absorbed and excreted in urine.

  Up to 10% of the sodium content of sodium phosphate and of sodium biphosphate enemas may be absorbed and excreted in urine.
- The lubricant laxative mineral oil, in its nonemulsified form, is not significantly absorbed; as much as one half of emulsified mineral oil may be absorbed.
- Stimulant laxatives are slightly absorbed and are metabolized in the liver. The metabolites are eliminated either in urine or—through the bile—in feces.

Combination products

AGORAL: mineral oil 28% and white phenolphthalein 1.3% in emulsion, with tragacanth, agar, egg albumin, acacia, and glycerin.
CASYLLIUM: psyllium husk powder 4.1 g, debittered fluidextract cascara 3 ml, and prune powder 1.2 g/6 g.
CORRECTOL: yellow phenolphthalein 64.8 mg and docusate sodium 100 mg.
DIALOSE: docusate sodium 100 mg and sodium carboxymethylcellulose 400 mg.
DIALOSE-PLUS: docusate sodium 100 mg and casanthranol 30 mg.
DORBANTYL: docusate sodium 50 mg and danthron 25 mg.
DORBANTYL FORTE: docusate sodium 100 mg and danthron 50 mg.
DOXAN-TABLETS: docusate sodium 60 mg and danthron 50 mg.
DOXIDAN♦: docusate calcium 60 mg and danthron 50 mg.
D-S-S PLUS: docusate sodium 100 mg and casanthranol 30 mg.
GENTLAX S: docusate sodium 50 mg and standardized senna concentrate 187 mg.
HALEY'S M-O: mineral oil (25%) and magnesium hydroxide.
HYDROCIL, FORTIFIED: blond psyllium coating 50% and casanthranol (with dextrose) 30 mg/6 g.
KONDREMUL WITH CASCARA♦: heavy mineral oil 55%, cascara sagrada extract 660 mg/15 ml, and Irish moss as emulsifier.
KONDREMUL WITH PHENOLPHTHALEIN♦: heavy mineral oil 55%, white phenolphthalein 147 mg/15 ml, and Irish moss as emulsifier.
PERI-COLACE♦ (capsules): docusate sodium 100 mg and casanthranol 30 mg.
PERI-COLACE (syrup): docusate sodium 60 mg and casanthranol 30 mg/15 ml.
SENOKOT WITH PSYLLIUM: psyllium 1 g and standardized senna concentrate 326 mg/teaspoonful.
STIMULAX: docusate sodium 250 mg and casanthranol 30 mg.

NAMES, INDICATIONS AND DOSAGES	SIDE EFFECTS
barley-malt extract Maltsupex **Constipation:** ADULTS: 4 tablets P.O. with meals and at bedtime for 4 days, then 2 to 4 tablets at bedtime; or 2 tablespoonfuls powder or liquid b.i.d. for 3 to 4 days, until stools become soft, then 1 to 2 tablespoonfuls at bedtime. CHILDREN OVER 2 MONTHS: ½ to 2 tablespoonfuls in milk or on cereal daily or b.i.d. INFANTS 1 OR 2 MONTHS: ½ tablespoonful daily with milk or cereal. To prevent constipation, may add 1 to 2 teaspoonfuls to each day's feeding.	**GI:** loose stools. **Other:** laxative dependence with frequent or long-term use.
bisacodyl Biscolax♦, Codylax, Dulcolax♦, Dulcolax Micro-enema♦♦, Fleet Bisacodyl, Rolax **Chronic constipation; preparation for delivery, surgery, or rectal or bowel examination:** ADULTS: 10 to 15 mg P.O. in evening or before breakfast. Up to 30 mg may be used for thorough evacuation needed for examinations or surgery. CHILDREN: 5 to 10 mg P.O. **Rectal:** ADULTS AND CHILDREN OVER 2 YEARS: 10 mg. ADULTS AND CHILDREN UNDER 2 YEARS: 5 mg. **Enema:** ADULTS: 1.25 oz. CHILDREN UNDER 6 YEARS: approximately ½ contents of micro enema.	**CNS:** muscle weakness in excessive use. **GI:** *nausea, abdominal cramps,* diarrhea in high doses, *burning sensation in rectum with suppositories.* **Metabolic:** alkalosis, hypokalemia, tetany, protein-losing enteropathy in excessive use. **Other:** laxative dependence in long-term or excessive use.
calcium polycarbophil Mitrolan **Constipation (tablets must be chewed before swallowing):** ADULTS: 1 g P.O. q.i.d. as required. Maximum 6 g in 24-hour period. CHILDREN 6 TO 12 YEARS: 500 mg P.O. t.i.d. as required. Maximum 3 g in 24-hour period. CHILDREN 3 TO 6 YEARS: 500 mg P.O. b.i.d. as required. Maximum 1.5 g in 24-hour period.	**GI:** abdominal fullness and increased flatus, intestinal obstruction. **Other:** laxative dependence in long-term or excessive use.
cascara sagrada **cascara sagrada aromatic fluidextract** **cascara sagrada fluidextract** **Acute constipation; preparation for bowel or rectal examination:** ADULTS: 325 mg cascara sagrada tablets P.O. h.s.; or 1 ml fluidextract daily; or 5 ml aromatic fluidextract daily.	**GI:** *nausea;* vomiting; diarrhea; loss of normal bowel function with excessive use; *abdominal cramps,* especially in severe constipation; malabsorption of nutrients; "cathartic colon" (syndrome resembling ulcerative colitis radiologically and pathologically) after chronic misuse; discoloration of rectal mucosa after long-term use.

♦ Available in U.S. and Canada. ♦♦ Available in Canada only.
All other products (no symbol) available in U.S. only. Italicized side effects are common or life-threatening.

INTERACTIONS AND SPECIAL CONSIDERATIONS

No significant interactions.

Special considerations:

• Contraindicated in abdominal pain, nausea, vomiting, or other symptoms of appendicitis or acute surgical abdomen, and in intestinal obstruction or ulceration, disabling adhesion, or difficulty swallowing.
• In patients with diabetes, carbohydrate content of approximately 14 g/tablespoon of liquid, 13 g/tablespoon of powder, and 0.6 g/tablet should be allowed for.
• Patient should take with at least 8 oz (240 ml) liquid.
• For short-term use. Before laxative is given, patient history of fluid intake, exercise, and diet should be obtained. Dietary sources of bulk include bran and other cereals, fresh fruit, and vegetables.
• Infants usually need diet change to increase bulk in addition to laxative.
• Laxative effect usually takes 12 to 24 hours; may be delayed 3 days.
• Bulk laxative; increases bulk and water content of stool.
• Not absorbed systemically; nontoxic.
• Reduces fecal pH. Especially useful in constipated postpartum mothers, debilitated patients, infants; in patients with chronic laxative abuse, irritable bowel syndrome, diverticular disease, and to empty colon before barium enema examination.

No significant interactions.

Special considerations:

• Contraindicated in abdominal pain, nausea, vomiting, or other symptoms of appendicitis or acute surgical abdomen, or in rectal fissures or ulcerated hemorrhoids.
• Patient should swallow enteric-coated tablet whole to avoid GI irritation. Should not be given with milk or antacids. Begins to act 6 to 12 hours after oral administration. Administration of drug should be timed so as not to interfere with scheduled activities or sleep.
• Soft, formed stool usually produced 15 to 60 minutes after rectal administration. Administration of drug should be timed so as not to interfere with scheduled activities or sleep.
• Tablets and suppositories may be used together to cleanse colon before and after surgery and before barium enema.
• For short-term treatment. Stimulant laxative, class of laxative most abused. Excessive use discouraged.
• Before laxative is given for constipation, patient history of fluid intake, exercise, and diet should be obtained. Dietary sources of bulk include bran and other cereals, fresh fruit, and vegetables.
• Store tablets and suppositories at temperature below 86° F. (30° C.).

No significant interactions.

Special considerations:

• Contraindicated in patients with signs of GI obstruction.
• Rectal bleeding or failure to respond to therapy may indicate need for surgery.
• Use for short-term treatment.
• Before laxative is given for constipation, patient history of fluid intake, exercise, and diet should be obtained. Dietary sources of bulk include bran and other cereals, fresh fruit, and vegetables.
• Patient should chew the tablets thoroughly and drink a full glass of water with each dose.
• Not absorbed systemically; nontoxic.
• Bulk laxative; increases bulk and water content of stool.
• Also used to treat diarrhea because it absorbs fecal water.

No significant interactions.

Special considerations:

• Contraindicated in abdominal pain, nausea, vomiting, or other symptoms of appendicitis or acute surgical abdomen; in acute surgical delirium, fecal impaction, intestinal obstruction or perforation. Use cautiously when rectal bleeding is present.
• Aromatic cascara fluidextract is less active and less bitter than nonaromatic fluidextract.
• Liquid preparations more reliable than solid dosage forms.
• Drug of choice among stimulant laxatives. For short-term treatment.
• Before laxative is given for constipation, patient history of fluid intake, exercise, and diet should be obtained. Dietary sources of bulk include bran and other cereals, fresh fruit, and vegetables.

(continued on following page)

NAMES, INDICATIONS AND DOSAGES	SIDE EFFECTS
cascara sagrada *(continued)* CHILDREN 2 TO 12 YEARS: ½ adult dose. CHILDREN UNDER 2 YEARS: ¼ adult dose.	**Metabolic:** hypokalemia, protein enteropathy, electrolyte imbalance in excessive use. **Other:** laxative dependence in long-term or excessive use.
castor oil Alphamul, Neoloid♦, Purge **Preparation for rectal or bowel examination, or surgery; acute constipation (rarely):** ADULTS: 15 to 60 ml P.O. as liquid or 1.25 to 3.7 mg P.O. as tablet. CHILDREN OVER 2 YEARS: 5 to 15 ml P.O. CHILDREN UNDER 2 YEARS: 1.25 to 7.5 ml P.O. INFANTS: up to 4 ml P.O. Increased dose produces no greater effect.	**GI:** *nausea;* vomiting; diarrhea; loss of normal bowel function with excessive use; *abdominal cramps,* especially in severe constipation; malabsorption of nutrients; "cathartic colon" (syndrome resembling ulcerative colitis radiologically and pathologically) in chronic misuse. May cause constipation after catharsis. **GU:** pelvic congestion in menstruating women. **Metabolic:** hypokalemia, protein enteropathy, other electrolyte imbalance in excessive use. **Other:** laxative dependence in long-term or excessive use.
danthron Dorbane♦, Duolax, Modane♦, Modane Mild♦ **Acute constipation, preparation for rectal or bowel examination, postsurgical and postpartum constipation:** ADULTS AND CHILDREN: 37.5 to 150 mg P.O. after or with evening meal.	**GI:** *nausea;* vomiting; diarrhea; loss of normal bowel function in excessive use; *abdominal cramps,* especially in severe constipation; malabsorption of nutrients; "cathartic colon" (syndrome resembling ulcerative colitis radiologically and pathologically) in chronic misuse; discoloration of rectal mucosa in long-term use. **Metabolic:** hypokalemia, protein enteropathy, electrolyte imbalance in excessive use. **Other:** laxative dependence in long-term or excessive use.
docusate calcium (formerly dioctyl calcium sulfosuccinate) Surfak♦ **docusate potassium (formerly dioctyl potassium sulfosuccinate)** Kasof **docusate sodium (formerly dioctyl sodium sulfosuccinate)** Bu-Lax, Colace, Comfolax, Disonate, Doctate, Doxinate, D.S.S., Laxinate, Regutol, Roctate **Stool softener:** ADULTS AND OLDER CHILDREN: 50 to 300 mg (docusate sodium) P.O. daily or 240 mg (docusate calcium and docusate potassium) P.O. daily until bowel movements are normal; or 5 ml	**EENT:** throat irritation. **GI:** bitter taste, mild abdominal cramping, diarrhea. **Other:** laxative dependence in long-term or excessive use.

♦ Available in U.S. and Canada. ♦♦ Available in Canada only.
All other products (no symbol) available in U.S. only. Italicized side effects are common or life-threatening.

INTERACTIONS AND SPECIAL CONSIDERATIONS

• May turn alkaline urine red-pink and acidic urine yellow-brown.
• Serum electrolytes should be monitored during prolonged use.

No significant interactions.

Special considerations:
• Contraindicated in ulcerative bowel lesions; during menstruation; in abdominal pain, nausea, vomiting, or other symptoms of appendicitis or acute surgical abdomen; in anal or rectal fissures, fecal impaction, intestinal obstruction or perforation. Use cautiously when rectal bleeding is present.
• Failure to respond may indicate acute condition requiring surgery.
• Should be taken with juice or carbonated beverage to mask oily taste. Ice held in mouth before taking drug will help prevent tasting it.
• Shake emulsion well. Store below 4.4° C. (40° F.). Don't freeze.
• Should be taken on empty stomach for best results.
• Produces complete evacuation after 3 hours. After castor oil has emptied bowel, patient will not have bowel movement for 1 to 2 days.
• Drug administration should be timed so that it doesn't interefere with scheduled activities or sleep.
• Serum electrolytes should be monitored during prolonged use.
• Generally used before diagnostic testing or therapy requiring thorough evacuation of GI tract.
• For short-term treatment. Not recommended for routine use; useful for acute constipation not responsive to milder laxatives.
• Before laxative is given for constipation, patient history of fluid intake, exercise, and diet should be obtained. Dietary sources of bulk include bran and other cereals, fresh fruit, and vegetables.
• Stimulant laxative.
• Increased intestinal motility lessens absorption of concomitantly administered oral drugs. Dosage should be rescheduled.

No significant interactions.

Special considerations:
• Contraindicated in abdominal pain, nausea, vomiting, or other symptoms of appendicitis or acute surgical abdomen; in intestinal obstruction or perforation; and in hepatic dysfunction. Use cautiously when rectal bleeding or fecal impaction is present.
• Given with fruit juice or carbonated beverage to mask oily taste.
• Should be given on empty stomach for best results.
• Produces complete evacuation of bowel in 6 to 24 hours. Patient will not have another bowel movement for 1 to 2 days. Administration of drug should be timed so that it doesn't interfere with scheduled activities or sleep.
• Generally used before diagnostic testing or therapy requiring thorough evacuation of GI tract.
• Agent of choice for cardiac patients; reduces strain of evacuation.
• For short-term treatment. Not recommended for routine use; useful for acute constipation not responsive to milder laxatives.
• Before laxative is given for constipation, patient history of fluid intake, exercise, and diet should be obtained. Dietary sources of bulk include bran and other cereals, fresh fruit, and vegetables.
• May discolor alkaline urine red-pink and acidic urine yellow-brown.
• Stimulant laxative.
• Serum electrolytes should be monitored during prolonged use.

No significant interactions.

Special considerations:
• Sodium salts: use cautiously in patients on sodium-restricted diets, or those with edema, congestive heart failure, renal dysfunction.
• Docusate sodium contains 5.17 mg sodium/100-mg capsule.
• Potassium salts: contraindicated in renal dysfunction.
• Liquid should be taken in milk, fruit juice, or infant formula to mask bitter taste.
• Not for use in treating existing constipation, but prevents constipation from developing.
• Laxative of choice in patients who should not strain during defecation, such as those recovering from myocardial infarction or rectal surgery; in disease of rectum and anus, which makes passage of firm stool difficult; or postpartum constipation.
• Acts within 24 to 48 hours to produce firm, semisolid stool.
• Dietary sources of bulk include bran and other cereals, fresh fruit, and vegetables.
• Emollient laxative or stool softener; doesn't stimulate intestinal peristaltic movements.
• Store at 15° to 30° C. (59° to 86° F.). Protect liquid from light.

(continued on following page)

NAMES, INDICATIONS AND DOSAGES	SIDE EFFECTS
docusate *(continued)* (250 mg) (docusate potassium) enema. CHILDREN OVER 12 YEARS: 2 ml (100 mg) (docusate potassium) enema. CHILDREN 6 TO 12 YEARS: 40 to 120 mg (docusate sodium) P.O. daily. CHILDREN 3 TO 6 YEARS: 20 to 60 mg (docusate sodium) P.O. daily. CHILDREN UNDER 3 YEARS: 10 to 40 mg (docusate sodium) P.O. daily. Higher doses are for initial therapy. Adjust dose to individual response. Usual dose in children and adults with minimal needs: 50 to 150 mg (docusate calcium) P.O. daily.	
glycerin **Constipation:** ADULTS AND CHILDREN OVER 6 YEARS: 3 g as a suppository; or 5 to 15 ml as an enema. CHILDREN UNDER 6 YEARS: 1 to 1.5 g as a suppository; or 2 to 5 ml as an enema.	**GI:** *cramping pain,* rectal discomfort, hyperemia of rectal mucosa.
lactulose Cephulac♦, Chronulac♦ **Treatment of constipation:** ADULTS: 15 to 30 ml P.O. daily. **To prevent and treat portal-systemic encephalopathy, including hepatic precoma and coma in patients with severe hepatic disease:** ADULTS: initially, 20 to 30 g P.O. (30 to 45 ml) t.i.d. or q.i.d., until 2 or 3 soft stools are produced daily. Usual dose is 60 to 100 g daily in divided doses. Can also be given by retention enema in at least 100 ml of fluid.	**GI:** abdominal cramps, belching, diarrhea, gaseous distention, flatulence.
magnesium salts Concentrated Milk of Magnesia, Magnesium Citrate, Magnesium Sulfate, Milk of Magnesia **Constipation, to evacuate bowel before surgery:** ADULTS AND CHILDREN OVER 6 YEARS: 15 g magnesium sulfate P.O. in glass of water; 10 to 20 ml concentrated milk of magnesia P.O.; or 15 to 30 ml milk of magnesia P.O.; or 5 to 10 oz magnesium citrate at bedtime. **Laxative:** ADULTS: 30 to 60 ml, usually h.s., Milk of Magnesia P.O. CHILDREN: 7.5 to 30 ml h.s. Milk of Magnesia P.O.	**GI:** *abdominal cramping, nausea.* **Metabolic:** fluid and electrolyte disturbances if used daily. **Other:** laxative dependence in long-term or excessive use.

♦ Available in U.S. and Canada. ♦♦ Available in Canada only.
All other products (no symbol) available in U.S. only. Italicized side effects are common or life-threatening.

INTERACTIONS AND SPECIAL CONSIDERATIONS

No significant interactions.

Special considerations:
- A hyperosmolar laxative used mainly to reestablish proper toilet habits in laxative-dependent patients.

No significant interactions.

Special considerations:
- Contraindicated in patients who need low-galactose diet. Use cautiously in diabetes mellitus.
- If diarrhea occurs dosage should be reduced and fluid loss replaced.
- If desired, minimize drug's sweet taste by diluting with water or fruit juice or giving with food.
- Store at room temperature, preferably below 30° C. (86° F.). Don't freeze.

No significant interactions.

Special considerations:
- Contraindicated in abdominal pain, nausea, vomiting, or other symptoms of appendicitis or acute surgical abdomen; in myocardial damage, heart block, imminent delivery, fecal impaction, rectal fissures, intestinal obstruction or perforation, renal disease. Use cautiously when rectal bleeding is present.
- Shake suspension well; take with large amount of water when used as laxative. When administering through nasogastric tube, tube should be placed properly and patent. After instillation, tube should be flushed with water to assure passage to stomach and maintain tube patency.
- Short-term; don't use longer than 1 week.
- When used as laxative, oral drugs should not be taken 1 to 2 hours before or after.
- Saline laxative; produces watery stool in 3 to 6 hours. Time drug administration not to interfere with scheduled activities or sleep.
- More potent than other saline laxatives.
- Before use for constipation, obtain patient history of fluid intake, exercise, and diet. Dietary sources of bulk include bran and other cereals, fresh fruit, and vegetables.
- Magnesium may accumulate in renal insufficiency.
- Chilling before use may make magnesium citrate more palatable.
- Frequent or prolonged use as a laxative may cause dependence. Monitor serum electrolytes during prolonged use.

NAMES, INDICATIONS AND DOSAGES	SIDE EFFECTS
methylcellulose Cellothyl, Cologel, Hydrolose, Syncelose **Chronic constipation:** ADULTS: 5 to 20 ml liquid P.O. t.i.d. with a glass of water; or 15 ml syrup P.O. morning and evening. CHILDREN: 5 to 10 ml P.O. daily or b.i.d.	**GI:** *nausea,* vomiting, diarrhea (all after excessive use); esophageal, gastric, small intestinal, or colonic strictures when drug is chewed or taken in dry form; *abdominal cramps,* especially in severe constipation. **Other:** laxative dependence in long-term or excessive use.
mineral oil Agoral Plain, Fleet Mineral Oil Enema, Kondremul Plain♦, Neo-Cultol, Petrogalar Plain, Saf-Tip Oil Retention Enema **Constipation; preparation for bowel studies or surgery:** ADULTS: 15 to 30 ml P.O., usually h.s.; or 4 oz enema. CHILDREN: 5 to 15 ml P.O. h.s.; or 1 to 2 oz enema.	**GI:** *nausea;* vomiting; diarrhea in excessive use; *abdominal cramps,* especially in severe constipation; decreased absorption of nutrients and fat-soluble vitamins, resulting in deficiency; slowed healing after hemorrhoidectomy; and increased risk of rectal infections due to seepage from rectum. **Other:** laxative dependence in long-term or excessive use.
phenolphthalein Alophen, Espotabs, Evac-U-Lac, Ex-Lax, Feen-A-Mint, Phenolax, Evac-U-Gen **Constipation:** ADULTS: 60 to 200 mg P.O., preferably h.s.	**GI:** diarrhea; *colic in large doses;* factitious nausea; vomiting; loss of normal bowel function in excessive use; *abdominal cramps,* especially in severe constipation; malabsorption of nutrients; "cathartic colon" (syndrome resembling ulcerative colitis radiologically and pathologically) in chronic misuse; reddish discoloration in alkaline feces. **Skin:** dermatitis, pruritus. **Other:** laxative dependence in long-term or excessive use.
psyllium Effersyllium Instant Mix, Hydrocil Instant Powder, Konsyl, L.A. Formula, Metamucil♦, Metamucil Instant Mix♦, Modane Bulk, Mucillium, Mucilose, Plain Hydrocil, Siblin♦, Syllact **Constipation; bowel management:** ADULTS: 1 to 2 rounded teaspoonfuls P.O. in full glass of liquid daily, b.i.d., or t.i.d., followed by second glass of liquid; or 1 packet P.O. dissolved in water daily, b.i.d., or t.i.d. CHILDREN OVER 6 YEARS: 1 level teaspoonful P.O. in ½ glass of liquid h.s.	**GI:** nausea, vomiting, diarrhea, all after excessive use; esophageal, gastric, small intestinal, or colonic strictures when drug taken in dry form; abdominal cramps, especially in severe constipation.

♦ Available in U.S. and Canada. ♦♦ Available in Canada only.
All other products (no symbol) available in U.S. only. Italicized side effects are common or life-threatening.

INTERACTIONS AND SPECIAL CONSIDERATIONS

No significant interactions.

Special considerations:

• Contraindicated in abdominal pain, nausea, vomiting, or other symptoms of appendicitis or acute surgical abdomen; and in intestinal obstruction or ulceration, disabling adhesion, or difficulty swallowing.

• Laxative effect usually takes 12 to 24 hours, but may be delayed 3 days.

• Patient should take drug with at least 8 oz of pleasant-tasting liquid to mask grittiness.

• Especially useful in postpartum constipation, chronic laxative abuse, irritable bowel syndrome, diverticular disease, colostomies, to empty colon before barium enema examinations, and in debilitated patients.

• For short-term treatment.

• Before laxative is given for constipation, patient history of fluid intake, exercise, and diet should be obtained. Dietary sources of bulk include bran and other cereals, fresh fruit, and vegetables.

• Not absorbed systemically; nontoxic.

• Bulk laxative; increases bulk and water content of stool.

• Patient should notify doctor in 1 week about response to therapy.

No significant interactions.

Special considerations:

• Contraindicated in abdominal pain, nausea, vomiting, or other symptoms of appendicitis or acute surgical abdomen; in fecal impaction, intestinal obstruction or perforation. Use cautiously in young children; in elderly or debilitated patients due to susceptibility to lipid pneumonitis through aspiration, absorption, and transport from intestinal mucosa; and in rectal bleeding. Enema contraindicated in children under 2 years.

• Drug should not be given with meals or immediately after, as it delays passage of food from stomach. More active on an empty stomach.

• A lubricant laxative.

• Should be given with fruit juices or carbonated drinks to disguise taste.

• Should be used when patient needs to ease the strain of evacuation.

• Before laxative is given for constipation, patient history of fluid intake, exercise, and diet should be obtained. Dietary sources of bulk include bran and other cereals, fresh fruit, and vegetables.

No significant interactions.

Special considerations:

• Contraindicated in abdominal pain, nausea, vomiting, or other symptoms of appendicitis or acute surgical abdomen; in fecal impaction, intestinal obstruction or perforation. Use cautiously in rectal bleeding.

• Laxative effect may last up to 3 to 4 days.

• Produces semisolid stool within 6 to 8 hours, with little or no griping. Administration of drug should be timed so that it doesn't interfere with scheduled activities or sleep.

• Patient with rash should avoid sun and discontinue use.

• Before laxative is given for constipation, patient history of fluid intake, exercise, and diet should be obtained. Dietary sources of bulk include bran and other cereals, fresh fruit, and vegetables.

• May discolor alkaline urine red-pink and acidic urine yellow-brown.

• Drug is available in many dosage forms. Most popular over-the-counter laxative; a frequent constituent of chewing gum and chocolate laxatives. Stimulant laxative, class of laxative most abused.

No significant interactions.

Special considerations:

• Contraindicated in abdominal pain, nausea, vomiting, or other symptoms of appendicitis; and in intestinal obstruction or ulceration, disabling adhesion, or difficulty swallowing.

• Metamucil Instant Mix (effervescent form) has a significant amount of sodium. Don't use for patients on sodium-restricted diets.

• All forms of Metamucil brand contain sugar. Different brands of psyllium should be used in patients with diabetes.

• Mix with at least 8 oz of cold, pleasant-tasting liquid to mask grittiness, and stir only a few seconds. Patient should drink it immediately or mixture will solidify; follow with additional glass of liquid.

• Short-term treatment; not for maintenance.

• Frequent use of laxatives can cause drug dependence for evacuation.

• Before use for constipation, obtain patient history of fluid intake, exercise, and diet. Dietary sources of bulk include bran and other cereals, fresh fruit, and vegetables.

• Laxative effect usually seen in 12 to 24 hours, but may be delayed 3 days.

• Bulk laxative; increases bulk and water content of stool. Highly refined, purified vegetable mucilloid; from seeds of platango plant.

• Not absorbed systemically; nontoxic. Especially useful in postpartum constipation, chronic laxative abuse, irritable bowel syndrome, diverticular disease, in combination with other laxatives to empty colon before barium enema examinations, and in debilitated patients.

NAMES, INDICATIONS AND DOSAGES	SIDE EFFECTS
senna Black Draught, Glysennid, Senokot, X-Prep **Acute constipation, preparation for bowel or rectal examination:** ADULTS: Dosage range for Senokot: 1 to 8 tablets P.O.; ½ to 4 teaspoonfuls of granules added to liquid; 1 to 2 suppositories h.s.; 1 to 4 teaspoonfuls syrup h.s. Black Draught: 7.5 to 15 ml. CHILDREN OVER 27 KG: ½ adult dose of tablets, granules, or syrup (except Black Draught tablets and granules not recommended for children). CHILDREN 1 MONTH TO 1 YEAR: 1.25 to 2.5 ml Senokot syrup P.O. h.s. X-Prep used solely as single dose for preradiographic bowel evacuation. Give ¾ oz powder dissolved in juice or 2.5 oz liquid between 2 and 4 p.m. on day before X-ray procedure. May be given in divided doses for elderly or debilitated patients.	**GI:** *nausea;* vomiting; diarrhea; loss of normal bowel function in excessive use; *abdominal cramps,* especially in severe constipation; malabsorption of nutrients; "cathartic colon" (syndrome resembling ulcerative colitis radiologically in chronic misuse; may cause constipation after catharsis); yellow, yellow-green cast feces, diarrhea in breast-feeding infants of mothers on senna; darkened pigmentation of rectal mucosa in long-term use, which is usually reversible within 4 to 12 months after stopping drug. **GU:** red-pink discoloration in alkaline urine; yellow-brown color to acid urine. **Metabolic:** hypokalemia, protein enteropathy, electrolyte imbalance with excessive use. **Other:** laxative dependence in long-term or excessive use.
sodium biphosphate Enemeez, Fleet Enema♦, Phospho-Soda, Saf-Tip Phosphate Enema **sodium phosphate** Sal-Hepatica **Constipation:** ADULTS: 5 to 20 ml liquid P.O. with water; or 4 g powder P.O. dissolved in warm water; or 20 to 46 ml solution mixed with 4 oz cold water; or 2 to 4.5 oz enema.	**GI:** *abdominal cramping.* **Metabolic:** fluid and electrolyte disturbances (hypernatremia, hyperphosphatemia) if used daily. **Other:** laxative dependence in long-term or excessive use.

♦ Available in U.S. and Canada. ♦♦ Available in Canada only.
All other products (no symbol) available in U.S. only. Italicized side effects are common or life-threatening.

INTERACTIONS AND SPECIAL CONSIDERATIONS

No significant interactions.

Special considerations:

- Contraindicated in ulcerative bowel lesions; in nausea, vomiting, abdominal pain, or other symptoms of appendicitis or acute surgical abdomen; in fecal impaction, intestinal obstruction, or perforation.
- For short-term treatment.
- More potent than cascara sagrada. Acts in 6 to 10 hours. X-Prep gives thorough, strong bowel action beginning in 6 hours.
- Most recommended stimulant laxative.
- Before laxative is given for constipation, patient history of fluid intake, exercise, and diet should be obtained. Dietary sources of bulk include bran and other cereals, fresh fruit, and vegetables.
- After X-Prep liquid is taken, diet should be confined to clear liquids.

No significant interactions.

Special considerations:

- Contraindicated in abdominal pain, nausea, vomiting, or other symptoms of appendicitis or acute surgical abdomen; in intestinal obstruction or perforation; edema; congestive heart failure; megacolon; impaired renal function; and in patients on salt-restricted diets.
- Failure to respond may indicate acute condition requiring surgery.
- Available in oral and rectal forms.
- Before laxative is given for constipation, patient history of fluid intake, exercise, and diet should be obtained. Dietary sources of bulk include bran and other cereals, fresh fruit, and vegetables.
- Saline laxative; up to 10% of sodium content may be absorbed.
- Enema form elicits response within 5 to 10 minutes.
- Used in preparation for barium enema and for fecal impaction.

48

Emetics and antiemetics

apomorphine hydrochloride
benzquinamide hydrochloride
buclizine hydrochloride
cyclizine hydrochloride
cyclizine lactate
dimenhydrinate
diphenidol
ipecac syrup
meclizine hydrochloride
prochlorperazine edisylate
prochlorperazine maleate
scopolamine
thiethylperazine maleate
trimethobenzamide hydrochloride

Emetics (apomorphine and ipecac) are organic compounds used in emergencies to remove poisons from the stomach. They induce vomiting and prevent extensive absorption. Although emetics should be given immediately, they may still be useful even if administration is delayed. However, they should not be used after ingestion of corrosives such as lye since further injury may result. The use of emetics, along with symptomatic and supportive care, can be lifesaving.

Antiemetics (the remaining drugs listed) relieve nausea and vomiting. They are clearly indicated whenever vomiting is severe enough to produce significant fluid, electrolyte, and nutrient losses. By preventing violent retching, they minimize injury to the esophagus and disruption of suture lines (as after intraocular surgery). However, over-the-counter antiemetics can be overused and abused.

Major uses

- Emetics induce vomiting after ingestion of toxic substances.
- Antiemetics are used to prevent and treat nausea, vomiting, and dizziness.

Mechanism of action

- Apomorphine acts directly on the chemoreceptor trigger zone in the medulla oblongata to induce vomiting.
- Ipecac syrup induces vomiting by acting locally on the gastric mucosa and centrally on the chemoreceptor trigger zone.
- Benzquinamide and trimethobenzamide may act on the chemoreceptor trigger zone to inhibit nausea and vomiting, but this is not certain.
- Buclizine, cyclizine, dimenhydrinate, and meclizine (antihistamine antiemetics) may affect neural pathways originating in the labyrinth to inhibit nausea and vomiting, but the exact mechanism of action is unknown.
- Diphenidol influences the chemoreceptor trigger zone to inhibit nausea and vomiting.
- Prochlorperazine and thiethylperazine (phenothiazine antiemetics) also act on the chemoreceptor trigger zone to inhibit nausea and vomiting, and in larger doses partially depress the vomiting center as well.
- Scopolamine reduces the excitability of labyrinth receptors, depressing conduction in vestibular pathways.

Absorption, distribution, metabolism, and excretion

- Apomorphine is poorly absorbed orally but well absorbed when administered by I.M. or subcutaneous injection. It is metabolized in the liver and excreted by the kidneys.
- Ipecac syrup is absorbed through the gastrointestinal tract; its metabolism and route of excretion, however, are unknown.
- Benzquinamide is rapidly absorbed after I.M. injection and rapidly distributed in body

THERAPEUTIC ACTIVITY OF EMETICS AND ANTIEMETICS

DRUG	ROUTE	ONSET	DURATION
Emetics			
apomorphine	parenteral	5 to 15 min	*
ipecac syrup	P.O.	20 to 30 min	*
Antiemetics			
benzquinamide	parenteral	15 to 30 min	3 to 4 hr
buclizine	P.O.	30 to 60 min	4 to 6 hr
cyclizine	I.M., P.O.	30 to 60 min	4 to 6 hr
dimenhydrinate	I.M., P.O., rectal	30 to 60 min	4 to 6 hr
diphenidol	parenteral, P.O.	30 to 40 min	4 to 6 hr
meclizine	P.O.	30 to 60 min	8 to 24 hr
prochlorperazine	parenteral	10 to 20 min	3 to 4 hr
	P.O.	30 to 40 min	3 to 4 hr (tablet) 10 to 12 hr (extended-release form)
	rectal	1 hr	3 to 4 hr
scopolamine	transdermal	2 to 8 hr	72 hr
thiethylperazine	P.O.	30 min	4 hr
trimethobenzamide	parenteral	15 to 35 min	2 to 3 hr
	P.O., rectal	10 to 40 min	3 to 4 hr

*Data not relevant

AN ALTERNATIVE FOR MOTION SICKNESS: SCOPOLAMINE COMES IN A TRANSDERMAL PATCH

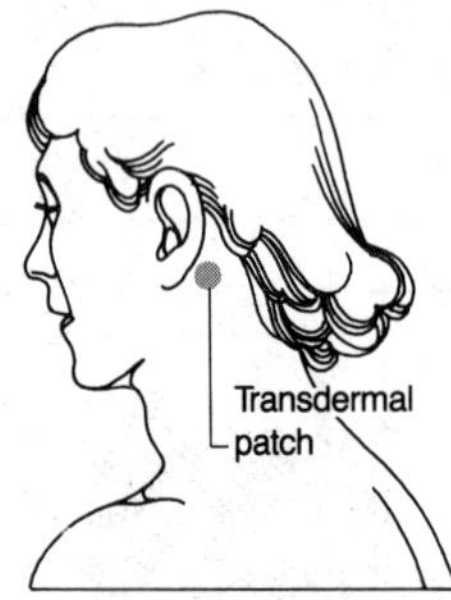

The more than 9 million persons who suffer from motion sickness now have another way to prevent it. Transderm-V (scopolamine), the first FDA-approved transdermal system, consists of a small patch that's worn behind the ear for sustained release of scopolamine. Although the anticholinergic scopolamine isn't new, the transdermal route of administration is.

Why the transdermal route for motion sickness?

- The group of nerve fibers in the inner ear's vestibular apparatus helps people maintain balance. But for some, motion increases the activity of these fibers, causing dizziness, nausea, and vomiting. Transderm-V helps reduce the activity of these inner ear fibers.
- The patch releases minute amounts of scopolamine that permeate the intact skin at a preprogrammed rate, minimizing side effects. Scopolamine is directly absorbed into the bloodstream, quickly achieving and maintaining an optimal dose for up to 72 hours. This prevents the nausea and vomiting of motion sickness.
- The patch is a flexible, adhesive disk of four layers, as shown in the illustration.

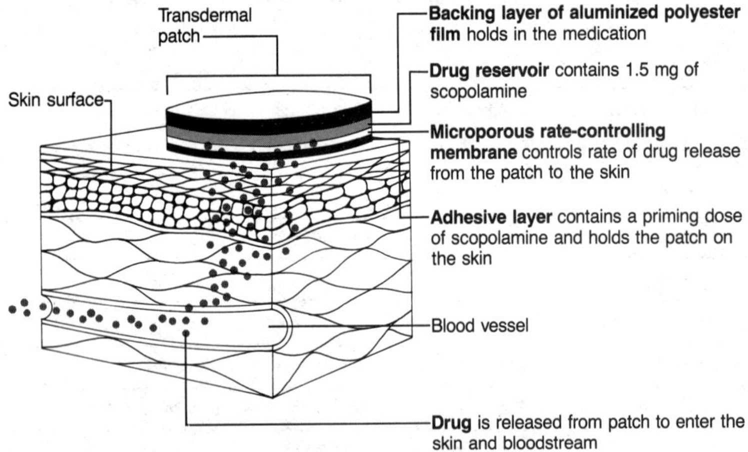

- The priming dose of scopolamine rapidly brings the blood level to the required steady-state level. Over the 3-day lifetime of the patch, the medication is delivered at a nearly constant rate from the patch to the skin to the blood.
- By diffusion, the drug passes through the membrane from the higher concentration inside the reservoir to the lower concentration outside the reservoir.
- The amount of drug delivered in the diffusion process is regulated by the membrane thickness, surface area and composition, and by the drug concentration on each side of the membrane.

Special considerations

Scopolamine should be used with caution in patients with glaucoma, pyloric obstruction, or urinary bladder neck obstruction. Some users experience dry mouth. However, drowsiness, which commonly occurs with higher doses of motion-sickness drugs, is minimized.

Transdermal administration systems have enormous potential, including treatment of such conditions as angina, high blood pressure, and asthma.

ARE MARIJUANA DERIVATIVES USEFUL AS ANTIEMETICS?

Anecdotal accounts that smoking marijuana prior to cancer chemotherapy treatments prevented nausea and vomiting led to the study of cannabinoid antiemetic properties. Investigational studies did indeed show that marijuana derivatives and synthetic tetrahydrocannabinol (THC) successfully reduce severe nausea and vomiting associated with chemotherapy. In several clinical studies, THC relieved chemotherapy-induced nausea and vomiting better than a placebo and equal to or better than prochlorperazine.

However, many patients experienced side effects, such as drowsiness, dry mouth, dizziness, decreased coordination, blurred vision, and decreased concentration. A few patients experienced depression, euphoria, tachycardia, and anxiety, but most patients preferred these side effects to chemotherapy-induced nausea and vomiting.

tissues, with highest concentration in the liver and kidneys. It is metabolized in the liver and eliminated in urine and feces.

- Buclizine, cyclizine, dimenhydrinate, and meclizine are well absorbed after either oral or parenteral administration. They are widely distributed in the tissues, metabolized in the liver, and excreted by the kidneys.
- Diphenidol is well absorbed after being given orally, distributed to most body tissues, and metabolized in the liver. It's eliminated in urine and feces.
- Prochlorperazine and thiethylperazine are well absorbed when given orally, parenterally, or rectally. Widely distributed, they are metabolized in the liver and eliminated either in urine or—through the bile—in feces.
- Scopolamine is completely and evenly absorbed transdermally. The drug is widely distributed and excreted unchanged in urine.
- Trimethobenzamide is well distributed to tissues, metabolized in the liver, and eliminated as both unchanged drug and metabolites in urine and feces.

Onset and duration

The table on p. 501 summarizes the therapeutic activity of the emetics and antiemetics.

Combination products

None.

NAMES, INDICATIONS AND DOSAGES	SIDE EFFECTS
apomorphine hydrochloride Controlled Substance Schedule II **To induce vomiting in poisoning:** ADULTS: 2 to 10 mg S.C. preceded by 200 to 300 ml water. Don't repeat. CHILDREN OVER 1 YEAR: 0.07 mg/kg S.C. preceded by up to 2 glasses of water. CHILDREN UNDER 1 YEAR: 0.07 mg/kg S.C. preceded by ½ to 1 glass of water.	**CNS:** *depression, euphoria,* restlessness, tremors. **CV:** *acute circulatory failure in elderly or debilitated patients,* tachycardia. **Other:** *depressed respiratory center in large or repeated doses.*
benzquinamide hydrochloride Emete-Con **Nausea and vomiting associated with anesthesia and surgery:** ADULTS: 50 mg I.M. (0.5 mg/kg to 1 mg/kg). May repeat in 1 hour, and thereafter q 3 to 4 hours, p.r.n.; or 25 mg (0.2 mg/kg to 0.4 mg/kg) I.V. as single dose, administered slowly.	**CNS:** *drowsiness,* fatigue, insomnia, restlessness, headache, excitation, tremors, twitching, dizziness. **CV:** sudden rise in blood pressure and transient arrhythmias (premature atrial and ventricular contractions, atrial fibrillation) after I.V. administration; hypertension; hypotension. **EENT:** dry mouth, salivation, blurred vision. **GI:** anorexia, nausea. **Skin:** urticaria, rash. **Other:** muscle weakness, flushing, hiccups, sweating, chills, fever. May mask signs of overdose of toxic agents or underlying conditions (intestinal obstruction, brain tumor).
buclizine hydrochloride Bucladin-S, Softran **Motion sickness (prevention):** ADULTS: 50 mg P.O. at least ½ hour before beginning travel. If needed, may repeat another 50 mg P.O. after 4 to 6 hours. **Nausea (treatment):** ADULTS: 50 mg P.O., up to 150 mg P.O. daily in severe cases. Maintenance dose is 50 mg b.i.d.	**CNS:** *drowsiness,* headache, dizziness, jitters. **EENT:** blurred vision, dry mouth. **GU:** urinary retention. **Other:** may mask symptoms of ototoxicity, intestinal obstruction, or brain tumor.
cyclizine hydrochloride **cyclizine lactate** Marezine, Marzine♦♦ **Motion sickness (prevention and treatment):** ADULTS: 50 mg P.O. (hydrochloride) ½ hour before travel, then q 4 to 6 hours, p.r.n., to maximum of 200 mg daily; or 50 mg I.M. (lactate) q 4 to 6 hours, p.r.n.	**CNS:** *drowsiness,* dizziness, auditory and visual hallucinations. **CV:** hypotension. **EENT:** blurred vision, dry mouth. **GI:** constipation. **GU:** urinary retention. **Other:** may mask symptoms of ototoxicity, brain tumor, or intestinal obstruction.

♦ Available in U.S. and Canada. ♦♦ Available in Canada only.
All other products (no symbol) available in U.S. only. Italicized side effects are common or life-threatening.

INTERACTIONS AND SPECIAL CONSIDERATIONS

No significant interactions.

Special considerations:
- Contraindicated in patients with hypersensitivity to narcotics; impending shock; corrosive poisoning; narcosis resulting from opiates, barbiturates, alcohol, or other CNS depressants; and in patients too inebriated to stand unaided. Use cautiously in children and in patients who are debilitated, have cardiac decompensation, or are predisposed to nausea and vomiting.
- Should not be given after ingestion of petroleum distillates (for example, kerosene or gasoline) or volatile oils; retching and vomiting may cause aspiration and lead to bronchospasm, pulmonary edema, or aspiration pneumonitis. Vegetable oil will delay absorption of these substances.
- Should not be given after ingestion of caustic substances, such as lye; additional injury to the esophagus and mediastinum can occur.
- Narcotic antagonists, such as naloxone, help stop vomiting and alleviate drowsiness.
- If delay in giving emetic is expected, activated charcoal should be given orally at once. When absorbable poison is ingested, activated charcoal should be given orally immediately after apomorphine hydrochloride.
- Vomiting occurs in 5 to 10 minutes in adults. If vomiting doesn't occur within 15 minutes, gastric lavage should begin. Apomorphine HCl is emetic of choice when rapid removal of poisons is necessary, and when identification of enteric-coated tablets or other ingested toxic material in vomitus is important. Stomach contents are usually expelled completely; vomitus may also contain material from upper portion of intestinal tract.
- Should not be administered if solution for injection is discolored or if precipitate is present.

No significant interactions.

Special considerations:
- I.V. use contraindicated in cardiovascular disease. Should not be given I.V. within 15 minutes of preanesthetic or cardiovascular drugs.
- For I.M. injection: give in large muscle mass; use deltoid area only if well developed; and aspirate syringe for I.M. injection to avoid inadvertent intravenous injection.
- Reconstituted solution stable for 14 days at room temperature. Store dry powder and reconstituted solution in light-resistant container.
- Blood pressure should be monitored frequently.
- Excellent substitute when prochlorperazine (Compazine) is contraindicated.

No significant interactions.

Special considerations:
- Patient should avoid driving and other activities that require alertness until CNS response to drug is established.
- Tablets may be placed in mouth and allowed to dissolve without water. May also be chewed or swallowed whole.

No significant interactions.

Special considerations:
- Use cautiously in patients with glaucoma, GU or GI obstruction, and in elderly males with possible prostatic hypertrophy.
- Patient should avoid driving and other activities that require alertness until CNS response to drug is determined.
- Classified as an antihistamine.
- Store in cool place. When stored at room temperature, injection may turn slightly yellow, but this color change does not indicate loss of potency.

(continued on following page)

NAMES, INDICATIONS AND DOSAGES	SIDE EFFECTS
cyclizine *(continued)* **Postoperative vomiting (prevention):** ADULTS: 50 mg I.M. (lactate) preoperatively or 20 to 30 minutes before expected termination of surgery; then postoperatively 50 mg I.M. (lactate) q 4 to 6 hours, p.r.n. **Motion sickness and postoperative vomiting:** CHILDREN 6 TO 12 YEARS: 3 mg/kg (lactate) I.M. divided t.i.d., or 25 mg (hydrochloride) P.O. q 4 to 6 hours p.r.n. to a maximum of 75 mg daily.	
dimenhydrinate Dimate, Dimen, Dimentabs, Dipendrate, Dramaject, Dramamine♦, Dramamine Junior, Dramocen, Dymenate, Eldodram, Gravol♦♦, Hydrate, Hypo-emesis, Marmine, Nauseal♦♦, Nauseatol♦♦, Novodimenate♦♦, Ram, Reidamine, Signate, Travamine♦♦, Trav-Arex, Traveltabs, Vertiban, Wehamine **Nausea, vomiting, dizziness of motion sickness (treatment and prevention):** ADULTS: 50 mg P.O. q 4 hours, or 100 mg q 4 hours if drowsiness is not objectionable; or 100 mg rectally daily or b.i.d. if oral route is not practical; or 50 mg I.M., p.r.n.; or 50 mg I.V. diluted in 10 ml NaCl solution, injected over 2 minutes. CHILDREN: 5 mg/kg P.O. or I.M. or rectally, divided q.i.d. Maximum 300 mg daily. Don't use in children less than 2 years old.	**CNS:** *drowsiness,* headache, incoordination, dizziness. **CV:** palpitations, hypotension. **EENT:** blurred vision, tinnitus, dry mouth and respiratory passages. **Other:** may mask symptoms of ototoxicity, brain tumor, or intestinal obstruction.
diphenidol Vontrol♦ **Peripheral (labyrinthine) dizziness; nausea and vomiting:** ADULTS: 25 to 50 mg P.O. q 4 hours, p.r.n., or 20 to 40 mg deep I.M. injection (for rapid control of acute symptoms), then another 20 mg I.M. after 1 hour if symptoms persist. Thereafter 20 to 40 mg I.M. q 4 hours, p.r.n., or 20 mg I.V. injected directly through venoclysis already in operation (for rapid control of acute symptoms). May inject another 20 mg I.V. after 1 hour if symptoms persist, then switch to P.O. or I.M. route. Total daily dosage should not exceed 300 mg. **Nausea and vomiting:** CHILDREN: 0.9 mg/kg P.O. or rectally, or 0.4 mg/kg I.M. Give children's doses no more frequently than q 4 hours unless symptoms persist after 1 dose. An oral or I.M. dose may be repeated after 1 hour. Thereafter, doses may be given p.r.n. Maximum children's dose 5.5 mg/kg P.O. daily; or 3.3 mg/kg I.M. daily.	**CNS:** drowsiness, dizziness, *confusion.* **CV:** transient hypotension; auditory and visual hallucinations, disorientation occur within 3 days of starting drug; subside within 3 days after stopping drug. **GI:** dry mouth, nausea, indigestion, heartburn. **Skin:** urticaria. **Other:** antiemetic effect may mask signs of overdose of drugs, or may obscure diagnosis of intestinal obstruction, brain tumor, or other conditions.

♦ Available in U.S. and Canada. ♦♦ Available in Canada only.
All other products (no symbol) available in U.S. only. Italicized side effects are common or life-threatening.

INTERACTIONS AND SPECIAL CONSIDERATIONS

No significant interactions.

Special considerations:
• Use cautiously in seizures, narrow-angle glaucoma, enlargement of prostate gland.
• Undiluted solution is irritating to veins; may cause sclerosis.
• Classified as an antihistamine.
• Patient should avoid driving and other activities that require alertness until CNS response to drug is determined.
• May mask ototoxicity of aminoglycoside antibiotics.
• Parenteral preparations should not be mixed with other drugs; incompatible with many solutions.

No significant interactions.

Special considerations:
• Contraindicated in anuria. Use cautiously in glaucoma, pyloric stenosis, pylorospasm, obstructive lesions of GI or GU tract, prostatic hypertrophy, or organic cardiospasm.
• I.V. use contraindicated in children and in patients with sinus tachycardia.
• Should not be given subcutaneously.
• Drug should be stopped if auditory or visual hallucinations, or disorientation or confusion occurs.
• Patient should be closely supervised. Patients are usually hospitalized when receiving this drug.
• Treatment of toxicity is symptomatic and supportive.
• Used in Ménière's disease, following middle and inner ear surgery, labyrinthine disturbances, and to control nausea and vomiting associated with infectious disease, malignancies, radiation sickness, general anesthetics, and antineoplastic agents.

NAMES, INDICATIONS AND DOSAGES	SIDE EFFECTS
ipecac syrup **To induce vomiting in poisoning:** ADULTS: 15 ml P.O., followed by 200 to 300 ml of water. CHILDREN 1 YEAR OR OLDER: 15 ml P.O., followed by about 200 ml of water or milk. CHILDREN UNDER 1 YEAR: 5 to 10 ml P.O., followed by about 200 ml of water or milk. May repeat dose once after 20 minutes, if necessary.	**CV:** *cardiac arrhythmias, atrial fibrillation, or fatal myocarditis* if drug is absorbed (e.g., if patient doesn't vomit within 30 minutes) or after ingestion of excessive dose.
meclizine hydrochloride Antivert♦, Bonamine♦♦, Bonine, Lamine, Roclizine, Vertrol, Whevert **Dizziness:** ADULTS: 25 to 100 mg P.O. daily in divided doses. Dose varies with patient response. **Motion sickness:** ADULTS: 25 to 50 mg P.O. 1 hour before travel, repeated daily for duration of journey.	**CNS:** *drowsiness,* fatigue. **EENT:** dry mouth, blurred vision. **Other:** may mask symptoms of ototoxicity, brain tumor, or intestinal obstruction.
prochlorperazine edisylate **prochlorperazine maleate** Compazine, Stemetil♦♦ **Preoperative nausea control:** ADULTS: 5 to 10 mg I.M. 1 to 2 hours before induction of anesthetic, repeat once in 30 minutes, if necessary; or 5 to 10 mg I.V. 15 to 30 minutes before induction of anesthetic (repeat once if necessary); or 20 mg/liter isotonic solution by I.V. infusion, added to infusion 15 to 30 minutes before induction. Maximum parenteral dose 40 mg daily. **Severe nausea, vomiting:** ADULTS: 5 to 10 mg P.O. t.i.d. or q.i.d.; or 15 mg sustained-release form P.O. on arising; or 10 mg sustained-release form P.O. q 12 hours; or 25 mg rectally b.i.d. or 5 to 10 mg I.M. injected deeply into upper outer quadrant of gluteal region. Repeat q 3 to 4 hours, p.r.n. CHILDREN 18 TO 39 KG: 2.5 mg P.O. or rectally t.i.d.; or 5 mg P.O. or rectally b.i.d. Maximum 15 mg daily; or 0.132 mg/kg deep I.M. injection. (Control usually obtained with 1 dose.) CHILDREN 14 TO 17 KG: 2.5 mg P.O. or rectally b.i.d. or t.i.d. Maximum 10 mg daily; or 0.132 mg/kg deep I.M. injection. (Control usually obtained with 1 dose.)	**Blood:** *transient leukopenia, agranulocytosis.* **CNS:** *extrapyramidal reactions (high incidence),* sedation (low incidence), pseudoparkinsonism, EEG changes, dizziness. **CV:** *orthostatic hypotension,* tachycardia, EKG changes. **EENT:** *ocular changes, blurred vision.* **GI:** *dry mouth, constipation.* **GU:** *urinary retention,* dark urine, menstrual irregularities, gynecomastia, inhibited ejaculation. **Hepatic:** *cholestatic jaundice.* **Metabolic:** hyperprolactinemia. **Skin:** *mild photosensitivity,* dermal allergic reactions, *exfoliative dermatitis.* **Other:** weight gain, increased appetite.

♦ Available in U.S. and Canada. ♦♦ Available in Canada only.
All other products (no symbol) available in U.S. only. Italicized side effects are common or life-threatening.

INTERACTIONS AND SPECIAL CONSIDERATIONS

Interactions:
ACTIVATED CHARCOAL: neutralized emetic effect. Don't give together but may give activated charcoal after vomiting has occurred.

Special considerations:
• Contraindicated in semicomatose or unconscious patients, and in those with severe inebriation, convulsions, shock, loss of gag reflex.
• Should not be given after ingestion of petroleum distillates (for example, kerosene or gasoline) or volatile oils; retching and vomiting may cause aspiration and lead to bronchospasm, pulmonary edema, or aspiration pneumonitis. Vegetable oil will delay absorption of these substances.
• Should not be given after ingestion of caustic substances, such as lye; additional injury to the esophagus and mediastinum can occur.
• Ipecac *syrup,* not single word "ipecac," should be clearly indicated to avoid confusion with fluidextract. Fluidextract is 14 times more concentrated and if advertently used instead of syrup may cause death.
• Induces vomiting within 30 minutes in more than 90% of patients; average time usually less than 20 minutes.
• Stomach is usually emptied completely; vomitus may contain some intestinal material as well.
• In antiemetic toxicity, ipecac syrup is usually effective if less than 1 hour has passed since ingestion of antiemetic.
• 1 oz of syrup should be readily available in the home when child becomes 1 year old for immediate use in case of emergency.
• No systemic toxicity with doses of 30 ml or less.
• If 2 doses do not induce vomiting, gastric lavage is necessary.

No significant interactions.

Special considerations:
• Patient should avoid driving and other activities that require alertness until CNS response to drug is determined.
• Antihistamine with a slower onset and longer duration of action than other antihistamine antiemetics.

Interactions:
ANTICHOLINERGICS, INCLUDING ANTIDEPRESSANT AND ANTI-PARKINSON AGENTS: increased anticholinergic activity, aggravated Parkinson-like symptoms. Use together cautiously.
ANTACIDS: inhibited absorption of oral phenothiazines. Separate antacid and phenothiazine dosage by at least 2 hours.
BARBITURATES: may decrease phenothiazine effect. Monitor patient for decreased antiemetic effect.

Special considerations:
• Contraindicated in phenothiazine hypersensitivity, coma, depression, CNS depression, bone marrow depression, subcortical damage; during pediatric surgery, use of spinal or epidural anesthetic or adrenergic blocking agents, alcohol usage. Use with caution in combination with other CNS depressants; in hepatic disease, arteriosclerosis or cardiovascular disease (may cause sudden drop in blood pressure), exposure to extreme heat or cold (including antipyretic therapy), respiratory disorders, hypocalcemia, vomiting in children, acutely ill or dehydrated children, convulsive disorders or severe reactions to insulin or electroshock therapy, suspected brain tumor or intestinal obstruction, glaucoma, or prostatic hypertrophy; in acutely ill or dehydrated children; and in elderly or debilitated patients.
• Should be stored in light-resistant container. Slight yellowing does not affect potency. Markedly discolored solutions should be discarded.
• Since drug has a very long duration of action, timed-release capsules have no significant advantage over ordinary oral dosage forms.
• Should be used only when vomiting can't be controlled by other measures, or when only a few doses are required. Medical supervision advised if more than 4 doses in 24-hour period needed.
• Not effective in motion sickness.
• Concentrate or injection solution on hands or clothing causes contact dermatitis.
• Concentrate should be diluted with tomato or fruit juice, milk, coffee, carbonated beverage, tea, water, soup, or pudding.
• CBC and liver function studies should be monitored during prolonged therapy. Patients should wear protective clothing when exposed to sunlight.
• Orthostatic hypotension possible.
• Should not be given subcutaneously or mixed in syringe with another drug. Should be given deep I.M.
• For symptoms and treatment of toxicity, see APPENDIX.

(continued on following page)

NAMES, INDICATIONS AND DOSAGES	SIDE EFFECTS
prochlorperazine *(continued)* CHILDREN 9 TO 13 KG: 2.5 mg P.O. or rectally daily or b.i.d. Maximum 7.5 mg daily; or 0.132 mg/kg deep I.M. injection. (Control usually obtained with 1 dose.)	
scopolamine Transderm-V **Prevention of nausea and vomiting associated with motion sickness:** ADULTS: One Transderm-V system (a circular flat unit) programmed to deliver 0.5 mg scopolamine over 3 days (72 hours), applied to the skin behind the ear several hours before the antiemetic is required. Not recommended for children.	**CNS:** *drowsiness,* restlessness, disorientation, confusion **EENT:** *dry mouth,* transient impairment of eye accommodation.
thiethylperazine maleate Torecan♦ **Nausea, vomiting:** ADULTS: 10 mg P.O., I.M., or rectally daily, b.i.d. or t.i.d.	**Blood:** *transient leukopenia, agranulocytosis.* **CNS:** *extrapyramidal reactions (high incidence),* sedation (low incidence), pseudoparkinsonism, EEG changes, dizziness. **CV:** *orthostatic hypotension,* tachycardia, EKG changes. **EENT:** *ocular changes, blurred vision.* **GI:** *dry mouth, constipation.* **GU:** *urinary retention,* dark urine, menstrual irregularities, gynecomastia, inhibited ejaculation. **Hepatic:** *cholestatic jaundice.* **Metabolic:** hyperprolactinemia. **Skin:** *mild photosensitivity,* dermal allergic reactions, *exfoliative dermatitis.* **Other:** weight gain, increased appetite.
trimethobenzamide hydrochloride Tigan **Nausea and vomiting (treatment):** ADULTS: 250 mg P.O. t.i.d. or q.i.d.; or 200 mg I.M. or rectally t.i.d. or q.i.d. **Postoperative nausea and vomiting (prevention):** ADULTS: 200 mg I.M. or rectally (single dose) before or during surgery; may repeat 3 hours after termination of anesthesia, p.r.n. CHILDREN 13 TO 40 KG: 100 to 200 mg P.O. or rectally t.i.d. or q.i.d. CHILDREN UNDER 13 KG: 100 mg rectally t.i.d. or q.i.d. Limited to prolonged vomiting of known etiology.	**CNS:** drowsiness, dizziness (in large doses). **CV:** hypotension. **GI:** diarrhea, exaggeration of preexisting nausea (in large doses). **Hepatic:** *liver toxicity.* **Local:** pain, stinging, burning, redness, swelling at I.M. injection site. **Skin:** skin hypersensitivity reactions. **Other:** antiemetic effect may mask signs of overdosage of toxic agents, or intestinal obstruction, brain tumor, or other conditions.

♦ Available in U.S. and Canada. ♦♦ Available in Canada only.
All other products (no symbol) available in U.S. only. Italicized side effects are common or life-threatening.

INTERACTIONS AND SPECIAL CONSIDERATIONS

No significant interactions.

Special considerations:
• Use cautiously in patients with glaucoma, pyloric obstruction, or urinary bladder neck obstruction.
• Hands should be washed and dried thoroughly before applying the system on dry skin behind the ear. After removing the system: discard it; then wash both the hands and application site thoroughly.
• If the system becomes displaced, it should be removed and replaced with another system on a fresh skin site in the postauricular area.
• A patient brochure is available with this product on request from the pharmacist.
• Patient should avoid driving and other activities that require alertness until CNS response to drug is determined.
• Sugarless hard candy may be helpful in minimizing dry mouth.
• Transderm-V is effective if applied 2 to 3 hours before experiencing motion, but more effective if used 12 hours before. Therefore, patient should apply system the night before a planned trip.
• Transdermal method of administration releases a controlled, therapeutic amount of scopolamine.

Interactions:
ANTICHOLINERGICS, INCLUDING ANTIDEPRESSANT AND ANTI-PARKINSON AGENTS: increased anticholinergic activity, aggravated Parkinson-like symptoms. Use together cautiously.
ANTACIDS: inhibited absorption of oral phenothiazines. Separate antacid and phenothiazine dosage by at least 2 hours.
BARBITURATES: may decrease phenothiazine effect. Monitor for decreased antiemetic effect.

Special considerations:
• Contraindicated in severe CNS depression, hepatic disease, coma, phenothiazine hypersensitivity.
• Should not be given I.V.
• For nausea and vomiting associated with anesthesia and surgery, deep I.M. injection should be given on or shortly before terminating anesthesia.
• Possibly effective in dizziness; not effective in motion sickness.
• Should be used only when vomiting can't be controlled by other measures, or when only a few doses are required.
• Patient should be warned about hypotension, and advised to stay in bed for 1 hour after receiving the drug.
• If drug gets on skin, should be washed off at once to prevent contact dermatitis.
• For symptoms and treatment of toxicity, see APPENDIX.

No significant interactions.

Special considerations:
• Contraindicated in children with viral illness (a possible cause of vomiting in children); may contribute to the development of Reye's syndrome, a potentially fatal acute childhood encephalopathy, characterized by fatty degeneration of the liver.
• Suppositories contraindicated in hypersensitivity to benzocaine hydrochloride or similar local anesthetic.
• Drug should be stopped if allergic skin reaction occurs.
• I.M. dose should be given by deep injection into upper outer quadrant of gluteal region to reduce pain and local irritation.
• Patient should be warned of the possibility of drowsiness and dizziness, and cautioned against driving and other activities that require alertness until CNS response to drug is determined.
• Suppositories should be stored in refrigerator.
• Has little or no value in preventing motion sickness; limited value as an antiemetic.

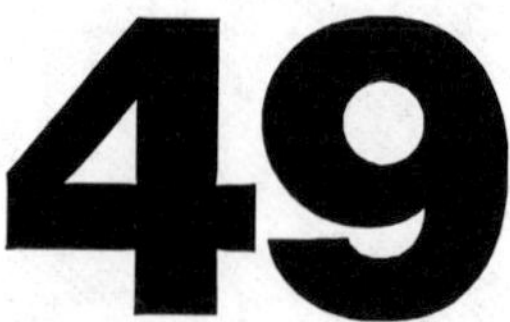

Gastrointestinal anticholinergics

Belladonna alkaloids
atropine sulfate
belladonna alkaloids
belladonna leaf
levorotatory alkaloids of belladonna
l-hyoscyamine sulfate

Quaternary anticholinergics
anisotropine methylbromide
clidinium bromide
diphemanil methylsulfate
glycopyrrolate
hexocyclium methylsulfate
homatropine methylbromide
isopropamide iodide
mepenzolate bromide
methantheline bromide
methscopolamine bromide
oxyphenonium bromide
propantheline bromide
tridihexethyl chloride

Tertiary synthetics (antispasmodics)
dicyclomine hydrochloride
methixene hydrochloride
oxyphencyclimine hydrochloride
thiphenamil hydrochloride

(All drugs are listed in alphabetical order in the tables that follow.)

Gastrointestinal (GI) anticholinergics may be used to relieve peptic ulcer pain; we lack evidence, however, that they heal peptic ulcers. Anticholinergics inhibit GI smooth muscle contraction and delay gastric emptying, thus enhancing the action of antacids. The anticholinergics should not be the sole basis of treatment, but rather part of a total therapeutic program.

Major uses
GI anticholinergics are therapeutic adjuncts for pain associated with peptic ulcers. They are also used to treat irritable colon (mucous colitis, spastic colon, and acute enterocolitis), other functional GI disorders, and neurogenic bowel disturbances, including splenic flexure syndrome and neurogenic colon.

Mechanism of action
- Belladonna alkaloids and quaternary anticholinergics block the actions of acetylcholine on the vagus nerve. (This blocking mechanism is known as competitive inhibition.) They decrease GI motility and inhibit gastric acid secretion.
- Tertiary synthetics exert a nonspecific direct spasmolytic action on smooth muscle. They also possess local anesthetic properties that may be partly responsible for the spasmolysis.

Absorption, distribution, metabolism, and excretion
- Belladonna alkaloids and tertiary synthetics are rapidly absorbed after oral administration. Because they readily cross the blood-brain barrier, they cause significant central nervous system (CNS) side effects. They are metabolized in the liver and eliminated both in urine and—through the bile—in feces.
- Quaternary anticholinergics are poorly and unreliably absorbed after oral administration. Since they *do not* cross the blood-brain barrier, their CNS side effects are negligible.

Onset and duration
Parenteral GI anticholinergics have a quicker onset and shorter duration than oral forms. Onset is usually 30 to 60 minutes, and duration 4 to 6 hours after oral administration.
- Belladonna alkaloids' effects usually last about 4 hours.

- Effects of the quaternary anticholinergics (except isopropamide) and the tertiary synthetics (except oxyphencyclimine) last 6 hours.
- Isopropamide and oxyphencyclimine have durations as long as 12 hours.

Combination products

BARBIDONNA TABLETS: atropine sulfate 0.025 mg, hyoscine hydrobromide 0.0074 mg, hyoscyamine hydrobromide or sulfate 0.1286 mg, and phenobarbital 16 mg.
BELLADENAL TABLETS♦: L-alkaloids of belladonna 0.25 mg and phenobarbital 50 mg.
BENTYL WITH PHENOBARBITAL SYRUP: dicyclomine hydrochloride 10 mg/5 ml, phenobarbital 15 mg/5 ml, and alcohol 19%.
BENTYL 10 MG WITH PHENOBARBITAL CAPSULES: dicyclomine hydrochloride 10 mg and phenobarbital 15 mg.
BENTYL 20 MG WITH PHENOBARBITAL TABLETS: dicyclomine hydrochloride 20 mg and phenobarbital 15 mg.
BUTIBEL ELIXIR: belladonna extract 15 mg/5 ml, butabarbital sodium 15 mg/5 ml, and alcohol 7%.
BUTIBEL TABLETS: belladonna extract 15 mg and butabarbital sodium 15 mg.
CANTIL WITH PHENOBARBITAL TABLETS: mepenzolate bromide 25 mg and phenobarbital 16 mg.
CHARDONNA-2: belladonna extract 15 mg and phenobarbital 15 mg.
COMBID SPANSULES♦: isopropamide iodide 5 mg and prochlorperazine maleate 10 mg.
DARICON PB TABLETS: oxyphencyclimine hydrochloride 5 mg and phenobarbital 15 mg.
DONNATAL ELIXIR♦: atropine sulfate 0.0194 mg/5 ml, hyoscine hydrobromide 0.0065 mg/5 ml, alcohol 23%, hyoscyamine hydrobromide or sulfate 0.1037 mg/5 ml and phenobarbital 16 mg/5 ml.
DONNATAL EXTENTABS♦: atropine sulfate 0.0582 mg, hyoscine hydrobromide 0.0195 mg, hyoscyamine sulfate 0.3111 mg, and phenobarbital 48.6 mg.
DONNATAL TABLETS AND CAPSULES♦: atropine sulfate 0.0194 mg, hyoscine hydrobromide 0.0065 mg, hyoscyamine hydrobromide or sulfate 0.1037 mg, phenobarbital 16 mg.
DONNATAL #2 TABLETS: atropine sulfate 0.0194 mg, hyoscine hydrobromide 0.0065 mg, hyoscyamine hydrobromide or sulfate 0.1037 mg, and phenobarbital 32.4 mg.
ENARAX 5 TABLETS: oxyphencyclimine hydrochloride 5 mg and hydroxyzine hydrochloride 25 mg.
KINESED TABLETS: atropine sulfate 0.02 mg, hyoscine hydrobromide 0.007 mg, hyoscyamine hydrobromide or sulfate 0.1 mg, and phenobarbital 16 mg.
LIBRAX CAPSULES: clidinium bromide 2.5 mg and chlordiazepoxide hydrochloride 5 mg.
MILPATH 200 TABLETS: tridihexethyl chloride 25 mg and meprobamate 200 mg.
MILPATH 400 TABLETS: tridihexethyl chloride 25 mg and meprobamate 400 mg.
PATHIBAMATE 200 TABLETS: tridihexethyl chloride 25 mg and meprobamate 200 mg.
PATHILON WITH PHENOBARBITAL TABLETS: tridihexethyl chloride 25 mg and phenobarbital 15 mg.
PRO-BANTHINE WITH PHENOBARBITAL TABLETS♦: propantheline bromide 15 mg and phenobarbital 15 mg.
ROBINUL PH TABLETS♦: glycopyrrolate 1 mg in addition to phenobarbital 16.2 mg.
VALPIN 50-PB TABLETS: anisotropine methylbromide 50 mg and phenobarbital 15 mg.
VISTRAX 10 TABLETS: oxyphencyclimine hydrochloride 10 mg and hydroxyzine hydrochloride 25 mg.

NAMES, INDICATIONS AND DOSAGES | SIDE EFFECTS

anisotropine methylbromide
Valpin 50

Adjunctive treatment of peptic ulcer:
ADULTS: 50 mg P.O. t.i.d. To be effective should be titrated to individual patient needs.

CNS: headache, insomnia, drowsiness, dizziness, *confusion or excitement in elderly patients,* nervousness, weakness.
CV: *palpitations,* tachycardia.
EENT: *blurred vision,* mydriasis, increased ocular tension, cycloplegia, photophobia.
GI: *dry mouth,* dysphagia, heartburn, loss of taste, nausea, vomiting, *paralytic ileus, constipation.*
GU: *urinary hesitancy and retention,* impotence.
Skin: urticaria, decreased sweating and possible anhidrosis, other dermal manifestations.
Other: fever, allergic reactions.
Overdosage may cause curare-like symptoms.

atropine sulfate

Adjunctive therapy in peptic ulcers, irritable bowel syndrome, neurogenic bowel disturbances, and functional gastrointestinal disorders:
ADULTS: 0.4 to 0.6 mg P.O. q 4 to 6 hours.
CHILDREN: the following dosages P.O. q 4 to 6 hours:
3 to 7 kg—0.1 mg (1/600 gr)
8 to 11 kg—0.15 mg (1/400 gr)
11 to 18 kg—0.2 mg (1/300 gr)
18 to 30 kg—0.3 mg (1/200 gr)
30 to 41 kg—0.4 mg (1/150 gr)
over 41 kg—0.4 to 0.6 mg (1/150 to 1/100 gr)

CNS: headache, insomnia, drowsiness, dizziness, *confusion or excitement in elderly patients,* nervousness, weakness.
CV: *palpitations,* tachycardia.
EENT: *blurred vision,* mydriasis, increased ocular tension, cycloplegia, photophobia.
GI: *dry mouth,* dysphagia, heartburn, loss of taste, nausea, vomiting, paralytic ileus.
GU: *urinary hesitancy and retention,* impotence.
Skin: urticaria, decreased sweating or anhidrosis, other dermal manifestations.
Other: fever, allergic reactions.
Overdosage may cause curare-like symptoms.

belladonna alkaloids

Adjunctive therapy in gastric, peptic, duodenal, or intestinal ulcers to control excess motor activity, hyperirritability or spasm of the gastrointestinal tract:
ADULTS: 0.4 to 0.8 mg (timed-release capsules) P.O. q 12 hours.

CNS: headache, insomnia, drowsiness, dizziness, *confusion or excitement in elderly patients,* nervousness, weakness.
CV: *palpitations,* tachycardia.
EENT: *blurred vision,* mydriasis, increased ocular tension, cycloplegia, photophobia.
GI: *dry mouth,* dysphagia, heartburn, loss of taste.
GU: *urinary hesitancy and retention,* impotence.
Skin: urticaria, decreased sweating or anhidrosis, other dermal manifestations.
Other: fever, allergic reactions.
Overdosage may cause curare-like symptoms.

belladonna leaf
(used to prepare extract, fluidextract, and tincture)
Belladonna Fluidextract, Belladonna Tincture USP

Adjunctive therapy for peptic ulcer, irritable bowel syndrome, functional gastrointestinal disorders, and neurogenic bowel disturbances:
ADULTS: 10.8 to 21.6 mg P.O. t.i.d. or q.i.d.

CNS: headache, insomnia, drowsiness, dizziness, *confusion or excitement in elderly patients,* nervousness, weakness.
CV: *palpitations,* tachycardia.
EENT: *blurred vision,* mydriasis, increased ocular tension, cycloplegia, photophobia.
GI: *dry mouth,* dysphagia, heartburn, loss of taste, *constipation,* nausea, vomiting.
GU: *urinary hesitancy and retention,* impotence.
Skin: urticaria, decreased sweating or anhidro-

◆ Available in U.S. and Canada. ◆◆ Available in Canada only.
All other products (no symbol) available in U.S. only. Italicized side effects are common or life-threatening.

INTERACTIONS AND SPECIAL CONSIDERATIONS

No significant interactions.

Special considerations:

• Contraindicated in narrow-angle glaucoma, obstructive uropathy, obstructive disease of the GI tract, severe ulcerative colitis, myasthenia gravis, hypersensitivity to anticholinergics, paralytic ileus, intestinal atony, unstable cardiovascular status in acute hemorrhage, and toxic megacolon. Use cautiously in autonomic neuropathy, hyperthyroidism, coronary artery disease, cardiac arrhythmias, congestive heart failure, hypertension, hiatal hernia associated with reflux esophagitis, hepatic or renal disease, ulcerative colitis, or in patients over 40 years because of increased incidence of glaucoma.
• Should be used with caution in hot or humid environments. Drug-induced heatstroke can develop.
• Should be given 30 minutes to 1 hour before meals.
• Smaller doses should be administered to the elderly.
• Patient's vital signs and urinary output should be monitored carefully.
• Patient should avoid driving and other hazardous activities if he is drowsy, dizzy, or has blurred vision; drink plenty of fluids to help prevent constipation; and report any skin rash or local eruption.
• Sugarless gum or hard candy may relieve mouth dryness.
• For symptoms and treatment of toxicity, see APPENDIX.

No significant interactions.

Special considerations:

• Contraindicated in narrow-angle glaucoma, obstructive uropathy, obstructive disease of GI tract, severe ulcerative colitis, myasthenia gravis, hypersensitivity to anticholinergics, paralytic ileus, intestinal atony, unstable cardiovascular status in acute hemorrhage, toxic megacolon. Use cautiously in autonomic neuropathy, hyperthyroidism, coronary artery disease, cardiac arrhythmias, congestive heart failure, hypertension, hiatal hernia associated with reflux esophagitis, hepatic or renal disease, ulcerative colitis, or in patients over 40 years because of increased incidence of glaucoma.
• Use with caution in hot, humid environments. Drug-induced heatstroke possible.
• Should be taken 30 minutes to 1 hour before meals and at bedtime. Bedtime dose can be larger and should be taken at least 2 hours after last meal of day.
• Smaller doses should be administered to the elderly.
• Patient's vital signs and urinary output should be monitored carefully.
• Patient should avoid driving and other hazardous activities if he is drowsy, dizzy, or has blurred vision; drink plenty of fluids to help prevent constipation; report any skin rash.
• Sugarless gum, hard candy, or pilocarpine syrup may relieve mouth dryness.
• Other anticholinergic drugs may increase vagal blockage.
• For symptoms and treatment of toxicity, see APPENDIX.

No significant interactions.

Special considerations:

• Contraindicated in narrow-angle glaucoma, obstructive uropathy, obstructive disease of GI tract, severe ulcerative colitis, myasthenia gravis, hypersensitivity to anticholinergics, paralytic ileus, intestinal atony, unstable cardiovascular status in acute hemorrhage, toxic megacolon. Use cautiously in autonomic neuropathy, hyperthyroidism, coronary artery disease, cardiac arrhythmias, congestive heart failure, hypertension, hiatal hernia with reflux esophagitis, hepatic or renal disease, ulcerative colitis, or in patients over 40 years because of increased incidence of glaucoma.
• Use with caution in hot or humid environments. Drug-induced heatstroke can develop.
• Smaller doses are required for the elderly.
• Patient's vital signs and urinary output should be monitored carefully.
• Patient should avoid driving and other hazardous activities if he is drowsy, dizzy, or has blurred vision; drink plenty of fluids to help prevent constipation; and report any skin rash.
• For symptoms and treatment of toxicity, see APPENDIX.

No significant interactions.

Special considerations:

• Contraindicated in narrow-angle glaucoma, obstructive uropathy, obstructive disease of GI tract, severe ulcerative colitis, myasthenia gravis, hypersensitivity to anticholinergics, paralytic ileus, intestinal atony, unstable cardiovascular status in acute hemorrhage, and toxic megacolon. Use cautiously in autonomic neuropathy, hyperthyroidism, coronary artery disease, cardiac arrhythmias, congestive heart failure, hypertension, hiatal hernia associated with reflux esophagitis, hepatic or renal disease, ulcerative colitis, or in patients over 40 years because of increased incidence of glaucoma.
• Should be taken 30 minutes to 1 hour before meals and at bedtime. Bedtime dose can be larger and should be taken at least 2 hours after last meal of day.
• Smaller doses are required for elderly.
• Caution should be used in hot or humid en-

(continued on following page)

NAMES, INDICATIONS AND DOSAGES	SIDE EFFECTS
belladonna leaf *(continued)* of the extract; 0.06 ml P.O. t.i.d. or q.i.d. of the Fluidextract; 0.6 to 1 ml t.i.d. or q.i.d. of tincture.	sis, other dermal manifestations. **Other:** fever, allergic reactions. Overdosage may cause curare-like symptoms.
clidinium bromide Quarzan **Adjunctive therapy for peptic ulcers:** Dosage should be individualized according to severity of symptoms and occurrence of side effects. ADULTS: 2.5 to 5 mg P.O. t.i.d. or q.i.d. before meals and at bedtime. GERIATRIC OR DEBILITATED PATIENTS: 2.5 mg P.O. t.i.d. before meals.	**CNS:** headache, insomnia, drowsiness, dizziness, *confusion or excitement in elderly patients,* nervousness, weakness. **CV:** *palpitations,* tachycardia. **EENT:** *blurred vision,* mydriasis, increased ocular tension, cycloplegia, photophobia. **GI:** *dry mouth,* dysphagia, heartburn, loss of taste, nausea, vomiting, *paralytic ileus, constipation.* **GU:** *urinary hesitancy and retention,* impotence. **Skin:** urticaria, decreased sweating or anhidrosis, other dermal manifestations. **Other:** fever, allergic reactions. Overdosage may cause curare-like symptoms.
dicyclomine hydrochloride Antispas, Bentyl, Bentylol♦♦, Cyclobec♦♦, Dibent, Dicen, Formulex♦♦, Menospasm♦♦, Nospaz, Or-Tyl, Rocyclo, Rotyl HCl, Stannitol, Viscerol♦♦ **Adjunctive therapy for peptic ulcers and other functional gastrointestinal disorders:** ADULTS: 10 to 20 mg P.O. t.i.d. or q.i.d.; 20 mg I.M. q 4 to 6 hours. CHILDREN: 10 mg P.O. t.i.d. or q.i.d. **Infant colic:** INFANTS: 5 mg P.O. t.i.d. or q.i.d. Always adjust dosage according to patient's needs and response.	**CNS:** *headache,* insomnia, drowsiness, *dizziness.* **CV:** *palpitations,* tachycardia. **GI:** nausea, *constipation,* vomiting, *paralytic ileus.* **GU:** urinary hesitancy and retention, impotence. **Skin:** urticaria, decreased sweating or anhidrosis, other dermal manifestations. **Other:** fever, allergic reactions. Overdosage may cause curare-like symptoms.
diphemanil methylsulfate Prantal **Adjunctive therapy in gastric hypersecretion associated with duodenal ulcer:** ADULTS: 100 to 200 mg P.O. q 4 to 6 hours, between meals (initial dose). Daily dosage should be adjusted according to response and tolerance. Maintenance dose: 50 to 100 mg q 4 to 6 hours.	**CNS:** headache, insomnia, drowsiness, dizziness, *confusion or excitement in elderly patients,* nervousness, weakness. **CV:** *palpitations,* tachycardia. **EENT:** *blurred vision,* mydriasis, increased ocular tension, cycloplegia, photophobia. **GI:** *dry mouth,* dysphagia, *constipation,* heartburn, loss of taste, nausea, vomiting, *paralytic ileus.* **GU:** *urinary hesitancy and retention,* impotence. **Skin:** urticaria, decreased sweating or anhidrosis, other dermal manifestations. **Other:** fever, allergic reactions. Overdosage may cause curare-like symptoms.

INTERACTIONS AND SPECIAL CONSIDERATIONS

vironments. Drug-induced heatstroke can develop.
• Patient's vital signs and urinary output should be monitored carefully.
• Patient should avoid driving and other hazardous activities if he is drowsy, dizzy, or has blurred vision; drink plenty of fluids to help prevent constipation; report any skin rash.
• Sugarless gum or hard candy may relieve mouth dryness.
• For symptoms and treatment of toxicity, see APPENDIX.

No significant interactions.

Special considerations:
• Contraindicated in narrow-angle glaucoma, obstructive uropathy, obstructive disease of GI tract, severe ulcerative colitis, myasthenia gravis, hypersensitivity to anticholinergics, paralytic ileus, intestinal atony, unstable cardiovascular status in acute hemorrhage, and toxic megacolon. Use cautiously in autonomic neuropathy, hyperthyroidism, coronary artery disease, cardiac arrhythmias, congestive heart failure, hypertension, hiatal hernia associated with reflux esophagitis, hepatic or renal disease, ulcerative colitis, or in patients over 40 years because of increased incidence of glaucoma.
• Should be taken 30 minutes to 1 hour before meals and at bedtime. Bedtime dose can be larger and should be taken at least 2 hours after last meal of day.
• Smaller doses are required for the elderly.
• Hot or humid environments require cautious use. Drug-induced heatstroke may develop.
• Patient's vital signs and urinary output should be monitored carefully.
• Patient should avoid driving and other hazardous activities if he is drowsy, dizzy, or has blurred vision; drink plenty of fluids to help prevent constipation; and report any skin rash or local eruption.
• Sugarless gum or hard candy may relieve mouth dryness.
• For symptoms and treatment of toxicity, see APPENDIX.

No significant interactions.

Special considerations:
• Contraindicated in obstructive uropathy, obstructive disease of GI tract, severe ulcerative colitis, myasthenia gravis, hypersensitivity to anticholinergics, paralytic ileus, intestinal atony, unstable cardiovascular status in acute hemorrhage, and toxic megacolon. Use cautiously in autonomic neuropathy, narrow-angle glaucoma, hyperthyroidism, coronary artery disease, cardiac arrhythmias, congestive heart failure, hypertension, hiatal hernia associated with reflux esophagitis, hepatic or renal disease, ulcerative colitis.
• Hot or humid environments require cautious use. Drug-induced heatstroke can develop.
• Should be taken 30 minutes to 1 hour before meals and at bedtime. Bedtime dose can be larger and should be taken at least 2 hours after last meal of day.
• Smaller doses are required for the elderly.
• Patient's vital signs and urinary output should be monitored carefully.
• Patient should avoid driving and other hazardous activities if he is drowsy, dizzy, or has blurred vision; drink plenty of fluids to help prevent constipation; and report any skin rash.
• Sugarless gum or hard candy may relieve mouth dryness.
• A synthetic tertiary derivative that is relatively free of atropine-like side effects.
• For symptoms and treatment of toxicity, see APPENDIX.

No significant interactions.

Special considerations:
• Contraindicated in narrow-angle glaucoma, obstructive uropathy, obstructive disease of GI tract, severe ulcerative colitis, myasthenia gravis, hypersensitivity to the anticholinergics, paralytic ileus, intestinal atony, unstable cardiovascular status in acute hemorrhage, and toxic megacolon. Use cautiously in autonomic neuropathy, hyperthyroidism, coronary artery disease, cardiac arrhythmias, congestive heart failure, hypertension, hiatal hernia associated with reflux esophagitis, hepatic or renal disease, ulcerative colitis, or in patients over 40 years because of increased incidence of glaucoma.
• Hot or humid environments require cautious use. Drug-induced heatstroke can develop.
• Should be taken 30 minutes to 1 hour before meals and at bedtime. Bedtime dose can be larger and should be taken at least 2 hours after last meal of day.
• Smaller doses are required for the elderly.
• Patient's vital signs and urinary output should be monitored carefully.
• Patient should avoid driving and other hazardous activities if he is drowsy, dizzy, or has blurred vision; drink plenty of fluids to help prevent constipation; and report any skin rash.
• Sugarless gum or hard candy may relieve mouth dryness.
• For symptoms and treatment of toxicity, see APPENDIX.

NAMES, INDICATIONS AND DOSAGES	SIDE EFFECTS
glycopyrrolate Robinul♦, Robinul Forte♦ **Adjunctive therapy in peptic ulcers and other gastrointestinal disorders:** ADULTS: 1 to 2 mg P.O. t.i.d. or 0.1 mg I.M. t.i.d. or q.i.d. Dosage should be individualized.	**CNS:** headache, insomnia, drowsiness, dizziness, *confusion or excitement in elderly patients,* nervousness, weakness. **CV:** *palpitations,* tachycardia. **EENT:** *blurred vision,* mydriasis, increased ocular tension, cycloplegia, photophobia. **GI:** *dry mouth,* dysphagia, *constipation,* heartburn, loss of taste, nausea, vomiting, *paralytic ileus.* **GU:** *urinary hesitancy and retention,* impotence. **Skin:** urticaria, decreased sweating or anhidrosis, other dermal manifestations. **Other:** fever, allergic reactions. Overdosage may cause curare-like symptoms.
hexocyclium methylsulfate Tral **Adjunctive therapy in peptic ulcer and other gastrointestinal disorders:** ADULTS: 25 mg q.i.d. before meals and h.s.	**CNS:** headache, insomnia, drowsiness, dizziness, *confusion or excitement in elderly patients,* nervousness, weakness. **CV:** *palpitations,* tachycardia. **EENT:** *blurred vision,* mydriasis, increased ocular tension, cycloplegia, photophobia. **GI:** *dry mouth,* dysphagia, heartburn, loss of taste, nausea, *constipation,* vomiting, *paralytic ileus.* **GU:** *urinary hesitancy and retention,* impotence. **Skin:** urticaria, decreased sweating or anhidrosis, other dermal manifestations. **Other:** fever, allergic reactions. Overdosage may cause curare-like symptoms.
homatropine methylbromide Ru-Spas No. 2 **Treatment of gastrointestinal spasm, hyperchlorhydria, and other mild spastic conditions of the bile ducts and gallbladder:** ADULTS: 2.5 to 5 mg t.i.d. to q.i.d. before meals and h.s.	**CNS:** headache, insomnia, drowsiness, dizziness, *confusion or excitement in elderly patients,* nervousness, weakness. **CV:** *palpitations,* tachycardia. **EENT:** *blurred vision,* mydriasis, increased ocular tension, cycloplegia, photophobia. **GI:** *dry mouth,* dysphagia, *constipation,* heartburn, loss of taste, nausea, vomiting, *paralytic ileus.* **GU:** *urinary hesitancy and retention,* impotence. **Skin:** urticaria, decreased sweating or anhidrosis, other dermal manifestations. **Other:** fever, allergic reactions. Overdosage may cause curare-like symptoms.
isopropamide iodide Darbid♦ **Adjunctive therapy for peptic ulcer, irritable bowel syndrome:** ADULTS AND CHILDREN OVER 12 YEARS: 5 mg P.O. q 12 hours. Some patients may require	**CNS:** headache, insomnia, drowsiness, dizziness, *confusion or excitement in elderly patients,* nervousness, weakness. **CV:** *palpitations,* tachycardia. **EENT:** *blurred vision,* mydriasis, increased ocular tension, cycloplegia, photophobia. **GI:** *dry mouth,* dysphagia, heartburn, loss of

INTERACTIONS AND SPECIAL CONSIDERATIONS

No significant interactions.

Special considerations:

• Contraindicated in narrow-angle glaucoma, obstructive uropathy, obstructive disease of GI tract, severe ulcerative colitis, myasthenia gravis, hypersensitivity to anticholinergics, paralytic ileus, intestinal atony, unstable cardiovascular status in acute hemorrhage, and toxic megacolon. Use cautiously in autonomic neuropathy, hyperthyroidism, coronary artery disease, cardiac arrhythmias, congestive heart failure, hypertension, hiatal hernia associated with reflux esophagitis, hepatic or renal disease, ulcerative colitis, or in patients over 40 years because of increased incidence of glaucoma.
• Hot or humid environments require cautious use. Drug-induced heatstroke can develop.
• Should be taken 30 minutes to 1 hour before meals.
• Smaller doses are required for the elderly.
• Patient's vital signs and urinary output should be monitored carefully.
• Patient should avoid driving and other hazardous activities if he is drowsy, dizzy, or has blurred vision; drink plenty of fluids to help prevent constipation; report any skin rash.
• Sugarless gum or hard candy may relieve mouth dryness.
• For symptoms and treatment of toxicity, see APPENDIX.

No significant interactions.

Special considerations:

• Contraindicated in narrow-angle glaucoma, obstructive uropathy, obstructive disease of GI tract, severe ulcerative colitis, myasthenia gravis, hypersensitivity to anticholinergics, paralytic ileus, intestinal atony, unstable cardiovascular status in acute hemorrhage, toxic megacolon. Use cautiously in autonomic neuropathy, hyperthyroidism, coronary artery disease, cardiac arrhythmias, congestive heart failure, hypertension, hiatal hernia associated with reflux esophagitis, hepatic or renal disease, ulcerative colitis, or in patients over 40 years because of increased incidence of glaucoma.
• Hot or humid environments require cautious use. Drug-induced heatstroke can develop.
• Should be taken 30 minutes to 1 hour before meals and at bedtime. Bedtime dose can be larger and should be taken at least 2 hours after last meal of day.
• Smaller doses are required for the elderly.
• Patient's vital signs and urinary output should be monitored carefully.
• Patient should avoid driving and other hazardous activities if he is drowsy, dizzy, or has blurred vision; drink plenty of fluids to help prevent constipation; and report any skin rash.
• Sugarless gum or hard candy may relieve mouth dryness.
• Tablets contain tartrazine dye. May cause allergy in susceptible patients.
• For symptoms and treatment of toxicity, see APPENDIX.

No significant interactions.

Special considerations:

• Contraindicated in narrow-angle glaucoma, obstructive uropathy, obstructive disease of GI tract, severe ulcerative colitis, myasthenia gravis, hypersensitivity to anticholinergics, paralytic ileus, intestinal atony, unstable cardiovascular status in acute hemorrhage, and toxic megacolon. Use cautiously in autonomic neuropathy, hyperthyroidism, coronary artery disease, cardiac arrhythmias, congestive heart failure, hypertension, hiatal hernia associated with reflux esophagitis, hepatic or renal disease, ulcerative colitis, or in patients over 40 years because of increased incidence of glaucoma.
• Hot or humid environments require cautious use. Drug-induced heatstroke can develop.
• Should be taken 30 minutes to 1 hour before meals and at bedtime. Bedtime dose can be larger and should be taken at least 2 hours after the last meal of the day.
• Smaller doses are required for the elderly.
• Patient's vital signs and urinary output should be monitored carefully.
• Patient should avoid driving and other hazardous activities if he is drowsy, dizzy, or has blurred vision; drink plenty of fluids to help prevent constipation; and report any skin rash.
• Sugarless gum or hard candy may relieve mouth dryness.
• For symptoms and treatment of toxicity, see APPENDIX.

No significant interactions.

Special considerations:

• Contraindicated in narrow-angle glaucoma, obstructive uropathy, obstructive disease of GI tract, severe ulcerative colitis, myasthenia gravis, hypersensitivity to anticholinergics, paralytic ileus, intestinal atony, unstable cardiovascular status in acute hemorrhage, toxic megacolon. Use cautiously in autonomic neuropathy, hyperthyroidism, coronary artery disease, cardiac arrhythmias, congestive heart failure, hypertension, hiatal hernia associated with reflux esophagitis, hepatic or renal disease, ulcerative colitis, or in patients over 40 years because of increased incidence of glaucoma.

(continued on following page)

NAMES, INDICATIONS AND DOSAGES	SIDE EFFECTS
isopropamide iodide *(continued)* 10 mg or more b.i.d. Dose should be individualized to patient's need.	taste, nausea, vomiting, *constipation, paralytic ileus.* **GU:** *urinary hesitancy and retention,* impotence. **Skin:** urticaria, decreased sweating or anhidrosis, other dermal manifestations, iodine skin rash. **Other:** fever, allergic reactions. Overdosage may cause curare-like symptoms.
levorotatory alkaloids of belladonna (as maleate salts) Bellafoline **Adjunctive therapy for peptic ulcer, irritable bowel syndrome, and functional gastrointestinal disorders:** ADULTS: 0.25 to 0.5 mg P.O. t.i.d.; or 0.125 to 0.5 mg S.C. daily or b.i.d. CHILDREN OVER 6 YEARS: 0.125 to 0.25 mg P.O. t.i.d.	**CNS:** headache, insomnia, drowsiness, dizziness, *confusion or excitement in elderly patients,* nervousness, weakness. **CV:** *palpitations,* tachycardia. **EENT:** *blurred vision,* mydriasis, increased ocular tension, cycloplegia, photophobia. **GI:** *dry mouth,* dysphagia, heartburn, loss of taste, *constipation, paralytic ileus.* **GU:** *urinary hesitancy and retention,* impotence. **Skin:** urticaria, decreased sweating or anhidrosis, other dermal manifestations. **Other:** fever, allergic reactions. Overdosage may cause curare-like symptoms.
l-hyoscyamine sulfate Anaspaz, Levsinex, Levsinex Time Caps **Treatment of gastrointestinal tract disorders due to spasm; adjunctive therapy for peptic ulcers:** ADULTS: 0.125 to 0.25 mg P.O. t.i.d. or q.i.d. before meals and at bedtime; sustained-release form 0.375 mg P.O. q 12 hours; or 0.25 to 0.5 mg (1 or 2 ml) I.M., I.V., or S.C. q 6 hours. (Substitute oral medication when symptoms are controlled.) CHILDREN 2 TO 10 YEARS: ½ adult dose P.O. CHILDREN UNDER 2 YEARS: ¼ adult dose P.O.	**CNS:** headache, insomnia, drowsiness, dizziness, *confusion or excitement in elderly patients,* nervousness, weakness. **CV:** *palpitations,* tachycardia. **EENT:** *blurred vision,* mydriasis, increased ocular tension, cycloplegia, photophobia. **GI:** *dry mouth,* dysphagia, *constipation,* heartburn, loss of taste, nausea, vomiting, *paralytic ileus.* **GU:** *urinary hesitancy and retention,* impotence. **Skin:** urticaria, decreased sweating or anhidrosis, other dermal manifestations. **Other:** fever, allergic reactions. Overdosage may cause curare-like symptoms.
mepenzolate bromide Cantil **Adjunctive therapy in treating peptic ulcer, irritable bowel syndrome, and neurologic bowel disturbances:** ADULTS: 25 to 50 mg P.O. q.i.d. with meals and at bedtime. Adjust dosage to individual patient's needs.	**CNS:** headache, insomnia, drowsiness, dizziness, *confusion or excitement in elderly patients,* nervousness, weakness. **CV:** *palpitations,* tachycardia. **EENT:** *blurred vision,* mydriasis, increased ocular tension, cycloplegia, photophobia. **GI:** *dry mouth,* dysphagia, heartburn, loss of taste, nausea, *constipation,* vomiting, *paralytic ileus.* **GU:** *urinary hesitancy and retention,* impotence. **Skin:** urticaria, decreased sweating or anhidrosis, other dermal manifestations. **Other:** fever, allergic reactions. Overdosage may cause curare-like symptoms.

INTERACTIONS AND SPECIAL CONSIDERATIONS

• Hot or humid environments require cautious use. Drug-induced heatstroke can develop.
• Should be taken 30 minutes to 1 hour before meals and at bedtime. Bedtime dose can be larger and should be taken at least 2 hours after the last meal of the day.
• Smaller doses are required for the elderly.
• Patient's vital signs and urinary output should be monitored carefully.
• Patient should avoid driving and other hazardous activities if he is drowsy, dizzy, or has blurred vision; drink plenty of fluids to help prevent constipation; and report any skin rash.
• Sugarless gum or hard candy may relieve mouth dryness.
• Single dose produces 10- to 12-hour antisecretory effect and gastrointestinal antispasmodic effect.
• Patient should discontinue 1 week before thyroid function studies.
• For symptoms and treatment of toxicity, see APPENDIX.

No significant interactions.

Special considerations:
• Contraindicated in narrow-angle glaucoma, obstructive uropathy, obstructive disease of GI tract, severe ulcerative colitis, myasthenia gravis, hypersensitivity to anticholinergics, paralytic ileus, intestinal atony, unstable cardiovascular status in acute hemorrhage, and toxic megacolon. Use cautiously in autonomic neuropathy, hyperthyroidism, coronary artery disease, cardiac arrhythmias, congestive heart failure, hypertension, hiatal hernia associated with reflux esophagitis, hepatic or renal disease, ulcerative colitis, or in patients over 40 years because of increased incidence of glaucoma.
• Hot or humid environments require cautious use. Drug-induced heatstroke can develop.
• Should be administered 30 minutes to 1 hour before meals.
• Smaller doses are required for the elderly.
• Patient's vital signs and urinary output should be monitored carefully.
• Patient should avoid driving and other hazardous activities if he is drowsy, dizzy, or has blurred vision; drink plenty of fluids to help prevent constipation; report any skin rash.
• Sugarless gum or sugarless hard candy may relieve mouth dryness.
• For symptoms and treatment of toxicity, see APPENDIX.

No significant interactions.

Special considerations:
• Contraindicated in narrow-angle glaucoma, obstructive uropathy, obstructive disease of GI tract, severe ulcerative colitis, myasthenia gravis, hypersensitivity to anticholinergics, paralytic ileus, intestinal atony, unstable cardiovascular status in acute hemorrhage, toxic megacolon. Use cautiously in autonomic neuropathy, hyperthyroidism, coronary artery disease, cardiac arrhythmias, congestive heart failure, hypertension, hiatal hernia associated with reflux esophagitis, hepatic or renal disease, ulcerative colitis, or in patients over 40 years because of the increased incidence of glaucoma.
• Hot or humid environments require cautious use. Drug-induced heatstroke can develop.
• Should be taken 30 minutes to 1 hour before meals and at bedtime. Bedtime dose can be larger and should be taken at least 2 hours after the last meal of the day.
• Smaller doses are required for the elderly.
• Patient's vital signs and urinary output should be monitored carefully.
• Patient should avoid driving and other hazardous activities if he is drowsy, dizzy, or has blurred vision; drink plenty of fluids to help prevent constipation; and report any skin rash.
• Sugarless gum or hard candy may relieve mouth dryness.
• For symptoms and treatment of toxicity, see APPENDIX.

No significant interactions.

Special considerations:
• Contraindicated in narrow-angle glaucoma, obstructive uropathy, obstructive disease of GI tract, severe ulcerative colitis, myasthenia gravis, hypersensitivity to anticholinergics, paralytic ileus, intestinal atony, unstable cardiovascular status in acute hemorrhage, toxic megacolon. Use cautiously in autonomic neuropathy, hyperthyroidism, coronary artery disease, cardiac arrhythmias, congestive heart failure, hypertension, hiatal hernia associated with reflux esophagitis, hepatic or renal disease, ulcerative colitis, or in those over 40 due to increased glaucoma.
• Hot or humid environments require cautious use. Drug-induced heatstroke can develop.
• Should be taken with meals and at bedtime.
• Smaller doses are required for the elderly.
• Patient's vital signs and urinary output should be monitored carefully.
• Patient should avoid driving and other hazardous activities if he is drowsy, dizzy, or has blurred vision; drink plenty of fluids to help prevent constipation; and report any skin rash.
• Sugarless gum or hard candy may relieve mouth dryness.
• For symptoms and treatment of toxicity, see APPENDIX.

NAMES, INDICATIONS AND DOSAGES	SIDE EFFECTS
methantheline bromide Banthine **Adjunctive therapy in peptic ulcer, pylorospasm, spastic colon, biliary dyskinesia, pancreatitis, and certain forms of gastritis:** ADULTS: 50 to 100 mg P.O. q 6 hours. CHILDREN OVER 1 YEAR: 12.5 to 50 mg q.i.d. CHILDREN UNDER 1 YEAR: 12.5 to 25 mg q.i.d.	**CNS:** headache, insomnia, drowsiness, dizziness, *confusion or excitement in elderly patients,* nervousness, weakness. **CV:** *palpitations,* tachycardia. **EENT:** *blurred vision,* mydriasis, increased ocular tension, cycloplegia, photophobia. **GI:** *dry mouth,* dysphagia, *constipation,* heartburn, loss of taste, nausea, vomiting, *paralytic ileus.* **GU:** *urinary hesitancy and retention,* impotence. **Skin:** urticaria, decreased sweating or anhidrosis, other dermal manifestations. **Other:** fever, allergic reactions. Overdosage may cause curare-like symptoms.
methixene hydrochloride Trest♦ **Adjunctive treatment of gastrointestinal disorders associated with hypermotility or spasm:** ADULTS: 1 or 2 mg P.O. t.i.d.	**CNS:** *headache,* insomnia, drowsiness, *dizziness.* **CV:** *palpitations,* tachycardia. **EENT:** *blurred vision,* mydriasis, increased ocular tension, cycloplegia, photophobia. **GI:** *constipation,* nausea, vomiting, *paralytic ileus.* **GU:** urinary hesitancy and retention, impotence. **Skin:** urticaria, decreased sweating or anhidrosis, other dermal manifestations. **Other:** fever, allergic reactions. Overdosage may cause curare-like symptoms.
methscopolamine bromide Pamine♦, Scoline **Adjunctive therapy in peptic ulcer:** ADULTS: 2.5 to 5 mg ½ hour before meals and h.s.	**CNS:** headache, insomnia, dizziness, *confusion or excitement in elderly patients,* nervousness, weakness. **CV:** *palpitations,* tachycardia. **EENT:** *blurred vision,* mydriasis, increased ocular tension, cycloplegia, photophobia. **GI:** *dry mouth,* dysphagia, *constipation,* heartburn, loss of taste, nausea, vomiting, *paralytic ileus.* **GU:** *urinary hesitancy and retention,* impotence. **Skin:** urticaria, decreased sweating or anhidrosis, other dermal manifestations. **Other:** fever, allergic reactions. Overdosage may cause curare-like symptoms.

♦ Available in U.S. and Canada. ♦♦ Available in Canada only.
All other products (no symbol) available in U.S. only. Italicized side effects are common or life-threatening.

INTERACTIONS AND SPECIAL CONSIDERATIONS

No significant interactions.

Special considerations:
• Contraindicated in narrow-angle glaucoma, obstructive uropathy, obstructive disease of GI tract, severe ulcerative colitis, myasthenia gravis, hypersensitivity to anticholinergics, paralytic ileus, intestinal atony, unstable cardiovascular status in acute hemorrhage, toxic megacolon. Use cautiously in autonomic neuropathy, hyperthyroidism, coronary artery disease, cardiac arrhythmias, congestive heart failure, hypertension, hiatal hernia associated with reflux esophagitis, hepatic or renal disease, ulcerative colitis, or in patients over 40 years because of the increased incidence of glaucoma.
• Hot or humid environments require cautious use. Drug-induced heatstroke can develop.
• Should be given 30 minutes to 1 hour before meals and at bedtime. Bedtime dose can be larger and should be given at least 2 hours after the last meal of the day.
• Smaller doses are required for the elderly.
• Patient also taking antihistamines may experience increased mouth dryness.
• Patient's vital signs and urinary output should be monitored carefully.
• Patient should avoid driving and other hazardous activities if he is drowsy, dizzy, or has blurred vision; drink plenty of fluids to help prevent constipation; and report any skin rash.
• Sugarless gum or hard candy may relieve mouth dryness.
• Therapeutic effects appear in 30 to 45 minutes; persist for 4 to 6 hours after oral administration.
• For symptoms and treatment of toxicity, see APPENDIX.

No significant interactions.

Special considerations:
• Contraindicated in narrow-angle glaucoma, obstructive uropathy, obstructive disease of the GI tract, severe ulcerative colitis, myasthenia gravis, hypersensitivity to anticholinergics, paralytic ileus, intestinal atony, unstable cardiovascular status in acute hemorrhage, and toxic megacolon. Use cautiously in autonomic neuropathy, hyperthyroidism, coronary artery disease, cardiac arrhythmias, congestive heart failure, hypertension, hiatal hernia associated with reflux esophagitis, hepatic or renal disease, ulcerative colitis, or in patients over 40 years because of the increased incidence of glaucoma.
• Hot or humid environments require cautious use. Drug-induced heatstroke can develop.
• Should be taken 30 minutes to 1 hour before meals.
• Smaller doses are required for the elderly.
• Patient's vital signs and urinary output should be monitored carefully.
• Patient should avoid driving and other hazardous activities if he is drowsy, dizzy, or has blurred vision; drink plenty of fluids to help prevent constipation; and report any skin rash.
• Sugarless gum or hard candy may relieve mouth dryness.
• Synthetic tertiary derivative that is relatively free of atropine-like side effect.
• For symptoms and treatment of toxicity, see APPENDIX.

No significant interactions.

Special considerations:
• Contraindicated in narrow-angle glaucoma, obstructive uropathy, obstructive disease of GI tract, severe ulcerative colitis, myasthenia gravis, hypersensitivity to anticholinergics, paralytic ileus, intestinal atony, unstable cardiovascular status in acute hemorrhage, toxic megacolon. Use cautiously in autonomic neuropathy, hyperthyroidism, coronary artery disease, cardiac arrhythmias, congestive heart failure, hypertension, hiatal hernia associated with reflux esophagitis, hepatic or renal disease, ulcerative colitis, or in patients over 40 years because of increased incidence of glaucoma.
• Hot or humid environments require cautious use. Drug-induced heatstroke can develop.
• Should be taken 30 minutes to 1 hour before meals and at bedtime. Bedtime dose can be larger and should be taken at least 2 hours after the last meal of the day.
• Smaller doses are required for the elderly.
• Patient's vital signs and urinary output should be monitored carefully.
• Patient should avoid driving and other hazardous activities if he is drowsy, dizzy, or has blurred vision; drink plenty of fluids to help prevent constipation; and report any skin rash.
• Sugarless gum or hard candy may relieve mouth dryness.
• For symptoms and treatment of toxicity, see APPENDIX.

NAMES, INDICATIONS AND DOSAGES	SIDE EFFECTS
oxyphencyclimine hydrochloride Daricon♦ **Adjunctive treatment of peptic ulcer:** ADULTS: 10 mg b.i.d. in the morning and h.s., or 5 mg b.i.d. or t.i.d.	**CNS:** *headache,* insomnia, drowsiness, *dizziness.* **CV:** *palpitations,* tachycardia. **EENT:** *blurred vision,* mydriasis, increased ocular tension, cycloplegia, photophobia. **GI:** *constipation,* nausea, vomiting, *paralytic ileus.* **GU:** urinary hesitancy and retention, impotence. **Skin:** urticaria, decreased sweating or anhidrosis, other dermal manifestations. **Other:** fever, allergic reactions. Overdosage may cause curare-like symptoms.
oxyphenonium bromide Antrenyl **Adjunctive treatment of peptic ulcer:** ADULTS: 10 mg P.O. q.i.d. for several days, then reduced according to patient response.	**CNS:** headache, insomnia, drowsiness, dizziness, *confusion or excitement in elderly patients,* nervousness, weakness. **CV:** *palpitations,* tachycardia. **EENT:** *blurred vision,* mydriasis, increased ocular tension, cycloplegia, photophobia. **GI:** *dry mouth,* dysphagia, *constipation,* heartburn, loss of taste, nausea, vomiting, *paralytic ileus.* **GU:** *urinary hesitancy and retention,* impotence. **Skin:** urticaria, decreased sweating or anhidrosis, other dermal manifestations. **Other:** fever, allergic reactions. Overdosage may cause curare-like symptoms.
propantheline bromide Banlin♦♦, Norpanth, Pro-Banthine♦, Propanthel♦♦, Robantaline, Ropanth, SK-Propantheline Bromide **Adjunctive treatment of peptic ulcer and irritable bowel syndrome, and other gastrointestinal disorders:** ADULTS: 15 mg P.O. t.i.d. before meals, and 30 mg at bedtime up to 60 mg q.i.d. For elderly patients, 7.5 mg P.O. t.i.d. before meals. When oral dosage not possible, 30 mg I.M. or I.V. q 6 hours, depending on individual response. Maintenance dose 15 mg I.M. q 6 hours.	**CNS:** headache, insomnia, drowsiness, dizziness, *confusion or excitement in elderly patients,* nervousness, weakness. **CV:** *palpitations,* tachycardia. **EENT:** *blurred vision,* mydriasis, increased ocular tension, cycloplegia, photophobia. **GI:** *dry mouth,* dysphagia, constipation, heartburn, loss of taste, nausea, vomiting, paralytic ileus. **GU:** *urinary hesitancy and retention,* impotence. **Skin:** urticaria, decreased sweating or anhidrosis, other dermal manifestations. **Other:** fever, allergic reactions. Overdosage may cause curare-like symptoms.

♦ Available in U.S. and Canada. ♦♦ Available in Canada only.
All other products (no symbol) available in U.S. only. Italicized side effects are common or life-threatening.

INTERACTIONS AND SPECIAL CONSIDERATIONS

No significant interactions.

Special considerations:

- Contraindicated in narrow-angle glaucoma, obstructive uropathy, obstructive disease of GI tract, severe ulcerative colitis, myasthenia gravis, hypersensitivity to anticholinergics, paralytic ileus, intestinal atony, unstable cardiovascular status in acute hemorrhage, toxic megacolon. Use cautiously in autonomic neuropathy, hyperthyroidism, coronary artery disease, cardiac arrhythmias, congestive heart failure, hypertension, hiatal hernia associated with reflux esophagitis, hepatic or renal disease, ulcerative colitis, or in patients over 40 years because of increased incidence of glaucoma.
- Hot or humid environments require cautious use. Drug-induced heatstroke can develop.
- Should be taken 30 minutes to 1 hour before breakfast and at bedtime.
- Smaller doses are required for the elderly.
- Patient's vital signs and urinary output should be monitored carefully.
- Patient should avoid driving and other hazardous activities if he is drowsy, dizzy, or has blurred vision; drink plenty of fluids to help prevent constipation; and report any skin rash.
- Sugarless gum or hard candy may relieve mouth dryness.
- Synthetic tertiary derivative that is relatively free of atropine-like side effects.
- For symptoms and treatment of toxicity, see APPENDIX.

No significant interactions.

Special considerations:

- Contraindicated in narrow-angle glaucoma, obstructive uropathy, obstructive disease of GI tract, severe ulcerative colitis, myasthenia gravis, hypersensitivity to anticholinergics, paralytic ileus, intestinal atony, unstable cardiovascular status in acute hemorrhage, toxic megacolon. Use cautiously in autonomic neuropathy, hyperthyroidism, coronary artery disease, cardiac arrhythmias, congestive heart failure, hypertension, hiatal hernia associated with reflux esophagitis, hepatic or renal disease, ulcerative colitis, or in patients over 40 years because of increased incidence of glaucoma.
- Hot or humid environments require cautious use. Drug-induced heatstroke can develop.
- Should be taken 30 minutes to 1 hour before meals and at bedtime. Bedtime dose can be larger and should be taken at least 2 hours after the last meal of the day.
- Smaller doses are required for the elderly.
- Patient's vital signs and urinary output should be monitored.
- Patient should avoid driving and other hazardous activities if he is drowsy, dizzy, or has blurred vision; drink plenty of fluids to help prevent constipation; and report any skin rash.
- Sugarless gum or hard candy may relieve mouth dryness.
- For symptoms and treatment of toxicity, see APPENDIX.

No significant interactions.

Special considerations:

- Contraindicated in narrow-angle glaucoma, obstructive uropathy, obstructive disease of GI tract, severe ulcerative colitis, myasthenia gravis, hypersensitivity to anticholinergics, paralytic ileus, intestinal atony, unstable cardiovascular status in acute hemorrhage, toxic megacolon. Use cautiously in autonomic neuropathy, hyperthyroidism, coronary artery disease, cardiac arrhythmias, congestive heart failure, hypertension, hiatal hernia associated with reflux esophagitis, hepatic or renal disease, ulcerative colitis, or in patients over 40 years because of the increased incidence of glaucoma.
- Hot or humid environments require cautious use. Drug-induced heatstroke can develop.
- Should be given 30 minutes to 1 hour before meals and at bedtime. Bedtime dose can be larger and should be given at least 2 hours after the last meal of the day.
- Smaller doses are required for the elderly.
- Patient's vital signs and urinary output should be monitored carefully.
- Patient should avoid driving and other hazardous activities if he is drowsy, dizzy, or has blurred vision; drink plenty of fluids to help prevent constipation; and report any skin rash.
- Sugarless gum or hard candy may relieve mouth dryness.
- For symptoms and treatment of toxicity, see APPENDIX.

NAMES, INDICATIONS AND DOSAGES	SIDE EFFECTS
thiphenamil hydrochloride Trocinate **Hypermotility and spasm of the gastrointestinal tract:** ADULTS: initially, 400 mg P.O. repeated in 4 hours, usually to maximum of 4 doses. Maintenance dose may be given at a reduced frequency of dosage.	**CNS:** headache, insomnia, drowsiness, dizziness, *confusion or excitement in elderly patients,* nervousness, weakness. **CV:** *palpitations,* tachycardia. **EENT:** *blurred vision,* mydriasis, increased ocular tension, cycloplegia, photophobia. **GI:** *dry mouth,* dysphagia, *constipation,* heartburn, loss of taste, nausea, vomiting, *paralytic ileus.* **GU:** *urinary hesitancy and retention,* impotence. **Skin:** urticaria, decreased sweating or anhidrosis, other dermal manifestations. **Other:** fever, allergic reactions. Overdosage may cause curare-like symptoms.
tridihexethyl chloride Pathilon **Adjunctive treatment of peptic ulcer, irritable bowel syndrome, and other gastrointestinal disorders:** ADULTS: initially, 25 to 50 mg P.O. t.i.d. before meals, and 50 mg h.s., increased to 75 mg q.i.d., if needed. With sustained-release capsules, 75 mg q 12 or q 6 hours. Maintenance dose usually half the therapeutic dose. Parenteral use: 10 to 20 mg I.V., I.M., or S.C. q 6 hours. Change to oral as soon as possible.	**CNS:** headache, insomnia, drowsiness, dizziness, *confusion or excitement in elderly patients,* nervousness, weakness. **CV:** *palpitations,* tachycardia. **EENT:** *blurred vision,* mydriasis, increased ocular tension, cycloplegia, photophobia. **GI:** *dry mouth,* dysphagia, *constipation,* heartburn, loss of taste, nausea, vomiting, *paralytic ileus.* **GU:** *urinary hesitancy and retention,* impotence. **Skin:** urticaria, decreased sweating or anhidrosis, other dermal manifestations. **Other:** fever, allergic reactions. Overdosage may cause curare-like symptoms.

INTERACTIONS AND SPECIAL CONSIDERATIONS

No significant interactions.

Special considerations:

- Contraindicated in narrow-angle glaucoma, obstructive uropathy, obstructive disease of GI tract, severe ulcerative colitis, myasthenia gravis, hypersensitivity to anticholinergics, paralytic ileus, intestinal atony, unstable cardiovascular status in acute hemorrhage, toxic megacolon. Use cautiously in autonomic neuropathy, hyperthyroidism, coronary artery disease, cardiac arrhythmias, congestive heart failure, hypertension, hiatal hernia associated with reflux esophagitis, hepatic or renal disease, ulcerative colitis, or in patients over 40 years because of increased incidence of glaucoma.
- Hot or humid environments require cautious use. Drug-induced heatstroke can develop.
- Smaller doses are required for the elderly.
- Patient's vital signs and urinary output should be monitored carefully.
- Patient should avoid driving and other hazardous activities if he is drowsy, dizzy, or has blurred vision; drink plenty of fluids to help prevent constipation; and report any skin rash.
- Sugarless gum or hard candy may relieve mouth dryness.
- For symptoms and treatment of toxicity, see APPENDIX.

No significant interactions.

Special considerations:

- Contraindicated in narrow-angle glaucoma, obstructive uropathy, obstructive disease of GI tract, severe ulcerative colitis, myasthenia gravis, hypersensitivity to anticholinergics, paralytic ileus, intestinal atony, unstable cardiovascular status in acute hemorrhage, toxic megacolon. Use cautiously in autonomic neuropathy, hyperthyroidism, coronary artery disease, cardiac arrhythmias, congestive heart failure, hypertension, hiatal hernia associated with reflux esophagitis, hepatic or renal disease, ulcerative colitis, or in patients over 40 years because of increased incidence of glaucoma.
- Hot or humid environments require cautious use. Drug-induced heatstroke can develop.
- Should be given 30 minutes to 1 hour before meals and at bedtime. Bedtime dose can be larger and should be given at least 2 hours after the last meal of the day.
- Smaller doses are required for the elderly.
- Patient's vital signs and urinary output should be monitored carefully.
- Patient should avoid driving and other hazardous activities if he is drowsy, dizzy, or has blurred vision; drink plenty of fluids to help prevent constipation; and report any skin rash.
- Sugarless gum or hard candy may relieve mouth dryness.
- For symptoms and treatment of toxicity, see APPENDIX.

50

Miscellaneous gastrointestinal drugs

choline
cimetidine
dexpanthenol
metoclopramide hydrochloride
sucralfate

The miscellaneous gastrointestinal (GI) drugs include lipotropic substances (choline), the histamine (H_2)-receptor antagonist cimetidine, the oral antiulcer drug sucralfate, the smooth muscle relaxant dexpanthenol, and metoclopramide.

Major uses

- Choline is essential for normal transport of lipids from the liver to the tissues and is used to treat hepatic fat transport disorders.
- Cimetidine is used to treat pathologic hypersecretory conditions, such as Zollinger-Ellison syndrome, and duodenal ulcer.
- Dexpanthenol is used prophylactically immediately after major abdominal surgery to reduce the risk of paralytic ileus. It is also used to treat intestinal atony (which can cause abdominal distention), postpartum or postoperative retention of gas, and postoperative delay in resumption of intestinal motility.
- Metoclopramide facilitates small bowel intubation and aids in radiologic examination. It is also used to treat diabetic gastroparesis.
- Sucralfate is used to treat duodenal ulcers.

Mechanism of action

- Choline promotes phospholipid turnover and enhances fat transport from the liver to the tissues, decreasing the liver's fat content.
- Cimetidine competitively inhibits the action of histamine at receptor sites of the parietal cells, decreasing gastric acid secretion.
- Dexpanthenol both stimulates and restores tone to intestinal smooth muscles.
- Metoclopramide stimulates motility of the upper GI tract by antagonizing dopamine's action.
- Sucralfate adheres to and protects the ulcer surface.

Absorption, distribution, metabolism, and excretion

- Choline is incompletely absorbed after oral administration since much of it is destroyed in the stomach by gastric acid. It is metabolized by the intestinal flora and eliminated in feces.
- Cimetidine is rapidly absorbed in the upper portion of the small intestine, widely distributed to all body tissues, metabolized in the liver, and excreted in urine.
- Dexpanthenol is given parenterally. It's completely absorbed, widely distributed, and converted in the blood to the active metabolite pantothenic acid. Most of the pantothenic acid is excreted unchanged in urine.
- Metoclopramide is immediately absorbed, widely distributed, metabolized in the liver, and excreted in urine.
- Sucralfate is only minimally absorbed and is excreted unchanged in the urine.

Onset and duration

- Choline's onset and duration of action are unknown.

UNDERSTANDING CIMETIDINE, THE *OTHER* ANTIHISTAMINE

When you hear the word antihistamine, you usually think of runny noses, clogged sinuses, and hay fever. But there's an antihistamine available that won't do a thing for the patient's allergy.

The *other* antihistamine—cimetidine (Tagamet)—decreases gastric acid secretion, providing excellent therapy for the patient with ulcers.

Two types of antihistamines

Antihistamines (technically referred to as histamine antagonists) were developed *to negate the effects of histamines.* Histamines, which occur naturally in the body,

- dilate capillaries and increase capillary permeability
- constrict bronchial smooth muscle in the lungs, and
- increase gastric acid secretion.

When classic antihistamines were developed in 1937, researchers initially thought these drugs would not only relieve allergy symptoms and inhibit histamine-induced smooth-muscle contraction in the lungs but would solve the problem of increased gastric acid secretion as well.

But classic antihistamines were ineffective in controlling gastric acid secretion, that is, they could not block the action of histamine in the stomach. Researchers then hypothesized that *more than one type of histamine receptor must exist.*

Two types of receptors

Physiologic substances (such as histamines) interact with cells to produce an anticipated response (such as increased gastric acid secretion). This response occurs at a specific site called the *receptor.* A drug (such as cimetidine) can modify the physiologic response by blocking the action of the physiologic substance. This drug is known as the *antagonist;* the physiologic substance, the *agonist* (see Chapter 2, PHARMACOLOGY, for more information on agonists and antagonists).

After years of study, researchers determined that indeed at least two different histamine receptors exist, each responding to its specific histamine antagonist. This is why classic antihistamines won't affect the patient's ulcers and cimetidine doesn't alleviate allergies.

H_1 and H_2 receptor antagonists

Classic antihistamines are labeled H_1 receptor antagonists and their receptors, H_1 receptors. Cimetidine is labeled an H_2 receptor antagonist; its receptors, H_2 receptors. Cimetidine is the only antihistamine currently marketed that effectively decreases gastric acid secretion.

Several other H_2 receptor antagonists have been studied, but thus far, however, they have proved ineffective, of low potency, or toxic.

- Cimetidine blood levels peak within 75 minutes after oral or parenteral administration. The drug has a half-life of about 2 hours. Its therapeutic action lasts 4 to 5 hours after oral or parenteral administration of 300 mg.
- Dexpanthenol takes 72 hours or longer to be effective. Its action lasts 4 to 12 hours.
- Metoclopramide acts within 1 to 3 minutes, and its effect lasts 1 to 2 hours after I.V. administration. After oral administration, it takes effect within 30 minutes; its action lasts 4 to 6 hours.
- Sucralfate begins to act within 1 hour; peak occurs in 1 to 3 hours and duration is 4 to 6 hours.

NAMES, INDICATIONS AND DOSAGES	SIDE EFFECTS
choline **Hepatic disorders and disturbed fat metabolism:** ADULTS AND CHILDREN: 650 to 750 mg P.O. daily.	**CNS:** dizziness. **GI:** irritation if taken on an empty stomach, nausea. **Metabolic:** ketosis after excessive dosages. **Other:** breath and body odor smelling like dead fish.
cimetidine Tagamet♦ **Duodenal ulcer (short-term treatment):** ADULTS AND CHILDREN OVER 16 YEARS: 300 mg P.O. q.i.d. with meals and h.s. for maximum therapy of 8 weeks. When healing occurs, stop treatment or give bedtime dose only to control nocturnal hypersecretion. Parenteral: 300 mg diluted to 20 ml with 0.9% normal saline solution or other compatible I.V. solution by I.V. push over 1 to 2 minutes q 6 hours. Or 300 mg diluted in 100 ml 5% dextrose solution or other compatible I.V. solution by I.V. infusion over 15 to 20 minutes q 6 hours. Or 300 mg I.M. q 6 hours (no dilution necessary). To increase dose, give 300 mg doses more frequently to maximum daily dose of 2,400 mg. **Duodenal ulcer prophylaxis:** ADULTS AND CHILDREN OVER 16 YEARS: 400 mg P.O. h.s. **Pathologic hypersecretory conditions (such as Zollinger-Ellison syndrome, systemic mastocytosis, and multiple endocrine adenomas):** ADULTS AND CHILDREN OVER 16 YEARS: 300 mg P.O. q.i.d. with meals and h.s.; adjust to individual needs. Maximum daily dose 2,400 mg. *Parenteral:* 300 mg diluted to 20 ml with 0.9% normal saline solution or other compatible I.V. solutions by I.V. push over 1 to 2 minutes q 6 hours. Or 300 mg diluted in 100 ml 5% dextrose solution or other compatible I.V. solution by I.V. infusion over 15 to 20 minutes q 6 hours. To increase dose, give 300 mg doses more frequently to maximum daily dose of 2,400 mg.	**Blood:** *agranulocytosis,* neutropenia, *thrombocytopenia, aplastic anemia.* **CNS:** mental confusion, dizziness, headaches. **CV:** bradycardia. **GI:** mild and transient diarrhea, perforation of chronic peptic ulcers after abrupt cessation of drug. **GU:** interstitial nephritis, *transient elevations in BUN and serum creatinine,* reduced sperm count. **Hepatic:** jaundice. **Skin:** acne-like rash, urticaria, *exfoliative dermatitis.* **Other:** hypersensitivity, muscle pain, mild gynecomastia after use longer than 1 month (but no change in endocrine function).

♦ Available in U.S. and Canada. ♦♦ Available in Canada only.
All other products (no symbol) available in U.S. only. Italicized side effects are common or life-threatening.

INTERACTIONS AND SPECIAL CONSIDERATIONS

No significant interactions.

Special considerations:

• Foods supplying choline include egg yolk, beef liver, legumes, vegetables, and milk. Average diet contains from 500 to 900 mg/day.
• Lipotropic agent.
• Used in many multivitamin preparations, but no evidence supplemental choline intake is more beneficial for long periods than an adequate diet.
• Synthesized by the body from serine, with methionine acting as a methyl donor in the reaction.
• Choline is no longer considered effective in treatment of hepatic disorders or disorders of lipid transport or metabolism.
• Investigative use in treatment of tardive dyskinesia: restores cholinergic tone and decreases choreic movements. Oral choline elevates brain choline and acetylcholine (the cholinergic neurotransmitter of the cholinergic nervous system) levels and restores cholinergic tone.
• Lecithin (available in health food stores) is a source of choline.

Interactions:

ANTACIDS: interfere with absorption of cimetidine. Separate cimetidine and antacids by at least 1 hour if possible.

Special considerations:

• Maintenance dosing for more than 12 months cannot be recommended. Long-term effects are not known.
• I.M. route of administration may be painful.
• I.V. solutions compatible for dilution with cimetidine: 0.9% sodium chloride, 5% and 10% dextrose (and combinations of these), lactated Ringer's solution, and 5% sodium bicarbonate injection. Should not be diluted with sterile water for injection.
• Hemodialysis reduces blood levels of cimetidine. Cimetidine dose should be scheduled at end of hemodialysis treatment.
• Up to 10 g overdosage has been reported without untoward effects.
• Neutropenia has been reported; however, these patients were also receiving other drugs or had disease states known to produce neutropenia.
• Effectiveness in treatment of gastric ulcers not as great as in duodenal ulcers. Cimetidine may prove useful but is still unapproved in pancreatic insufficiency, short bowel syndrome, psoriasis, prevention and treatment of GI bleeding, relief of symptoms and acid sensitivity in reflux esophagitis, and prevention of gastric inactivation of oral enzyme preparations by gastric acid and pepsin.
• Taking tablets with meals will ensure a more consistent therapeutic effect.
• Large parenteral doses should be avoided in patients with asthma.
• Blue dye in Tagamet tablets may produce a false-positive Hemoccult test for blood in gastric juice. This can be avoided by administering the tablet at least 15 minutes before gastric juice is obtained by aspiration.
• Elderly patients more susceptible to cimetidine-induced mental confusion. Dose should be decreased in the elderly and in patients with renal insufficiency.
• I.V. cimetidine often used in critically ill patients prophylactically to prevent GI bleeding.
• Cimetidine is being used investigationally to treat chronic hives.
• When cimetidine is administered I.V. in 100 ml of diluent solution, it should not be infused so rapidly that circulatory overload is produced.
• Available in liquid form (300 mg/5 ml).

NAMES, INDICATIONS AND DOSAGES	SIDE EFFECTS
dexpanthenol Ilopan♦, Intrapan, Motilyn♦♦, Tonestat **Postoperative abdominal distention (resulting from flatus retention):** ADULTS AND CHILDREN: 250 to 500 mg I.M., repeat in 2 hours and again q 6 hours until distention is relieved. May require therapy for 48 to 72 hours or longer. Or, 500 mg infused slow I.V. drip in glucose or lactated Ringer's solution. **Treatment and postoperative prevention of paralytic ileus:** ADULTS AND CHILDREN: 500 mg I.M., repeat in 2 hours; then q 4 to 6 hours until distention is relieved. May require therapy for 48 to 72 hours or longer.	**Blood:** prolonged bleeding time. **GI:** excessive passage of flatus with increased doses or prolonged use, increased frequency of bowel movements, hyperperistalsis.
metoclopramide hydrochloride Maxeran♦♦, Reglan♦ **To facilitate small bowel intubation and to aid in radiologic examinations:** ADULTS: 10 mg (2 ml) I.V. as a single dose over 1 to 2 minutes. CHILDREN 6 TO 14 YEARS: 2.5 to 5 mg (0.5 to 1 ml). CHILDREN UNDER 6 YEARS: 0.1 mg/kg. **Delayed gastric emptying secondary to diabetic gastroparesis:** ADULTS: 10 mg P.O. 30 minutes before meals and at bedtime for 2 to 8 weeks, depending on response.	**CNS:** restlessness, *drowsiness,* fatigue, *lassitude,* insomnia, headache, dizziness, extrapyramidal symptoms. **GI:** nausea, bowel disturbances.
sucralfate Carafate **Short-term (up to 8 weeks) treatment of duodenal ulcer:** ADULTS: 1 g P.O. q.i.d. 1 hour before meals and at bedtime.	**CNS:** dizziness, sleepiness. **GI:** *constipation,* nausea, gastric discomfort, diarrhea.

INTERACTIONS AND SPECIAL CONSIDERATIONS

No significant interactions.

Special considerations:
• Contraindicated in hemophilia.
• I.V. solution should always be diluted.
• Dexpanthenol use shouldn't delay treatment of mechanical ileus if present.
• A smooth muscle stimulant; used postoperatively against delayed resumption of intestinal motility. Also used as adjunctive treatment of peripheral neuritis and lupus erythematosus.
• Hypokalemia may cause a decreased response. If this occurs, potassium supplements should be started. Increased doses of dexpanthenol may be needed.
• May also be useful during laxative withdrawal after long-term use.
• 12 hours should elapse between administration of parasympathomimetics and dexpanthenol.

Interactions:
ANTICHOLINERGICS, NARCOTIC ANALGESICS: antagonize effects of metoclopramide. Use together cautiously.

Special considerations:
• Contraindicated whenever stimulation of GI motility might be dangerous (hemorrhage, obstruction, perforation), and in pheochromocytoma and epilepsy.
• Speeds gastric emptying by stimulating smooth muscle in upper GI tract.
• If I.V. injection is too rapid, a transient but intense feeling of anxiety and restlessness, followed by drowsiness, occurs.
• Patient should avoid activities requiring alertness for 2 hours after taking drug.
• Oral form should be taken with meals.
• Injectable form may be useful as an antiemetic following chemotherapy.

Interactions:
ANTACIDS: may decrease binding of drug to gastroduodenal mucosa, impairing effectiveness. Should not be taken within 30 minutes of each other.

Special considerations:
• No known contraindications.
• Symptomatic improvement doesn't preclude possibility of gastric cancer.
• Drug is minimally absorbed. Incidence of side effects is low.
• For best results sucralfate should be taken on an empty stomach (1 hour before each meal and at bedtime).
• Pain and ulcer symptoms may subside within first few weeks of therapy. However, for complete healing, patient should continue prescribed regimen.
• Patient should be monitored for severe, persistent constipation.
• Studies suggest that drug's as effective as cimetidine in healing duodenal ulcers.
• Drug has been used to treat gastric ulcers, but effectiveness of this use is still under investigation.
• Drug contains aluminum, but isn't classified as an antacid.

51

Corticosteroids

Glucocorticoids
beclomethasone dipropionate
betamethasone
betamethasone acetate and betamethasone sodium phosphate
betamethasone disodium phosphate
betamethasone sodium phosphate
cortisone acetate
dexamethasone
dexamethasone acetate
dexamethasone sodium phosphate
hydrocortisone
hydrocortisone acetate
hydrocortisone retention enema
hydrocortisone sodium phosphate
hydrocortisone sodium succinate
methylprednisolone
methylprednisolone acetate
methylprednisolone sodium succinate
paramethasone acetate
prednisolone
prednisolone acetate
prednisolone sodium phosphate
prednisolone tebutate
prednisone
triamcinolone
triamcinolone acetonide
triamcinolone diacetate
triamcinolone hexacetonide

Mineralocorticoids
desoxycorticosterone acetate
desoxycorticosterone pivalate
fludrocortisone acetate

(All drugs are listed in alphabetical order in the tables that follow.)

Corticosteroids are hormones produced naturally by the adrenal cortex. The corticosteroids described in this chapter are organic or synthetic compounds used to treat adrenocortical disorders, produce immunosuppression, and reduce inflammation. They are divided into three groups on the basis of their primary physiologic actions:
• *Glucocorticoids* produce organic effects regulating carbohydrate, fat, and protein metabolism; they also have anti-inflammatory activity.
• *Mineralocorticoids* produce inorganic effects regulating electrolyte and water metabolism.
• *Adrenal androgens and estrogens* produce sex hormonal effects. (For a complete discussion of these, see Chapter 52, ANDROGENS AND ANABOLIC STEROIDS, and Chapter 54, ESTROGENS.)

Major uses
• Glucocorticoids have several uses, including:
—treatment of adrenal insufficiency (Addison's disease)
—treatment of hypercalcemia resulting from breast cancer, multiple myeloma, sarcoidosis, or vitamin D intoxication (but not hyperparathyroidism)
—topical treatment of dermatologic and ocular inflammations, such as exfoliative dermatitis, uncontrollable eczema, cutaneous sarcoidosis, and Stevens-Johnson syndrome
—systemic or inhalation therapy for respiratory diseases, including status asthmaticus, refractory bronchial asthma, berylliosis, Löffler's syndrome, and lipid pneumonitis
—relief of inflammation in rheumatic fever, rheumatoid arthritis, collagen diseases (systemic lupus erythematosus, dermatomyositis, and periarteritis nodosa), and nephrotic syndrome (They do not affect the progression of these diseases.)
—suppression of inflammatory reaction in allergic dermatoses, food and drug allergies, asthma, ulcerative colitis, and vasculitis
—diagnosis of endocrine disorders such as Cushing's syndrome and certain adrenocortical tumors

RELATIVE POTENCY OF SELECTED GLUCOCORTICOIDS

DRUG	ANTI-INFLAMMATORY POTENCY (in mg equivalent to 5 mg prednisone)	MINERALOCORTICOID POTENCY (salt-retaining potency)	DURATION
betamethasone	0.6	0	48 hr or more
cortisone acetate	25	1	12 hr or less
dexamethasone	0.75	0	48 hr or more
hydrocortisone	20	1	12 hr or less
methylprednisolone	4	0.5	24 to 36 hr
paramethasone	2	0	24 to 36 hr
prednisolone	5	0.8	24 to 36 hr
prednisone	5	0.8	24 to 36 hr
triamcinolone	4	0	24 to 36 hr

Short-term therapy (less than 7 days) with moderate doses (40 mg or less) of prednisone or equivalent produces few side effects and may be abruptly discontinued. Long-term (more than 1 week) or high-dose therapy must be discontinued gradually or acute adrenal insufficiency may result.

To minimize adrenal insufficiency, the daily dose should be administered before 9 a.m.

—emergency treatment of shock and anaphylactic reactions
—immunosuppression and relief of inflammation in organ and tissue transplants to prevent rejection
—adjunctive treatment of leukemias, lymphomas, and myelomas
—relief of cerebral edema resulting from either neurosurgical procedures or brain tumors.

• Mineralocorticoids are used to treat adrenal insufficiency (Addison's disease) in combination with glucocorticoids.

Desoxycorticosterone, supplemented with extracts containing adrenocortical steroids, may be therapeutic for recurrent hypoglycemia.

Fludrocortisone is used to treat salt-losing forms of adrenogenital syndrome (congenital adrenal hyperplasia) after electrolyte balance is restored.

Mechanism of action

The chart on page 536 summarizes the sites and mechanisms of action of the corticosteroids.

CORTICOSTEROIDS: HOW THEY WORK

CLASSIFICATION	WHAT IS INFLUENCED	MECHANISM OF ACTION
Adrenal androgens and estrogens	Primary and secondary sex organs	Sex hormonal effects
Glucocorticoids	Fat metabolism	Induce lipogenesis, increasing adipose tissue formation; in high doses, cause fat redistribution with loss of fat from extremities and accumulation in neck, cheeks, and back.
	Protein metabolism	Increase protein catabolism, decrease use of amino acids for protein synthesis, and convert amino acids to glucose, resulting in accelerated protein breakdown and muscle weakness and wasting. Interference with wound healing, suppression of immune response, temporary growth arrest, and osteoporosis may also be related to protein catabolism.
	Carbohydrate metabolism	Convert amino acids to glucose and decrease peripheral utilization of glucose, raising blood glucose level, which in turn triggers insulin release from the pancreas. Prolonged glucocorticoid treatment in patients with controlled diabetes may result in resistance to exogenous insulin and necessitate adjustment of insulin levels.
	Inflammatory process	Interfere with histamine synthesis; inhibit fibroblast formation, collagen disposition, and capillary proliferation; inhibit microvascular dilation and increased capillary permeability in response to tissue injury; block plasma exudation, migration of polymorphonuclear leukocytes into inflamed area, and phagocytosis; stabilize cell membrane and inhibit release of proteolytic enzymes, preventing normal inflammatory response; exert antilymphocytic action in treatment of some neoplasms.
	Miscellaneous	Potentiate vasoconstricting effect of norepinephrine in treatment of shock; suppress pituitary ACTH release, leading to adrenocortical suppression; lower blood calcium levels by antagonizing vitamin D effects on calcium absorption from the bowel and by decreasing calcium reabsorption from bone in multiple myeloma.
Mineralocorticoids	Kidneys	Increase sodium reabsorption and potassium and hydrogen secretion at distal segment of renal tubules.
	Blood volume	Secondary to the increased sodium retention, there's a corresponding increase in water retention. This results in increased plasma volume and elevated blood pressure.

PATIENT-TEACHING AID

HOW TO USE BECLOMETHASONE DIPROPIONATE AEROSOL PROPERLY

Dear Patient:

Taking beclomethasone dipropionate aerosol (BDA) regularly will greatly reduce the symptoms associated with your asthma. BDA is different from some other asthma medications in that you'll have to take it every day, even when you're feeling fine.

First, learn how to inhale this drug properly. By following these instructions, you'll get the best results:

• Shake the canister well and remove the cap.
• Exhale completely.
• Put the canister in your mouth, and make sure your tongue is underneath the mouthpiece.
• Tilt your head back slightly.
• Breathe in slowly but deeply while you depress the top of the canister completely.
• Take the canister out of your mouth, but be sure you hold your breath for as long as you can.
• Release your breath very slowly.

If you're instructed to inhale the aerosol more than once, wait 1 minute between inhalations. Then, follow the instructions from the beginning. When you're finished, rinse your mouth or gargle. And make sure you keep the canister clean.

Follow the doctor's instructions about taking other medications when you're taking BDA.

Absorption, distribution, metabolism, and excretion

• Most corticosteroids are efficiently absorbed from the gastrointestinal tract. Desoxycorticosterone, however, is not dependably absorbed orally and therefore is administered only parenterally.
• Water-soluble esters (for example, hydrocortisone sodium succinate and dexamethasone sodium phosphate) achieve rapid and high blood levels when given parenterally.
• Aqueous suspensions and solutions in oil are slowly absorbed by I.M. injection.
• Corticosteroids are rapidly distributed to all body tissues, metabolized in the liver, and excreted in urine.

Onset and duration

• Oral corticosteroids usually begin to act within 6 hours.
• Aqueous suspensions and solutions in oil have slow onset after I.M. administration; they produce low, prolonged blood levels (days to weeks).
• Aqueous solutions given I.V. have a rapid onset.
• Implanted compressed pellets (desoxycorticosterone acetate) provide 6 to 8 months of steroid therapy.
• Some glucocorticoids (for example, betamethasone and dexamethasone) have a prolonged duration of action (more than 48 hours).

Because they have such a long duration of action, they should not be used in alternate-day therapy.

Combination products

None.

NAMES, INDICATIONS AND DOSAGES	SIDE EFFECTS
beclomethasone dipropionate Beclovent♦, Vanceril♦ **Steroid-dependent asthma:** ADULTS: 2 to 4 inhalations t.i.d. or q.i.d. Maximum 20 inhalations daily. CHILDREN 6 TO 12 YEARS: 1 to 2 inhalations t.i.d. or q.i.d. Maximum 10 inhalations daily.	**EENT:** hoarseness, fungal infections of mouth and throat. **GI:** dry mouth.
betamethasone Betnelan♦♦, Celestone♦ **betamethasone acetate and betamethasone sodium phosphate** Celestone Soluspan♦ **betamethasone disodium phosphate** Betnesol♦♦ **betamethasone sodium phosphate** Celestone Phosphate **Severe inflammation or immunosuppression:** ADULTS: 0.6 to 7.2 mg P.O. daily; or 0.5 to 9 mg (sodium phosphate) I.M., I.V., or into joint or soft tissue daily; or 1.5 to 12 mg (sodium phosphate-acetate suspension) into joint or soft tissue q 1 to 2 weeks, p.r.n.	Most side effects of corticosteroids are dose- or duration-dependent. **CNS:** *euphoria, insomnia,* psychotic behavior, pseudotumor cerebri. **CV:** *congestive heart failure,* hypertension, edema. **EENT:** cataracts, glaucoma. **GI:** *peptic ulcer,* gastrointestinal irritation, increased appetite. **Metabolic:** *possible hypokalemia, hyperglycemia and carbohydrate intolerance,* growth suppression in children. **Skin:** delayed wound healing, acne, various skin eruptions. **Other:** muscle weakness, pancreatitis, hirsutism, susceptibility to infections. Acute adrenal insufficiency may follow increased stress (infection, surgery, trauma) or abrupt withdrawal after long-term therapy. **Withdrawal symptoms:** rebound inflammation, fatigue, weakness, arthralgia, fever, dizziness, lethargy, depression, fainting, orthostatic hypotension, dyspnea, anorexia, hypoglycemia. *Sudden withdrawal may be fatal.*
cortisone acetate Cortistan, Cortone Acetate♦ **Adrenal insufficiency, allergy, inflammation:** ADULTS: 25 to 300 mg P.O. or I.M. daily or on alternate days. Doses highly individualized, depending on severity of disease.	Most side effects of corticosteroids are dose- or duration-dependent. **CNS:** *euphoria, insomnia,* psychotic behavior, pseudotumor cerebri. **CV:** *congestive heart failure,* hypertension, edema. **EENT:** cataracts, glaucoma. **GI:** *peptic ulcer,* gastrointestinal irritation, increased appetite. **Metabolic:** *possible hypokalemia, hyperglycemia and carbohydrate intolerance,* growth suppression in children. **Skin:** delayed wound healing, acne, various skin eruptions. **Local:** atrophy at I.M. injection sites. **Other:** muscle weakness, pancreatitis, hirsutism, susceptibility to infections. Acute adrenal insufficiency may follow increased stress (infection, surgery, trauma) or abrupt withdrawal after long-term therapy. **Withdrawal symptoms:** rebound inflammation, fatigue, weakness, arthralgia, fever, dizziness, lethargy, depression, fainting, ortho-

♦ Available in U.S. and Canada. ♦♦ Available in Canada only.
All other products (no symbol) available in U.S. only. Italicized side effects are common or life-threatening.

INTERACTIONS AND SPECIAL CONSIDERATIONS

No significant interactions.

Special considerations:

• Contraindicated in status asthmaticus. Not for asthma controlled by bronchodilators or other noncorticosteroids, or for nonasthmatic bronchial diseases.
• Oral therapy should be tapered slowly. Acute adrenal insufficiency and death have occurred in patients with asthma who changed abruptly from oral corticosteroids to beclomethasone.
• During times of stress (trauma, surgery, infection), systemic corticosteroids may be needed to prevent adrenal insufficiency in previously steroid-dependent patients.
• Patient should carry a card indicating his need for supplemental systemic glucocorticoids during stress.
• Patient requiring bronchodilator should use it several minutes before beclomethasone.
• Don't store near heat or open flame.
• Glucocorticoid with potent antiinflammatory action.
• Oral fungal infections can be prevented by following inhalations with a glass of water.

Interactions:

BARBITURATES, PHENYTOIN, RIFAMPIN: decreased corticosteroid effect. Corticosteroid dose may need to be increased.
INDOMETHACIN, ASPIRIN: increased risk of GI distress and bleeding. Give together cautiously.

Special considerations:

• Contraindicated in systemic fungal infections. Use cautiously in patients with GI ulceration or renal disease, hypertension, osteoporosis, varicella, vaccinia, exanthema, diabetes mellitus, Cushing's syndrome, thromboembolic disorders, seizures, myasthenia gravis, congestive heart failure, tuberculosis, ocular herpes simplex, hypoalbuminemia, emotional instability, or psychotic tendencies.
• Should not be used for alternate-day therapy.
• Adrenal suppression may last up to 1 year after drug stopped. Drug dosage should gradually be reduced after long-term therapy. Patient should not stop drug abruptly or without doctor's consent.
• Should always be titrated to lowest effective dose.
• To prevent muscle atrophy, should be given by deep I.M. injection.
• Blood and urine sugars, along with serum potassium, should be monitored regularly.
• Patients who are on long-term therapy should be alert for cushingoid symptoms.
• Infection is possible, especially after steroid withdrawal.
• Patient should carry a card indicating his need for supplemental glucocorticoids during stress.
• Should be given with milk or food to reduce gastric irritation.
• Glucocorticoid with little mineralocorticoid effect.
• Additional potassium depletion is possible, especially in patients who receive diuretics or amphotericin B.
• Immunizations may show decreased antibody response.
• Patient should be weighed daily. Sudden weight gain may occur.
• Patients using glucose oxidase reagent sticks instead of tablets should be checked for glycosuria.

Interactions:

BARBITURATES, PHENYTOIN, RIFAMPIN: decreased corticosteroid effect. Corticosteroid dose may need to be increased.
INDOMETHACIN, ASPIRIN: increased risk of GI distress and bleeding. Give together cautiously.

Special considerations:

• Contraindicated in systemic fungal infections. Use cautiously in patients with GI ulceration or renal disease, hypertension, osteoporosis, varicella, vaccinia, exanthema, diabetes mellitus, Cushing's syndrome, thromboembolic disorders, seizures, myasthenia gravis, congestive heart failure, tuberculosis, ocular herpes simplex, hypoalbuminemia, emotional instability, or psychotic tendencies.
• Drug dosage should gradually be reduced after long-term therapy. Patient should not discontinue drug abruptly or without doctor's consent.
• Should always be titrated to lowest effective dose.
• Patient may need salt-restricted diet and potassium supplement.
• I.M. route causes slow onset of action; should not be used in acute conditions where rapid effect required. May be used on a b.i.d. schedule matching diurnal variation.
• Glucocorticoid with potent mineralocorticoid effect; sudden weight gain or edema may occur.
• Infection is possible, especially after steroid withdrawal.
• Drug of choice for replacement therapy in adrenal insufficiency.
• Should not be used for alternate-day therapy.
• Serum electrolytes and blood and urine sugars should be monitored.
• Patients on long-term therapy should be alert for cushingoid symptoms.
• Should be given with milk or food to reduce gastric irritation.
• Patient should carry a card indicating his need for supplemental glucocorticoids during stress.
• Not for I.V. use.
• Additional potassium depletion from diuretics

(continued on following page)

NAMES, INDICATIONS AND DOSAGES	SIDE EFFECTS
cortisone acetate *(continued)*	static hypotension, dyspnea, anorexia, hypoglycemia. *Sudden withdrawal may be fatal.*
desoxycorticosterone acetate Doca Acetate, Percorten Acetate **desoxycorticosterone pivalate** Percorten Pivalate **Adrenal insufficiency (partial replacement), salt-losing adrenogenital syndrome:** ADULTS: 2 to 5 mg (acetate) I.M. daily; or 25 to 100 mg (pivalate) I.M. q 4 weeks. Or implant 1 pellet for each 0.5 mg of the daily injected maintenance dose. Pellets last for 8 to 12 months.	**CV:** *sodium and water retention,* hypertension, cardiac hypertrophy, edema. **Metabolic:** *hypokalemia.*
dexamethasone Decadron♦, Dexasone♦♦, Dexone, Dezone, Hexadrol, SK-Dexamethasone **dexamethasone acetate** Decadron-LA, Decameth-LA, Dexacen-LA, Dexasone-LA **dexamethasone sodium phosphate** Decadron Phosphate, Decaject, Decameth, Dexacen-4, Dexasone, Dexone, Dezone, Hexadrol Phosphate♦, Savacort-D, Solurex **Cerebral edema:** ADULTS: initially, 10 mg (phosphate) I.V., then 4 to 6 mg I.M. q 6 hours for 2 to 4 days, then taper over 5 to 7 days. CHILDREN: 0.2 mg/kg P.O. daily in divided doses. **Inflammatory conditions, allergic reactions, neoplasias:** ADULTS: 0.25 to 4 mg P.O. b.i.d., t.i.d., or q.i.d.; or 4 to 16 mg (acetate) I.M. into joint or soft tissue q 1 to 3 weeks; or 0.8 to 1.6 mg (acetate) into lesions q 1 to 3 weeks. **Shock:** ADULTS: 1 to 6 mg/kg (phosphate) I.V. single dose; or 40 mg I.V. q 2 to 6 hours, p.r.n. **Dexamethasone suppression test:** 0.5 mg P.O. q 6 hours for 48 hours.	Most side effects of corticosteroids are dose- or duration-dependent. **CNS:** *euphoria, insomnia,* psychotic behavior, pseudotumor cerebri. **CV:** *congestive heart failure,* hypertension, edema. **EENT:** cataracts, glaucoma. **GI:** *peptic ulcer,* gastrointestinal irritation, increased appetite. **Metabolic:** *possible hypokalemia, hyperglycemia and carbohydrate intolerance,* growth suppression in children. **Skin:** delayed wound healing, acne, various skin eruptions. **Local:** atrophy at I.M. injection sites. **Other:** muscle weakness, pancreatitis, hirsutism, susceptibility to infections. Acute adrenal insufficiency may follow increased stress (infection, surgery, trauma) or abrupt withdrawal after long-term therapy. **Withdrawal symptoms:** rebound inflammation, fatigue, weakness, arthralgia, fever, dizziness, lethargy, depression, fainting, orthostatic hypotension, dyspnea, anorexia, hypoglycemia. *Sudden withdrawal may be fatal.*
fludrocortisone acetate Florinef♦ **Adrenal insufficiency (partial replacement), salt-losing adrenogenital syndrome:** ADULTS: 0.1 to 0.2 mg P.O. daily.	**CV:** *sodium and water retention,* hypertension, cardiac hypertrophy, edema. **Metabolic:** hypokalemia.

INTERACTIONS AND SPECIAL CONSIDERATIONS

and amphotericin B is possible.
• Immunizations may show decreased antibody response.

No significant interactions.

Special considerations:
• Contraindicated in hypertension, congestive heart failure, cardiac disease. Use cautiously in Addison's disease. Patients may have exaggerated side effects.
• Has no anti-inflammatory effect.
• Most potent mineralocorticoid. Has little glucocorticoid effect.
• Use with glucocorticoid for full treatment of adrenal insufficiency.
• Significant weight gain, edema, hypertension, or cardiac symptoms may occur; drug may have to be stopped.
• Injection is sesame oil solution. Dose should be withdrawn from container with 19G needle, but given with 23G needle and injected in upper outer quadrant of buttocks. Not for I.V. use.
• Sodium and potassium levels and fluid intake should be monitored. Patient may need salt-restricted diet and potassium supplement.
• Additional potassium depletion is possible, especially in patients who receive diuretics or amphotericin B.

Interactions:
BARBITURATES, PHENYTOIN, RIFAMPIN: decreased corticosteroid effect. Corticosteroid dose may need to be increased.
INDOMETHACIN, ASPIRIN: increased risk of GI distress and bleeding. Give together cautiously.

Special considerations:
• Contraindicated in systemic fungal infections and for alternate-day therapy. Use cautiously in patients with GI ulceration or renal disease, hypertension, osteoporosis, varicella, vaccinia, exanthema, diabetes mellitus, Cushing's syndrome, thromboembolic disorders, seizures, myasthenia gravis, metastatic cancer, congestive heart failure, tuberculosis, ocular herpes simplex, hypoalbuminemia, emotional instability or psychotic tendencies, and in children.
• Drug dosage should gradually be reduced after long-term therapy. Patient should not discontinue drug abruptly or without doctor's consent.
• Should always be titrated to lowest effective dose.
• Patient's weight, blood pressure, and serum electrolytes should be monitored.
• Patient should carry a card indicating his need for supplemental systemic glucocorticoids during stress, especially as dose is decreased.
• Signs of early adrenal insufficiency: fatigue, muscular weakness, joint pain, fever, anorexia, nausea, dyspnea, dizziness, fainting.
• May mask or exacerbate infections.
• Possible depression or psychotic episodes, notably in high-dose therapy.
• Patient's skin may develop petechiae and ecchymoses.
• Patients with diabetes may need increased insulin; urine should be monitored for sugar.
• Growth in infants and children on long-term therapy should be monitored.
• I.M. injection should be given deep into gluteal muscle. Subcutaneous injection should be avoided, as atrophy and sterile abscesses may occur.
• Oral dose should be given with food when possible.
• Patients on long-term therapy should be alert for cushingoid symptoms.
• Additional potassium depletion is possible, especially in patients who receive diuretics or amphotericin B.
• Immunizations may show decreased antibody response.
• Hospital guidelines should be followed when dexamethasone suppression test is being performed.

No significant interactions.

Special considerations:
• Contraindicated in hypertension, congestive heart failure, cardiac disease. Use cautiously in Addison's disease.
• Patient's blood pressure, serum electrolytes, and weight should be monitored.
• Mild peripheral edema is common.
• Unless contraindicated, salt-restricted diet rich in potassium and protein recommended. Potassium supplement may be needed.
• Has potent mineralocorticoid effects. Little glucocorticoid effect with usual doses.
• Used with cortisone or hydrocortisone in adrenal insufficiency.
• Additional potassium depletion from diuretics and amphotericin B possible.

NAMES, INDICATIONS AND DOSAGES	SIDE EFFECTS
hydrocortisone Cortef♦, Hydrocortone♦ **hydrocortisone acetate** Cortef Acetate, Cortril Acetate, Hydrocortone Acetate **hydrocortisone retention enema** Cortenema, Rectoid **hydrocortisone sodium phosphate** Hydrocortone Phosphate **hydrocortisone sodium succinate** A-Hydrocort, S-Cortilean♦♦, Solu-Cortef♦, Solu-Ject♦♦ **Severe inflammation, adrenal insufficiency:** ADULTS: 5 to 30 mg P.O. b.i.d., t.i.d., or q.i.d. (as much as 80 mg P.O. q.i.d. may be given in acute situations); or initially, 100 to 250 mg (succinate) I.M. or I.V., then 50 to 100 mg I.M., as indicated; or 15 to 240 mg (phosphate) I.M. or I.V. q 12 hours; or 5 to 75 mg (acetate) into joints and soft tissue. Dose varies with size of joint. Often local anesthetics are injected with dose. **Shock:** ADULTS: 500 mg to 2 g (succinate) q 2 to 6 hours. CHILDREN: 0.16 to 1 mg/kg (phosphate or succinate) I.M. or I.V. b.i.d. or t.i.d. **Adjunctive treatment of ulcerative colitis and proctitis:** ADULTS: 1 enema (100 mg) nightly for 21 days.	Most side effects of corticosteroids are dose- or duration-dependent. **CNS:** *euphoria, insomnia,* psychotic behavior, pseudotumor cerebri. **CV:** *congestive heart failure,* hypertension, edema. **EENT:** cataracts, glaucoma. **GI:** *peptic ulcer,* gastrointestinal irritation, increased appetite. **Metabolic:** *possible hypokalemia, hyperglycemia and carbohydrate intolerance,* growth suppression in children. **Skin:** delayed wound healing, acne, various skin eruptions. **Other:** muscle weakness, pancreatitis, hirsutism, susceptibility to infections. Acute adrenal insufficiency may occur with increased stress (infection, surgery, trauma) or abrupt withdrawal after long-term therapy. **Withdrawal symptoms:** rebound inflammation, fatigue, weakness, arthralgia, fever, dizziness, lethargy, depression, fainting, orthostatic hypotension, dyspnea, anorexia, hypoglycemia. *Sudden withdrawal may be fatal.*
methylprednisolone Medrol♦ **methylprednisolone acetate** Depo-Medrol♦, D-Med, Medralone, Methydrol-40, Pre-Dep, Rep-Pred **methylprednisolone sodium succinate** A-Methapred, Solu-Medrol♦ **Severe inflammation or immunosuppression:** ADULTS: 2 to 60 mg P.O. in 4 divided doses; or 40 to 80 mg (acetate) daily, I.M. or 10 to 250 mg (succinate) I.M. or I.V. q 4 hours; or 4 to 30 mg (acetate) into joints and soft tissue, p.r.n. CHILDREN: 117 mcg to 1.66 mg/kg (succinate) I.V. in 3 or 4 divided doses. **Shock:** 100 to 250 mg (succinate) I.V. at 2- to 6-hour intervals.	Most side effects of corticosteroids are dose- or duration-dependent. **CNS:** *euphoria, insomnia,* psychotic behavior, pseudotumor cerebri. **CV:** *congestive heart failure,* hypertension, edema. **EENT:** cataracts, glaucoma. **GI:** *peptic ulcer,* gastrointestinal irritation, increased appetite. **Metabolic:** *possible hypokalemia, hyperglycemia and carbohydrate intolerance,* growth suppression in children. **Skin:** delayed wound healing, acne, various skin eruptions. **Other:** muscle weakness, pancreatitis, hirsutism, susceptibility to infections. Acute adrenal insufficiency may occur with increased stress (infection, surgery, trauma) or abrupt withdrawal after long-term therapy. **Withdrawal symptoms:** rebound inflammation, fatigue, weakness, arthralgia, fever, dizziness, lethargy, depression, fainting, orthostatic hypotension, dyspnea, anorexia, hypoglycemia. *Sudden withdrawal may be fatal.*

INTERACTIONS AND SPECIAL CONSIDERATIONS

Interactions:
BARBITURATES, PHENYTOIN, RIFAMPIN: decreased corticosteroid effect. Corticosteroid dose may need to be increased.
INDOMETHACIN, ASPIRIN: increased risk of GI distress and bleeding. Give together cautiously.

Special considerations:
- Contraindicated in systemic fungal infections. Use cautiously in patients with GI ulceration or renal disease, hypertension, osteoporosis, varicella, vaccinia, exanthema, diabetes mellitus, Cushing's syndrome, thromboembolic disorders, seizures, myasthenia gravis, metastatic cancer, congestive heart failure, tuberculosis, ocular herpes simplex, hypoalbuminemia, emotional instability or psychotic tendencies, and in children.
- Drug dosage should be gradually reduced after long-term therapy. Patient should not discontinue drug abruptly or without doctor's consent.
- Should always be titrated to lowest effective dose.
- Glucocorticoid and mineralocorticoid effect.
- Patient's weight, blood pressure, and serum electrolytes should be monitored.
- May mask or exacerbate infections.
- Stress (fever, trauma, surgery, emotional problems) may increase adrenal insufficiency. Dose may have to be increased.
- Patient should carry a card identifying his need for supplemental systemic glucocorticoids during stress.
- Signs of early adrenal insufficiency: fatigue, muscular weakness, joint pain, fever, anorexia, nausea, dyspnea, dizziness, fainting.
- Depression or psychotic episodes may occur, notably in high-dose therapy.
- Patient's skin may develop petechiae or ecchymoses.
- Patients with diabetes may need increased insulin; monitor urine for sugar.
- Growth in infants and children on long-term therapy should be monitored.
- I.M. injection should be given deep into gluteal muscle. Subcutaneous injection should be avoided, as atrophy and sterile abscesses may occur.
- Unless contraindicated, salt-restricted diet rich in potassium and protein recommended. Potassium supplement may be needed. Additional potassium depletion from diuretics and amphotericin B possible.
- Oral dose should be given with food when possible.
- Patients on long-term therapy should be alert for cushingoid symptoms.
- Acetate form not for I.V. use.
- Enema may produce same systemic effects as other forms of hydrocortisone. If enema therapy must exceed 21 days, administration should be gradually discontinued by reducing administration to every other night for 2 or 3 weeks.
- Immunizations may show decreased antibody response.
- Solu-Cortef should not be confused with Solu-Medrol.
- Not for alternate-day therapy.

Interactions:
BARBITURATES, PHENYTOIN, RIFAMPIN: decreased corticosteroid effect. Corticosteroid dose may need to be increased.
INDOMETHACIN, ASPIRIN: increased risk of GI distress and bleeding. Give together cautiously.

Special considerations:
- Contraindicated in systemic fungal infections. Use cautiously in patients with GI ulceration or renal disease, hypertension, osteoporosis, varicella, vaccinia, exanthema, diabetes mellitus, Cushing's syndrome, thromboembolic disorders, seizures, myasthenia gravis, metastatic cancer, congestive heart failure, tuberculosis, ocular herpes simplex, hypoalbuminemia, emotional instability, or psychotic tendencies.
- Drug dosage should gradually be reduced after long-term therapy. Patient should not discontinue drug abruptly or without doctor's consent.
- Should always be titrated to lowest effective dose.
- Glucocorticoid with little mineralocorticoid effect.
- Reconstituted solutions should be discarded after 48 hours.
- Acetate salt should not be used when immediate onset of action needed.
- Dermal atrophy may occur with large doses of acetate salt. Multiple small injections should be given into lesions.
- Patient's weight, blood pressure, serum electrolytes, and sleep patterns should be monitored. Euphoria may initially interfere with sleep, but patient generally adjusts to the medication after 1 to 3 weeks.
- May mask or exacerbate infections.
- Patient should carry a card identifying his need for supplemental systemic glucocorticoids during stress.
- Signs of early adrenal insufficiency: fatigue, muscular weakness, joint pain, fever, anorexia, nausea, dyspnea, dizziness, fainting.
- Possible depression or psychotic episodes, notably in high-dose therapy.
- Patients with diabetes may need increased insulin; monitor urine for sugar.
- I.M. injection should be given deep into gluteal muscle. Subcutaneous injection should be avoided, as atrophy and sterile abscesses may occur.
- Unless contraindicated, salt-restricted diet rich in potassium and protein recommended.

(continued on following page)

NAMES, INDICATIONS AND DOSAGES	SIDE EFFECTS
methylprednisolone *(continued)*	
paramethasone acetate Haldrone **Inflammatory conditions:** ADULTS: 0.5 to 6 mg P.O. t.i.d. or q.i.d. CHILDREN: 58 to 800 mcg/kg daily divided t.i.d. or q.i.d.	Most side effects of corticosteroids are dose- or duration-dependent. **CNS:** *euphoria, insomnia,* psychotic behavior, pseudotumor cerebri. **CV:** *congestive heart failure,* hypertension, edema. **EENT:** cataracts, glaucoma. **GI:** *peptic ulcer,* gastrointestinal irritation, increased appetite. **Metabolic:** *possible hypokalemia, hyperglycemia and carbohydrate intolerance,* growth suppression in children. **Skin:** delayed wound healing, acne, various skin eruptions. **Other:** muscle weakness, pancreatitis, hirsutism, susceptibility to infections. Acute adrenal insufficiency may occur with increased stress (infection, surgery, trauma) or abrupt withdrawal after long-term therapy. **Withdrawal symptoms:** rebound inflammation, fatigue, weakness, arthralgia, fever, dizziness, lethargy, depression, fainting, orthostatic hypotension, dyspnea, anorexia, hypoglycemia. *Sudden withdrawal may be fatal.*
prednisolone Cordrol, Delta-Cortef♦, Predoxine, Ropredlone, Ster 5, Sterane **prednisolone acetate** **prednisolone sodium phosphate** **prednisolone tebutate** Hydeltra-TBA, Metalone-TBA **Severe inflammation or immunosuppression:** ADULTS: 2.5 to 15 mg P.O. b.i.d., t.i.d., or q.i.d.; 2 to 30 mg I.M. (acetate, phosphate), or I.V. (phosphate) q 12 hours; or 2 to 30 mg (phosphate) into joints, lesions, and soft tissue; or 4 to 40 mg (tebutate) into joints and lesions; or 0.25 to 1 ml (acetate-phosphate suspension) into joints weekly, p.r.n.	Most side effects of corticosteroids are dose- or duration-dependent. **CNS:** *euphoria, insomnia,* psychotic behavior, pseudotumor cerebri. **CV:** *congestive heart failure,* hypertension, edema. **EENT:** cataracts, glaucoma. **GI:** *peptic ulcer,* gastrointestinal irritation, increased appetite. **Metabolic:** *possible hypokalemia, hyperglycemia and carbohydrate intolerance,* growth suppression in children. **Skin:** delayed wound healing, acne, various skin eruptions. **Other:** muscle weakness, pancreatitis, hirsutism, susceptibility to infections. Acute adrenal insufficiency may occur with increased stress (infection, surgery, trauma) or abrupt withdrawal after long-term therapy. **Withdrawal symptoms:** rebound inflammation, fatigue, weakness, arthralgia, fever, dizziness, lethargy, depression, fainting, orthostatic hypotension, dyspnea, anorexia, hypoglycemia. *Sudden withdrawal may be fatal.*

INTERACTIONS AND SPECIAL CONSIDERATIONS

Potassium supplement may be needed. Additional potassium depletion from diuretics and amphotericin B possible.
• Give oral dose with food if possible.
• I.V. dose should be given slowly over 1 minute; in shock, massive I.V. doses should be given over 3 to 15 minutes to prevent cardiac arrhythmias and circulatory collapse.
• Patients on long-term therapy should be alert for cushingoid symptoms.
• Acetate form not for I.V. use.
• Solu-Medrol should not be confused with Solu-Cortef.
• Immunizations may show decreased antibody response.
• May be used for alternate-day therapy.

Interactions:
BARBITURATES, PHENYTOIN, RIFAMPIN: decreased corticosteroid effect. Corticosteroid dose may need to be increased.
INDOMETHACIN, ASPIRIN: increased risk of GI distress and bleeding. Give together cautiously.

Special considerations:
• Contraindicated in systemic fungal infections and alternate-day therapy. Use cautiously in patients with GI ulceration or renal disease, hypertension, osteoporosis, varicella, vaccinia, exanthema, diabetes mellitus, Cushing's syndrome, thromboembolic disorders, seizures, myasthenia gravis, metastatic cancer, congestive heart failure, tuberculosis, ocular herpes simplex, hypoalbuminemia, emotional instability or psychotic tendencies.
• Gradually reduce drug dosage after long-term therapy. Always titrate to lowest effective dose. Patient should not discontinue drug abruptly or without doctor's consent.
• Glucocorticoid with little mineralocorticoid effect.
• Patient's weight, blood pressure, and serum electrolytes should be monitored.
• May mask or exacerbate infections.
• Patient should carry a card identifying his need for supplemental systemic glucocorticoids during stress.
• Signs of early adrenal insufficiency: fatigue, muscular weakness, joint pain, fever, anorexia, nausea, dyspnea, dizziness, fainting.
• Possible depression or psychotic episodes, notably in high-dose therapy.
• Patients with diabetes may need increased insulin; urine should be monitored for sugar.
• Growth in infants and children on long-term therapy needs monitoring.
• Unless contraindicated, salt-restricted diet rich in potassium and protein recommended. Potassium supplement may be needed. Additional potassium depletion from diuretics or amphotericin B is possible.
• Oral dose should be given with food when possible, especially if GI irritation occurs.
• Patients on long-term therapy should be alert for cushingoid symptoms.
• Immunizations may show decreased antibody response.

Interactions:
BARBITURATES, PHENYTOIN, RIFAMPIN: decreased corticosteroid effect. Corticosteroid dose may need to be increased.
INDOMETHACIN, ASPIRIN: increased risk of GI distress and bleeding. Give together cautiously.

Special considerations:
• Contraindicated in systemic fungal infections. Use cautiously in patients with GI ulceration or renal disease, hypertension, osteoporosis, varicella, vaccinia, exanthema, diabetes mellitus, Cushing's syndrome, thromboembolic disorders, seizures, myasthenia gravis, metastatic cancer, congestive heart failure, tuberculosis, ocular herpes simplex, hypoalbuminemia, emotional instability, or psychotic tendencies.
• Gradually reduce drug dosage after long-term therapy. Always titrate to lowest effective dose. Patient should not discontinue drug abruptly or without doctor's consent.
• Glucocorticoid with slight mineralocorticoid action.
• Prednisolone salts (acetate, sodium phosphate, sodium succinate, and tebutate) are used parenterally less often than other corticosteroids that have more potent anti-inflammatory action.
• May be used for alternate-day therapy.
• Patient's weight, blood pressure, and serum electrolytes should be monitored.
• Patient should carry a card identifying his need for supplemental systemic glucocorticoids during stress.
• Signs of early adrenal insufficiency: fatigue, muscular weakness, joint pain, fever, anorexia, nausea, dyspnea, dizziness, fainting.
• Depression or psychotic episodes possible, notably in high-dose therapy.
• Patients with diabetes may need increased insulin; urine should be monitored for sugar.
• I.M. injection should be given deep into gluteal muscle. Subcutaneous injection should be avoided, as atrophy and sterile abscesses may occur. Acetate form not for I.V. use.
• Unless contraindicated, salt-restricted diet rich in potassium and protein recommended. Potassium supplement may be needed. Additional potassium depletion from diuretics or amphotericin B is possible.
• Give oral dose with food if possible.
• Possible cushingoid symptoms with long use.
• Immunizations may show decreased antibody response. May mask or exacerbate infections.

NAMES, INDICATIONS AND DOSAGES	SIDE EFFECTS
prednisone Colisone◆◆, Deltasone◆, Fernisone, Meticorten, Orasone, Prednicen-M, SK-Prednisone, Sterapred **Severe inflammation or immunosuppression:** ADULTS: 2.5 to 15 mg P.O. b.i.d., t.i.d., or q.i.d. Maintenance dose given once daily or every other day. CHILDREN: 0.14 to 2 mg/kg daily P.O. divided q.i.d.	Most side effects of corticosteroids are dose- or duration-dependent. **CNS:** *euphoria, insomnia,* psychotic behavior, pseudotumor cerebri. **CV:** *congestive heart failure,* hypertension, edema. **EENT:** cataracts, glaucoma. **GI:** *peptic ulcer,* gastrointestinal irritation, increased appetite. **Metabolic:** *possible hypokalemia, hyperglycemia and carbohydrate intolerance,* growth suppression in children. **Skin:** delayed wound healing, acne, various skin eruptions. **Other:** muscle weakness, pancreatitis, hirsutism, susceptibility to infections. Acute adrenal insufficiency may occur with increased stress (infection, surgery, trauma) or abrupt withdrawal after long-term therapy. **Withdrawal symptoms:** rebound inflammation, fatigue, weakness, arthralgia, fever, dizziness, lethargy, depression, fainting, orthostatic hypotension, dyspnea, anorexia, hypoglycemia. *Sudden withdrawal may be fatal.*
triamcinolone Aristocort◆, Kenacort◆, Spencort, Tricilone **triamcinolone acetonide** Kenalog◆ **triamcinolone diacetate** Amcort, Aristocort Parenteral Forte, Cenocort Forte, Cino-40, Tracilon, Triam-Forte, Tristoject **triamcinolone hexacetonide** Aristospan◆ **Severe inflammation or immunosuppression:** ADULTS: 4 to 48 mg P.O. daily divided b.i.d., t.i.d., or q.i.d., or 40 mg I.M. (diacetate or acetonide) weekly; or 5 to 48 mg (diacetate or acetonide) into lesions; or 2 to 40 mg (diacetate or acetonide) into joints and soft tissue; or up to 0.5 mg (hexacetonide) per square inch of affected skin intralesional; or 2 to 20 mg (hexacetonide) intra-articular or intrasynovial into soft tissue or into joint or lesion. Often, a local anesthetic is injected into the joint with triamcinolone.	Most side effects of corticosteroids are dose- or duration-dependent. **CNS:** *euphoria, insomnia,* psychotic behavior, pseudotumor cerebri. **CV:** *congestive heart failure,* hypertension, edema. **EENT:** cataracts, glaucoma. **GI:** *peptic ulcer,* gastrointestinal irritation, increased appetite. **Metabolic:** *possible hypokalemia, hyperglycemia and carbohydrate intolerance,* growth suppression in children. **Skin:** delayed wound healing, acne, various skin eruptions. **Other:** muscle weakness, pancreatitis, hirsutism, susceptibility to infections. Acute adrenal insufficiency may occur with increased stress (infection, surgery, trauma) or abrupt withdrawal after long-term therapy. **Withdrawal symptoms:** rebound inflammation, fatigue, weakness, arthralgia, fever, dizziness, lethargy, depression, fainting, orthostatic hypotension, dyspnea, anorexia, hypoglycemia. *Sudden withdrawal may be fatal.*

INTERACTIONS AND SPECIAL CONSIDERATIONS

Interactions:

BARBITURATES, PHENYTOIN, RIFAMPIN: decreased corticosteroid effect. Corticosteroid dose may need to be increased.

INDOMETHACIN, ASPIRIN: increased risk of GI distress and bleeding. Give together cautiously.

Special considerations:

- Contraindicated in systemic fungal infections. Use cautiously in patients with GI ulceration or renal disease, hypertension, osteoporosis, varicella, vaccinia, exanthema, diabetes mellitus, Cushing's syndrome, thromboembolic disorders, seizures, myasthenia gravis, metastatic cancer, congestive heart failure, tuberculosis, ocular herpes simplex, hypoalbuminemia, emotional instability, or psychotic tendencies.
- Drug dosage should gradually be reduced after long-term therapy. Patient should not discontinue drug abruptly or without doctor's consent.
- Should always be titrated to lowest effective dose.
- Patient's blood pressure, sleep patterns, and serum potassium levels should be monitored.
- Patient should be weighed daily; sudden weight gain possible.
- May mask or exacerbate infections.
- Patient should carry a card identifying his need for supplemental systemic glucocorticoids during stress.
- Signs of early adrenal insufficiency: fatigue, muscular weakness, joint pain, fever, anorexia, nausea, dyspnea, dizziness, fainting.
- Depression or psychotic episodes possible, notably in high-dose therapy.
- Patients with diabetes may need increased insulin; urine should be monitored for sugar.
- Growth in infants and children on long-term therapy should be monitored.
- Salt-restricted diet rich in potassium and protein recommended. Potassium supplement may be needed. Additional potassium depletion from diuretics and amphotericin B is possible.
- Unless contraindicated, oral dose should be given with food when possible, to reduce GI irritation.
- May be used for alternate-day therapy.
- Patients on long-term therapy should be alert for cushingoid symptoms.
- Immunizations may show decreased antibody response.

Interactions:

BARBITURATES, PHENYTOIN, RIFAMPIN: decreased corticosteroid effect. Corticosteroid dose may need to be increased.

INDOMETHACIN, ASPIRIN: increased risk of GI distress and bleeding. Give together cautiously.

Special considerations:

- Contraindicated in systemic fungal infections. Use cautiously in patients with GI ulceration or renal disease, hypertension, osteoporosis, varicella, vaccinia, exanthema, diabetes mellitus, Cushing's syndrome, thromboembolic disorders, seizures, myasthenia gravis, metastatic cancer, congestive heart failure, tuberculosis, ocular herpes simplex, hypoalbuminemia, emotional instability, or psychotic tendencies.
- Drug dosage should gradually be reduced after long-term therapy. Patient should not discontinue drug abruptly or without doctor's consent.
- Should always be titrated to lowest effective dose.
- Patient's weight, blood pressure, and serum electrolytes should be monitored.
- May mask or exacerbate infections.
- Patient should carry a card identifying his need for supplemental systemic glucocorticoids during stress.
- Signs of early adrenal insufficiency: fatigue, muscular weakness, joint pain, fever, anorexia, nausea, dyspnea, dizziness, fainting.
- Mild peripheral edema is common.
- Depression or psychotic episodes possible, notably in high-dose therapy.
- Patients with diabetes may need increased insulin; monitor urine for sugar.
- I.M. injection should be given deep into gluteal muscle. Subcutaneous injection should be avoided, as atrophy and sterile abscesses may occur.
- Unless contraindicated, salt-restricted diet rich in potassium and protein recommended. Potassium supplement may be needed. Additional potassium depletion from diuretics and amphotericin B is possible.
- Oral dose should be given with food when possible, to reduce GI irritation.
- Glucocorticoid with very little mineralocorticoid effect.
- Unused diluted suspension should be discarded within 7 days.
- Diluents that contain preservatives should not be used. Flocculation may occur.
- Patients on long-term therapy should be alert for cushingoid symptoms.
- Immunizations may show decreased antibody response.
- Not for alternate-day therapy.
- No forms for I.V. use. Hexacetonide not for I.V. or I.M. use.

52

Androgens and anabolic steroids

danazol
ethylestrenol
fluoxymesterone
methandrostenolone
methyltestosterone
nandrolone decanoate
nandrolone phenpropionate
oxandrolone
oxymetholone
stanozolol
testosterone
testosterone cypionate
testosterone enanthate
testosterone propionate

Androgens (danazol, fluoxymesterone, methyltestosterone, and testosterone and its salts) include both the organic and the synthetic steroids that stimulate growth of the male accessory sex organs, promoting development of secondary sex characteristics such as facial and body hair, deep voice, and skeletal muscle. Testosterone, the primary natural androgen in humans, is produced by the interstitial cells of the testes under the stimulation of luteinizing hormone (LH) from the pituitary. A smaller amount of testosterone is secreted by the adrenal cortex in both sexes and by the ovaries in females.

Anabolic steroids (ethylestrenol, methandrostenolone, nandrolone decanoate, nandrolone phenpropionate, oxandrolone, oxymetholone, and stanozolol) are synthetic compounds structurally related to testosterone. They promote tissue-building and reverse tissue-depleting processes. They have an advantage over testosterone, its esters, and synthetic androgens when anabolic rather than androgenic activity is desired. Despite their preponderant anabolic properties, their residual androgenic activity may produce some virilization in female patients if large doses are administered for long periods.

Major uses

• *Androgens in androgen-deficient males* combat hypogonadism of either primary origin (for example, Klinefelter's syndrome or myotonic dystrophy) or secondary origin (for example, pituitary tumors or pituitary insufficiency, and selective gonadotropin deficiencies, such as eunuchoidism).

They're also used to treat oligospermia and impotence.

• *Androgens in women* prevent postpartum breast pain and engorgement in non–breast-feeding mothers (lactation is not suppressed).

They may also palliate androgen-responsive, advanced inoperable breast cancer in patients who have been in menopause for more than 1 year but less than 5 years, or who have an estrogen-dependent tumor.

They're also used to treat certain gynecologic conditions (for example, uterine hemorrhage, dysmenorrhea, and menopausal syndrome).

Danazol, a synthetic androgen, is therapeutic for fibrocystic breast disease. It is also used to treat refractory endometriosis.

• Anabolic steroids promote weight gain in patients who are underweight due to predisposing catabolic states. An adequate dietary regimen should be established to maximize tissue building.

Anabolic steroids also correct corticosteroid catabolism and reverse the profound negative nitrogen balance that occurs in corticosteroid therapy.

As adjunctive therapy, they may be effective in senile and postmenopausal osteoporosis as well as refractory anemias associated with chronic disease.

Mechanism of action

• Androgens are simply exogenous replacements that stimulate target tissues to develop normally in androgen-deficient males.

• Anabolic steroids stimulate cellular protein synthesis in debilitated patients. The resulting positive nitrogen balance promotes anabolism. They also promote a sense of well-being in debilitated patients. This may encourage the patient to eat more and gain weight. They improve calcium balance and decrease bone resorption. They also enhance erythropoiesis by stimulating secretion of renal or extrarenal erythropoietin and by directly stimulating heme synthesis, an action potentiated by erythropoietin.

Absorption, distribution, metabolism, and excretion

• Testosterone and its derivatives are well absorbed from the gastrointestinal tract. However, since most of these drugs undergo rapid degradation in the liver (because of first-pass effect), they are not effective when given orally. Administering testosterone buccally or sublingually circumvents the drug's hepatic degradation.

• Methyltestosterone and fluoxymesterone resist hepatic metabolism because they are alkylated in the 17-alpha position and are therefore the only orally active agents.

• Testosterone cypionate and enanthate are dissolved in oil and injected intramuscularly.

• All androgens and anabolic steroids are metabolized in the liver and excreted primarily by the kidneys.

Onset and duration

• Onset of the androgens and anabolic steroids is difficult to determine because subjective response varies. Hematologic and other objective responses are not apparent for at least 3 months.

• Nandrolone decanoate and phenpropionate given I.M. have durations of 3 to 4 weeks and 1 to 2 weeks, respectively.

• Testosterone cypionate and enanthate have effects that last as long as 4 weeks.

• Testosterone propionate dissolved in oil has a shorter action than the other two ester analogs; however, its 2- to 3-day duration supplies the effect of daily injections of testosterone alone.

• Subcutaneous implantation of testosterone pellets prolongs action up to 6 months.

Combination products

DELADUMONE INJECTION (oil)♦: testosterone enanthate 90 mg, estradiol valerate 4 mg, and chlorobutanol 0.5%.

DEPO-TESTADIOL (oil): testosterone cypionate 50 mg, estradiol cypionate 2 mg, and chlorobutanol 0.5%.

FORMATRIX: conjugated estrogens 1.25 mg, methyltestosterone 10 mg, and ascorbic acid 400 mg.

GYNETONE .02: ethinyl estradiol 0.02 mg and methyltestosterone 5 mg.

LACTOSTAT (oil)♦♦: testosterone enanthate benzilic acid hydrazone 300 mg, estradiol dienanthate 15 mg, and estradiol benzoate 6 mg.

PREMARIN WITH METHYLTESTOSTERONE♦: conjugated estrogens 0.625 mg and methyltestosterone 5 mg.

NAMES, INDICATIONS AND DOSAGES	SIDE EFFECTS
danazol Cyclomen♦♦, Danocrine **Endometriosis:** WOMEN: 400 mg P.O. b.i.d. uninterrupted for 3 to 6 months; may continue for 9 months. **Fibrocystic breast disease:** WOMEN: 100 to 400 mg P.O. daily in 2 divided doses uninterrupted for 2 to 6 months. **Prevention of hereditary angioedema:** ADULTS: 200 mg P.O. 2 to 3 times a day, continued until favorable response is achieved. Then dosage should be decreased by half at 1- to 3-month intervals.	**Androgenic:** acne, edema, *weight gain, hirsutism,* hoarseness, clitoral enlargement, *decrease in breast size,* changes in libido, male-pattern baldness, *oiliness of skin or hair.* **CNS:** dizziness, headache, sleep disorders, fatigue, tremor, irritability, excitation, lethargy, mental depression, chills, paresthesias. **CV:** elevated blood pressure. **EENT:** visual disturbances. **GI:** gastric irritation, nausea, vomiting, diarrhea, constipation, change in appetite. **GU:** hematuria. **Hepatic:** jaundice. **Hypoestrogenic:** flushing; sweating; vaginitis, including itching, dryness, burning, and vaginal bleeding; nervousness, emotional lability. **Other:** muscle cramps or spasms.
ethylestrenol Maxibolin♦ **Promote weight gain and combat tissue depletion, refractory anemias, catabolic effects of corticosteroid therapy, osteoporosis, prolonged immobilization, and debilitated states:** ADULTS: 4 to 8 mg P.O. daily, reduced to minimum levels at first evidence of clinical response. CHILDREN: 1 to 3 mg P.O. daily; highly individualized. A single course of therapy in both adults and children should not exceed 6 weeks; may be reinstituted after 4-week interval.	**Androgenic:** in females—*acne, edema, oily skin, weight gain, hirsutism, hoarseness,* clitoral enlargement, changes in libido. In males—prepubertal: premature epiphyseal closure, acne, priapism, growth of body and facial hair, phallic enlargement; postpubertal: testicular atrophy, oligospermia, decreased ejaculatory volume, impotence, gynecomastia, epididymitis. **CV:** edema. **GI:** gastroenteritis, nausea, vomiting, diarrhea, constipation, change in appetite. **GU:** bladder irritability. **Hepatic:** jaundice. **Hypoestrogenic:** in females—flushing; sweating; vaginitis with itching, drying, burning, or bleeding; menstrual irregularities. **Other:** hypercalcemia.
fluoxymesterone Android-F, Halotestin♦, Oratestin♦♦, Oratestryl **Hypogonadism and impotence due to testicular deficiency:** ADULTS: 2 to 10 mg P.O. daily. **Palliation of breast cancer in women:** 15 to 30 mg P.O. daily in divided doses. All dosages should be individualized and reduced to minimum when effect is noted. **Postpartum breast engorgement:** 2.5 mg P.O. followed by 5 to 10 mg daily for 5 days.	**Androgenic:** in females—*acne, edema, oily skin, weight gain, hirsutism, hoarseness,* clitoral enlargement, change in libido. In males—prepubertal: premature epiphyseal closure, acne, priapism, growth of body and facial hair, phallic enlargement; postpubertal: testicular atrophy, oligospermia, decreased ejaculatory volume, impotence, gynecomastia, epididymitis. **CV:** edema. **GI:** gastroenteritis, nausea, vomiting, constipation, change in appetite, diarrhea. **GU:** bladder irritability. **Hepatic:** jaundice. **Hypoestrogenic:** in females—flushing; sweating; vaginitis with itching, drying, burning, or bleeding; menstrual irregularities; emotional lability.

♦ Available in U.S. and Canada. ♦♦ Available in Canada only.
All other products (no symbol) available in U.S. only. Italicized side effects are common or life-threatening.

INTERACTIONS AND SPECIAL CONSIDERATIONS

No significant interactions.

Special considerations:

- Contraindicated in patients with undiagnosed abnormal genital bleeding; impaired renal, cardiac, or hepatic function. Use cautiously in patients with epilepsy or migraine headache.
- Should be used with diet high in calories and protein unless contraindicated.
- Patient should be monitored closely for signs of virilization. Some androgenic effects, such as deepening of voice, may not be reversible upon discontinuation of drug.
- Patient who is taking danazol for fibrocystic disease should examine breasts regularly. If breast nodule enlarges during treatment, patient should call doctor immediately.
- Patient should wear cotton underwear only.
- Washing after intercourse is recommended to decrease the risk of vaginitis.

No significant interactions.

Special considerations:

- Contraindicated in patients with prostatic hypertrophy with obstruction; carcinoma of male breast; hypercalcemia; prostatic cancer; cardiac, hepatic, or renal decompensation; nephrosis; premature infants. Use cautiously in prepubertal males; patients with diabetes or coronary disease; patients taking ACTH, corticosteroids, or anticoagulants.
- Hypercalcemic symptoms may be difficult to distinguish from symptoms of condition being treated unless anticipated and thought of as a symptom cluster. Hypercalcemia is particularly likely to occur in patients with metastatic breast cancer and may indicate bone metastases.
- Females should report menstrual irregularities; therapy should be discontinued pending etiologic determination.
- Virilizing effects may be irreversible despite prompt discontinuation of therapy. Benefits should be weighed against effects.
- Boys under age 7 should be closely monitored for precocious development of male sexual characteristics.
- In children: therapy should be preceded by X-ray of wrist bones to establish level of bone maturation. During treatment, bone maturation may proceed more rapidly than linear growth; dosage should be intermittent and X-rays taken periodically.
- Edema is generally controllable with salt restriction and/or diuretics. Weight should be checked routinely.
- Jaundice is possible. Dose adjustment may reverse condition. If liver function studies are abnormal, therapy should be discontinued.
- Patient on concomitant anticoagulant therapy may develop ecchymotic areas, petechiae, abnormal bleeding. Monitor prothrombin time.
- Hypoglycemia is possible in patients with diabetes. Dosage of antidiabetic drug may need adjustment.
- Use with diet high in calories and protein unless contraindicated.
- Anabolic steroids may alter many laboratory studies during therapy and for 2 to 3 weeks after therapy is stopped.
- The patient, family members, and a dietitian should be involved in developing a dietary regimen suitable to the anorexic or debilitated patient.

No significant interactions.

Special considerations:

- Contraindicated in patients with prostatic hypertrophy with obstruction; carcinoma of male breast; prostatic cancer; cardiac, hepatic, or renal decompensation; nephrosis; hypercalcemia. Use cautiously in prepubertal males; patients with diabetes or coronary disease; and patients taking ACTH, corticosteroids, or anticoagulants.
- Hypercalcemic symptoms may be difficult to distinguish from symptoms associated with condition being treated unless anticipated and thought of as a symptom cluster. Hypercalcemia is particularly likely to occur in patients with metastatic breast cancer and may indicate bone metastases.
- In patient on drug for palliation of breast cancer, virilization usually occurs at dosage used. Patient should report androgenic effects immediately. Stopping drug will prevent further androgenic changes but will probably not reverse those already existing.
- When used in breast cancer, subjective effects may not be seen for about 1 month; objective symptoms not for 3 months.
- Females should report menstrual irregularities; therapy should be discontinued pending etiologic determination.
- Edema is generally controllable with salt restriction and/or diuretics.
- Jaundice is possible. Dose adjustment may reverse condition. If liver function studies are

(continued on following page)

NAMES, INDICATIONS AND DOSAGES	SIDE EFFECTS

fluoxymesterone
(continued)

Other: hypercalcemia.

---

methandrostenolone
Danabol♦♦, Dianabol

Senile and postmenopausal osteoporosis:
ADULTS: initially 5 mg P.O. daily. Maintenance 2.5 to 5 mg P.O. daily.

Anabolic effect:
ADULTS: 5 to 10 mg P.O. daily.

Severe debilitation:
ADULTS: 10 to 20 mg P.O. daily for 3 weeks, reduced to 5 to 10 mg P.O. daily for maintenance.

Severe maturational delay when growth hormone is unavailable:
CHILDREN: (postpubertal) up to 0.05 mg/kg P.O. daily.
Intermittent therapy is recommended in prolonged use.

Androgenic: in females—*acne, edema, oily skin, weight gain, hirsutism, hoarseness,* clitoral enlargement, changes in libido. In males—prepubertal: premature epiphyseal closure, acne, priapism, growth of body and facial hair, phallic enlargement; postpubertal: testicular atrophy, oligospermia, decreased ejaculatory volume, impotence, gynecomastia, epididymitis.
CV: edema.
EENT: burning of tongue.
GI: gastroenteritis, nausea, vomiting, change in appetite, diarrhea, anorexia, constipation.
GU: bladder irritability.
Hepatic: jaundice.
Hypoestrogenic: in females—flushing; sweating; vaginitis with itching, drying, burning, or bleeding; menstrual irregularities.
Other: hypercalcemia.

---

methyltestosterone
Android-5, Android-10, Metandren♦, Oreton-Methyl, Testred, Virilon

ADULTS:
Breast engorgement of non–breast-feeding mothers: 80 mg P.O. daily, or 40 mg buccal daily for 3 to 5 days.

Breast cancer in women 1 to 5 years postmenopausal: 200 mg P.O. daily; or 100 mg buccal daily.

Eunuchoidism and eunuchism, male climacteric symptoms: 10 to 40 mg P.O. daily; or 5 to 20 mg buccal daily.

Postpubertal cryptorchidism: 30 mg P.O. daily; or 15 mg buccal daily.

Androgenic: in females—*acne, edema, oily skin, weight gain, hirsutism, hoarseness,* clitoral enlargement, changes in libido. In males—prepubertal: premature epiphyseal closure, acne, priapism, growth of body and facial hair, phallic enlargement; postpubertal: testicular atrophy, oligospermia, decreased ejaculatory volume, impotence, gynecomastia, epididymitis.
CV: edema.
GI: gastroenteritis, constipation, nausea, vomiting, diarrhea, change in appetite.
GU: bladder irritability.
Hepatic: jaundice.
Hypoestrogenic: in females—flushing; sweating; vaginitis with itching, drying, burning, or bleeding; menstrual irregularities.
Local: irritation of oral mucosa with buccal administration.
Other: hypercalcemia.

---

nandrolone decanoate
Deca-Durabolin♦, Deca-Hybolin
nandrolone phenpropionate
Anabolin, Anorolone, Durabolin♦, Nandrolin

Severe debility or disease states, refractory anemias (decanoate):
ADULTS: 100 to 200 mg I.M. weekly. Therapy should be intermittent.

Androgenic: in females—*acne, edema, oily skin, weight gain, hirsutism, hoarseness,* clitoral enlargement, decreased or increased libido. In males—prepubertal: premature epiphyseal closure, acne, priapism, growth of body and facial hair, phallic enlargement; postpubertal: testicular atrophy, oligospermia, decreased ejaculatory volume, impotence, gynecomastia, epididymitis.

INTERACTIONS AND SPECIAL CONSIDERATIONS

abnormal, therapy should be discontinued.
• Patient on concomitant anticoagulant therapy may develop ecchymotic areas, petechiae, or abnormal bleeding. Monitor prothrombin time.
• Hypoglycemia is possible in patients with diabetes. Dosage of antidiabetic drug may need adjustment.
• Use with diet high in calories and protein unless contraindicated.

No significant interactions.

Special considerations:
• Contraindicated in prostatic hypertrophy with obstruction; carcinoma of male breast; prostatic cancer; cardiac, hepatic, or renal decompensation; nephrosis; and in premature infants. Use cautiously in prepubertal males; patients with diabetes or coronary disease; patients taking ACTH, corticosteroids, or anticoagulants.
• Hypercalcemic symptoms may be difficult to distinguish from symptoms of condition being treated unless anticipated and thought of as a cluster. Hypercalcemia is particularly likely to occur with metastatic breast cancer and may indicate bone metastases. Therapy should be discontinued.
• Females should report menstrual irregularities; therapy should be discontinued pending etiologic determination.
• Virilizing effects may be irreversible despite prompt stopping of therapy.
• In children, therapy should be preceded by X-ray of wrist bones to establish level of bone maturation. During treatment, bone maturation may proceed more rapidly than linear growth; dosage should be intermittent and X-rays taken periodically.
• Edema is generally controllable with salt restriction and/or diuretics.
• Jaundice is possible. Dose adjustment may reverse condition. If liver function studies are abnormal, therapy should be discontinued.
• Patients on concomitant anticoagulant therapy may develop ecchymotic areas, petechiae, or abnormal bleeding. Prothrombin time should be monitored.
• Hypoglycemia is possible in patients with diabetes. Dosage of antidiabetic drug may need adjustment.
• May lower fasting blood sugar in both diabetic and nondiabetic patients.
• Does not enhance athletic ability.
• Anabolic steroids may alter many laboratory studies during therapy and for 2 to 3 weeks after therapy is stopped.

No significant interactions.

Special considerations:
• Contraindicated in women of childbearing potential (possible masculinization of female infant); in elderly, asthenic males who may react adversely to androgen overstimulation; and in hypercalcemia; cardiac, hepatic, or renal decompensation; prostatic or breast cancer in males; benign prostatic hypertrophy with obstruction; conditions aggravated by fluid retention; hypertension; and in premature infants. Use cautiously in myocardial infarction or coronary artery disease.
• Treatment of breast cancer usually restricted to patients 1 to 5 years postmenopausal.
• Edema is generally controllable with salt restriction and/or diuretics.
• Periodic serum cholesterol and calcium determinations, and cardiac and liver function studies recommended. Jaundice is possible.
• In metastatic breast cancer, hypercalcemia may indicate progression of bone metastases.
• Therapeutic response in breast cancer is usually apparent within 3 months. Therapy should be stopped if signs of disease progression appear.
• Enhances hypoglycemia; patient should know signs of hypoglycemia and report them immediately if they occur.
• Patients receiving concomitant anticoagulants may develop ecchymoses, petechiae, and abnormal bleeding.
• Signs of virilization in females should be promptly reported.
• Use with diet high in calories and protein unless contraindicated.
• Buccal tablets twice as potent as oral tablets. Patient should avoid eating, drinking, chewing, or smoking while buccal tablet is in place. Tablet is not to be swallowed. Tablet requires 30 to 60 minutes to dissolve. Patient should change tablet absorption site with each dose to minimize risk of buccal irritation.
• Does not enhance athletic ability.

No significant interactions.

Special considerations:
• Contraindicated in prostatic hypertrophy with obstruction; male breast and prostatic cancer; cardiac, hepatic, or renal decompensation; nephrosis; and in premature infants. Use cautiously in prepubertal males; patients with diabetes or coronary disease; patients taking ACTH, corticosteroids, or anticoagulants.
• Drug should be injected deep I.M., preferably into upper outer quadrant of gluteal muscle in adults.
• Serum cholesterol should be monitored in cardiac patients.
• Hypercalcemia is most likely to occur in patients with breast cancer; these patients should have quantitative urinary and serum calcium

(continued on following page)

NAMES, INDICATIONS AND DOSAGES	SIDE EFFECTS
nandrolone *(continued)* **Tissue-building (decanoate):** ADULTS: 50 to 100 mg I.M. q 3 to 4 weeks. CHILDREN 2 TO 13 YEARS: 25 to 50 mg I.M. q 3 to 4 weeks. **Severe debility or disease states (phenpropionate):** ADULTS: 50 to 100 mg I.M. weekly. CHILDREN 2 TO 13 YEARS: 12.5 to 25 mg I.M. q 2 to 4 weeks. CHILDREN UNDER 2 YEARS: 12.5 mg I.M. q 2 to 4 weeks. Therapy should be intermittent, based on therapeutic response. **Tissue building and/or erythropoietic effects (phenpropionate):** ADULTS: 25 to 50 mg I.M. weekly.	**CV:** edema. **GI:** gastroenteritis, nausea, vomiting, diarrhea, change in appetite. **GU:** bladder irritability. **Hepatic:** jaundice. **Hypoestrogenic:** in females—flushing; sweating; vaginitis with itching, drying, burning, or bleeding; menstrual irregularities with large doses. **Local:** pain at injection site, induration. **Other:** hypercalcemia, hypercalciuria.
oxandrolone Anavar **To combat catabolic effects of corticosteroid therapy, osteoporosis, prolonged immobilization and debilitated states:** ADULTS: 2.5 mg P.O. b.i.d., t.i.d., or q.i.d.; up to 20 mg daily for 2 to 4 weeks. CHILDREN: 0.25 mg/kg daily P.O. for 2 to 4 weeks. Continuous therapy should not exceed 3 months.	**Androgenic:** in females—*acne, edema, oily skin, weight gain, hirsutism, hoarseness,* clitoral enlargement, decreased or increased libido. In males—prepubertal: premature epiphyseal closure, acne, priapism, growth of body and facial hair, phallic enlargement; postpubertal: testicular atrophy, oligospermia, decreased ejaculatory volume, impotence, gynecomastia, epididymitis. **CV:** edema. **GI:** gastroenteritis, nausea, vomiting, constipation or diarrhea, change in appetite. **GU:** bladder irritability. **Hepatic:** jaundice. **Hypoestrogenic:** in females—flushing; sweating; vaginitis with itching, drying, burning, or bleeding; menstrual irregularities. **Other:** hypercalcemia.
oxymetholone Adroyd♦, Anapolon 50♦♦ **Aplastic anemia:** ADULTS AND CHILDREN: 1 to 5 mg/kg P.O. daily. Dose highly individualized; response not immediate. Trial of 3 to 6 months required. **Osteoporosis, catabolic conditions:** ADULTS: 5 to 15 mg P.O. daily, or up to 30 mg P.O. daily. CHILDREN OVER 6 YEARS: up to 10 mg P.O. daily. CHILDREN UNDER 6 YEARS: 1.25 mg P.O. daily or up to q.i.d. Continuous therapy should	**Androgenic:** in females—*acne, edema, oily skin, weight gain, hirsutism, hoarseness,* clitoral enlargement, decreased or increased libido, male-pattern hair loss. In males—prepubertal: premature epiphyseal closure, acne, priapism, growth of body and facial hair, phallic enlargement; postpubertal: testicular atrophy, oligospermia, decreased ejaculatory volume, impotence, gynecomastia, epididymitis. **CV:** edema. **GI:** gastroenteritis, nausea, vomiting, constipation, diarrhea, change in appetite. **GU:** bladder irritability. **Hepatic:** jaundice. **Hypoestrogenic:** in females—flushing; sweat-

INTERACTIONS AND SPECIAL CONSIDERATIONS

level determinations.

- Females should report menstrual irregularities; therapy should be discontinued pending etiologic determination.
- Virilizing effects may be irreversible despite prompt discontinuation of therapy.
- Boys under age 7 should be closely observed for precocious development of male sexual characteristics.
- In children, therapy should be preceded by X-ray of wrist bones to establish level of bone maturation. During treatment, bone maturation may proceed more rapidly than linear growth; dosage should be intermittent and X-rays taken periodically.
- Edema is generally controllable with salt restrictions and/or diuretics.
- Jaundice is possible. Dose adjustment may reverse condition. If liver function studies are abnormal, therapy should be discontinued.
- Patients receiving concomitant anticoagulant therapy may develop ecchymotic areas, petechiae, or abnormal bleeding. Prothrombin time should be monitored.
- Hypoglycemia is possible in patients with diabetes. Dosage of antidiabetic drug may need adjustment.
- Use with diet high in calories and protein unless contraindicated.
- Does not enhance athletic ability.
- Considered an adjunctive therapy.
- Anabolic steroids may alter many laboratory studies during therapy and for 2 to 3 weeks after therapy is stopped.

No significant interactions.

Special considerations:

- Contraindicated in prostatic hypertrophy with obstruction; prostatic and male breast cancer; cardiac, hepatic, or renal decompensation; nephrosis; and in premature infants. Use cautiously in prepubertal males; patients with diabetes or coronary disease; patients taking ACTH, corticosteroids, or anticoagulants.
- Hypercalcemia symptoms may be difficult to distinguish from symptoms of condition being treated unless anticipated and thought of as a cluster. Hypercalcemia most likely to occur with metastatic breast cancer and may indicate bone metastases.
- Females should report menstrual irregularities; therapy should be discontinued pending etiologic determination.
- Virilizing effects may be irreversible despite prompt stopping of therapy. Benefits should be weighed against effects.
- Boys under age 7 should be closely observed for precocious development of male sexual characterisitics.
- In children, therapy should be preceded by X-ray of wrist bones to establish level of bone maturation. During treatment, bone maturation may proceed more rapidly than linear growth; dosage should be intermittent and X-rays taken periodically.
- Edema is generally controllable with salt restriction and/or diuretics.
- Jaundice is possible. Dose adjustment may reverse condition. Periodic liver function studies are recommended.
- Patient on concomitant anticoagulant therapy may develop ecchymotic areas, petechiae, or abnormal bleeding. Monitor prothrombin time.
- Hypoglycemia is possible in patients with diabetes. Change of dosage in antidiabetic drug may be required.
- Use with diet high in calories and protein unless contraindicated.
- Does not enhance athletic ability.
- Anabolic steroids may alter many laboratory studies during therapy and for 2 to 3 weeks after therapy is stopped.

No significant interactions.

Special considerations:

- Contraindicated in prostatic hypertrophy with obstruction; prostatic and male breast cancer; cardiac, hepatic, or renal decompensation; nephrosis; and in premature infants. Use cautiously in prepubertal males; patients with diabetes or coronary diseases; patients taking ACTH, corticosteroids, or anticoagulants.
- Hypercalcemia symptoms may be difficult to distinguish from symptoms of condition being treated unless anticipated and thought of as a cluster. Hypercalcemia most likely to occur in metastatic breast cancer and may indicate bone metastases.
- Supportive treatment of anemias (transfusions, correction of iron, folic acid, vitamin B_{12}, or pyroxidine deficiency). Should be taken 3 to 6 months for response.
- Effects in osteoporosis usually seen in 4 to 6 weeks.
- Virilizing effects may be irreversible despite prompt stopping of therapy. Benefits should be weighed against effects.
- Boys under age 7 should be closely observed for precocious development of male sexual characteristics.
- Females should report menstrual irregularities; therapy should be discontinued pending

(continued on following page)

NAMES, INDICATIONS AND DOSAGES	SIDE EFFECTS
oxymetholone *(continued)* not exceed 30 days in children; 90 days in any patient.	ing; vaginitis with itching, drying, burning, or bleeding; menstrual irregularities. **Other:** hypercalcemia.
stanozolol Winstrol♦ **To increase hemoglobin in some cases of aplastic anemia:** ADULTS: 2 mg P.O. t.i.d. CHILDREN 6 TO 12 YEARS: up to 2 mg P.O. t.i.d. CHILDREN UNDER 6 YEARS: 1 mg P.O. b.i.d. Therapy should be intermittent.	**Androgenic:** in females—*acne, edema, oily skin, weight gain, hirsutism, hoarseness,* clitoral enlargement, decreased or increased libido. In males—prepubertal: premature epiphyseal closure, acne, priapism, growth of body and facial hair, phallic enlargement; postpubertal: testicular atrophy, oligospermia, decreased ejaculatory volume, impotence, gynecomastia, epididymitis. **CV:** edema. **GI:** gastroenteritis, nausea, vomiting, constipation, diarrhea, change in appetite. **GU:** bladder irritability. **Hypoestrogenic:** in females—flushing; sweating; vaginitis with itching, drying, burning or bleeding; menstrual irregularities. **Other:** hypercalcemia.
testosterone Android-T, Andronaq, Histerone, Malogen♦, Oreton, Testoject **Eunuchoidism, eunuchism, male climacteric symptoms:** ADULTS: 10 to 25 mg I.M. 2 to 5 times weekly; or 2 to 6 pellets (75 mg each) implanted subcutaneously q 3 to 6 months. **Breast engorgement of non–breast-feeding mothers:** 25 to 50 mg I.M. daily for 3 to 4 days, starting at delivery. **Breast cancer in women 1 to 5 years postmenopausal:** 100 mg I.M. 3 times weekly as long as improvement maintained.	**Androgenic:** in females—*acne, edema, oily skin, weight gain, hirsutism, hoarseness,* clitoral enlargement, decreased or increased libido. In males—prepubertal: premature epiphyseal closure, acne, priapism, growth of body and facial hair, phallic enlargement; postpubertal: testicular atrophy, oligospermia, decreased ejaculatory volume, impotence, gynecomastia, epididymitis. **CV:** edema. **GI:** gastroenteritis, nausea, vomiting, constipation, diarrhea, change in appetite. **GU:** bladder irritability. **Hepatic:** jaundice. **Hypoestrogenic:** in females—flushing; sweating; vaginitis with itching, drying, burning, or bleeding; menstrual irregularities. **Local:** pain at injection site, induration, irritation and sloughing with pellet implantation, edema. **Other:** hypercalcemia.

♦ Available in U.S. and Canada. ♦♦ Available in Canada only.
All other products (no symbol) available in U.S. only. Italicized side effects are common or life-threatening.

INTERACTIONS AND SPECIAL CONSIDERATIONS

etiologic determination.
- In children, therapy should be preceded by X-ray of wrist bones to establish level of bone maturation. During treatment, bone maturation may proceed more rapidly than linear growth; dosage should be intermittent and X-rays taken periodically. Epiphyseal development may continue 6 months after stopping therapy.
- Edema is generally controllable with salt restriction and/or diuretics.
- Jaundice is possible. Dose adjustment may reverse condition. If liver function studies are abnormal, therapy should be discontinued.
- Patient on concomitant anticoagulant therapy may develop ecchymotic areas, petechiae, or abnormal bleeding. Monitor prothrombin time.
- Hypoglycemia may develop in patients with diabetes. Change of dosage in antidiabetic drug may be required.
- Use with diet high in calories and protein unless contraindicated.
- Does not enhance athletic ability.
- Anabolic steroids may alter many laboratory studies during therapy and for 2 to 3 weeks after therapy is stopped.

No significant interactions.

Special considerations:
- Contraindicated in prostatic hypertrophy with obstruction; prostatic and male breast cancer; cardiac, hepatic, or renal decompensation; nephrosis; and in premature infants. Use cautiously in prepubertal males; patients with diabetes or coronary disease; patients taking ACTH, corticosteroids, or anticoagulants.
- Hypercalcemia symptoms may be difficult to distinguish from symptoms of condition being treated unless anticipated and thought of as a cluster. Hypercalcemia most likely to occur in metastatic breast cancer and may indicate bone metastases.
- Females should report menstrual irregularities; therapy should be discontinued pending etiologic determination.
- Smaller dose (2 mg b.i.d.) is used in females to avoid virilizing effects. Virilizing effects may be irreversible despite prompt stopping of therapy. Benefits should be weighed against effects.
- Boys under age 7 should be closely observed for precocious development of male sexual characteristics.
- In children, therapy should be preceded by X-ray of wrist bones to establish level of bone maturation. During treatment, bone maturation may proceed more rapidly than linear growth; dosage should be intermittent and X-rays taken periodically.
- Edema is generally controllable with salt restriction and/or diuretics.
- Jaundice is possible. Dose adjustment may reverse condition. Liver function studies should be checked regularly. If abnormal, therapy should be discontinued.
- Patient on concomitant anticoagulant therapy may develop ecchymotic areas, petechiae, or abnormal bleeding. Monitor prothrombin time.
- Hypoglycemia may develop in patients with diabetes. Change of dosage in antidiabetic drug may be required.
- Use with diet high in calories and protein unless contraindicated.
- Should be administered before or with meals to minimize GI distress.
- Serum cholesterol should be monitored in cardiac patients.
- Does not enhance athletic ability.
- Anabolic steroids may alter many laboratory studies during therapy and for 2 to 3 weeks after therapy is stopped.

No significant interactions.

Special considerations:
- Contraindicated in women of childbearing potential (possible masculinization of female infant); in elderly, asthenic males who may react adversely to androgen overstimulation; and in hypercalcemia; cardiac, hepatic, or renal decompensation; prostatic or breast cancer in males; benign prostatic hypertrophy with obstruction; conditions aggravated by fluid retention; hypertension; and in premature infants. Use cautiously in myocardial infarction or coronary artery disease, and in prepubertal males.
- Edema is generally controllable with salt restriction and/or diuretics.
- Periodic liver function studies should be performed.
- In metastatic breast cancer, hypercalcemia usually indicates progression of bone metastases.
- Therapeutic response in breast cancer is usually apparent within 3 months. If signs of disease progression appear, therapy should be stopped.
- Enhances hypoglycemia; patient should report signs of hyperinsulinism.
- Males should report priapism, reduced ejaculatory volume, and gynecomastia. Drug should be withdrawn if these occur.
- Virilization in females requires reevaluation of treatment.
- Prepubertal males should be monitored by X-ray for rate of bone maturation.
- Use with diet high in calories and protein unless contraindicated.
- Drug should be injected deep into upper outer quadrant of gluteal muscle.
- Irritation and sloughing with pellet implantation.
- Patients on concomitant anticoagulant therapy may develop ecchymotic areas, petechiae, or abnormal bleeding. Monitor prothrombin time.

(continued on following page)

NAMES, INDICATIONS AND DOSAGES	SIDE EFFECTS

testosterone
(continued)

testosterone cypionate
Andro-Cyp, Androgen-860, D-Test, Depotest, Depo-Test, Depo-Testosterone♦, Durandro, Duratest, Jactatest, Malogen Cyp
testosterone enanthate
Android-T, Andryl, Arderone, Delatestryl♦, Everone, Malogen LA, Malogex♦♦, Span-Test, Testate, Testone LA, Testostroval-P.A.
testosterone propionate
Androlan, Androlin, Malogen in Oil♦♦, Oreton Propionate, Testex, Vulvan

Eunuchism, eunuchoidism, deficiency after castration and male climacteric:
ADULTS: 200 to 400 mg (cypionate or enanthate) I.M. q 4 weeks.

Oligospermia:
ADULTS: 100 to 200 mg (cypionate or enanthate) I.M. q 4 to 6 weeks for development and maintenance of testicular function.

Eunuchism and eunuchoidism, male climacteric, impotence:
ADULTS: 10 to 25 mg (propionate) I.M. 2 to 4 times weekly; or 5 to 20 mg buccal daily (strictly individualized).

Breast engorgement of non–breast-feeding mothers: 40 mg (propionate) buccal daily, for 3 to 5 days starting at delivery.

Metastatic breast cancer in women: 50 to 100 mg (propionate) I.M. 3 times weekly; or 100 mg buccal daily as long as improvement maintained.

Postpubertal cryptorchidism:
15 mg (propionate) buccal daily.

Androgenic: in females—*acne, edema, oily skin, weight gain, hirsutism, hoarseness,* clitoral enlargement, changes in libido. In males—prepubertal: premature epiphyseal closure, acne, priapism, growth of body and facial hair, phallic enlargement; postpubertal: testicular atrophy, oligospermia, decreased ejaculatory volume, impotence, gynecomastia, epididymitis.
CV: edema.
GI: gastroenteritis, nausea, vomiting, constipation, diarrhea, change in appetite.
GU: bladder irritability.
Hepatic: jaundice.
Local: pain at injection site, induration, postinjection furunculosis.
Other: hypercalcemia.

♦ Available in U.S. and Canada. ♦♦ Available in Canada only.
All other products (no symbol) available in U.S. only. Italicized side effects are common or life-threatening.

INTERACTIONS AND SPECIAL CONSIDERATIONS

• Implantation of pellets may take place in physician's office in a minor surgical procedure with aseptic precautions observed.

• Many laboratory studies may be altered during therapy and for 2 to 3 weeks after therapy is stopped.

No significant interactions.

Special considerations:

• Contraindicated in women of childbearing potential (possible masculinization of female infant); in elderly, asthenic males who may react adversely to androgen overstimulation; and in hypercalcemia; cardiac, hepatic, or renal decompensation; prostatic or breast cancer in males; benign prostatic hypertrophy with obstruction; conditions aggravated by fluid retention; hypertension; and in premature infants. Use cautiously in myocardial infarction or coronary artery disease, and in prepubertal males.

• Periodic liver function studies should be performed.

• In metastatic breast cancer, hypercalcemia usually indicates progression of bone metastases.

• Response in breast cancer is usually apparent within 3 months. If signs of disease progression appear, therapy should be stopped.

• Enhances hypoglycemia; patient should report signs of hypoglycemia immediately if they occur.

• Males should report priapism, reduced ejaculatory volume, and gynecomastia. Drug should be withdrawn if they occur.

• Ecchymoses and petechiae may appear with concomitant anticoagulants. Prothrombin time should be monitored.

• Should be injected deep into upper outer quadrant of gluteal muscle and soreness at site reported; possibility of postinjection furunculosis.

• Virilization in females requires reevaluation of treatment.

• Prepubertal males should be monitored by X-ray for rate of bone maturation.

• Edema is generally controllable with salt restriction and/or diuretics.

• Use with diet high in calories and protein unless contraindicated.

• Good oral hygiene decreases possibility of irritation from buccal tablet. Patient shouldn't eat, drink, chew, or smoke while tablet is in place.

• Daily requirements best administered in divided doses.

• May alter many laboratory studies during therapy and for 2 to 3 weeks after therapy is stopped.

53

Oral contraceptives

estrogen with progestogen

Oral contraceptives are one of the most popular and effective forms of birth control used today. Although they're convenient to use, they may produce serious side effects in women predisposed to certain risk factors.

Currently, two recognized classes of oral contraceptives are being marketed: an estrogen-progestogen combination and a progestogen-only minipill. The combination tablet contains a synthetic estrogen compound (ethinyl estradiol or mestranol) and a synthetic progestogen (ethynodiol diacetate, norethindrone, norethindrone acetate, norethynodrel, or norgestrel). It is taken for 21 days of the menstrual cycle (usually days 5 through 24). Natural steroids aren't used because large doses are required to achieve the same pharmacologic effect as the synthetics.

The progestogen-only pill contains either norethindrone or norgestrel and is taken once daily every day of the menstrual cycle. (For complete information on progestogen-only contraceptives, see Chapter 55, PROGESTOGENS.)

The minipill is not widely used because it frequently causes menstrual irregularities. Although slightly less effective than the combination product, it may suffice for the patient who has to avoid the use of estrogen or for whom pregnancy is not life-threatening.

In choosing an appropriate oral contraceptive, the doctor must weigh the side effects of the high-dose combinations against the possibly weaker action of the low-dose combinations. In general, the more estrogen and progestogen in the preparation, the more serious, frequent, and fast-acting the side effects. The lower the hormonal concentration, the less effective the preparation, especially in a woman taking drugs that increase metabolism and thus lower the blood levels of estrogens. A woman who misses taking a pill may have a greater risk of failure with a low-dose than with a high-dose preparation.

Generally, oral contraceptives that contain the smallest effective quantity of hormone and produce the fewest side effects are preferable. This usually means a product with 50 mcg or less of estrogen.

Major uses

Oral contraceptives are used to prevent pregnancy. High-dose estrogen-progestogen combinations are usually used to treat such menstrual cycle disorders as endometriosis and hypermenorrhea.

Estrogen with progestogen is also commonly used to treat hormone-induced acne, but it's often ineffective.

Mechanism of action

Oral contraceptives inhibit ovulation through a negative feedback mechanism directed at the hypothalamus. They may also prevent transport of the ovum through the fallopian tubes.

• Estrogen suppresses secretion of follicle-stimulating hormone, blocking follicular development and ovulation.

• Progestogen suppresses luteinizing hormone secretion so ovulation can't occur even if the follicle develops. Progestogen thickens cervical mucus, which interferes with sperm migration, and causes endometrial changes that prevent implantation of the fertilized ovum.

PATIENT-TEACHING AID

CHOOSING A METHOD OF CONTRACEPTION

Dear Patient:

Before you decide on a method of contraception, ask your doctor to explain the advantages and disadvantages of each method. Since each woman's contraceptive needs vary, your doctor can help by properly assessing your life-style, answering your questions, and considering your needs.

If you choose an oral contraceptive, follow these guidelines:

- Determine that oral contraceptives are safe for you. Your doctor is the best person to help you make this decision. Always remain under a doctor's care while you're on the pill. *Remember:* if you have thromboembolic disease, you *should not* take the pill.
- Take the medication as prescribed. If you miss *one* pill, take it as soon as you remember. If you miss *two* consecutive pills, take two pills a day for the next two days. If you miss *three or more* consecutive pills, stop treatment and use another contraceptive for the rest of the cycle (month). Then, begin again, according to your doctor's directions.
- Remember to use an alternate method of contraception for the first 7 days after you begin taking the pill. Also, if you stop taking the pill for any reason, use an alternate contraceptive method.
- Call your doctor if you notice any side effects like nausea, headache, dizziness, or swelling.
- Recognize that the pill increases your susceptibility to vaginal infections. Call your doctor if you notice any vaginal discharge, itching, or pain.
- Schedule a Pap test semiannually and a complete physical examination yearly.
- Contact your doctor if you miss your menstrual period. If you miss two consecutive periods, your doctor may advise you to stop taking the pill until he can determine whether or not you may be pregnant.
- Consult your doctor if you wish to discontinue therapy, especially if you plan to become pregnant. He may advise you not to become pregnant for 2 or more months *after* discontinuing the pill.

Absorption, distribution, metabolism, and excretion

Oral contraceptives are rapidly and completely absorbed from the GI tract and distributed to all body tissues. They are metabolized in the liver and excreted in urine.

Onset and duration

As contraceptives begun on day 5 of the menstrual cycle, these drugs theoretically provide complete protection, if taken on schedule. However, alternative protection is recommended for at least the first 7 days of therapy since ovulation and conception are still possible during this time.

Duration of effect is about 1 day; hence strict compliance is necessary to ensure effectiveness. For complex endocrine, metabolic, and acne disorders, several months of treatment may be needed to obtain a satisfactory response.

NAMES, INDICATIONS AND DOSAGES

estrogen with progestogen

Brevicon, Demulen♦, Enovid, Enovid-E, Loestrin 1/20, Loestrin 1.5/30♦, Lo/Ovral, Min-Ovral♦♦, Modicon, Norinyl 1 + 35, Norinyl 1 + 50♦, Norinyl 1 + 80♦, Norinyl 2 mg♦, Norlestrin♦, Ortho-Novum 1/50♦, Ortho-Novum 1/80♦, Ortho-Novum 2 mg♦, Ovcon 35, Ovcon 50, Ovral, Ovulen♦

Contraception:

WOMEN: 1 tablet P.O. daily, beginning on day 5 of menstrual cycle (first day of menstrual flow is day 1). With 20- and 21-tablet packages, new dosing cycle begins 7 days after last tablet taken. With 28-tablet packages, dosage is 1 tablet daily without interruption; extra tablets are placebos or contain iron.

If only 1 or 2 doses are missed, dosage may continue on schedule. If 3 or more doses are missed, remaining tablets in monthly package must be discarded and another contraceptive method substituted. If next menstrual period doesn't begin on schedule, rule out pregnancy before starting new dosing cycle. If menstrual period begins, start new dosing cycle 7 days after last tablet was taken. If all doses have been taken on schedule and 1 menstrual period is missed, continue dosing cycle. If 2 consecutive menstrual periods are missed, pregnancy test is required before new dosing cycle is started.

Hypermenorrhea:

WOMEN: use high-dose combinations only. Dose same as for contraception.

Endometriosis:

WOMEN: Cyclic therapy: 1 tablet Ortho-Novum 10 mg P.O. daily for 20 days from day 5 to day 24 of menstrual cycle.

Suppressive therapy: Enovid 5 mg or 10 mg—1 tablet P.O. daily for 2 weeks starting on day 5 of menstrual cycle. Continue without interruption for 6 to 9 months, increasing dose by 5 to 10 mg q 2 weeks, up to 20 mg daily. Up to 40 mg daily may be needed if breakthrough bleeding occurs.

SIDE EFFECTS

CNS: *headache, dizziness,* depression, libido changes, lethargy, migraine.
CV: *thromboembolism,* hypertension, edema.
EENT: worsening of myopia or astigmatism, intolerance to contact lenses.
GI: *nausea,* vomiting, abdominal cramps, bloating, diarrhea, constipation, anorexia, changes in appetite, weight gain, *bowel ischemia.*
GU: *breakthrough bleeding,* dysmenorrhea, amenorrhea, cervical erosion or abnormal secretions, enlargement of uterine fibromas, vaginal candidiasis.
Hepatic: gallbladder disease, cholestatic jaundice, liver tumors.
Metabolic: hyperglycemia, hypercalcemia, folic acid deficiency.
Skin: rash, acne, seborrhea, oily skin, erythema multiforme.
Other: *breast tenderness,* enlargement, secretion.
Adverse effects may be more serious, frequent, and rapid in onset with high-dose than with low-dose combinations.

♦ Available in U.S. and Canada. ♦♦ Available in Canada only.
All other products (no symbol) available in U.S. only. Italicized side effects are common or life-threatening.

INTERACTIONS AND SPECIAL CONSIDERATIONS

Interactions:

AMPICILLIN, TETRACYCLINE, BARBITURATES, ANTICONVULSANTS, RIFAMPIN: may diminish contraceptive effectiveness. Use supplemental form of contraception.

Special considerations:

- Contraindicated in thromboembolic disorders, cerebrovascular or coronary artery disease, myocardial infarction, known or suspected cancer of breasts or reproductive organs, benign or malignant hepatic tumors, undiagnosed abnormal vaginal bleeding, known or suspected pregnancy, lactation; and in adolescents with incomplete epiphyseal closure. Contraindicated in women 35 years or older who smoke over 15 cigarettes a day, and in all women over age 40. Use cautiously in hypertension, mental depression, migraine, epilepsy, asthma, diabetes mellitus, amenorrhea, scanty or irregular periods, fibrocystic breast disease, family history (mother, grandmother, sister) of breast or genital tract cancer, renal or gallbladder disease. Development or worsening of these conditions should be reported. Prolonged therapy inadvisable in women who plan to become pregnant.
- If 1 menstrual period is missed and tablets have been taken on schedule, patient should continue taking them. If 2 consecutive menstrual periods are missed, patient should stop drug and have pregnancy test. Progestogens may cause birth defects if taken early in pregnancy.
- Missed doses in midcycle greatly increase likelihood of pregnancy.
- Headache, nausea, dizziness, breast tenderness, spotting, and breakthrough bleeding are common at first. These should diminish after 3 to 6 dosing cycles (months). However, breakthrough bleeding in patients taking high-dose estrogen-progestogen combinations for menstrual disorders may require dosage adjustment.
- Patient should immediately report abdominal pain; numbness, stiffness or pain in legs or buttocks; pressure or pain in chest; shortness of breath; severe headache; visual disturbances, such as blind spots, blurriness, or flashing lights; undiagnosed vaginal bleeding or discharge; 2 consecutive missed menstrual periods; lumps in the breast; swelling of hands or feet; severe pain in the abdomen (tumor rupture in the liver).
- Patient should take tablets at same time each day; nighttime dosing may reduce nausea and headaches.
- Semiannual Pap tests and annual gynecologic examinations are essential while taking estrogen-progestogen combinations.
- The patient should know the signs and symptoms of gallbladder disease.
- Delay in achieving pregnancy is possible when pill is discontinued.
- The patient should be taught how to perform a breast self-examination.
- The patient should be advised of increased risks associated with simultaneous use of cigarettes and oral contraceptives.
- Many laboratory tests are affected by oral contraceptives; some are: increase in serum bilirubin, alkaline phosphatase, SGOT, SGPT, and protein-bound iodine; decrease in glucose tolerance and urinary excretion of 17-hydroxycorticosteroids (17-OHCS).
- Estrogens and progestogens may alter glucose tolerance, thus changing requirements for antidiabetic drugs.
- The patient should weigh herself at least twice a week and report any sudden weight gain or edema.
- Many doctors recommend that women not become pregnant within 2 months after stopping the pill. The patient should be advised to check with her doctor about how soon pregnancy may be attempted after hormonal therapy is stopped.
- The same drug should not be taken for longer than 18 months without reevaluation.
- Many doctors advise women on the pill for extended time (5 years or more) to stop drug and use other birth control methods in order to periodically reassess patient while off hormone therapy.

54

Estrogens

chlorotrianisene
dienestrol
diethylstilbestrol
diethylstilbestrol diphosphate
esterified estrogens
estradiol
estradiol cypionate
estradiol valerate
estrogenic substances, conjugated
estrone
ethinyl estradiol
quinestrol

Estrogens are organic compounds that occur naturally in humans and animals; they are also produced synthetically. They can be chemically classified as either steroidal or nonsteroidal estrogens. Steroidal estrogens include all natural estrogens (estradiol, estriol, and estrone), esters of natural estrogens (estradiol cypionate, estradiol valerate, and esterified estrogens), a conjugate of natural estrogens (conjugated estrogenic substances), and a semisynthetic estrogen (ethinyl estradiol). Nonsteroidal estrogens comprise the synthetic estrogens (chlorotrianisene, dienestrol, diethylstilbestrol, diethylstilbestrol diphosphate, and quinestrol). Estrogens have been traditionally described as agents that produce estrus, whether or not they are derived from the ovaries. Secreted mainly by the ovarian follicles, they are also secreted in large amounts by the placenta, in smaller quantities by the testes, and—in both sexes—by the adrenal cortex.

The reproductive physiochemistry of estrogens in women parallels that of testosterone in men. Estrogens promote growth and development of the vagina, uterus, and fallopian tubes; enlargement of the breasts; molding of the body contours; and closure of the epiphyses of the long bones. They also promote growth of axillary and pubic hair, and pigmentation of the skin of the nipples and genital region. They stimulate estrus and produce changes in the genital tract and mammary glands during pregnancy.

Metabolic activities: Estrogens reduce blood cholesterol by altering lipid metabolism, exert a protein anabolic action, and promote sodium and water retention.

Major uses

Estrogens have the following uses:

• As replacement therapy, they're used in menopause, pituitary failure to stimulate development of secondary sex characteristics, and postoperative radical hysterectomy.

They are used to treat atrophic changes in the lower genital tract (as in atrophic vaginitis or pruritus vulvae), which are caused by chronic estrogen deficiency.

They can also initiate menstrual periods and relieve secondary amenorrhea (as in female hypogonadism, female castration, and primary ovarian failure).

• They relieve postpartum breast engorgement.

• They are used in the palliation and inhibition of androgen-dependent primary tumors with soft tissue metastases (for example, inoperable cancer of the prostate and breast in males and inoperable postmenopausal breast carcinoma in females).

• They provide contraception (in combination with progestogen). Their use as a contraceptive is described in greater detail in Chapter 53, ORAL CONTRACEPTIVES.

Mechanism of action

• Estrogens replace endogenous hormones to maintain normal hormonal balance.
• They suppress lactation by inhibiting prolactin secretion from the anterior pituitary.
• They antagonize the action of androgens that stimulate growth of tumor tissue.
• As oral contraceptives, estrogens suppress gonadotropin output from the anterior pi-

GUIDELINES FOR PATIENTS ON ESTROGEN THERAPY

• Any discomforting side effects, such as the following, should be reported:
—Mood changes, especially depression
—Thrombophlebitis (warmth or pain in the calf)
—Excessive fluid retention
—Jaundice
—Excessive nausea and vomiting
—Dizziness and frequent headaches (which point to elevated blood pressure)
—Loss of scalp hair
—Hirsutism
—Indigestion after eating fatty foods, or stomach pain.

• Gynecologic visits should be scheduled regularly—at least once a year. (Visits should include a pelvic examination, a Pap test, and a breast examination.)

• Breast self-examination should be performed monthly.

• Bleeding after estrogen withdrawal is expected. In the postmenopausal woman, bleeding is pseudomenstruation and does not mean fertility has been restored.

• A patient with diabetes should make frequent urine checks for sugar and acetone.

Because there's some controversy concerning a link between estrogen and cancer, the patient may wish to discuss her concerns with her doctor. Follow-up examinations should be scheduled to carefully monitor this risk.

Estrogen—specifically diethylstilbestrol—is used to *treat* some cancers. The patient should understand this mode of therapy.

tuitary by a negative feedback effect. (Their mechanism of action is described in greater detail in Chapter 53.)

Absorption, distribution, metabolism, and excretion
Estrogens are readily absorbed from the gastrointestinal tract, distributed to all body tissues, metabolized in the liver, and excreted primarily in urine. Small amounts are also eliminated—through the bile—in feces.

• Estradiol is rapidly metabolized (oxidized) in the liver to estrone, which is subsequently converted to estriol.

• Ethinyl estradiol is well absorbed when given orally. Most of it is metabolized in the liver. Because metabolism is slow, the drug retains its high intrinsic potency.

Onset and duration

• Estrogens begin to act immediately.

• Oral estrogens (except chlorotrianisene) have a short duration of action; daily doses are usually needed. Chlorotrianisene is a long-acting drug because it's stored in and released only gradually from adipose tissue.

• Parenteral estrogens have a longer duration of action than the oral preparations; their effect may last several days.

Combination products
MENRIUM 5-2♦: chlordiazepoxide 5 mg and esterified estrogens 0.2 mg.
MENRIUM 5-4♦: chlordiazepoxide 5 mg and esterified estrogens 0.4 mg.
MILPREM-200: conjugated estrogens 0.45 mg and meprobamate 200 mg.
See Chapter 53 for oral contraceptives and other estrogen combinations.

NAMES, INDICATIONS AND DOSAGES	SIDE EFFECTS
chlorotrianisene Tace♦ MEN: **Prostatic cancer:** 12 to 25 mg P.O. daily. NON-BREAST-FEEDING MOTHERS: **Postpartum breast engorgement:** 72 mg P.O. b.i.d. for 2 days; or 50 mg q 6 hours for 6 doses; or 12 mg q.i.d. for 7 days. Start dosing within 8 hours after delivery. WOMEN: **Menopausal symptoms:** 12 to 25 mg P.O. daily for 30 days or cyclic (3 weeks on, 1 week off). **Female hypogonadism:** 12 to 25 mg P.O. for 21 days, followed by 1 dose of progesterone 100 mg I.M. or 5 days of oral progestogen given concurrently with last 5 days of chlorotrianisene (i.e., medroxyprogesterone 5 to 10 mg). **Atrophic vaginitis:** 12 to 25 mg P.O. daily for 30 to 60 days.	**CNS:** headache, dizziness, chorea, migraine, depression, libido changes. **CV:** thrombophlebitis; *thromboembolism;* hypertension; edema; *increased risk of stroke, pulmonary embolism, and myocardial infarction.* **EENT:** worsening of myopia or astigmatism, intolerance to contact lenses. **GI:** *nausea,* vomiting, abdominal cramps, bloating, diarrhea, constipation, anorexia, increased appetite, excessive thirst, weight changes. **GU:** breakthrough bleeding, altered menstrual flow, dysmenorrhea, amenorrhea, cervical erosion or abnormal secretions, enlargement of uterine fibromas, vaginal candidiasis; *in males: gynecomastia, testicular atrophy, impotence.* **Hepatic:** cholestatic jaundice. **Metabolic:** hyperglycemia, hypercalcemia, folic acid deficiency. **Skin:** melasma, urticaria, acne, seborrhea, oily skin, hirsutism or loss of hair. **Other:** leg cramps, purpura, breast changes (tenderness, enlargement, secretion).
dienestrol Dienestrol Cream♦ Available in combination with sulfanilamide and aminacrine as AVC/Dienestrol, cream or suppositories POSTMENOPAUSAL WOMEN: **Atrophic vaginitis and kraurosis vulvae:** 1 to 2 applicatorfuls of cream daily for 2 weeks, then half that dose for 2 more weeks; or 1 to 2 vaginal suppositories daily for 1 month, as directed. **Atrophic and senile vaginitis and kraurosis vulvae when complicated by infection:** 1 applicatorful AVC/Dienestrol cream intravaginally daily or b.i.d. for 1 to 2 weeks, then every other day for 1 to 2 weeks.	**GU:** vaginal discharge; with excessive use, uterine bleeding. **Local:** increased discomfort, burning sensation. Systemic effects possible. **Other:** breast tenderness.
diethylstilbestrol DES, Stibilium♦♦ **diethylstilbestrol diphosphate** Honvol♦♦, Stilphostrol WOMEN: **Atrophic vaginitis or kraurosis vulvae:** 0.1 to 1 mg as suppository daily for 10 to 14 days concurrently with oral therapy; or up to 5 mg weekly as suppository. **Hypogonadism, castration, primary ovarian failure:** 0.2 to 0.5 mg P.O. daily. **Menopausal symptoms:** 0.1 to 2 mg P.O. daily in cycles of 3 weeks on and 1 week off. **Postcoital contraception ("morning-after pill"):** 25 mg P.O. b.i.d. for 5 days, starting within 72 hours after coitus. **Postpartum breast engorgement:** 5 mg P.O. daily or t.i.d. up to total dose of 30 mg. MEN: **Prostatic cancer:** 1 to 3 mg P.O. daily, initially; may be reduced to 1 mg P.O. daily, or	**CNS:** headache, dizziness, chorea, depression, lethargy. **CV:** *thrombophlebitis; thromboembolism;* hypertension; edema; *increased risk of stroke, pulmonary embolism, and mycardial infarction.* **EENT:** worsening of myopia or astigmatism, intolerance to contact lenses. **GI:** *nausea,* vomiting, abdominal cramps, bloating, diarrhea, constipation, anorexia, increased appetite, excessive thirst, weight changes. **GU:** breakthrough bleeding, altered menstrual flow, dysmenorrhea, amenorrhea, cervical erosion, altered cervical secretions, enlargement of uterine fibromas, vaginal candidiasis, loss of libido; *in males:* gynecomastia, testicular atrophy, impotence. **Hepatic:** cholestatic jaundice. **Metabolic:** hyperglycemia, hypercalcemia, folic acid deficiency. **Skin:** melasma, urticaria, acne, seborrhea, oily skin, hirsutism or loss of hair.

♦ Available in U.S. and Canada. ♦♦ Available in Canada only.
All other products (no symbol) available in U.S. only. Italicized side effects are common or life-threatening.

INTERACTIONS AND SPECIAL CONSIDERATIONS

No significant interactions.

Special considerations:

- Contraindicated in thrombophlebitis or thromboembolic disorders; cancer of breast, reproductive organs, or genitals; undiagnosed abnormal genital bleeding. Use cautiously in hypertension, asthma, mental depression, bone diseases, blood dyscrasias, gallbladder disease, migraine, seizures, diabetes mellitus, amenorrhea, heart failure, hepatic or renal dysfunction, and family history (mother, grandmother, sister) of breast or genital tract cancer. Development or worsening of these conditions may require stopping drug.
- FDA regulations require that female patients receive package insert explaining possible estrogen side effects before first dose. Verbal explanation should be provided also.
- Patient should report immediately abdominal pain; pain, numbness, or stiffness in legs or buttocks; pressure or pain in chest; shortness of breath; severe headaches; visual disturbances, such as blind spots, flashing lights, blurriness; undiagnosed vaginal bleeding or discharge; breast lumps; swelling of hands or feet; yellow skin and sclera; dark urine; and light-colored stools.
- Male patients on long-term therapy should be alert for possible gynecomastia and impotence, which will disappear when therapy is terminated.
- Not used for menstrual disorders because duration of action is very long.
- Pathologist should be advised of estrogen therapy when specimen sent.
- Patients with diabetes should report positive urine tests so antidiabetic medication dose can be adjusted.
- Female patients should be taught how to perform routine breast self-examination.
- Patient on cyclic therapy for postmenopausal symptoms should know that although withdrawal bleeding may occur during week off drug, fertility has not been restored. Pregnancy is not possible since she has not ovulated.

No significant interactions.

Special considerations:

- Contraindicated in thrombophlebitis or thromboembolic disorders; cancer of breast, reproductive organs, or genitals; undiagnosed abnormal genital bleeding. Use cautiously in menstrual irregularities or endometriosis.
- Prolonged therapy with estrogen-containing products is contraindicated.
- FDA regulations require that female patients receive package insert explaining possible estrogen side effects before first dose. Verbal explanation should be provided also.
- Systemic reactions possible with normal intravaginal use and should be monitored closely.
- Patient should not exceed dose.
- Withdrawal bleeding may be precipitated if estrogen is suddenly stopped.
- Patient should know how to insert suppositories or cream.

No significant interactions.

Special considerations:

- Contraindicated in thrombophlebitis or thromboembolic disorders; undiagnosed abnormal genital bleeding. Use cautiously in hypertension, asthma, mental depression, bone disease, migraine, seizures, blood dyscrasias, diabetes mellitus, gallbladder disease, amenorrhea, heart failure, hepatic or renal dysfunction, and family history (mother, grandmother, sister) of breast or genital tract cancer. Development or worsening of these conditions may require stopping drug.
- FDA regulations require that all female patients receive package insert explaining possible estrogen side effects before first dose. Verbal explanation should be provided also.
- Only 25 mg tablet approved by FDA as the "morning-after pill." To be effective it must be taken within 72 hours after coitus.
- Patient should stop taking drug immediately if she becomes pregnant, since it can affect the fetus adversely.
- Patient should report immediately abdominal pain; pain, numbness, or stiffness in legs or buttocks; pressure or pain in chest; shortness of breath; severe headache; visual disturbances, such as blind spots, flashing lights, or blurriness; undiagnosed vaginal bleeding or discharge; breast lumps; swelling of hands or feet; yellow sclera or skin; dark urine or light-colored stools.
- Pathologist should be advised of estrogen therapy when specimen sent to laboratory.
- Patients with diabetes should report positive urine tests so antidiabetic medication dose can be adjusted.
- High incidence of gross nonmalignant genital changes in offspring of women taking drug during pregnancy. Female offspring also have higher than normal risk of developing cervical and vaginal adenocarcinoma. Male offspring may have higher than normal risk of developing testicular tumors.

(continued on following page)

NAMES, INDICATIONS AND DOSAGES	SIDE EFFECTS
diethylstilbestrol *(continued)* 5 mg I.M. twice weekly initially, followed by up to 4 mg I.M. twice weekly. Or 50 to 200 mg (diphosphate) P.O. t.i.d.; or 0.25 to 1 g I.V. daily for 5 days, then once or twice weekly. MEN AND POSTMENOPAUSAL WOMEN: **Breast cancer:** 15 mg P.O. daily.	**Other:** leg cramps, breast tenderness or enlargement.
esterified estrogens Amnestrogen, Climestrone♦♦, Estabs, Estratab, Menest, Menotrol♦♦, Ms-Med, Neo-Estrone♦♦ MEN: **Prostatic cancer:** 1.25 to 2.5 mg P.O. t.i.d. MEN AND POSTMENOPAUSAL WOMEN: **Breast cancer:** 10 mg P.O. t.i.d. for 3 or more months. WOMEN: **Hypogonadism, castration, primary ovarian failure:** 2.5 mg daily to t.i.d. in cycles of 3 weeks on, 1 week off. **Menopausal symptoms:** average 0.3 to 3.75 mg P.O. daily in cycles of 3 weeks on, 1 week off.	**CNS:** headache, dizziness, chorea, depression, libido changes, lethargy. **CV:** thrombophlebitis; *thromboembolism;* hypertension; edema; *increased risk of stroke, pulmonary embolism, and myocardial infarction.* **EENT:** worsening of myopia or astigmatism, intolerance to contact lenses. **GI:** *nausea,* vomiting, abdominal cramps, bloating, diarrhea, constipation, anorexia, increased appetite, weight changes. **GU:** breakthrough bleeding, altered menstrual flow, dysmenorrhea, amenorrhea, cervical erosion, altered cervical secretions, enlargement of uterine fibromas, vaginal candidiasis; *in males:* gynecomastia, testicular atrophy, impotence. **Hepatic:** cholestatic jaundice. **Metabolic:** hyperglycemia, hypercalcemia, folic acid deficiency. **Skin:** melasma, rash, acne, hirsutism or hair loss, seborrhea, oily skin. **Other:** breast changes (tenderness, enlargement, secretion).
estradiol Estrace♦ **estradiol cypionate** D-Est 5, Depo-Estradiol Cypionate, Depogen, Duraestrin, E-Ionate P.A., Estro-Cyp **estradiol valerate** Ardefem, Delestrogen♦♦, Dioval♦, Duragen, Estate, Estradiol L.A., Estraval, Rep Estra, Reposo-E, Retestrin, Valergen WOMEN: **Menopausal symptoms, hypogonadism, castration, primary ovarian failure:** 1 to 2 mg P.O. daily, in cycles of 21 days on and 7 days off, or cycles of 5 days on and 2 days off; or 0.2 to 1 mg I.M. weekly. **Kraurosis vulvae:** 1 to 1.5 mg I.M. once or more per week. **Menopausal symptoms:** 1 to 5 mg (cypionate) I.M. q 3 to 4 weeks. Or 5 to 20 mg (valerate) I.M., repeated once after 2 to 3 weeks **Postpartum breast engorgement:** 10 to 25 mg (valerate) I.M. at end of first stage of labor. MEN: **Prostatic cancer:** 25 mg S.C. pellet implants (Progynon) q 3 to 4 months, or 50 mg q 4 to 6 months. Or 30 mg (valerate) I.M. q 1 to 2 weeks.	**CNS:** headache, dizziness, chorea, depression, libido changes, lethargy. **CV:** thrombophlebitis, *thromboembolism,* hypertension, edema. **EENT:** worsening of myopia or astigmatism, intolerance to contact lenses. **GI:** *nausea,* vomiting, abdominal cramps, bloating, diarrhea, constipation, anorexia, increased appetite, weight changes. **GU:** breakthrough bleeding, altered menstrual flow, dysmenorrhea, amenorrhea, cervical erosion, altered cervical secretions, enlargement of uterine fibromas, vaginal candidiasis; *in males:* gynecomastia, testicular atrophy, impotence. **Hepatic:** cholestatic jaundice. **Metabolic:** hyperglycemia, hypercalcemia, folic acid deficiency. **Skin:** melasma, urticaria, acne, seborrhea, oily skin, hirsutism or hair loss. **Other:** breast changes (tenderness, enlargement, secretion), leg cramps.

♦ Available in U.S. and Canada. ♦♦ Available in Canada only.
All other products (no symbol) available in U.S. only. Italicized side effects are common or life-threatening.

INTERACTIONS AND SPECIAL CONSIDERATIONS

• Increased number of cardiovascular deaths reported in men taking diethylstilbestrol tablet (5 mg daily) for prostatic cancer long-term. This effect not associated with 1 mg daily dose.
• Male patients on estrogen therapy should know that side effects such as gynecomastia and impotence will disappear when therapy ends.
• Female patients should be taught how to perform routine breast self-examination.
• Patient on cyclic therapy for postmenopausal symptoms should know that although withdrawal bleeding may occur during week off drug, fertility has not been restored. Pregnancy is not possible since she has not ovulated.
• Use of estrogens associated with increased risk of endometrial cancer. Possible increased risk of breast cancer.

No significant interactions.

Special considerations:
• Contraindicated in thrombophlebitis or thromboembolic disorders; undiagnosed abnormal genital bleeding. Use cautiously in history of hypertension, mental depression, gallbladder disease, migraine, seizure, diabetes mellitus, amenorrhea, or family history (mother, grandmother, sister) of breast or genital tract cancer. Development or worsening of these conditions may necessitate discontinuing drug.
• FDA regulations require that female patients receive package insert explaining possible estrogen side effects before first dose. Verbal explanation should be provided also.
• Patient should report immediately abdominal pain; pain, numbness, or stiffness in legs or buttocks; pressure or pain in chest; shortness of breath; severe headaches; visual disturbances, such as blind spots, flashing lights, or blurriness; undiagnosed vaginal bleeding or discharge; breast lumps; swelling of hands or feet; yellow skin or sclera; dark urine or light-colored stools.
• Pathologist should be advised of estrogen therapy when specimen sent to laboratory.
• Patients with diabetes should report positive urine tests so antidiabetic medication dose can be adjusted.
• Patient on cyclic therapy for postmenopausal symptoms should know that although she may experience withdrawal bleeding during week off drug, fertility has not been restored. Pregnancy cannot occur since she has not ovulated.
• Female patients should be taught how to perform routine breast self-examination.
• Male patients on estrogen therapy should understand that side effects such as gynecomastia and impotence will disappear when therapy ends.

No significant interactions.

Special considerations:
• Contraindicated in thrombophlebitis or thromboembolic disorders; cancer of breast or reproductive organs; undiagnosed abnormal genital bleeding. Use cautiously in hypertension, mental depression, bone diseases, blood dyscrasias, migraine, seizures, diabetes mellitus, amenorrhea, heart failure, hepatic or renal dysfunction, or family history (mother, grandmother, sister) of breast or genital tract cancer. Development or worsening of these conditions may require stopping drug.
• FDA regulations require that female patients receive package insert explaining possible estrogen side effects before first dose. Verbal explanation should be provided also.
• Patient should report immediately abdominal pain; pain, numbness, or stiffness in legs or buttocks; pressure or pain in chest; shortness of breath; severe headaches; visual disturbances, such as blind spots, flashing lights, or blurriness; undiagnosed vaginal bleeding or discharge; breast lumps; swelling of hands or feet; yellow skin or sclera; dark urine or light-colored stools.
• Risk of endometrial cancer is increased in postmenopausal women who take estrogens for more than 1 year.
• Patients with diabetes should report positive urine tests so antidiabetic medication dose can be adjusted.
• Pathologist should be advised of estrogen therapy when specimen sent to laboratory.
• Estradiol available as aqueous suspension or solution in peanut oil.
• Estradiol cypionate available as solution in cottonseed oil or vegetable oil.
• Estradiol valerate available as solution in castor oil, sesame oil, and vegetable oil. Patient should be checked for allergy.
• Before injection, drug should be well dispersed by rolling vial between palms. Drug should be injected deep I.M. into large muscle.
• Male patient should know that possible side effects of gynecomastia and impotence disappear after termination of therapy.
• Female patients should be taught how to perform routine breast self-examination.
• Patient on cyclic therapy for postmenopausal symptoms should understand that although withdrawal bleeding may occur during week off drug, fertility has not been reinstated. Pregnancy cannot occur since she has not ovulated.

NAMES, INDICATIONS AND DOSAGES	SIDE EFFECTS
estrogenic substances, conjugated Estrocon, Premarin♦, Sodestrin-H WOMEN: **Abnormal uterine bleeding (hormonal imbalance):** 25 mg I.V. or I.M. Repeat in 6 to 12 hours. **Breast cancer (at least 5 years after menopause):** 10 mg P.O. t.i.d. for 3 months or more. **Castration, primary ovarian failure, and osteoporosis:** 1.25 mg P.O. daily in cycles of 3 weeks on, 1 week off. **Hypogonadism:** 2.5 mg P.O. b.i.d. or t.i.d. for 20 consecutive days each month. **Menopausal symptoms:** 0.3 to 1.25 mg P.O. daily in cycles of 3 weeks on, 1 week off. **Postpartum breast engorgement:** 3.75 mg P.O. q 4 hours for 5 doses or 1.25 mg q 4 hours for 5 days. MEN: **Prostatic cancer:** 1.25 to 2.5 mg P.O. t.i.d.	**CNS:** headache, dizziness, chorea, depression, libido changes, lethargy. **CV:** thrombophlebitis; *thromboembolism;* hypertension; edema; *increased risk of stroke, pulmonary embolism, and myocardial infarction.* **EENT:** worsening of myopia or astigmatism, intolerance to contact lenses. **GI:** *nausea,* vomiting, abdominal cramps, bloating, diarrhea, constipation, anorexia, increased appetite, weight changes. **GU:** breakthrough bleeding, altered menstrual flow, dysmenorrhea, amenorrhea, cervical erosion, altered cervical secretions, enlargement of uterine fibromas, vaginal candidiasis; *in males:* gynecomastia, testicular atrophy, impotence. **Hepatic:** cholestatic jaundice. **Metabolic:** hyperglycemia, hypercalcemia, folic acid deficiency. **Skin:** melasma, urticaria, acne, seborrhea, oily skin, flushing (when given rapidly I.V.), hirsutism or loss of hair. **Other:** breast changes (tenderness, enlargement, secretion), leg cramps.
estrone Foygen, Gravigen, Ogen♦, Theelin WOMEN: **Atrophic vaginitis:** 0.2 mg intravaginal suppository daily or apply cream to vagina once nightly. **Hypogonadism, castration, ovarian failure:** 1.25 to 7.5 mg P.O. daily for 20 consecutive days each month; or 0.1 to 2 mg I.M. weekly. **Menopausal symptoms:** 0.625 to 5 mg P.O. daily in cycle of 3 weeks on, 1 week off; or 0.1 to 0.5 mg I.M. 2 to 3 times weekly. MEN: **Prostatic cancer:** 2 to 4 mg I.M. 2 to 3 times weekly.	**CNS:** headache, dizziness, chorea, depression, libido changes, lethargy. **CV:** thrombophlebitis, *thromboembolism,* hypertension, edema. **EENT:** worsening of myopia or astigmatism, intolerance to contact lenses. **GI:** *nausea,* vomiting, abdominal cramps, bloating, diarrhea, constipation, anorexia, increased appetite, weight changes. **GU:** breakthrough bleeding, altered menstrual flow, dysmenorrhea, amenorrhea, cervical erosion, altered cervical secretions, enlargement of uterine fibromas, vaginal candidiasis; *in males:* gynecomastia, testicular atrophy, impotence. **Hepatic:** cholestatic jaundice. **Metabolic:** hyperglycemia, hypercalcemia, folic acid deficiency. **Skin:** melasma, urticaria, acne, seborrhea, oily skin, hirsutism or hair loss. **Other:** breast changes (tenderness, enlargement, secretion), leg cramps.
ethinyl estradiol Estinyl♦, Feminone WOMEN: **Breast cancer (at least 5 years after menopause):** 1 mg P.O. t.i.d. **Hypogonadism:** 0.05 mg daily to t.i.d. for 2 weeks a month, followed by 2 weeks progesterone therapy; continue for 3 to 6 monthly dosing cycles, followed by 2 months off. **Menopausal symptoms:** 0.02 to 0.05 mg P.O.	**CNS:** headache, dizziness, chorea, depression, libido changes, lethargy. **CV:** thrombophlebitis, *thromboembolism,* hypertension, edema. **EENT:** worsening of myopia or astigmatism, intolerance to contact lenses. **GI:** *nausea,* vomiting, abdominal cramps, bloating, diarrhea, constipation, anorexia, increased appetite, weight changes. **GU:** breakthrough bleeding, altered menstrual flow, dysmenorrhea, amenorrhea, cervical ero-

INTERACTIONS AND SPECIAL CONSIDERATIONS

No significant interactions.

Special considerations:

- Contraindicated in thrombophlebitis or thromboembolic disorders; undiagnosed abnormal genital bleeding. Use cautiously in hypertension, gallbladder disease, bone diseases, blood dyscrasias, migraine, seizures, diabetes mellitus, amenorrhea, heart failure, hepatic or renal dysfunction, or family history (mother, grandmother, sister) of breast or genital tract cancer. Development or worsening of these conditions may require stopping drug.
- FDA regulations require that female patients receive package insert explaining possible estrogen side effects before first dose. Verbal explanation should be provided also.
- Patient should report any unusual symptoms immediately, especially abdominal pain; pain, numbness, or stiffness in legs or buttocks; pressure or pain in chest; shortness of breath; severe headaches; visual disturbances, such as blind spots, flashing lights, or blurriness; undiagnosed vaginal bleeding or discharge; breast lumps; swelling of hands or feet; yellow skin or sclera; dark urine or light-colored stools.
- I.M. or I.V. use preferred for rapid treatment of dysfunctional uterine bleeding or reduction of surgical bleeding.
- Should be refrigerated before reconstituting and agitated gently after diluent added.
- Pathologist should be advised of estrogen therapy when specimen sent to laboratory.
- Patients with diabetes should report positive urine tests so antidiabetic medication dose can be adjusted.
- Use associated with increased risk of endometrial cancer. Possible increased risk of breast cancer.
- Female patients should be taught how to perform routine breast self-examination.
- Patient on cyclic therapy for postmenopausal symptoms should understand that although withdrawal bleeding may occur during week off drug, fertility has not been restored. Pregnancy cannot occur since she has not ovulated.
- Male patients should know that possible side effects of gynecomastia and impotence disappear after termination of therapy.

No significant interactions.

Special considerations:

- Contraindicated in thrombophlebitis or thromboembolic disorders; cancer of breast or reproductive organs; undiagnosed abnormal genital bleeding. Use cautiously in hypertension, mental depression, migraine, seizures, diabetes mellitus, amenorrhea, hepatic or renal dysfunction, or family history (mother, grandmother, sister) of breast or genital tract cancer. Development or worsening of these may require stopping drug.
- I.V. use contraindicated.
- FDA regulations require that female patients receive package insert explaining possible estrogen side effects before first dose. Verbal explanation should be provided also.
- Patient should report any unusual symptoms immediately, especially abdominal pain; pain, numbness, or stiffness in legs or buttocks; pressure or pain in chest; shortness of breath; severe headaches; visual disturbances, such as blind spots, flashing lights, or blurriness; undiagnosed vaginal bleeding or discharge; breast lumps; swelling of hands or feet.
- Oil preparation may become cloudy if chilled. Solution should be warmed until clear before use. Also available in aqueous suspension.
- Pathologist should be advised of estrogen therapy when specimen sent to laboratory.
- Patients with diabetes should report positive urine test so antidiabetic medication dose can be adjusted.
- Female patients should be taught how to perform routine breast self-examination.
- Use of estrogens associated with increased risk of endometrial cancer. Possible increased risk of breast cancer.
- Patient on cyclic therapy for postmenopausal symptoms should understand that although withdrawal bleeding may occur during week off drug, fertility has not been restored. Pregnancy cannot occur since she has not ovulated.
- Male patients should know that possible side effects of gynecomastia and impotence disappear after termination of therapy.

No significant interactions.

Special considerations:

- Contraindicated in thrombophlebitis or thromboembolic disorders; undiagnosed abnormal genital bleeding. Use cautiously in hypertension, mental depression, bone diseases, migraine, seizures, blood dyscrasias, diabetes mellitus, amenorrhea, heart failure, hepatic or renal dysfunction, or family history (mother, grandmother, sister) of breast or genital tract cancer. Development or worsening of these conditions may require stopping drug.
- FDA regulations require that female patients receive package insert explaining possible estrogen side effects before first dose. Verbal explanation should be provided also.
- Patient should report any unusual symptoms immediately, especially abdominal pain; pain, numbness, or stiffness in legs or buttocks; pressure or pain in chest; shortness of breath; severe headaches; visual disturbances, such as blind

(continued on following page)

NAMES, INDICATIONS AND DOSAGES	SIDE EFFECTS
ethinyl estradiol *(continued)* daily for cycles of 3 weeks on, 1 week off. **Postpartum breast engorgement:** 0.5 to 1 mg P.O. daily for 3 days, then taper over 7 days to 0.1 mg and discontinue. MEN: **Prostatic cancer:** 0.15 to 2 mg P.O. daily.	sion, altered cervical secretions, enlargement of uterine fibromas, vaginal candidiasis; *in males:* gynecomastia, testicular atrophy, impotence. **Hepatic:** cholestatic jaundice. **Metabolic:** hyperglycemia, hypercalcemia, folic acid deficiency. **Skin:** melasma, urticaria, acne, seborrhea, oily skin, hirsutism or hair loss. **Other:** breast changes (tenderness, enlargement, secretion), leg cramps.
quinestrol Estrovis WOMEN: **Moderate-to-severe vasomotor symptoms associated with menopause, and for atrophic vaginitis, kraurosis vulvae, female hypogonadism, female castration, and primary ovarian failure**—100-mcg tablet once daily for 7 days, followed by 100 mcg weekly as maintenance dose beginning 2 weeks after start of treatment. Dosage may be increased to 200 mcg weekly.	**CNS:** headache, dizziness, chorea, migraine, depression, libido changes. **CV:** thrombophlebitis; *thromboembolism;* hypertension; edema; *increased risk of stroke, pulmonary embolism, and myocardial infarction.* **EENT:** worsening of myopia or astigmatism, intolerance to contact lenses. **GI:** *nausea,* vomiting, abdominal cramps, bloating, diarrhea, constipation, anorexia, increased appetite, excessive thirst, weight changes. **GU:** breakthrough bleeding, altered menstrual flow, dysmenorrhea, amenorrhea, cervical erosion or abnormal secretions, enlargement of uterine fibromas, vaginal candidiasis. **Hepatic:** cholestatic jaundice. **Metabolic:** hyperglycemia, hypercalcemia, folic acid deficiency. **Skin:** melasma, urticaria, acne, seborrhea, oily skin, hirsutism or loss of hair. **Other:** leg cramps, purpura, breast changes (tenderness, enlargement, secretion).

INTERACTIONS AND SPECIAL CONSIDERATIONS

spots, flashing lights, or blurriness; undiagnosed vaginal bleeding or discharge; breast lumps; swelling of hands or feet; yellow skin or sclera; dark urine or light-colored stools.
- Pathologist should be advised of estrogen therapy when specimen sent to laboratory.
- Patients with diabetes should report positive urine test so antidiabetic medication dose can be adjusted.
- Female patients should be taught how to perform routine breast self-examination.
- Use of estrogens associated with increased risk of endometrial cancer. Possible increased risk of breast cancer.
- Patient on cyclic therapy for postmenopausal symptoms should understand that although withdrawal bleeding may occur during week off drug, fertility has not been restored. Pregnancy cannot occur since she has not ovulated.
- Male patients should know that possible side effects of gynecomastia and impotence disappear after termination of therapy.

No significant interactions.

Special considerations:
- Contraindicated in thrombophlebitis or thromboembolic disorders; cancer of breast or reproductive organs; undiagnosed abnormal genital bleeding. Use cautiously in patients with hypertension, mental depression, migraine, seizures, diabetes mellitus, amenorrhea, hepatic or renal dysfunction, or family history (mother, grandmother, sister) of breast or genital tract cancer. Development or worsening of these may require discontinuation of the drug.
- FDA regulations require that female patients receive package insert explaining possible estrogen side effects before first dose. Verbal explanation should be provided also.
- Patient should report immediately: abdominal pain; pain, numbness, or stiffness in legs or buttocks; pressure or pain in chest; shortness of breath; severe headaches; visual disturbances, such as blind spots, flashing lights, or blurriness; vaginal bleeding or discharge; breast lumps; swelling of hands or feet; yellow skin or sclera; dark urine or light-colored stools.
- Pathologist should be advised of estrogen therapy when specimen sent to laboratory.
- Patients with diabetes should report positive urine test so antidiabetic medication dose can be adjusted.
- Attempts to discontinue medication should be made at 3- to 6-month intervals.
- Similar in effectiveness to conjugated estrogens in treatment of postmenopausal symptoms. Biggest advantage is that quinestrol can be taken once a week.
- Use of estrogens associated with increased risk of endometrial cancer. Possible increased risk of breast cancer.
- Patients on replacement therapy for postmenopausal symptoms should know that although menstrual-like bleeding or spotting may occur, fertility has not been restored.
- Female patients should know how to perform breast self-examination.
- Possible side effects of gynecomastia and impotence in male patients disappear after termination of therapy.

55

Progestogens

hydroxyprogesterone caproate
medroxyprogesterone acetate
norethindrone
norethindrone acetate
norgestrel
progesterone

The natural hormone progesterone and its synthetic derivatives are called progestogens or progestins; they produce the characteristic endometrial changes that favor pregnancy (gestation). Progesterone is secreted mainly by the corpus luteum after ovulation (during the last half of the menstrual cycle). Large amounts, however, are also secreted by the placenta. Smaller quantities are produced by both the mature follicle before ovulation (during the first half of the menstrual cycle) and the adrenal cortex.

Progestogens trigger glandular and vascular development, which results in the endometrial swelling essential for implantation of the fertilized ovum. If implantation doesn't occur, the sharp drop in the progesterone level at the end of the menstrual cycle helps start menstruation.

Progestogens also relax uterine smooth muscle. During pregnancy, increased progesterone secretion prevents premature uterine contractions and allows the pregnancy to continue to term. Along with estrogen, progestogens aid growth and development of the alveolar duct system in the mammary glands.

Progestogens also promote protein catabolism and sodium and water retention.

Major uses

Progestogens relieve dysfunctional uterine bleeding, amenorrhea, and dysmenorhea.

- Norethindrone and norethindrone acetate are used to treat endometriosis.
- Norethindrone, norethindrone acetate, and norgestrel are used alone or in combination with estrogens in oral contraceptives.

Mechanism of action

- Progestogens mimic the body's production of progesterone to reestablish a normal menstrual cycle in patients with amenorrhea.
- They promote glandular and vascular development of the endometrium by restoring progesterone levels.
- Progestogens suppress ovulation possibly by inhibiting pituitary gonadotropin secretion. They also form a thick cervical mucus that is relatively impermeable to sperm.

Absorption, distribution, metabolism, and excretion

Progestogens are rapidly absorbed, distributed to all tissues, metabolized in the liver, and excreted in urine.

Onset and duration

Onset and duration vary with the disorder, the progestogen given, and use of an estrogen (that is, whether the progestogen is administered with, after, or without an estrogen). Generally, however, onset is fastest when estrogens are given first; duration is longest when the slow-release ("depot") forms (injection in oil, for example) are used.

HOW PROGESTERONE AFFECTS THE PREGNANT WOMAN

Progesterone, meaning *for gestation,* is secreted in large amounts by the placenta during pregnancy. It promotes these necessary adaptations in the pregnant woman:

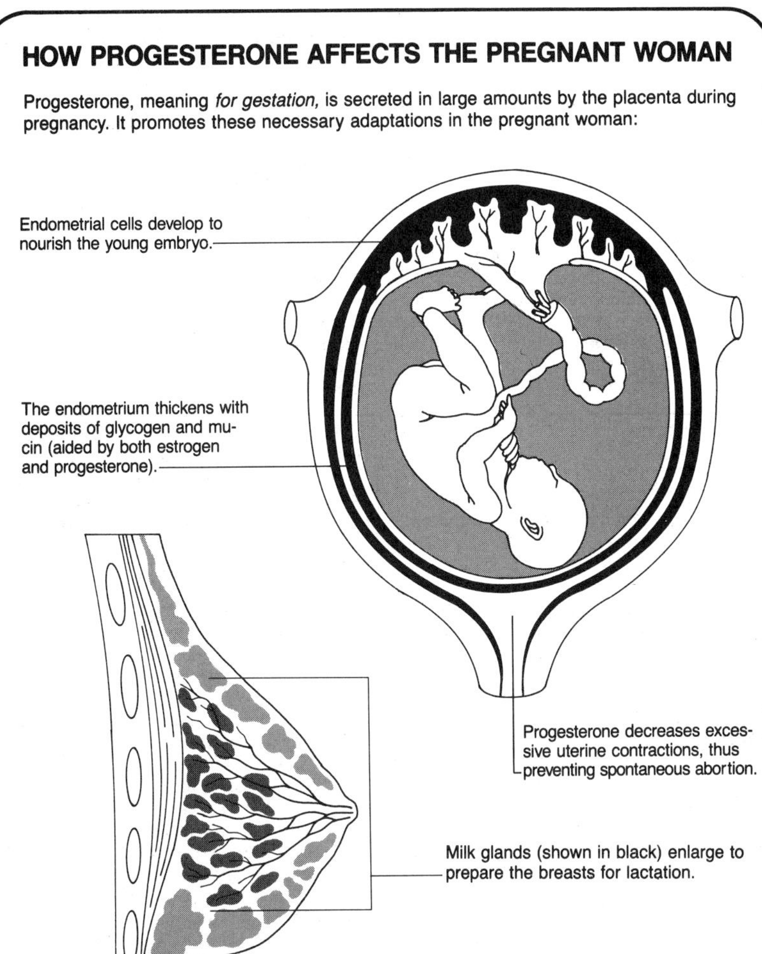
Endometrial cells develop to nourish the young embryo.
The endometrium thickens with deposits of glycogen and mucin (aided by both estrogen and progesterone).
Progesterone decreases excessive uterine contractions, thus preventing spontaneous abortion.
Milk glands (shown in black) enlarge to prepare the breasts for lactation.

NAMES, INDICATIONS AND DOSAGES	SIDE EFFECTS
hydroxyprogesterone caproate Curretab, Delalutin♦, Dura-Lutin WOMEN: **Menstrual disorders:** 125 to 375 mg I.M. q 4 weeks. Stop after 4 cycles. **Uterine cancer:** 1 to 5 g I.M. weekly.	**CNS:** dizziness, migraine headache, lethargy, depression. **CV:** hypertension, thrombophlebitis, *pulmonary embolism, edema.* **GI:** nausea, vomiting, abdominal cramps. **GU:** breakthrough bleeding, dysmenorrhea, amenorrhea; cervical erosion or abnormal secretions; uterine fibromas; vaginal candidiasis. **Hepatic:** cholestatic jaundice. **Local:** irritation and pain at injection site. **Metabolic:** hyperglycemia. **Skin:** melasma, rash. **Other:** breast tenderness, enlargement, or secretion; decreased libido.
medroxyprogesterone acetate Amen, Depo-Provera♦, Provera♦ WOMEN: **Abnormal uterine bleeding due to hormonal imbalance:** 5 to 10 mg P.O. daily for 5 to 10 days beginning on the 16th day of cycle. If patient has received estrogen—10 mg P.O. daily for 10 days beginning on 16th day of cycle. **Secondary amenorrhea:** 5 to 10 mg P.O. daily for 5 to 10 days.	**CNS:** dizziness, migraine headache, lethargy, depression. **CV:** hypertension, thrombophlebitis, *pulmonary embolism, edema.* **GI:** nausea, vomiting, abdominal cramps. **GU:** breakthrough bleeding, dysmenorrhea, amenorrhea; cervical erosion or abnormal secretions; uterine fibromas, vaginal candidiasis. **Hepatic:** cholestatic jaundice. **Metabolic:** hyperglycemia, decreased libido. **Skin:** melasma, rash. **Other:** breast tenderness, enlargement, or secretion.
norethindrone Norlutin♦, Nor-Q.D. WOMEN: **Amenorrhea; abnormal uterine bleeding:** 5 to 20 mg P.O. daily on days 5 to 25 of menstrual cycle. **Endometriosis:** 10 mg P.O. daily for 14 days, then increase by 5 mg P.O. daily q 2 weeks up to 30 mg daily.	**CNS:** dizziness, migraine headache, lethargy, depression. **CV:** hypertension, thrombophlebitis, *pulmonary embolism, edema.* **GI:** nausea, vomiting, abdominal cramps. **GU:** breakthrough bleeding, dysmenorrhea, amenorrhea; cervical erosion or abnormal secretions; uterine fibromas; vaginal candidiasis. **Hepatic:** cholestatic jaundice. **Metabolic:** hyperglycemia, decreased libido. **Skin:** melasma, rash. **Other:** breast tenderness, enlargement, or secretion.
norethindrone acetate Norlutate♦ WOMEN: **Amenorrhea, abnormal uterine bleeding:** 2.5 to 10 mg P.O. daily on days 5 to 25 of menstrual cycle. **Endometriosis**—5 mg P.O. daily for 14 days, then increase by 2.5 mg daily q 2 weeks up to 15 mg daily.	**CNS:** dizziness, migraine headache, lethargy, depression. **CV:** hypertension, thrombophlebitis, *pulmonary embolism, edema.* **GI:** nausea, vomiting, abdominal cramps. **GU:** breakthrough bleeding, dysmenorrhea, amenorrhea; cervical erosion or abnormal secretions; uterine fibromas; vaginal candidiasis. **Hepatic:** cholestatic jaundice. **Metabolic:** hyperglycemia, decreased libido. **Skin:** melasma, rash. **Other:** breast tenderness, enlargement, or secretion.

INTERACTIONS AND SPECIAL CONSIDERATIONS

No significant interactions.

Special considerations:

• Contraindicated in thromboembolic disorders, breast cancer, undiagnosed abnormal vaginal bleeding, severe hepatic disease, missed abortion, or pregnancy. Use cautiously when diabetes mellitus, seizure disorder, migraine, cardiac or renal disease, asthma, or mental illness is present.
• FDA regulations require that before receiving first dose patients read package insert explaining possible progestogen side effects. A verbal explanation should be provided also. Patient should report any unusual symptoms immediately and should stop drug and call doctor if visual disturbances or migraine occurs.
• Should not be used as test for pregnancy; drug may cause birth defects and masculinization of female fetus.
• Edema and weight gain are likely.
• Oil solutions (sesame oil and castor oil) should be given deep I.M. in gluteal muscle.
• Preliminary estrogen treatment usually needed in menstrual disorders.
• Effect lasts 7 to 14 days.
• For I.M. use only.
• Patient should be taught how to perform a breast self-examination.

No significant interactions.

Special considerations:

• Contraindicated in thromboembolic disorders, breast cancer, undiagnosed abnormal vaginal bleeding, pregnancy, missed abortion, hepatic dysfunction. Use cautiously when diabetes mellitus, seizure disorder, migraine, cardiac or renal disease, asthma, or mental illness is present.
• FDA regulations require that before receiving first dose patients read package insert explaining possible progestogen side effects. A verbal explanation should be provided also. Patient should report any unusual symptoms immediately and should stop drug and call doctor if visual disturbances or migraine occurs.
• Should not be used as test for pregnancy; drug may cause birth defects and masculinization of female fetus.
• Patient should be taught how to perform a breast self-examination.

No significant interactions.

Special considerations:

• Contraindicated in thromboembolic disorders, breast cancer, undiagnosed abnormal vaginal bleeding, severe hepatic disease, missed abortion, or pregnancy. Use cautiously when diabetes mellitus, seizure disorder, migraine, cardiac or renal disease, asthma, or mental illness is present.
• Should not be used as test for pregnancy; drug may cause birth defects and masculinization of female fetus.
• FDA regulations require that before receiving first dose patients read package insert explaining possible progestogen side effects. A verbal explanation should also be provided. Patient should report any unusual symptoms immediately and should stop drug and call doctor if visual disturbances or migraine occurs.
• Patient may develop edema.
• Preliminary estrogen treatment usually needed in menstrual disorders.
• Patient should be taught how to perform a breast self-examination.

No significant interactions.

Special considerations:

• Contraindicated in thromboembolic disorders, breast cancer, undiagnosed abnormal vaginal bleeding, severe hepatic disease, missed abortion, or pregnancy. Use cautiously when diabetes mellitus, seizure disorder, migraine, cardiac or renal disease, asthma, or mental illness is present.
• FDA regulations require that before receiving first dose patients read package insert explaining possible progestogen side effects. A verbal explanation should also be provided. Patient should report any unusual symptoms immediately and should stop drug and call doctor if visual disturbances or migraine occurs.
• Should not be used as test for pregnancy; drug may cause birth defects and masculinization of female fetus.
• Preliminary estrogen treatment usually needed in menstrual disorders.
• Twice as potent as norethindrone.
• Patient should be taught how to perform a breast self-examination.

NAMES, INDICATIONS AND DOSAGES	SIDE EFFECTS
norgestrel Ovrette WOMEN: **Contraception:** 1 tablet P.O. daily.	**CNS:** cerebral thrombosis or hemorrhage, migraine headache, lethargy, depression. **CV:** hypertension, thrombophlebitis, *pulmonary embolism, edema.* **GI:** nausea, vomiting, abdominal cramps, gallbladder disease. **GU:** *breakthrough bleeding, change in menstrual flow,* dysmenorrhea, spotting, amenorrhea; cervical erosion, vaginal candidiasis. **Hepatic:** cholestatic jaundice. **Skin:** melasma, rash. **Other:** breast tenderness, enlargement, or secretion.
progesterone Profac-O, Progelan, Progestasert♦, Progestilin♦♦, Progestin WOMEN: **Amenorrhea:** 5 to 10 mg I.M. daily for 6 to 8 days. **Dysfunctional uterine bleeding:** 5 to 10 mg I.M. daily for 6 doses. **Contraception (as an intrauterine device):** Progestasert system inserted into uterine cavity. Replace after 1 year.	**CNS:** dizziness, migraine headache, lethargy, depression. **CV:** hypertension, thrombophlebitis, *pulmonary embolism, edema.* **GI:** nausea, vomiting, abdominal cramps. **GU:** breakthrough bleeding, dysmenorrhea, amenorrhea; cervical erosion or abnormal secretions; uterine fibromas; vaginal candidiasis. **Hepatic:** cholestatic jaundice. **Local:** pain at injection site. **Metabolic:** hyperglycemia, decreased libido. **Skin:** melasma, rash. **Other:** breast tenderness, enlargement, or secretion.

INTERACTIONS AND SPECIAL CONSIDERATIONS

No significant interactions.

Special considerations:

- Contraindicated in thromboembolic disorders, breast cancer, undiagnosed abnormal vaginal bleeding, severe hepatic disease, missed abortion, or pregnancy. Use cautiously when diabetes mellitus, seizure disorder, migraine, cardiac or renal disease, asthma, or mental illness is present.
- FDA regulations require that before receiving first dose patients read package insert explaining possible progestogen effects. A verbal explanation should also be provided. Patient should report any unusual symptoms immediately and should stop drug and call doctor if visual disturbances, migraine, or numbness or tingling in limbs occurs.
- Patient should take pill every day even if menstruating. Pill should be taken at the same time every day.
- Progestogen—only oral contraceptive known as mini-pill.
- Patient should be taught how to perform a breast self-examination.
- Women using oral contraceptives should be advised of the increased risk of serious cardiovascular side effects associated with heavy cigarette smoking (15 or more cigarettes per day). These risks are quite marked in women over 35 years.
- Risk of pregnancy increases with each tablet missed. A patient who misses one tablet should take it as soon as she remembers; she should then take the next tablet at the regular time. A patient who misses two tablets should take one as soon as she remembers and then take the next regular dose at the usual time; she should use a nonhormonal method of contraception in addition to norgestrel until 14 tablets have been taken. A patient who misses three or more tablets should discontinue the drug and use a nonhormonal method of contraception until after her menses. If her menstrual period does not occur within 45 days, pregnancy testing is necessary.
- Patient should report immediately excessive bleeding or bleeding between menstrual cycles.

No significant interactions.

Special considerations:

- Contraindicated in thromboembolic disorders, breast cancer, undiagnosed abnormal vaginal bleeding, severe hepatic disease, or missed abortion. Use cautiously when diabetes mellitus, seizure disorder, migraine, cardiac or renal disease, asthma, or mental illness is present.
- FDA regulations require that before receiving first dose patients read package insert explaining possible progestogen side effects. A verbal explanation should also be provided. Patient should report any unusual symptoms immediately and should stop drug and call doctor if visual disturbances or migraine occurs.
- Oil solutions (peanut oil or sesame oil) should be given deep I.M.
- A progesterone-containing IUD (Progestasert) available that releases 65 mcg progesterone daily for 1 year.
- Patient with Progestasert IUD should be taught how to check for proper IUD placement, and informed that she may experience cramps for several days after insertion and menstrual periods may be heavier. Patient should report excessively heavy menses and bleeding between menses to the doctor.
- Patient with Progestasert IUD should be informed that the progesterone supply is depleted in 1 year and the device must be changed. Pregnancy risk increases after 1 year if patient relies on progesterone-depleted device for contraception.
- Patients considering IUD contraception should be advised of side effects, including uterine perforation, increased risk of infection, pelvic inflammatory disease, ectopic pregnancy, abdominal cramping, increased menstrual flow, and expulsion of the device.
- Preliminary estrogen treatment is usually needed in menstrual disorders.
- Patient should be taught how to perform a breast self-examination.

56

Gonadotropins

chorionic gonadotropin, human
menotropins

Gonadotropins are hormones that stimulate both male and female gonads. Human chorionic gonadotropin (HCG) originates in the placenta. Human menopausal gonadotropin (HMG or menotropins) is an extract of both luteinizing hormone (LH) and follicle-stimulating hormone (FSH), two gonadotropins that originate in the pituitary gland.

HCG and HMG are the only commercially available gonadotropins. They're purified preparations obtained from the urine of pregnant and postmenopausal women, respectively.

LH and FSH are only available investigationally.

Major uses

HCG and HMG induce ovulation in infertile women when anovulation is not due primarily to ovarian failure.

- HCG is used to treat cryptorchidism not due to anatomic obstruction. Stimulation of androgen secretion by HCG leads to the development of secondary sex characteristics and may promote testicular descent.
- HCG is also therapeutic for hypogonadism secondary to pituitary deficiency in males.

Mechanism of action

- HCG, when given on the day after the last dose of HMG, serves as a substitute for LH to stimulate ovulation of an HMG-prepared follicle.
- HCG also promotes secretion of gonadal steroid hormones by stimulating production of androgen by the interstitial cells of the testes (Leydig's cells).
- HMG, administered to women without primary ovarian failure, mimics FSH in inducing follicular growth, and LH in aiding follicular maturation.

Absorption, distribution, metabolism, and excretion

Gonadotropins are administered I.M. because oral doses are destroyed by digestive enzymes. They're distributed throughout the body, with highest concentrations in the ovaries and testes.

- HCG is partly degraded in the body but is largely excreted in urine.
- HMG is not excreted and is believed to undergo total degradation in the body.

Onset and duration

Gonadotropin blood levels peak 6 hours after injection.

EVALUATING AND SUPPORTING PATIENTS ON INFERTILITY THERAPY

Gonadotropins are used to induce ovulation in anovulatory women. When ovulatory dysfunction has been demonstrated, gonadotropins are initially given in sufficient doses to induce follicular growth and maturation.

Before treatment, a thorough gynecologic and endocrinologic evaluation is made of the patient, which includes:

- determination of urine gonadotropin levels to rule out primary ovarian failure. (Urine gonadotropin levels vary according to a woman's age. Gonadotropin hormone secretion begins at puberty, signaling onset of sexual maturation. Normally, gonadotropin secretion increases at a steady rate, as reflected in total urine gonadotropin levels, until menopause, and then it begins to decline.)
- meticulous physical examination to rule out pathologic conditions of the uterus and fallopian tubes, pregnancy, endometrial cancer, and other organic causes of abnormal bleeding.
- similar evaluation of the patient's sexual partner. (Approximately 15% of all couples face infertility, from multiple causes. In the population at large, more female abnormalities than male abnormalities are responsible for infertility.)

Before treatment

- The patient should be provided with the support she needs. Many women appear anxious and tense. The natural desire to achieve motherhood combined with societal pressure places a great deal of stress on the infertile woman. The patient who decides to *discontinue* therapy also needs special support.
- The patient should know that support groups are available to help her through the trauma of infertility. She should be advised of her alternatives, which include adoption or artificial insemination, if her partner is infertile.
- The actions and side effects of the drug she's taking should be explained.
- The patient should be advised that gonadotropin-induced ovulation may be expensive, difficult to achieve, and likely to produce multiple birth.

Duration of action varies widely, as the half-lives of these agents range from 4 to 70 hours.

Combination products
None.

NAMES, INDICATIONS AND DOSAGES	SIDE EFFECTS
chorionic gonadotropin, human Android HCG, Antuitrin-S♦, A.P.L.♦, Chorex, Follutein, Glukor, Libigen, Pregnyl, Stemultrolin **Anovulation and infertility:** WOMEN: 10,000 units I.M. 1 day after last dose of menotropins. **Hypogonadism:** MEN: 500 to 1,000 units I.M. 3 times weekly for 3 weeks, then twice weekly for 3 weeks; or 4,000 units I.M. 3 times weekly for 6 to 9 months, then 2,000 units 3 times weekly for 3 more months. **Nonobstructive cryptorchidism:** BOYS 4 TO 9 YEARS: 5,000 units I.M. every other day for 4 doses.	**CNS:** headache, fatigue, irritability, restlessness, depression. **GU:** early puberty (growth of testes, penis, pubic and axillary hair; voice change; down on upper lip; growth of body hair). **Local:** *pain at injection site.* **Other:** gynecomastia, edema.
menotropins Pergonal **Anovulation:** WOMEN: 75 IU (international units) each FSH and LH I.M. daily for 9 to 12 days, followed by 10,000 units chorionic gonadotropin I.M. 1 day after last dose of menotropins. Repeat for 1 to 3 menstrual cycles until ovulation occurs. **Infertility with ovulation:** 75 IU each of FSH and LH I.M. daily for 9 to 12 days, followed by 10,000 units chorionic gonadotropin I.M. 1 day after last dose of menotropins. Repeat for 2 menstrual cycles and then increase to 150 IU each FSH and LH I.M. daily for 9 to 12 days, followed by 10,000 units chorionic gonadotropin I.M. 1 day after last dose of menotropins. Repeat for 2 menstrual cycles. Menotropins are available in ampuls containing 75 IU each FSH and LH.	**Blood:** hemoconcentration with fluid loss into abdomen. **GI:** nausea, vomiting, diarrhea. **GU:** *ovarian enlargement with pain and abdominal distention,* multiple births, ovarian hyperstimulation syndrome (sudden ovarian enlargement, ascites with or without pain, or pleural effusion). **Other:** fever.

INTERACTIONS AND SPECIAL CONSIDERATIONS

No significant interactions.

Special considerations:

• Contraindicated in pituitary hypertrophy or tumor, prostatic cancer, and early puberty (usual onset between 10 and 13 years of age). Use cautiously in epilepsy, migraine, asthma, cardiac or renal disease.
• Not for obesity control.
• When used with menotropins to induce ovulation, multiple births possible.
• In infertility, daily intercourse should be encouraged from day before chorionic gonadotropin is given until ovulation occurs.
• Genitalia of boys should be inspected for signs of early puberty; drug may be discontinued if early puberty occurs.

No significant interactions.

Special considerations:

• Contraindicated in high urinary gonadotropin levels, thyroid or adrenal dysfunction, pituitary tumor, abnormal uterine bleeding, ovarian cysts or enlargement, and pregnancy.
• Possibility of multiple births.
• In infertility daily intercourse should be encouraged from day before chorionic gonadotropin is given until ovulation occurs.
• Should be reconstituted with 1 to 2 ml sterile saline injection and used immediately.

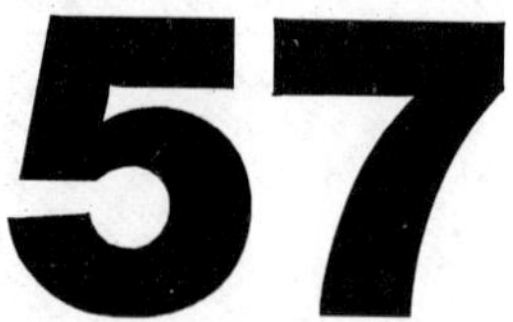

Antidiabetic agents and glucagon

acetohexamide
chlorpropamide
glucagon
insulins
tolazamide
tolbutamide

Antidiabetic drugs supply exogenous insulin or stimulate production of endogenous insulin in patients with diabetes mellitus. Endogenous insulin, produced by beta cells of the pancreatic islets of Langerhans, and commercial insulin, obtained from beef and pork pancreases, *lower* glucose levels. Synthetic antidiabetic drugs (sulfonylureas including acetohexamide, chlorpropamide, tolazamide, and tolbutamide) are given orally to stimulate insulin secretion in patients with diabetes who have some beta cell function. They have no value in patients with no functional beta cell tissue. Glucagon, a hormone normally produced by alpha cells of the pancreatic islets, *raises* blood glucose levels by stimulating glycogenolysis and glyconeogenesis. It thus reverses insulin-induced hypoglycemia in patients with adequate hepatic glycogen stores.

Major uses

- Glucagon is used in emergencies to reverse insulin-induced hypoglycemia in patients with diabetes mellitus.
- Insulin supplements or replaces endogenous insulin in the treatment of diabetes mellitus, especially the juvenile-onset (insulin-dependent) form. It's used in maturity-onset (non–insulin-dependent) diabetes mellitus if oral sulfonylureas are ineffective.
- Sulfonylureas are used to treat maturity-onset diabetes mellitus that is inadequately controlled by diet alone. Chlorpropamide is also used to treat diabetes insipidus.

Mechanism of action

- Glucagon raises blood glucose levels by promoting catalytic depolymerization of hepatic glycogen to glucose.
- Insulin increases glucose transport across muscle and fat cell membranes to reduce blood glucose levels. It promotes conversion of glucose to its storage form, glycogen; triggers amino acid uptake and conversion to protein in muscle cells and inhibits protein degradation; stimulates triglyceride formation and inhibits release of free fatty acids from adipose tissue; and stimulates lipoprotein lipase activity, which converts circulating lipoproteins to fatty acids.
- Sulfonylureas stimulate insulin release from the pancreatic beta cells and reduce glucose output by the liver. Chlorpropamide also exerts an antidiuretic effect in patients with pituitary-deficient diabetes insipidus.

Absorption, distribution, metabolism, and excretion

- Glucagon is rapidly absorbed after parenteral administration, metabolized mainly in the liver, and excreted in urine.
- Insulin, because it is destroyed in the gastrointestinal tract, is generally administered by subcutaneous injection. It is absorbed directly from the injection site into the bloodstream. Absorption rate depends on insulin type, concentration, dose, volume, vascularity at the injection site, and the patient's physical activity pattern. Vigorous exercise, for example, accelerates absorption and metabolism from an injection in the thigh but not from an injection in the arm. Insulin is distributed throughout extracellular fluid and metabolized in the liver (primary site) and in the kidneys and muscles (secondary sites).

THERAPEUTIC ACTIVITY OF ANTIDIABETIC DRUGS AND GLUCAGON

DRUG	ONSET	PEAK	DURATION	REMARKS
Rapid-acting insulins				
prompt insulin zinc suspension (semilente)	1 to 2 hr	4 to 7 hr	12 to 16 hr	Glycosuria most likely nocturnally. Hypoglycemia most likely 10 a.m. to lunchtime.
regular insulin	30 to 60 min	2 to 3 hr	5 to 7 hr	
Intermediate-acting insulins				
insulin zinc suspension (lente)	1 to 2 hr	8 to 12 hr	24 to 28 hr	Glycosuria most likely before lunch. Hypoglycemia most likely 3 p.m. to dinnertime.
globin zinc insulin	2 hr	8 to 16 hr	18 to 24 hr	
isophane insulin suspension (NPH)	1 to 2 hr	8 to 12 hr	24 to 28 hr	
Long-acting insulins				
extended insulin zinc suspension (ultralente)	4 to 8 hr	18 to 24 hr	> 36 hr	Glycosuria most likely before lunch and at bedtime. Hypoglycemia most likely 2 a.m. to breakfast.
protamine zinc insulin suspension (PZI)	4 to 8 hr	14 to 24 hr	> 36 hr	
Sulfonylureas				
acetohexamide	1 hr	4 to 5 hr	12 to 24 hr	
chlorpropamide	1 hr	3 to 6 hr	40 to 60 hr	
tolazamide	4 to 6 hr	4 to 6 hr	10 to 14 hr	
tolbutamide	1 hr	4 to 6 hr	6 to 12 hr	
glucagon	15 to 30 min	—	1 to 1½ hr	

Only small quantities of insulin are excreted in urine.

• Of the sulfonylureas, acetohexamide and tolazamide are metabolized to active metabolites and excreted in urine. Chlorpropamide is excreted in urine, primarily unchanged. Tolbutamide is metabolized to inactive metabolites and excreted in urine.

NAMES, INDICATIONS AND DOSAGES	SIDE EFFECTS

acetohexamide
Dimelor♦♦, Dymelor

Stable, maturity-onset nonketotic diabetes mellitus uncontrolled by diet alone and previously untreated:
ADULTS: initially, 250 mg P.O. daily before breakfast; may increase dose q 5 to 7 days (by 250 to 500 mg) as needed to maximum 1.5 g daily, divided b.i.d. to t.i.d. before meals.

To replace insulin therapy: if insulin dose is less than 20 units daily, insulin may be stopped and oral therapy started with 250 mg P.O. daily, before breakfast, increased as above if needed. If insulin dose is 20 to 40 units daily, start oral therapy with 250 mg P.O. daily, before breakfast, while reducing insulin dose 25% to 30% daily or every other day, depending on response to oral therapy.

Blood: *bone marrow aplasia.*
GI: nausea, heartburn, vomiting.
Metabolic: sodium loss, *hypoglycemia.*
Skin: rash, pruritus, facial flushing.
Other: hypersensitivity reactions.

chlorpropamide
Chloromide♦♦, Chloronase♦♦, Diabinese♦, Novopropamide♦♦, Stabinol♦♦

Stable, maturity-onset nonketotic diabetes mellitus uncontrolled by diet alone and previously untreated:
ADULTS: 250 mg P.O. daily with breakfast or in divided doses if GI disturbances occur. First dosage increase may be made after 5 to 7 days due to extended duration of action, then dose may be increased q 3 to 5 days by 50 to 125 mg, if needed, to maximum 750 mg daily. Start with dose of 100 to 125 mg in older patients.

To change from insulin to oral therapy: if insulin dose less than 40 units daily, insulin may be stopped and oral therapy started as above. If insulin dose is 40 units or more daily, start oral therapy as above with insulin dose reduced 50%. Further insulin reductions should be made according to the patient's response.

Blood: *bone marrow aplasia.*
GI: nausea, heartburn, vomiting.
GU: tea-colored urine.
Metabolic: prolonged hypoglycemia, *dilutional hyponatremia.*
Skin: rash, pruritus, facial flushing.
Other: *hypersensitivity reactions.*

glucagon

Coma of insulin-shock therapy:
ADULTS: 0.5 to 1 mg S.C., I.M., or I.V. 1 hour after coma develops; may repeat within 25 minutes, if necessary. In very deep coma, also

GI: nausea, vomiting.
Other: hypersensitivity.

♦ Available in U.S. and Canada. ♦♦ Available in Canada only.
All other products (no symbol) available in U.S. only. Italicized side effects are common or life-threatening.

INTERACTIONS AND SPECIAL CONSIDERATIONS

Interactions:
ALCOHOL, CORTICOSTEROIDS, DEXTROTHYROXINE, ESTROGENS, GLUCAGON, RIFAMPIN, THIAZIDE DIURETICS, THYROXINE: decreased hypoglycemic response. Monitor blood glucose.
ANABOLIC STEROIDS, CLOFIBRATE, GUANETHIDINE, HALOFENATE, MAO INHIBITORS, PHENYLBUTAZONE, SALICYLATES, SULFONAMIDES, ORAL ANTICOAGULANTS: increased hypoglycemic activity. Monitor blood glucose.
METOPROLOL, PROPRANOLOL, CLONIDINE: prolonged hypoglycemic effect and masked symptoms of hypoglycemia. Use together cautiously.

Special considerations:
• Contraindicated in treatment of juvenile, growth-onset, brittle, and severe diabetes; in diabetes mellitus adequately controlled by diet; in maturity-onset diabetes complicated by ketosis, acidosis, diabetic coma; Raynaud's gangrene; renal or hepatic impairment; thyroid or other endocrine dysfunction. Use cautiously in patients with sulfonamide hypersensitivity.
• Patient should understand nature of the disease; importance of following therapeutic regimen and adhering to specific diet, weight reduction, exercise, personal hygiene, and avoiding infection; how and when to test for glycosuria and ketonuria; recognition of hypoglycemia and hyperglycemia.
• Therapy relieves symptoms but doesn't cure disease.
• Patient transferring from another oral sulfonylurea antidiabetic drug usually needs no transition period.
• Patient transferring from insulin therapy to an oral antidiabetic should be monitored for urinary glucose and ketones at least 3 times a day; patient may require hospitalization during transition.
• During periods of increased stress, such as infection, fever, surgery, or trauma, patient may require insulin therapy. Patient should be monitored closely for hyperglycemia in these situations.
• Patient should avoid moderate-to-large intake of alcohol; disulfiram reaction possible.
• For symptoms and treatment of toxicity, see APPENDIX.

Interactions:
ALCOHOL, CORTICOSTEROIDS, DEXTROTHYROXINE, GLUCAGON, RIFAMPIN, THIAZIDE DIURETICS: decreased hypoglycemic response. Monitor blood glucose.
ANABOLIC STEROIDS, CHLORAMPHENICOL, CLOFIBRATE, GUANETHIDINE, HALOFENATE, MAO INHIBITORS, PHENYLBUTAZONE, SALICYLATES, SULFONAMIDES, ORAL ANTICOAGULANTS: increased hypoglycemic activity. Monitor blood glucose.
METOPROLOL, PROPRANOLOL, CLONIDINE: prolonged hypoglycemic effect and masked symptoms of hypoglycemia. Use together cautiously.

Special considerations:
• Contraindicated in the treatment of juvenile, growth-onset, brittle, and severe diabetes.
• Contraindicated in diabetes mellitus adequately controlled by diet and in maturity-onset diabetes complicated by fever, ketosis, acidosis, diabetic coma; major surgery; severe trauma; Raynaud's gangrene; renal or hepatic impairment; thyroid or other endocrine dysfunction. Use cautiously in patients with sulfonamide hypersensitivity.
• Patient should understand nature of the disease; importance of following therapeutic regimen and adhering to specific diet, weight reduction, exercise, personal hygiene, avoiding infection; how and when to test for glycosuria and ketonuria; and recognition of and intervention for hypoglycemia and hyperglycemia.
• Therapy relieves symptoms but does not cure the disease.
• Side effects, especially hypoglycemia, may be more frequent or severe than with some other sulfonylurea drugs (acetohexamide, tolazamide, and tolbutamide) because of its long duration of effect (36 hours).
• If hypoglycemia occurs, patient should be monitored closely for a minimum of 3 to 5 days.
• Patient transferring from another oral sulfonylurea antidiabetic drug usually needs no transition period.
• Patient transferring from insulin therapy to an oral antidiabetic should be monitored for urinary glucose and ketones at least t.i.d.; patient may require hospitalization during transition.
• Drug may accumulate in patients with renal insufficiency.
• Patient should avoid moderate-to-large intake of alcohol; disulfiram reaction possible.
• Signs of impending renal insufficiency: dysuria, anuria, and hematuria.
• For symptoms and treatment of toxicity, see APPENDIX.

Interactions:
PHENYTOIN: inhibited glucagon-induced insulin release. Use cautiously.

Special considerations:
• Glucagon should be used only under medical supervision.
• Patients with hypoglycemic juvenile or unstable diabetes usually do not respond to glucagon. Should be given dextrose I.V. instead.
• Patient should be aroused from coma as quickly as possible and given additional carbohydrates

(continued on following page)

NAMES, INDICATIONS AND DOSAGES	SIDE EFFECTS

glucagon
(continued)

give glucose 10% to 50% I.V. for faster response. When patient responds, give additional carbohydrate immediately.

Severe insulin-induced hypoglycemia during diabetic therapy:
ADULTS AND CHILDREN: 0.5 to 1 mg S.C., I.M., or I.V.; may repeat q 20 minutes for 2 doses, if necessary. If coma persists, give glucose 10% to 50% I.V.

---

insulins
regular insulin
Actrapid, Beef Regular Iletin II (acid neutral CZI), Insulin-Toronto (beef or pork)♦♦, Pork Regular Iletin II, Velosulin
regular insulin concentrated
Regular (concentrated) Iletin
prompt insulin zinc suspension
Semilente Iletin, Semilente Insulin♦, Semitard
isophane insulin suspension (NPH)
Beef NPH Iletin II, Insulatard NPH, Lentard, NPH Iletin, NPH Insulin♦♦, Pork NPH Iletin II
insulin zinc suspension
Beef Lente Iletin, Beef Lente Iletin II, Lente Iletin, Lente Insulin♦, Pork Lente Iletin II
globin zinc insulin
protamine zinc insulin suspension (PZI)
Beef Protamine Zinc Iletin II, Pork Protamine Zinc Iletin II, Protamine Zinc Iletin
extended insulin zinc suspension
Ultralente Iletin, Ultralente Insulin♦, Ultratard

Diabetic ketoacidosis (use regular insulin only):
ADULTS: 25 to 150 units I.V. stat, then additional doses may be given q 1 hour based on blood sugar levels until patient is out of acidosis; then give S.C. q 6 hours thereafter.
Alternative dosage schedule: 50 to 100 units I.V. and 50 to 100 units S.C. stat; additional doses may be given q 2 to 6 hours based on blood sugar levels; or 0.33 units/kg I.V. bolus, followed by 7 to 10 units/hour I.V. by continuous infusion. Continue infusion until blood sugar drops to 250 mg%, then start S.C. insulin q 6 hours.
CHILDREN: 0.5 to 1 unit/kg divided into 2 doses, 1 given I.V. and the other S.C., followed by 0.5 to 1 unit/kg I.V. q 1 to 2 hours; or 0.1 unit/kg I.V. bolus, then 0.1 unit/kg/hour continuous I.V. infusion until blood sugar drops to 250 mg%, then start S.C. insulin.
Preparation of infusion: add 100 units regular insulin and 1 g albumin to 100 ml 0.9% saline solution. Insulin concentration will be 1 unit/ml. (The albumin will adsorb to plastic, preventing loss of the insulin to plastic.)

Metabolic: *hypoglycemia, hyperglycemia (rebound, or Somogyi, effect).*
Skin: urticaria.
Local: *lipoatrophy, lipohypertrophy,* itching, swelling, redness, stinging, warmth at site of injection.
Other: *anaphylaxis.*

♦ Available in U.S. and Canada. ♦♦ Available in Canada only.
All other products (no symbol) available in U.S. only. Italicized side effects are common or life-threatening.

INTERACTIONS AND SPECIAL CONSIDERATIONS

to prevent secondary hypoglycemic reactions.
• For I.V. drip infusion, glucagon is compatible with dextrose solution but forms a precipitate in chloride solutions.
• Patient and family should understand proper glucagon administration, recognition of hypoglycemia, and urgency of calling doctor immediately in emergencies.
• May be used as diagnostic aid in radiologic examination of the stomach, duodenum, small bowel, and colon when a hypotonic state is advantageous.
• May be stored for 3 months at 2° to 15° C. (35.6° to 59° F.) after reconstitution.

Interactions:
METOPROLOL, PROPRANOLOL: hyperglycemia or hypoglycemia may occur. Symptoms of hypoglycemia may be masked. Use together cautiously.
ALCOHOL, CORTICOSTEROIDS, DEXTROTHYROXINE, ESTROGENS, GLUCAGON, RIFAMPIN, THIAZIDE DIURETICS, THYROXINE: decreased insulin response. Monitor blood glucose.
ANABOLIC STEROIDS, CLOFIBRATE, GUANETHIDINE, HALOFENATE, MAO INHIBITORS, PHENYLBUTAZONE, SALICYLATES, SULFONAMIDES, ORAL ANTICOAGULANTS: increased insulin response. Monitor for blood glucose.

Special considerations:
• Only regular insulin should be used in patients with circulatory collapse, diabetic ketoacidosis, or hyperkalemia. Regular insulin concentrated should not be used I.V. Intermediate or long-acting insulins should not be used for coma or other emergency requiring rapid drug action.
• During 1980, more purified forms of insulin became available. (These are called "new" insulin and are so labeled.) These new, highly purified forms may require dosage adjustment in patients previously stabilized on insulin. Patient should be made aware of this and observe closely until dosage is established.
• Accuracy of measurement is very important, especially with regular insulin concentrated. Aids such as magnifying sleeve, dose magnifier, or cornwall syringe may help improve accuracy.
• With regular insulin concentrated, a deep secondary hypoglycemic reaction may occur 18 to 24 hours after injection.
• Dosage is always expressed in USP units.
• Regular, intermediate, and long-acting insulin may be mixed to meet patient's needs. All components should have same concentration.
• Store insulin in a cool area. Refrigeration is desirable but not essential, except with regular insulin concentrated.
• Insulin that has changed color should not be used.
• Check expiration date on vial before contents are used.
• Administration route is subcutaneous because absorption rate and pain are less than with I.M. injections. Ketosis-prone juvenile-onset, severely ill, and newly diagnosed patients with diabetes with very high blood sugar levels may require hospitalization and I.V. treatment with regular fast-acting insulin. Patients with diabetes who are ketosis-resistant may be treated as outpatients with intermediate-acting insulin and instructions on how to alter dosage according to self-performed urine glucose determinations. Some patients, primarily pregnant or brittle diabetics, may use a dextrometer to do fingerstick blood glucose tests at home.
• Site should not be rubbed after injection. Injection sites should be rotated to avoid overuse of one area. However, patients with unstable diabetes may achieve better control if injection site is rotated within same anatomic region.
• To mix insulin suspension, vial should be swirled gently or rotated between palms or between palm and thigh. Should not be shaken vigorously, which causes bubbling and air in syringe.
• Insulin requirements increase, sometimes drastically, in pregnant patients who are diabetic, then decline immediately postpartum.
• Therapy relieves symptoms but doesn't cure the disease.
• Patient should understand nature of the disease, importance of following therapeutic regimen and specific diet, weight reduction, exercise, personal hygiene, avoiding infection, and timing of injection and eating. Urine tests are essential guides to dosage and success of therapy. Patient should know how to recognize hypoglycemic symptoms because insulin-induced hypoglycemia is hazardous and may cause brain damage if prolonged; most side effects are self-limiting and temporary.
• Patient should wear medical I.D. always; carry ample insulin supply and syringes on trips; have carbohydrates (lump of sugar or candy) on hand for emergency; take note of time zone changes for dose schedule when traveling.
• Marijuana may increase insulin requirements.
• U-80 strength no longer certified by Food and Drug Administration. Instruct patient in use of U-100 strength.
• Some patients may develop insulin resistance and require large insulin doses to control symp-

(continued on following page)

NAMES, INDICATIONS AND DOSAGES	SIDE EFFECTS
insulins *(continued)* **Ketosis-prone and juvenile-onset diabetes mellitus, diabetes mellitus inadequately controlled by diet and oral hypoglycemics:** ADULTS AND CHILDREN: therapeutic regimen prescribed by doctor and adjusted according to patient's blood and urine glucose concentrations.	
tolazamide Tolinase **Stable, maturity-onset nonketotic diabetes mellitus uncontrolled by diet alone and previously untreated:** ADULTS: initially, 100 mg P.O. daily with breakfast if fasting blood sugar (FBS) under 200 mg%; or 250 mg if FBS is over 200 mg%. May adjust dose at weekly intervals by 100 to 250 mg. Maximum dose 500 mg b.i.d. before meals. ELDERLY OR DEBILITATED PATIENTS: increase dose by 50 to 125 mg at weekly intervals. **To change from insulin to oral therapy:** if insulin dose under 20 units daily, insulin may be stopped and oral therapy started at 100 mg P.O. daily with breakfast. If insulin dose is 20 to 40 units daily, insulin may be stopped and oral therapy started at 250 mg P.O. daily with breakfast. If insulin dose is over 40 units daily, decrease insulin dose 50% and start oral therapy at 250 mg P.O. daily with breakfast. Increase doses as above.	**Blood:** *bone marrow aplasia.* **GI:** nausea, vomiting. **Metabolic:** hypoglycemia. **Skin:** rash, urticaria, facial flushing. **Other:** hypersensitivity reactions.
tolbutamide Mellitol♦♦, Mobenol♦♦, Neo-Dibetic♦♦, Novobutamide♦♦, Oramide♦♦, Orinase♦, SK-Tolbutamide, Tolbutone♦♦ **Stable, maturity-onset nonketotic diabetes mellitus uncontrolled by diet alone and previously untreated:** ADULTS: initially, 1 to 2 g P.O. daily as single dose or divided b.i.d. to t.i.d. May adjust dose to maximum 3 g daily. **To change from insulin to oral therapy:** if insulin dose is under 20 units daily, insulin may be stopped and oral therapy started at 1 to 2 g daily. If insulin dose is 20 to 40 units daily, insulin dose is reduced 30% to 50% and oral therapy started as above. If insulin dose is over 40 units daily, insulin dose is decreased 20% and oral therapy started as above. Further reductions in insulin dose are based on patient's response to oral therapy.	**Blood:** *bone marrow aplasia.* **GI:** nausea, heartburn. **Metabolic:** hypoglycemia. **Skin:** rash, pruritus, facial flushing. **Other:** hypersensitivity reactions.

♦ Available in U.S. and Canada. ♦♦ Available in Canada only.
All other products (no symbol) available in U.S. only. Italicized side effects are common or life-threatening.

INTERACTIONS AND SPECIAL CONSIDERATIONS

toms of diabetes. U-500 insulin is available for such patients as Purified Pork Iletin Regular Insulin, U500. Although every pharmacy may not normally stock it, it is readily available. Patient should notify pharmacist several days before refill of prescription is needed. Nurse should give hospital pharmacy sufficient notice before needing to refill in-house prescription. U-500 insulin must never be stored in same area with other insulin preparations due to danger of severe overdose if given accidentally to other patients. U-500 insulin must be administered with a U-100 syringe since no syringes are made for this drug.

• For symptoms and treatment of toxicity, see APPENDIX.

Interactions:

ALCOHOL, CORTICOSTEROIDS, DEXTROTHYROXINE, ESTROGENS, GLUCAGON, RIFAMPIN, THIAZIDE DIURETICS, THYROXINE: decreased hypoglycemic response. Monitor blood glucose.

ANABOLIC STEROIDS, CLOFIBRATE, GUANETHIDINE, HALOFENATE, MAO INHIBITORS, PHENYLBUTAZONE, SALICYLATES, SULFONAMIDES, ORAL ANTICOAGULANTS: increased hypoglycemic activity. Monitor blood glucose.

METOPROLOL, PROPRANOLOL, CLONIDINE: prolonged hypoglycemic effect and masked symptoms of hypoglycemia. Use together cautiously.

Special considerations:

• Contraindicated in juvenile, growth-onset, and severe diabetes mellitus; diabetes mellitus adequately controlled by diet; in maturity-onset diabetes mellitus complicated by fever, ketosis, acidosis, or coma; major surgery; severe trauma; Raynaud's gangrene; renal or hepatic impairment; thyroid or other endocrine dysfunction. Use cautiously in patients with sulfonamide hypersensitivity and in elderly, debilitated, or malnourished patients.

• Patient should understand nature of the disease; importance of following therapeutic regimen and specific diet, weight reduction, exercise, personal hygiene, avoiding infection; how and when to test for glycosuria and ketonuria; and recognition of hypoglycemia and hyperglycemia.

• Therapy relieves symptoms but doesn't cure the disease.

• Patient transferring from another oral sulfonylurea antidiabetic drug usually needs no transition period.

• Patient transferring from insulin therapy to an oral hypoglycemic should test urine for glucose and ketones at least 3 times a day; hospitalization may be required during the transition.

• Patient should avoid moderate-to-large intake of alcohol; disulfiram reaction possible.

• For symptoms and treatment of toxicity, see APPENDIX.

Interactions:

ALCOHOL, CORTICOSTEROIDS, DEXTROTHYROXINE, ESTROGENS, GLUCAGON, RIFAMPIN, THIAZIDE DIURETICS, THYROXINE: decreased hypoglycemic response. Monitor blood glucose.

ANABOLIC STEROIDS, CHLORAMPHENICOL, CLOFIBRATE, GUANETHIDINE, HALOFENATE, MAO INHIBITORS, PHENYLBUTAZONE, SALICYLATES, SULFONAMIDES, ORAL ANTICOAGULANTS: increased hypoglycemic activity. Monitor blood glucose.

METOPROLOL, PROPRANOLOL, CLONIDINE: prolonged hypoglycemic effect and masked symptoms of hypoglycemia. Use together cautiously.

Special considerations:

• Contraindicated in juvenile, growth-onset, brittle, and severe diabetes; diabetes mellitus adequately controlled by diet; in maturity-onset diabetes mellitus complicated by fever, ketosis, acidosis, or coma; major surgery; severe trauma; Raynaud's gangrene; renal or hepatic impairment; thyroid or other endocrine dysfunction; or pregnancy. Use cautiously in sulfonamide hypersensitivity.

• Patient should understand nature of the disease; importance of following therapeutic regimen and specific diet, weight reduction, exercise, personal hygiene, and avoiding infection; how and when to test for glycosuria and ketonuria; and recognition of hypoglycemia and hyperglycemia.

• Therapy relieves symptoms but doesn't cure the disease.

• Patient transferring from another oral sulfonylurea antidiabetic drug usually needs no transition period.

• Patient transferring from insulin therapy to an oral hypoglycemic should test urine for glucose and ketones at least 3 times a day; hospitalization may be required during the transition.

• Patient should avoid moderate-to-large intake of alcohol; disulfiram reaction possible.

• For symptoms and treatment of toxicity, see APPENDIX.

58

Thyroid hormones

levothyroxine sodium (T_4 or L-thyroxine sodium)
liothyronine sodium (T_3)
liotrix
thyroglobulin
thyroid USP (desiccated)
thyrotropin (thyroid-stimulating hormone or TSH)

The thyroid preparations described in this chapter are used as replacement therapy in patients with diminished or absent thyroid function.

Thyroid hormones are produced and stored in the follicles of the thyroid gland. Their synthesis and release are regulated by *thyrotropin,* also known as thyroid-stimulating hormone (TSH), which is secreted by the anterior pituitary gland. Increased blood levels of thyroid hormones inhibit release of pituitary TSH. Through this negative feedback mechanism, they homeostatically control further increases in thyroid hormone.

Thyroid extract is the prototype of the substances used to treat hypothyroidism. This substance, the desiccated thyroid gland of animals, contains T_3 (liothyronine) and T_4 (tetraiodothyronine or thyroxine), as well as other organic materials. *Thyroglobulin* is a purified extract of a hog's thyroid gland that is standardized on the basis of iodine content and metabolic activity. Thyroid USP (desiccated) is a cleaned, dried, and powdered thyroid gland obtained from animal (usually hog) sources.

Major uses

Thyroid hormones prevent goiter and hypothyroidism in patients receiving antithyroid drugs for thyrotoxicosis. They are also used to treat confirmed hypothyroidism and supply replacement therapy in primary and secondary myxedema, myxedema coma, cretinism, and simple nontoxic goiter.

• Thyroglobulin and thyroid USP are used to treat certain thyrotropin-dependent carcinomas of the thyroid.

• Thyrotropin is used in combination with radioactive iodine in treatment of thyroid tumors and is also used in differential diagnosis of subclinical hypothyroidism and low thyroid reserve.

Mechanism of action

Thyroid hormones stimulate the metabolism of all body tissues by accelerating the rate of cellular oxidation. They enhance carbohydrate and protein biosynthesis by glyconeogenesis, which increases the mobilization and utilization of glycogen stores. They also affect lipid metabolism by decreasing cholesterol levels in the liver and blood.

• Thyrotropin stimulates the uptake of radioactive iodine in patients with thyroid carcinoma. It also promotes thyroid hormone production by the anterior pituitary.

Absorption, distribution, metabolism, and excretion

• Levothyroxine, liothyronine, thyroglobulin, and thyroid USP are efficiently absorbed from the gastrointestinal tract. Liothyronine is better absorbed, however, than levothyroxine.

• Levothyroxine, well distributed to all body tissues, is partially metabolized in the liver. Both the metabolite and the unchanged hormone are passed into the bile. The metabolite is eliminated in feces; the small amount of free levothyroxine is recycled to the liver.

• Liothyronine's metabolism is unclear. Liothyronine releases iodine into the body tissues.

THERAPEUTIC EFFECTIVENESS OF THYROID HORMONES

DRUG	EQUIVALENT DOSE	CONTENTS	RELATIVE DURATION	
levothyroxine	100 mcg	T_4	Long (once-daily dosing possible)	
liothyronine	25 mcg	T_3	Short (multiple doses must be given daily)	
liotrix	Either Euthroid-1 or Thyrolar-1	T_4 and T_3 in 4:1 ratio	Intermediate	(Those with higher T_4 concentration are longer-acting; those with lower T_4 concentration are shorter-acting.)
thyroglobulin	65 mg	T_4 and T_3 in 2.5:1 ratio	Intermediate	
thyroid USP	65 mg	T_4 and T_3 in variable ratios	Intermediate	

The thyroid then uses this iodine for synthesis of additional levothyroxine and liothyronine. Some of the iodine released by liothyronine is either excreted in urine or eliminated through the bile in feces.

Onset and duration

- Full onset of levothyroxine, liotrix, thyroglobulin, and thyroid USP takes 1 to 3 weeks, although a response may be noted after several days.
- Levothyroxine generally has the slowest onset (several days), and a half-life of 6½ days. It has a long duration: its action may persist for weeks after therapy is terminated.
- Liothyronine has a relatively rapid onset of action (a few hours), and its half-life is less than 3 days. Its action persists for several days.

Combination products

EUTHROID-½: levothyroxine sodium 30 mcg and liothyronine sodium 7.5 mcg.
EUTHROID-1: levothyroxine sodium 60 mcg and liothyronine sodium 15 mcg.
EUTHROID-2: levothyroxine sodium 120 mcg and liothyronine sodium 30 mcg.
EUTHROID-3: levothyroxine sodium 180 mcg and liothyronine sodium 45 mcg.
THYROLAR-¼: levothyroxine sodium 12.5 mcg and liothyronine sodium 3.1 mcg.
THYROLAR-½♦: levothyroxine sodium 25 mcg and liothyronine sodium 6.25 mcg.
THYROLAR-1♦: levothyroxine sodium 50 mcg and liothyronine sodium 12.5 mcg.
THYROLAR-2♦: levothyroxine sodium 100 mcg and liothyronine sodium 25 mcg.
THYROLAR-3♦: levothyroxine sodium 150 mcg and liothyronine sodium 37.5 mcg.

NAMES, INDICATIONS AND DOSAGES	SIDE EFFECTS

levothyroxine sodium (T_4 or L-thyroxine sodium)

Eltroxin♦♦, Levoid, Levothroid, Noroxine, Synthroid♦

Cretinism in children younger than 1 year:
Initially, 0.025 to 0.05 mg P.O. daily, increased by 0.05 mg P.O. q 2 to 3 weeks to total daily dose 0.1 to 0.4 mg P.O.

Myxedema coma:
ADULTS: 0.2 to 0.5 mg I.V. If no response in 24 hours, additional 0.1 to 0.3 mg I.V. After condition stabilized, oral maintenance.

Thyroid hormone replacement:
ADULTS: initially, 0.025 to 0.1 mg P.O. daily, increased by 0.05 to 0.1 mg P.O. q 1 to 4 weeks until desired response. Maintenance dose 0.1 to 0.4 mg daily.
CHILDREN: initially, maximum 0.05 mg P.O. daily, gradually increased by 0.025 to 0.05 mg P.O. q 1 to 4 weeks until desired response.

Side effects of thyroid hormones are extensions of their pharmacologic properties and reflect patient sensitivity to them.
Signs of overdosage:
CNS: *nervousness, insomnia, tremor.*
CV: *tachycardia, palpitations, arrhythmias, angina pectoris,* hypertension.
GI: change in appetite, nausea, diarrhea.
Other: headache, leg cramps, weight loss, sweating, heat intolerance, fever, menstrual irregularities.

liothyronine sodium (T_3)

Cytomel♦, Cytomine

Cretinism:
CHILDREN 3 YEARS AND OLDER: 50 to 100 mcg P.O. daily.
CHILDREN UNDER 3 YEARS: 5 mcg P.O. daily, increased by 5 mcg q 3 to 4 days until desired response occurs.

Myxedema:
ADULTS: initially 5 mcg daily, increased by 5 to 10 mcg q 1 or 2 weeks. Maintenance dose 50 to 100 mcg daily.

Nontoxic goiter:
ADULTS: initially, 5 mcg P.O. daily; may be increased by 12.5 to 25 mcg daily q 1 to 2 weeks. Usual maintenance dose 75 mcg daily.
ELDERLY: initially, 5 mcg P.O. daily, increased by 5-mcg increments at weekly intervals until desired response.
CHILDREN: initially, 5 mcg P.O. daily, increased by 5-mcg increments at weekly intervals until desired response.

Thyroid hormone replacement:
ADULTS: initially, 25 mcg P.O. daily, in-

Side effects of thyroid hormones are extensions of their pharmacologic properties and reflect patient sensitivity to them.
CNS: hyperirritability, *nervousness, insomnia,* twitching, *tremors,* headache.
CV: increased cardiac output, *tachycardia,* cardiac arrhythmias, *angina pectoris,* increased blood pressure, *cardiac decompensation and collapse.*
GI: diarrhea, abdominal cramps, vomiting.
Other: weight loss, heat intolerance, hyperhidrosis, menstrual irregularities; in infants and children—accelerated rate of bone maturation.

INTERACTIONS AND SPECIAL CONSIDERATIONS

Interactions:
CHOLESTYRAMINE: levothyroxine absorption impaired. Separate doses by 4 to 5 hours.
I.V. PHENYTOIN: free thyroid released. Monitor for tachycardia.

Special considerations:
- Contraindicated in myocardial infarctions, thyrotoxicosis (except with antithyroid drugs), or uncorrected adrenal insufficiency (thyroid hormones increase tissue demand for adrenocortical hormone and may cause acute adrenal crisis). Use with extreme caution in angina pectoris, hypertension, or other cardiovascular disorders; renal insufficiency; or ischemic states.
- Use carefully in myxedema; patients unusually sensitive to thyroid hormone. Dose varies widely among patients; should start at lowest dose and titrate in higher doses according to patient's symptoms and laboratory data until euthyroid state is reached.
- Rapid replacement in patients with arteriosclerosis may precipitate angina, coronary occlusion, or stroke. Use cautiously in such patients.
- Patients with coronary artery disease who must receive thyroid should be observed carefully for possible coronary insufficiency if catecholamines must be given.
- Potentially dangerous; not indicated to relieve vague symptoms, such as physical and mental sluggishness, irritability, depression, nervousness, ill-defined pains; to treat obesity in euthyroid persons; to treat metabolic insufficiency not associated with thyroid insufficiency; or to treat menstrual disorders or male infertility, unless associated with hypothyroidism.
- When changing from levothyroxine to liothyronine, levothyroxine should be stopped before beginning liothyronine. Should be increased in small increments after residual effects of levothyroxine have disappeared. When changing from liothyronine to levothyroxine, levothyroxine should be started several days before liothyronine is withdrawn to avoid relapse.
- Patient should immediately report signs of overdosage: chest pain (especially in elderly), palpitations, sweating, or nervousness. Chest pain, dyspnea, and tachycardia may signal aggravated cardiovascular disease and require clinical reevaluation.
- Patient should take thyroid hormones regularly, at the same time each day, to maintain constant hormone levels.
- Morning dosage prevents insomnia.
- Pulse rate and blood pressure should be monitored.
- Should be protected from moisture and light, and I.V. dose prepared immediately before injection.
- Thyroid hormones alter thyroid function study results. Prothrombin time should be monitored; patients taking these hormones usually require less anticoagulant. Patients should report unusual bleeding and bruising.
- Patients taking levothyroxine who need to have radioactive iodine uptake studies must discontinue drug 4 weeks before test.

Interactions:
CHOLESTYRAMINE: liothyronine absorption impaired. Separate doses by 4 to 5 hours.
I.V. PHENYTOIN: free thyroid released. Monitor for tachycardia.

Special considerations:
- Contraindicated in myocardial infarction, thyrotoxicosis (except with antithyroid drugs), or uncorrected adrenal insufficiency (thyroid hormones increase tissue demand for adrenocortical hormone and may cause acute adrenal crisis). Use with extreme caution in angina pectoris, hypertension, or other cardiovascular disorders; renal insufficiency; or ischemic states.
- Rapid replacement in patients with arteriosclerosis may precipitate angina, coronary occlusion, or stroke. Use cautiously in such patients.
- Patients with coronary artery disease who must receive thyroid should be observed carefully for possible coronary insufficiency if catecholamines must be given.
- Use carefully in myxedema; patients unusually sensitive to thyroid hormone.
- Potentially dangerous; not indicated to relieve vague symptoms, such as physical and mental sluggishness, irritability, depression, nervousness, and ill-defined aches and pains; to treat obesity in euthyroid persons; to treat metabolic insufficiency; or to treat menstrual disorders or male infertility, unless associated with hypothyroidism.
- When changing from levothyroxine to liothyronine, levothyroxine should be stopped before beginning liothyronine. Should be increased in small increments after residual effects of levothyroxine have disappeared. When changing from liothyronine to levothyroxine, levothyroxine should be started several days before liothyronine is withdrawn to avoid relapse.
- Patient should immediately report signs of overdosage: chest pain (especially in elderly), palpitations, sweating, or nervousness. Chest pain, dyspnea, and tachycardia may signal aggravated cardiovascular disease and require clinical reevaluation.
- Patient should take thyroid hormones regularly, at the same time each day, to maintain constant hormone levels.
- Morning dosage prevents insomnia.
- Pulse rate and blood pressure should be monitored.
- Thyroid hormones alter thyroid function study results. Prothrombin time should be monitored; patients taking these hormones may require less

(continued on following page)

NAMES, INDICATIONS AND DOSAGES	SIDE EFFECTS
liothyronine sodium *(continued)* creased by 12.5 to 25 mcg q 1 to 2 weeks until satisfactory response. Usual maintenance dose 25 to 75 mcg daily.	
liotrix Euthroid, Thyrolar♦ **Hypothyroidism:** Dosages must be individualized to approximate the deficit in the patient's thyroid secretion. ADULTS AND CHILDREN: initially, 15 to 30 mg P.O. daily, increasing by 15 to 30 mg q 1 to 2 weeks to desired response; increments in children's dose q 2 weeks. ELDERLY: initially, 15 to 30 mg. Usual adult dose doubled q 6 to 8 weeks to desired response.	Side effects of thyroid hormones are extensions of their pharmacologic properties and reflect patient sensitivity to them. **CNS:** hyperirritability, *nervousness, insomnia,* twitching, *tremors.* **CV:** increased cardiac output, *tachycardia,* cardiac arrhythmia, *angina pectoris,* increased blood pressure, *cardiac decompensation and collapse.* **GI:** diarrhea, abdominal cramps, vomiting. **Other:** weight loss, menstrual irregularities, heat intolerance, hyperhidrosis; infants and children—accelerated rate of bone maturation.
thyroglobulin Proloid♦ **Cretinism and juvenile hypothyroidism:** CHILDREN 1 YEAR AND OLDER: dosage may approach adult dose (60 to 180 mg P.O. daily), depending on response. CHILDREN 4 TO 12 MONTHS: 60 to 80 mg P.O. daily. CHILDREN 1 TO 4 MONTHS: initially, 15 to 30 mg P.O. daily, increased at 2-week intervals. Usual maintenance dose 30 to 45 mg P.O. daily. **Hypothyroidism or myxedema:** ADULTS: initially, 15 to 30 mg P.O. daily, increased by 15 to 30 mg at 2-week intervals until desired response. Usual maintenance dose 60 to 180 mg P.O. daily, as a single dose. ELDERLY: initially 7.5 to 15 mg P.O. daily; the dose is doubled at 6- to 8-week intervals until desired response is obtained.	Side effects of thyroid hormones are extensions of their pharmacologic properties and reflect patient sensitivity to them. **CNS:** hyperirritability, *nervousness, insomnia,* twitching, *tremors,* headache. **CV:** increased cardiac output, *tachycardia,* cardiac arrhythmias, *angina pectoris,* increased blood pressure, *cardiac decompensation and collapse.* **GI:** diarrhea, abdominal cramps, vomiting. **Other:** weight loss, heat intolerance, hyperhidrosis, menstrual irregularities; in infants and children—accelerated rate of bone maturation.

INTERACTIONS AND SPECIAL CONSIDERATIONS

anticoagulant. Patients should report unusual bleeding and bruising.

• Patients taking liothyronine who need to have radioactive iodine uptake studies must discontinue drug 7 to 10 days before test.

Interactions:

CHOLESTYRAMINE: liotrix absorption impaired. Separate doses by 4 to 5 hours.

I.V. PHENYTOIN: free thyroid released. Monitor for tachycardia.

Special considerations:

• Contraindicated in myocardial infarction, thyrotoxicosis (except with antithyroid drugs), or uncorrected adrenal insufficiency (thyroid hormones increase tissue demand for adrenocortical hormone and may cause acute adrenal crisis). Use with extreme caution in angina pectoris, hypertension, or other cardiovascular disorders; renal insufficiency; or ischemic states.

• Rapid replacement in patients with arteriosclerosis may precipitate angina, coronary occlusion, or stroke. Use cautiously in such patients.

• Use carefully in myxedema; patients are unusually sensitive to thyroid hormone.

• Patients with coronary artery disease who must receive thyroid should be observed carefully for possible coronary insufficiency if catecholamines must be given. Also, should be observed carefully during surgery, since cardiac arrhythmias can be precipitated.

• Potentially dangerous; not indicated to relieve vague symptoms, such as physical and mental sluggishness, irritability, depression, nervousness, ill-defined pains; to treat obesity in euthyroid persons; to treat metabolic insufficiency not associated with thyroid insufficiency; or to treat menstrual disorders or male infertility, unless associated with hypothyroidism.

• Patient should take thyroid hormones regularly, at the same time each day, preferably before breakfast, to maintain constant hormone levels.

• Patient should immediately report signs of overdosage: chest pain (especially in elderly), palpitations, sweating, or nervousness. Chest pain, dyspnea, and tachycardia may signal aggravated cardiovascular disease and require clinical reevaluation.

• The two commercially prepared liotrix drugs contain different amounts of each ingredient; do not change from one brand to the other without considering the differences in potency: Thyrolar-½ contains 25 mcg T_4 and 6.25 mcg T_3; Euthroid-½ contains 30 mcg T_4 and 7.5 mcg T_3.

• Pulse rate and blood pressure should be monitored.

• Protect from heat, light, and moisture.

• Thyroid hormones alter thyroid function study results. Prothrombin time should be monitored; patients taking these hormones usually require less anticoagulant. Patients should report unusual bleeding and bruising.

Interactions:

CHOLESTYRAMINE: thyroglobulin absorption impaired. Separate doses by 4 to 5 hours.

I.V. PHENYTOIN: free thyroid released. Monitor for tachycardia.

Special considerations:

• Contraindicated in myocardial infarction, thyrotoxicosis (except with antithyroid drugs), or uncorrected adrenal insufficiency (thyroid hormones increase tissue demand for adrenocortical hormone and may cause acute adrenal crisis). Use with extreme caution in angina pectoris, hypertension, or other cardiovascular disorders; renal insufficiency; or ischemic states.

• Patients with coronary artery disease who must receive thyroid should be observed carefully for possible coronary insufficiency if catecholamines must be given.

• Use carefully in myxedema; patients unusually sensitive to thyroid hormone.

• Potentially dangerous; not indicated to relieve vague symptoms, such as physical and mental sluggishness, irritability, depression, nervousness, ill-defined pains; to treat obesity in euthyroid persons; to treat metabolic insufficiency not associated with thyroid insufficiency; or to treat menstrual disorders or male infertility, unless associated with hypothyroidism.

• Patient should take thyroid hormones regularly, at the same time each day, to maintain constant hormone levels.

• Patient should immediately report signs of overdosage: chest pain (especially in elderly), palpitations, sweating, or nervousness. Chest pain, dyspnea, and tachycardia may signal aggravated cardiovascular disease and require clinical reevaluation.

• Morning dosage prevents insomnia.

• Pulse rate and blood pressure should be monitored.

• Thyroid hormones alter thyroid function study results. Prothrombin time should be monitored; patients taking these hormones usually require less anticoagulant. Patients should report unusual bleeding and bruising.

NAMES, INDICATIONS AND DOSAGES	SIDE EFFECTS

thyroid USP (desiccated)
Dathroid, Delcoid, S-P-T, Thyrar, Thyro-Teric

Adult hypothyroidism:
ADULTS: initially, 60 mg P.O. daily, increased by 60 mg q 30 days until desired response. Usual maintenance dose 60 to 180 mg P.O. daily, as a single dose.
ELDERLY: 7.5 to 15 mg P.O. daily; dose is doubled at 6- to 8-week intervals.

Adult myxedema:
ADULTS: 16 mg P.O. daily. May double dose q 2 weeks to maximum 120 mg.

Cretinism and juvenile hypothyroidism:
CHILDREN 1 YEAR AND OLDER: dosage may approach adult dose (60 to 180 mg) daily, depending on response.
CHILDREN 4 TO 12 MONTHS: 30 to 60 mg P.O. daily.
CHILDREN 1 TO 4 MONTHS: initially, 15 to 30 mg P.O. daily, increased at 2-week intervals. Usual maintenance dose 30 to 45 mg P.O. daily.

Side effects of thyroid hormones are extensions of their pharmacologic properties and reflect patient sensitivity to them.
CNS: *hyperirritability, nervousness, insomnia,* twitching, tremors, headache.
CV: increased cardiac output, *tachycardia,* cardiac arrhythmias, *angina pectoris,* increased blood pressure, *cardiac decompensation and collapse.*
GI: diarrhea, abdominal cramps, vomiting.
Other: weight loss, heat intolerance, hyperhidrosis, menstrual irregularities; in infants and children—accelerated rate of bone maturation.

thyrotropin
Thyrotron♦♦, Thytropar♦

Diagnosis of thyroid cancer remnant with ^{131}I after surgery: 10 international units I.M. or S.C. for 3 to 7 days.

Differential diagnosis of primary and secondary hypothyroidism: 10 units I.M. or S.C. for 1 to 3 days.

In PBI or ^{131}I uptake determinations for differential diagnosis of subclinical hypothyroidism or low thyroid reserve: 10 units I.M. or S.C.

Therapy for thyroid carcinoma (local or metastatic) with ^{131}I: 10 units I.M. or S.C. for 3 to 8 days.

To determine thyroid status of patient receiving thyroid: 10 units I.M. or S.C. for 1 to 3 days.

CNS: headache.
CV: *tachycardia,* atrial fibrillation, *angina pectoris, congestive failure,* hypotension.
GI: nausea, vomiting.
Other: thyroid hyperplasia (large doses), fever, menstrual irregularities, allergic reactions (postinjection flare, urticaria, *anaphylaxis).*

INTERACTIONS AND SPECIAL CONSIDERATIONS

Interactions:
CHOLESTYRAMINE: thyroid absorption impaired. Separate doses by 4 to 5 hours.
I.V. PHENYTOIN: free thyroid released. Monitor for tachycardia.

Special considerations:
- Contraindicated in myocardial infarction, thyrotoxicosis (except with antithyroid drugs), or uncorrected adrenal insufficiency (thyroid hormones increase tissue demand for adrenocortical hormone and may cause acute adrenal crisis). Use with extreme caution in angina pectoris, hypertension, or other cardiovascular disorders; renal insufficiency; or ischemic states.
- Use carefully in myxedema; patients are unusually sensitive to thyroid hormone.
- Patients with coronary artery disease who must receive thyroid should be observed carefully for possible coronary insufficiency if catecholamines must be given.
- Potentially dangerous; not indicated to relieve vague symptoms, such as physical and mental sluggishness, irritability, depression, nervousness, ill-defined pains; to treat obesity in euthyroid persons; to treat metabolic insufficiency not associated with thyroid insufficiency; or to treat menstrual disorders or male infertility, unless associated with hypothyroidism.
- Patient should take thyroid hormones regularly, at the same time each day, to maintain constant hormone levels.
- Patient should immediately report signs of overdosage: chest pain (especially in elderly), palpitations, sweating, or nervousness. Chest pain, dyspnea, and tachycardia may signal aggravated cardiovascular disease and require clinical reevaluation.
- Morning dosage prevents insomnia.
- Pulse rate and blood pressure should be monitored.
- In children, the sleeping pulse and basal morning temperature are guides to treatment.
- Thyroid hormones alter thyroid function study results. Prothrombin time should be monitored; patients taking these hormones usually require less anticoagulant. Patients should report unusual bleeding and bruising.

No significant interactions.

Special considerations:
- Contraindicated in coronary thrombosis and untreated Addison's disease. Use cautiously in angina pectoris, cardiac failure, hypopituitarism, adrenocortical suppression.
- Purified thyrotropic hormone (TSH) is isolated from bovine anterior pituitary. It stimulates the formation and secretion of thyroid hormone and increases thyroidal uptake of iodine: may cause thyroid hyperplasia.
- Diagnostic use: to identify subclinical hypothyroidism or low thyroid reserve, to evaluate need for thyroid therapy, to distinguish between primary and secondary hypothyroidism, and to detect thyroid remnants and metastases of thyroid carcinoma.
- Therapeutic use: management of certain types of thyroid carcinoma and resulting metastases, and in conjunction with radioactive ^{131}I to enhance the uptake of ^{131}I by the thyroid.
- Three-day dosage schedule may be used in long-standing pituitary myxedema or with prolonged use of thyroid medication.
- For treatment of anaphylaxis, see APPENDIX.

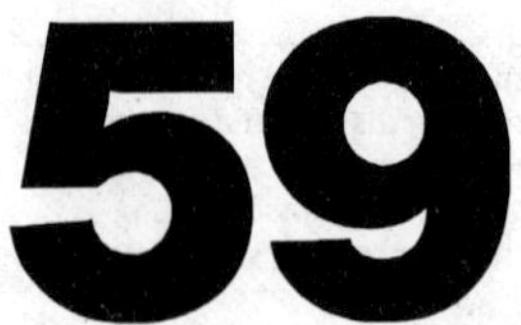

Thyroid hormone antagonists

iodine
radioactive iodine (sodium iodide) ^{131}I
methimazole
propylthiouracil (PTU)

Thyroid hormone antagonists, or antithyroid agents, are used to treat hyperthyroidism. Some antagonists, such as iodine and the thionamines (methimazole and propylthiouracil), have reversible effects and may be used in a young patient or one in whom hyperthyroidism is not necessarily permanent. They do not permanently affect the thyroid gland, but control hormone production until spontaneous remission of hyperthyroidism occurs.

Radiation therapy (with radioactive iodine) and thyroidectomy (partial or total) are definitive treatments for hyperthyroidism. Both procedures are reserved for adult patients who may not respond to milder agents. Unfortunately, radiation therapy and surgical treatment carry a long-term risk of hypothyroidism.

Major uses

- Iodine, methimazole, and propylthiouracil are used to treat hyperthyroidism (Graves' disease, multinodular goiter, and thyroiditis) in children, pregnant women, patients in whom thyroidectomy is contraindicated, and those in whom the condition is not necessarily permanent. These agents also help prepare patients for thyroidectomy and are effective for thyrotoxic crisis.
- Iodine combats lethal thyrotoxic crisis in adults and neonates. It is used preoperatively to decrease vascularity of the thyroid gland.
- Radioactive iodine is usually therapeutic for hyperthyroidism in adults when surgical treatment is contraindicated. However, it is not used in pregnant women.

Radioactive iodine is also used as a diagnostic tracer in thyroid function disorders and as a therapeutic adjunct after thyroidectomy for thyroid cancer. It causes ablation of any residual thyroid tissue. It can also be used to treat thyroid cancer metastases.

Mechanism of action

- Iodine inhibits thyroid hormone formation by blocking iodotyrosine and iodothyronine synthesis. It also limits iodide transport into the thyroid gland and blocks thyroid hormone release.
- Radioactive iodine limits thyroid hormone secretion by destroying thyroid tissue. The affinity of thyroid tissue for radioactive iodine facilitates uptake of the drug by cancerous thyroid tissue that has metastasized to other sites in the body.
- The thionamines inhibit oxidation of iodine in the thyroid gland, blocking iodine's ability to combine with tyrosine to form thyroxine. They may also prevent the coupling of monoiodotyrosine and diiodotyrosine to form thyroxine and triiodothyronine.

Absorption, distribution, metabolism, and excretion

- Methimazole and propylthiouracil are readily absorbed from the gastrointestinal tract and metabolized in the liver. Their metabolites are excreted in urine; however, 35% of propylthiouracil is excreted unchanged.
- Radioactive iodine in high concentrations is trapped in the thyroid gland within 30 minutes of oral administration and incorporated into the thyroid follicles; it is excreted in urine.

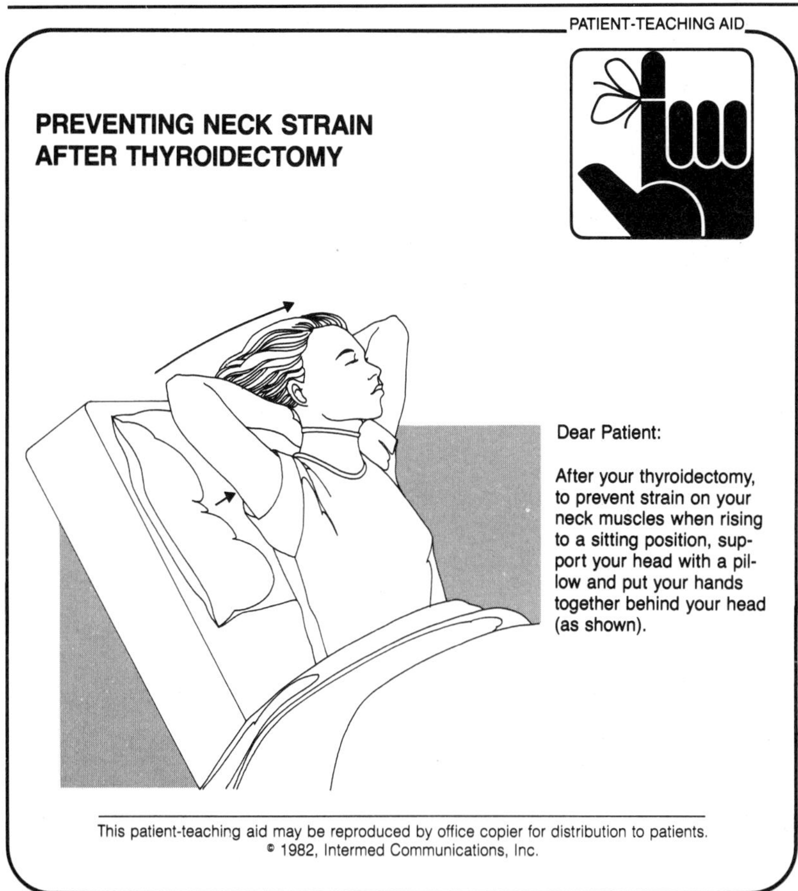

PATIENT-TEACHING AID
PREVENTING NECK STRAIN
AFTER THYROIDECTOMY
Dear Patient:
After your thyroidectomy, to prevent strain on your neck muscles when rising to a sitting position, support your head with a pillow and put your hands together behind your head (as shown).
This patient-teaching aid may be reproduced by office copier for distribution to patients.
© 1982, Intermed Communications, Inc.

Onset and duration

• Radioactive iodine's action may not begin for weeks; however, temporary but potentially serious thyrotoxic reactions may occur during the first few days of treatment. Radioactive iodine has a half-life of 8 days.

• The thionamines' onset may not be apparent for days or weeks—until the stored supply of thyroid hormones is depleted. The half-life of propylthiouracil is 2 hours; that of methimazole, 6 to 9 hours. After correction of the abnormally high metabolic rate (as in hyperthyroidism), the half-lives of these drugs may increase, necessitating lower doses. Patients with severe hyperthyroidism respond most rapidly, usually within 1 or 2 days.

NAMES, INDICATIONS AND DOSAGES	SIDE EFFECTS
iodine Potassium Iodide Solution, USP; Sodium Iodide, USP; Strong Iodine Solution, USP (Lugol's Solution), containing 5% iodine and 10% potassium iodide **Preparation for thyroidectomy:** ADULTS AND CHILDREN: Strong Iodine Solution, USP, 0.1 to 0.3 ml t.i.d., or Potassium Iodide Solution, USP, 5 drops in water t.i.d. after meals for 2 to 3 weeks before surgery. **Thyrotoxic crisis:** ADULTS AND CHILDREN: Strong Iodine Solution, USP, 1 ml in water P.O. t.i.d. after meals in refractory cases; Sodium Iodide, USP, 250 to 500 mg (or up to 2 g) daily, slow I.V. infusion with antithyroid drugs and propranolol.	**EENT:** acute rhinitis, inflammation of salivary glands, periorbital edema, conjunctivitis, hyperemia. **GI:** burning, irritation, *nausea,* vomiting, *metallic taste.* **Skin:** acneiform rash, mucous membrane ulceration. **Other:** fever, frontal headache; with I.V. use (sodium iodide): acute iodism, *colloidoclastic shock,* pulmonary edema.
radioactive iodine (sodium iodide) ^{131}I **Hyperthyroidism:** ADULTS: usual dose is 4 to 10 millicuries P.O. Dose based on estimated weight of thyroid gland and thyroid uptake. Treatment may be repeated after 6 weeks, according to serum thyroxine levels. **Thyroid cancer:** ADULTS: 50 to 150 millicuries P.O. Dose based on estimated malignant thyroid tissue and metastatic tissue as determined by total body scan. Dose may be repeated according to clinical status.	**EENT:** *feeling of fullness in neck,* metallic taste, "radiation mumps." **Endocrine:** hypothyroidism, radiation thyroiditis. **GU:** possible increased risk of birth defects in offspring after sufficient ^{131}I dose for thyroid ablation following cancer surgery. **Other:** possible increased risk of developing leukemia later in life after sufficient ^{131}I dose for thyroid ablation following cancer surgery.
methimazole Tapazole **Hyperthyroidism:** ADULTS: 5 mg P.O. t.i.d. if mild; 10 to 15 mg P.O. t.i.d. if moderately severe; and 20 mg P.O. t.i.d. if severe. Continue until patient euthyroid, then start maintenance dose of 5 mg daily to t.i.d. Maximum dose 150 mg daily. CHILDREN: 0.4 mg/kg/day divided q 8 hours. Continue until patient euthyroid, then start maintenance dose of 0.2 mg/kg/day divided q 8 hours. **Preparation for thyroidectomy:** ADULTS AND CHILDREN: same doses as for	**Blood:** *agranulocytosis,* leukopenia, granulopenia, thrombocytopenia (appear to be dose-related). **CNS:** headache, drowsiness, vertigo. **GI:** diarrhea, nausea, vomiting (may be dose-related). **Hepatic:** jaundice. **Skin:** rash, urticaria, skin discoloration. **Other:** arthralgia, myalgia, salivary gland enlargement, loss of taste, drug fever, lymphadenopathy.

INTERACTIONS AND SPECIAL CONSIDERATIONS

Interactions:
LITHIUM CARBONATE: hypothyroidism may occur. Use with caution.

Special considerations:
• Contraindicated in tuberculosis, iodide hypersensitivity, hyperkalemia, after meals that contain excessive starch; in laryngeal edema, swelling of salivary glands.
• Generally I.V. route should be used only if patient is vomiting or cannot receive anything by mouth. Some prefer I.V. route to prevent GI side effects, especially during critical time at beginning of treatment.
• Oral doses should be diluted in water, milk, or fruit juice, and given after meals to prevent gastric irritation, to hydrate the patient, and to mask the very salty taste.
• Patient should ask doctor about using iodized salt or eating shellfish during treatment. Iodine-rich foods may not be permitted.
• Sudden withdrawal may precipitate thyroid storm.
• Store in light-resistant container.
• Iodides should be given through straw to prevent tooth discoloration.
• Usually given with other antithyroid drugs.

Interactions:
LITHIUM CARBONATE: hypothyroidism may occur. Use with caution.

Special considerations:
• Contraindicated in pregnancy and lactation unless used to treat thyroid cancer.
• All antithyroid medications, thyroid preparations, and iodine-containing preparations should be stopped 1 week before ^{131}I dose. If medications are not stopped, patient may receive thyroid-stimulating hormone for 3 days before ^{131}I dose. When treating women of childbearing age, dose should be given during menstruation or within 7 days after menstruation.
• After therapy for hyperthyroidism, patient should not resume antithyroid drugs, but should continue propranolol or other drugs used to treat symptoms of hyperthyroidism until onset of full ^{131}I effect (usually 6 weeks).
• Thyroid function should be monitored with serum thyroxine levels.
• After dose for hyperthyroidism, patient's urine and saliva are slightly radioactive for 24 hours; vomitus is highly radioactive for 6 to 8 hours. Full radiation precautions should be instituted during this time. Patient should use appropriate disposal methods when coughing and expectorating.
• After dose for thyroid cancer, patient's urine, saliva, and perspiration remain radioactive for 3 days. Patient should be isolated and the following precautions observed: pregnant personnel should not take care of patient; disposable eating utensils and linens should be used; all urine should be saved in lead containers for 24 to 48 hours so amount of radioactive material excreted can be determined. Patient should drink as much fluid as possible for 48 hours after drug administration to facilitate excretion. Contact with patient should be limited to 30 minutes per shift per person the first day. Time may be increased to 1 hour second day and longer on third day.
• If patient is discharged less than 7 days after ^{131}I dose for thyroid cancer, he should avoid close, prolonged contact with small children (for example, holding children on lap), and not sleep in same room with spouse for 7 days after treatment due to increased risk of thyroid cancer in persons exposed to ^{131}I. Patient may use same bathroom facilities as rest of family. However, pets should not be allowed to drink from toilet for 7 days (increased risk of thyroid cancer).

No significant interactions.

Special considerations:
• Use cautiously in pregnancy. Pregnant women may require less drug as pregnancy progresses. Thyroid function studies should be monitored closely. Thyroid may be added to regimen. Drugs may be stopped during last few weeks of pregnancy.
• Mental depression, cold intolerance, and hard nonpitting edema are signs of hypothyroidism. Dose may need to be adjusted.
• CBC should be monitored periodically to detect impending leukopenia, thrombocytopenia, and agranulocytosis.
• Patient should report immediately fever, sore throat, or mouth sores (possible signs of developing agranulocytosis). Agranulocytosis can develop too rapidly to be detected by periodic blood cell counts. He should also report immediately any skin eruptions (sign of hypersensitivity).
• Drug should be stopped if severe rash or enlarged cervical lymph nodes develop.
• Patient should ask doctor about using iodized salt or eating shellfish during treatment.
• Patient should avoid over-the-counter cough medicines; many contain iodine.
• Should be taken with meals to reduce GI side effects.
• Store in light-resistant container.

(continued on following page)

NAMES, INDICATIONS AND DOSAGES	SIDE EFFECTS
methimazole *(continued)* hyperthyroidism until patient is euthyroid; then iodine may be added for 10 days before surgery. **Thyrotoxic crisis:** ADULTS AND CHILDREN: same doses as for hyperthyroidism, with concomitant iodine therapy and propranolol.	
propylthiouracil (PTU) Propyl-Thyracil♦♦ **Hyperthyroidism:** ADULTS: 100 mg P.O. t.i.d.; up to 300 mg q 8 hours have been used in severe cases. Continue until patient euthyroid, then start maintenance dose of 100 mg daily to t.i.d. CHILDREN OVER 10 YEARS: 100 mg P.O. t.i.d. Continue until patient euthyroid, then start maintenance dose of 25 mg t.i.d. to 100 mg b.i.d. CHILDREN 6 TO 10 YEARS: 50 to 150 mg P.O. divided doses q 8 hours. **Preparation for thyroidectomy:** ADULTS AND CHILDREN: same doses as for hyperthyroidism, then iodine may be added 10 days before surgery. **Thyrotoxic crisis:** ADULTS AND CHILDREN: same doses as for hyperthyroidism, with concomitant iodine therapy and propranolol.	**Blood:** *agranulocytosis,* leukopenia, thrombocytopenia (appear to be dose-related). **CNS:** headache, drowsiness, vertigo. **EENT:** visual disturbances. **GI:** diarrhea, *nausea, vomiting* (may be dose-related). **Hepatic:** jaundice. **Skin:** rash, urticaria, skin discoloration, pruritus. **Other:** arthralgia, myalgia, salivary gland enlargement, loss of taste, drug fever, lymphadenopathy.

INTERACTIONS AND SPECIAL CONSIDERATIONS

No significant interactions.

Special considerations:
- Use cautiously in pregnancy. Pregnant women may require less drug as pregnancy progresses. Thyroid function studies should be monitored closely. Thyroid may be added to regimen. Drugs may be stopped during last few weeks of pregnancy.
- Mental depression, cold intolerance, and hard nonpitting edema are signs of hypothyroidism. Dose may need to be adjusted.
- CBC should be monitored periodically to detect impending leukopenia, thrombocytopenia, and agranulocytosis.
- Patient should report immediately fever, sore throat, or mouth sores (possible signs of developing agranulocytosis), and any skin eruptions (sign of hypersensitivity). Agranulocytosis can develop too rapidly to be detected by periodic blood cell counts.
- Drug should be stopped if severe rash or enlarged cervical lymph nodes develop.
- Patient should ask doctor about using iodized salt or eating shellfish during treatment.
- Patient should avoid over-the-counter cough medicines; iodine in many.
- Should be taken with meals to reduce GI side effects.
- Store in light-resistant container.

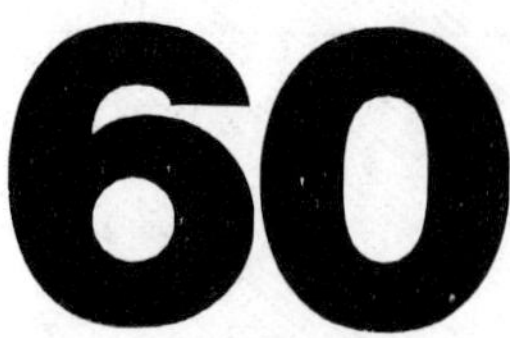

Pituitary hormones

corticotropin (ACTH)
cosyntropin
desmopressin acetate
lypressin
somatotropin (human growth hormone)
vasopressin (antidiuretic hormone)
vasopressin tannate

The pituitary hormones fall into three groups according to use: Corticotropin and cosyntropin are used to diagnose primary adrenal insufficiency; somatotropin spurs growth in patients with pituitary growth deficiency; and vasopressin and its synthetic derivatives desmopressin acetate and lypressin regulate water balance in patients with diabetes insipidus. All these hormones are either natural pituitary extracts or synthetic derivatives.

The pituitary gland is the most complex endocrine structure in the body. Its two major divisions are the anterior lobe (adenohypophysis) and the posterior lobe (neurohypophysis). Except for melanocyte-stimulating hormone—which is not commercially available—and somatotropin, the anterior lobe secretes tropic (primary) hormones that activate other organs (target glands) to secrete their characteristic hormones, called genic (secondary) hormones.

Extract from the posterior lobe may be divided into two active components: vasopressin (primarily associated with pressor and antidiuretic activities) and oxytocin (primarily associated with pronounced uterine-contracting and milk-releasing action). (See Chapter 105, OXYTOCICS, for a detailed description of oxytocin.)

Major uses

- Corticotropin and cosyntropin act as screening agents for primary adrenal insufficiency.
- Desmopressin, lypressin, and vasopressin combat symptoms of central diabetes insipidus.
- Somatotropin is used to treat growth impairment due to growth hormone deficiency.

Mechanism of action

- Corticotropin and cosyntropin, by replacing the body's own tropic hormone, stimulate the adrenal cortex to secrete its entire spectrum of hormones.
- Desmopressin, lypressin, and vasopressin increase the permeability of the renal tubular epithelium to adenosine monophosphate and water; the epithelium promotes reabsorption of water and produces a concentrated urine (antidiuretic hormone effect).
- Lypressin and vasopressin cause contraction of smooth muscle in the vascular bed (vasopressor effect). Vasopressin also causes contraction of smooth muscle in the gastrointestinal (GI) tract.
- Somatotropin stimulates linear growth in patients with pituitary growth deficiency by various mechanisms. These include facilitating intracellular transport of amino acids;

increasing intestinal absorption and urinary excretion of calcium; increasing renal tubular reabsorption of phosphorus and decreasing that of calcium; promoting synthesis of collagen and chondroitin, which form cartilage; and inhibiting intracellular glucose metabolism.

Absorption, distribution, metabolism, and excretion

- Corticotropin is destroyed in the GI tract after oral administration but is well absorbed parenterally. The parenteral form is well distributed and inactivated in body tissues and excreted in urine.
- Cosyntropin is destroyed by the proteolytic enzymes of the GI tract and so must be given either I.M. or I.V. It is inactivated in the tissues and excreted in urine.
- Desmopressin and lypressin, because they are inactivated in the GI tract by the enzyme trypsin, are given intranasally. Absorption through the nasal mucosa is adequate but decreases in nasal congestion, rhinitis, and upper respiratory tract infection.

  Desmopressin and lypressin are distributed throughout the extracellular fluid, metabolized in the liver and kidneys, and excreted in urine.
- Somatotropin is destroyed in the GI tract after oral administration but is well distributed to the body tissues after I.M. administration. It is metabolized in the liver and excreted in urine.
- Vasopressin tannate in oil is absorbed more slowly than the aqueous solution. Vasopressin is distributed throughout the extracellular fluid, metabolized in the liver and kidneys, and excreted in urine.

Onset and duration

- Corticotropin begins to work within 5 minutes and lasts 3 to 25 hours, depending on dose and route of administration.
- Cosyntropin, as reflected by plasma cortisol levels, has an onset within 5 minutes, peaks within 1 hour, and lasts 4 hours.
- Desmopressin and lypressin take effect within 1 hour. Desmopressin peaks in 1 to 5 hours and lasts 8 to 20 hours. Lypressin lasts 3 to 8 hours.
- Somatotropin takes effect immediately; its action lasts several days.
- Vasopressin (aqueous solution) goes to work within 1 hour and lasts 2 to 8 hours when given subcutaneously, and 6 to 12 hours when given I.V.
- Vasopressin tannate becomes effective within 1 hour and lasts 48 to 72 hours after I.M. injection.

Combination products

None.

NAMES, INDICATIONS AND DOSAGES	SIDE EFFECTS
corticotropin (ACTH) Acthar♦, Acton "X"♦♦, Cortigel-80, Cortrophin Gel, Cortrophin Zinc, Duracton♦♦, H.P. Acthar Gel **Diagnostic test of adrenocortical function:** ADULTS: up to 80 units I.M. or S.C. in divided doses; or a single dose of repository form; or 10 to 25 units (aqueous form) in 500 ml dextrose 5% in water I.V. over 8 hours, between blood samplings. Individual dosages generally vary with adrenal glands' sensitivity to stimulation as well as with specific disease. Infants and younger children require larger doses per kilogram than do older children and adults. **For therapeutic use:** ADULTS: 40 units S.C. or I.M. in 4 divided doses (aqueous); 40 units q 12 to 24 hours (gel or repository form).	**CNS:** *convulsions, dizziness,* papilledema, headache, *euphoria, insomnia,* mood swings, personality changes, depression, psychosis. **EENT:** cataracts, glaucoma. **GI:** *peptic ulcer with perforation and hemorrhage,* pancreatitis, abdominal distention, ulcerative esophagitis, nausea, vomiting. **GU:** menstrual irregularities. **Metabolic:** *sodium and fluid retention,* calcium and potassium loss, hypokalemic alkalosis, negative nitrogen balance. **Skin:** *impaired wound healing,* thin fragile skin, petechiae, ecchymoses, facial erythema, increased sweating, acne, hyperpigmentation, allergic skin reactions, hirsutism. **Other:** muscle weakness, steroid myopathy, loss of muscle mass, osteoporosis, vertebral compression fractures, cushingoid state, suppression of growth in children, *activation of latent diabetes mellitus,* progressive increase in antibodies, and loss of ACTH stimulatory effect.
cosyntropin Cortrosyn♦, Synacthen Depot♦♦ **Diagnostic test of adrenocortical function:** ADULTS AND CHILDREN: 0.25 to 1 mg I.M. or I.V. (unless label prohibits I.V. administration) between blood samplings. CHILDREN YOUNGER THAN 2 YEARS: 0.125 mg I.M. or I.V.	**Skin:** pruritus. **Other:** flushing.
desmopressin acetate DDAVP **Nonnephrogenic diabetes insipidus, temporary polyuria and polydipsia associated with pituitary trauma:** ADULTS: 0.1 to 0.4 ml intranasally daily in 1 to 3 doses. Adjust morning and evening doses separately for adequate diurnal rhythm of water turnover. CHILDREN 3 MONTHS TO 12 YEARS: 0.05 to 0.3 ml intranasally daily in 1 or 2 doses.	**CNS:** headache. **CV:** slight rise in blood pressure at high dosage. **EENT:** nasal congestion, rhinitis. **GI:** nausea. **GU:** vulval pain. **Other:** flushing.
lypressin Diapid **Nonnephrogenic diabetes insipidus:** ADULTS AND CHILDREN: 1 or 2 sprays (approximately 2 USP posterior pituitary pressor units per spray) in either or both nostrils q.i.d. and an additional dose at bedtime, if needed, to prevent nocturia. If usual dosage is inadequate, increase frequency rather than number of sprays.	**CNS:** headache, dizziness. **EENT:** nasal congestion or ulceration, irritation, pruritus of nasal passages, rhinorrhea, conjunctivitis. **GI:** heartburn due to drip of excess spray into pharynx, abdominal cramps, frequent bowel movements. **GU:** possible transient fluid retention due to overdose. **Skin:** hypersensitivity reaction.

♦ Available in U.S. and Canada. ♦♦ Available in Canada only.
All other products (no symbol) available in U.S. only. Italicized side effects are common or life-threatening.

INTERACTIONS AND SPECIAL CONSIDERATIONS

No significant interactions.

Special considerations:

• Contraindicated in scleroderma, osteoporosis, systemic fungal infections, ocular herpes simplex, recent surgery, peptic ulcer, congestive heart failure, hypertension, sensitivity to pork and pork products, concomitant smallpox vaccination, adrenocortical hyperfunction or primary insufficiency, or Cushing's syndrome. Use with caution in pregnant women or breast-feeding mothers and in women of childbearing age; patients being immunized; latent tuberculosis or tuberculin reactivity; hypothyroidism, cirrhosis, infection (use anti-infective therapy during and after ACTH treatment); acute gouty arthritis (limit ACTH treatment to a few days and use conventional therapy during and for several days after ACTH treatment); emotional instability or psychotic tendencies; diabetes; abscess; pyogenic infections; renal insufficiency; myasthenia gravis.
• ACTH treatment should be preceded by verification of adrenal responsiveness and testing for hypersensitivity and allergic reactions.
• ACTH should be adjunctive; not sole therapy. Oral agents are preferred for long-term therapy.
• Unusual stress may require additional use of rapidly acting corticosteroids. ACTH dosage should be reduced gradually when reduction is possible to minimize induced adrenocortical insufficiency, and therapy should be reinstituted if stressful situation (trauma, surgery, severe illness) occurs shortly after stopping drug.
• Hypoadrenalism may develop in neonates of ACTH-treated mothers.
• Low-sodium, high-potassium intake counteracts edema; high-protein diet inhibits nitrogen loss; and lowered ACTH dosage and administration of sedatives counteract psychotic changes.
• ACTH may mask signs of chronic disease and decrease host resistance and ability to localize infection.
• Weight changes, fluid exchange, and resting blood pressures should be monitored until minimal effective dose is achieved.
• Reconstituted solution should be refrigerated and used within 24 hours.
• For gel administration: warm to room temperature; draw into large needle; give slowly deep I.M. with 21G or 22G needle. Patient should be warned that injection is painful.

No significant interactions.

Special considerations:

• Use cautiously in hypersensitivity to natural corticotropin.
• Drug is synthetic duplication of the biologically active part of the ACTH molecule. It is less likely to produce sensitivity than natural ACTH from animal sources.

No significant interactions.

Special considerations:

• Use with caution in patients with coronary artery insufficiency or hypertensive cardiovascular disease.
• Fluid intake should be adjusted to reduce risk of water intoxication and sodium depletion, especially in very young or old patients.
• Dosage should be titrated to allow patient sufficient sleep.
• Should be given intranasally only.
• Overdose may cause oxytocic or vasopressor activity. Drug should be withheld until effects subside. Furosemide may be used if fluid retention is excessive.
• Not effective in nephrogenic diabetes insipidus.
• Some patients may have difficulty measuring and inhaling drug into nostrils, and should be taught correct method of administration.

No significant interactions.

Special considerations:

• Should be used with caution in patients with coronary artery disease.
• Particularly useful if diabetes insipidus is unresponsive to other therapy, or if antidiuretic hormones of animal origin cause adverse reactions.
• Nasal congestion, allergic rhinitis, or upper respiratory infections may diminish drug absorption and require larger dose or adjunctive therapy.
• Inadvertent inhalation of spray may cause tightness in chest, coughing, transient dyspnea.
• Patients sensitive to antidiuretic hormone should be tested for sensitivity to lypressin.
• A uniform, well-diffused spray is administered by holding bottle upright while patient in vertical position holds head upright.
• Patient should carry the medication with him at all times because of its fairly short duration.

NAMES, INDICATIONS AND DOSAGES	SIDE EFFECTS

somatotropin (human growth hormone)
Asellacrin, Crescormon

Growth failure due to pituitary growth hormone deficiency:
CHILDREN: 2 IU (1 ml) I.M. 3 times weekly, with a minimum of 48 hours between injections. Double dose if growth doesn't exceed 1″ in 6 months, or recheck diagnosis. Discontinue when epiphyses close, patient achieves satisfactory adult height, or patient fails to respond.

GU: excess calcium in urine.
Metabolic: hyperglycemia.

vasopressin (antidiuretic hormone)
Pitressin Synthetic♦
vasopressin tannate
Pitressin Tannate

Nonnephrogenic, nonpsychogenic diabetes insipidus:
ADULTS: 5 to 10 units I.M. or S.C. b.i.d. to q.i.d., p.r.n.; or intranasally (spray or cotton balls) in individualized doses, based on response. For chronic therapy, inject 2.5 to 5 units Pitressin Tannate in oil suspension I.M. or S.C. every 2 to 3 days.
CHILDREN: 2.5 to 10 units I.M. or S.C. b.i.d. to q.i.d., p.r.n.; or intranasally (spray or cotton balls) in individualized doses. For chronic therapy, inject 1.25 to 2.5 units Pitressin Tannate in oil suspension I.M. or S.C. every 2 to 3 days.

Postoperative abdominal distention:
ADULTS: 5 units (aqueous) I.M. initially, then q 3 to 4 hours, increasing dose to 10 units, if needed. Reduce dose for children proportionately.

To expel gas before abdominal X-ray:
ADULTS: inject 10 units S.C. at 2 hours, then again at 30 minutes before X-ray. Enema before first dose may also help to eliminate gas.

Upper GI tract hemorrhage (intra-arterial):
ADULTS: 0.2 to 0.4 units/minute. Do not use Tannate in oil suspension.

CNS: tremor, dizziness, headache.
CV: *angina in patients with vascular disease,* vasoconstriction. Large doses may cause hypertension, electrocardiographic changes.
GI: abdominal cramps, nausea, vomiting, diarrhea, intestinal hyperactivity.
GU: uterine cramps, anuria.
Skin: circumoral pallor.
Other: water intoxication (drowsiness, listlessness, headache, confusion, weight gain), hypersensitivity reactions (urticaria, angioneurotic edema, bronchoconstriction, fever, rash, wheezing, dyspnea, *anaphylaxis),* sweating.

INTERACTIONS AND SPECIAL CONSIDERATIONS

No significant interactions.

Special considerations:
• Contraindicated in patients with closed epiphyses or intracranial lesions. Use with caution in patients with diabetes or with family history of diabetes mellitus. Regular testing for glycosuria should be done.
• Subcutaneous administration not recommended.
• Should be used only by doctors experienced in treating patients with pituitary growth hormonal deficiency.
• Concurrent thyroid hormone or androgen therapy may accelerate epiphyseal closure and limit duration of somatropin treatment.
• Bone age progression should be monitored annually.
• Store powder at or below room temperature.
• Reconstitute with 5 ml of bacteriostatic water per 10-IU vial. Refrigerate unused portion; discard after 1 month. Injection sites should be rotated.

Interactions:
LITHIUM, DEMECLOCYCLINE: reduced antidiuretic activity. Use together cautiously.
CHLORPROPAMIDE: increased antidiuretic response. Use together cautiously.

Special considerations:
• Contraindicated in chronic nephritis with nitrogen retention. Use cautiously in children, elderly persons, pregnant women, and patients with epilepsy, migraine, asthma, cardiovascular disease, or fluid overload.
• Vasopressin tannate should never be injected in oil I.V.
• Should never be injected during first stage of labor; may cause ruptured uterus.
• Specific gravity of urine should be monitored. Intake and output should be monitored to aid evaluation of drug effectiveness.
• Before I.M. injection dose is withdrawn, tannate in oil should be placed in warm water for 10 to 15 minutes and then shaken thoroughly to make suspension uniform. Small brown particles must be seen in suspension. Absolutely dry syringe used to avoid dilution.
• Should be given with 1 to 2 glasses of water to reduce side effects and to improve therapeutic response.
• To prevent convulsions, coma, and death, patient should be observed closely for early signs of water intoxication.
• Overhydration more likely with long-acting tannate oil suspension than with aqueous vasopressin solution.
• Minimum effective dose should be used to reduce side effects.
• May be used for transient polyuria due to antidiuretic hormone deficiency related to neurosurgery or head injury.
• Synthetic desmopressin is sometimes preferred because of longer duration and less frequent side effects.
• Patient with abdominal distention should be questioned about passage of flatus and stool.
• Blood pressure of patient on vasopressin should be monitored twice daily. Excessively elevated blood pressure or lack of response to drug may be indicated by hypotension.
• For treatment of anaphylaxis, see APPENDIX.

61

Parathyroid and parathyroid-like agents

calcifediol
calcitonin (Salmon)
calcitriol
dihydrotachysterol (AT-10)
etidronate disodium
parathyroid hormone (PTH)

The major regulatory hormone of the parathyroid glands is parathyroid hormone (PTH); its secretion is indirectly related to the concentration of calcium ions in the blood. In humans, the serum calcium level is regulated within narrow limits (10 ± 1 mg/100 ml). A decrease in this concentration stimulates release of endogenous PTH that in turn lowers serum phosphate and raises serum calcium concentrations.

Calcifediol, calcitriol, and dihydrotachysterol, the activated forms of vitamin D, are like PTH in that they stimulate transport of calcium from bone to blood, raising serum calcium and lowering PTH.

Calcitonin is a hormone secreted by the parafollicular cells of the thyroid gland. It immediately lowers higher-than-normal serum calcium levels.

Etidronate, a synthetic compound, acts primarily on the bones to lower serum calcium levels, but it has little effect on PTH levels.

The body has an exceptional capacity to ensure normal serum calcium levels. Normally, calcium homeostasis is regulated by the kidneys and gastrointestinal (GI) tract. Alternative regulating mechanisms may maintain homeostasis levels at the expense of bone.

Major uses

- Calcifediol and calcitriol are used to treat hypocalcemia in patients undergoing hemodialysis.
- Calcitonin reduces serum calcium levels in acute hypercalcemia.
- Calcitonin and etidronate combat Paget's disease (osteitis deformans).
- Dihydrotachysterol is effective against hypocalcemia in renal failure.
- PTH is used in the diagnosis of hypoparathyroidism.
- Dihydrotachysterol and PTH are used to combat hypocalcemia associated with hypoparathyroidism.

Mechanism of action

- Calcifediol, calcitriol, and dihydrotachysterol stimulate calcium absorption from the GI tract and promote secretion of calcium from bone to blood, thereby raising serum calcium levels; they may also increase urinary excretion of inorganic phosphate.
- Calcitonin and etidronate decrease osteoclastic activity by inhibiting osteocytic osteolysis. They also decrease mineral release and matrix or collagen breakdown in bone.
- PTH enhances phosphate excretion by inhibiting renal tubular reabsorption of phosphate, mobilizing bone calcium and increasing GI absorption of calcium.

Absorption, distribution, metabolism, and excretion

- Calcifediol, calcitriol, dihydrotachysterol, and etidronate are absorbed from the GI tract. Calcifediol, calcitriol, and dihydrotachysterol are metabolized in the liver and

THYROIDECTOMY? CHECK POSTOPERATIVELY

In 100 patients with thyroidectomies, you may see one case of post-thyroidectomy hypoparathyroidism. The incidence of hypoparathyroidism is especially high in patients who have had radical thyroidectomy for cancer. Symptoms begin about 24 hours after surgery. To detect this disorder, watch for:

- Chvostek's or Trousseau's sign
- hypocalcemia
- dystonia
- choreoathetoid movement
- grand mal seizures
- tetany
- paresthesias (especially circumoral)
- impaired cognitive function
- depression
- psychological changes (especially in older patients) such as irritability and emotional lability.

eliminated—through the bile—in feces. Etidronate, as the unchanged drug, is primarily excreted in the urine; a small amount, however, is eliminated in feces.

• Calcitonin and PTH are well absorbed after subcutaneous or I.M. administration. Because they're destroyed in the GI tract, they must be given parenterally. Calcitonin is metabolized by the kidneys and excreted in urine.

Onset and duration

• Calcifediol and calcitriol become effective in about 2 hours. Maximal hypercalcemic effect of calcifediol and calcitriol occurs in 10 hours. Duration of action of these activated vitamin D compounds is about 3 to 5 days.

• Calcitonin's onset after I.V. administration is 15 minutes; its duration is 30 minutes to 12 hours. After I.M. or subcutaneous injection, onset is 4 hours and duration is 8 to 24 hours.

• Dihydrotachysterol begins to work several hours after administration. Maximal hypercalcemic effect of this drug occurs within 1 week if a loading dose is used and within 2 weeks if a loading dose is not used. Serum calcium level drops markedly within 4 to 5 days after therapy is stopped, and the drug's effect completely disappears after 2 weeks.

• Etidronate begins to work after 1 to 3 months. Maximal therapeutic activity occurs in about 6 months.

• PTH, after I.M. or subcutaneous injection, raises serum calcium level within 4 hours; the level peaks in 12 to 18 hours. Duration of action is 20 to 24 hours.

After I.V. administration, PTH begins to work within 15 minutes, and serum calcium level rises in 1 hour. Duration of action is much shorter with I.V. administration than with the I.M. or subcutaneous form.

Combination products

None.

NAMES, INDICATIONS AND DOSAGES	SIDE EFFECTS
calcifediol Calderol **Treatment and management of metabolic bone disease associated with chronic renal failure:** ADULTS: initially, 300 to 350 mcg P.O. weekly, given on a daily or alternate-day schedule. Dosage may be increased at 4-week intervals. Optimal dose must be carefully determined for each patient.	Vitamin D intoxication associated with hypercalcemia: **CNS:** headache, somnolence. **EENT:** conjunctivitis, photophobia, rhinorrhea. **GI:** nausea, vomiting, constipation, metallic taste, dry mouth. **GU:** polyuria. **Other:** weakness, bone and muscle pain.
calcitonin (Salmon) Calcimar♦ **Paget's disease of bone (osteitis deformans):** ADULTS: initially, 100 MRC units daily, S.C. or I.M. Maintenance: 50 to 100 units daily or every other day. **Hypercalcemia:** ADULTS: 100 to 400 MRC units I.M. once or twice daily.	**CNS:** headaches. **GI:** transient nausea with or without vomiting, diarrhea. **GU:** transient diuresis. **Metabolic:** hyperglycemia. **Local:** inflammation at injection site, skin rashes. **Other:** *facial flushing;* hypocalcemia; swelling, tingling, and tenderness of hands; unusual taste sensation; *anaphylaxis.*
calcitriol (1, 25-dihydroxycholecalciferol) Rocaltrol **Management of hypocalcemia in patients undergoing chronic dialysis:** ADULTS: initially, 0.25 mcg daily. Dosage may be increased by 0.25 mcg/day at 2- to 4-week intervals. Maintenance: 0.25 mcg every other day up to 0.5 to 1.25 mcg daily.	Vitamin D intoxication associated with hypercalcemia: **CNS:** headache, somnolence. **EENT:** conjunctivitis, photophobia, rhinorrhea. **GI:** nausea, vomiting, constipation, metallic taste, dry mouth. **GU:** polyuria. **Other:** weakness, bone and muscle pain.

INTERACTIONS AND SPECIAL CONSIDERATIONS

Interactions:
CHOLESTYRAMINE: may impair absorption of calcifediol. Monitor calcium levels.

Special considerations:
• Contraindicated in hypercalcemia or vitamin D toxicity. All preparations containing vitamin D should be withheld in patients taking calcifediol. Use cautiously in patients on digitalis because hypercalcemia may precipitate cardiac arrhythmias.
• Serum calcium should be monitored; serum calcium times serum phosphate should not exceed 70. During titration, serum calcium levels should be determined at least weekly. If hypercalcemia occurs, calcifediol should be discontinued but resumed after serum calcium returns to normal.
• Patient should receive adequate daily intake of calcium—1,000 mg RDA.
• Patient should adhere to diet and calcium supplementation, and avoid nonprescription drugs.
• Most patients respond to doses between 50 and 100 mcg daily or between 100 and 200 mcg on alternate days.

No significant interactions.

Special considerations:
• Contraindicated in hypersensitivity to gelatin diluent used to prepare drug. Not recommended for breast-feeding mothers, or women who are or may become pregnant. Safe use in children not established.
• Periodic serum alkaline phosphatase and 24-hour urine hydroxyproline levels should be determined to evaluate drug effect.
• Skin test is usually done before beginning therapy.
• Systemic allergic reactions possible since hormone is protein. Epinephrine should be kept available when calcitonin is administered.
• Patients with good initial clinical response to calcitonin who suffer relapse should be evaluated for antibody formation response to the hormone protein.
• Patient in whom calcitonin loses its hypocalcemic activity should be advised that further medication or increased dosages will be of no value.
• Patient should be taught aseptic method of preparing and administering injection; important to rotate injection sites.
• Facial flushing and warmth occur in 20% to 30% of all patients within minutes of injection; usually last about 1 hour.
• Signs of hypocalcemic tetany during therapy: muscle twitching, tetanic spasms, and convulsions if hypocalcemia is severe.
• Calcium levels should be monitored closely. Signs of hypercalcemic relapse: bone pain, renal calculi, polyuria, anorexia, nausea, vomiting, thirst, constipation, lethargy, bradycardia, muscle hypotonicity, pathologic fracture, psychosis, and coma.
• Periodic examinations of urine sediment advisable.
• Actually derived from the thyroid gland, not the parathyroid.
• Solution should be refrigerated.

No significant interactions.

Special considerations:
• Contraindicated in hypercalcemia or vitamin D toxicity. All preparations containing vitamin D should be withheld in patients taking calcitriol. Not recommended in breast-feeding mothers. Use cautiously in patients on digitalis; hypercalcemia may precipitate cardiac arrhythmias.
• Serum calcium should be monitored; serum calcium times serum phosphate should not exceed 70. During titration, serum levels should be determined twice weekly. If hypercalcemia occurs, calcitriol should be discontinued but resumed after serum calcium returns to normal. Patient should receive adequate daily intake of calcium, 1,000 mg RDA.
• Protect from heat and light.
• Patient should adhere to diet and calcium supplementation and avoid unapproved nonprescription drugs.
• Patients should not use magnesium-containing antacids while taking this drug.
• Patients should report to doctor immediately any of the following symptoms: weakness, nausea, vomiting, dry mouth, constipation, muscle or bone pain, or metallic taste—early symptoms of vitamin D intoxication.
• Although this drug is a vitamin, it must not be taken by anyone for whom it was not prescribed, due to its potentially serious toxicities.
• Most potent form of vitamin D available.

NAMES, INDICATIONS AND DOSAGES	SIDE EFFECTS
dihydrotachysterol (AT-10) Hytakerol ♦ **Familial hypophosphatemia:** ADULTS AND CHILDREN: 0.5 to 2 mg P.O. daily. Maintenance: 0.3 to 1.5 mg daily. **Hypocalcemia associated with hypoparathyroidism and pseudohypoparathyroidism:** ADULTS: initially, 0.8 to 2.4 mg P.O. daily for several days. Maintenance: 0.2 to 2 mg daily, as required for normal serum calcium levels. Average dose 0.6 mg daily. CHILDREN: initially, 1 to 5 mg for several days. Maintenance: 0.5 to 1.5 mg daily, as required for normal serum calcium levels. **Renal osteodystrophy in chronic uremia:** ADULTS: 0.1 to 0.6 mg P.O. daily.	Vitamin D intoxication associated with hypercalcemia: **CNS:** headache, somnolence. **EENT:** conjunctivitis, photophobia, rhinorrhea. **GI:** nausea, vomiting, constipation, metallic taste, dry mouth. **GU:** polyuria. **Other:** weakness, bone and muscle pain.
etidronate disodium Didronel **Symptomatic Paget's disease:** ADULTS: 5 mg/kg/day P.O. as a single dose 2 hours before a meal with water or juice. Patient should not eat for 2 hours after dose. May give up to 10 mg/kg/day in severe cases. Maximum dose 20 mg/kg/day. **Heterotopic ossification in spinal cord injuries:** ADULTS: 20 mg/kg/day for 2 weeks, then 10 mg/kg/day for 10 weeks. Total treatment period 12 weeks. **Heterotopic ossification after total hip replacement:** ADULTS: 20 mg/kg/day for 1 month prior to total hip replacement and for 3 months afterward.	**GI:** (seen most frequently at 20 mg/kg/day) diarrhea, increased frequency of bowel movements, nausea. **Other:** increased or recurrent bone pain at pagetic sites, pain at previously asymptomatic sites, increased risk of fracture, elevated serum phosphate.
parathyroid hormone (PTH) Para-thor-mone, Paroidin **Acute hypoparathyroidism with tetany:** ADULTS: 20 to 40 units S.C., I.M., or I.V. q 12 hours. INFANTS: (with transient congenital idiopathic true hypoparathyroidism) 25 to 50 units I.M. q 12 hours for 1 to 3 days.	**Allergic:** *anaphylactic reactions* (parathyroid hormone is a foreign protein). **CNS:** headache, vertigo. **GI:** anorexia, nausea, vomiting, abdominal cramps, diarrhea. **Other:** hypercalcemia (muscle weakness, bone and flank pain), lethargy, tinnitus, ataxia.

♦ Available in U.S. and Canada. ♦♦ Available in Canada only.
All other products (no symbol) available in U.S. only. Italicized side effects are common or life-threatening.

INTERACTIONS AND SPECIAL CONSIDERATIONS

No significant interactions.

Special considerations:
• Contraindicated in hypercalcemia, hypocalcemia associated with renal insufficiency and hyperphosphatemia, renal stones, hypersensitivity to vitamin D, and in breast-feeding mothers.
• Serum and urine calcium levels should be monitored. Hypercalcemia is possible.
• Adequate dietary calcium intake is necessary; usually supplemented with 10 to 15 g oral calcium lactate or gluconate daily.
• Hypercalcemia reactions may occur. Early signs of hypercalcemia include thirst, headache, vertigo, tinnitus, anorexia.
• 1 mg equal to 120,000 units ergocalciferol (vitamin D_2).
• Store in tightly closed, light-resistant containers. Don't refrigerate.

No significant interactions.

Special considerations:
• Use cautiously in enterocolitis and impaired renal function.
• Therapy should not last more than 6 months. After 3 months, may be resumed if needed. Should not be given longer than 3 months at doses above 10 mg/kg/day.
• Should not be given with food, milk, or antacids; may reduce absorption.
• Renal function should be monitored before and during therapy.
• Drug effect should be monitored by serum alkaline phosphatase and urine hydroxyproline excretion (both lowered if therapy effective).
• Improvement may not occur for up to 3 months but may continue for months after drug stopped. Good nutrition important, especially diet high in calcium and vitamin D.

No significant interactions.

Special considerations:
• Contraindicated in hypercalcemia, hypercalciuria, tetany unrelated to parathyroid failure; and by I.V. administration when serum calcium levels are above normal. Use cautiously in sarcoidosis, renal or cardiac disease, and in digitalized patients.
• Rarely used because calcium salts often effective alone.
• Subcutaneous injections may produce moderate inflammatory reaction.
• Therapy lasts only a few days; patients may soon become refractory to treatment due to parathyroid-initiated production of antihormone antibodies.
• If given I.V., patient should be skin-tested for sensitivity; if positive, patient should be desensitized.
• Epinephrine injection should be kept available when parathyroid hormone is given.
• Serum calcium and serum phosphate levels, and intake and output should be monitored.
• Hypoparathyroidism, calcium deficiency, and drug-induced hypercalcemia may occur. Chvostek's and Trousseau's signs should be tested for.
• Use seizure precautions in patients with calcium deficiency: padded rails, soft light, no irritating noises until normal calcium level is restored.
• Should not be diluted with saline solution as a precipitate will form.
• Store ampules at 2° to 8° C. (36° to 46° F.); do not freeze.

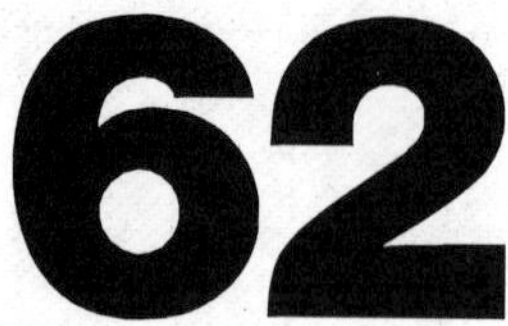

Diuretics

Thiazide diuretics
bendroflumethiazide
benzthiazide
chlorothiazide
cyclothiazide
hydrochlorothiazide
hydroflumethiazide
methyclothiazide
polythiazide
trichlormethiazide

Thiazide-like diuretics
chlorthalidone
metolazone
quinethazone

Loop diuretics
ethacrynate sodium
ethacrynic acid
furosemide

Carbonic anhydrase inhibitors
acetazolamide
acetazolamide sodium
dichlorphenamide
ethoxzolamide
methazolamide

Miscellaneous diuretics
amiloride hydrochloride
mannitol
mercaptomerin sodium
spironolactone
triamterene
urea (carbamide)

(All drugs are listed in alphabetical order in the tables that follow.)

Diuretics reduce the body's total volume of water and salt by increasing their urinary excretion. This occurs mainly because diuretics impair sodium chloride reabsorption in the renal tubules. Diuretics can be classified according to chemical structure (thiazide and thiazide-like drugs), location of salt- and water-depleting effect on the kidney's nephrons (loop diuretics), and pharmacologic activity (carbonic anhydrase inhibitors and miscellaneous drugs with other mechanisms).

Major uses
The matrix on the opposite page indicates the major uses of the diuretics.

Mechanism of action
- The thiazide and thiazide-like diuretics increase urinary excretion of sodium and water by inhibiting sodium reabsorption in the cortical diluting site of the ascending loop of Henle. They also increase urinary excretion of chloride, potassium, and—to a lesser extent—bicarbonate ions.
- Loop diuretics inhibit reabsorption of sodium and chloride at the proximal portion of the ascending loop of Henle, enhancing water excretion. These very potent diuretics can be effective in patients with markedly reduced glomerular filtration rates (in whom other diuretics usually fail).
- Carbonic anhydrase inhibitors, by enzymatic blocking, promote renal excretion of sodium, potassium, bicarbonate, and water. Bicarbonate ion excretion makes urine alkaline; blood bicarbonate levels are accordingly reduced, leading to metabolic acidosis. In this condition, carbonic anhydrase inhibitors become less effective as diuretics. (Carbonic anhydrase inhibitors also decrease secretion of aqueous humor in the eye, thus lowering intraocular pressure; this mechanism is unrelated to their diuretic action.)

℞ MAJOR USES OF DIURETICS

	thiazide diuretics	thiazide-like diuretics	loop diuretics	carbonic anhydrase inhibitors	amiloride	mannitol	mercaptomerin	spironolactone	triamterene	urea	
Treatment of essential hypertension	•	•	•		•		•	•	•		
Treatment of edema associated with congestive heart failure, cirrhosis of liver, and renal disease	•	•	•		•		•	•	•		
Treatment of pulmonary edema			•								
Reduction of intracranial pressure in hydrocephalus				•		•				•	
Reduction of intraocular pressure				•		•				•	
Treatment of open-angle glaucoma (as adjunct)				•							
Prophylaxis for epilepsy (as adjunct)				•							
Treatment of primary aldosteronism								•			
Potentiation of effects of mercurial diuretics				•							

• Among miscellaneous diuretics, mannitol increases the osmotic pressure of glomerular filtrate, inhibiting tubular reabsorption of water and electrolytes. Mercaptomerin works mainly in the ascending limb of the loop of Henle where the mercuric (Hg^{++}) ion interferes with renal tubular transport of chloride. During the ensuing diuresis, sodium, chloride, and water are excreted without profound potassium depletion. Diuresis is enhanced by acidifying agents. Spironolactone antagonizes the hormone aldosterone at the distal tubule, increasing excretion of sodium and water but sparing potassium. Amiloride and triamterene depress sodium reabsorption and potassium secretion by direct action on the distal segment of the uriniferous tubule. This reduces potassium excretion. Urea rapidly increases blood tonicity, which results in passage of fluid from the tissue (including the brain) to the blood.

DIURETICS: PRINCIPAL SITES OF ACTION

Diuretics increase the urinary excretion of water and salt by impairing sodium chloride reabsorption in the renal tubules.

NEPHRON UNIT

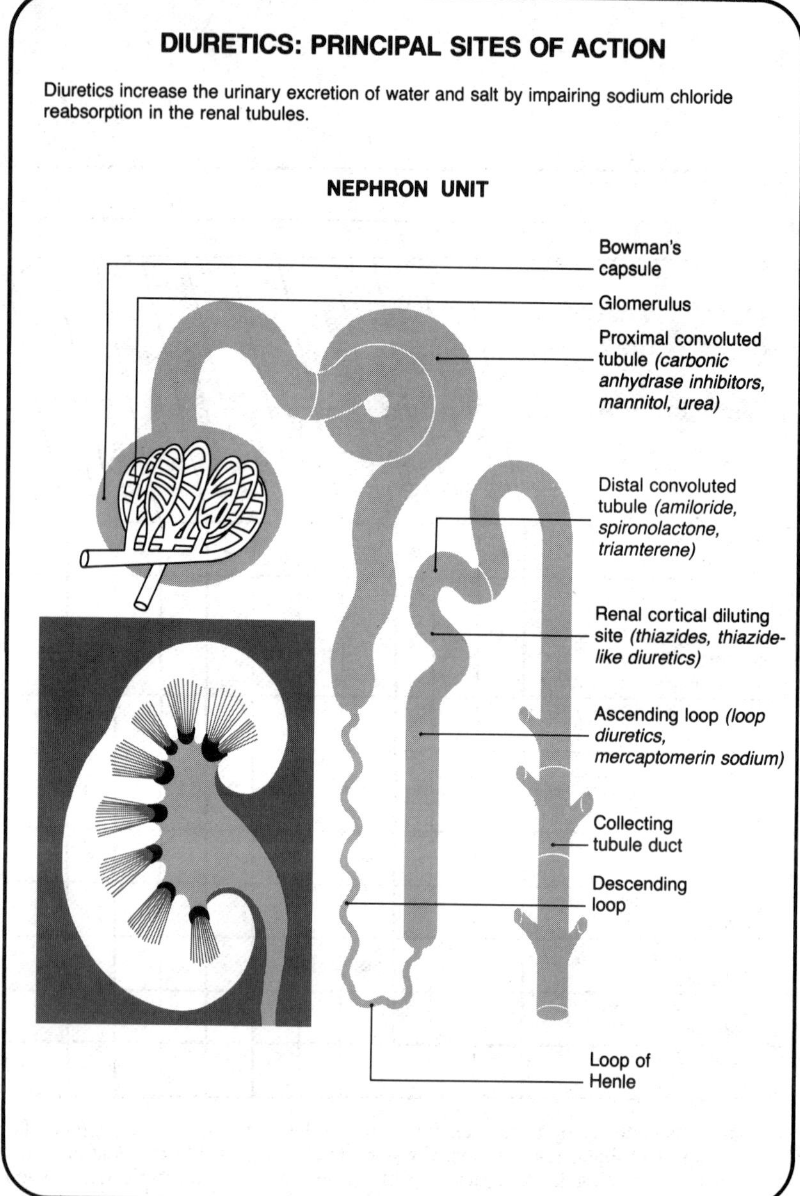

Absorption, distribution, metabolism, and excretion

• Thiazides and thiazide-like diuretics are all well absorbed from the gastrointestinal (GI) tract; these diuretics are well distributed to the body tissues; and they are excreted primarily unchanged in urine.

• Among loop diuretics ethacrynic acid is rapidly absorbed after oral administration, metabolized in the liver, and excreted by the kidneys. Ethacrynate sodium is administered parenterally. Its metabolism and excretion are the same as ethacrynic acid's.

Furosemide is partially (about 60%) absorbed from the GI tract; a small amount is metabolized. Both metabolite and unchanged drug are excreted in urine.

• Carbonic anhydrase inhibitors are absorbed from the GI tract after oral administration and are distributed throughout body tissue.

Acetazolamide is excreted unchanged in urine, but other carbonic anhydrase inhibitors are partially metabolized and eliminated in both urine and feces.

• Among miscellaneous diuretics, mannitol remains in the extracellular fluid, is filtered by the glomeruli, and is excreted unchanged in urine.

Mercaptomerin is completely absorbed after I.M. or subcutaneous injection, distributed mainly to the kidneys, metabolized in the liver, and excreted almost entirely in urine.

Spironolactone is absorbed from the GI tract, distributed to body tissues, metabolized in the liver, and eliminated in both urine and feces.

Amiloride and triamterene are absorbed from the GI tract, partially bound to plasma proteins, distributed to body tissues, and rapidly excreted unchanged in urine.

Urea is well absorbed after oral administration, but it's seldom given orally because of its unpleasant taste. After I.V. administration, it's distributed to intracellular and extracellular fluids, including cerebrospinal fluid. It's hydrolyzed in the GI tract by bacterial ureases and excreted by the kidneys.

Onset and duration

• Thiazides and thiazide-like diuretics begin to act 1 to 2 hours after oral administration. Most of them have a duration of action of 12 to 24 hours, but several act as long as 36 to 72 hours. Intravenous chlorothiazide takes effect within 15 minutes after administration and has a duration of 2 hours.

• Among loop diuretics, ethacrynic acid begins to act 30 minutes after oral administration and has a duration of up to 12 hours. Ethacrynate sodium, after I.V. administration, begins to act within 5 minutes. Its duration is 2 hours.

• Carbonic anhydrase inhibitors begin to act 1 to 3 hours after oral administration and have a duration of 8 to 12 hours. Acetazolamide (timed-release form), however, acts as long as 24 hours, and methazolamide acts up to 18 hours. After I.V. administration, acetazolamide has an onset within 2 minutes and a duration of 4 to 5 hours.

Furosemide, after oral administration, begins to act in 30 to 60 minutes and has a duration of 6 to 8 hours. After I.V. administration, its onset occurs within 5 minutes, and it has a duration of 2 hours. After I.M. injection, it begins to act within 30 minutes and has a duration of 6 to 8 hours.

• Among miscellaneous diuretics, mannitol begins to act 15 to 30 minutes after I.V. administration; diuresis occurs in 1 to 3 hours. Duration is 4 to 6 hours, but it may reduce cerebrospinal fluid pressure for up to 8 hours.

Mercaptomerin begins to act 1 to 3 hours after I.M. or subcutaneous injection; its duration is 12 to 24 hours.

Spironolactone's onset occurs gradually over 2 to 3 days, but a loading dose may be used for faster effect. The drug continues to act for 2 to 3 days.

Amiloride and triamterene begin to act in 2 to 4 hours and have a duration of up to 24 hours. Maximal therapeutic effect may not occur during the first few days of therapy.

Urea begins to act 1 to 2 hours after I.V. administration and has a duration of 3 to 10 hours.

Combination products

ALDACTAZIDE♦: spironolactone 25 mg and hydrochlorothiazide 25 mg.
DYAZIDE♦: triamterene 50 mg and hydrochlorothiazide 25 mg.

NAMES, INDICATIONS AND DOSAGES	SIDE EFFECTS
acetazolamide Acetazolam♦♦, Diamox♦, Diamox Sequels♦, Hydrazol **acetazolamide sodium** Diamox Parenteral♦ **Narrow-angle glaucoma:** ADULTS: 250 mg q 4 hours; or 250 mg b.i.d. P.O., I.M., or I.V. for short-term therapy. **Edema, in congestive heart failure:** ADULTS: 250 to 375 mg P.O., I.M., or I.V. daily in a.m. CHILDREN: 5 mg/kg daily in a.m. **Epilepsy:** CHILDREN: 8 to 30 mg/kg daily P.O., I.M., or I.V. in divided doses. **Open-angle glaucoma:** ADULTS: 250 mg daily to 1 g P.O., I.M., or I.V. divided q.i.d.	**Blood:** *aplastic anemia,* hemolytic anemia, leukopenia. **CNS:** drowsiness, paresthesias. **EENT:** transient myopia. **GI:** nausea, vomiting, anorexia. **GU:** crystalluria, renal calculi. **Metabolic:** *hyperchloremic acidosis,* hypokalemia, asymptomatic hyperuricemia. **Skin:** rash.
amiloride hydrochloride Midamor **Hypertension; or edema associated with congestive heart failure, usually in patients who are also taking thiazide or other potassium-wasting diuretics:** ADULTS: Usual dosage is 5 mg P.O. daily. Dosage may be increased to 10 mg daily, if necessary. As much as 20 mg daily can be given.	**CNS:** *headache,* weakness, dizziness. **CV:** orthostatic hypotension. **GI:** *nausea, anorexia, diarrhea, vomiting,* abdominal pain, constipation. **GU:** *impotence.* **Metabolic:** *hyperkalemia.*
bendroflumethiazide Naturetin♦ **Edema, hypertension:** ADULTS: 5 to 20 mg P.O. daily or b.i.d. in divided doses. CHILDREN: initially, 0.1 to 0.4 mg/kg daily in 1 or 2 doses. Maintenance: 0.05 to 0.1 mg/kg daily in 1 or 2 doses.	**Blood:** *aplastic anemia, agranulocytosis,* leukopenia, thrombocytopenia. **CV:** *volume depletion and dehydration,* orthostatic hypotension. **GI:** anorexia, nausea, pancreatitis. **Hepatic:** hepatic encephalopathy. **Metabolic:** *hypokalemia, asymptomatic hyperuricemia, hyperglycemia and impairment of glucose tolerance,* fluid and electrolyte imbalances including dilutional hyponatremia and hypochloremia, metabolic alkalosis, hypercalcemia, gout. **Skin:** dermatitis, photosensitivity, rash. **Other:** hypersensitivity reactions such as pneumonitis and vasculitis.
benzthiazide Aquapres, Aqua-Scrip, Aquasec, Aquatag, Diretic, Exna♦, Hydrex, Lemazide, Marazide, Proaqua, Ridema, S-Aqua, Urazide	**Blood:** *aplastic anemia, agranulocytosis,* leukopenia, thrombocytopenia. **CV:** *volume depletion and dehydration,* orthostatic hypotension. **GI:** anorexia, nausea, pancreatitis. **Hepatic:** hepatic encephalopathy.

♦ Available in U.S. and Canada. ♦♦ Available in Canada only.
All other products (no symbol) available in U.S. only. Italicized side effects are common or life-threatening.

INTERACTIONS AND SPECIAL CONSIDERATIONS

No significant interactions.

Special considerations:

• Contraindicated in long-term therapy for chronic noncongestive narrow-angle glaucoma; also in depressed sodium or potassium blood serum levels, renal or hepatic disease or dysfunction, adrenal gland failure, and hyperchloremic acidosis. Use cautiously in respiratory acidosis, emphysema, chronic pulmonary disease, or in patients receiving other diuretics.
• Intake and output and electrolytes, especially serum potassium, should be monitored. When used in diuretic therapy, high-potassium diet advised.
• Patient should be weighed daily; rapid weight loss may cause hypotension.
• Diuretic effect decreased when acidosis occurs but can be reestablished by withdrawing drug for several days and then restarting, or by utilizing intermittent administration schedules.
• 500-mg vial should be reconstituted with at least 5 ml sterile water for injection and used within 24 hours of reconstitution.
• I.M. injection painful because of alkalinity of solution. Direct I.V. administration preferred (100 to 500 mg/minute).
• Elderly patients are especially susceptible to excessive diuresis.
• May cause false-positive urine protein test results by alkalinizing the urine.
• A carbonic anhydrase inhibitor. Its acidotic effects limit usefulness for daily treatment of edema.

No significant interactions.

Special considerations:

• Contraindicated with elevated serum potassium levels (greater than 5.5 mEq/liter). Don't administer to patients receiving other potassium-sparing diuretics, such as spironolactone and triamterene. Also contraindicated in anuria.
• Use cautiously in patients with renal impairment, because potassium retention is increased.
• Risk of hyperkalemia is greater when a potassium-wasting drug is not taken concurrently. When amiloride is taken this way, daily potassium levels should be monitored.
• Amiloride should be discontinued immediately if potassium level exceeds 6.5 mEq/liter.
• Patient should avoid excessive ingestion of potassium-rich foods.
• Amiloride should be taken with or after meals to prevent nausea.

Interactions:

CHOLESTYRAMINE, COLESTIPOL: intestinal absorption of thiazides decreased. Keep doses as separate as possible.
DIAZOXIDE: increased antihypertensive, hyperglycemic, hyperuricemic effects. Use together cautiously.

Special considerations:

• Contraindicated in anuria and in hypersensitivity to other thiazides or other sulfonamide-derived drugs. Use cautiously in severe renal disease and impaired hepatic function.
• Intake and output, weight, serum electrolytes, serum creatinine, and BUN levels should be monitored regularly. Not effective if these levels are more than twice normal.
• Serum potassium levels should be monitored; muscle weakness and cramps are signs of hypokalemia. Patients on digitalis have an increased risk of digitalis toxicity due to potassium-depleting side effect of this diuretic. May require high-potassium diet or potassium-sparing diuretic.
• Foods rich in potassium include citrus fruits, bananas, tomatoes, dates, and apricots.
• Blood sugar should be monitored and insulin requirements checked in patients with diabetes. Severe hyperglycemia may be treated with oral antidiabetic agents.
• Blood uric acid levels should be monitored, especially in patients with a history of gout.
• Patient should take in a.m. to prevent nocturia.
• Elderly patients are especially susceptible to excessive diuresis.
• In hypertension, therapeutic response may be delayed several days.
• A thiazide diuretic.
• Thiazides should be discontinued before studies for parathyroid function are performed.
• For treatment of anaphylaxis, see APPENDIX.

Interactions:

CHOLESTYRAMINE, COLESTIPOL: intestinal absorption of thiazides decreased. Keep doses as separate as possible.
DIAZOXIDE: increased antihypertensive, hyperglycemic, hyperuricemic effects. Use together cautiously.

Special considerations:

• Contraindicated in anuria; hypersensitivity to other thiazides or other sulfonamide-derived drugs. Use cautiously in severe renal disease and

(continued on following page)

NAMES, INDICATIONS AND DOSAGES	SIDE EFFECTS
benzthiazide *(continued)* **Edema:** ADULTS: 50 to 200 mg P.O. daily or in divided doses. CHILDREN: 1 to 4 mg/kg daily in 3 divided doses. **Hypertension:** ADULTS: 50 mg P.O. daily b.i.d., t.i.d., or q.i.d., adjusted to patient's response.	**Metabolic:** *hypokalemia, asymptomatic hyperuricemia, hyperglycemia and impairment of glucose tolerance,* fluid and electrolyte imbalances including dilutional hyponatremia and hypochloremia, metabolic alkalosis, hypercalcemia, gout. **Skin:** dermatitis, photosensitivity, rash. **Other:** hypersensitivity reactions such as pneumonitis and vasculitis.
chlorothiazide Diuril♦, Ro-Chlorozide, SK-Chlorothiazide **Diuresis:** CHILDREN OVER 6 MONTHS: 20 mg/kg P.O. or I.V. daily in divided doses. CHILDREN UNDER 6 MONTHS: may require 30 mg/kg P.O. or I.V. daily in 2 divided doses. **Edema, hypertension:** ADULTS: 500 mg to 2 g P.O. or I.V. daily or in 2 divided doses.	**Blood:** *aplastic anemia, agranulocytosis,* leukopenia, thrombocytopenia. **CV:** *volume depletion and dehydration,* orthostatic hypotension. **GI:** anorexia, nausea, pancreatitis. **Hepatic:** hepatic encephalopathy. **Metabolic:** *hypokalemia, asymptomatic hyperuricemia, hyperglycemia and impairment of glucose tolerance,* fluid and electrolyte imbalances including dilutional hyponatremia and hypochloremia, metabolic alkalosis, hypercalcemia, gout. **Skin:** dermatitis, photosensitivity, rash. **Other:** hypersensitivity reactions such as pneumonitis and vasculitis.
chlorthalidone Hygroton♦, Novothalidone♦♦, Uridon♦♦ **Edema, hypertension:** ADULTS: 25 to 100 mg P.O. daily, or 100 mg 3 times weekly or on alternate days. Occasionally, up to 200 mg daily may be needed. CHILDREN: 2 mg/kg P.O. 3 times weekly.	**Blood:** *aplastic anemia, agranulocytosis,* leukopenia, thrombocytopenia. **CV:** *volume depletion and dehydration,* orthostatic hypotension. **GI:** anorexia, nausea, pancreatitis. **GU:** impotence. **Hepatic:** hepatic encephalopathy. **Metabolic:** *hypokalemia, asymptomatic hyperuricemia, hyperglycemia and impairment of glucose tolerance,* fluid and electrolyte imbalances including dilutional hyponatremia and hypochloremia, metabolic alkalosis, hypercalcemia, gout. **Skin:** dermatitis, photosensitivity, rash. **Other:** hypersensitivity reactions such as pneumonitis and vasculitis.

♦ Available in U.S. and Canada. ♦♦ Available in Canada only.
All other products (no symbol) available in U.S. only. Italicized side effects are common or life-threatening.

INTERACTIONS AND SPECIAL CONSIDERATIONS

impaired hepatic function.

• Intake and output, weight, serum electrolytes, and serum potassium levels should be monitored regularly. Muscle weakness and cramps are signs of hypokalemia. Patients on digitalis have an increased risk of digitalis toxicity due to the potassium-depleting side effect of this diuretic. May require high-potassium diet or potassium-sparing diuretic.
• Foods rich in potassium include citrus fruits, bananas, tomatoes, dates, and apricots.
• Serum creatinine and BUN levels should be monitored regularly. Not effective if these levels are more than twice normal.
• Blood sugar should be monitored and insulin requirements checked in patients with diabetes. Severe hyperglycemia may be treated with oral antidiabetic agents.
• Blood uric acid levels should be monitored, especially in patients with a history of gout.
• Patient should take in a.m. to prevent nocturia.
• Elderly patients are especially susceptible to excessive diuresis.
• In hypertension, therapeutic response may be delayed several days.
• A thiazide diuretic.
• For treatment of anaphylaxis, see APPENDIX.

Interactions:

CHOLESTYRAMINE, COLESTIPOL: intestinal absorption of thiazides decreased. Keep doses as separate as possible.

DIAZOXIDE: increased antihypertensive, hyperglycemic, hyperuricemic effects. Use together cautiously.

Special considerations:

• Contraindicated in anuria; hypersensitivity to other thiazides or other sulfonamide-derived drugs; impaired hepatic function; progressive hepatic disease. Use cautiously in severe renal disease.
• Intake and output, weight, serum electrolytes, and serum potassium levels should be monitored regularly. Muscle weakness and cramps are signs of hypokalemia. Patients on digitalis have an increased risk of digitalis toxicity due to the potassium-depleting effect of this diuretic. May require high-potassium diet or potassium-sparing diuretic.
• Foods rich in potassium include citrus fruits, tomatoes, bananas, dates, and apricots.
• Blood sugar should be monitored and insulin requirements checked in patients with diabetes. Severe hyperglycemia may be treated with oral antidiabetic agents.
• Serum creatinine and BUN levels should be monitored regularly. Not effective if these levels are more than twice normal.
• Blood uric acid levels should be monitored, especially in patients with a history of gout.
• Decreased calcium excretion and progressive renal impairment possible.
• Only injectable thiazide. For I.V. use only—not I.M. or subcutaneously. Should be reconstituted with 18 ml of sterile water for injection/500-mg vial. Reconstituted solutions may be stored at room temperature up to 24 hours. Compatible with intravenous dextrose or sodium chloride solutions.
• I.V. infiltration should be avoided; can be very painful.
• Should be given in a.m. to prevent nocturia.
• In hypertension, therapeutic response may be delayed several days.
• Elderly patients especially susceptible to excessive diuresis.
• A thiazide diuretic.
• The only thiazide available in liquid form.
• Thiazides should be stopped before tests for parathyroid function are performed.
• For treatment of anaphylaxis, see APPENDIX.

Interactions:

CHOLESTYRAMINE, COLESTIPOL: intestinal absorption of thiazides decreased. Keep doses as separate as possible.

DIAZOXIDE: increased antihypertensive, hyperglycemic, hyperuricemic effects. Use together cautiously.

Special considerations:

• Contraindicated in anuria; hypersensitivity to thiazides or other sulfonamide-derived drugs. Use cautiously in severe renal disease, progressive hepatic disease, impaired hepatic function.
• Intake and output, weight, serum electrolytes, and serum potassium levels should be monitored regularly. Muscle weakness and cramps are signs of hypokalemia. Patients on digitalis have an increased risk of digitalis toxicity due to the potassium-depleting effect of this diuretic. May require high-potassium diet or potassium-sparing diuretic.
• Foods rich in potassium include citrus fruits, tomatoes, bananas, dates, and apricots.
• Serum creatinine and BUN levels should be monitored regularly. Not effective if these levels are more than twice normal.
• Blood uric acid levels should be monitored, especially in patients with a history of gout.
• Blood sugar should be monitored and insulin requirements checked in patients with diabetes. Severe hyperglycemia may be treated with oral antidiabetic agents.
• In hypertension, therapeutic response may be delayed several days.
• Should be given in a.m. to prevent nocturia.
• Elderly patients are especially susceptible

(continued on following page)

NAMES, INDICATIONS AND DOSAGES	SIDE EFFECTS

chlorthalidone
(continued)

cyclothiazide
Anhydron

Edema:

ADULTS: 1 to 2 mg P.O. daily. May be used on alternate days as maintenance dose.

CHILDREN: 0.02 to 0.04 mg/kg P.O. daily.

Hypertension:

ADULTS: 2 mg P.O. daily; up to 2 mg b.i.d. or t.i.d.

Blood: *aplastic anemia, agranulocytosis,* leukopenia, thrombocytopenia.
CV: *volume depletion and dehydration,* orthostatic hypotension.
GI: anorexia, nausea, pancreatitis.
Hepatic: hepatic encephalopathy.
Metabolic: *hypokalemia, asymptomatic hyperuricemia, hyperglycemia and impairment of glucose tolerance,* fluid and electrolyte imbalances including dilutional hyponatremia and hypochloremia, metabolic alkalosis, hypercalcemia, gout.
Skin: dermatitis, photosensitivity, rash.
Other: hypersensitivity reactions such as pneumonitis and vasculitis.

dichlorphenamide
Daranide♦, Oratrol

Adjunct in glaucoma:

ADULTS: initially, 100 to 200 mg P.O., followed by 100 mg q 12 hours until desired response obtained. Maintenance: 25 to 50 mg P.O. daily b.i.d. or t.i.d. Give miotics concomitantly.

Blood: *aplastic anemia,* hemolytic anemia, leukopenia.
CNS: drowsiness, paresthesias.
EENT: transient myopia.
GI: nausea, vomiting, anorexia.
GU: crystalluria, renal calculi.
Metabolic: *hyperchloremic acidosis,* hypokalemia, asymptomatic hyperuricemia.
Skin: rash.

ethacrynate sodium
Sodium Edecrin

ethacrynic acid
Edecrin♦

Acute pulmonary edema:

ADULTS: 50 to 100 mg of ethacrynate sodium I.V. slowly over several minutes.

Edema:

ADULTS: 50 to 200 mg P.O. daily. Refractory cases may require up to 200 mg b.i.d.

CHILDREN: initial dose 25 mg P.O., cautiously, increased in 25-mg increments daily until desired effect is obtained.

Blood: *agranulocytosis,* thrombocytopenia.
CV: *volume depletion and dehydration, orthostatic hypotension.*
EENT: transient deafness with too rapid I.V. injection.
GI: abdominal discomfort and pain, diarrhea.
Metabolic: *hypokalemia; hypochloremic alkalosis; asymptomatic hyperuricemia; fluid and electrolyte imbalances including dilutional hyponatremia and hypochloremia, hypocalcemia, hypomagnesemia;* hyperglycemia and impairment of glucose tolerance.
Skin: dermatitis.

INTERACTIONS AND SPECIAL CONSIDERATIONS

to excessive diuresis.
• A thiazide-like diuretic.
• For treatment of anaphylaxis, see APPENDIX.

Interactions:
CHOLESTYRAMINE, COLESTIPOL: intestinal absorption of thiazides decreased. Keep doses as separate as possible.
DIAZOXIDE: increased antihypertensive, hyperglycemic, hyperuricemic effects. Use together cautiously.

Special considerations:
• Contraindicated in anuria; hypersensitivity to other thiazides or other sulfonamide-derived drugs. Use cautiously in severe renal disease, impaired hepatic function, progressive hepatic disease.
• Intake and output, weight, serum electrolytes, and serum potassium levels should be monitored regularly. Muscle weakness and cramps are signs of hypokalemia. Patients on digitalis have an increased risk of digitalis toxicity due to the potassium-depleting effect of this diuretic. May require high-potassium diet or potassium-sparing diuretic.
• Foods rich in potassium include citrus fruits, tomatoes, bananas, dates, and apricots.
• Blood sugar should be monitored and insulin requirements checked in patients with diabetes. Severe hyperglycemia may be treated with oral antidiabetic agents.
• Serum creatinine and BUN levels should be monitored regularly. Not effective if these levels are more than twice normal.
• Blood uric acid levels should be monitored, especially in patients with a history of gout.
• In hypertension, therapeutic response may be delayed several days.
• Patient should take in a.m. to prevent nocturia.
• Elderly patients are especially susceptible to excessive diuresis.
• A thiazide diuretic.
• For treatment of anaphylaxis, see APPENDIX.

No significant interactions.

Special considerations:
• Contraindicated in hepatic insufficiency, renal failure, adrenocortical insufficiency, hyperchloremic acidosis, depressed sodium or potassium levels, severe pulmonary obstruction with inability to increase alveolar ventilation, Addison's disease. Long-term use contraindicated in severe, absolute, or chronic noncongestive narrow-angle glaucoma. Use cautiously in respiratory acidosis, monitoring blood pH and blood gases.
• Electrolytes should be monitored, especially serum potassium in initial treatment. Usually no problem in long-term glaucoma therapy unless risk of hypokalemia from other causes; potassium supplements may be necessary.
• May cause false-positive results in urine protein tests.
• Drug should be taken everyday for glaucoma but intermittently for edema.
• Patient with glaucoma should be evaluated for eye pain to make sure drug is effective in decreasing intraocular pressure.
• A carbonic anhydrase inhibitor.

Interactions:
AMINOGLYCOSIDE ANTIBIOTICS: potentiated ototoxic side effects of both ethacrynic acid and aminoglycosides. Use together cautiously.

Special considerations:
• Contraindicated in patients with anuria and in infants. Use cautiously in electrolyte abnormalities. If electrolyte imbalance, azotemia, or oliguria develops, may require discontinuing drug.
• Intake and output, weight, serum electrolytes, and serum potassium levels should be monitored regularly. Muscle weakness and cramps are signs of hypokalemia and may require high-potassium diet or potassium-sparing diuretic.
• Foods rich in potassium include citrus fruits, tomatoes, bananas, dates, and apricots.
• Patients also on digitalis have an increased risk of digitalis toxicity due to the potassium-depleting effect of this diuretic.
• I.V. injection painful; may cause thrombophlebitis. Should not be given subcutaneously or I.M. Should be given slowly through tubing of running infusion over several minutes.
• Salt and potassium chloride supplement may be needed during therapy.
• Vacuum vial should be reconstituted with 50 ml of 5% dextrose injection or NaCl injection and unused solution discarded after 24 hours. Cloudy or opalescent solutions should not be used.
• Elderly patients are especially susceptible to excessive diuresis.
• Oral doses should be taken in a.m. to prevent nocturia.
• Blood uric acid levels should be monitored, especially in patients with history of gout.
• May potentiate effects of the anticoagulant warfarin; patients receiving both drugs should be monitored carefully.
• A loop diuretic, especially strong.

NAMES, INDICATIONS AND DOSAGES	SIDE EFFECTS
ethoxzolamide Ethamide **Edema (from congestive heart failure):** ADULTS: 62.5 to 125 mg P.O. daily in a.m. for 3 consecutive days each week or every other day. Refractory cases may require 250 mg/day. **Glaucoma:** ADULTS: 62.5 to 250 mg P.O. b.i.d., t.i.d., or q.i.d. Give miotics concomitantly.	**Blood:** *aplastic anemia,* hemolytic anemia, leukopenia. **CNS:** drowsiness, paresthesias. **EENT:** transient myopia. **GI:** nausea, vomiting, anorexia. **GU:** crystalluria, renal calculi. **Metabolic:** *hyperchloremic acidosis,* hypokalemia, asymptomatic hyperuricemia. **Skin:** rash.
furosemide Lasix♦, Novosemide♦♦, Uritol♦♦ **Acute pulmonary edema:** ADULTS: 40 mg I.V. injected slowly; then 40 mg I.V. in 1 to 1½ hours if needed. **Edema:** ADULTS: 20 to 80 mg P.O. daily in a.m., second dose can be given in 6 to 8 hours; carefully titrated up to 600 mg daily if needed; or 20 to 40 mg I.M. or I.V. Increase by 20 mg q 2 hours until desired response is achieved. I.V. dose should be given slowly over 1 to 2 minutes. INFANTS AND CHILDREN: 2 mg/kg daily; dose increased by 1 to 2 mg/kg in 6 to 8 hours if needed; carefully titrated up to 6 mg/kg daily if needed. **Hypertensive crisis, acute renal failure:** ADULTS: 100 to 200 mg I.V. over 1 to 2 minutes. **Chronic renal failure:** ADULTS: initially, 80 mg P.O. daily. Increase by 80 to 120 mg daily until desired response is achieved.	**Blood:** *agranulocytosis,* thrombocytopenia. **CV:** *volume depletion and dehydration, orthostatic hypotension.* **EENT:** transient deafness with too rapid I.V. injection. **GI:** abdominal discomfort and pain. **Metabolic:** *hypokalemia; hypochloremic alkalosis; asymptomatic hyperuricemia, fluid and electrolyte imbalances including dilutional hyponatremia and hypochloremia, hypocalcemia, hypomagnesemia;* hyperglycemia and impairment of glucose tolerance. **Skin:** dermatitis.

INTERACTIONS AND SPECIAL CONSIDERATIONS

No significant interactions.

Special considerations:

• Contraindicated in hyperchloremic acidosis, renal failure, hepatic insufficiency, adrenal failure, depressed sodium or potassium blood levels, and long-term therapy for chronic noncongestive narrow-angle glaucoma. Use with caution in advanced pulmonary disease, respiratory acidosis, and concomitantly with other diuretics.

• Electrolytes, especially serum potassium, should be monitored; high-potassium diet recommended. Intake and output, and weight should be monitored.

• May cause false-positive results in urine protein tests.

• Dehydration, especially in elderly patients, is possible.

• Drug should be taken every day for glaucoma but intermittently for edema. Patient should comply with prescribed dosage and schedule to lessen chance of metabolic acidosis.

• Patient with glaucoma should be evaluated for eye pain to make sure drug is effective in decreasing intraocular pressure.

• A carbonic anhydrase inhibitor. When used on a daily basis for edema, its acidotic effects limits its usefulness.

Interactions:

AMINOGLYCOSIDE ANTIBIOTICS: potentiated ototoxicity. Use together cautiously.

CHLORAL HYDRATE: sweating, flushing with I.V. furosemide. Observe patient.

CLOFIBRATE: enhanced furosemide effects. Use cautiously.

INDOMETHACIN: inhibited diuretic response. Use cautiously.

Special considerations:

• Use cautiously in cardiogenic shock complicated by pulmonary edema, anuria, hepatic coma, or electrolyte imbalances. Drug is not routinely administered to women of childbearing age because its safety in pregnancy hasn't been established.

• Potent loop diuretic; can lead to profound water and electrolyte depletion. Blood pressure and pulse rate during rapid diuresis should be monitored.

• Sulfonamide-sensitive patients may have allergic reaction to furosemide.

• If oliguria or azotemia increases or develops, may require stopping drug.

• Serum electrolytes, BUN, and CO_2 should be monitored frequently.

• Serum potassium levels should be monitored. Muscle weakness and cramps are signs of hypokalemia. Patients also on digitalis have an increased risk of digitalis toxicity due to the potassium-depleting effect of this diuretic. May require high-potassium diet.

• Foods rich in potassium include citrus fruits, tomatoes, bananas, dates, and apricots.

• Blood sugar levels should be monitored in patients with diabetes. Severe hyperglycemia may be treated with oral antidiabetic agents.

• Blood uric acid levels should be monitored, especially in patients with a history of gout.

• I.V. doses should be given over 1 to 2 minutes. Doses over 100 mg should be given at 10 mg/minute to prevent tinnitus associated with rapid infusion of large doses. In decreased renal function, I.V. doses should be given at rate of 10 mg/minute or less.

• Parenteral route not recommended in infants and children unless oral dosage form is not practical.

• I.M. injection causes transient pain; can be moderated by using "Z" track to limit leakage into subcutaneous tissues.

• Oral and I.M. preparations should be given in a.m. to prevent nocturia. Second doses should be given in early afternoon.

• Elderly patients are especially susceptible to excessive diuresis, with potential for circulatory collapse and thromboembolic complications.

• Store tablets in light-resistant container to prevent discoloration (doesn't affect potency). Discolored (yellow) injectable preparation should not be used. Oral furosemide solution should be stored in the refrigerator to ensure stability of the drug.

• Promotes calcium excretion. I.V. furosemide often used to treat hypercalcemia.

• Patients taking furosemide should be advised to stand slowly to prevent dizziness, and to limit alcohol intake and strenuous exercise in hot weather since these exacerbate orthostatic hypotension.

• Patients should report immediately ringing in ears, severe abdominal pain, or sore throat and fever; may indicate furosemide toxicity.

• Patients receiving furosemide therapy at home should be discouraged from storing different types of medication in the same container. This increases the risk of drug errors, especially for patients taking both furosemide and digoxin, since the most popular strengths of these drugs pills are white tablets approximately equal in size.

• To prepare parenteral furosemide for I.V. infusion, drug should be mixed with 5% dextrose in water, 0.9% sodium chloride solution, or lactated Ringer's solution. Prepared infusion solution should be used within 24 hours.

NAMES, INDICATIONS AND DOSAGES	SIDE EFFECTS
hydrochlorothiazide Chlorzide, Diuchlor-H♦♦, Diu-Scrip, Esidrix♦, Hydrid♦♦, HydroAquil♦♦, Hydro Diuril♦, Hydromal, Hydro-Z-25, Hydro-Z-50, Hydrozide♦♦, Hyperetic, Kenazide, Lexor, Neo-Codema♦♦, Novohydrazide♦♦, Oretic, Ro-Hydrazide, Urozide♦♦, Zide **Edema:** ADULTS: initially, 25 to 100 mg P.O. daily or intermittently for maintenance to minimize electrolyte imbalance. CHILDREN OVER 6 MONTHS: 2.2 mg/kg P.O. daily divided b.i.d. CHILDREN UNDER 6 MONTHS: up to 3.3 mg/kg P.O. daily divided b.i.d. **Hypertension:** ADULTS: 25 to 100 mg P.O. daily or divided dosage. Daily dosage increased or decreased according to blood pressure.	**Blood:** *aplastic anemia, agranulocytosis,* leukopenia, thrombocytopenia. **CV:** *volume depletion and dehydration,* orthostatic hypotension. **GI:** anorexia, nausea, pancreatitis. **Hepatic:** hepatic encephalopathy. **Metabolic:** *hypokalemia, asymptomatic hyperuricemia, hyperglycemia and impairment of glucose tolerance,* fluid and electrolyte imbalances including dilutional hyponatremia and hypochloremia, metabolic alkalosis, hypercalcemia, gout. **Skin:** dermatitis, photosensitivity, rash. **Other:** hypersensitivity reactions such as pneumonitis and vasculitis.
hydroflumethiazide Diucardin♦, Saluron **Edema:** ADULTS: 25 mg to 200 mg P.O. daily in divided doses. Maintenance doses may be on intermittent or alternate-day schedule. CHILDREN: 1 mg/kg P.O. daily. **Hypertension:** ADULTS: 50 to 100 mg P.O. daily or b.i.d.	**Blood:** *aplastic anemia, agranulocytosis,* leukopenia, thrombocytopenia. **CV:** *volume depletion and dehydration,* orthostatic hypotension. **GI:** anorexia, nausea, pancreatitis. **Hepatic:** hepatic encephalopathy. **Metabolic:** *hypokalemia, asymptomatic hyperuricemia, hyperglycemia and impairment of glucose tolerance,* fluid and electrolyte imbalances including dilutional hyponatremia and hypochloremia, metabolic alkalosis, hypercalcemia, gout. **Skin:** dermatitis, photosensitivity, rash. **Other:** hypersensitivity reactions such as pneumonitis and vasculitis.
mannitol Osmitrol♦ ADULTS AND CHILDREN OVER 12 YEARS: **Test dose for marked oliguria or suspected inadequate renal function:** 200 mg/kg or 12.5 g as a 15% or 20% solution I.V. over 3 to 5 minutes. Response adequate if 30 to 50 ml urine/hour is excreted over 2 to 3 hours. **Treatment of oliguria:** 50 to 100 g I.V. as a 15% to 20% solution over 90 minutes to several hours. **Prevention of oliguria or acute renal failure:** 50 to 100 g I.V. of a concentrated (5% to 25%) solution. Exact concentration is determined by fluid requirements. **Edema:** 100 g as a 10% to 20% solution over 2- to 6-hour period. **To reduce intraocular pressure or intracranial pressure:** 1.5 to 2 g/kg as a 15% to 25%	**CNS:** rebound increase in intracranial pressure 8 to 12 hours after diuresis, headache, confusion. **CV:** *transient expansion of plasma volume during infusion causing circulatory overload and pulmonary edema,* tachycardia, anginalike chest pain. **EENT:** blurred vision, rhinitis. **GI:** thirst, nausea, vomiting. **GU:** urinary retention. **Metabolic:** *fluid and electrolyte imbalances, water intoxication, cellular dehydration.*

♦ Available in U.S. and Canada. ♦♦ Available in Canada only.
All other products (no symbol) available in U.S. only. Italicized side effects are common or life-threatening.

INTERACTIONS AND SPECIAL CONSIDERATIONS

Interactions:
CHOLESTYRAMINE, COLESTIPOL: intestinal absorption of thiazides decreased. Keep doses as separate as possible.
DIAZOXIDE: increased antihypertensive, hyperglycemic, hyperuricemic effects. Use together cautiously.

Special considerations:
• Contraindicated in anuria; hypersensitivity to other thiazides or other sulfonamide derivatives. Use cautiously in severe renal disease, impaired hepatic function, progressive hepatic disease.
• Intake and output, weight, serum electrolytes, and serum potassium levels should be monitored regularly. Muscle weakness and cramps are signs of hypokalemia. Patients also on digitalis have an increased risk of digitalis toxicity due to the potassium-depleting effect of this diuretic. May require high-potassium diet or potassium-sparing diuretic.
• Foods rich in potassium include citrus fruits, tomatoes, bananas, dates, and apricots.
• Serum creatinine and BUN levels should be monitored regularly. Not effective if these levels are more than twice normal.
• Blood uric acid levels should be monitored, especially in patients with a history of gout.
• Insulin requirements should be checked in patients with diabetes. Oral antidiabetic agents may be used to treat severe hyperglycemia.
• In hypertension, therapeutic response may be delayed several days.
• Patient should take in a.m. to prevent nocturia.
• Elderly patients are especially susceptible to excessive diuresis.
• A thiazide diuretic.
• For treatment of anaphylaxis, see APPENDIX.

Interactions:
CHOLESTYRAMINE, COLESTIPOL: intestinal absorption of thiazides decreased. Keep doses as separate as possible.
DIAZOXIDE: increased antihypertensive, hyperglycemic, hyperuricemic effects. Use together cautiously.

Special considerations:
• Contraindicated in anuria; hypersensitivity to other thiazides or other sulfonamide-derived drugs. Use cautiously in severe renal disease, impaired hepatic function, progressive hepatic disease.
• Intake and output, weight, serum electrolytes, and serum potassium levels should be monitored regularly. Muscle weakness and cramps are signs of hypokalemia. Patients also on digitalis have an increased risk of digitalis toxicity due to the potassium-depleting effects of this diuretic. May require high-potassium diet or potassium-sparing diuretic.
• Foods rich in potassium include citrus fruits, tomatoes, bananas, dates, and apricots.
• Serum creatinine and BUN levels should be monitored regularly. Not effective if these levels are more than twice normal.
• Blood uric acid levels should be monitored, especially in patients with history of gout.
• Insulin requirements should be checked in patients with diabetes. Oral antidiabetic agents may be used to treat severe hyperglycemia.
• Patient should take in a.m. to prevent nocturia.
• In hypertension, therapeutic response may be delayed several days.
• Elderly patients are especially susceptible to excessive diuresis.
• A long-acting thiazide diuretic.
• For treatment of anaphylaxis, see APPENDIX.

No significant interactions.

Special considerations:
• Contraindicated in anuria, severe pulmonary congestion, frank pulmonary edema, severe congestive heart disease, severe dehydration, metabolic edema, progressive renal disease or dysfunction, progressive heart failure during administration, active intracranial bleeding except during craniotomy.
• Vital signs (including CVP) should be monitored at least hourly; intake and output hourly (watch for increasing oliguria). Weight, renal function, fluid balance, serum and urine sodium and potassium levels should be monitored daily.
• Solution often crystallizes, especially at low temperatures. To redissolve, bottle should be warmed in hot water bath and shaken vigorously. Should be cooled to body temperature before given. Concentrations greater than 15% have greater tendency to crystallize. Solution with undissolved crystals should not be used.
• Infusions should always be given I.V. via an in-line filter.
• Infiltration should be avoided, and inflammation, edema, and potential necrosis monitored.
• For maximum pressure reduction before surgery, should be given 1 to 1½ hours preoperatively.
• Can be used to measure glomerular filtration rate.
• Frequent mouth care or fluids as permitted to relieve thirst recommended.
• Foley catheter is inserted in comatose or incontinent patients because therapy is based on strict evaluation of intake and output. In patients with Foley catheters, an hourly urometer collection bag should be used to facilitate accurate evaluation of output.

(continued on following page)

NAMES, INDICATIONS AND DOSAGES	SIDE EFFECTS
mannitol *(continued)* solution I.V. over 30 to 60 minutes. **To promote diuresis in drug intoxication:** 5% to 10% solution continuously up to 200 g I.V., while maintaining 100 to 500 ml urinary output/hour and a positive fluid balance.	
mercaptomerin sodium Thiomerin Sodium♦ **Edema:** ADULTS: 125 to 250 mg I.M. or S.C. daily. Maintenance with 1 to 2 times weekly dose. CHILDREN: 125 mg/m² I.M.	**Blood:** *agranulocytosis,* leukopenia. **CNS:** dizziness, confusion, headache. **CV:** volume depletion and dehydration, orthostatic hypotension. **Metabolic:** *fluid and electrolyte imbalances including dilutional hyponatremia and hypochloremia, metabolic alkalosis,* asymptomatic hyperuricemia. **Local:** pain on injection. **Other:** signs of mercury toxicity (albuminuria, hematuria, renal casts, stomatitis, metallic taste, colitis).
methazolamide Neptazane **Glaucoma (open-angle, or preoperatively in obstructive or narrow-angle):** ADULTS: 50 to 100 mg b.i.d. or t.i.d.	**Blood:** *aplastic anemia,* hemolytic anemia, leukopenia. **CNS:** drowsiness, paresthesias. **EENT:** transient myopia. **GI:** nausea, vomiting, anorexia. **GU:** crystalluria, renal calculi. **Metabolic:** *hyperchloremic acidosis,* hypokalemia, asymptomatic hyperuricemia. **Skin:** rash.
methyclothiazide Aquatensen, Duretic♦♦, Enduron **Edema, hypertension:** ADULTS: 2.5 to 10 mg P.O daily.	**Blood:** *aplastic anemia, agranulocytosis,* leukopenia, thrombocytopenia. **CV:** *volume depletion and dehydration,* orthostatic hypotension. **GI:** anorexia, nausea, pancreatitis. **Hepatic:** hepatic encephalopathy. **Metabolic:** *hypokalemia, asymptomatic hyperuricemia, hyperglycemia and impairment of glucose tolerance,* fluid and electrolyte imbalances including dilutional hyponatremia and hypochloremia, metabolic alkalosis, hypercalcemia, gout. **Skin:** dermatitis, photosensitivity, rash. **Other:** hypersensitivity reactions such as pneumonitis and vasculitis.

♦ Available in U.S. and Canada. ♦♦ Available in Canada only.
All other products (no symbol) available in U.S. only. Italicized side effects are common or life-threatening.

INTERACTIONS AND SPECIAL CONSIDERATIONS

• An osmotic diuretic.

No significant interactions.

Special considerations:
• Contraindicated in renal insufficiency and acute or subacute nephritis. Use cautiously in impaired hepatic function.
• Rarely used; agents available with less severe side effects.
• Mercurial diuretic. Testing for mercury hypersensitivity with 0.5 ml 24 hours before initiating therapy is advised. Patient may develop signs of mercurialism.
• Urine should be monitored for albumin, blood cells, and casts. Weight and serum electrolyte levels, especially potassium, should be monitored regularly and a high-potassium diet provided.
• Should be given in a.m. for diuresis within 1 to 2 hours.
• For I.M. or subcutaneous injection, rotate site, massage gently; avoid edematous or adipose tissue, and areas of poor circulation. Should not be used I.V.
• Good oral hygiene important to limit or prevent stomatitis.
• Elderly patients are more susceptible to excessive dehydration with potential for circulatory collapse or thromboembolic phenomena.
• For symptoms and treatment of anaphylaxis, see APPENDIX.

No significant interactions.

Special considerations:
• Contraindicated in severe or absolute glaucoma; for long-term use in chronic noncongestive narrow-angle glaucoma; and in patients with depressed sodium or potassium serum levels, renal or hepatic disease or dysfunction, adrenal gland dysfunction, and hyperchloremic acidosis. Use cautiously in respiratory acidosis, emphysema, chronic lung disease.
• Intake and output, weight, and serum electrolytes should be monitored frequently.
• May cause false-positive urine protein test results by alkalinizing urine.
• A carbonic anhydrase inhibitor.
• Elderly patients are especially susceptible to excessive diuresis.
• Diuretic effect decreases in acidosis.
• Drug should be taken every day for glaucoma but intermittently for edema. Patient should be cautioned to comply with prescribed dosage and schedule to lessen risk of metabolic acidosis.
• Patient with glaucoma should be evaluated for eye pain to make sure drug is effective in decreasing intraocular pressure.

Interactions:
CHOLESTYRAMINE, COLESTIPOL: intestinal absorption of thiazides decreased. Keep doses as separate as possible.
DIAZOXIDE: increased antihypertensive, hyperglycemic, hyperuricemic effects. Use together cautiously.

Special considerations:
• Contraindicated in renal decompensation; anuria; hypersensitivity to other thiazides or other sulfonamide-derived drugs. Use cautiously in potassium depletion, renal disease or dysfunction, impaired hepatic function, progressive hepatic disease.
• Intake and output, weight, serum electrolytes, and serum potassium levels should be monitored regularly. Muscle weakness and cramps are signs of hypokalemia. Patients also on digitalis have an increased risk of digitalis toxicity due to the potassium-depleting effect of this diuretic. May require high-potassium diet or potassium-sparing diuretic.
• Foods rich in potassium include citrus fruits, tomatoes, bananas, dates, and apricots.
• Insulin requirements should be checked in patients with diabetes. Oral antidiabetic agents may be used to treat severe hyperglycemia.
• Serum creatinine and BUN levels should be monitored regularly. Not effective if these levels are more than twice normal.
• Blood uric acid levels should be monitored, especially in patients with a history of gout.
• In hypertension, therapeutic response may be delayed several days.
• Patient should take in a.m. to prevent nocturia.
• Elderly patients are especially susceptible to excessive diuresis.
• A thiazide diuretic.
• For treatment of anaphylaxis, see APPENDIX.

NAMES, INDICATIONS AND DOSAGES	SIDE EFFECTS
metolazone Diulo, Zaroxolyn♦ **Edema (heart failure):** ADULTS: 5 to 10 mg P.O. daily. **Edema (renal disease):** ADULTS: 5 to 20 mg P.O. daily. **Hypertension:** ADULTS: 2.5 to 5 mg P.O. daily. Maintenance dose determined by patient's blood pressure.	**Blood:** *aplastic anemia, agranulocytosis,* leukopenia, thrombocytopenia. **CV:** *volume depletion and dehydration,* orthostatic hypotension. **GI:** anorexia, nausea, pancreatitis. **Hepatic:** hepatic encephalopathy. **Metabolic:** *hypokalemia, asymptomatic hyperuricemia, hyperglycemia and impairment of glucose tolerance,* fluid and electrolyte imbalances including dilutional hyponatremia and hypochloremia, metabolic alkalosis, hypercalcemia, gout. **Skin:** dermatitis, photosensitivity, rash. **Other:** hypersensitivity reactions such as pneumonitis and vasculitis.
polythiazide Renese♦ **Hypertension:** ADULTS: 2 to 4 mg P.O. daily. **Edema (heart failure, renal failure):** ADULTS: 1 to 4 mg P.O. daily.	**Blood:** *aplastic anemia, agranulocytosis,* leukopenia, thrombocytopenia. **CV:** *volume depletion and dehydration,* orthostatic hypotension. **GI:** anorexia, nausea, pancreatitis. **Hepatic:** hepatic encephalopathy. **Metabolic:** *hypokalemia, asymptomatic hyperuricemia, hyperglycemia and impairment of glucose tolerance,* fluid and electrolyte imbalances including dilutional hyponatremia and hypochloremia, metabolic alkalosis, hypercalcemia, gout. **Skin:** dermatitis, photosensitivity, rash. **Other:** hypersensitivity reactions such as pneumonitis and vasculitis.
quinethazone Aquamox♦♦, Hydromox **Edema:** ADULTS: 50 to 100 mg P.O. daily or 50 mg P.O. b.i.d. Occasionally, up to 150 to 200 mg P.O. daily may be needed.	**Blood:** *aplastic anemia, agranulocytosis,* leukopenia, thrombocytopenia. **CV:** *volume depletion and dehydration,* orthostatic hypotension. **GI:** anorexia, nausea, pancreatitis. **Hepatic:** *hepatic encephalopathy.* **Metabolic:** *hypokalemia, asymptomatic hyperuricemia, hyperglycemia and impairment of glucose tolerance,* fluid and electrolyte imbalances including dilutional hyponatremia and hypochloremia, metabolic alkalosis, hypercalcemia, gout. **Skin:** dermatitis, photosensitivity, rash. **Other:** hypersensitivity reactions such as pneumonitis and vasculitis.

INTERACTIONS AND SPECIAL CONSIDERATIONS

Interactions:

CHOLESTYRAMINE, COLESTIPOL: intestinal absorption of thiazides decreased. Keep doses as separate as possible.

DIAZOXIDE: increased antihypertensive, hyperglycemic, hyperuricemic effects. Use together cautiously.

Special considerations:

- Contraindicated in anuria; hepatic coma or precoma; hypersensitivity to thiazides or other sulfonamide-derived drugs. Use cautiously in hyperuricemia or gout, and severely impaired renal function.
- Intake and output, weight, serum electrolytes, and serum potassium levels should be monitored regularly. Muscle weakness and cramps are signs of hypokalemia. Patients on digitalis may have an increased risk of digitalis toxicity due to the potassium-depleting effect of this diuretic. May require high-potassium diet or potassium-sparing diuretic.
- Foods rich in potassium include citrus fruits, tomatoes, bananas, dates, and apricots.
- Insulin requirements should be checked in patients with diabetes. Oral antidiabetic agents may be used to treat severe hyperglycemia.
- Blood uric acid levels should be checked, especially in patients with a history of gout.
- In hypertension, therapeutic response may be delayed several days.
- Patient should take in a.m. to prevent nocturia.
- Elderly patients are especially susceptible to excessive diuresis.
- A thiazide-related diuretic. However, unlike thiazide diuretics, metolazone is effective in patients with decreased renal function.
- Used as an adjunct in furosemide-resistant edema.

Interactions:

CHOLESTYRAMINE, COLESTIPOL: intestinal absorption of thiazides decreased. Keep doses as separate as possible.

DIAZOXIDE: increased antihypertensive, hyperglycemic, hyperuricemic effects. Use together cautiously.

Special considerations:

- Contraindicated in anuria; hypersensitivity to other thiazides or other sulfonamide-derived drugs. Use cautiously in severe renal disease, impaired hepatic function, allergies.
- Intake and output, weight, serum electrolytes, and serum potassium levels should be monitored regularly. Muscle weakness and cramps are signs of hypokalemia. Patients also on digitalis may have an increased risk of digitalis toxicity due to the potassium-depleting effect of this diuretic. May require high-potassium diet or potassium-sparing diuretic.
- Foods rich in potassium include citrus fruits, tomatoes, bananas, dates, and apricots.
- Serum creatinine and BUN levels should be monitored regularly. Not effective if these levels are more than twice normal.
- Monitor blood uric acid levels, especially in patients with a history of gout.
- Insulin requirements should be checked in patients with diabetes. Oral antidiabetic agents may be used to treat severe hyperglycemia.
- In hypertension, therapeutic response may be delayed several days.
- Patient should take in a.m. to prevent nocturia.
- Elderly patients are especially susceptible to excessive diuresis.
- A long-acting thiazide diuretic.
- For treatment of anaphylaxis, see APPENDIX.

Interactions:

CHOLESTYRAMINE, COLESTIPOL: intestinal absorption of thiazides decreased. Keep doses as separate as possible.

DIAZOXIDE: increased antihypertensive, hyperglycemic, hyperuricemic effects. Use together cautiously.

Special considerations:

- Contraindicated in anuria; hypersensitivity to quinethazones, thiazides, or other sulfonamide-derived drugs. Use cautiously in severe renal disease, impaired hepatic function, allergies.
- Intake and output, weight, serum electrolytes, and serum potassium levels should be monitored regularly. Muscle weakness and cramps are signs of hypokalemia. Patients also on digitalis have an increased risk of digitalis toxicity due to the potassium-depleting effect of this diuretic. Patients taking this drug may require high-potassium diet or potassium-sparing diuretic.
- Foods rich in potassium include citrus fruits, tomatoes, bananas, dates, and apricots.
- Serum creatinine and BUN levels should be monitored regularly. Not effective if these levels are more than twice normal.
- Insulin requirements should be checked in patients with diabetes. Oral antidiabetic agents may be used to treat severe hyperglycemia.
- Blood uric acid levels should be monitored, especially in patients with a history of gout.
- In hypertension, therapeutic response may be delayed several days.
- Patient should take in a.m. to prevent nocturia.
- Elderly patients are especially susceptible to excessive diuresis.
- A long-acting sulfonamide similar to thiazide diuretics.
- For treatment of anaphylaxis, see APPENDIX.

NAMES, INDICATIONS AND DOSAGES	SIDE EFFECTS
spironolactone Aldactone♦, Altex **Edema:** ADULTS: 25 to 200 mg P.O. daily in divided doses. CHILDREN: initially, 3.3 mg/kg P.O. daily in divided doses. **Hypertension:** ADULTS: 50 to 100 mg P.O. daily in divided doses. **Treatment of diuretic-induced hypokalemia:** ADULTS: 25 to 100 mg P.O. daily when oral potassium supplements are considered inappropriate. **Detection of primary hyperaldosteronism:** ADULTS: 400 mg P.O. daily for 4 days (short test) or for 3 to 4 weeks (long test). If hypokalemia and hypertension are corrected, a presumptive diagnosis of primary hyperaldosteronism is made.	**CNS:** headache. **GI:** anorexia, nausea, diarrhea. **Metabolic:** *hyperkalemia,* dehydration, hyponatremia, transient rise in BUN, acidosis. **Skin:** urticaria. **Other:** gynecomastia in males, breast soreness and menstrual disturbances in females.
triamterene Dyrenium♦ **Diuresis:** ADULTS: initially, 100 mg P.O. b.i.d. after meals. Total daily dosage should not exceed 300 mg.	**Blood:** megaloblastic anemia related to low folic acid levels. **CNS:** dizziness. **CV:** hypotension. **EENT:** sore throat. **GI:** dry mouth, nausea, vomiting. **Metabolic:** *hyperkalemia,* dehydration, hyponatremia, transient rise in BUN, acidosis. **Skin:** photosensitivity, rash. **Other:** *anaphylaxis,* muscle cramps.
trichlormethiazide Diurese, Metahydrin, Naqua, Rochlomethiazide, Trichlorex **Edema:** ADULTS: 1 to 4 mg P.O. daily or in 2 divided doses. **Hypertension:** ADULTS: 2 to 4 mg P.O. daily.	**Blood:** *aplastic anemia, agranulocytosis,* leukopenia, thrombocytopenia. **CV:** *volume depletion and dehydration,* orthostatic hypotension. **GI:** anorexia, nausea, pancreatitis. **Hepatic:** hepatic encephalopathy. **Metabolic:** *hypokalemia, asymptomatic hyperuricemia, hyperglycemia and impairment of glucose tolerance,* fluid and electrolyte imbalances including dilutional hyponatremia and hypochloremia, metabolic alkalosis, hypercalcemia, gout. **Skin:** dermatitis, photosensitivity, rash. **Other:** hypersensitivity reactions such as pneumonitis and vasculitis.

INTERACTIONS AND SPECIAL CONSIDERATIONS

Interactions:
ASPIRIN: possible blocked spironolactone effect. Watch for diminished spironolactone response.

Special considerations:
• Contraindicated in anuria, acute or progressive renal insufficiency, hyperkalemia. Use cautiously in fluid or electrolyte imbalances, impaired renal function, and hepatic disease.
• Serum potassium levels, electrolytes, intake and output, weight, and blood pressure should be monitored regularly.
• Potassium-sparing diuretic; useful as an adjunct to other diuretic therapy. Less potent diuretic than thiazide and loop types. Diuretic effect delayed 2 to 3 days when used alone.
• Maximum antihypertensive response may be delayed up to 2 weeks.
• Patient should avoid excessive ingestion of potassium-rich foods.
• Elderly patients are more susceptible to excess diuresis.
• Protect drug from light.
• Breast cancer reported in some patients taking spironolactone, but cause-and-effect relationship not confirmed. Should not be taken indiscriminately.
• Patient should take drug with meals to enhance absorption.
• Concomitant potassium supplement can lead to serious hyperkalemia.

No significant interactions.

Special considerations:
• Contraindicated in anuria, severe or progressive renal disease or dysfunction, severe hepatic disease, hyperkalemia. Use cautiously in impaired hepatic function, diabetes mellitus, pregnancy or lactation.
• Blood dyscrasias possible.
• BUN and serum potassium and electrolytes should be monitored.
• A potassium-sparing diuretic, useful as an adjunct to other diuretic therapy. Less potent than thiazide and loop diuretics. Full diuretic effect delayed 2 to 3 days.
• Patients should avoid excessive ingestion of potassium-rich foods.
• Medication should be taken after meals to prevent nausea.
• Should be withdrawn gradually to prevent excessive rebound potassium excretion.
• Concomitant potassium supplement can lead to serious hyperkalemia.
• For treatment of anaphylaxis, see APPENDIX.

Interactions:
CHOLESTYRAMINE, COLESTIPOL: intestinal absorption of thiazides decreased. Keep doses as separate as possible.
DIAZOXIDE: increased antihypertensive, hyperglycemic, hyperuricemic effects. Use together cautiously.

Special considerations:
• Contraindicated in anuria; hypersensitivity to other thiazides or other sulfonamide-derived drugs. Use cautiously in severe renal disease and impaired hepatic function.
• Intake and output, weight, serum electrolytes, and serum potassium levels should be monitored regularly. Muscle weakness and cramps are signs of hypokalemia. Patients also on digitalis have an increased risk of digitalis toxicity due to the potassium-depleting effect of this diuretic. May require high-potassium diet or potassium-sparing diuretic.
• Foods rich in potassium include citrus fruits, tomatoes, bananas, dates, and apricots.
• Serum creatinine and BUN levels should be monitored regularly. Not effective if these levels are more than twice normal.
• Insulin requirements should be checked in patients with diabetes. Oral antidiabetic agents may be used to treat severe hyperglycemia. Blood sugar should be monitored.
• Blood uric acid levels should be monitored, especially in patients with a history of gout.
• In hypertension, therapeutic response may be delayed several days.
• Patient should take in a.m. to prevent nocturia.
• Elderly patients are especially susceptible to excessive diuresis.
• A long-acting thiazide diuretic.
• For treatment of anaphylaxis, see APPENDIX.

NAMES, INDICATIONS AND DOSAGES	SIDE EFFECTS
urea (carbamide) Ureaphil **Intracranial or intraocular pressure:** ADULTS: 1 to 1.5 g/kg as a 30% solution by slow I.V. infusion over 1 to 2.5 hours. CHILDREN OVER 2 YEARS: 0.5 to 1.5 g/kg slow I.V. infusion. CHILDREN UNDER 2 YEARS: as little as 0.1 g/kg slow I.V. infusion. Maximum 4 ml/minute. Maximum adult daily dose 120 g. To prepare 135 ml 30% solution, mix contents of 40-g vial of urea with 105 ml dextrose 5% or 10% in water or 10% invert sugar in water. Each ml of 30% solution provides 300 mg urea.	**CNS:** *headache.* **CV:** tachycardia, volume expansion. **GI:** *nausea, vomiting.* **Metabolic:** sodium and potassium depletion. **Local:** irritation or necrotic sloughing may occur with extravasation.

INTERACTIONS AND SPECIAL CONSIDERATIONS

No significant interactions.

Special considerations:

- Contraindicated in severely impaired renal function, marked dehydration, frank hepatic failure, active intracranial bleeding. Use cautiously in pregnancy, lactation, cardiac disease, hepatic impairment, or sickle cell damage with CNS involvement.
- For I.V. administration avoid rapid infusion: may cause hemolysis or increased capillary bleeding; avoid extravasation: may cause reactions ranging from mild irritation to necrosis.
- Should not be administered through the same infusion as blood.
- Should not be infused into leg veins: may cause phlebitis or thrombosis, especially in the elderly.
- Hyponatremia or hypokalemia (muscle weakness, lethargy) may indicate electrolyte depletion before serum levels are reduced.
- Adequate hydration should be maintained and fluid and electrolyte balance monitored.
- In renal disease, BUN should be monitored frequently.
- Indwelling urethral catheter should be used in comatose patients to assure bladder emptying. An hourly urometer collection bag should be used to facilitate accurate evaluation of diuresis.
- If satisfactory diuresis does not occur in 6 to 12 hours, urea should be discontinued and renal function reevaluated.
- Only freshly reconstituted urea should be used for I.V. infusion; solution becomes ammonia upon oxidation when standing.
- Should be used within minutes of reconstitution.

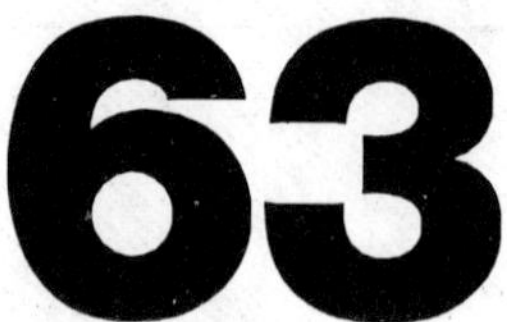

Electrolytes and replacement solutions

calcium chloride
calcium gluceptate
calcium gluconate
calcium lactate
dextrans (low molecular weight)
dextrans (high molecular weight)
hetastarch
magnesium sulfate
potassium acetate
potassium bicarbonate
potassium chloride
potassium gluconate
potassium phosphate
Ringer's injection
Ringer's injection, lactated
sodium chloride

Maintaining proper fluid and electrolyte balance is one of the most critical goals of total patient care. Electrolytes and replacement solutions help maintain homeostasis by replacing specific fluid or electrolyte deficiencies.

Major uses and mechanism of action
Electrolytes and replacement solutions replace and maintain specific anion or cation levels.
• Dextrans and hetastarch are mainly used to expand plasma volume and provide fluid replacement.

Absorption, distribution, metabolism, and excretion
• All electrolytes and replacement solutions are immediately absorbed by the I.V. route. All these preparations (except calcium salts) are excreted by the kidneys.
• Oral forms of calcium are readily absorbed from the duodenum and proximal jejunum at pH 5.0 to 7.0, if parathyroid hormone and vitamin D levels are adequate. Calcium salts are eliminated mainly in feces and to a lesser degree in urine.
• Potassium is slowly but completely absorbed from the gastrointestinal tract.

Onset and duration
• Calcium, when given I.V., raises blood levels immediately; levels return to normal in 30 minutes to 2 hours.
• Dextrans and hetastarch expand plasma volume several minutes after the infusion ends; maximal duration of action is 24 hours.
• Magnesium sulfate's onset occurs 30 minutes after I.V. administration; 1 hour after I.M. administration. Duration is 3 to 4 hours by either route.
• Potassium's onset and duration vary according to the form used. Oral sugar-coated tablets containing potassium chloride embedded in a wax matrix release the drug slowly (1 to 2 hours); doses are repeated every 8 to 12 hours. Liquid potassium preparations are absorbed much faster than the tablets (usually within 30 minutes) and are also excreted faster.

I.V. potassium chloride is infused directly into the systemic circulation. Excretion of I.V. potassium is rapid.
• Ringer's injection solution and sodium chloride solutions replace electrolytes as soon as they're infused into the bloodstream. Requirements for repeated doses vary greatly from patient to patient.

Combination products
BI-K: 20 mEq potassium (as potassium gluconate and potassium citrate) per 15 ml.

TREATING HYPOKALEMIA

Hypokalemia occurs when a patient's serum potassium level falls below 3.5 mEq/liter. The most common cause of hypokalemia is drug therapy, particularly the use of diuretics. Both thiazide and loop diuretics cause mild-to-moderate hypokalemia in many patients.

When hypokalemia occurs, it's often accompanied by hypochloremic alkalosis. Potassium chloride (KCl) oral solution may be prescribed, although it's not very palatable. It can be mixed with beverages, but if the patient still can't tolerate any of the products, slow-release preparations, such as Slow-K and Kaon-Cl, are available. These preparations contain KCl in a wax matrix. However, these are more expensive than most forms of liquid KCl and may cause small bowel ulceration.

Some doctors advocate potassium-rich foods, such as bananas and orange juice, as the sole source of potassium replacement. But these natural sources of potassium are expensive, high in calories and sugar, and usually adequate only for very mild cases.

Salt substitutes containing KCl may be an effective dietary supplement for a hypokalemic patient, but they should be used sparingly when taken with other forms of potassium.

Some doctors prescribe potassium-sparing diuretics, such as triamterene and spironolactone. These diuretics cause potassium to be retained rather than excreted.

CALCIUM-SANDOZ FORTE♦♦: calcium lactate-gluconate 2.94 g, calcium carbonate 0.3 g, elemental sodium 275.8 mg; provides 500 mg elemental calcium.
DUO-K: 20 mEq potassium, 3.4 mEq chloride (from potassium gluconate and potassium chloride).
GRAMCAL♦♦: calcium lactate-gluconate 3,080 mg, calcium carbonate 1,500 mg, and potassium 390 mg; provides 1,000 mg of elemental calcium.
KAOCHLOR-EFF: 20 mEq potassium, 20 mEq chloride (from potassium chloride, potassium citrate, potassium bicarbonate, and betaine hydrochloride).
KEFF: 20 mEq each potassium and chloride (potassium chloride, potassium carbonate, potassium bicarbonate, and betaine hydrochloride).
KLORVESS: 20 mEq each potassium and chloride (from potassium chloride, potassium bicarbonate, and l-lysine mono-hydrochloride).
KOLYUM: 20 mEq potassium, 3.4 mEq chloride (from potassium gluconate and potassium chloride).
NEUTRA-PHOS: phosphorus 250 mg, sodium 164 mg, potassium 278 mg (from dibasic and monobasic sodium and potassium phosphate).
POTASSIUM-SANDOZ♦♦: potassium chloride 600 mg and potassium bicarbonate 400 mg (provides 12 mEq potassium and 8 mEq chloride).
POTASSIUM TRIPLEX: 45 mEq potassium (from potassium acetate, potassium bicarbonate, and potassium citrate) per 15 ml.
THERMOTABS: 450 mg sodium chloride, 30 mg potassium chloride, 18 mg calcium carbonate, and 200 mg dextrose.
TRIKATES: 45 mEq potassium (from potassium acetate, potassium bicarbonate, and potassium citrate) per 15 ml.

NAMES, INDICATIONS AND DOSAGES	SIDE EFFECTS

calcium chloride
calcium gluceptate
calcium gluconate
calcium lactate

Hypocalcemia, hypocalcemic tetany, hypocalcemia during exchange transfusions, cardiac resuscitation for inotropic effect when epinephrine has failed; magnesium intoxication; hypoparathyroidism:

ADULTS AND CHILDREN: initially 500 mg to 1 g elemental calcium I.V., with further dosage based on serum calcium determinations.

Dosage with calcium chloride (1 g [10 ml] yields 13.5 mEq Ca^{++}):

Magnesium intoxication:

ADULTS AND CHILDREN: initially 500 mg I.V., with further doses based on calcium and magnesium determination.

Cardiac arrest: 0.5 to 1 g I.V., not to exceed 1 ml/minute; or 200 to 800 mg into the ventricular cavity.

Hypocalcemia: 500 mg to 1 g I.V. at intervals of 1 to 3 days, determined by serum calcium levels.

Dosage with calcium gluconate (1 g [10 ml] yields 4.5 mEq Ca^{++}):

Hypocalcemia:

ADULTS: 500 mg to 1 g I.V., repeated q 1 to 3 days p.r.n. as determined by serum calcium levels. Further doses depend on serum calcium determination.

CHILDREN: 500 mg/kg I.V. daily.

Rate of infusion should not exceed 0.5 ml/minute.

Dosage with calcium gluceptate (1.1 g [5 ml] yields 4.5 mEq Ca^{++}) and calcium salts (18 mg [1 ml] yields 0.898 mEq Ca^{++}):

Hypocalcemia:

ADULTS: initially 5 to 20 ml I.V., with further doses based on serum calcium determinations. If I.V. injection is impossible, 2 to 5 ml I.M. Average adult oral dose, 1 to 2 g/day P.O. in divided doses, t.i.d. or q.i.d. Average oral dose for children, 45 to 65 mg/kg P.O. daily, in divided doses, t.i.d. or q.i.d.

During exchange transfusions:

ADULTS AND CHILDREN: 0.5 ml I.V. after each 100 ml blood exchanged.

Side effects:

CNS: from I.V. use, tingling sensations, sense of oppression or heat waves; with rapid I.V. injection, syncope.
CV: mild fall in blood pressure; with rapid I.V. injection, vasodilation, *bradycardia, cardiac arrhythmias, and cardiac arrest.*
GI: with oral ingestion, irritation, hemorrhage, *constipation;* with I.V. administration, chalky taste; with oral calcium chloride, gastrointestinal hemorrhage, nausea, vomiting, thirst, abdominal pain.
GU: hypercalcemia, polyuria, renal calculi.
Skin: local reaction if calcium salts given I.M.: burning, necrosis, sloughing of tissue, cellulitis, soft tissue calcification.
Local: with S.C. injection, pain and irritation; *with I.V., venous irritation.*

dextrans

(low molecular weight dextrans)
Dextran 40, Gentran 40, LMVD, Rheomacrodex♦

Plasma volume expansion:

Dosage of 10% solution by I.V. infusion depends on amount of fluid loss.

First 500 ml of Dextran 40 may be infused

Side effects:

Blood: *decreased level of hemoglobin and hematocrit;* with higher doses, increased bleeding time.
GI: nausea, vomiting.
GU: tubular stasis and blocking, increased viscosity of urine.
Hepatic: increased SGPT and SGOT levels.
Skin: hypersensitivity reaction, urticaria.
Other: *anaphylaxis.*

INTERACTIONS AND SPECIAL CONSIDERATIONS

Interactions:
CARDIOTONIC GLYCOSIDES: increased digitalis toxicity; administer calcium very cautiously (if at all) to digitalized patients.

Special considerations:
• Contraindicated in ventricular fibrillation, hypercalcemia, renal calculi. Use cautiously in patients with sarcoidosis and renal or cardiac disease, and in digitalized patients. Use calcium chloride cautiously in cor pulmonale, respiratory acidosis, or respiratory failure.
• EKG should be monitored when calcium is given I.V. Such injections should not exceed 0.7 to 1.5 mEq/minute. Injection should be stopped if patient complains of discomfort. Following I.V. injection, patient should remain recumbent for a short while.
• I.M. injection should be given in the gluteal region, adults; lateral thigh, infants. I.M. route used only in emergencies when no I.V. route available.
• Blood calcium levels should be monitored frequently.
• Hypercalcemia may result after large doses in chronic renal failure.
• I.V. route generally recommended in children, but not by scalp vein (can cause tissue necrosis).
• Solutions should be warmed to body temperature before administration.
• Calcium chloride and calcium gluconate should be given I.V. only.
• Severe necrosis and sloughing of tissues follow extravasation. Calcium gluconate is less irritating to veins and tissues than calcium chloride.
• If GI upset occurs, oral calcium products should be given 1 to 1½ hours after meals.
• Oxalic acid (found in rhubarb and spinach), phytic acid (in bran and whole cereals), and phosphorus (in milk and dairy products) may interfere with absorption of calcium.
• Crash carts usually contain both gluconate and chloride. Doctor should specify which form he wants administered.

No significant interactions.

Special considerations:
• Contraindicated in marked hemostatic defects; marked cardiac decompensation or pulmonary edema; renal disease with severe oliguria or anuria; or extreme dehydration. Use cautiously in active hemorrhage: may cause additional blood loss. Patient's hydration status should be evaluated before administration.
• Hazardous when given to patients with heart failure, especially if in saline solution. Dextrose solution required instead.
• Works as plasma expander via colloidal osmotic effect, thereby drawing fluid from interstitial to intravascular space. Provides plasma expansion slightly greater than volume infused. Circulatory overload possible.

(continued on following page)

NAMES, INDICATIONS AND DOSAGES	SIDE EFFECTS
dextrans *(continued)* rapidly with central venous pressure monitoring. Infuse remaining dose slowly. Total daily dose not to exceed 2 g/kg body weight. If therapy continued past 24 hours, do not exceed 1 g/kg daily. Continue for no longer than 5 days. **Reduction of blood sludging:** 500 ml of 10% solution by I.V. infusion.	
dextrans (high molecular weight dextrans) Dextran 70, Dextran 75♦, Gentran 75, Macrodex♦ **Plasma expander:** ADULTS: usual dose 30 g (500 ml of 6% solution) I.V. In emergency situations, may be administered at rate of 1.2 to 2.4 g (20 to 40 ml)/minute. In normovolemic or nearly normovolemic patients, rate of infusion should not exceed 240 mg (4 ml)/minute. Total dose during first 24 hours not to exceed 1.2 g/kg; actual dose depends on amount of fluid loss and resultant hemoconcentration, and must be determined for each patient.	**Blood:** *decreased level of hemoglobin and hematocrit;* with doses of 15 ml/kg body weight, prolonged bleeding time and significant suppression of platelet function. **GI:** nausea, vomiting. **GU:** increased specific gravity and viscosity of urine, tubular stasis and blocking. **Hepatic:** increased SGPT and SGOT levels. **Skin:** hypersensitivity reaction, urticaria. **Other:** fever, arthralgia, nasal congestion, *anaphylaxis.*
hetastarch Hespan, Volex **Plasma expander:** ADULTS: 500 to 1,000 ml I.V. dependent on amount of blood lost and resultant hemoconcentration. Total dosage usually not to exceed 1,500 ml/day. Up to 20 ml/kg/hour may be used in hemorrhagic shock.	**CNS:** headaches. **CV:** peripheral edema of lower extremities. **EENT:** periorbital edema. **GI:** nausea, vomiting. **Skin:** urticaria. **Other:** wheezing, mild fever.
magnesium sulfate **Hypomagnesemia:** ADULTS: 1 g, or 8.12 mEq, of 50% solution (2 ml) I.M. q 6 hours for 4 doses, depending on serum magnesium level. **Severe hypomagnesemia (serum magnesium 0.8 mEq/liter or less, with symptoms):** 6 g, or 50 mEq, of 50% solution I.V. in 1 liter of solution over 4 hours. Subsequent doses depend on serum magnesium levels. **Magnesium supplementation in hyperalimentation:** ADULTS: 8 to 24 mEq/day added to hyperalimentation solution. CHILDREN OVER 6 YEARS: 2 to 10 mEq/day added to hyperalimentation solution. Each 2 ml of 50% solution contains 1 g, or 8.12 mEq, magnesium sulfate.	**CNS:** toxicity: weak or absent deep-tendon reflexes, flaccid paralysis, hypothermia, drowsiness, respiratory depression or paralysis; hypocalcemia (perioral paresthesias, twitching carpopedal spasm, tetany, and seizures). **CV:** slow, weak pulse; cardiac arrhythmias (hypocalcemia); hypotension. **Skin:** flushing, sweating.

♦ Available in U.S. and Canada. ♦♦ Available in Canada only.
All other products (no symbol) available in U.S. only. Italicized side effects are common or life-threatening.

INTERACTIONS AND SPECIAL CONSIDERATIONS

• Urine flow rate should be monitored during administration. If oliguria or anuria occurs or is not relieved by infusion, dextran should be stopped and osmotic diuretic given.
• Hydration should be assessed before starting therapy; otherwise, urine or serum osmolarity should be used, because urine specific gravity is affected by urine dextran concentration.
• Hemoglobin and hematocrit should not fall below 30% by volume.
• Blood samples should be drawn *before* starting infusion.
• Most anaphylactoid reactions occur during early phase of infusion.
• May interfere with analysis of blood grouping, crossmatching, bilirubin, blood glucose, and protein.
• Store at constant 25° C. (77° F.). May precipitate in storage but can be heated to dissolve if necessary.

No significant interactions.

Special considerations:
• Contraindicated in marked hemostatic defects; marked cardiac decompensation or pulmonary edema; renal disease with severe oliguria or anuria; and extreme dehydration. Use cautiously in active hemorrhage; may cause additional blood loss.
• Hazardous when given to patients with heart failure, especially if in saline solution. Dextrose solution required instead.
• Works as plasma expander via colloidal osmotic effect, thereby drawing fluid from interstitial to intravascular space. Provides plasma expansion slightly greater than volume infused. Circulatory overload possible.
• Urine flow rate should be monitored during administration. If oliguria or anuria occurs or is not relieved by infusion, dextran should be stopped and osmotic diuretic given.
• Hydration should be assessed before starting therapy; otherwise, urine or serum osmolarity should be used, because urine specific gravity is affected by the urine dextran concentration.
• Hemoglobin and hematocrit should not fall below 30% by volume.
• Blood samples should be drawn *before* starting infusion.
• Most anaphylactoid reactions occur during early phase of infusion.
• May interfere with analysis of blood grouping, crossmatching, bilirubin, blood glucose, and protein.
• May precipitate in storage but can be heated to dissolve if necessary.
• Dextran 70 and Dextran 75 can be used interchangeably. Differ significantly from Dextran 40—should not be interchanged.

No significant interactions.

Special considerations:
• Contraindicated in severe bleeding disorders or with severe congestive heart failure and renal failure with oliguria and anuria.
• To avoid circulatory overload, patients with impaired renal function should be monitored carefully.
• Drug should be discontinued if allergic or sensitivity reactions occur. If necessary, an antihistamine should be administered.
• Hetastarch is *not* a substitute for blood or plasma.
• Available in 500-ml I.V. infusion bottles.

No significant interactions.

Special considerations:
• Contraindicated in impaired renal function, myocardial damage, heart block, and in actively progressing labor. Use parenteral magnesium with extreme caution in patients receiving digitalis preparations. Treating magnesium toxicity with calcium in such patients could cause serious alterations in cardiac conduction; heart block may result.
• Maximum infusion rate 150 mg/minute. Rapid drip causes feeling of heat.
• I.V. calcium reverses magnesium intoxication.
• Vital signs should be monitored every 15 minutes when drug given I.V. for severe hypomagnesemia. Respiratory depression and signs of heart block are possible. Respirations should be more than 16/minute before dose is given.
• Intake and output should be monitored. Output should be 100 ml or more during 4-hour period before dose.
• Knee jerk and patellar reflexes should be tested before each additional dose. If absent, no more magnesium should be given until reflexes return; otherwise, patient may develop temporary respiratory failure and need cardiopulmonary resuscitation or I.V. administration of calcium.
• Magnesium levels should be checked after repeated doses.
• Newborns of toxemic mothers receiving drug within 24 hours before delivery may develop magnesium toxicity, including neuromuscular and respiratory depression.

NAMES, INDICATIONS AND DOSAGES	SIDE EFFECTS
potassium acetate **Potassium replacement:** I.V. should be used for life-threatening hypokalemia or when oral replacement not feasible. Give no more than 20 mEq/hour in concentration of 40 mEq/liter or less. Total 24-hour dose should not exceed 150 mEq (3 mEq/kg in children). Potassium replacement should be done with EKG monitoring and frequent serum K^+ determinations. **Prevention of hypokalemia:** ADULTS AND CHILDREN: 20 mEq P.O. daily, in divided doses b.i.d., t.i.d., or q.i.d. **Potassium depletion:** ADULTS AND CHILDREN: usual dose 40 to 100 mEq P.O. daily, in divided doses b.i.d., t.i.d., or q.i.d.	*Signs of hyperkalemia:* **CNS:** paresthesias of the extremities, listlessness, mental confusion, weakness or heaviness of legs, flaccid paralysis. **CV:** *peripheral vascular collapse with fall in blood pressure, cardiac arrhythmias,* heart block, possible cardiac arrest, EKG changes (prolonged P-R intervals; wide QRS; ST segment depression; tall, tented T waves). **GI:** nausea, vomiting, abdominal pain, diarrhea, bowel ulceration. **GU:** oliguria. **Skin:** cold skin, gray pallor.
potassium bicarbonate K-Lyte, K-Lyte DS **Hypokalemia:** 25 mEq or 50 mEq tablet dissolved in water 1 to 4 times a day.	**CNS:** paresthesias of the extremities, listlessness, mental confusion, weakness or heaviness of legs, flaccid paralysis. **CV:** *cardiac arrhythmias,* EKG changes (prolonged P-R interval; wide QRS; ST segment depression; tall, tented T waves). **GI:** *nausea, vomiting, abdominal pain,* diarrhea, ulcerations, hemorrhage, obstruction, perforation.
potassium chloride K-Lor, K-Lyte/Cl, K-10♦, Kaochlor 10%, Kaochlor S-F 10%, Kaon, Kaon-Cl, Kaon-Cl 20%, Kato Powder, KayCiel♦, Klor-10%, Kloride, Klorvess, Klotrix, K Tab, SK-Potassium Chloride, Slow K♦ **Hypokalemia:** 40 to 100 mEq P.O. divided into 3 to 4 doses daily for treatment; 20 mEq for prevention. Further dose based on serum potassium determinations. I.V. route when oral replacement not feasible or when hypokalemia life-threatening. Usual dose 20 mEq/hour in concentration of 40 mEq/liter or less. Total daily dose not to exceed 150 mEq (3 mEq/kg in children). Potassium replacement should be done only with EKG monitoring and frequent serum K^+ determinations.	*Signs of hyperkalemia:* **CNS:** paresthesias of the extremities, listlessness, mental confusion, weakness or heaviness of limbs, flaccid paralysis. **CV:** *peripheral vascular collapse with fall in blood pressure, cardiac arrhythmias, heart block, possible cardiac arrest,* EKG changes (prolonged P-R interval; wide QRS; ST segment depression; tall, tented T waves). **GI:** *nausea, vomiting, abdominal pain,* diarrhea, GI ulcerations (possible stenosis, hemorrhage, obstruction, perforation). **GU:** oliguria. **Skin:** cold skin, gray pallor.

♦ Available in U.S. and Canada. ♦♦ Available in Canada only.
All other products (no symbol) available in U.S. only. Italicized side effects are common or life-threatening.

INTERACTIONS AND SPECIAL CONSIDERATIONS

No significant interactions.

Special considerations:

• Contraindicated in severe renal impairment with oliguria, anuria, azotemia; untreated Addison's disease; acute dehydration, hyperkalemia, hyperkalemic form of familial periodic paralysis, and conditions associated with extensive tissue breakdown. Use cautiously in patients with cardiac disease, in patients receiving potassium-sparing diuretics, and in those with renal impairment.
• Monitor EKG, serum potassium level, renal function, BUN, serum creatinine, and intake and output. Potassium should never be given postoperatively until urine flow is established.
• Diluted solution should be given slowly; potentially fatal hyperkalemia may result from too rapid infusion.
• Infusion site should be checked for pain and redness. Large-bore needle reduces local irritation.
• Parenteral potassium given by infusion only; never I.V. push or I.M.
• Signs of GI ulceration: obstruction, hemorrhage, pain, distention, severe vomiting, bleeding.
• Potassium acetate powder should be reconstituted with liquids; given after meals with a full glass of water or fruit juice to minimize GI irritation.
• To prevent serious hyperkalemia, potassium deficits must be replaced gradually.

No significant interactions.

Special considerations:

• Contraindicated in severe renal impairment with oliguria, anuria, azotemia, and untreated Addison's disease; also in acute dehydration, hyperkalemia, hyperkalemic familial periodic paralysis, and conditions associated with extensive tissue breakdown. Use with caution in patients with cardiac disease and in those receiving potassium-sparing diuretics.
• Serum potassium level, BUN, serum creatinine, and intake and output should be monitored.
• Switching potassium products requires medical supervision.
• Potassium bicarbonate tablets should be dissolved in 6 to 8 oz of cold water.
• Should be taken with meals and sipped slowly over a 5- to 10-minute period.
• Potassium bicarbonate cannot be given instead of potassium chloride.
• Potassium bicarbonate does not correct hypokalemic alkalosis.
• Available in lime or orange flavor.

No significant interactions.

Special considerations:

• Contraindicated in severe renal impairment with oliguria, anuria, azotemia, and untreated Addison's disease; also in acute dehydration, hyperkalemia, hyperkalemic form of familial periodic paralysis, and conditions associated with extensive tissue breakdown. Use with caution in patients with cardiac disease and in those receiving potassium-sparing diuretics.
• Potassium should not be given during immediate postoperative period until urine flow is established.
• Parenteral potassium given by infusion only; never I.V. push or I.M.
• Dilute solution should be given slowly; potentially fatal hyperkalemia may result from too rapid infusion.
• Oral potassium supplements should be given with extreme caution because their many forms deliver varying amounts of potassium. Products should never be switched without a doctor's order. Patient should report if he tolerates one product better than another.
• Sugar-free liquid available (Kaochlor S-F 10%).
• Patient should sip liquid potassium slowly to minimize GI irritation.
• Patient should take with or after meals with full glass of water or fruit juice to lessen GI distress.
• Powders should be completely dissolved before giving.
• Enteric-coated tablets not recommended due to potential GI bleeding and small bowel ulcerations.
• Tablets in wax matrix sometimes lodge in esophagus and cause ulceration in cardiac patients who have esophageal compression due to enlarged left atrium. In such patients and in those with esophageal stasis or obstruction, liquid form is recommended.
• Often used orally with diuretics that cause potassium excretion. Potassium chloride most useful since diuretics waste chloride ion. Hypokalemic alkalosis treated best with potassium chloride.
• EKG, serum potassium levels, and other electrolytes should be monitored during therapy.

NAMES, INDICATIONS AND DOSAGES	SIDE EFFECTS
potassium gluconate Kaon Liquid, Kaon Tablets♦, Potassium Rougier♦♦ **Hypokalemia:** 40 to 100 mEq P.O. divided into 3 to 4 doses daily for treatment; 20 mEq/day for prevention. Further dose based on serum potassium determinations.	**CNS:** paresthesias of the extremities, listlessness, mental confusion, weakness or heaviness of legs, flaccid paralysis. **CV:** cardiac arrhythmias, EKG changes (prolonged P-R interval; wide QRS; ST segment depression; tall, tented T waves). **GI:** *nausea, vomiting, abdominal pain,* diarrhea, GI ulcerations with oral products (especially enteric-coated tablets); ulcerations may be accompanied by stenosis, hemorrhage, obstruction, perforation.
potassium phosphate **Hypokalemia:** I.V. should be used when oral replacement not feasible or when hypokalemia life-threatening. Dosage up to 20 mEq/hour in concentration of 60 mEq/liter or less. Total daily dose not to exceed 150 mEq. Should be done only with EKG monitoring and frequent serum K^+ determinations. Average P.O. dose: 40 to 100 mEq. **Hypophosphatemia:** 3 mM/ml is administered I.V. after diluting in a larger volume of fluid. Dosage is adjusted according to individual needs of patient.	*Signs of hyperkalemia:* **CNS:** paresthesias, listlessness, confusion, weakness or heaviness of legs, flaccid paralysis; hypocalcemia—perioral paresthesias, twitching, carpopedal spasm, tetany, and seizures. **CV:** *peripheral vascular collapse with fall in blood pressure, cardiac arrhythmias, heart block, possible cardiac arrest,* EKG changes (prolonged P-R interval; wide QRS; ST segment depression; tall, tented T waves). **GI:** nausea, vomiting, abdominal pain, diarrhea. **GU:** oliguria. **Skin:** cold skin, gray pallor. **Other:** soft tissue calcification.
Ringer's injection **Fluid and electrolyte replacement:** ADULTS AND CHILDREN: dose highly individualized, but generally 1.5 to 3 liters (2% to 6% body weight) infused I.V. over 18 to 24 hours.	**CV:** fluid overload.
Ringer's injection, lactated (Hartmann's solution, Ringer's lactate solution) **Fluid and electrolyte replacement:** ADULTS AND CHILDREN: dose highly individualized, but generally 1.5 to 3 liters (2% to 6% body weight) infused I.V. over 18 to 24 hours.	**CV:** fluid overload.
sodium chloride **Highly individualized fluid and electrolyte replacement in hyponatremia due to electrolyte loss or in severe salt depletion:** 400 ml of 3% or 5% solutions only with frequent electrolyte determination and by slow I.V.; *with 0.45% solution:* 3% to 8% of body weight, as needed, over 18 to 24 hours; *with 0.9% solution:* 2% to 6% of body weight, as needed, over 18 to 24 hours. **Management of "heat cramp":** ADULTS: 1 g P.O. with every glass of water.	**CV:** aggravation of congestive heart failure; edema and pulmonary edema if too much given or given too rapidly. **Metabolic:** hypernatremia and aggravation of existing acidosis with excessive infusion; serious electrolyte disturbance, loss of potassium.

♦ Available in U.S. and Canada. ♦♦ Available in Canada only.
All other products (no symbol) available in U.S. only. Italicized side effects are common or life-threatening.

INTERACTIONS AND SPECIAL CONSIDERATIONS

No significant interactions.

Special considerations:
• Contraindicated in severe renal impairment with oliguria, anuria, azotemia, and untreated Addison's disease; also in acute dehydration, hyperkalemia, hyperkalemic form of familial periodic paralysis, and conditions associated with extensive tissue breakdown. Use with caution in patients with cardiac disease and in those receiving potassium-sparing diuretics.
• Serum potassium level, BUN, serum creatinine, and intake and output should be monitored.
• Oral potassium supplements should be given with extreme caution because their many forms deliver varying amounts of potassium. Patient should report if one product is tolerated better than another so brand and dosage can be changed.
• Patient should sip liquid potassium slowly to minimize GI irritation.
• Take with or after meals with full glass of water or fruit juice to lessen GI distress.
• Potassium gluconate does not correct hypokalemic hypochloremic alkalosis.
• Enteric-coated tablets not recommended: possible GI bleeding, small-bowel ulcerations.
• EKG, serum potassium, and other electrolytes should be monitored during therapy.

No significant interactions.

Special considerations:
• Contraindicated in severe renal impairment with oliguria, anuria, azotemia, and untreated Addison's disease; also in acute dehydration, hyperkalemia, hyperkalemic form of familial periodic paralysis, extensive tissue damage, and hypocalcemia. Use with caution in patients with cardiac disease and in those receiving potassium-sparing diuretics.
• Potassium should never be given postoperatively until urine flow is established.
• EKG should be monitored for indications of tissue potassium levels; plasma potassium and calcium levels as well as BUN and creatinine should be monitored for renal function; inorganic phosphorus levels and intake and output should also be monitored.
• Dilute solution should be given slowly; potentially fatal hyperkalemia may result from too rapid an infusion.
• Parenteral potassium given by infusion only; never I.V. push or I.M.
• Powder should be reconstituted in juice and taken after meals.

No significant interactions.

Special considerations:
• Contraindicated in renal failure, except as emergency volume expander. Use cautiously in congestive heart failure, circulatory insufficiency, renal dysfunction, hypoproteinemia, or pulmonary edema.
• Ringer's injection contains sodium, 147 mEq/liter; potassium, 4 mEq/liter; calcium, 4.5 mEq liter; and chloride, 155.5 mEq/liter. This electrolyte content insufficient to treat severe electrolyte deficiencies, but does provide electrolyte levels about equal to those of blood. May be given with dextrose infusion, other carbohydrates, or sodium lactate.

No significant interactions.

Special considerations:
• Contraindicated in renal failure, except as emergency volume expander. Use cautiously in CHF, circulatory insufficiency, renal dysfunction, hypoproteinemia, and pulmonary edema.
• Ringer's injection, lactated, contains sodium, 130 mEq/liter; potassium, 4 mEq/liter; calcium, 2.7 mEq/liter; chloride, 109.7 mEq/liter; and lactate, 27 mEq/liter.
• Approximates more closely the electrolyte concentration in blood plasma than Ringer's injection. May be given with dextrose infusion.

No significant interactions.

Special considerations:
• Use with caution in congestive heart failure, circulatory insufficiency, renal dysfunction, hypoproteinemia.
• 3% and 5% solutions should be infused very slowly and with caution to avoid pulmonary edema. Should be used only for critical situations and patient observed constantly.
• Concentrates available for addition to parenteral nutrient solutions. These small volumes of parenterals should not be confused with sodium chloride injection isotonic 0.9%. *Read label carefully.*
• Serum electrolytes should be monitored during therapy.

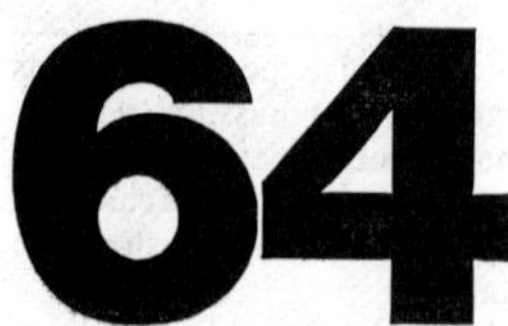

Potassium-removing resin

sodium polystyrene sulfonate

Potassium-removing resin is used to lower dangerously elevated serum potassium levels.

This drug is generally used, with other modes of therapy, to treat renal failure. It is too slow acting to be used alone or in an emergency hyperkalemic situation.

Major uses

Potassium-removing resin is used to treat hyperkalemia. It is effective in *chronic* renal failure.

Because sodium polystyrene sulfonate is relatively slow acting and gives a variable response, it should not be used as primary treatment of either acute renal failure or burns with rapid tissue breakdown.

Mechanism of action

The potassium-removing resin exchanges sodium ions for potassium ions in the intestine: 1 g of sodium polystyrene sulfonate is exchanged for 0.5 to 1 mEq of potassium. The resin is then eliminated. Much of the exchange capacity is used for cations other than potassium (calcium and magnesium) and possibly for fats and proteins.

Absorption, distribution, metabolism, and excretion

The potassium-removing resin is distributed through the intestine (especially the large intestine) and eliminated in feces.

Onset and duration

- Intestinal ion exchange requires about 6 hours.
- Action of the potassium-removing resin is slow and unpredictable. Because therapeutic effect isn't evident for 2 to 24 hours, sodium polystyrene sulfonate is most useful when either potassium levels aren't life-threatening or other measures (such as glucose-insulin infusions) have reduced the immediate danger of hyperkalemia.

MANAGING HYPERKALEMIA

It's time to watch dietary potassium when serum potassium concentrations rise above 5.5 mEq/liter, causing severe muscle weakness, paralysis, abdominal distention, diarrhea, oliguria, and anuria.

Potassium excess (hyperkalemia) may develop in patients with inadequate renal function; adrenocortical insufficiency; increased potassium load, as in severe tissue damage, metabolic acidosis, or overtreatment with potassium salts; and in those taking potassium-sparing diuretics.

One way to control hyperkalemia is to limit dietary intake of potassium. The patient-teaching aid for a low-potassium diet can be used as a guide for patients in measuring and minimizing potassium intake.

PATIENT-TEACHING AID

SUGGESTIONS FOR A LOW-POTASSIUM DIET

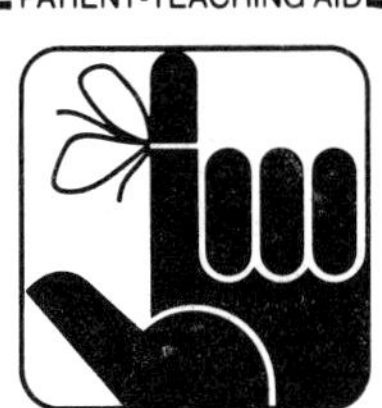

Dear Patient:

The doctor has asked you to go on a low-potassium diet because your body retains too much of this mineral. Here's a list showing the amount of potassium in 100-gram portions (approximately 3½ oz) of some foods you can eat. Buy or borrow a food scale to weigh your portions.

Avoid high-potassium foods, such as milk, potatoes and potato chips, bananas, dried fruit, catsup, pickles, nuts, chocolate, and peanut butter. Limit your intake of meats and eggs. You can reduce the potassium content of vegetables by boiling them for a long period in large amounts of water. Keep track of what you eat, and be sure the total daily amount of potassium doesn't exceed your doctor's recommendation (usually 2 grams or 2,000 milligrams).

DAIRY PRODUCTS	mg/100 g
Cheese, cheddar	82
Cheese, cream	85
Eggs	98
Butter	23

FRUITS AND VEGETABLES	
Applesauce	65
Blueberries	81
Cranberry juice	10
Pears, canned	84
Pineapple, canned	96
Beans, snap	95
Corn, canned	97
Peas, canned	96

MEAT, FISH, POULTRY	mg/100 g
	approx. 350

BREAD AND CEREAL	
Rice	28
Noodles	44
Macaroni	61
Bread, cracked wheat	134
Bread, white	105
Bread, rye	115
Oatmeal	61
Cornflakes	120
Corn grits	11
Farina	188

Combination products
None.

NAMES, INDICATIONS AND DOSAGES	SIDE EFFECTS
sodium polystyrene sulfonate Kayexalate ♦ **Hyperkalemia:** ADULTS: 15 g daily to q.i.d. in water or sorbitol (3 to 4 ml/g of resin). CHILDREN: 1 g of resin for each mEq of potassium to be removed. *Oral administration* preferred since drug should remain in intestine for at least 6 hours; otherwise, consider nasogastric administration. *Nasogastric administration:* mix dose with appropriate medium: aqueous suspension or diet appropriate for renal failure; instill in plastic tube. *Rectal administration:* ADULTS: 30 to 50 g/100 ml of sorbitol q 6 hours as warm emulsion deep into sigmoid colon (20 cm). In persistent vomiting or paralytic ileus, high retention enema of sodium polystyrene sulfonate (30 g) suspended in 200 ml of 10% methylcellulose, 10% dextrose, or 25% sorbitol solution.	**GI:** *constipation,* fecal impaction (in elderly), anorexia, gastric irritation, nausea, vomiting, *diarrhea (with sorbitol emulsions).* **Other:** *hypokalemia,* hypocalcemia, hypomagnesemia, sodium retention.

INTERACTIONS AND SPECIAL CONSIDERATIONS

Interactions:
ANTACIDS AND LAXATIVES (NONABSORBABLE CATION-DONATING TYPE, INCLUDING MAGNESIUM HYDROXIDE): systemic alkalosis, reduced potassium exchange capability. Don't use together.

Special considerations:
• Use with caution in elderly patients and in those on digitalis therapy, with severe congestive heart failure, severe hypertension, and marked edema.
• Treatment may result in potassium deficiency. Serum potassium should be monitored at least once daily. Usually stopped when potassium level is reduced to 4 or 5 mEq/liter. Other signs of hypokalemia: irritability, confusion, cardiac arrhythmias, EKG changes, severe muscle weakness and sometimes paralysis, and digitalis toxicity in digitalized patients.
• Symptoms of other electrolyte deficiencies (magnesium, calcium) should be monitored for, since drug is nonselective. Serum calcium determination should be monitored in patients receiving sodium polystyrene therapy for more than 3 days. Supplementary calcium may be needed.
• Sodium overload is possible. About ⅓ of resin's sodium stays in body.
• Only fresh suspensions should be used, stirred just before use, and unused portions discarded after 24 hours.
• Resin should not be heated: this will impair effectiveness of drug. Resin should be mixed with water or sorbitol only for P.O. administration; should *never* be mixed with orange juice (high K^+ content) to disguise taste.
• Chilling oral suspension recommended for greater palatability.
• If sorbitol is given, it may be mixed with resin suspension.
• Solid form may be considered. Resin cookie recipe is available; perhaps pharmacist or dietitian can supply.
• Possible constipation in oral or nasogastric administration. Sorbitol should be used (10 to 20 ml of 70% syrup every 2 hours as needed) to produce 1 or 2 watery stools daily.
• Polystyrene resin should be mixed only with water and sorbitol for oral or rectal use. Other vehicles (that is, mineral oil) not recommended for rectal administration to prevent impactions. Ion exchange requires aqueous medium. Sorbitol content prevents impaction.
• Fecal impaction may be prevented in the elderly by administering resin rectally. Cleansing enema given before rectal administration. Retention for 6 to 10 hours is ideal, but 30 to 60 minutes is acceptable.
• Rectal dose should be prepared at room temperature and emulsion stirred gently during administration.
• For rectal dose: insert 20 cm of #28 French rubber tube into sigmoid colon; tape tube in place. Alternatively, consider a Foley catheter with a 30-ml ballloon inflated distal to anal sphincter to aid in retention. This is especially helpful for patients with poor sphincter control (for example, after cerebrovascular accident). Use gravity flow. Drain returns constantly through Y-tube connection. When giving rectally, patient should be in knee-chest position or with hips on pillow for a while if back-leakage occurs.
• Should flush with 50 to 100 ml of nonsodium fluid after rectal administration.
• If hyperkalemia is severe, more drastic modalities can be added; for example, dextrose 50% with regular insulin I.V. push. Polystyrene resin should not be depended on solely to lower serum potassium levels in severe hyperkalemia.

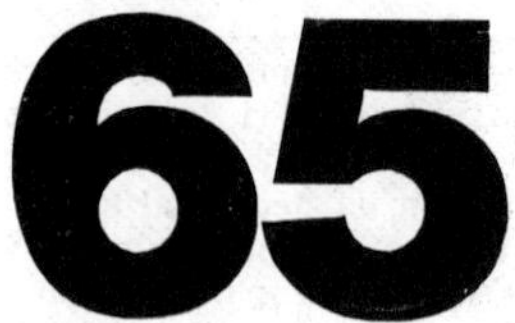

Hematinics

ferrocholinate
ferrous fumarate
ferrous gluconate
ferrous sulfate
iron dextran

Hematinics are iron-containing compounds that increase both the hemoglobin level and the number of red blood cells (RBCs). Iron is necessary for formation of hemoglobin, which transports oxygen within the RBCs from the lungs to the tissues. Iron deficiency, reflected by decreased hemoglobin synthesis and decreased red cell production, may result from blood loss or from inadequate iron intake during accelerated growth or pregnancy. Although many expensive forms of iron therapy are available, ferrous sulfate is the cheapest and most effective.

Major uses

Iron preparations supplement depleted stores, thereby arresting anemia. As a daily dietary supplement, 10 to 18 mg of elemental iron for adults and 4 to 8 mg for children are sufficient. Patients with iron deficiency may require 90 to 200 mg of elemental iron daily.

Mechanism of action

After absorption into the blood, iron is immediately bound to transferrin. Transferrin carries iron to bone marrow, where it's used to synthesize hemoglobin. Some iron is also used to synthesize myoglobin or other nonhemoglobin heme units.

Absorption, distribution, metabolism, and excretion

• The absorption of iron is complex and influenced by many factors, including the iron salt given, iron stores in the body, degree of erythropoiesis, drug dose, and diet.

Absorption occurs mainly in the duodenum after oral administration, although a small amount is absorbed in the proximal jejunum. Healthy persons absorb about 10% of the iron present in their diets, whereas patients with iron deficiency may absorb as much as 30% of dietary iron in an attempt to replace body stores of this element.

When given therapeutically, ferrous form of iron is better absorbed orally than ferric form. In iron deficiency, as much as 60% of iron dose is absorbed. When total body stores of iron are large, absorption is less. After I.M. injection, 60% of the iron is absorbed after 3 days; up to 90% after 1 to 3 weeks. If given I.V., all iron is absorbed at once.

• Iron is distributed in the bone marrow (2,400 mg) and in the liver (800 mg in males, 300 mg in females). The remainder is bound to plasma proteins and contained in muscles (myoglobin) and certain enzymes.

• Iron metabolism is a closed system: the body conserves and reuses most of the iron that's liberated by hemoglobin destruction.

• Elimination of iron is minimal; 500 mcg to 2 mg are lost daily, primarily as cells exfoliated from the skin, gastrointestinal mucosa, nails, and hair. Only trace amounts of iron are secreted in bile or excreted in sweat. Women normally lose 12 to 30 mg of iron during each menstrual period.

Onset and duration

With therapeutic doses of iron salts, symptoms of iron deficiency usually improve within

HOW TO INJECT IRON SOLUTIONS

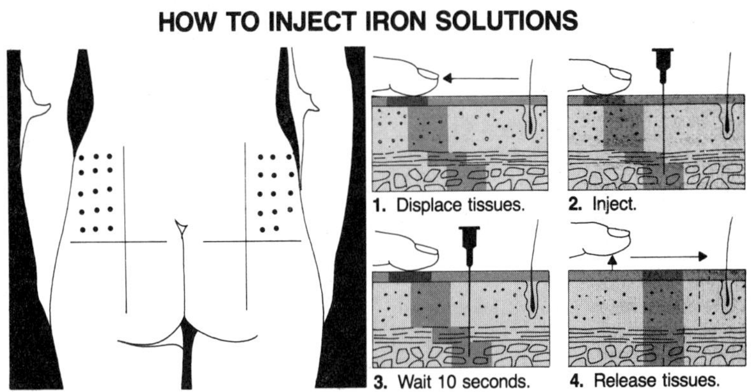
1. Displace tissues. 2. Inject. 3. Wait 10 seconds. 4. Release tissues.

For I.M. injections of iron solutions, use the Z-track technique to prevent subcutaneous irritation and discoloration from leaking medication. Follow these guidelines:

- Choose a 19G or 20G, 2″ or 3″ needle, depending on the patient's size.
- After drawing up the solution, allow 0.5 cc of air into the syringe. Then change to a fresh needle to prevent tracking iron solution through to subcutaneous tissue.
- Select an injection site in the upper outer quadrant of buttocks only. If the patient is standing, have him bear weight on the leg opposite the site; if he's in bed, place him in lateral position, with injection site up.
- Displace the skin, fat, and muscle at the site firmly to one side. Cleanse the area and insert the needle.
- Aspirate to check for entry into a blood vessel. Inject the medication and the air bubble in the syringe slowly.
- Wait 10 seconds, pull the needle straight out, and release the tissues to seal off the needle track.
- Apply direct pressure to the site, but don't massage it. To increase the absorption rate, encourage physical activity, like walking. But caution your patient against exercising vigorously for 15 to 30 minutes, and against wearing tight-fitting clothes that could force medication into subcutaneous tissue and cause irritation.
- For subsequent injections, alternate buttocks.

2 to 3 days. Peak reticulocytosis (formation of young red cells) occurs in 5 to 10 days, and hemoglobin level rises after 2 to 4 weeks. Normal hemoglobin values are usually attained in 2 months, unless blood loss continues.

Combination products

FERMALOX: ferrous sulfate 200 mg, and magnesium hydroxide and dried aluminum hydroxide gel 200 mg.
FERRO-SEQUELS: iron (as fumarate) 50 mg and docusate sodium 100 mg.
SIMRON: iron (as gluconate) 10 mg and polysorbate 20, 400 mg.

NAMES, INDICATIONS AND DOSAGES	SIDE EFFECTS

ferrocholinate
Chel-Iron, Firon, Kelex

Iron deficiency:
ADULTS: 333-mg tablet P.O. t.i.d.
CHILDREN: 6 mg/kg P.O. daily in divided doses t.i.d.

Prevention of iron deficiency:
CHILDREN: 1 mg/kg P.O. daily as single or divided dose.

GI: *nausea,* vomiting, *constipation, black stools.*
Other: stained tooth enamel.

ferrous fumarate
Eldofe, F&B Caps, Farbegen, Feco-T, Feostat, Feroton♦♦, Ferranol, Ferrofume♦♦, Fersamal♦♦, Fumasorb, Fumerin, Hematon♦♦, Hemocyte, Ircon, Laud-Iron, Maniron, Novofumar♦♦, Palafer♦♦, Palmiron, Span-FF, Toleron

Iron deficiency states:
ADULTS: 200 mg P.O. daily t.i.d. or q.i.d.

GI: *nausea,* vomiting, *constipation, black stools.*
Other: stained tooth enamel.

ferrous gluconate
Entron, Fergon♦, Ferralet, Ferrous-G, Fertinic♦♦, Novoferrogluc♦♦

Iron deficiency:
ADULTS: 200 to 600 mg P.O., t.i.d.
CHILDREN 6 TO 12 YEARS: 300 to 900 mg P.O. daily.
CHILDREN UNDER 6 YEARS: 100 to 300 mg P.O. daily.
1 tablet contains 320 mg ferrous gluconate (37 mg elemental iron).
5 ml of elixir contains 300 mg ferrous gluconate (35 mg elemental iron).

GI: *nausea,* vomiting, *constipation, black stools.*
Other: elixir may stain teeth.

ferrous sulfate
Arne Modified Caps, Feosol, Fer-In-Sol♦, Fero-Grad♦♦, Fero-Gradumet, Ferolix, Ferospace, Ferralyn, Fesofor♦♦, Irospan, Mol-Iron, Novo-ferrosulfa♦♦, Slow-Fe♦♦, Telefon

Iron deficiency:
ADULTS: 750 mg to 1.5 g P.O. daily divided t.i.d.; or 225 to 525 mg P.O. sustained-release

GI: *nausea,* vomiting, *constipation, black stools.*
Other: elixir may stain teeth.

♦ Available in U.S. and Canada. ♦♦ Available in Canada only.
All other products (no symbol) available in U.S. only. Italicized side effects are common or life-threatening.

INTERACTIONS AND SPECIAL CONSIDERATIONS

Interactions:
ANTACIDS, CHOLESTYRAMINE RESIN, PANCREATIC EXTRACTS, VITAMIN E: decreased iron absorption. Separate doses if possible.
CHLORAMPHENICOL: watch for delayed response to iron therapy.
VITAMIN C: may increase iron absorption. Beneficial drug interaction.

Special considerations:
• Contraindicated in hemosiderosis, hemochromatosis, and hemolytic anemia. Usually contraindicated in peptic ulcer or ulcerative colitis. Use cautiously on long-term basis.
• GI upset related to dose. Between-meal dosing preferable but can be given with some foods although absorption may be decreased. Enteric-coated products reduce GI upset but also reduce amount of iron absorbed.
• Iron is toxic; parents should be aware of iron poisoning in children.
• Liquid preparations should be diluted in juice (preferably orange juice) or water, but not in milk or antacids. Tablets should be taken with orange juice to promote iron absorption.
• Constipation is possible. Patient should follow dietary measures to prevent constipation.
• Hemoglobin and reticulocyte counts should be monitored during therapy.
• To avoid staining teeth, liquid iron preparations should be taken with glass straw.

Interactions:
ANTACIDS, CHOLESTYRAMINE RESIN, PANCREATIC EXTRACTS, VITAMIN E: decreased iron absorption. Separate doses if possible.
CHLORAMPHENICOL: watch for delayed response to iron therapy.
VITAMIN C: may increase iron absorption. Beneficial drug interaction.

Special considerations:
• Contraindicated in peptic ulcer, regional enteritis, ulcerative colitis, hemosiderosis, and hemochromatosis. Use cautiously on long-term basis and in patients with anemia.
• GI upset related to dose. Between-meal dosing preferable but can be given with some foods although absorption may be decreased. Enteric-coated products reduce GI upset but also reduce amount of iron absorbed.
• Iron is toxic; parents should be aware of iron poisoning in children.
• Tablets should be taken with juice or water, but not in milk or antacids. Should be taken with orange juice to promote iron absorption.
• To avoid staining teeth, liquid iron preparations should be taken with glass straw.
• Patient should follow dietary measures to prevent constipation.
• Hemoglobin and reticulocyte counts should be monitored during therapy.
• Combination products—Simron, Ferro-Sequels, Ferocyl, Fer-Regules—contain stool softeners to help prevent constipation. Fermalox contains antacids to help relieve GI upset, if present; this product not recommended unless absolutely necessary because of decreased iron absorption.

Interactions:
ANTACIDS, CHOLESTYRAMINE RESIN, PANCREATIC EXTRACTS, VITAMIN E: decreased iron absorption. Separate doses if possible.
CHLORAMPHENICOL: watch for delayed response to iron therapy.
VITAMIN C: may increase iron absorption. Beneficial drug interaction.

Special considerations:
• Contraindicated in peptic ulcer, regional enteritis, ulcerative colitis, hemosiderosis, and hemochromatosis. Use cautiously on long-term basis and in patients with anemia.
• GI upset related to dose. Between-meal dosing preferable but can be given with some foods although absorption may be decreased. Enteric-coated products reduce GI upset but also reduce amount of iron absorbed.
• Iron is toxic; parents should be aware of iron poisoning in children.
• Liquid preparations should be diluted in juice (preferably orange juice) or water, but not in milk or antacids. Tablets should be taken with orange juice to promote absorption.
• To avoid staining teeth, liquid preparation should be taken with glass straw.
• Patient should follow dietary measures to prevent constipation.
• Hemoglobin and reticulocyte counts should be monitored during therapy.

Interactions:
ANTACIDS, CHOLESTYRAMINE RESIN, PANCREATIC EXTRACTS, VITAMIN E: decreased iron absorption. Separate doses if possible.
CHLORAMPHENICOL: watch for delayed response to iron therapy.
VITAMIN C: may increase iron absorption. Beneficial drug interaction.

Special considerations:
• Contraindicated in peptic ulcer, ulcerative colitis, regional enteritis, hemosiderosis, and hemochromatosis. Use cautiously on long-term basis and in patients with anemia.
• GI upset related to dose. Between-meal dosing preferable but can be given with some foods although absorption may be decreased. Enteric-coated products reduce GI upset but also reduce

(continued on following page)

NAMES, INDICATIONS AND DOSAGES	SIDE EFFECTS
ferrous sulfate *(continued)* preparations once daily or q 12 hours. CHILDREN 6 TO 12 YEARS: 600 mg P.O. daily in divided doses. **Prophylaxis for iron deficiency anemia:** PREGNANT WOMEN: 300 to 600 mg P.O. daily in divided doses. PREMATURE OR UNDERNOURISHED INFANTS: 3 to 6 mg/kg P.O. daily in divided doses.	
iron dextran Hematran, Hydextran, Imferon♦, K-FeRON **Iron deficiency anemia:** ADULTS: I.M. or I.V. injections of iron are advisable only for patients for whom oral administration is impossible or ineffective. Test dose (0.5 ml) required before administration. *I.M. (by Z-track):* inject 0.5 ml test dose. If no reactions, next daily dose should ordinarily not exceed 0.5 ml (25 mg) for infants under 5 kg; 1 ml (50 mg) for children under 9 kg; 2 ml (100 mg) for patients under 50 kg; 5 ml (250 mg) for patients over 50 kg. *I.V. push:* inject 0.5 ml test dose. If no reactions, within 2 to 3 days the dosage may be raised to 2 ml/day I.V., 1 ml/minute undiluted and infused slowly until total dose is achieved. No single dose should exceed 100 mg of iron. *I.V. infusion:* dosages are expressed in terms of elemental iron. Dilute in 250 to 1,000 ml of normal saline solution; dextrose increases local vein irritation. Infuse test dose of 25 mg slowly over 5 minutes. If no reaction occurs in 5 minutes, infusion may be started. Infuse total dose slowly over approximately 6 to 12 hours. 1 ml iron dextran = 50 mg elemental iron.	**CNS:** headache, transitory paresthesias, arthralgia, myalgia, dizziness, malaise, syncope. **CV:** *hypotensive reaction, peripheral vascular flushing with overly rapid I.V. administration, tachycardia.* **GI:** nausea, vomiting, metallic taste, transient loss of taste perception. **Local:** *soreness and inflammation at injection site (I.M.); brown skin discoloration at injection site (I.M.); local phlebitis at injection site (I.V.).* **Skin:** rash, urticaria. **Other:** *anaphylaxis.*

♦ Available in U.S. and Canada. ♦♦ Available in Canada only.
All other products (no symbol) available in U.S. only. Italicized side effects are common or life-threatening.

INTERACTIONS AND SPECIAL CONSIDERATIONS

amount of iron absorbed.
- Iron is toxic; parents should be aware of iron poisoning in children.
- Liquid preparations should be diluted in juice (preferably orange juice) or water, but not in milk or antacids. Tablets should be taken with orange juice to promote iron absorption.
- Patient should follow dietary measures to prevent constipation.
- Hemoglobin and reticulocyte counts should be monitored during therapy.

No significant interactions.

Special considerations:
- Contraindicated in all anemias other than iron deficiency anemia. Use with extreme caution in patients with impaired hepatic function and rheumatoid arthritis.
- Vital signs should be monitored for drug reaction. Reactions are varied and severe, ranging from pain, inflammation, and myalgia to hypotension, shock, and death.
- Should be injected deeply into upper outer quadrant of buttock—never into arm or other exposed area—with a 2″ to 3″, 19G or 20G needle. Z-track technique should be used to avoid leakage into subcutaneous tissue and tattooing of skin.
- Hemoglobin concentration, hematocrit, and reticulocyte count should be determined periodically.
- I.V. recommended in these situations: insufficient muscle mass for deep intramuscular injection; impaired absorption from muscle due to stasis or edema; possibility of uncontrolled intramuscular bleeding from trauma (as may occur in hemophilia); and when massive and prolonged parenteral therapy is indicated (as may be necessary in cases of chronic substantial blood loss).
- Patient should rest 15 to 30 minutes after I.V. administration.
- In some hospitals, only doctor may administer iron I.V.
- Not removed by hemodialysis.
- For treatment of anaphylaxis, see APPENDIX.

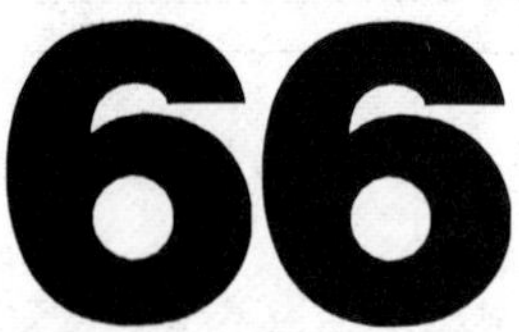

Anticoagulants and heparin antagonist

anisindione
dicumarol
heparin calcium
heparin sodium
phenindione
phenprocoumon
protamine sulfate
warfarin potassium
warfarin sodium

Anticoagulants are given to patients at risk of developing clots (thromboses). These drugs are also used to prevent clot enlargement or fragmentation (thromboembolism).

Oral anticoagulants include the coumarin derivatives (dicumarol, phenprocoumon, warfarin potassium, and warfarin sodium) and the indandione derivatives (anisindione and phenindione). Heparin sodium, a parenteral anticoagulant, is antagonized by protamine sulfate.

Heparin, the coumarin derivatives, and the indandione derivatives impede clotting by preventing fibrin formation.

Major uses

All anticoagulants are used to treat pulmonary emboli and deep vein thrombosis (DVT) and to reduce thrombus formation after myocardial infarction.

- Heparin is administered subcutaneously in low doses (minidoses) to prevent DVT and pulmonary embolism as well.
- Oral anticoagulants are also used in rheumatic heart disease with valvular damage and in atrial arrhythmias that obstruct hemodynamics.
- Protamine sulfate neutralizes the effects of heparin.

Mechanism of action

- Heparin accelerates formation of an antithrombin III-thrombin complex. It inactivates thrombin and prevents conversion of fibrinogen to fibrin.
- The oral anticoagulants inhibit vitamin K–dependent activation of clotting factors II, VII, IX, and X, which are formed in the liver.
- Protamine sulfate, a strong base, forms a physiologically inert complex with heparin sodium, a strong acid.

Absorption, distribution, metabolism, and excretion

- Heparin is not absorbed from the gastrointestinal (GI) tract and must be administered parenterally. Although absorption after subcutaneous injection varies greatly among patients, heparin is generally well absorbed and is usually administered by this route.

Heparin is distributed widely in the blood.

Although heparin's metabolism is not completely clear, most of the drug seems to be removed from circulation by the reticuloendothelial cells. However, some heparin is probably metabolized by the liver. A small fraction of the drug is excreted unchanged in urine.

- The oral anticoagulants anisindione, phenindione, phenprocoumon, and warfarin salts are well absorbed from the GI tract; dicumarol is incompletely absorbed.

Oral anticoagulants are 98% bound to plasma proteins, primarily albumin, and are widely distributed in body tissues.

THERAPEUTIC ACTIVITY

THERAPEUTIC ACTIVITY OF ORAL ANTICOAGULANTS

DRUG	PEAK PROTHROMBIN TIME	DURATION
anisindione	1 to 3 days	1 to 6 days
dicumarol	1 to 3 days	2 to 10 days
phenindione	½ to 3 days	1 to 5 days
phenprocoumon	1½ to 3 days	7 to 14 days
warfarin salts*	½ to 3 days	2 to 5 days

*Potassium and sodium salts

They are largely metabolized in the liver, secreted into the bile as inactive metabolites, reabsorbed, and excreted in the urine.
• Protamine's metabolism and excretion are unclear.

Onset and duration
• Heparin sodium begins to act immediately, with peak effects occurring within minutes. Clotting time returns to normal within 2 to 6 hours.
• Oral anticoagulants are detectable in the blood within 1 hour after administration, and blood levels usually peak within 12 hours. However, oral anticoagulants require 1 to 3 days to produce therapeutic anticoagulation, even though they alter prothrombin time the first day of therapy. The average course of therapy is 3 to 6 months, but the anticoagulants should be used for the shortest period necessary. Durations vary from 1 to 14 days.
• Protamine sulfate neutralizes heparin within 5 minutes after I.V. administration.

Combination products
None.

NAMES, INDICATIONS AND DOSAGES	SIDE EFFECTS
anisindione Miradon **Treatment of pulmonary emboli; prevention and treatment of deep vein thrombosis, myocardial infarction, rheumatic heart disease with heart valve damage, atrial arrhythmias:** ADULTS: 300 mg P.O. first day, 200 mg P.O. second day, 100 mg P.O. third day. Maintenance dose: 25 to 250 mg daily based on prothrombin times.	**Blood:** *hemorrhage with excessive dosage, agranulocytosis,* leukopenia, leukocytosis, eosinophilia. **CNS:** headache. **CV:** myocarditis, tachycardia. **EENT:** conjunctivitis, blurred vision, paralysis of ocular accommodation. **GI:** diarrhea, sore mouth and throat. **GU:** *nephropathy with renal tubular necrosis,* albuminuria. **Hepatic:** jaundice. **Skin:** *rash, severe exfoliative dermatitis.* **Other:** *fever.*
dicumarol Dufalone♦♦ **Treatment of pulmonary emboli; prevention and treatment of deep vein thrombosis, myocardial infarction, rheumatic heart disease with heart valve damage, atrial arrhythmias:** ADULTS: 200 to 300 mg P.O. on first day, 25 to 200 mg P.O. daily thereafter, based on prothrombin times.	**Blood:** *hemorrhage with excessive dosage,* leukopenia, *agranulocytosis.* **GI:** anorexia, nausea, vomiting, cramps, *diarrhea,* mouth ulcers. **GU:** hematuria. **Skin:** dermatitis, urticaria, alopecia, *rash.* **Other:** *fever.*

INTERACTIONS AND SPECIAL CONSIDERATIONS

Interactions:

ALLOPURINOL, CLOFIBRATE, DEXTROTHYROXINE, THYROID DRUGS, HEPARIN, ANABOLIC STEROIDS, DISULFIRAM, PARA-AMINOSALICYLIC ACID, GLUCAGON, INHALATION ANESTHETICS, SULFONAMIDES: increased prothrombin time. Monitor patient carefully. Consider anticoagulant dose reduction.

ETHACRYNIC ACID, INDOMETHACIN, MEFENAMIC ACID, OXYPHENBUTAZONE, PHENYLBUTAZONE, SALICYLATES: increased prothrombin time; ulcerogenic effects. Don't use together.

ANTIPYRINE, CARBAMAZEPINE, ANTACIDS, GRISEOFULVIN, HALOPERIDOL, PARALDEHYDE, RIFAMPIN: decreased prothrombin time. Monitor patient carefully.

PHENYTOIN, GLUTETHIMIDE, CHLORAL HYDRATE, TRICLOFOS SODIUM, ALCOHOL, DIURETICS: increased or decreased prothrombin time. Avoid use if possible, or monitor patient carefully.

BARBITURATES: inhibition of hypoprothrombinemic effect of anticoagulants. If barbiturates are withdrawn, reduce anticoagulant dose; inhibition may last for weeks after anticoagulant is withdrawn, but fatal hemorrhage can occur when inhibiting effect disappears.

CHOLESTYRAMINE: decreased response when administered too close together. Administer 6 hours after oral anticoagulants.

Special considerations:

- Contraindicated in hemophilia, thrombocytopenic purpura, leukemia with pronounced bleeding tendency, open wounds or ulcers, impaired hepatic or renal function, severe hypertension, acute nephritis, subacute bacterial endocarditis. Use cautiously in pregnancy or lactation, during menstruation, during use of any drainage tube in any orifice, and in any patient in whom slight bleeding is dangerous. Use with extreme caution (if at all) in psychiatric, debilitated, or cachectic patients.
- Caution should be used when adding or stopping any drug for patient receiving anticoagulants. May change the clotting status and result in hemorrhage.
- Fever and skin rash signal severe complications.
- Drug should be taken at same time daily. Complying with recommended dosage and keeping follow-up appointments are important. Patient should carry a card that identifies him as a potential bleeder.
- Patient should be inspected regularly for bleeding gums, bruises on arms or legs, petechiae, nosebleeds, melena, tarry stools, hematuria, hematemesis. Patient and family should report these signs to doctor at once.
- Patient should avoid over-the-counter products containing aspirin, other salicylates, or drugs that may interact with anisindione.
- Because onset of action is delayed, heparin sodium is often given during first few days of treatment. When heparin is being given simultaneously, blood for prothrombin time (PT) should not be drawn within 5 hours after I.V. heparin administration.
- Dose given depends on PT; usually PT maintained at 1.5 to 2 times normal. Numerical PT values depend on procedure and reagents used in individual laboratory.
- Patient should notify doctor if menstrual flow is heavier than usual. May require adjusting dose.
- Patient should use electric razor when shaving to avoid scratching skin, and brush teeth with a soft toothbrush.
- Alkaline urine may turn red-orange.
- An indandione derivative.
- Duration of action 1.5 to 5 days.
- Light-to-moderate alcohol intake does not significantly affect prothrombin times.
- For symptoms and treatment of toxicity, see APPENDIX.

Interactions:

ALLOPURINOL, CLOFIBRATE, DEXTROTHYROXINE, THYROID DRUGS, HEPARIN, ANABOLIC STEROIDS, DISULFIRAM, PARA-AMINOSALICYLIC ACID, GLUCAGON, INHALATION ANESTHETICS, SULFONAMIDES: increased prothrombin time. Monitor patient carefully. Consider anticoagulant dose reduction.

ETHACRYNIC ACID, INDOMETHACIN, MEFENAMIC ACID, OXYPHENBUTAZONE, PHENYLBUTAZONE, SALICYLATES: increased prothrombin time; ulcerogenic effects. Don't use together.

ANTIPYRINE, CARBAMAZEPINE, ANTACIDS, GRISEOFULVIN, HALOPERIDOL, PARALDEHYDE, RIFAMPIN: decreased prothrombin time. Monitor patient carefully.

PHENYTOIN, GLUTETHIMIDE, CHLORAL HYDRATE, TRICLOFOS SODIUM: increased or decreased prothrombin time. Avoid use if possible, or monitor patient carefully.

BARBITURATES: inhibition of hypoprothrombinemic effect of anticoagulants. If barbiturates are withdrawn, reduce anticoagulant dose; inhibition may last weeks after anticoagulant is withdrawn, but fatal hemorrhage can occur when inhibiting effect disappears.

CHOLESTYRAMINE: decreased response when administered too close together. Administer 6 hours after oral anticoagulants.

Special considerations:

- Contraindicated in hemophilia, thrombocytopenic purpura, leukemia with pronounced bleeding tendency, open wounds or ulcers, impaired hepatic or renal function, severe hypertension, acute nephritis, subacute bacterial endocarditis. Use cautiously in pregnancy or lactation, during menstruation, during use of any

(continued on following page)

NAMES, INDICATIONS AND DOSAGES	SIDE EFFECTS

dicumarol
(continued)

---

heparin calcium
Calciparine
heparin sodium
Hepalean♦♦, Lipo-Hepin, Liquaemin Sodium, Panheprin

Treatment of deep vein thrombosis, myocardial infarction:
ADULTS: initially, 5,000 to 7,500 units I.V. push, then adjust dose according to partial thromboplastin time (PTT) results and give dose I.V. q 4 hours (usually 4,000 to 5,000 units); or 5,000 to 7,500 units I.V. bolus, then 1,000 units/hour by I.V. infusion pump. Wait 8 hours following bolus dose, and adjust hourly rate according to PTT.

Treatment of pulmonary embolism:
ADULTS: initially, 7,500 to 10,000 units I.V. push, then adjust dose according to PTT results and give dose I.V. q 4 hours (usually 4,000 to 5,000 units); or 7,500 to 10,000 units I.V. bolus, then 1,000 units/ hour by I.V. infusion pump. Wait 8 hours following bolus dose, and adjust hourly rate according to PTT.

Prophylaxis of embolism:
ADULTS: 5,000 units S.C. q 12 hours.

Open heart surgery:
ADULTS: (total body perfusion) 150 to 300 units/kg continuous I.V infusion.

Treatment of pulmonary emboli; prevention and treatment of deep vein thrombosis:
CHILDREN: initially, 50 units/kg I.V. drip. Maintenance dose 100 units/kg I.V. drip q 4 hours. Constant infusion: 20,000 units/m^2 daily. Dosages adjusted according to PTT.

Blood: *hemorrhage with excessive dosage, overly prolonged clotting time, thrombocytopenia.*
Local: irritation, mild pain.
Other: hypersensitivity reactions including chills, fever, pruritus, rhinitis, burning of feet, conjunctivitis, lacrimation, arthralgia, urticaria.

INTERACTIONS AND SPECIAL CONSIDERATIONS

drainage tube, and in any patient in whom slight bleeding is dangerous. Use with extreme caution (if at all) in psychiatric, debilitated, or cachectic patients.
• Caution should be used when adding or stopping any drug for patient receiving anticoagulants. May change clotting status and result in hemorrhage.
• Fever and skin rash signal severe complications.
• Drug should be taken at same time daily. Complying with recommended dosage and keeping follow-up appointments are important. Patient should carry a card that identifies him as a potential bleeder.
• Patient should be inspected regularly for bleeding gums, bruises on arms or legs, petechiae, nosebleeds, melena, tarry stools, hematuria, hematemesis. Patient and family should report these signs to doctor immediately.
• Patient should avoid over-the-counter products containing aspirin, other salicylates, or drugs that may interact with dicumarol.
• Because onset of action is delayed, heparin sodium is often given during first few days of treatment. When heparin is being given simultaneously, blood for prothrombin time (PT) should not be drawn within 5 hours after I.V. heparin administration.
• Dose given depends on PT; usually PT maintained at 1.5 to 2 times normal. PT values depend on procedure and reagents used in individual laboratory.
• Patient should notify doctor if menstrual flow is heavier than usual. May require adjusting dose.
• Patient should use electric razor when shaving to avoid scratching skin, and brush teeth with a soft toothbrush.
• May turn alkaline urine red-orange.
• Duration of action 2 to 6 days.
• Light-to-moderate alcohol intake does not significantly affect prothrombin times.
• For symptoms and treatment of toxicity, see APPENDIX.

Interactions:
SALICYLATES: increased anticoagulant effect. Don't use together.
ANTICOAGULANTS, ORAL: additive anticoagulation. Monitor prothrombin time and partial thromboplastin time.

Special considerations:
• Conditionally contraindicated in active bleeding, blood dyscrasias or bleeding tendencies such as hemophilia, thrombocytopenia, or hepatic disease with hypoprothrombinemia; suspected intracranial hemorrhage; suppurative thrombophlebitis; inaccessible ulcerative lesions (especially of GI tract); open ulcerative wounds; extensive denudation of skin; ascorbic acid deficiency and other conditions causing increased capillary permeability; during or after brain, eye, or spinal cord surgery; during continuous tube drainage of stomach or small intestine; in subacute bacterial endocarditis; shock; advanced kidney disease; threatened abortion; severe hypertension. Although the use of heparin is clearly hazardous in these conditions, the decision to use it depends on the comparative risk in failure to treat the coexisting thromboembolic disorder.
• Should be used cautiously during menstruation; in mild hepatic or renal disease; alcoholism; in patients in occupations with the risk of physical injury; immediately postpartum; and in patients with history of allergies, asthma, or GI ulcers.
• PTT should be measured carefully and regularly. Anticoagulation present when PTT values are 1½ to 2 times control values.
• Drug requirements are higher in early phases of thrombogenic diseases and febrile states; lower when patient becomes stabilized.
• Patient should be inspected regulary for bleeding gums, bruises on arms or legs, petechiae, nosebleeds, melena, tarry stools, hematuria, hematemesis. Patient and family should report these signs to doctor immediately.
• Patient should avoid over-the-counter medications containing aspirin, other salicylates, or drugs that may interact with heparin.
• Heparin comes in various concentrations. Check order and vial.
• Low-dose injections given sequentially between iliac crest in lower abdomen deep into subcutaneous fat. Inject drug slowly subcutaneously into fat pad. Leave needle in place for 10 seconds; withdraw needle. Alternate site every 12 hours—right for a.m., left for p.m.
• After subcutaneous injection, don't massage; watch for signs of bleeding at injection site; rotate sites.
• Constant I.V. infusions require regular checking, even when pumps are in good working order, to prevent overdosage or underdosage.
• I.M. administration not recommended.
• I.V. administration preferred because of long-term effect and irregular absorption when given subcutaneously. Whenever possible, I.V. heparin should be administered by infusion pump to provide maximum safety.
• Concentrated heparin solutions (greater than 100 units/ml) can irritate blood vessels.
• I.V. team or laboratory personnel should use pressure dressings after taking blood.
• To avoid or minimize hematomas, excessive I.M. injections of other drugs not recommended.
• Elderly patients should usually start at lower doses.
• When I.V. intermittent therapy is utilized, blood should always be drawn ½ hour before

(continued on following page)

NAMES, INDICATIONS AND DOSAGES	SIDE EFFECTS
heparin *(continued)* Heparin dosing is highly individualized, depending upon disease state, age, renal and hepatic status.	
phenindione Danilone♦♦, Eridione, Hedulin **Treatment of pulmonary emboli; prevention and treatment of deep vein thrombosis, myocardial infarction, rheumatic heart disease with heart valve damage, atrial arrhythmias:** ADULTS: 300 mg P.O. first day; 200 mg P.O. second day. Maintenance dose: 50 to 150 mg daily, based on prothrombin times.	**Blood:** *hemorrhage with excessive dosage, agranulocytosis,* leukopenia, leukocytosis, eosinophilia. **CNS:** headache. **CV:** myocarditis, tachycardia. **EENT:** conjunctivitis, blurred vision, paralysis of ocular accommodation. **GI:** diarrhea, sore mouth and throat. **GU:** *nephropathy with renal tubular necrosis,* albuminuria. **Hepatic:** jaundice. **Skin:** *rash, severe exfoliative dermatitis.* **Other:** *fever.*
phenprocoumon Liquamar, Marcumar♦♦ **Treatment of pulmonary emboli; prevention and treatment of deep vein thrombosis, myocardial infarction, rheumatic heart disease**	**Blood:** *hemorrhage with excessive dosage, agranulocytosis,* leukopenia. **GI:** paralytic ileus and intestinal obstruction (both resulting from hemorrhage), nausea, vomiting, cramps, diarrhea, mouth ulcers. **GU:** nephropathy, hematuria.

♦ Available in U.S. and Canada. ♦♦ Available in Canada only.
All other products (no symbol) available in U.S. only. Italicized side effects are common or life-threatening.

INTERACTIONS AND SPECIAL CONSIDERATIONS

next scheduled dose to avoid falsely elevated PTT.
• Blood for PTT can be drawn any time after 8 hours of initiation of continuous I.V. heparin therapy. Blood for PTT should never be drawn from the I.V. tubing of the heparin infusion, or from vein of infusion. Falsely elevated PTT will result. Blood should always be drawn from opposite arm.
• Should be given on time, not skipping a dose. If I.V. is out, should be restarted as soon as possible, and dose rescheduled immediately.
• Other drugs should never be piggybacked into an infusion line while heparin infusion is running. Many antibiotics and other drugs inactivate heparin. Heparin should never be mixed in syringe with any drug when bolus therapy is used.
• Abrupt withdrawal may cause increased coagulability. Usually, heparin therapy is followed by oral anticoagulants for prophylaxis.
• For symptoms and treatment of toxicity, see APPENDIX.

Interactions:
ALLOPURINOL, CLOFIBRATE, DEXTROTHYROXINE, THYROID DRUGS, HEPARIN, ANABOLIC STEROIDS, DISULFIRAM, PARA-AMINOSALICYLIC ACID, GLUCAGON, INHALATION ANESTHETICS, SULFONAMIDES: increased prothrombin time. Monitor patient carefully. Consider anticoagulant dose reduction.
ETHACRYNIC ACID, INDOMETHACIN, MEFENAMIC ACID, OXYPHENBUTAZONE, PHENYLBUTAZONE, SALICYLATES: increased prothrombin time; ulcerogenic effects. Don't use together.
ANTIPYRINE, CARBAMAZEPINE, ANTACIDS, GRISEOFULVIN, HALOPERIDOL, PARALDEHYDE, RIFAMPIN: decreased prothrombin time. Monitor patient carefully.
PHENYTOIN, GLUTETHIMIDE, CHLORAL HYDRATE, TRICLOFOS SODIUM, ALCOHOL, DIURETICS: increased or decreased prothrombin time. Avoid use if possible, or monitor patient carefully.
BARBITURATES: inhibition of hypoprothrombinemic effect of anticoagulants. If barbiturates are withdrawn, reduce anticoagulant dose; inhibition may last weeks after anticoagulant is withdrawn, but fatal hemorrhage can occur when inhibiting effect disappears.
CHOLESTYRAMINE: decreased response when administered too close together. Administer 6 hours after oral anticoagulants.

Special considerations:
• Contraindicated in hemophilia, thrombocytopenic purpura, leukemia with pronounced bleeding tendency, open wounds or ulcers, impaired hepatic or renal function, severe hypertension, acute nephritis, and subacute bacterial endocarditis. Use cautiously in pregnancy or lactation, during menstruation, during use of any drainage tube in any orifice, and in any patient in whom slight bleeding is dangerous. Use with extreme caution (if at all) in psychiatric, debilitated, or cachectic patients.
• Caution should be used when adding or stopping any drug. May cause alteration in clotting status and result in hemorrhage.
• Fever and skin rash signal severe complications.
• Drug should be taken at same time daily. Patient should comply with recommended dosage, keep follow-up appointments, and carry a card that identifies him as a potential bleeder.
• Patient should be inspected regularly for bleeding gums, bruises on arms or legs, petechiae, nosebleeds, melena, tarry stools, hematuria, hematemesis. Patient and family should report these signs to doctor immediately.
• Patient should avoid over-the-counter products containing aspirin, other salicylates, or drugs that may interact with phenindione.
• Because onset of action is delayed, heparin sodium is often given during first few days of treatment. When heparin is being given simultaneously, blood for prothrombin times should not be drawn within 5 hours after I.V. heparin administration.
• Dose given depends on prothrombin times (PT); usually PT maintained at 1.5 to 2 times normal. Numerical PT values depend on procedure and reagents used in individual laboratory.
• Patient should notify doctor if menstrual flow is heavier than usual. May require adjusting dose.
• Patient should use electric razor when shaving to avoid scratching skin, and brush teeth with a soft toothbrush.
• Alkaline urine may turn red-orange.
• Duration of action is 2 to 4 days.
• Light-to-moderate alcohol intake does not significantly affect prothrombin times.
• For symptoms and treatment of toxicity, see APPENDIX.

Interactions:
ALLOPURINOL, CLOFIBRATE, DEXTROTHYROXINE, THYROID DRUGS, HEPARIN, ANABOLIC STEROIDS, DISULFIRAM, PARA-AMINOSALICYLIC ACID, GLUCAGON, INHALATION ANESTHETICS, SULFINPYRAZONE, SULINDAC, SULFONAMIDES: increased prothrombin time. Monitor patient carefully. Consider anticoagulant dose reduction.
ETHACRYNIC ACID, INDOMETHACIN, MEFENAMIC ACID, OXYPHENBUTAZONE, PHENYLBUTAZONE, SALICYLATES: increased prothrom-

(continued on following page)

NAMES, INDICATIONS AND DOSAGES	SIDE EFFECTS
phenprocoumon *(continued)* **with heart valve damage, atrial arrhythmias:** ADULTS: initially, 24 mg P.O. Maintenance dose: 0.75 to 6 mg daily, based on prothrombin time.	**Skin:** *rash,* alopecia, necrosis. **Other:** *fever*.
protamine sulfate **Heparin overdose:** ADULTS: dosage based on venous blood coagulation studies, generally 1 mg for each 78 to 95 units of heparin. Give diluted to 1% (10 mg/ml) slow I.V. injection over 1 to 3 minutes. Maximum 50 mg/10 minutes.	**CV:** fall in blood pressure, bradycardia. **Other:** transitory flushing, feeling of warmth, dyspnea.
warfarin potassium Athrombin-K♦ **warfarin sodium** Coumadin♦, Panwarfin, Warfilone Sodium♦♦, Warnerin Sodium♦♦ **Treatment of pulmonary emboli; prevention and treatment of deep vein thrombosis, myocardial infarction, rheumatic heart disease with heart valve damage, atrial arrhythmias:** ADULTS: 10 to 15 mg P.O. for 3 days, then dosage based on daily prothrombin times (PT). Usual maintenance dose 2 to 10 mg P.O. daily. Alternate regimen: initially, 40 to 60 mg P.O.	**Blood:** *hemorrhage with excessive dosage,* leukopenia. **GI:** paralytic ileus, intestinal obstruction (both resulting from hemorrhage), diarrhea, vomiting, cramps, nausea. **GU:** excessive uterine bleeding. **Skin:** dermatitis, urticaria, *rash,* necrosis, alopecia. **Other:** *fever*.

INTERACTIONS AND SPECIAL CONSIDERATIONS

bin time; ulcerogenic effects. Don't use together.
ANTIPYRINE, CARBAMAZEPINE, ANTACIDS, GRISEOFULVIN, HALOPERIDOL, PARALDEHYDE, RIFAMPIN: decreased prothrombin time. Monitor patient carefully.
PHENYTOIN, GLUTETHIMIDE, CHLORAL HYDRATE, TRICLOFOS SODIUM: increased or decreased prothrombin time. Avoid use if possible, or monitor patient carefully.
BARBITURATES: inhibition of hypoprothrombinemic effect of anticoagulants. If barbiturates are withdrawn, reduce anticoagulant dose; inhibition may last for weeks after anticoagulant is withdrawn, but fatal hemorrhage can occur when inhibiting effect disappears.
CHOLESTYRAMINE: decreased response when administered too close together. Administer 6 hours after oral anticoagulants.

Special considerations:
- Contraindicated in hemophilia, thrombocytopenic purpura, leukemia with pronounced bleeding tendency, open wounds or ulcers, impaired hepatic or renal function, severe hypertension, acute nephritis, and subacute bacterial endocarditis. Use cautiously in pregnancy or lactation, during menstruation, during use of any drainage tube in any orifice, and in any patient in whom slight bleeding is dangerous. Use with extreme caution (if at all) in psychiatric, debilitated, or cachectic patients.
- Caution should be used when adding or stopping any drug for patient receiving anticoagulants. May change the clotting status and result in hemorrhage.
- Fever and skin rash signal severe complications.
- Drug should be taken at same time daily. Patient should comply with recommended dosage, keep follow-up appointments, and carry a card that identifies him as a potential bleeder.
- Periodic blood and liver function studies required.
- Patient should be inspected regularly for bleeding gums, bruises on arms or legs, petechiae, nosebleeds, melena, tarry stools, hematuria, hematemesis. Patient and family should report these signs to doctor immediately.
- Patient should avoid over-the-counter products containing aspirin, other salicylates, or drugs that may interact with phenprocoumon.
- Because onset of action is delayed, heparin sodium is often given during first few days of treatment. When heparin is being given simultaneously, blood for prothrombin times should not be drawn within 5 hours after I.V. heparin administration.
- Dose given depends on prothrombin times (PT); usually PT maintained at 1.5 to 2 times normal. Numerical PT values depend on procedure and reagents used in individual laboratory.
- Patient should notify doctor if menstrual flow is heavier than usual. May require adjusting dose.
- Patient should use electric razor when shaving to avoid scratching skin, and brush teeth with a soft toothbrush.
- Alkaline urine may turn orange-red.
- A coumarin derivative.
- Duration of action is 7 to 14 days.
- Light-to-moderate alcohol intake does not significantly affect prothrombin times.
- For symptoms and treatment of toxicity, see APPENDIX.

No significant interactions.

Special considerations:
- Use cautiously in patients who are hypersensitive to fish or after cardiac surgery.
- Should be given slowly to reduce side effects, and equipment kept available to treat shock.
- Patient should be monitored continually; vital signs checked frequently.
- Spontaneous bleeding (heparin rebound) possible, especially in patients undergoing dialysis and in those who have had cardiac surgery.
- Protamine sulfate may act as anticoagulant in very high doses.
- 1 mg of protamine neutralizes 78 to 95 units of heparin.
- Heparin antagonist.

Interactions:
ALLOPURINOL, CLOFIBRATE, DEXTROTHYROXINE, THYROID DRUGS, HEPARIN, ANABOLIC STEROIDS, CIMETIDINE, DISULFIRAM, PARA-AMINOSALICYLIC ACID, GLUCAGON, INHALATION ANESTHETICS, METRONIDAZOLE SULFINPYRAZONE, SULINDAC, SULFONAMIDES: increased prothrombin time. Monitor patient carefully for bleeding. Consider anticoagulant dose reduction.
ETHACRYNIC ACID, INDOMETHACIN, MEFENAMIC ACID, OXYPHENBUTAZONE, PHENYLBUTAZONE, SALICYLATES: increased prothrombin time; ulcerogenic effects. Don't use together.
GRISEOFULVIN, HALOPERIDOL, PARALDEHYDE, RIFAMPIN: decreased prothrombin time. Monitor patient carefully.
GLUTETHIMIDE, CHLORAL HYDRATE, TRICLOFOS SODIUM: increased or decreased prothrombin time. Avoid use if possible, or monitor patient carefully.
BARBITURATES: inhibition of hypoprothrombinemic effect of anticoagulants. If barbiturates are withdrawn, reduce anticoagulant dose; inhibition may last weeks after anticoagulant is withdrawn, but fatal hemorrhage can occur when inhibiting effect disappears.
CHOLESTYRAMINE: decreased response when

(continued on following page)

NAMES, INDICATIONS AND DOSAGES	SIDE EFFECTS
warfarin *(continued)* daily; then 2 to 10 mg daily based on PT determinations. Warfarin sodium also available for I.V. use (50 mg/vial). Reconstitute with sterile water for injection. I.V. form rarely used and may be in periodic short supply.	

INTERACTIONS AND SPECIAL CONSIDERATIONS

administered too close together. Administer 6 hours after oral anticoagulants.

Special considerations:
• Contraindicated in bleeding or hemorrhagic tendencies resulting from open wounds, visceral cancer, GI ulcers, severe hepatic or renal disease, severe uncontrolled hypertension, subacute bacterial endocarditis, vitamin K deficiency; after recent operations in eye, brain, or spinal cord. Use cautiously in diverticulitis, colitis, mild or moderate hypertension, mild or moderate hepatic or renal disease; lactation; in presence of drainage tubes in any orifice; with regional or in lumbar block anesthesia; or in any condition increasing risk of hemorrhage.
• Breast-feeding infants of mothers on drug may develop unexpected bleeding.
• PT determinations essential for proper control. High incidence of bleeding when PT exceeds 2½ times control values. Usually PT maintained at 1.5 to 2 times normal.
• May divide large doses to reduce GI distress.
• Should be taken at same time daily. Patient should comply with recommended dosage, keep follow-up appointments, and carry a card that identifies him as a potential bleeder.
• Elderly patients and patients in renal or hepatic failure are especially sensitive to warfarin effect.
• Half-life of warfarin is 36 to 44 hours.
• Warfarin effect can be neutralized by vitamin K injections.
• Patient should be inspected regularly for bleeding gums, bruises on arms or legs, petechiae, nosebleeds, melena, tarry stools, hematuria, hematemesis. Patient and family should report these signs to doctor at once.
• Patient should avoid over-the-counter products containing aspirin, other salicylates, or drugs that may interact with warfarin potassium or warfarin sodium.
• Because onset of action is delayed, heparin sodium is often given during first few days of treatment. When heparin is being given simultaneously, blood should not be drawn for prothrombin times within 5 hours after I.V. heparin administration.
• Fever and skin rash signal severe complications.
• Patient should notify doctor if menstrual flow is heavier than usual. May require adjusting dose.
• Patient should use electric razor when shaving to avoid scratching skin, and brush teeth with a soft toothbrush.
• Best oral anticoagulant when patient must receive antacids or phenytoin.
• Light-to-moderate alcohol intake does not significantly affect prothrombin times.
• Possibly effective in treatment of transient cerebral ischemic attacks.
• For symptoms and treatment of toxicity, see APPENDIX.

67

Hemostatics

absorbable gelatin sponge
aminocaproic acid
antihemophilic factor (AHF)
carbazochrome salicylate
Factor IX complex
microfibrillar collagen hemostat
negatol
oxidized cellulose
thrombin

Hemostatics, which arrest blood flow or reduce capillary bleeding, should be used cautiously to avoid the risk of redundant clotting. Although all these agents stop excessive bleeding, each has a specific indication in clotting. An accurate diagnosis of the cause of excessive bleeding should be established quickly. If the bleeding results from a specific hereditary deficiency (hemophilia A), diagnosis and treatment may be relatively simple; conversely, multiple acquired deficiencies may be difficult to diagnose and respond poorly to treatment.

The hemostatics antihemophilic factor and Factor IX complex are administered systemically to overcome specific coagulation defects in various forms of hemophilia. They are prepared as concentrates from human blood. The other systemically administered hemostatic agent, aminocaproic acid, augments clotting by inhibiting fibrinolysis.

Absorbable gelatin sponge, carbazochrome, microfibrillar collagen, oxidized cellulose, negatol, and thrombin are applied locally to control surface bleeding and capillary oozing.

Major uses

- Absorbable gelatin sponge, microfibrillar collagen hemostat, and oxidized cellulose are hemostatic adjuncts in various surgical procedures. Absorbable gelatin sponge also aids healing of decubitus ulcers.
- Aminocaproic acid is used to arrest excessive bleeding resulting from hyperfibrinolysis. It is also an antidote for both streptokinase and urokinase toxicity.
- Antihemophilic factor corrects hemophilia A (Factor VIII deficiency).
- Carbazochrome salicylate corrects excessive capillary permeability during surgical treatment for conditions accompanied by excessive oozing.
- Factor IX complex, which contains factors II, VII, IX, and X, is used to treat hemophilia B (Factor IX deficiency, or Christmas disease) and also combats anticoagulant overdose.
- Negatol, which acts as a styptic and hemostatic, is used for oral ulcers and cervical bleeding.
- Thrombin controls bleeding from tissue parenchyma, cancellous bone, and dental sockets; during nasal and laryngeal surgical procedures, plastic surgery, and skin-grafting procedures; and in acute gastrointestinal hemorrhages.

Mechanism of action

- Absorbable gelatin sponge and oxidized cellulose absorb and hold many times their weight in blood. Absorbable gelatin sponge also provides a framework for growth of granulation tissue.
- Aminocaproic acid inhibits plasminogen activator substances. To a lesser degree, it blocks antiplasmin activity by inhibiting fibrinolysis.
- Antihemophilic factor and Factor IX complex directly replace deficient clotting factors.
- Carbazochrome salicylate decreases capillary permeability.
- Microfibrillar collagen hemostat attracts and aggregates platelets.

UNDERSTANDING INHERITANCE PATTERNS OF HEMOPHILIA

1

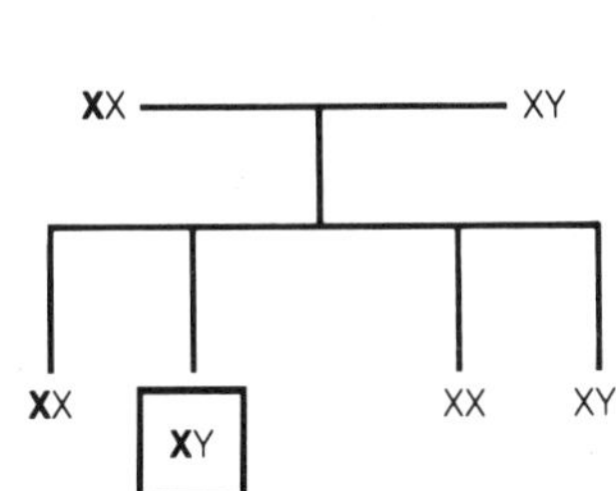

2

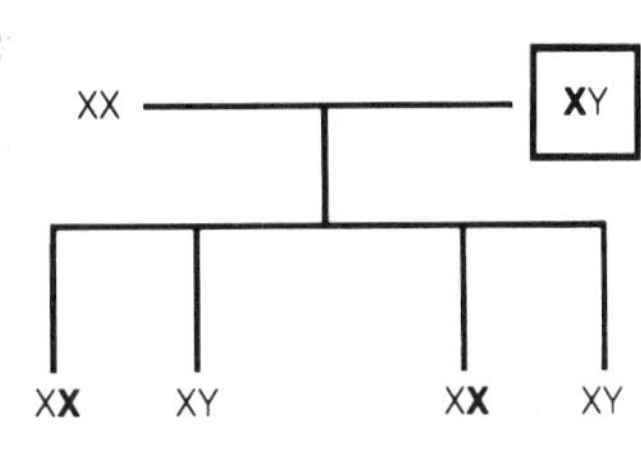

Illustration 1: A female carrier (**X**X) marries a normal male (XY). Their daughters have a 50% chance of being carriers (**X**X) and a 50% chance of being normal (XX). If the couple has sons, each son has a 50% chance of being hemophiliac (**X**Y) and a 50% chance of being normal (XY).

Illustration 2: A normal female (XX) marries a hemophiliac (**X**Y). All the daughters are carriers (X**X**) and all the sons are normal (XY).

- Negatol is an astringent and protein denaturant.
- Thrombin clots to form fibrin in the presence of fibrinogen.

Absorption, distribution, metabolism, and excretion
- Aminocaproic acid is rapidly absorbed after oral administration and excreted mostly unmetabolized in urine.
- Antihemophilic factor and Factor IX complex are distributed to the plasma after I.V. administration. They are metabolized and excreted as normal physiologic substances.
- The topical agents aren't absorbed and therefore aren't distributed, metabolized, or excreted.

Onset and duration
- Aminocaproic acid begins to act almost immediately after oral or parenteral administration and reaches peak levels within 1 to 2 hours. Rapid excretion and short duration require either repeated oral doses at 1- to 2-hour intervals or continuous I.V. infusion.
- Antihemophilic factor and Factor IX complex begin to act immediately. Their durations are related to the level of factor deficiency and the presence of Factor VIII and Factor IX antibodies.
- Thrombin's onset and duration depend on concentration. For example, 5,000 units of thrombin/5 ml normal saline solution clot an equal volume of blood in less than 1 second and clot 1 liter of blood in less than 1 minute.
- Onset and duration of the other topical agents depend on the amount used, extent of blood saturation, and type of tissue bed.

NAMES, INDICATIONS AND DOSAGES	SIDE EFFECTS
absorbable gelatin sponge Gelfoam ADULTS: **Decubitus ulcers:** place aseptically deep into ulcer. Don't disturb or remove; may add extra p.r.n. **To provide hemostasis in surgery (adjunct):** apply saturated with isotonic NaCl injection or thrombin solution. Hold in place for 10 to 15 seconds. When bleeding is controlled, allow material to remain in place.	None reported.
aminocaproic acid Amicar♦ **Excessive bleeding resulting from hyperfibrinolysis:** ADULTS: initially, 5 g P.O. or slow I.V. infusion, followed by 1 to 1.25 g hourly until bleeding is controlled. Maximum dose 30 g daily.	**Blood:** generalized thrombosis. **CNS:** dizziness, malaise, headache. **CV:** hypotension, bradycardia, arrhythmia (with rapid I.V. infusion). **EENT:** tinnitus, nasal stuffiness, conjunctival suffusion. **GI:** nausea, cramps, diarrhea. **Skin:** rash. **Other:** malaise.
antihemophilic factor (AHF) Actif VIII, Antihemophilic Globulin (AHG), Factorate, Hemofil, Humafac, Koate, Profilate **Hemophilia A (Factor VIII deficiency):** ADULTS AND CHILDREN: 10 to 20 units/kg I.V. push or infusion q 8 to 24 hours. Maintenance doses may be less. Infusion rate usually 10 to 20 ml reconstituted solution per 3 minutes. Dosage varies with individual needs.	**CNS:** headache, paresthesias, clouding or loss of consciousness. **CV:** tachycardia, hypotension, possible intravascular hemolysis in patients with blood types A, B, or AB. **EENT:** disturbed vision. **GI:** nausea, vomiting. **Skin:** erythema, urticaria. **Other:** *chills, fever, backache, flushing,* constriction in chest; hypersensitivity.
carbazochrome salicylate Adrenosem Salicylate **Surgery with excessive capillary bleeding or oozing:** ADULTS AND CHILDREN OVER 12 YEARS: 10 mg I.M. preoperatively on night before surgery and with on-call medication, and 5 mg P.O. or I.M. postoperatively q 2 to 4 hours. CHILDREN UNDER 12 YEARS: 5 mg I.M. preoperatively on night before surgery and with on-call medication, and 2.5 mg P.O. or I.M. postoperatively q 2 to 4 hours.	**Local:** pain at I.M. injection site.
Factor IX complex Konyne, Proplex **Factor IX deficiency (hemophilia B or Christmas disease), anticoagulant overdosage:** ADULTS AND CHILDREN: units required equal 0.6 × body weight in kg × percentage of desired increase of Factor IX level, by slow I.V. infusion or I.V. push. Dosage is highly individid-	**CNS:** headache. **CV:** *thromboembolic reactions,* possible intravascular hemolysis in patients with blood types A, B, AB. **Other:** *transient fever, chills, flushing, tingling,* hypersensitivity.

♦ Available in U.S. and Canada. ♦♦ Available in Canada only.
All other products (no symbol) available in U.S. only. Italicized side effects are common or life-threatening.

INTERACTIONS AND SPECIAL CONSIDERATIONS

No significant interactions.

Special considerations:
• Contraindicated in frank infection, as sole hemostatic agent in abnormal bleeding, or in postpartum bleeding or hemorrhage.
• Overpacking should be avoided when placed into body cavities or closed tissue spaces.
• Systemically absorbed within 4 to 6 weeks; no need to remove.

Interactions:
ORAL CONTRACEPTIVES: increased probability of hypercoagulability. Use together cautiously.

Special considerations:
• Contraindicated in active intravascular clotting. Use cautiously in thrombophlebitis, or cardiac, hepatic, or renal disease.
• Coagulation studies, heart rhythm, and blood pressure should be monitored.
• Also used as antidote for streptokinase or urokinase toxicity; not beneficial in the treatment of thrombocytopenia.
• Solution should be diluted with sterile water for injection, normal saline injection, 5% dextrose in water, or Ringer's injection.

No significant interactions.

Special considerations:
• Use cautiously in neonates, infants, and patients with hepatic disease, because of susceptibility to hepatitis, which may be transmitted in antihemophilic factor.
• Blood should be typed and crossmatched to treat possible hemorrhage.
• Vital signs should be monitored regularly, and baseline pulse rate taken before I.V. administration. Significant pulse rate increases require flow rate reduction or discontinuation of drug.
• Patient should be monitored for allergic reactions.
• For I.V. use only. Plastic syringe should be used; drug may interact with glass syringe, causing binding of ground-glass surface.
• Concentrate should be refrigerated until ready to use, but not after reconstituted. Refrigeration after reconstitution may cause the active ingredient to precipitate. Before reconstituting, concentrate and diluent bottles should be warmed to room temperature. To mix drug, vial should be rolled gently between hands. Reconstituted solution unstable; should be used within 3 hours, and stored away from heat. Should not be shaken or mixed with other I.V. solutions.
• Coagulation studies should be monitored before and during therapy.

No significant interactions.

Special considerations:
• Contraindicated in hypersensitivity to salicylates.
• Patient history concerning allergies, especially to salicylates, should be obtained.
• Has no effect on blood-clotting time, prothrombin time, or vitamin K level.

No significant interactions.

Special considerations:
• Contraindicated in hepatic disease, intravascular coagulation, or fibrinolysis. Use cautiously in neonates and infants because of susceptibility to hepatitis, which may be transmitted with Factor IX complex.
• Blood should be typed and crossmatched to treat possible hemorrhage. If given to patients with types A, B, AB, intravascular hemolysis may occur.
• Patient should be monitored for allergic reactions and vital signs checked regularly.
• Rapid infusion should be avoided. If tingling sensation, fever, chills, or headache develop during I.V. infusion, flow rate should be decreased.

(continued on following page)

NAMES, INDICATIONS AND DOSAGES	SIDE EFFECTS
Factor IX complex *(continued)* ualized, depending on degree of deficiency, level of Factor IX desired, weight of patient, and severity of bleeding.	
microfibrillar collagen hemostat Avitene **To provide hemostasis in surgery (adjunct):** ADULTS AND CHILDREN: amount depends on severity of bleeding. Compress area with dry sponges. Apply to bleeding site for 1 to 5 minutes. Remove excess. Reapply if needed.	**Blood:** hematoma. **Local:** exacerbation of wound dehiscence, abscess formation, foreign body reaction, adhesion formation. **Other:** enhanced infection in contaminated wounds, mediastinitis, hypersensitivity.
negatol Negatan **Cervical bleeding:** WOMEN: insert 1″ gauze dipped in 1:10 dilution in cervical canal. If tolerated, may increase to full-strength solution. After 24 hours: remove pack; 2 qt dilute negatol or vinegar douche. **Oral ulcers:** ADULTS AND CHILDREN: apply to dried lesion with applicator, leave for 1 minute, then neutralize with large amounts of water.	**Local:** *burning sensation.* **Skin:** erythema, superficial desquamation when applied to skin.
oxidized cellulose Oxycel♦, Surgicel **To provide hemostasis in surgery (adjunct):** ADULTS AND CHILDREN: apply with sterile technique, p.r.n. Remove after hemostasis, if possible, with dry sterile forceps. Leave in place if necessary.	**CNS:** headache when used as packing for epistaxis, or after rhinologic procedures or application to surface wounds. **EENT:** sneezing, epistaxis or stinging, burning when used as packing for rhinologic procedures; nasal membrane necrosis or septal perforation. **Local:** encapsulation of fluid, foreign body reaction, burning or stinging after application to surface wounds. **Other:** possible prolongation of drainage in cholecystectomies.
thrombin Fibrindex **Bleeding from parenchymatous tissue; cancellous bone; dental sockets; nasal, laryngeal, and plastic surgery; and skin-grafts:** ADULTS: apply 100 units/ml of sterile isotonic NaCl solution or sterile distilled water to bleeding area where clotting needed (may apply dry powder in bone surgery); in major bleeding, apply 1,000 to 2,000 units/ml sterile isotonic NaCl solution. Avoid sponging after application. **GI hemorrhage:** ADULTS: give 2 oz of milk, followed by 2 oz of milk containing 10,000 to 20,000 units thrombin. Repeat t.i.d. for 4 to 5 days or until bleeding is controlled.	**Systemic:** hypersensitivity and fever.

INTERACTIONS AND SPECIAL CONSIDERATIONS

• For I.V. administration: reconstitute with 20 ml sterile water for injection for each vial of lyophilized drug. Keep refrigerated until ready to use; warm to room temperature before reconstituting. Use within 3 hours of reconstitution. Unstable in solution. Don't shake, refrigerate, or mix reconstituted solution with other I.V. solutions. Store away from heat.

No significant interactions.

Special considerations:
• Contraindicated in closure of skin incisions; it may interfere with healing.
• Not for injection.
• Should not be spilled on nonbleeding surfaces.
• Should not be diluted; always applied dry.
• Adheres to wet gloves, instruments, or tissue surfaces. Should be handled and applied with smooth, dry forceps, directly to bleeding site.

No significant interactions.

Special considerations:
• Turns vaginal membrane grayish.
• When used in vagina, patient should wear a perineal pad to prevent soiling of clothing.
• When used for oral ulcers, topical anesthetic may be applied first to prevent burning sensation.
• Area to be treated should always be clean and dry.
• Astringent, styptic. and protein denaturant; highly acidic.

No significant interactions.

Special considerations:
• Contraindicated in controlling hemorrhage from large arteries; in nonhemorrhagic, serous, oozing surfaces; in implantation in bone defects.
• Should not be packed or wadded unless it will be removed after hemostasis. Don't apply too tightly when used as wrap sheet in vascular surgery; apply loosely against bleeding surface.
• Always remove after hemostasis when used in laminectomies or near optic nerve chain.
• This product should not be autoclaved.
• Use only amount needed to produce hemostasis; remove excess before surgical closure.
• Use minimum in urologic procedures.
• In large wounds, skin edges should not be overlapped.
• Should be removed using sterile technique from open wounds after hemostasis. Should not be removed without first irrigating material; otherwise, fresh bleeding may occur.
• Should not be moistened. Hemostatic effect is greater when applied dry.
• Should not be used for permanent packing in fractures because it may result in cyst formation.

No significant interactions.

Special considerations:
• Contraindicated in hypersensitivity to thrombin or bovine products.
• Patient history of reactions to thrombin or bovine products should be obtained.
• Vital signs should be monitored regularly.
• Blood should be typed and crossmatched to treat possible hemorrhage.
• Topical thrombin should not be injected or allowed to enter large blood vessels. I.V. injection may cause death because of severe intravascular clotting.
• May be used with absorbable gelatin sponge but not with oxidized cellulose. Sponge labeling should be consulted before use.
• Stomach acids should be neutralized before oral use in GI hemorrhage.
• Should be kept refrigerated, preferably frozen, until ready to use. Unstable in solution. Should be used within 24 hours of reconstitution, discarded after 48 hours, and stored away from heat.
• Broken down by diluted acid, alkali, and salts of heavy metals.

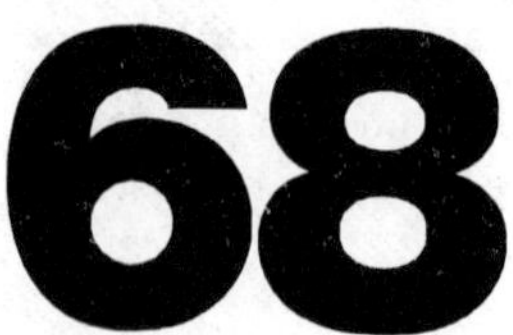

Blood derivatives

normal serum albumin
plasma protein fraction

Normal serum albumin and plasma protein fraction are made from pooled normal human blood, plasma, or serum; albumin is also obtained from human placentas. Both preparations furnish means for stabilizing the body's hemodynamic mechanisms in hypovolemic shock or hypoproteinemia, or both.

Current techniques allow separation of freshly donated whole blood into its component fractions: human red cells (packed red cells), plasma, platelets, granulocytes, $Rh_o(D)$ immune human globulin, albumin, and plasma protein. Because each component can correct a particular hematologic deficiency, use of whole blood is seldom needed. Whole blood is indicated only when a patient has lost considerable quantities of blood within a short time.

Component transfusion—the technique of administering specific components rather than whole blood to a patient—has several advantages. In addition to providing deficiency-specific therapy, the technique expands the potential usefulness of a single blood donation and helps ease the chronic shortage of blood. The risk of viral hepatitis and exposure to sensitizing agents or drugs in blood are also reduced.

Major uses

The blood derivatives act as plasma expanders in hypovolemic shock caused by burns, trauma, sepsis, or surgical procedures. They are also used to treat hypoproteinemia associated with malnutrition, toxemia of pregnancy, or prematurity.

- Normal serum albumin 25% is used to treat hypoproteinemia associated with hepatic cirrhosis and nephrotic syndrome.

Mechanism of action

- Normal serum albumin 25% furnishes an intravascular oncotic pressure in a ratio of 5:1. This causes a migration of fluid from the interstitial space to the circulation and causes a slight increase in plasma protein concentration.
- Normal serum albumin 5% and plasma protein fraction supply colloid to the blood and expand plasma volume.

Absorption, distribution, metabolism, and excretion

Since these blood derivatives are given only by the I.V. route, absorption is complete; they are rapidly distributed in the blood.

Onset and duration

Adequate patient response to normal serum albumin usually occurs within 15 to 30 minutes. Duration of therapy with albumin and plasma protein fraction varies not only with the patient but also with the abnormality or condition that is being treated.

HOW BURN DAMAGE AFFECTS FLUID BALANCE

Osmosis and diffusion maintain a delicate balance of body fluid distribution (70% intracellular fluid; 30% extracellular fluid, consisting of 6% in the plasma and 24% in the interstitial fluid) in the healthy adult.

With severe burn injury, huge amounts of fluids shift out of the blood into the interstitial space in the first 24 to 48 hours. This shift is called burn shock.

Burn damage increases capillary permeability. This increase and the inflammatory process cause the fluid leakage into the interstitial space. Since water, electrolyte, and albumin molecules are small, more of these are lost from the vascular space than blood cells (red, white, and platelets) or large protein molecules, like globulins, which remain in the vessels.

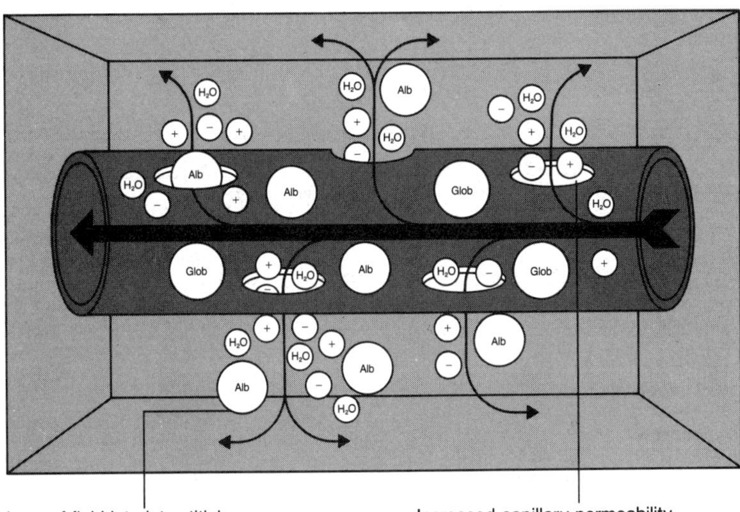

NAMES, INDICATIONS AND DOSAGES	SIDE EFFECTS

normal serum albumin 5%
Albuconn 5%, Albuminar 5%, Albuspan 5%, Albutein 5%, Buminate 5%, Plasbumin 5%
normal serum albumin 25%
Albuconn 25%, Albuminar 25%, Albumisol 25%, Buminate 25%, Plasbumin 25%

Shock:
ADULTS: initially, 500 ml (5% solution) by I.V. infusion, repeat q 30 minutes, p.r.n. Dose varies with patient's condition and response.
CHILDREN: 25% to 50% adult dose in nonemergency.

Hypoproteinemia:
ADULTS: 1,000 to 1,500 ml 5% solution by I.V. infusion daily, maximum rate 5 to 10 ml/minute; or 25 to 100 g 25% solution by I.V. infusion daily, maximum rate 3 ml/minute. Dose varies with patient's condition and response.

Burns: dosage varies according to extent of burn and patient's condition. Generally maintain plasma albumin at 2 to 3 g/100 ml.

Hyperbilirubinemia:
INFANTS: 1 g albumin (4 ml 25%)/kg before transfusion.

CV: *vascular overload after rapid infusion,* hypotension, altered pulse rate.
GI: increased salivation, nausea, vomiting.
Skin: urticaria.
Other: chills, fever, altered respiration.

---

plasma protein fraction
Plasmanate, Plasmatein, Protenate

Shock:
ADULTS: varies with patient's condition and response, but usual dose is 250 to 500 ml (12.5 to 25 g protein), usually not faster than 10 ml/minute.
CHILDREN: 22 to 33 ml/kg I.V. infused at rate of 5 to 10 ml/minute.

Hypoproteinemia:
ADULTS: 1,000 to 1,500 ml I.V. daily. Maximum infusion rate 8 ml/minute.

CNS: headache.
CV: variable effects on blood pressure after rapid infusion or intra-arterial administration; *vascular overload after rapid infusion.*
GI: nausea, vomiting, hypersalivation.
Skin: erythema, urticaria.
Other: flushing, chills, fever, back pain, dyspnea.

♦ Available in U.S. and Canada. ♦♦ Available in Canada only.
All other products (no symbol) available in U.S. only. Italicized side effects are common or life-threatening.

INTERACTIONS AND SPECIAL CONSIDERATIONS

No significant interactions.

Special considerations:
• Contraindicated in severe anemia and heart failure. Use cautiously in low cardiac reserve, absence of albumin deficiency, restricted salt intake.
• No more than 250 g should be given in 48 hours.
• Possible hemorrhage or shock if used after surgery or injury.
• Vital signs should be monitored carefully.
• Patient may develop vascular overload (heart failure or pulmonary edema).
• Patient should be properly hydrated before infusion of solution.
• Rapid I.V. infusion should be avoided. Specific rate is individualized according to patient's age, condition, and diagnosis.
• For I.V. administration: dilute with sterile water for injection, 0.9% NaCl, or 5% dextrose injection. Use solution promptly: contains no preservatives. Discard unused solution.
• Cloudy solutions or those containing sediment should not be used; solution should be clear amber color.
• Freezing may cause the bottle to break. Storage instructions on bottle should be followed.
• One volume of 25% albumin is equivalent to 5 volumes of 5% albumin in producing hemodilution and relative anemia.
• This product is very expensive, and random supply shortages occur often.
• Intake and output, hemoglobin, hematocrit, and serum protein and electrolytes should be monitored during therapy.

No significant interactions.

Special considerations:
• Contraindicated in patients with severe anemia or heart failure, and in patients undergoing cardiac bypass. Use cautiously in hepatic or renal failure, low cardiac reserve, restricted salt intake.
• Blood pressure should be monitored. Infusion should be slowed or stopped if sudden hypotension occurs.
• Vital signs should return to normal gradually; should be monitored hourly.
• Patient may develop vascular overload (heart failure or pulmonary edema).
• Intake and output should be monitored. Decreased urinary output possible.
• Expiration date on container should be checked before using, and solutions discarded in containers that have been opened for more than 4 hours. Solution contains no preservatives.
• Solutions that are cloudy, contain sediment, or have been frozen should not be used.
• If patient is dehydrated, additional fluids should be given either orally or I.V.
• No more than 250 g (5,000 ml 5%) should be given in 48 hours.
• Contains 130 to 160 mEq sodium/liter.

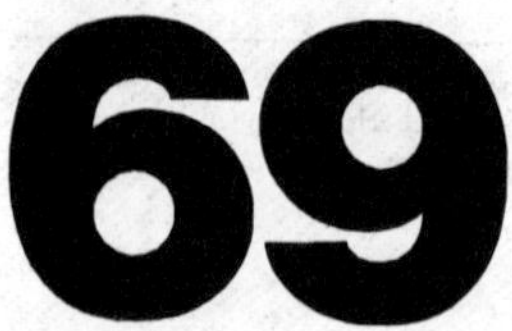

Thrombolytic enzymes

streptokinase
urokinase

Thrombolytic enzymes are effective in treating acute and extensive episodes of thrombotic disorders. Before administering these enzymes, however, be aware of the increased risk of hemorrhage that attends their use. Although major bleeding is a possible complication of treatment, bruising and oozing of blood at the incision site and surgical trauma are more likely. Because of the inherent risk of hemorrhage, thrombolytic enzyme therapy should be initiated only by doctors skilled in its use and under close laboratory monitoring.

Major uses
Streptokinase and urokinase are used to treat acute, massive pulmonary emboli. Streptokinase is also used to dissolve acute, extensive deep vein thrombi and acute arterial thromboemboli.

Mechanism of action
Both streptokinase and urokinase activate plasminogen and convert it to plasmin, which degrades fibrin clots, fibrinogen, and other plasma proteins.

- Streptokinase activates plasminogen in a two-step process. Plasminogen and streptokinase form a complex that exposes the plasminogen-activating site. Plasminogen is converted to plasmin by cleavage of the peptide bond.
- Urokinase activates plasminogen by directly cleaving peptide bonds at two different sites.

Absorption, distribution, metabolism, and excretion
Streptokinase and urokinase are administered only by I.V. infusion and are distributed throughout the body. Their metabolism and excretion have not been fully elucidated.

Onset and duration
Streptokinase and urokinase begin to act immediately. They must be infused at a constant dosage level to maintain therapeutic effectiveness. Their action ceases when the I.V. infusion is discontinued, but residual effects on coagulation may last as long as 12 hours.

Combination products
None.

HOW DRUGS ACTIVATE THE FIBRINOLYTIC SYSTEM

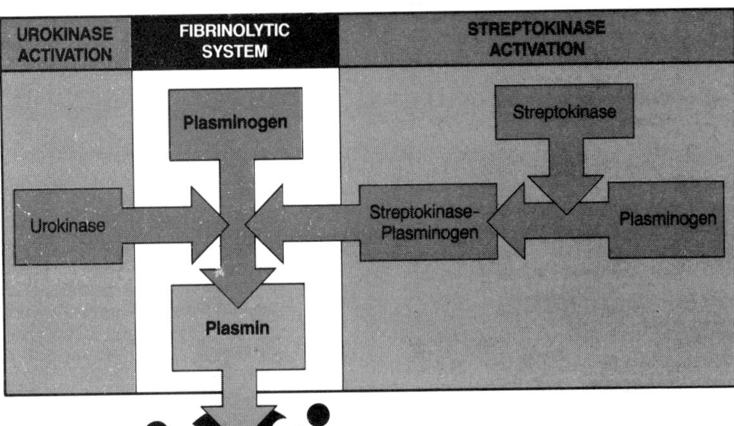

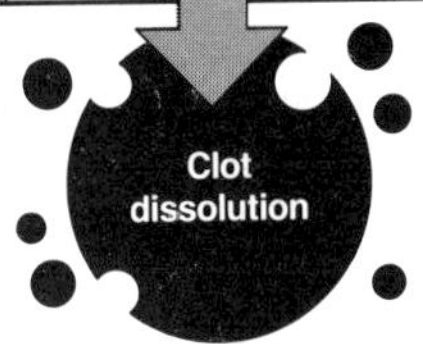

When blood begins to form a clot, the natural mechanism for dissolving this clot is also initiated.

The mechanism for dissolving clotted blood when it's no longer needed is called the fibrinolytic system. Its physiologic stimuli are kinases, activated Factor XII, and certain tissue activators. They activate plasminogen to form plasmin, the proteolytic enzyme that dissolves a clot's fibrin threads.

When undesirable clots form, the fibrinolytic system's anticoagulant action can be hastened with the thrombolytic drugs streptokinase and urokinase.

These drugs imitate the system's natural activators. Urokinase reacts directly with plasminogen to create the lysing agent plasmin; streptokinase joins plasminogen in a complex that then reacts with plasminogen to form plasmin. This activated plasmin then dissolves the clot.

Adapted with permission from Philip P. Gerbino and Sanford J. Shattil, "Prevention and Treatment of Pulmonary Embolism," *U.S. Pharmacist,* 5:5:H-1, May 1980.

NAMES, INDICATIONS AND DOSAGES	SIDE EFFECTS

streptokinase
Kabikinase, Streptase

Arteriovenous cannula occlusion:
ADULTS: 250,000 IU in 2 ml I.V. solution by I.V. pump infusion into each occluded limb of the cannula over 25 to 35 minutes. Clamp off cannula for 2 hours. Then aspirate contents of cannula; flush with saline solution and reconnect.

Venous thrombosis, pulmonary embolism, and arterial thrombosis and embolism:
ADULTS: loading dose—250,000 IU I.V. infusion over 30 minutes; sustaining dose—100,000 IU/hour I.V. infusion for 72 hours for deep vein thrombosis and 100,000 IU/hour over 24 to 72 hours by I.V. infusion pump for pulmonary embolism.

Blood: *bleeding, decreased hematocrit.*
CV: transient lowering or elevation of blood pressure.
EENT: periorbital edema.
Local: *phlebitis at injection site.*
Skin: urticaria.
Other: *hypersensitivity to drug, anaphylaxis,* musculoskeletal pain, minor breathing difficulty, bronchospasms, angioneurotic edema.

urokinase
Abbokinase, Breokinase, Win-Kinase

Lysis of acute massive pulmonary emboli and lysis of pulmonary emboli accompanied by unstable hemodynamics:
ADULTS: for I.V. infusion only by constant infusion pump that will deliver a total volume of 195 ml.

Priming dose—4,400 IU/kg/hour of urokinase-normal saline solution admixture given over 10 minutes. Follow with 4,400 IU/kg/hour for 12 to 24 hours. Total volume should not exceed 200 ml. Follow therapy with continuous I.V. infusion of heparin, then oral anticoagulants.

Blood: *bleeding, decreased hematocrit.*
Local: *phlebitis at injection site.*
Other: hypersensitivity (not as frequent as streptokinase), musculoskeletal pain, bronchospasm, *anaphylaxis.*

♦ Available in U.S. and Canada. ♦♦ Available in Canada only.
All other products (no symbol) available in U.S. only. Italicized side effects are common or life-threatening.

INTERACTIONS AND SPECIAL CONSIDERATIONS

Interactions:

ANTICOAGULANTS: concurrent use with streptokinase not recommended. Reversing effects of oral anticoagulants must be considered before beginning therapy; heparin must be stopped and its effect allowed to diminish.

ASPIRIN, INDOMETHACIN, PHENYLBUTAZONE, DRUGS AFFECTING PLATELET ACTIVITY: increased risk of bleeding. Do not use together.

Special considerations:

• Contraindicated in ulcerative wounds, active internal bleeding, and recent cerebrovascular accident or trauma with possible internal injuries; visceral or intracranial malignancy; ulcerative colitis; diverticulitis; severe hypertension; acute or chronic hepatic or renal insufficiency; uncontrolled hypocoagulation; chronic pulmonary disease with cavitation; subacute bacterial endocarditis or rheumatic valvular disease; recent cerebral embolism, thrombosis, or hemorrhage. Contraindicated within 10 days after intra-arterial diagnostic procedure, liver or kidney biopsy, lumbar puncture, thoracentesis, paracentesis, cutdowns, or surgery.

• Should be used cautiously when treating arterial emboli that originate from left side of heart because of danger of cerebral infarction.

• I.M. injections contraindicated during streptokinase therapy.

• Before initiating therapy, draw blood to determine partial thromboplastin time and prothrombin time. Rate of I.V. infusion depends on thrombin time and streptokinase resistance.

• Recent streptococcal infection or streptokinase treatment may require higher loading dose.

• I.V. solution: reconstitute each vial with 5 ml sodium chloride for injection. Further dilute to 45 ml. Don't shake; roll gently to mix. Use within 24 hours. Store at room temperature.

• Monitor patient for excessive bleeding; if evident, therapy should be stopped. Pretreatment with heparin or drugs affecting platelets causes high risk of bleeding. Crossmatched and typed packed red cells and whole blood should be available to treat possible hemorrhage. Aminocaproic acid and corticosteroids treat adverse reactions not responding to blood replacement.

• Before using streptokinase to clear an occluded arteriovenous cannula, flushing with heparinized saline solution should be tried.

• Bruising more likely during therapy.

• Keep puncture sites to a minimum; use pressure dressing on sites for at least 15 minutes.

• Vital signs should be monitored frequently.

• Patient may develop hypersensitivity.

• Heparin by continuous infusion is usually started within an hour after stopping streptokinase. Use infusion pump to give heparin.

• For use only by doctors with wide experience in managing thrombotic disease with clinical and laboratory monitoring.

• Used investigationally to treat acute myocardial infarction. Streptokinase prevents primary or secondary thrombus formation in the microcirulation surrounding the necrotic area.

• For treatment of anaphylaxis, see APPENDIX.

Interactions:

ANTICOAGULANTS: concurrent use with urokinase is not recommended. Reversing effects of oral anticoagulants must be considered before beginning therapy; heparin must be stopped and its effect allowed to diminish.

ASPIRIN, INDOMETHACIN, PHENYLBUTAZONE, DRUGS AFFECTING PLATELET ACTIVITY: increased risk of bleeding. Do not use together.

Special considerations:

• Contraindicated in ulcerative wounds, active internal bleeding, and cerebrovascular accident; recent trauma with possible internal injuries; visceral or intracranial malignancy; pregnancy and first 10 days postpartum; ulcerative colitis; diverticulitis; severe hypertension; acute or chronic hepatic or renal insufficiency; uncontrolled hypocoagulation; chronic pulmonary disease with cavitation; subacute bacterial endocarditis or rheumatic valvular disease; and recent cerebral embolism, thrombosis, or hemorrhage. Contraindicated within 10 days after intra-arterial diagnostic procedure, liver or kidney biopsy, lumbar puncture, thoracentesis, paracentesis, cutdowns, or surgery.

• I.M. injections are contraindicated during urokinase therapy.

• I.V. solution: add 5.2 ml sterile water for injection. Dilute more with 0.9% saline solution before infusion. Avoid bacteriostatic water for injection to reconstitute; contains preservatives.

• Monitor for bleeding. Pretreatment with drugs affecting platelets carry high risk of bleeding. Crossmatched, typed red cells, whole blood may be needed for possible hemorrhage. Aminocaproic acid and corticosteroids treat adverse reactions unresponsive to blood replacement.

• Patient may develop hypersensitivity.

• Vital signs should be monitored.

• Keep puncture sites to a minimum; use pressure dressing on sites for at least 15 minutes.

• Heparin by continuous infusion usually started within an hour after urokinase has been stopped. Use infusion pump to administer heparin.

• Bruising during therapy more likely.

• For use only by doctors with wide experience in managing thrombotic disease with clinical and laboratory monitoring.

• For treatment of anaphylaxis, see APPENDIX.

70

Implications of chemotherapy

Antineoplastic drugs destroy cancer cells by interfering with neoplastic cell growth and division. They block the supply or utilization of essential cellular building blocks or interrupt the process of cell division known as the cell cycle. The cell cycle consists of five specific phases. Antineoplastic drugs that destroy cells only at a specific point in the cell cycle are called cell cycle specific; those that affect the cells at any phase of the cell cycle are called cell cycle nonspecific.

Because of the toxic effects these drugs have on normal as well as cancerous cells, chemotherapy is most effective during the early stages of a tumor's growth, when fewer cancer cells are present. At this time, when the patient is not debilitated and overwhelmed by his disease, he is better able to combat the drug's toxic effects.

In a solid tumor, chemotherapy may be used with surgery and/or radiation therapy, usually after the tumor mass has been reduced. Therapy that combines antineoplastics and surgery is less successful when the malignancy is extensive or metastatic.

Chemotherapy alone is the treatment of choice in hematologic malignancies, such as leukemia or lymphatic tumors with no localized focus of disease. Chemotherapy has been successful in treating certain lymphatic and leukemic diseases, commonly producing remissions of many years. Thousands of children who would have died within a year of diagnosis more than 15 years ago have now reached adulthood disease-free due to advances in chemotherapy.

Adjuvant chemotherapy is often administered after surgery or radiation of the primary lesion—even to patients showing no clinical evidence of disease—to destroy any remaining cancer cells and prevent local or metastatic recurrent disease.

Combination therapy

In the early 1950s methotrexate and nitrogen mustard were the only antineoplastic agents used; combination therapy wasn't tried until the late 1960s. Today, more than 30 cancer chemotherapeutic drugs are available and more than 50 others are being investigated.

Drug therapy seldom comprises a single agent; most cancer chemotherapy regimens combine at least three drugs. Combination therapy can triple or quadruple single-agent response rates, while minimizing toxicity.

Drugs are combined to delay the development of neoplastic cells resistant to specific antineoplastics. Also, drugs that act in different parts of the cell cycle or by different mechanisms can be used together synergistically. Furthermore, the highest tolerable dose of each drug may be used if drugs with different, rather than overlapping, side effects are combined. An example is the combination of prednisone and vincristine in the treatment of acute lymphocytic leukemia (ALL) in children. When these medications are used together for the initial treatment of ALL, the complete remission (CR) rate is higher than 90%. If either drug were used singly, the CR rate would be only about 50%.

In some cancers, such as leukemia, different antineoplastic agents are administered in a specific order to achieve optimal results. For instance, one drug may induce remission but not maintain it, so this drug is then followed by another more effective at maintaining the remission. Higher remission and survival rates are the goals of combination therapy.

Toxic effects of chemotherapy

Chemotherapy affects rapidly dividing cells. Unfortunately, the doses needed to obtain maximum therapeutic response are quite toxic. Actively dividing normal cells—such as bone marrow, skin, gastrointestinal (GI) mucosa, hair follicles, and fetal tissue—are the ones that are most susceptible to toxicity.

Patients should know the side effects that may occur with their medications and the measures that can alleviate them. Patients should be able to recognize potentially life-threatening side effects. Close monitoring and good patient care can prevent or minimize many side effects and make patients more comfortable.

The benefits of using chemotherapy in pregnant or lactating women should be weighed against the risks of probable teratogenicity, mutagenicity, and carcinogenicity in fetuses or infants. For the same reasons, some oncologists discourage men receiving chemotherapy from fathering children during treatment and for several months afterward. Most doctors advise women to avoid pregnancy during therapy.

Bone marrow depression

Bone marrow depression is usually the dose-limiting factor of an antineoplastic. Leukopenia and thrombocytopenia are indications of bone marrow depression. When a patient's WBC count falls below 4,000 cells/mm³, the dosage of most antineoplastics is reduced by 50%. Further dosage reductions are made as subsequent counts drop. When the WBC count falls below 2,500 cells/mm³, or the platelet count falls below 80,000 cells/mm³, all drugs except bleomycin are sometimes withheld. After the bone marrow recovers (WBC more than 4,000 cells/mm³ and platelet count more than 120,000 cells/mm³), therapy is resumed.

The patient should be carefully monitored for bone marrow depression, keeping the following in mind:

- The patient should know how to read a thermometer. He should take his temperature at home once daily in the late afternoon and report any temperature of 101° F. (38.3° C.) or higher to the doctor or nurse. Antipyretics, such as acetaminophen, mask fever and should not be taken unless ordered.
- The patient should avoid aspirin or any medication containing aspirin while on chemotherapy. Aspirin interferes with the clotting process.
- The patient should understand the importance of reporting for scheduled blood counts. Infection possible when the absolute granulocyte count falls below 1,000 cells/mm³.
- Prepare injection sites with iodophor or similar solutions to help prevent infection.
- Signs of infection, such as increased temperature, cough, sore throat, mouth sores, and burning on urination, should be reported immediately.
- Administering suppositories or I.M. injections should be avoided, and rectal temperatures shouldn't be taken if platelets fall below 50,000 cells/mm³. When platelets are at this level, the patient should use an electric razor and soft-bristled toothbrush to prevent injuring skin, which could lead to hemorrhage.
- The patient should report any signs of decreased platelet count, such as petechiae, ecchymoses, easy bruising, hematuria, bleeding from gums, or epistaxis. Antineoplastic destruction of platelets can cause spontaneous bleeding that is difficult to stop.
- Special care is required in watching for bone marrow depression in patients undergoing concurrent radiation therapy, as this may potentiate the problem. Myelosuppression is generally cumulative with antineoplastic agents, so a patient doesn't tolerate subsequent courses of treatment as well as the first.

Nausea and vomiting

Nausea, vomiting, and anorexia are common side effects of most chemotherapeutic agents.

Antineoplastics rapidly stimulate the brain's chemoreceptor trigger zone, which affects the vomiting center. Here are some guidelines for good patient care:

- Nausea and vomiting may increase with anxiety, so chemotherapy should be administered in a pleasant atmosphere.
- Good hydration should be maintained, especially before an antineoplastic is given. The patient may not be able to keep down food for several days after treatment, and dehydration must be prevented. Fluid—2 to 3 liters—should be forced daily. Carbonated beverages, Popsicles, and gelatin desserts are usually well tolerated. Carbonated beverages may also reduce nausea.
- Signs of dehydration: poor skin turgor, dryness; significant weight loss during treatment; signs of electrolyte imbalance. Supplemental I.V. therapy may be needed.
- When a fluid deficit is known, vital signs should be monitored closely.
- Elevated BUN is possible. Remnants of neoplastic cells are excreted through the kidneys and may affect the patient's renal function. Fluid intake and output, including emesis, should be recorded. Drug excretion depends on good urine output.
- Lotion may be applied to dry skin and water-soluble lubricant to dry lips.
- Each patient should be treated individually. Some patients prefer a light meal before receiving chemotherapy, whereas others prefer not to eat.
- Giving an antiemetic and small amounts of bland food 30 to 60 minutes *before* administering antineoplastics may help reduce nausea and vomiting. An antiemetic is more effective when given before rather than after chemotherapy. (Some oncologists request patients to start taking antiemetics 24 hours before treatment.)
- If a patient vomits after receiving an antineoplastic drug orally, it should be reported immediately; the drug may be lost and dosage may need to be adjusted.
- To speed recovery and lessen toxicity during the treatment course, the patient should eat well and drink sufficient fluids despite anorexia. The dietitian may be able to work out a diet the patient likes. (He's most likely to accept food that does not have an overpowering aroma.) The patient's family may bring his favorite soups or stews, or other foods that can be warmed easily. Mealtimes should be flexible and care that may tire the patient should be postponed until after he has eaten.
- If the patient develops a nutritional deficiency from chemotherapy, some dietary supplements should be requested and the dietitian asked to add more calories and protein to the patient's menu. Freezing the supplements and serving them like ice cream in sundaes and milk shakes may make them more palatable.

Diarrhea and constipation

Diarrhea and constipation are GI side effects of some antineoplastic agents. Diarrhea is due to the direct irritation of bowel mucosa caused by the death of rapidly dividing cells that line the GI tract. Constipation is an early symptom of central nervous system toxicity (neurotoxicity) resulting from drug therapy. Try to prevent diarrhea and constipation to avoid further irritation of the lower GI tract. Here's what you can do:

- If the patient has diarrhea, he should be given small feedings and decreased roughage; if he is constipated, he should be given increased roughage in his diet. A laxative, antidiarrheal, or stool softener should be ordered as needed.
- The patient should have access to a bathroom. If he's too weak to walk, a bedpan should be placed within his reach. After each bowel movement, the perianal area should be cleaned and dried. Protective cream should be applied to irritated skin.
- The patient should be observed for dehydration. Body fluids and electrolytes are lost with diarrhea. Electrolytes should be monitored.
- Fluid intake should be encouraged. I.V. therapy may be needed to replace lost fluids.
- Diarrhea should be recorded as output. Taking temperature rectally should be avoided as this may further irritate rectal mucosa.

Alopecia

Alopecia is common with certain antineoplastic drugs, and many patients find it distressing. Antineoplastics damage hair follicles perhaps even more than they do malignant cells. With many drugs, a patient may lose some or all of his hair, including scalp hair, eyelashes, eyebrows, and underarm and pubic hair.

HOW TO ANSWER PATIENTS' QUESTIONS ABOUT CHEMOTHERAPY

Before speaking to the patient about chemotherapy, assess his knowledge of his illness. He may not recognize or accept his illness as cancer. For instance, he may speak of "my tumor." Only after he himself tells you he has cancer should you use this word. If needed, modify the following answers to use the patient's own terms for his illness.

What is chemotherapy?

Chemotherapy literally means treatment with chemicals. However, it's commonly accepted to mean drug treatment of cancer.

Is there more than one type of chemotherapy?

Yes. Many drugs can be given many ways (orally, by injection into a muscle or subcutaneous tissue, or by intravenous infusion). One that is correct for you and your condition will be selected.

Will it hurt?

Not usually. However, with some intravenous drugs, you may experience a temporary burning or cold sensation. You will be told this beforehand, so you won't be alarmed if it happens.

How long will each treatment take?

This will depend on the kind and number of drugs. Some drugs are given directly into the vein; others are given with a running I.V. solution; still others are added to an I.V. solution and dripped in over a specified time. Ask your doctor or nurse how long the treatment will take.

Will I have to be hospitalized?

Most drugs can be given in your doctor's office or at a hospital's outpatient department. But if you are taking a drug that requires close medical supervision, you may have to be hospitalized.

How long will I have to take these drugs and how often?

Check with your doctor or nurse for a time estimate. Usually, the duration of treatment varies from several months to 2 years, depending on the type of cancer, the types and number of drugs, and your response to the drugs (including adverse reactions). Most drugs are given weekly or monthly. Between times, you may take an oral form at home.

Will I be sick when I have chemotherapy?

Everyone responds differently. With many of the drugs, you may experience nausea or vomiting. If you do, you will be given another drug to relieve it.

Will I be able to continue working or taking care of my family?

Again, this depends on the kind of cancer and response to treatment. You will probably be able to resume normal activities without problems. But if you feel a little tired after treatment, relax for the rest of the day.

May I have alcoholic drinks while I'm undergoing chemotherapy?

Usually, a cocktail or glass of wine will not be harmful, but ask your doctor.

Will my diet be restricted?

No. As long as you're not having any problems eating normally, continue to do so. If you have any problems, your doctor may suggest a diet change. You may tolerate chemotherapy better if you eat a light meal before and after the procedure. Also, increase your fluid intake by two to four glasses daily before, during, and after chemotherapy.

Should I discontinue other drugs I'm taking?

Tell your doctor about all other drugs you're taking, how much and how often. He needs to know this because some drugs can interfere with your chemotherapy. Examples of such drugs are anticoagulants, antibiotics, aspirin, barbiturates, diuretics, hormones, cough medicines, and medications for diabetes and high blood pressure. Your prescriptions should be adjusted as needed.

Is chemotherapy really worthwhile?

Patients *really do benefit* from chemotherapy with increased chances of survival and enhanced quality of life. Ultimately based on your condition and the kind of chemotherapy, only you and your family can decide how worthwhile it is for you.

• If the patient is receiving a drug that generally causes alopecia, he should know that this side effect is likely. His hair should begin to grow back about 8 weeks after therapy is stopped. With some drugs, new hair may grow even during maintenance therapy. However, the new hair may be a different texture or color. The patient may obtain a hairpiece, scarf, hat, or a ski cap before treatment begins.
• Hair loss usually begins several days after chemotherapy is given and may continue for several weeks. Once hair loss starts, some patients prefer to shave their heads rather than lose hair gradually. Some patients may experience hair thinning only.
• Usually, ice bags and scalp tourniquets don't prevent hair loss. Also, they may counteract the chemotherapy's effectiveness in blood-borne tumors. Their use is therefore not appropriate for some tumors and in the presence of metastatic disease.

Stomatitis
Inflammation of the buccal mucosa may occur with most antineoplastics but is most commonly associated with the antimetabolites and antibiotics. Remember:
• The patient should have all dental work completed before beginning chemotherapy, to reduce possible infection or bleeding. Ill-fitting dentures are potentially irritating and should be replaced before therapy begins. Denture fit should be checked periodically as patient's weight fluctuates.
• Good mouth care should be encouraged before and during treatment to help prevent oral side effects. Mucosal deterioration begins when more than 6 hours pass without good mouth care. Patient should use soft rayon-tipped swabs for mouth care. (Lemon-glycerin swabs should not be used because they dry the mouth.)
• To prevent gum irritation, the patient should use a soft-bristled toothbrush and dental floss unless he has thrombocytopenia. If platelet count falls below 50,000 cells/mm^3, he should discontinue brushing and flossing and use a mouth rinse frequently instead.
• The patient should cleanse his mouth by rinsing with hydrogen peroxide and water (1:6 solution) three to four times daily. If the peroxide is irritating, the patient may rinse with normal saline solution alone or with 1 teaspoon baking soda mixed with 1 liter normal saline solution, four times daily.
• If pain is a problem, the doctor may prescribe Benylin Elixir and Kaopectate (1:1) to be used as a mouthwash every 4 hours.
• To further reduce discomfort, the patient may use Xylocaine Viscous as an oral rinse before he eats. For severe mucositis, dilute Xylocaine Viscous 2% with equal part water.
• The patient with candidiasis may use nystatin suspension (mouthwash), vaginal tablets as lozenges, or flavored nystatin ice pops.
• The patient may apply a water-soluble lubricant such as KY jelly to treat or prevent cracked, dry lips.
• Soothing foods, such as milk products and Popsicles, should be encouraged. The patient should avoid tart, spicy, or rough-textured foods if his mouth becomes irritated or inflamed. The dietary staff should provide a soft, palatable diet to help prevent anorexia.
• Erythema of buccal mucosa may be an early symptom of bone marrow toxicity. Antineoplastic dosage should be lowered or the drug stopped to prevent oral ulceration. If stopped, therapy may be started again, at a lower dose, about 7 to 10 days after the ulcer heals. The patient should report ulcerations to the doctor or nurse.

Hyperuricemia
Hyperuricemia is a common problem in newly treated patients with hematologic malignancies, such as leukemia and lymphomas. Massive cell destruction releases purines,

COMMON TERMS IN CANCER CARE

BLOOD-RELATED TERMS

Absolute granulocyte count: the number of granulocytes (mostly neutrophils) per mm^3. To calculate, multiply % Polys times WBC. For example, WBC = 5,000/mm^3 Polys = 60%: 5,000 × 60% = 3,000.

Leukopenia: decrease in circulating WBCs (leukocytes)

Nadir: point at which blood counts (WBC or platelets) reach their lowest level as a result of chemotherapy (usually 7 to 10 days after dose). The patient is then at greatest risk of developing complications, such as infections.

Neutropenia: decrease in circulating neutrophils

Neutrophils: (polymorphonuclear leukocytes, PMNs, or Polys): the most important type of white cell for fighting acute infections

Pancytopenia: decreased level of all blood components –WBC, platelets, granulocytes

Thrombocytopenia: decrease in circulating platelets

SIDE EFFECTS

Cystitis: inflammation of the urinary bladder. Bleeding may develop (hemorrhagic cystitis)

Extravasation: leakage of fluid (or drug) out of the vein into surrounding tissue

Myelosuppression: suppression of bone marrow function

Stomatitis: inflammation of mucous membranes of the mouth; often appears as white patches on oral mucosa

TYPES OF THERAPY

Adjuvant therapy: chemotherapy and radiation therapy used in addition to surgery even though there is no evidence of metastasis and the patient is asymptomatic

Immunotherapy: administration of preformed antibodies (serum or gamma globulin) to produce or enhance immunity

Supportive therapy: treatment given with systemic chemotherapy (steroids, radiation, antibiotics, blood, etc.)

RESPONSE RATE

Complete (CR): complete disappearance of all measurable and evaluable disease

Partial (PR): 50% decrease of all measurable and evaluable disease except for hepatomegaly, in which only a 30% decrease is needed

No change: less than 50% decrease in all measurable and evaluable disease

Progression: appearance of any new lesions, or increase by 25% of any previously measurable disease

which convert to uric acid. The uric acid may precipitate into crystals in the kidneys and lead to renal failure. To minimize the risk of hyperuricemia:

- Force three liters of fluid daily; monitor intake and output; monitor serum uric acid and serum creatinine levels.
- Allopurinol prevents uric acid from forming. It should be ordered and started 24 hours before chemotherapy is initiated and continued throughout treatment.

Advances in cancer therapy

Researchers are constantly refining protocols; developing new, more effective drugs and methods of administering them; and searching for new solutions to the cancer problem. Synthetic antineoplastics, Interferon research, intra-arterial chemotherapy, and immunotherapy are examples of these continuing efforts.

71

Alkylating agents

busulfan
carmustine (BCNU)
chlorambucil
cisplatin (cis-platinum)
cyclophosphamide
dacarbazine (DTIC)
lomustine (CCNU)
mechlorethamine hydrochloride (nitrogen mustard)
melphalan
pipobroman
thiotepa
uracil mustard

Alkylating agents are anticancer or antitumor drugs developed from nitrogen mustard or its derivatives as a result of military research. Because these compounds produce bone marrow depression and atrophy of lymphoid tissue, they were first used to treat malignant lymphomas and leukemias. But since the introduction of mechlorethamine, the first nitrogen mustard, an intensive search for more potent and less toxic agents has been underway. Alkylating agents act during any phase of cellular activity, giving them an advantage over more specific antineoplastics, which are effective only during a single phase. This makes their toxicity nonspecific.

Major uses
Alkylating agents are used to treat carcinomas, sarcomas, lymphomas, and leukemias. They're also used to treat polycythemia vera.

Mechanism of action
Alkylating agents cross-link strands of cellular DNA, causing an imbalance of growth that leads to cell death.

Absorption, distribution, metabolism, and excretion
Busulfan, chlorambucil, cyclophosphamide, lomustine, melphalan, pipobroman, and uracil mustard are absorbed from the gastrointestinal tract after oral administration. All

HOW ALKYLATING AGENTS AFFECT DNA

Alkylating agents settle in the cell nucleus, where they attack DNA by binding its chains together or by breaking them apart (see diagram). They act at all phases of the cell cycle and so are called cell-cycle nonspecific agents.

Because of their inability to selectively attack cancer cells, they also affect other rapidly dividing cells, such as those in the gastrointestinal mucosa, hair follicles, and bone marrow.

Consequently, their common side effects include gastrointestinal irritation, alopecia, and pancytopenia.

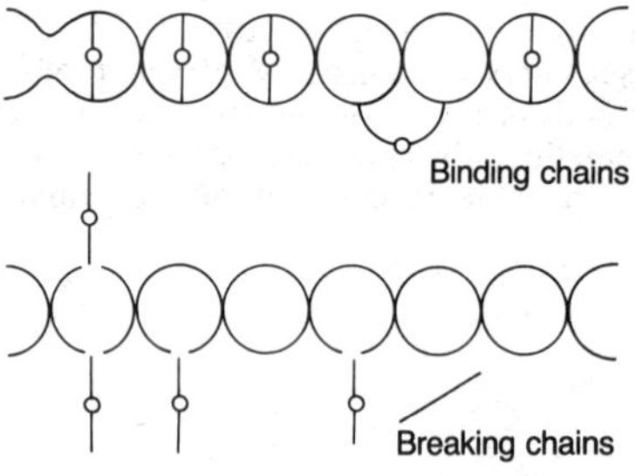

CISPLATIN: A BREAKTHROUGH FOR THE CANCER PATIENT

Cisplatin (Platinol) is a new and very effective intravenous drug for cancer. As the name implies, cisplatin (also called cis-platinum) is a derivative of the heavy metal platinum. Although it's officially approved to treat only testicular and ovarian tumors, cisplatin may also be prescribed for both bladder and head and neck cancer, as well as for other primary tumors.

Cisplatin is especially effective because it works well together with other chemotherapeutic drugs. Before the advent of cisplatin, testicular and ovarian tumors resisted most attempts at chemotherapy. But when cisplatin is combined with vinblastine (Velban, Velbe) and bleomycin (Blenoxane) for testicular cancer, the response rate is between 84% and 100%. When combined with doxorubicin (Adriamycin) for ovarian cancer, the response rate is between 50% and 92%.

Common side effects

When cisplatin is given by I.V. push or by a rapid infusion (taking less than 2 hours), the patient will almost always experience severe nausea and vomiting. Symptoms usually begin within an hour. The vomiting usually subsides within 24 to 36 hours, but the patient may be nauseated for several days. When the infusions run over a longer period, these symptoms are still present but are milder.

Administration tips

To prepare the drug for administration, reconstitute each vial with sterile water for injection. (Keep unreconstituted cisplatin refrigerated, but store the reconstituted drug at room temperature; if refrigerated, it may precipitate.) When adding the reconstituted cisplatin to the I.V. container, be sure to dilute it with either normal or half-normal saline solution to prolong the drug's stability. You don't have to protect the container from light when infusing the cisplatin solution.

Aluminum reacts with cisplatin, making cisplatin lose its potency. Therefore, don't use I.V. sets, catheters, or needles that contain aluminum when preparing or administering cisplatin.

DON'T USE THESE PRODUCTS WHEN PREPARING OR ADMINISTERING CISPLATIN

A partial list of aluminum-containing products

Disposable needles

Jelco disposable needle 22-1½"—
HRI 8003-002305 and
HRI 8003-002307

Monoject (Sherwood) #200 and #250 disposable needle 20-1"

I.V. administration sets

McGaw Disposable SECONDARY SET for use with ADDit I.V.®
Primary Sets V 1903

Travenol 2CO418 Add-A-Line™ secondary medication set, 86 cm (34") long

other alkylating agents must be administered parenterally.

- All alkylating agents are distributed widely to body tissues. Carmustine, lomustine, and thiotepa diffuse into the cerebrospinal fluid and cross the blood-brain barrier.
- All alkylating agents except thiotepa are metabolized in the liver and excreted in the urine as either active or inactive metabolites. Thiotepa is excreted unchanged by the kidneys.

Onset and duration

Therapeutic activity varies with the alkylating agent, disease, and patient response.

NAMES, INDICATIONS AND DOSAGES	SIDE EFFECTS
busulfan Myleran♦ **Chronic myelocytic (granulocytic) leukemia:** ADULTS: 4 to 6 mg P.O. daily up to 8 mg P.O. daily until WBC falls to 10,000/mm^3; stop drug until WBC rises to 50,000/mm^3, then resume treatment as before; or 4 to 8 mg P.O. daily until WBC falls to 10,000 to 20,000/mm^3, then reduce daily dose as needed to maintain WBC at this level (usually 2 mg daily). CHILDREN: 0.06 to 0.12 mg/kg or 2.3 to 4.6 mg/m^2/day P.O.; adjust dose to maintain WBC at 20,000/mm^3, but never less than 10,000/mm^3.	**Blood:** WBC falling after about 10 days and continuing to fall for 2 weeks after stopping drug; *thrombocytopenia,* pancytopenia, anemia. **GI:** nausea, vomiting, diarrhea, cheilosis, glossitis. **GU:** amenorrhea, testicular atrophy, impotence. **Metabolic:** Addison-like wasting syndrome, profound hyperuricemia due to increased cell lysis. **Skin:** transient hyperpigmentation, anhidrosis. **Other:** gynecomastia; alopecia; *irreversible pulmonary fibrosis, commonly termed "busulfan lung."*
carmustine (BCNU) BiCNU♦ **Brain, colon, and stomach cancer; Hodgkin's disease; non-Hodgkin's lymphomas; melanomas; multiple myeloma; and hepatoma:** ADULTS: 100 mg/m^2 I.V. by slow infusion daily for 2 days; repeat q 6 weeks if platelets are above 100,000/mm^3 and WBC is above 4,000/mm^3. Dose is reduced 50% when WBC less than 2,000/mm^3 and platelets less than 25,000/mm^3. *Alternate therapy*—200 mg/m^2 I.V. slow infusion as a single dose, repeated q 6 to 8 weeks; or 40 mg/m^2 I.V. slow infusion for 5 consecutive days, repeated q 6 weeks.	**Blood:** *cumulative bone marrow depression, delayed 4 to 6 weeks, lasting 1 to 2 weeks; leukopenia; thrombocytopenia.* **GI:** *nausea, which lasts 2 to 6 hours after giving (can be severe); vomiting.* **Hepatic:** hepatotoxicity. **Metabolic:** possible hyperuricemia in lymphoma patients when rapid cell lysis occurs. **Local:** *intense pain at infusion site.* **Other:** *pulmonary fibrosis.*
chlorambucil Leukeran♦ **Chronic lymphocytic leukemia, lymphosarcoma, giant follicular lymphoma, Hodgkin's disease, ovarian carcinoma, mycosis fungoides:** ADULTS: 0.1 to 0.2 mg/kg P.O. daily for 3 to 6 weeks, then adjust for maintenance (usually 2 mg daily). CHILDREN: 0.1 to 0.2 mg/kg/day or 4.5 mg/m^2/day P.O. as single dose or in divided doses.	**Blood:** leukopenia, delayed up to 3 weeks, lasting up to 10 days after last dose; thrombocytopenia; anemia; myelosuppression (usually moderate, gradual, and rapidly reversible). **Metabolic:** hyperuricemia. **Skin:** *exfoliative dermatitis.* **Other:** allergic febrile reactions.
cisplatin (cis-platinum) Platinol **Adjunctive therapy in metastatic testicular cancer:** ADULTS: 20 mg/m^2 I.V. daily for 5 days. Repeat every 3 weeks for 3 cycles or longer. **Adjunctive therapy in metastatic ovarian cancer:** 100 mg/m^2 I.V. Repeat every 4 weeks; or 50 mg/m^2 I.V. every 3 weeks with concurrent doxorubicin HCl therapy. Give as I.V. infusion in 2 liters normal saline solution with 37.5 g	**Blood:** *reversible myelosuppression in 25% to 30% of patients, leukopenia, thrombocytopenia,* anemia; nadirs in circulating platelets and leukocytes on days 18 to 23, with recovery by day 39. **CNS:** peripheral neuritis, loss of taste, seizures. **EENT:** *tinnitus, hearing loss.* **GI:** *nausea, vomiting, beginning 1 to 4 hours after dose and lasting 24 hours; diarrhea.* **GU:** *more prolonged and severe renal toxicity with repeated courses of therapy.* **Other:** anaphylactoid reaction.

INTERACTIONS AND SPECIAL CONSIDERATIONS

No significant interactions.

Special considerations:

- Use cautiously in patients recently given other myelosuppressive drugs or radiation treatment, and in those with depressed neutrophil or platelet counts.
- Infection (fever, sore throat) is possible.
- Side effects may be delayed for 4 to 6 months.
- Persistent cough, progressive dyspnea with alveolar exudate may result from drug toxicity, not pneumonia.
- Uric acid and CBC should be monitored.
- Patient response usually begins within 1 to 2 weeks (increased appetite, sense of well-being, decreased total leukocyte count, reduction in size of spleen).
- Can cause false-positive cytology in all body secretions.
- Anticoagulants should be used cautiously. Bleeding is possible.
- All I.M. injections should be avoided when platelets are low.

No significant interactions.

Special considerations:

- To reduce pain on infusion, should be further diluted or infusion rate slowed.
- Signs of infection and bone marrow toxicity (fever, sore throat, anemia, fatigue, easy bruising, nose or gum bleeds, melena) are possible. Temperature should be taken daily.
- Uric acid and CBC should be monitored.
- To reduce nausea, antiemetic should be given before administering.
- Should not be mixed with other drugs during administration.
- To reconstitute: dissolve 100 mg carmustine in 3 ml absolute alcohol; dilute solution with 27 ml sterile water for injection. Resultant solution contains 3.3 mg carmustine/ml in 10% alcohol. Dilute in normal saline solution or dextrose 5% in water for I.V. infusion; give at least 250 ml over 1 to 2 hours.
- Reconstituted solution may be stored in refrigerator for 24 hours.
- If powder liquefies or appears oily, it is sign of decomposition; should be discarded.
- Can cause false-positive cytology in all body secretions.
- To prevent hyperuricemia with resulting uric acid nephropathy, allopurinol may be used with adequate hydration and alkalinization of urine. Urine should be screened for stones.
- Contact with skin should be avoided, as carmustine will cause a brown stain. If drug comes into contact with skin, should be washed off thoroughly.
- Anticoagulants should be used cautiously. Bleeding is possible.
- All I.M. injections should be avoided when platelets are low.

No significant interactions.

Special considerations:

- Myelosuppression reversible up to cumulative dose of 6.5 mg/kg.
- Uric acid and CBC should be monitored.
- To prevent hyperuricemia with resulting uric acid nephropathy, allopurinol may be used with adequate hydration and alkalinization of urine. Urine should be screened for stones.
- Can cause false-positive cytology in all body secretions.
- I.M. injections should be avoided when platelets are low.
- Anticoagulants should be used cautiously. Bleeding is possible.

No significant interactions.

Special considerations:

- Contraindicated in preexisting renal impairment, myelosuppression, and hearing impairment.
- Patient should be hydrated with normal saline solution before drug is given, and urine output of 100 ml/hour maintained for 4 consecutive hours before therapy and for 24 hours after therapy.
- Aluminum needles should not be used for reconstitution or administration of cis-platinum; a black precipitate may form.
- Mannitol may be given as 12.5 g I.V. bolus before starting cis-platinum infusion; followed by infusion of mannitol at rate up to 10 g/hour p.r.n. to maintain urine output during and 6 to 24 hours after cis-platinum infusion.
- Dose should not be repeated unless platelets are over 100,000/mm^3, WBC is over 4,000/mm^3, creatinine is under 1.5 mg%, or BUN is under 25 mg%.
- CBC, platelets, and renal function studies

(continued on following page)

NAMES, INDICATIONS AND DOSAGES	SIDE EFFECTS

cisplatin
(continued)

mannitol over 6 to 8 hours.

Note: Prehydration and mannitol diuresis may reduce renal toxicity and ototoxicity significantly.

cyclophosphamide
Cytoxan♦, Procytox♦♦

Breast, colon, head, neck, lung, ovarian, and prostatic cancer; Hodgkin's disease; chronic lymphocytic leukemia; chronic myelocytic leukemia; acute lymphoblastic leukemia; neuroblastoma; retinoblastoma; non-Hodgkin's lymphomas; multiple myeloma; mycosis fungoides; sarcomas:

ADULTS: 40 to 50 mg/kg P.O. or I.V. in single dose or in 2 to 5 daily doses, then adjust for maintenance; or 2 to 4 mg/kg P.O. daily for 10 days, then adjust for maintenance. Maintenance dose 1.5 to 3 mg/kg/day P.O.; or 10 to 15 mg/kg q 7 to 10 days I.V.; or 3 to 5 mg/kg twice weekly I.V.

CHILDREN: 2 to 8 mg/kg/day or 60 to 250 mg/m²/day P.O. or I.V. for 6 days (dose depends on susceptibility of neoplasm); divide oral dosages; give I.V. dosages once weekly. Maintenance dose 2 to 5 mg/kg or 50 to 150 mg/m² twice weekly P.O.

Blood: *leukopenia,* nadir between days 8 to 15, recovery in 17 to 28 days; thrombocytopenia; anemia.
CV: *cardiotoxicity* (with very high doses and in combination with doxorubicin).
GI: anorexia; *nausea and vomiting beginning within 6 hours, lasting 4 hours;* stomatitis; mucositis.
GU: gonadal suppression (may be irreversible), *hemorrhagic cystitis,* bladder fibrosis, sterility, nephrotoxicity.
Metabolic: hyperuricemia; syndrome of inappropriate ADH secretion (with high doses).
Other: *alopecia in 50% of patients, especially with high doses;* secondary malignancies, *pulmonary fibrosis (high doses).*

dacarbazine (DTIC)
DTIC-Dome♦

Hodgkin's disease, metastatic malignant melanoma, neuroblastoma, sarcomas:

ADULTS: 2 to 4.5 mg/kg or 70 to 160 mg/m² I.V. daily for 10 days, then repeat q 4 weeks as tolerated; or 250 mg/m² I.V. daily for 5 days, repeated at 3-week intervals.

Blood: *WBC falling for up to 5 weeks, recovering in 2 weeks; thrombocytopenia.*
GI: *severe nausea and vomiting begin within 1 to 3 hours in 90% of patients, last 1 to 12 hours; anorexia.*
Local: severe pain if I.V. infiltrates or if solution is too concentrated; tissue damage.
Other: *flulike syndrome* (fever, malaise, myalgia beginning 7 days after treatment stopped and possibly lasting 7 to 21 days), alopecia.

lomustine (CCNU)
CeeNU♦

Brain, colon, lung, and renal cell cancer; Hodgkin's disease; lymphomas; melanomas; multiple myeloma:

ADULTS AND CHILDREN: 130 mg/m² P.O. as single dose q 6 weeks. Reduce dose according to bone marrow depression. Repeat doses should not be given until WBC is more than 4,000/mm³

Blood: *leukopenia, delayed up to 6 weeks, lasting 1 to 2 weeks; thrombocytopenia, delayed up to 4 weeks, lasting 1 to 2 weeks.*
GI: *nausea and vomiting beginning within 4 to 5 hours, lasting 24 hours;* stomatitis.
Other: alopecia.

♦ Available in U.S. and Canada. ♦♦ Available in Canada only.
All other products (no symbol) available in U.S. only. Italicized side effects are common or life-threatening.

INTERACTIONS AND SPECIAL CONSIDERATIONS

should be monitored before initial and subsequent doses.
• Patient should report tinnitus immediately to prevent permanent hearing loss. Audiometry recommended before and during treatment.
• Nausea and vomiting may be severe and protracted (up to 24 hours.) Antiemetics can be started 24 hours before therapy. Intake and output should be monitored. I.V. hydration should be continued until patient can tolerate adequate oral intake.
• For I.V. administration: reconstitute with sterile water for injection; stable for 8 hours at room temperature; don't refrigerate.
• Given with bleomycin and vinblastine for testicular cancer and with doxorubicin HCl for ovarian cancer.
• Also used in treatment of advanced bladder cancer.
• Renal toxicity becomes more severe with repeated doses. Renal function must return to normal before next dose can be given.
• I.M. injections should be avoided when platelets are low.

Interactions:
CORTICOSTEROIDS, CHLORAMPHENICOL: reduced activity of cyclophosphamide. Use cautiously.
ALLOPURINOL: may produce excessive cyclophosphamide effect. Monitor for enhanced toxicity.

Special considerations:
• Use cautiously in severe leukopenia, thrombocytopenia, malignant cell infiltration of bone marrow, recent radiation therapy or chemotherapy, hepatic or renal disease.
• Male and female patients should practice contraception while taking this drug and for 4 months after; drug is potentially teratogenic.
• Uric acid, CBC, and renal and hepatic functions should be monitored.
• To reduce nausea, antiemetic should be given before administering.
• Fluid (3 liters daily) should be pushed to prevent hemorrhagic cystitis. Drug should not be given at bedtime, since voiding is too infrequent to avoid cystitis. If hemorrhagic cystitis occurs, drug is stopped. Cystitis can occur months after therapy has been stopped.
• Reconstituted solution is stable 6 days refrigerated or 24 hours at room temperature.
• Can cause false-positive cytology in all body secretions.
• I.M. injections should be avoided when platelets are low.
• Can be given by direct I.V. push into a running I.V. line or by infusion in normal saline solution or dextrose 5% in water.
• To prevent hyperuricemia with resulting uric acid nephropathy, patient should be kept well hydrated and urine alkalinized.
• Alopecia is likely to occur.
• Anticoagulants should be used cautiously. Bleeding is possible.
• Has been used successfully to treat many nonmalignant conditions.

No significant interactions.

Special considerations:
• Lower dose required if renal function or bone marrow is impaired, and drug should be stopped if WBC falls to 3,000/mm³ or platelets drop to 100,000/mm³.
• Temperature should be taken daily. Infection is possible.
• Uric acid and CBC should be monitored.
• Refrigerated solution should be discarded after 72 hours; room temperature solution after 8 hours.
• Can cause false-positive cytology in all body secretions.
• I.M. injections should be avoided when platelets are low.
• I.V. infusion should be given in 50 to 100 ml dextrose 5% in water over 30 minutes. May dilute further or slow infusion to decrease pain at infusion site. Drug infiltration should be avoided.
• For Hodgkin's disease, usually given with bleomycin, vinblastine, doxorubicin.
• Anticoagulants should be used cautiously. Bleeding is possible.
• Antiemetics administered before giving dacarbazine may help decrease nausea. Nausea and vomiting usually subside after several doses.

No significant interactions.

Special considerations:
• Should be given 2 to 4 hours after meals. To avoid nausea, antiemetic should be given before administering.
• May be useful in cancer involving CNS, since cerebrospinal fluid level equals 30% to 50% of plasma level 1 hour after administration.
• Blood counts should be monitored weekly. Should not be given more often than every 6 weeks; bone marrow toxicity is cumulative and delayed.
• Uric acid and CBC should be monitored.
• Can cause false-positive cytology in all body secretions.
• I.M. injection should be avoided when platelets are low.
• For Hodgkin's disease, usually given with mechlorethamine.

(continued on following page)

NAMES, INDICATIONS AND DOSAGES	SIDE EFFECTS

lomustine
(continued)

and platelet count is more than 100,000/mm³.

---

mechlorethamine hydrochloride (nitrogen mustard)
Mustargen♦

Breast, lung, and ovarian cancer; Hodgkin's disease; non-Hodgkin's lymphomas; lymphosarcoma:
ADULTS: 0.4 mg/kg or 10 mg/m² I.V. as single or divided dose q 3 to 6 weeks. Give through running I.V. infusion. Dose reduced in prior radiation or chemotherapy to 0.2 to 0.4 mg/kg. Dose based on ideal or actual body weight, whichever is less.

Neoplastic effusions:
ADULTS: 10 to 20 mg intracavitarily.

Blood: *nadir of leukopenia, thrombocytopenia, myelosuppression occuring by days 4 to 10, lasting 10 to 21 days;* mild anemia begins in 2 to 3 weeks, possibly lasting 7 weeks.
EENT: tinnitus, *metallic taste,* immediately after dose; deafness in high doses.
GI: *nausea, vomiting, and anorexia begin within minutes, last 8 to 24 hours.*
Metabolic: hyperuricemia.
Local: *thrombophlebitis, sloughing, severe irritation if drug extravasates or touches skin.*
Other: *alopecia,* may precipitate herpes zoster.

---

melphalan
Alkeran♦

Multiple myeloma, malignant melanoma, testicular seminoma, reticulum cell sarcoma, osteogenic sarcoma, breast and ovarian cancer:
ADULTS: 6 mg P.O. daily for 2 to 3 weeks, then stop drug for up to 4 weeks or until WBC and platelets stop dropping and begin to rise again; resume with maintenance dose of 2 to 4 mg daily. Stop drug if WBC below 3,000/mm³ or platelets below 100,000/mm³.
Alternate therapy—0.15 mg/kg/day P.O. for 7 days, wait for WBC and platelets to recover, then resume with 0.05 mg/kg/day P.O.

Blood: *thrombocytopenia, leukopenia, agranulocytosis.*
GI: anorexia, nausea, vomiting.
Other: *pneumonitis.*

---

pipobroman
Vercyte♦

Polycythemia vera:
ADULTS AND CHILDREN OVER 15 YEARS: 1 mg/kg P.O. daily for 30 days; may increase to 1.5 to 3 mg/kg P.O. daily until hematocrit reduced to 50% to 55%, then 0.1 to 0.2 mg/kg daily maintenance.

Chronic myelocytic leukemia:
ADULTS AND CHILDREN OVER 15 YEARS: 1.5 to 2.5 mg/kg P.O. daily until WBC drops to 10,000/mm³, then start maintenance 7 to 175 mg daily. Stop drug if WBC below 3,000/mm³ or platelets below 150,000/mm³.

Blood: *leukopenia and thrombocytopenia, delayed up to 4 weeks or longer.*
GI: nausea, vomiting, cramping, diarrhea, anorexia.
Skin: rash.

♦ Available in U.S. and Canada. ♦♦ Available in Canada only.
All other products (no symbol) available in U.S. only. Italicized side effects are common or life-threatening.

INTERACTIONS AND SPECIAL CONSIDERATIONS

- Anticoagulants should be used cautiously. Bleeding is possible.
- Can cause alopecia, but hair will grow back.

No significant interactions.

Special considerations:

- Use cautiously in severe anemia, depressed neutrophil or platelet counts, and in patients recently treated with radiation or chemotherapy.
- Contact with skin or mucous membranes should be avoided. If contact occurs, skin should be washed with copious amounts of water.
- Giving antiemetic before drug not always effective in reducing nausea.
- I.V. infiltration should be avoided. If drug extravasates, cold compresses should be applied.
- When given intracavitarily, patient should be turned from side to side every 15 minutes to 1 hour to distribute drug.
- Uric acid and CBC should be monitored.
- Severe herpes zoster may require stopping drug.
- Very unstable solution. Should be prepared immediately before infusion and used within 15 minutes. Unused solution should be discarded.
- To prevent hyperuricemia with resulting uric acid nephropathy, allopurinol may be given; patient should be kept well hydrated and urine alkalinized.
- Can cause false-positive cytology in all body secretions.
- I.M. injections should be avoided when platelets are low.
- One of the most effective drugs in treatment of Hodgkin's disease.
- Has been used topically in treatment of mycosis fungoides.
- Anticoagulants should be used cautiously. Bleeding is possible.

No significant interactions.

Special considerations:

- Not recommended in severe leukopenia, thrombocytopenia, or anemia; chronic lymphocytic leukemia; or suppurative inflammation.
- To reduce nausea, antiemetic should be given before administering.
- Uric acid and CBC should be monitored.
- Can cause false-positive cytology in all body secretions.
- I.M. injections should be avoided when platelets are low.
- May need dose reduction in renal impairment.
- Drug of choice in multiple myeloma.
- Anticoagulants should be used cautiously. Bleeding is possible.

No significant interactions.

Special considerations:

- Contraindicated in bone marrow depression.
- WBC and platelet count should be done until desired response or toxicity occurs (platelets less than 150,000/mm^3 or WBC less than 3,000/mm^3).
- CBC should be monitored.
- Anticoagulants should be used cautiously. Bleeding is possible.

NAMES, INDICATIONS AND DOSAGES	SIDE EFFECTS

thiotepa
Thiotepa♦

ADULTS AND CHILDREN OVER 12 YEARS:
Breast, lung, and ovarian cancer; Hodgkin's disease; lymphomas: 0.2 mg/kg I.V. daily for 5 days; then maintenance dose of 0.2 mg/kg I.V. q 1 to 3 weeks.

Bladder tumor: 60 mg in 60 ml water instilled in bladder once weekly for 4 weeks.

Neoplastic effusions: 10 to 15 mg intracavitarily, p.r.n. Stop drug or decrease dosage if WBC below 4,000/mm^3 or if platelets below 150,000/mm^3.

Blood: *leukopenia begins within 5 to 30 days; thrombocytopenia; neutropenia.*
GI: nausea, vomiting, anorexia.
GU: amenorrhea, decreased spermatogenesis.
Metabolic: hyperuricemia.
Skin: hives, rash.
Local: intense pain at administration site.
Other: headache, fever, tightness of throat, dizziness.

uracil mustard

Chronic lymphocytic and myelocytic leukemia; Hodgkin's disease; non-Hodgkin's lymphomas of the histiocytic and lymphocytic types; reticulum cell sarcoma; lymphomas; mycosis fungoides; polycythemia vera; cancer of ovaries, cervix, and lungs:
ADULTS: 1 to 2 mg P.O. daily for 3 months or until desired response or toxicity; maintenance 1 mg daily for 3 out of 4 weeks until optimum response or relapse; or 3 to 5 mg P.O. for 7 days not to exceed total dose 0.5 mg/kg, then 1 mg daily until response, then 1 mg daily 3 out of 4 weeks.

Blood: bone marrow depression, delayed 2 to 4 weeks; *thrombocytopenia; leukopenia;* anemia.
CNS: irritability, nervousness, mental cloudiness and depression.
GI: *nausea, vomiting, diarrhea, epigastric distress,* abdominal pain, anorexia.
Metabolic: hyperuricemia.
Skin: pruritus, dermatitis, hyperpigmentation, alopecia.

♦ Available in U.S. and Canada. ♦♦ Available in Canada only.
All other products (no symbol) available in U.S. only. Italicized side effects are common or life-threatening.

INTERACTIONS AND SPECIAL CONSIDERATIONS

No significant interactions.

Special considerations:

- Use cautiously in bone marrow depression, chronic lymphocytic leukemia, renal or hepatic dysfunction.
- WBC and RBC counts should be done weekly for at least 3 weeks after last dose. Patient should report even mild infections.
- GU side effects reversible in 6 to 8 months.
- May require use of local anesthetic at injection site if intense pain occurs.
- For bladder instillation: dehydrate patient 8 to 10 hours before therapy; instill drug into bladder by catheter; ask patient to retain solution for 2 hours. Volume may be reduced to 30 ml if discomfort is too great with 60 ml. Patient should be repositioned every 15 minutes for maximum area contact.
- Toxicity delayed and prolonged because drug binds to tissue and stays in body several hours.
- Uric acid and CBC should be monitored.
- Dry powder should be refrigerated and protected from light.
- Only sterile water for injection should be used to reconstitute. Refrigerated solution stable 5 days.
- To prevent hyperuricemia with resulting uric acid nephropathy, allopurinol may be given; patient should be kept well hydrated, and urine alkalinized.
- Can cause false-positive cytology in all body secretions.
- I.M. injections should be avoided when platelets are low.
- Can be given by all parenteral routes, including direct injection into tumor.
- Anticoagulants should be used cautiously. Bleeding is possible.
- When drug therapy is initiated, female patients should be advised that amenorrhea is possible.

No significant interactions.

Special considerations:

- Not recommended in severe thrombocytopenia, aplastic anemia or leukopenia, acute leukemias.
- Should be given at bedtime to reduce nausea.
- Patient may develop ecchymoses, easy bruising, petechiae.
- Uric acid should be monitored, and regular platelet count done. CBC should be done 1 to 2 times weekly for 4 weeks; then 4 weeks after stopping drug.
- Drug should not be given within 2 to 3 weeks after maximum bone marrow depression from past radiation or chemotherapy.
- To prevent hyperuricemia and resulting uric acid nephropathy, allopurinol can be given; patient should be kept hydrated, and urine alkalinized.
- Can cause false-positive cytology in all body secretions.
- I.M. injections should be avoided when platelets are low.
- Anticoagulants should be used cautiously. Bleeding is possible.

72

Antimetabolites

azathioprine
cytarabine
floxuridine
fluorouracil
hydroxyurea
mercaptopurine
methotrexate
methotrexate sodium
thioguanine

Antimetabolites, the first group of antineoplastics designed specifically as antitumor agents, function in one of two ways—as replacements for cellular components or as enzyme inhibitors. When they replace a necessary component in a cellular compound, the resulting cell product fails to function, blocking cell division. When antimetabolites inhibit a key enzyme reaction, they interfere with cellular metabolism.

Antimetabolites can be grouped as folic acid antagonists (methotrexate and methotrexate sodium); purine antagonists (azathioprine, mercaptopurine, and thioguanine); and pyrimidine antagonists (cytarabine, floxuridine, and fluorouracil). Hydroxyurea also functions as an antimetabolite but cannot be assigned to any group.

Major uses

Antimetabolites, with the exception of azathioprine, are used to treat carcinomas (mostly of the breast and gastrointestinal tract), trophoblastic tumors such as choriocarcinomas and hydatidiform moles, medulloblastomas, and osteogenic sarcomas.

• Azathioprine produces immunosuppression in renal transplants and is also indicated in the treatment of severe, active rheumatoid arthritis when other measures aren't effective.

Mechanism of action

All the antimetabolites interfere with DNA synthesis as follows:

• Azathioprine, mercaptopurine, and thioguanine inhibit purine synthesis.
• Cytarabine, floxuridine, and fluorouracil inhibit pyrimidine synthesis.
• Hydroxyurea inhibits ribonucleotide reductase.
• Methotrexate prevents reduction of folic acid to tetrahydrofolate by binding to dihydrofolate reductase.

Absorption, distribution, metabolism, and excretion

• Azathioprine, hydroxyurea, mercaptopurine, methotrexate, and thioguanine are well absorbed when given orally.
• Cytarabine, floxuridine, and fluorouracil are not absorbed after oral administration and must be given parenterally. However, fluorouracil can be administered orally in local treatment of some gastrointestinal carcinomas.

HOW ANTIMETABOLITES AFFECT THE CELL CYCLE

Antimetabolites are cell cycle–specific antineoplastics. Like all antineoplastics, by interrupting protein synthesis they prevent cells—including cancer cells—from reproducing and surviving.

A cell's various proteins are manufactured at specific points during the cell cycle, which is divided in these distinct phases:

- **phase G_1:** the period immediately before DNA synthesis (at this time, the cell may also become dormant, a state designated G_0)
- **phase S:** DNA synthesis
- **phase G_2:** RNA synthesis
- **phase M:** mitosis (prophase, metaphase, anaphase, and telophase).

The duration of a cell's life cycle differs according to its tissue of origin, but on the average the process—excluding mitosis—takes 10 hours.

Antimetabolites act during the entire cell cycle but are most effective during phase S. They are divided into folic acid antagonists (which interfere with biosynthetic enzymes), and purine and pyrimidine antagonists (which take the place of normal components during both DNA and RNA synthesis). Antimetabolites destroy healthy cells as well as those that are diseased; their limited toxicity can be attributed to the different rates at which different cells grow. The degree of their toxicity is such, however, that they have the narrowest range of application of all antineoplastics.

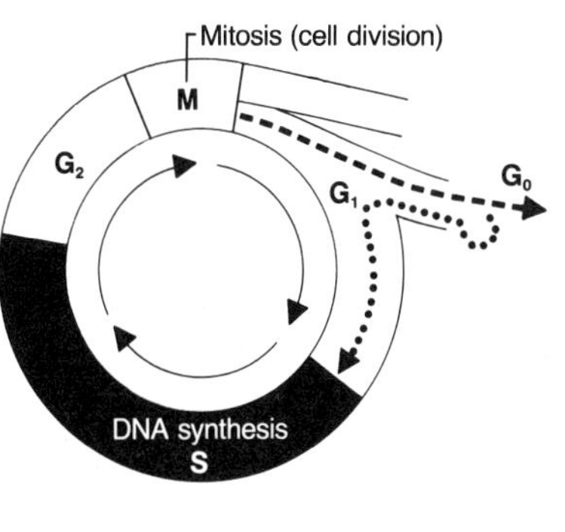

• All antimetabolites are distributed widely in body tissues and fluids, metabolized in the liver, and excreted in urine, largely as inactive metabolites.

Onset and duration
Therapeutic activity varies with the antimetabolite, disease, and patient response.

Combination products
None.

NAMES, INDICATIONS AND DOSAGES	SIDE EFFECTS
azathioprine Imuran ♦ **Immunosuppression in renal transplants:** ADULTS AND CHILDREN: initially, 3 to 5 mg/kg P.O. daily. Maintain at 1 to 2 mg/kg/day (dose varies considerably according to patient response). **Treatment of severe, refractory rheumatoid arthritis:** ADULTS: initially, 1 mg/kg taken as a single dose or as 2 doses. If patient response not satisfactory after 6 to 8 weeks, dosage may be increased by 0.5 mg/kg/day (up to a maximum of 2.5 mg/kg/day) at 4-week intervals.	**Blood:** *leukopenia, bone marrow depression,* anemia, pancytopenia, thrombocytopenia. **GI:** nausea, vomiting, anorexia, pancreatitis, ascites, steatorrhea, mouth ulceration, esophagitis. **Hepatic:** hepatoxicity, jaundice. **Skin:** rash. **Other:** *immunosuppression (possibly profound),* arthralgia, muscle wasting, alopecia, pancreatitis.
cytarabine (ARA-C, cytosine arabinoside) Cytosar-U ♦ **Acute myelocytic and other acute leukemias:** ADULTS AND CHILDREN: 2 to 3 mg/kg (100 mg/m²) I.V. or S.C. b.i.d. for 7 days; 2 to 3 mg/kg (100 mg/m²) daily for 7 days by 24-hour continuous infusion; or 10 to 30 mg/m² intrathecally, up to 3 times weekly. Maintenance 2 to 3 mg/kg I.V. or S.C. b.i.d. for 5 days.	**Blood:** WBC nadir 5 to 7 days after drug stopped; *leukopenia, anemia, thrombocytopenia,* reticulocytopenia; platelet nadir occurring on day 10; *megaloblastosis.* **GI:** *nausea, vomiting,* diarrhea, dysphagia; reddened area at juncture of lips, followed by sore mouth, oral ulcers in 5 to 10 days; high dose given via rapid I.V. may cause projectile vomiting. **Hepatic:** hepatotoxicity (usually mild and reversible). **Other:** flulike syndrome.
floxuridine FUDR **Brain, breast, head, neck, liver, gallbladder, and bile duct cancer:** ADULTS: 0.1 to 0.6 mg/kg daily by intra-arterial infusion (use pump for continuous, uniform rate); or 0.4 to 0.6 mg/kg daily into hepatic artery.	**Blood:** *leukopenia, anemia,* thrombocytopenia. **CNS:** cerebellar ataxia, vertigo, nystagmus, convulsions, depression, hemiplegia, hiccups, lethargy. **EENT:** blurred vision. **GI:** *stomatitis, cramps, nausea, vomiting, diarrhea, bleeding, enteritis.* **Skin:** *erythema,* dermatitis, pruritus, rash.
fluorouracil (5-fluorouracil) Adrucil, 5-FU **Colon, rectal, breast, ovarian, cervical, bladder, liver, and pancreatic cancer:** ADULTS: 12.5 mg/kg I.V. daily for 3 to 5 days q 4 weeks; or 15 mg/kg weekly for 6 weeks. (Doses recommended based on lean body weight.)	**Blood:** *leukopenia, thrombocytopenia,* anemia. WBC nadir 9 to 14 days after first dose; platelet nadir in 7 to 14 days. **GI:** *stomatitis, GI ulcer may precede leukopenia, nausea, vomiting in 30% to 50% of patients; diarrhea.* **Skin:** *dermatitis,* hyperpigmentation (especially in Blacks), nail changes, pigmented palmar creases.

♦ Available in U.S. and Canada. ♦♦ Available in Canada only.
All other products (no symbol) available in U.S. only. Italicized side effects are common or life-threatening.

INTERACTIONS AND SPECIAL CONSIDERATIONS

Interactions:
ALLOPURINOL: impaired inactivation of azathioprine. Decrease azathioprine dose to ¼ or ⅓ normal dose.

Special considerations:
• Use cautiously in hepatic or renal dysfunction.
• Patient may develop clay-colored stools, dark urine, pruritus, yellow skin, sclera, and increased alkaline phosphatase, bilirubin, SGOT, and SGPT.
• In renal homotransplants, drug should be started 1 to 5 days before surgery.
• Hemoglobin, WBC, and platelet count should be done at least once a week; more often at beginning of treatment. Drug should be stopped immediately when WBC is less than 3,000/mm^3 to prevent extension to irreversible bone marrow depression.
• This is a potent immunosuppressant. Patient should report even mild infections (coryza, fever, sore throat, malaise).
• Patient should avoid conception during and up to 4 months after stopping therapy.
• Alopecia may occur.
• I.M. injections should be avoided in patients with severely depressed platelet counts (thrombocytopenia) to prevent bleeding.
• When used to treat refractory rheumatoid arthritis, it may take up to 12 weeks to be effective.

No significant interactions.

Special considerations:
• Contraindicated in inadequate bone marrow reserve. Use cautiously in renal or hepatic disease and after other chemotherapy or radiation therapy.
• Patient may develop infection (leukoplakia, fever, sore throat).
• Excellent mouth care can help prevent oral side effects.
• Intake and output should be monitorerd carefully. High fluid intake should be maintained and allopurinol given to avoid urate nephropathy in leukemia induction therapy.
• Uric acid, CBC with platelets, and hepatic function should be monitored.
• Preservative-free water required for intrathecal use.
• Optimum schedule is continuous infusion.
• To reduce nausea, antiemetic should be given before administering.
• Dry powder should be stored in refrigerator; refrigerated, reconstituted solution stable 12 hours. Cloudy reconstituted solution should be discarded.
• I.M. injections should be avoided in patients with severely depressed platelet count (thrombocytopenia) to prevent bleeding.
• Therapy should be modified or discontinued if polymorphonuclear granulocyte count is 1,000/mm^3 or if platelet count is 50,000/mm^3.

No significant interactions.

Special considerations:
• Use cautiously in poor nutritional state, bone marrow depression, or serious infection. Use cautiously following high-dose pelvic irradiation or use of alkylating agent, and in impaired hepatic or renal function.
• Severe skin and GI side effects require stopping drug. Use of antacid eases but probably won't prevent GI distress.
• Excellent mouth care can help prevent oral side effects.
• Intake and output, CBC, and renal and hepatic function should be monitored.
• Drug should be discontinued if WBC falls below 3,500/mm^3 or if platelet count below 100,000/mm^3.
• Therapeutic effect may be delayed 1 to 6 weeks.
• Should be reconstituted with sterile water for injection; diluted further in 5% dextrose in water or normal saline for actual infusion. Infusion pump should always be used.
• I.M. injections of any drugs should be avoided in patients with thrombocytopenia to prevent bleeding.
• Refrigerated solution stable no more than 2 weeks.
• Precautions for catheter line care should be observed in arterial perfused area. Line should be checked for bleeding, blockage, displacement, or leakage.

No significant interactions.

Special considerations:
• Use cautiously following major surgery, in poor nutritional state, serious infections, bone marrow depression. Use cautiously following high-dose pelvic irradiation or use of alkylating agents, in impaired hepatic or renal function, or in widespread neoplastic infiltration of bone marrow.
• Stomatitis and diarrhea are signs of toxicity. Topical oral anesthetic may be used to soothe lesions. Should be discontinued if diarrhea occurs.
• Antiemetic should be given before administering to reduce GI side effects.
• WBC and platelet counts should be done daily. Drug should be stopped when WBC is less than

(continued on following page)

NAMES, INDICATIONS AND DOSAGES	SIDE EFFECTS
fluorouracil *(continued)* Maximum single recommended dose is 800 mg, although higher single doses (up to 1.5 g) have been used. The injectable form has been given orally but is not recommended.	**Other:** *alopecia in 5% to 20% of patients, weakness, malaise.*
hydroxyurea Hydrea **Melanoma; resistant chronic myelocytic leukemia; recurrent, metastatic, or inoperable ovarian cancer:** ADULTS: 80 mg/kg P.O. as single dose q 3 days; or 20 to 30 mg/kg P.O. daily.	**Blood:** *leukopenia,* thrombocytopenia, anemia, *megaloblastosis; dose-limiting and dose-related bone marrow depression, with rapid recovery.* **CNS:** drowsiness. **GI:** *anorexia, nausea, vomiting, diarrhea,* stomatitis. **GU:** increased BUN, serum creatinine. **Metabolic:** hyperuricemia. **Skin:** rash, pruritus.
mercaptopurine Purinethol♦ **Acute lymphoblastic leukemia (in children), acute myeloblastic leukemia, chronic myelocytic leukemia:** ADULTS: 80 to 100 mg/m² P.O. daily as a single dose up to 5 mg/kg/day. CHILDREN: 70 mg/m² P.O. daily. Usual maintenance for adults and children: 1.5 to 2.5 mg/kg/day.	**Blood:** *decreased RBC; leukopenia, thrombocytopenia, bone marrow hypoplasia; all may persist several days after drug is stopped.* **GI:** *nausea, vomiting, and anorexia in 25% of patients;* painful oral ulcers. **Hepatic:** *jaundice, hepatic necrosis.* **Metabolic:** hyperuricemia.
methotrexate **methotrexate sodium** Mexate **Trophoblastic tumors (choriocarcinoma, hydatidiform mole):** ADULTS: 15 to 30 mg P.O. or I.M. daily for 5 days. Repeat after 1 or more weeks, according to response or toxicity. **Acute lymphoblastic and lymphatic leukemia:** ADULTS AND CHILDREN: 3.3 mg/m² P.O., I.M., or I.V. daily for 4 to 6 weeks or until remission occurs; then 20 to 30 mg/m² P.O. or I.M. twice weekly. **Meningeal leukemia:** ADULTS AND CHILDREN: 0.2 to 0.5 mg/kg intrathecally q 2 to 5 days until cerebrospinal	**Blood:** WBC and platelet nadir occurring on day 7; anemia, *leukopenia, thrombocytopenia* (all dose-related). **CNS:** *arachnoiditis within hours of intrathecal use;* subacute neurotoxicity which may begin a few weeks later; necrotizing demyelinating leukoencephalopathy a few years later. **GI:** *stomatitis* (common); *diarrhea leading to hemorrhagic enteritis and intestinal perforation.* **GU:** *tubular necrosis.* **Hepatic:** hepatic dysfunction leading to cirrhosis or hepatic fibrosis. **Metabolic:** hyperuricemia. **Skin:** exposure to sun may aggravate psoriatic lesions, rash, photosensitivity. **Other:** alopecia; *pulmonary interstitial infiltrates;* long-term use in children may cause osteoporosis.

♦ Available in U.S. and Canada. ♦♦ Available in Canada only.
All other products (no symbol) available in U.S. only. Italicized side effects are common or life-threatening.

INTERACTIONS AND SPECIAL CONSIDERATIONS

3,500/mm³. Ecchymoses, petechiae, easy bruising, and anemia are possible. Drug should be stopped if platelets are less than 100,000/mm³.
• Skin and ocular side effects reversible when drug is stopped. Patient should use highly protective sun blockers to avoid inflammatory erythematous dermatitis.
• Therapeutic concentrations don't reach cerebrospinal fluid.
• Slowing infusion rate so it takes from 2 to 8 hours lessens toxicity but also lessens efficacy compared with rapid injection.
• Intake and output, CBC, and renal and hepatic functions should be monitored.
• Fluorouracil should not be refrigerated.
• Don't use cloudy solution. If crystals form, redissolve by warming.
• Sometimes ordered as 5-FU. The number 5 is part of the drug name and should not be confused with dosage units.
• Sometimes administered via hepatic arterial infusion in treatment of hepatic metastases.
• Alopecia may occur but is reversible.
• Excessive I.M. injections should be avoided in patients with thrombocytopenia to prevent bleeding.
• Fluorouracil toxicity is delayed for 1 to 3 weeks.

No significant interactions.

Special considerations:
• Use cautiously following other chemotherapy or radiation therapy.
• Use with caution in renal dysfunction. Should be discontinued if WBC is less than 2,500/mm³ or if platelet count is less than 100,000/mm³.
• If patient can't swallow capsule, he may empty contents into water and take immediately.
• Intake and output should be monitored, and patient kept hydrated.
• BUN, uric acid, and serum creatinine should be monitored regularly.
• Drug passes blood-brain barrier.
• Auditory and visual hallucinations and blood toxicity possible when decreased renal function exists.
• May exacerbate postirradiation erythema.
• I.M. injections should be avoided when platelets are low.

Interactions:
ALLOPURINOL: slowed inactivation of mercaptopurine. Decrease mercaptopurine to ¼ or ⅓ normal dose.

Special considerations:
• Use cautiously following chemotherapy or radiation therapy, in depressed neutrophil or platelet count, impaired hepatic or renal function.
• Bleeding and infection are possible.
• Hepatic dysfunction reversible when drug is stopped. Patient may develop jaundice, clay-colored stools, frothy dark urine. Drug should be stopped if liver tenderness occurs.
• Weekly blood counts should be done; precipitous fall possible.
• Intake and output should be monitored, and fluids (3 liters daily) pushed.
• Sometimes ordered as 6-mercaptopurine or 6-MP. The number 6 is part of drug name and does not signify number of dosage units.
• Improvement may take 2 to 4 weeks or longer.
• GI side effects less common in children than in adults.
• I.M. injections should be avoided when platelets are low.

Interactions:
ALCOHOL: increased hepatotoxicity; warn patient not to drink alcoholic beverages.
PROBENECID, PHENYLBUTAZONE, SALICYLATES, SULFONAMIDES: increased methotrexate toxicity; don't use together if possible.

Special considerations:
• Use cautiously in impaired hepatic or renal function, bone marrow depression, aplasia, leukopenia, thrombocytopenia, anemia. Use cautiously in infection, peptic ulcer, ulcerative colitis, and in very young, old, or debilitated patients.
• Patient should avoid conception during and immediately after therapy because of possible abortion or congenital anomalies.
• GI side effects may require stopping drug.
• Rash, redness, or ulcerations in mouth or pulmonary side effects may signal serious complications.
• Uric acid should be monitored.
• Intake and output should be monitored daily; fluids forced (2 to 3 liters daily); and thirst and urinary frequency checked.
• Urine should be alkalinized by giving $NaHCO_3$ tablets to prevent precipitation of drug, especially with high doses. Urine pH should be maintained at more than 6.5. Dose should be reduced if BUN 20 to 30 mg% or creatinine 1.2 to 2 mg%, and drug stopped if BUN more than 30 mg% or creatinine more than 2 mg%.
• Increases in SGOT, SGPT, alkaline phosphatase should be watched; may signal hepatic dysfunction.
• Patient may develop bleeding (especially GI) and infection.
• Patient should use highly protective sun blocker

(continued on following page)

NAMES, INDICATIONS AND DOSAGES	SIDE EFFECTS
methotrexate *(continued)* fluid is normal. Use only 20-, 50-, or 100-mg vials of powder with no preservatives, and dilute to concentration of 1 mg/ml using 0.9% NaCl injection *without* preservatives. Use only new vials of drug and diluent. Use immediately. **Burkitt's lymphoma (Stage I or Stage II):** ADULTS: 10 to 25 mg P.O. daily for 4 to 8 days with 1-week rest intervals. **Burkitt's lymphoma (Stage III):** ADULTS: up to 1 g/m²/day with cyclophosphamide and prednisolone. **Lymphosarcoma (Stage III):** ADULTS: 0.625 to 2.5 mg/kg daily P.O., I.M., or I.V. **Mycosis fungoides:** ADULTS: 2.5 to 10 mg P.O. daily or 50 mg I.M. weekly; or 25 mg I.M. twice weekly. **Psoriasis:** ADULTS: 10 to 25 mg P.O., I.M., or I.V. as single weekly dose. To detect idiosyncratic reactions, 5 to 10 mg test dose recommended 1 week before methotrexate regimen.	
thioguanine Lanvis♦♦ **Acute leukemia, chronic granulocytic leukemia:** ADULTS AND CHILDREN: initially, 2 mg/kg/day P.O. (usually calculated to nearest 20 mg); then increased gradually to 3 mg/kg/day if no toxic effects occur.	**Blood:** *leukopenia,* anemia, *thrombocytopenia* (occurs slowly over 2 to 4 weeks). **GI:** nausea, vomiting, stomatitis, diarrhea, anorexia. **Hepatic:** hepatotoxicity, jaundice. **Metabolic:** hyperuricemia.

INTERACTIONS AND SPECIAL CONSIDERATIONS

when exposed to sun.
• Temperature should be taken daily, and cough, dyspnea, and cyanosis watched for; corticosteroids may help reduce pulmonary side effects.
• Leucovorin rescue: leucovorin calcium (folinic acid) is given within 4 hours of administration of methotrexate and is usually continued 24 to 72 hours. Should not be confused with folic acid. This rescue technique is effective against systemic toxicity but does not interfere with the tumor cells' absorption of the methotrexate.
• I.M. injections should be avoided in patients with thrombocytopenia.

No significant interactions.

Special considerations:
• Use cautiously in renal or hepatic dysfunction.
• Drug should be stopped if hepatotoxicity or liver tenderness occurs. Patient may develop jaundice; may reverse if drug stopped promptly.
• CBC should be done daily during induction, then weekly during maintenance therapy.
• Serum uric acid should be monitored.
• Sometimes ordered as 6-thioguanine. The number 6 is part of drug name and does not signify dosage units.
• I.M. injections should be avoided when platelets are low.

73

Antibiotic antineoplastic agents

bleomycin sulfate
dactinomycin (actinomycin D)
daunorubicin hydrochloride
doxorubicin hydrochloride
mithramycin
mitomycin
procarbazine hydrochloride

Antibiotic antineoplastics are isolated from naturally occurring microorganisms that inhibit bacterial growth. But unlike the anti-infective drugs that they're related to, antibiotic antineoplastics can disrupt the functioning of both the host's cells and bacterial cells. Although procarbazine hydrochloride is not an antibiotic, it's included in this chapter because it acts in a similar manner.

Major uses

- Bleomycin, dactinomycin, doxorubicin, mitomycin, and procarbazine are used mainly to treat carcinomas, sarcomas, and lymphomas.
- Daunorubicin is used to treat acute leukemias.
- Mithramycin is used specifically to treat testicular carcinoma and hypercalcemia from various causes.

Mechanism of action

- Bleomycin inhibits deoxyribonucleic acid (DNA) synthesis and causes scission of DNA strands.
- Dactinomycin, daunorubicin, doxorubicin, and mithramycin interfere with DNA-dependent ribonucleic acid (RNA) synthesis by intercalation.
- Mithramycin also inhibits osteocytic activity, blocking calcium and phosphorus resorption from bone.
- Mitomycin acts like an alkylating agent, cross-linking strands of DNA. This causes an imbalance of cell growth, leading to cell death.
- Procarbazine inhibits DNA, RNA, and protein synthesis.

Absorption, distribution, metabolism, and excretion

- Procarbazine is well absorbed after oral administration. All the other drugs must be given parenterally.
- All are distributed to most body tissues and organs, especially the liver, spleen, kidneys, lungs, and heart.
- Mithramycin is the only drug that crosses the blood-brain barrier in significant amounts.
- The drugs are generally metabolized in the liver. Their inactive metabolites are eliminated in urine or through the bile in feces.

Onset and duration

Therapeutic activity varies with the drug, disease, and patient response.

Combination products

None.

ANTHRACYCLINE THERAPY: A PROGRESS REPORT

The presently available anthracyclines—doxorubicin and daunorubicin—effectively treat:

- acute leukemia
- Hodgkin's disease
- non-Hodgkin's lymphomas
- breast cancer
- sarcomas.

But, unfortunately, these drugs are corrosive when extravasated, and may present side effects such as:

- hematopoietic suppression
- nausea and vomiting
- alopecia
- and most important, *cardiomyopathy.*

Cardiomyopathy is the treatment-limiting toxicity associated with anthracycline therapy: The higher the total dose of anthracycline given, the greater the chance of toxicity. So the doctor has to choose between escalating the risk of cardiac toxicity and stopping this cancer therapy.

Recently, however, an effort has been made to seek out the ultimate anthracycline drug—one that works effectively with reduced side effects, particularly less cardiac toxicity. Although hundreds of anthracyclines have been developed, no currently approved anthracycline achieves the ideal. However, soon any one of the following investigational-use anthracyclines may be available for your patients:

DRUG	MAJOR USE	ADVANTAGES	ADVERSE REACTIONS	SPECIAL CONSIDERATIONS
aclacinomycin A	Acute leukemias	Less cardiac toxicity and mutagenicity than doxorubicin at equivalent dose levels	None reported	Greatest therapeutic potential of all the anthracyclines for your patient
carubicin	Soft-tissue sarcomas	Alopecia and extravasation problems are rare. No instances of cardiomyopathy.	Arrhythmias in 5% of patients	Well absorbed after oral or subcutaneous administration
zorubicin	Acute leukemias	Higher doses than daunorubicin possible without cardiac toxicity, but stronger therapeutic effect is questionable	Chills, fever, urticarial reactions	Use immediately after preparation

NAMES, INDICATIONS AND DOSAGES	SIDE EFFECTS
bleomycin sulfate Blenoxane♦ Dosage and indications may vary. Check patient's protocol with doctor. **Cervical, esophageal, head, neck, and testicular cancer:** ADULTS: 10 to 20 units/m^2 I.V., I.M., or S.C. 1 or 2 times weekly to total 300 to 400 units. **Hodgkin's disease:** 10 to 20 units/m^2 I.V., I.M., or S.C. 1 or 2 times weekly. After 50% response, maintenance 1 unit I.M. or I.V. daily or 5 units I.M. or I.V. weekly. **Lymphomas:** first 2 doses should be 5 units or less, and patient should be monitored for any allergic reaction. If no reaction occurs, then follow above dosing schedule.	**CNS:** hyperesthesia of scalp and fingers, headache. **GI:** *stomatitis in 22% to 50% of patients, prolonged anorexia in 13% of patients, nausea, vomiting,* diarrhea. **Skin:** *erythema, vesiculation, and hardening and discoloration of palmar and plantar skin in 8% of patients;* desquamation of hands, feet, and pressure areas; *hyperpigmentation; acne.* **Other:** *alopecia,* swelling of interphalangeal joints, *pulmonary fibrosis in 10% of patients, pulmonary side effects (fine rales, fever, dyspnea), leukocytosis and nonproductive cough, allergic reaction (fever up to 106° F. [41.1° C.], with chills up to 5 hours after injection; anaphylaxis in 1% to 6% of patients).*
dactinomycin (actinomycin D) Cosmegen♦ Dosage and indications may vary. Check patient's protocol with doctor. **Melanomas, sarcomas, trophoblastic tumors in women, testicular cancer:** ADULTS: 500 mcg I.V. daily for 5 days; wait 2 to 4 weeks and repeat; or 2 mg I.V. single weekly dose for 3 weeks; wait for bone marrow recovery, then repeat in 3 to 4 weeks. **Wilms' tumor, rhabdomyosarcoma:** CHILDREN: 15 mcg/kg I.V. daily for 5 days. Maximum dose 500 mcg daily. Wait for marrow recovery.	**Blood:** anemia, *leukopenia, thrombocytopenia, pancytopenia.* **GI:** *anorexia, nausea, vomiting,* abdominal pain, diarrhea, *stomatitis.* **Skin:** *erythema;* desquamation; *hyperpigmentation of skin, especially in previously irradiated areas; acne-like eruptions (reversible).* **Local:** phlebitis, severe damage to soft tissue. **Other:** reversible alopecia.
daunorubicin hydrochloride Cerubidine♦ Dosage and indications may vary. Check patient's protocol with doctor. **Remission induction in acute nonlymphocytic leukemia (myelogenous, monocytic, erythroid) in adults:** *As a single agent:* 60 mg/m^2/day I.V. on days 1, 2, 3 q 3 to 4 weeks. *In combination:* 45 mg/m^2/day I.V. on days 1, 2, 3 of the first course and on days 1, 2 of subsequent courses with cytosine arabinoside infusions. *Note:* Dose should be reduced if hepatic function is impaired.	**Blood:** *bone marrow depression* (lowest blood counts 10 to 14 days after administration). **CV:** *cardiomyopathy (dose-related), EKG changes, arrhythmias,* pericarditis, myocarditis. **GI:** *nausea, vomiting, stomatitis, esophagitis,* anorexia, diarrhea. **Skin:** rash. **Local:** *severe cellulitis or tissue slough if drug extravasates.* **Other:** *generalized alopecia,* fever, chills.
doxorubicin hydrochloride Adriamycin♦ Dosage and indications may vary. Check pa-	**Blood:** *leukopenia, especially agranulocytosis, during days 10 to 15, with recovery by day 21; thrombocytopenia.* **CV:** *cardiac depression, seen in such EKG*

INTERACTIONS AND SPECIAL CONSIDERATIONS

No significant interactions.

Special considerations:
- Use cautiously in renal or pulmonary impairment.
- Drug concentrates in keratin of squamous epithelium. To prevent linear streaking, adhesive dressings should not be used on skin.
- Allergic reactions may be delayed 6 to 15 hours, especially in lymphoma.
- Chest X-rays should be taken and lungs checked.
- Pulmonary function studies should be performed to establish baseline. Drug should be stopped if pulmonary function study shows a marked decline.
- Pulmonary side effects common in patients over 70 years and in patients who receive a total dose of more than 400 mg.
- Alopecia may occur.
- Refrigerated, reconstituted solution stable 4 weeks; at room temperature, stable 2 weeks. Solutions prepared in ampules should be discarded if not used immediately.
- Fatal pulmonary fibrosis occurs in 1% of patients, especially when cumulative dose exceeds 400 mg.
- Bleomycin-induced fever is common; may be treated with antipyretics.

No significant interactions.

Special considerations:
- Contraindicated in renal, hepatic, or bone marrow impairment; viral infection; or during chickenpox or herpes zoster infection. Use cautiously in metastatic testicular tumors, in combination therapy with chlorambucil and methotrexate therapy. Extreme bone marrow and GI toxicity can occur with this combined therapy.
- Stomatitis, diarrhea, leukopenia, thrombocytopenia may require stopping therapy.
- Antiemetic should be given before administering to reduce nausea.
- Renal and hepatic functions should be monitored.
- CBCs should be monitored daily and platelet counts every third day.
- Bleeding is possible.
- Alopecia may occur but is usually reversible.
- Only sterile water (without preservatives) should be used as diluent for injection.
- Should be administered through a running I.V. infusion. Infiltration should be avoided.

Interactions:
HEPARIN: don't mix. May form a precipitate.

Special considerations:
- Use cautiously in myelosuppression and impaired cardiac function.
- Signs of congestive heart failure or cardiomyopathy require immediate drug discontinuation. May be prevented by limiting cumulative dose to 550 mg/m²; 450 mg/m² when patient has been receiving radiation therapy that encompasses the heart or any other cardiotoxic agent.
- EKG should be monitored before treatment, monthly during therapy.
- High resting pulse signals cardiac side effects.
- *Extravasation should be avoided;* drug should be injected into tubing of freely flowing I.V. Drug should *never* be given I.M. or subcutaneously.
- CBC and hepatic function should be monitored.
- Urine may be red for 1 to 2 days; this is a normal side effect, not hematuria.
- Alopecia may occur, but it's usually reversible.
- A scalp tourniquet or ice bag should not be used to prevent alopecia. May compromise effectiveness of drug.
- Nausea and vomiting may be very severe and last 24 to 48 hours.
- Refrigerated, reconstituted solution stable for at least 36 hours; 24 hours at room temperature. Optimally, solution should be used within 8 hours of preparation.
- Reddish color looks very similar to doxorubicin (Adriamycin). *The two drugs should not be confused.*

No significant interactions.

Special considerations:
- Use cautiously in myelosuppression and impaired cardiac function.
- Drug should be stopped or rate of infusion slowed if tachycardia develops.
- Signs of congestive heart failure or cardio-

(continued on following page)

NAMES, INDICATIONS AND DOSAGES	SIDE EFFECTS
doxorubicin hydrochloride *(continued)* tient's protocol with doctor. **Bladder, breast, cervical, head, neck, liver, lung, ovarian, prostatic, stomach, testicular, and thyroid cancer; Hodgkin's disease; acute lymphoblastic and myeloblastic leukemia; Wilms' tumor; neuroblastomas; lymphomas; sarcomas:** ADULTS: 60 to 75 mg/m² I.V. as single dose q 3 weeks; or 30 mg/m² I.V. in single daily dose, days 1 to 3 of 4-week cycle. Maximum cumulative dose 550 mg/m².	*changes as sinus tachycardia, T-wave flattening, ST segment depression, voltage reduction; arrhythmias in 11% of patients; cardiomyopathy (sometimes with pulmonary edema) with mortality of 30% to 75%.* **GI:** *nausea, vomiting,* diarrhea, *stomatitis,* esophagitis. **GU:** enhancement of cyclophosphamide-induced bladder injury, red urine. **Skin:** *hyperpigmentation of skin, especially in previously irradiated areas.* **Local:** *severe cellulitis or tissue slough if drug extravasates.* **Other:** hyperpigmentation of nails and dermal creases, *complete alopecia within 3 to 4 weeks;* hair may regrow 2 to 5 months after drug is stopped.
mithramycin Mithracin Dosage and indications may vary. Check patient's protocol with doctor. **Hypercalcemia:** ADULTS: 25 mcg/kg I.V. daily for 1 to 4 days. **Testicular cancer:** ADULTS: 25 to 30 mcg/kg I.V. daily for up to 8 to 10 days (based on ideal body weight). I.V. infusions should be in 5% dextrose in water or 0.9% normal saline solution (1,000 ml over 4 to 6 hours).	**Blood:** *thrombocytopenia; bleeding syndrome, from epistaxis to generalized hemorrhage; facial flushing.* **GI:** *nausea, vomiting,* anorexia, diarrhea, stomatitis. **GU:** proteinuria; increased BUN, serum creatinine. **Metabolic:** *decreased serum calcium,* potassium, and phosphorus. **Skin:** periorbital pallor, usually the day before toxic symptoms occur. **Local:** extravasation causes irritation, cellulitis.
mitomycin Mutamycin♦ **Breast, colon, head, neck, lung, pancreatic, and stomach cancer; malignant melanoma:** ADULTS: 2 mg/m² I.V. daily for 5 days. Stop drug for 2 days, then repeat dose for 5 more days; or 20 mg/m² as a single dose. Repeat cycle 6 to 8 weeks. Stop drug if WBC less than 4,000/mm³ or platelets less than 75,000/mm³.	**Blood:** *thrombocytopenia, leukopenia* (may be delayed up to 8 weeks). **CNS:** paresthesias. **GI:** nausea, vomiting, anorexia, stomatitis. **Local:** desquamation, induration, pruritus, *pain at site of injection.* Extravasation causes cellulitis, ulceration, sloughing. **Other:** *alopecia.*
procarbazine hydrochloride Matulane, Natulan♦♦ **Hodgkin's disease, lymphomas, brain and lung cancer:** ADULTS: 100 to 150 mg/m² P.O. for 10 days until WBC falls below 4,000/mm³ or platelets fall below 100,000/mm³. After bone marrow recovers, resume maintenance dose 50 to 100 mg P.O. daily. CHILDREN: 50 mg P.O. daily for first week, then 100 mg/m² until response or toxicity occurs. Maintenance dose is 50 mg P.O. daily after bone marrow recovery.	**Blood:** bleeding tendency, *leukopenia,* anemia. **CNS:** nervousness, depression, insomnia, nightmares, *hallucinations,* confusion. **EENT:** retinal hemorrhage, nystagmus, photophobia. **GI:** *nausea, vomiting, anorexia,* stomatitis, dry mouth, dysphagia, diarrhea, constipation. **Skin:** dermatitis. **Other:** alopecia, pleural effusion.

♦ Available in U.S. and Canada. ♦♦ Available in Canada only.
All other products (no symbol) available in U.S. only. Italicized side effects are common or life-threatening.

INTERACTIONS AND SPECIAL CONSIDERATIONS

myopathy require immediate drug discontinuation. May be prevented by limiting cumulative dose to 550 mg/m^2; 450 mg/m^2 when patient is also receiving cyclophosphamide.
• EKG should be monitored before treatment and monthly during therapy.
• High resting pulse signals cardiac side effects.
• *Extravasation should be avoided;* drug should be injected into tubing of freely flowing I.V.; *never* given I.M. or subcutaneously.
• CBC and hepatic function should be monitored.
• Urine will be red for 1 to 2 days.
• Dose should be reduced in hepatic dysfunction.
• Alopecia will occur. A scalp tourniquet or application of ice may decrease alopecia. However, should *not* be used if treating leukemias or other neoplasms where tumor stem cells may be present in scalp.
• Refrigerated, reconstituted solution stable 48 hours; at room temperature, stable 24 hours.
• If cumulative dose exceeds 550 mg/m^2 body surface area, 30% of patients develop cardiac side effects, which begin 2 weeks to 6 months after stopping drug.
• Dose should be decreased if serum bilirubin is increased: 50% dose when bilirubin is 1.2 to 3 mg/100 ml; 25% dose when bilirubin is greater than 3 mg/100 ml.
• Esophagitis very common in patients who have also received radiation therapy.
• Reddish color looks very similar to daunorubicin. *The two drugs should not be confused.*

No significant interactions.

Special considerations:
• Contraindicated in thrombocytopenia and in coagulation and bleeding disorders. Use cautiously in renal, hepatic, or bone marrow impairment.
• Slow infusion reduces nausea that develops with I.V. push.
• LDH, SGOT, SGPT, alkaline phosphatase, BUN, creatinine, potassium, calcium, and phosphorus should be monitored.
• Platelet count and prothrombin time should be monitored before and during therapy.
• Bleeding is possible.
• Antiemetic should be given before administering to reduce nausea.
• Extravasation should be avoided. If I.V. infiltrates, it should be stopped immediately and ice packs should be applied. Then I.V. should be restarted.
• Contact with skin or mucous membranes should be avoided.
• Therapeutic effect in hypercalcemia may not be seen for 24 to 48 hours; may last 3 to 15 days.
• Precipitous drop in calcium possible. Patient should be monitored for tetany, carpopedal spasm, Chvostek's sign, muscle cramps; serum calcium levels should be checked.
• Lyophilized powder should be stored in refrigerator. Remains stable after reconstitution for 24 hours; 48 hours in refrigerator.

No significant interactions.

Special considerations:
• Use cautiously when platelet count is less than 75,000/mm^3, WBC is less than 4,000/mm^3, in coagulation or bleeding disorders, serious infections, impaired renal function.
• CBC and blood studies should be continued at least 7 weeks after therapy is stopped. Bleeding is possible.
• Alopecia may occur but is usually reversible.
• Reconstituted solution stable 1 week at room temperature, 2 weeks refrigerated.
• Dosage and indications may vary. Check patient's protocol with doctor.

Interactions:
ALCOHOL: disulfiram(Antabuse)-like reaction. Warn patient not to drink alcohol.

Special considerations:
• Use cautiously in inadequate bone marrow reserve, leukopenia, thrombocytopenia, anemia, impaired hepatic or renal function.
• Bleeding is possible.
• Alopecia may occur.
• Patient should not drink alcoholic beverages while taking this drug.
• Dosage and indications may vary. Check patient's protocol with doctor.

74

Antineoplastics altering hormone balance

aminoglutethimide
dromostanolone propionate
megestrol acetate
mitotane
tamoxifen citrate
testolactone

Synthetic sex hormones such as dromostanolone propionate, megestrol acetate, and testolactone counterbalance the tumor-stimulating effects of endogenous sex hormones. Tamoxifen citrate is not a synthetic hormone, but an estrogen antagonist. Aminoglutethimide and mitotane, which are also not hormones, are useful in managing cancer of the adrenal cortex.

These drugs are especially useful in treating cancer because they inhibit neoplastic growth in specific tissues without directly causing cytotoxicity.

Estrogens and androgens are also used as hormone manipulators in the treatment of cancer. (See Chapter 52, ANDROGENS AND ANABOLIC STEROIDS, and Chapter 54, ESTROGENS, for specific information.)

Major uses

- Aminoglutethimide and mitotane are palliatives in inoperable adrenocortical carcinoma.
- Dromostanolone, tamoxifen, and testolactone are used as palliatives in postmenopausal metastatic breast cancer.
- Megestrol is a palliative in both breast and endometrial cancer.

Mechanism of action

- Aminoglutethimide inhibits the synthesis of glucocorticoids, mineralocorticoids, and other steroids.
- Dromostanolone, megestrol, and testolactone change the tumor's hormonal environment and alter the neoplastic process.
- Mitotane selectively destroys adrenocortical tissue and hinders extra-adrenal metabolism of cortisol.
- Tamoxifen acts as an estrogen antagonist.

Absorption, distribution, metabolism, and excretion

Most of the drugs are well absorbed after oral administration and distributed widely in body tissues.

- Mitotane is partially absorbed when given orally (about 40%); dromostanolone must be given I.M.

All the drugs are metabolized in the liver and excreted in urine.

Onset and duration

Therapeutic activity varies with the drug, disease, and patient response.

Combination products

None.

HOW ESTROGEN ANTAGONISTS WORK

Estrogen antagonists, such as tamoxifen, bring about the death of estrogen-dependent tumors by preventing estrogen from nourishing tumor cells.

This occurs in two ways. First, through the process of competitive inhibition, tamoxifen binds with estrogen receptors in the cell cytoplasm, reducing the number of available receptors. Second, tamoxifen causes the estrogen that does enter the tumor cell nucleus to alter protein synthesis, thereby interfering with tumor cell division.

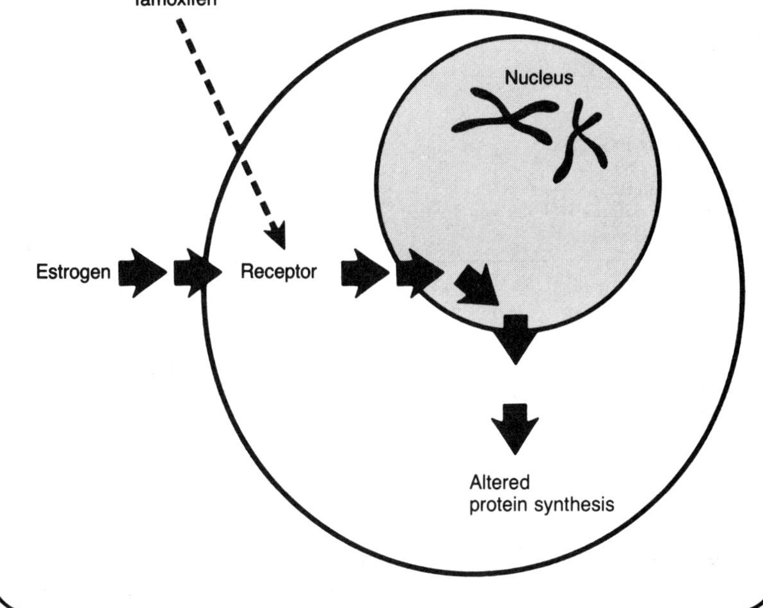

NAMES, INDICATIONS AND DOSAGES	SIDE EFFECTS
aminoglutethimide Cytadren **Suppression of adrenal function in Cushing's syndrome and adrenal cancer:** ADULTS: 250 mg P.O. q.i.d. at 6-hour intervals. Dosage may be increased in increments of 250 mg daily every 1 to 2 weeks to a maximum total daily dose of 2 g.	**Blood:** transient leukopenia, *severe pancytopenia.* **CNS:** *drowsiness,* headache, dizziness. **CV:** hypotension, tachycardia **Endocrine:** adrenal insufficiency, masculinization, hirsutism. **GI:** *nausea, anorexia.* **Skin:** *morbilliform skin rash,* pruritis, urticaria. **Other:** fever, myalgia.
dromostanolone propionate Drolban **Advanced, inoperable metastatic breast cancer, 1 to 5 years postmenopausal:** WOMEN: 100 mg deep I.M. 3 times weekly.	**GU:** clitoral enlargement. **Metabolic:** hypercalcemia. **Skin:** acne. **Other:** *virilism (deepened voice, facial hair growth), which may be intense after long-term treatment;* edema, pain at injection site.
megestrol acetate Megace♦ **Breast cancer:** WOMEN: 40 mg P.O. q.i.d. **Endometrial cancer:** WOMEN: 40 to 320 mg P.O. daily in divided doses.	None reported.
mitotane Lysodren♦ **Inoperable adrenocortical cancer:** ADULTS: 9 to 10 g P.O. daily, divided t.i.d. to q.i.d. If severe side effects appear, reduce dose until maximum tolerated dose is achieved (varies from 2 to 16 g/day but is usually 8 to 10 g/day).	**CNS:** *depression, somnolence, vertigo;* brain damage and dysfunction in long-term, high-dose therapy. **GI:** *severe nausea, vomiting,* diarrhea, anorexia. **Metabolic:** adrenal insufficiency. **Skin:** dermatitis.
tamoxifen citrate Nolvadex♦ **Advanced premenopausal and postmenopausal breast cancer:** WOMEN: 10 to 20 mg P.O. b.i.d.	**Blood:** transient fall in WBC or platelets. **GI:** nausea in 10% of patients, vomiting, anorexia. **GU:** vaginal discharge and bleeding. **Skin:** rash. **Other:** temporary bone or tumor pain, hot flashes in 7% of patients. Brief exacerbation of pain from osseous metastases.

♦ Available in U.S. and Canada. ♦♦ Available in Canada only.
All other products (no symbol) available in U.S. only. Italicized side effects are common or life-threatening.

INTERACTIONS AND SPECIAL CONSIDERATIONS

No significant interactions.

Special considerations:

- May cause adrenal hypofunction, especially under stressful conditions such as surgery, trauma, or acute illness. Patients may need hydrocortisone and mineralocorticoid supplements in these situations. Patients should be monitored carefully.
- Blood pressure should be checked frequently. Patient should stand up slowly to minimize orthostatic hypotension.
- May cause a decrease in thyroid hormone production. Thyroid function studies should be monitored.
- Baseline hematologic studies should be performed and CBC monitored periodically.
- Drug can cause drowsiness and dizziness. Patient should avoid activities that require alertness and good psychomotor coordination until response to drug has been determined.
- Skin rash that persists for more than 5 to 8 days should be reported. Drowsiness, nausea, and loss of appetite will diminish within 2 weeks after start of aminoglutethimide therapy. However, patient should report persistent symptoms.
- Also used to produce a medical adrenalectomy in patients who have metastatic breast cancer.

No significant interactions.

Special considerations:

- Contraindicated by any route other than I.M.; and in breast cancer in males and premenopausal women. Use cautiously in hepatic disease, cardiac decompensation, nephritis, nephrosis, and prostatic cancer.
- If severe hypercalcemia develops or disease accelerates, drug should be stopped.
- Therapeutic effect may be delayed 8 to 12 weeks.
- Do not store in refrigerator; drug precipitates at cold temperatures.
- Virilizing effects and skin and libido changes are possible in female patients.

No significant interactions.

Special considerations:

- Use cautiously in patients with history of thrombophlebitis.
- Adequate trial is 2 months. Therapeutic response isn't immediate.

No significant interactions.

Special considerations:

- Use cautiously in hepatic disease.
- Drug should be stopped if shock or trauma occurs. Use of corticosteroids may avoid acute adrenocortical insufficiency.
- Behavioral and neurologic signs should be assessed and recorded for baseline data daily throughout therapy.
- Antiemetic should be given before administering to reduce nausea.
- Obese patients may need higher dosage and may have longer-lasting side effects, since drug distributes mostly to body fat.
- Because of possible CNS side effects, patient should be warned to avoid hazardous tasks requiring mental alertness or physical coordination.
- Effectiveness can be monitored by reduction in pain, weakness, anorexia.
- Adequate trial is at least 3 months, but therapy can continue if clinical benefits are observed.

No significant interactions.

Special considerations:

- Use cautiously in preexisting leukopenia and thrombocytopenia.
- Analgesic used to relieve pain.
- WBC and platelet counts should be monitored.
- Acts as an anti-estrogen. Best results in patients with positive estrogen receptors.
- Side effects are usually minor and are well tolerated.
- Acute exacerbation of bone pain during tamoxifen therapy usually indicates drug will produce good response.
- Currently used to treat breast cancer in males.

NAMES, INDICATIONS AND DOSAGES	SIDE EFFECTS
testolactone Teslac♦ **Advanced postmenopausal breast cancer:** WOMEN: 100 mg deep I.M 3 times weekly; or 250 mg P.O. q.i.d.	**Local:** pain, inflammation at injection site. **Metabolic:** hypercalcemia.

INTERACTIONS AND SPECIAL CONSIDERATIONS

No significant interactions.

Special considerations:

- Contraindicated in breast cancer in males and not recommended in premenopausal females.
- Adequate trial is 3 months. Therapeutic response isn't immediate.
- Fluids and electrolytes should be monitored, especially calcium levels.
- Immobilized patients more prone to hypercalcemia. Exercise may prevent it. Fluids should be pushed to aid calcium excretion.
- Vial should be shaken vigorously before drawing up injection. Should not be refrigerated.
- 1.5″ needle used to inject dose into upper outer quadrant of gluteal region. Injection sites should be rotated.
- No advantage over testosterone, except less virilization.
- Higher than recommended doses do not increase incidence of remission.

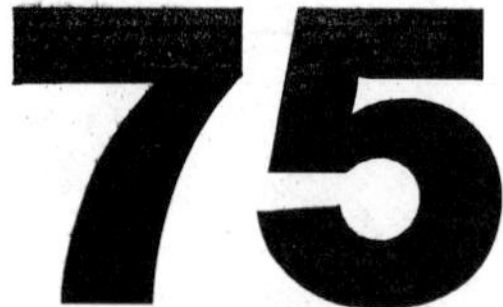

Vinca alkaloids, podophyllin derivatives, and asparaginase

asparaginase (L-asparaginase)
etoposide (VP-16)
vinblastine sulfate (VLB)
vincristine sulfate
vindesine sulfate
VM-26 (teniposide)

Vinblastine, vincristine, and vindesine are used as palliative treatment of various malignant neoplastic conditions. Closely related derivatives of the periwinkle plant, they are referred to as vinca alkaloids.

The podophyllin derivatives etoposide (VP-16) and VM-26 (teniposide) are used for the same purpose as the vinca alkaloids.

Asparaginase, derived from *Escherichia coli* and a number of other sources, is usually given in combination with other antineoplastic drugs.

Major uses

All the drugs furnish supplemental or adjunctive therapy for acute lymphocytic leukemia. • Podophyllin derivatives and vinca alkaloids are used as palliative therapy for lymphomas, leukemias, sarcomas, and some carcinomas.

BACKGROUND ON VINCA ALKALOIDS

The vinca alkaloids, commonly used in cancer treatment, are derived from the periwinkle *(Vinca rosea),* a species of myrtle. The beneficial properties of the periwinkle have been described in folklore.

In 1949, an alleged activity as an oral hypoglycemic agent prompted research on crude extracts from the plant. Working with periwinkle extracts, in 1958, Noble and co-workers were unable to back up the claims for hypoglycemic activity in laboratory animals. They did, however, see granulocytopenia and bone marrow suppression in rats—effects that led to the extraction and purification of an active alkaloid, originally termed vincaleukoblastine. Other investigations by Johnson and associates supplemented this work.

A frequent side effect with vinca alkaloid usage is peripheral neuropathy, especially prevalent in fingers and hands. This side effect generally subsides several weeks after drug treatment is discontinued.

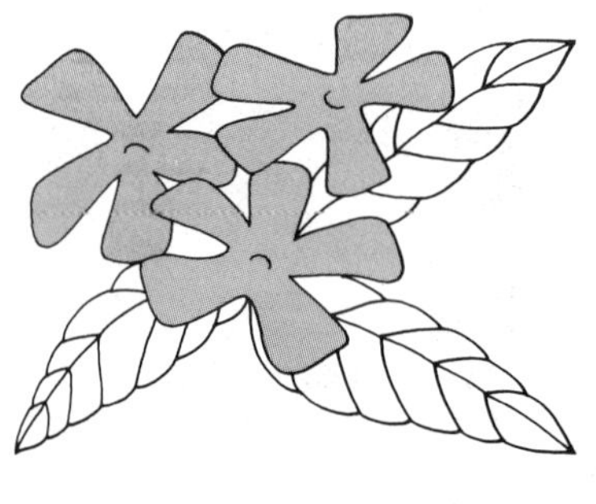

DRUG ALERT

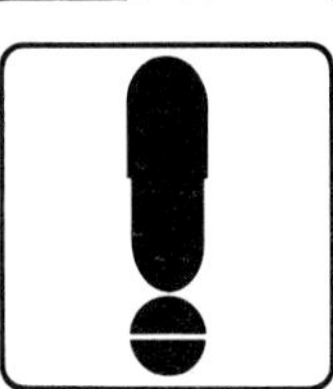

WATCH FOR VINCRISTINE NEUROTOXICITY

Vincristine causes neural damage, so the patient on this drug should report early symptoms of neural drug toxicity, such as constipation, tingling, numbness and tremors in his extremities.

A later effect of neurotoxicity is loss of deep tendon reflexes. The patient's reflexes should be checked regularly, especially the Achilles tendon. By the time the patient has difficulty heel-walking or rising from chairs, the damage is severe.

Although the drug may be discontinued, side effects can persist up to 2 years. Some effects may be permanent.

Mechanism of action

- Asparaginase destroys the amino acid asparagine, which is needed for protein synthesis in acute lymphocytic leukemia. This leads to death of the leukemic cell.
- Podophyllin derivatives and vinca alkaloids all arrest metaphase in mitosis, blocking cell division.

Absorption, distribution, metabolism, and excretion

- Although all the drugs are rapidly cleared from the blood and distributed in body tissues, they penetrate the blood-brain barrier poorly.
- Asparaginase is well absorbed after I.M. injection; it can also be administered I.V. Its metabolism and route of excretion are unknown. Only trace amounts are excreted in urine.
- Podophyllin derivatives and vinca alkaloids are given I.V. only. They are extensively metabolized in the liver and eliminated both in urine and—through the bile—in feces.

Onset and duration

Therapeutic activity varies with the drug, disease, and patient response.

Combination products

None.

NAMES, INDICATIONS AND DOSAGES	SIDE EFFECTS

asparaginase (or L-asparaginase)
Elspar

Acute lymphocytic leukemia (when used along with other drugs):
ADULTS AND CHILDREN: 1,000 international units (IU)/kg I.V. daily for 10 days, injected over 30 minutes or by slow I.V. push; or 6,000 IU/m^2 I.M. at intervals specified in protocol.
Sole induction agent—200 IU/kg I.V. daily for 28 days.

Blood: *hypofibrinogenemia* and depression of other clotting factors, thrombocytopenia, *leukopenia,* depression of serum albumin.
GI: *vomiting (may last up to 24 hours), anorexia, nausea,* cramps, weight loss.
GU: *azotemia,* renal failure, uric acid nephropathy, glycosuria, polyuria.
Hepatic: elevated SGOT, SGPT; *hepatotoxicity.*
Metabolic: elevated alkaline phosphatase and bilirubin (direct and indirect); increase or decrease in total lipids; *hyperglycemia; increased blood ammonia.*
Skin: *rash, urticaria.*
Other: *hemorrhagic pancreatitis, anaphylaxis (relatively common).*

etoposide (VP-16)

Small cell carcinoma of the lung, acute nonlymphocytic leukemia, lymphosarcoma, Hodgkin's disease, testicular carcinoma:
ADULTS: 45 to 75 mg/m^2/day I.V. for 3 to 5 days repeated q 3 to 5 weeks; or 200 to 250 mg/m^2 I.V. weekly; or 125 to 140 mg/m^2/day I.V. 3 times a week q 5 weeks.

Blood: *myelosuppression (dose-limiting), leukopenia,* thrombocytopenia.
CV: hypotension from rapid infusion.
GI: nausea and vomiting.
Local: infrequent phlebitis.
Other: occasional headache and fever, *alopecia, anaphylaxis* (rare).

vinblastine sulfate (VLB)
Velban, Velbe♦♦

Breast or testicular cancer, generalized Hodgkin's disease, choriocarcinoma, lymphosarcoma, neuroblastoma, mycosis fungoides, histiocytosis:
ADULTS AND CHILDREN: 0.1 mg/kg or 3.7 mg/m^2 I.V. weekly or q 2 weeks. May be increased to maximum dose (adults) of 0.5 mg/kg or 18.5 mg/m^2 I.V. weekly according to response. Dose should not be repeated if WBC less than 4,000/mm^3.

Blood: *leukopenia* (nadir days 4 to 10 and lasts another 7 to 14 days), *thrombocytopenia.*
CNS: depression, *paresthesias, peripheral neuropathy and neuritis, numbness, loss of deep tendon reflexes, muscle pain and weakness.*
EENT: pharyngitis.
GI: *nausea, vomiting, stomatitis,* ulcer and bleeding, *constipation, ileus, anorexia, weight loss,* abdominal pain.
GU: oligospermia, aspermia, urinary retention.
Skin: dermatitis, vesiculation.
Local: *irritation, phlebitis,* cellulitis, necrosis if I.V. extravasates.
Other: reversible alopecia in 5% to 10% of patients; *pain in tumor site,* low fever.

INTERACTIONS AND SPECIAL CONSIDERATIONS

No significant interactions.

Special considerations:
• Contraindicated in pancreatitis and in previous hypersensitivity unless desensitized. Use cautiously in preexisting hepatic dysfunction.
• Should be administered in hospital setting with close supervision.
• Should not be used as sole agent to induce remission unless combination therapy is inappropriate. Not recommended for maintenance therapy.
• Risk of hypersensitivity increases with repeated doses. Patient may be desensitized, but this doesn't rule out risk of allergic reactions. Routine administration of 2-unit I.V. test dose may identify high-risk patients.
• I.V. administration of asparaginase with or immediately before vincristine or prednisone may increase toxicity reactions.
• I.V. injection should be given over 30-minute period through a running infusion of sodium chloride injection or 5% dextrose injection.
• For I.M. injection, dose should be limited at single injection site to 2 ml.
• Due to vomiting, patient may need parenteral fluids for 24 hours or until oral fluids are tolerated.
• Blood count and bone marrow levels should be monitored. Bone marrow regeneration may take 5 to 6 weeks.
• Uric acid nephropathy is possible. Occurrence prevented by increasing fluid intake and alkalinization of urine. Allopurinol may be ordered.
• Patient may develop signs of bleeding, such as petechiae and melena.
• Blood sugar should be monitored and urine tested for sugar before and during therapy. Signs of hyperglycemia, such as glycosuria and polyuria, are possible.
• Should be reconstituted with 2 to 5 ml sterile water for injection or sodium chloride injection.
• Vial should not be shaken; may cause loss of potency. Cloudy solutions should not be used.
• Unopened dry powder should be refrigerated. Reconstituted solution stable 6 hours at room temperature, 24 hours refrigerated.
• Epinephrine, diphenhydramine, and I.V. corticosteroids should be available to treat anaphylaxis.
• For treatment of anaphylaxis, see APPENDIX.

No significant interactions.

Special considerations:
• Intraperitoneal, intrapleural, and intrathecal administration of this drug is contraindicated.
• Drug should be given by slow I.V. infusion (over at least 30 minutes) to prevent severe hypotension.
• Patients receiving drug over less than 2 hours should be in the recumbent position.
• Blood pressure should be monitored before infusion and at 30-minute intervals during infusion. Systolic blood pressure that falls below 90 mmHg should be reported and infusion should be stopped.
• Drug should *not* be diluted in 5% dextrose in water due to physical incompatibility (precipitate will form).
• Drug must be diluted to a concentration of 1 mg/ml or less with normal saline solution before administration. Cloudy solutions should be discarded.
• Solutions containing 1 mg/ml stable for 30 minutes; 0.4 mg/ml stable 3 hours; 0.2 mg/ml stable 6 hours.
• Diphenhydramine, hydrocortisone, epinephrine, and airway should be available in case of an anaphylactic reaction.
• CBC should be monitored. Bone marrow depression is possible.
• An investigational drug.

No significant interactions.

Special considerations:
• Contraindicated in severe leukopenia and bacterial infection. Use cautiously in jaundice or hepatic dysfunction.
• Antiemetic should be given before administering to reduce nausea.
• Drug should be stopped if stomatitis occurs.
• Laxatives should be given as needed. Stool softeners may be used prophylactically.
• If dose is repeated more frequently than every 7 days, severe leukopenia will develop.
• Less neurotoxic than vincristine.
• Should be injected directly into vein or tubing of running I.V. over 1 minute. May also be given in 50 ml dextrose in water or normal saline solution and infused over 15 minutes. If extravasation occurs, infusion should be stopped. Ice packs should be applied on and off every 2 hours for 24 hours.
• Alopecia may occur but is usually reversible.
• Adequate trial 12 weeks; therapeutic response isn't immediate.
• 10-mg vial should be reconstituted with 10 ml of sodium chloride injection or sterile water. This yields 1 mg/ml.
• Reconstituted solution should be refrigerated and discarded after 30 days.
• Vinblastine should not be confused with vincristine or the investigational agent vindesine.

NAMES, INDICATIONS AND DOSAGES	SIDE EFFECTS
vincristine sulfate Oncovin♦ **Acute lymphoblastic and other leukemias, Hodgkin's disease, lymphosarcoma, reticulum cell sarcoma, neuroblastoma, rhabdomyosarcoma, Wilms' tumor, osteogenic and other sarcomas, lung and breast cancer:** ADULTS: 1 to 2 mg/m² I.V. weekly. CHILDREN: 1.5 to 2 mg/m² I.V. weekly. Maximum single dose (adults and children) is 2 mg.	**Blood:** rapidly reversible mild anemia and leukopenia. **CNS:** *peripheral neuropathy*, sensory loss, *deep tendon reflex loss, paresthesias, wrist and foot drop*, ataxia, cranial nerve palsies (headache, *jaw pain*, hoarseness, vocal cord paralysis, visual disturbances), *muscle weakness and cramps*, depression, agitation, insomnia; neurotoxicities may be permanent. **EENT:** diplopia, optic and extraocular neuropathy, ptosis. **GI:** *constipation, cramps*, ileus that mimics surgical abdomen, *nausea, vomiting*, anorexia, *stomatitis*, weight loss, dysphagia. **GU:** urinary retention. **Local:** *phlebitis*, cellulitis. **Other:** *reversible alopecia (up to 71% of patients).*
vindesine sulfate Eldesine, DAVA **Acute lymphoblastic leukemia, breast cancer, malignant melanoma, lymphosarcoma, non–small cell lung carcinoma:** ADULTS: 3 to 4 mg/m² I.V. q 7 to 14 days, or continuous I.V. infusion 1.2 to 1.5 mg/m²/day for 5 days every 3 weeks.	**Blood:** *leukopenia, thrombocytopenia.* **CNS:** *paresthesias, decreased deep tendon reflex, muscle weakness.* **GI:** *constipation, abdominal cramping*, nausea, vomiting. **Local:** *phlebitis*, necrosis on extravasation. **Other:** *alopecia*, jaw pain, fever with continuous infusions.
VM-26 (teniposide) **Hodgkin's and non-Hodgkin's lymphomas, acute lymphocytic leukemia, bladder carcinoma:** ADULTS: 50 to 100 mg/m² I.V. once or twice weekly for 4 to 6 weeks, or 40 to 50 mg/m²/day I.V. for 5 days repeated every 3 to 4 weeks.	**Blood:** *myelosuppression (dose-limiting), leukopenia*, some thrombocytopenia. **CV:** hypotension from rapid infusion. **GI:** nausea and vomiting. **Local:** *phlebitis*, extravasation. **Other:** alopecia (rare), *anaphylaxis* (rare).

♦ Available in U.S. and Canada. ♦♦ Available in Canada only.
All other products (no symbol) available in U.S. only. Italicized side effects are common or life-threatening.

INTERACTIONS AND SPECIAL CONSIDERATIONS

No significant interactions.

Special considerations:

- Use cautiously in jaundice or hepatic dysfunction, neuromuscular disease, infection, or with other neurotoxic drugs.
- Because of neurotoxicity, drug should not be given more than once a week. Children more resistant to neurotoxicity than adults.
- Should be given directly into vein or tubing of running I.V. slowly over 1 minute. May also be given in 50 ml dextrose in water or normal saline solution and infused over 15 minutes. If drug infiltrates, ice packs should be applied on and off every 2 hours for 24 hours.
- Depression of Achilles tendon reflex, numbness, tingling, foot or wrist drop, difficulty in walking, ataxia, slapping gait, and ability to walk on heels should be checked. Patient needs support when walking.
- Bowel function should be monitored. Stool softener, laxative, or water should be given before dosing. Constipation may be an early sign of neurotoxicity.
- Should be reconstituted with sodium chloride injection, normal saline solution, or sterile water.
- Reconstituted solution should be refrigerated and discarded after 14 days.
- Alopecia may occur but is usually reversible.
- Vincristine should not be confused with vinblastine or the investigational agent vindesine.

No significant interactions.

Special considerations:

- Drug should not be given as a continuous infusion unless patient has a central I.V. line.
- To prevent paralytic ileus, patient should force fluids, increase ambulation, and use stool softeners.
- Patient should report signs of neurotoxicity: numbness and tingling of extremities, jaw pain, constipation (may be early sign of neurotoxicity).
- Patient should be assessed for depression of Achilles tendon reflex, foot or wrist drop, slapping gait (late signs of neurotoxicity).
- Neuropathy may be assessed by recording patient signatures before each course of therapy and observing for deterioration of handwriting.
- CBC should be monitored.
- Extravasation should be avoided. Drug is a painful vesicant. 10 ml normal saline solution flush should be given before drug to test vein patency, and 10 ml normal saline solution flush to remove any remaining drug from tubing after drug is given.
- When reconstituted with the 10 ml diluent provided or normal saline solution, the drug is stable for 2 weeks under refrigeration.
- Vindesine should not be mixed with other drugs; compatibility with other drugs has not yet been determined.
- An investigational drug.

No significant interactions.

Special considerations:

- May be diluted for infusion in either 5% dextrose in water or normal saline solution, but cloudy solutions should be discarded.
- Should be infused over 45 to 90 minutes to prevent hypotension.
- Solutions containing 0.5 to 2 mg/ml are stable for 4 hours. Solutions containing 0.1 to 0.2 mg/ml are stable for 6 hours.
- Blood pressure should be monitored before infusion and at 30-minute intervals during infusion. Systolic blood pressure that falls below 90 mmHg should be reported and infusion should be stopped.
- Diphenhydramine, hydrocortisone, epinephrine, and airway should be available in case of an anaphylactic reaction.
- CBC should be monitored. Bone marrow depression is possible.
- Extravasation should be avoided.
- Drug may be given by local bladder instillation as a treatment for bladder cancer.
- An investigational drug.

76

Ophthalmic anti-infectives

bacitracin
benzalkonium chloride
boric acid
chloramphenicol
chlortetracycline hydrochloride
erythromycin
gentamicin sulfate
idoxuridine (IDU)
natamycin
neomycin sulfate
polymyxin B sulfate
silver nitrate 1%
sulfacetamide sodium
tetracycline hydrochloride
tobramycin
trifluridine
vidarabine

Ophthalmic anti-infectives have antibacterial, antiviral, or antifungal activity. Most are antibiotics, but others, such as boric acid and benzalkonium chloride, are not. Although sulfacetamide sodium belongs to this group, other antibiotics have largely replaced it, except for use in minor infections. Idoxuridine, trifluridine, and vidarabine are specific antiviral agents. These agents are available as solutions, suspensions, or ointments.

Major uses

- Bacitracin, chloramphenicol, chlortetracycline, erythromycin, gentamicin, neomycin, polymyxin B, sulfacetamide, tetracycline, and tobramycin are used to treat surface infections of the conjunctiva or cornea caused by such microorganisms as *Chlamydia trachomatis, Pseudomonas,* and *Staphylococcus.*
- Benzalkonium chloride is a weak bactericide used as a wetting solution and a preservative; it also facilitates transcorneal penetration of other ophthalmic drugs.
- Boric acid is a bacteriostatic and fungistatic irrigating solution.
- Idoxuridine, trifluridine, and vidarabine are used to treat acute keratoconjunctivitis or recurrent epithelial keratitis caused by herpes simplex types I and II.
- Natamycin is used to treat ophthalmic fungal infections.
- Silver nitrate is used to prevent gonorrheal ophthalmia neonatorum.

Mechanism of action

- Bacitracin, chloramphenicol, erythromycin, gentamicin, neomycin, polymyxin B, the tetracyclines, and tobramycin inhibit protein synthesis in susceptible microorganisms.
- Benzalkonium chloride increases corneal permeability, enabling greater penetration of other drugs.
- Boric acid's mechanism of action is unknown.
- Idoxuridine, trifluridine, and vidarabine interfere with DNA synthesis.
- Natamycin increases fungal cell membrane permeability.
- Silver nitrate causes protein denaturation, which prevents gonorrheal ophthalmia neonatorum.
- Sulfacetamide prevents uptake of para-aminobenzoic acid, a metabolite of bacterial folic acid synthesis.

Absorption, distribution, metabolism, and excretion

- Bacitracin, chloramphenicol, and neomycin penetrate the cornea and conjunctiva, and are excreted by the nasolacrimal system.
- Benzalkonium chloride and silver nitrate do not penetrate intraocularly.

• Boric acid and idoxuridine are poorly absorbed topically.
• Chloramphenicol penetrates the aqueous humor; both chloramphenicol and gentamicin are excreted through the nasolacrimal system.
• Erythromycin, gentamicin, polymyxin B, the tetracyclines, and tobramycin penetrate poorly through an intact cornea but well through corneal abrasions.
• Natamycin does not reach measurable levels in deeper corneal layers unless there's a defect in the epithelium.
• Sulfacetamide's intraocular penetration varies.
• Trifluridine and vidarabine are found in trace amounts in the aqueous humor after topical application to a cornea with an epithelial defect or inflammation, but neither drug is significantly absorbed systemically.

Onset and duration

As a rule, ophthalmic anti-infectives are administered often—sometimes as frequently as every 2 hours. Onset and duration vary according to the condition and patient response. Therefore, dosage should be adjusted accordingly.

Combination products

BLEPHAMIDE LIQUIFILM SUSPENSION: sodium sulfacetamide 10%, prednisolone acetate 0.2%, and phenylephrine hydrochloride 0.12%.
CETAPRED OINTMENT♦: sodium sulfacetamide 10% and prednisolone acetate 0.25%.
CHLOROMYCETIN HYDROCORTISONE OPHTHALMIC♦: chloramphenicol 1.25% and hydrocortisone acetate 2.5%.
CHLOROMYXIN OPHTHALMIC♦: chloramphenicol 10 mg and polymyxin B sulfate 5,000 units.
CHLOROPTIC-P S.O.P.: chloramphenicol 1% and prednisolone alcohol 0.5%.
CORTISPORIN OPHTHALMIC OINTMENT♦: polymyxin B sulfate 5,000 units, bacitracin zinc 400 units, neomycin sulfate 0.5%, and hydrocortisone 1%.
ISOPTO CETAPRED SUSPENSION♦: sulfacetamide 10% and prednisolone acetate 0.25%.
MAXITROL OPHTHALMIC OINTMENT/SUSPENSION♦: dexamethasone 0.1%, neomycin sulfate 3.5 mg, and polymyxin B sulfate 6,000 units.
MYCITRACIN OPHTHALMIC: polymyxin B sulfate 5,000 units, neomycin sulfate 5 mg, and bacitracin 500 units.
NEO-CORTEF OPHTHALMIC♦: hydrocortisone 0.5% or 1.5% and neomycin sulfate 0.5%.
NEODECADRON OPHTHALMIC OINTMENT: dexamethasone phosphate 0.5% and neomycin sulfate 0.5%.
NEO-DELTA CORTEF SUSPENSION: prednisolone acetate 0.25%; neomycin sulfate 0.5%.
NEO-MEDROL OINTMENT: methylprednisolone 0.1% and neomycin sulfate 0.5%.
NEOSPORIN OPHTHALMIC OINTMENT♦: polymyxin B sulfate 5,000 units, neomycin sulfate 5 mg, and bacitracin zinc 100 units/g.
OPTIMYD SOLUTION: prednisolone phosphate 0.5% and sodium sulfacetamide 10%.
POLYSPORIN OPHTHALMIC OINTMENT: neomycin sulfate 5 mg, polymyxin B sulfate 10,000 units, and bacitracin zinc 500 units.
SULFAPRED OPHTHALMIC SUSPENSION: sodium sulfacetamide 10%, prednisolone acetate 0.25%, and phenylephrine HCl 0.125%.
VASOCIDIN OINTMENT: sodium sulfacetamide 10%, prednisolone acetate 0.2%, and phenylephrine HCl 0.125%.

NAMES, INDICATIONS AND DOSAGES	SIDE EFFECTS
bacitracin Baciguent Ophthalmic Ointment♦ **Ocular infections:** ADULTS AND CHILDREN: apply small amount into conjunctival sac several times a day or p.r.n. until favorable response is observed.	**Eye:** slowed corneal wound healing, temporary visual haze. **Other:** overgrowth of nonsusceptible organisms.
benzalkonium chloride Spensomide, Zephiran♦ **To increase transcorneal penetration of drugs:** ADULTS AND CHILDREN: 1:5,000 to 1:2,000 concentration used in some irrigating solutions for its antiseptic as well as its surface-active qualities. **To sterilize ophthalmic solutions:** use 1:5,000 concentration. An ingredient in germicidal cleaning solutions for contact lens.	**Eye:** toxic to abraded cornea and to endothelial cells of cornea if introduced into anterior chamber.
boric acid Blinx, Collyrium, Neo-Flo **For irrigation following tonometry, gonioscopy, foreign body removal, or use of fluorescein; used to soothe and cleanse the eye; used in conjunction with contact lens:** ADULTS: irrigate eye with 2% solution or apply 5% or 10% ointment, p.r.n.	*Note:* toxic if absorbed from abraded skin areas, granulating wounds, or ingestion.
chloramphenicol Antibiopto, Chloromycetin Ophthalmic♦, Chloroptic Ophthalmic♦, Chloroptic S.O.P., Econochlor Ophthalmic, Fenicol♦♦, Isopto Fenicol♦♦, Nova-Phenicol♦♦, Ophthoclor Ophthalmic, Pentamycetin♦♦ **Surface bacterial infection involving conjunctiva or cornea:** ADULTS AND CHILDREN: instill 2 drops of solution in eye q 1 hour until condition improves, or instill q.i.d., depending on severity of infection. Apply small amount of ointment to lower conjunctival sac at bedtime as supplement to drops. May use ointment alone by applying a small amount of ointment to lower conjunctival sac q 3 to 6 hours or more frequently, if necessary. Continue until condition improves.	*Note:* systemic adverse reactions have not been reported with short-term topical use. **Blood:** *bone marrow hypoplasia with prolonged use.* **Eye:** optic atrophy in children, stinging or burning of eye after instillation. **Other:** overgrowth of nonsusceptible organisms; hypersensitivity, including itching and burning eye, dermatitis, angioedema.

♦ Available in U.S. and Canada. ♦♦ Available in Canada only.
All other products (no symbol) available in U.S. only. Italicized side effects are common or life-threatening.

INTERACTIONS AND SPECIAL CONSIDERATIONS

Interactions:
HEAVY METALS (SILVER NITRATE): inactivate bacitracin. Don't use together.

Special considerations:
• Use cautiously in patients with hereditary predisposition to antibiotic hypersensitivity.
• Patient should avoid sharing washcloths and towels with family members and should always wash hands before and after applying ointment.
• Eye area should be cleansed of excessive exudate before application.
• Patient should watch for signs of sensitivity, such as itching lids or constant burning. Patient should stop drug and notify doctor immediately.
• Compliance with recommended therapy is important.
• Tip of tube should not touch any part of eye or surrounding tissue.
• Solution not commercially available but may be prepared by pharmacy. May be stored up to 3 weeks in refrigerator.
• Bactericidal or bacteriostatic, depending on concentration and infection.
• Store in tightly closed, light-resistant container.
• Patient should not share eye medication. If a family member develops similar symptoms, he should contact the doctor.

Interactions:
FLUORESCEIN: destroys benzalkonium chloride antibacterial activity. May cause corneal staining. Don't use together.
SULFONAMIDES (OPHTHALMIC): incompatible. Don't apply at same time.

Special considerations:
• A straight benzalkonium chloride solution should never be prepared for use in eye.
• Patient should avoid sharing washcloths and towels with family members.
• Concentrations greater than 1:5,000 should not be used in the eye; may be irritating.
• Patient should watch for signs of sensitivity, such as itching lids or constant burning. Patient should stop drug and notify doctor immediately.
• Applicator should not be touched to eye or surrounding tissue.
• Hands should always be washed before and after applying drug.
• Eye area should be cleansed of excessive exudate before application.
• Present in majority of combination topical eye preparations commercially available.
• Patient should not share eye medication. If a family member develops similar symptoms, he should contact the doctor.

Interactions:
POLYVINYL ALCOHOL (LIQUIFILM): may form insoluble complex. Check with pharmacy on contents in eye drugs and contact lens wetting solutions.

Special considerations:
• Contraindicated in eye abrasions.
• Should not be applied to abraded cornea or skin.
• Lethal dose is 5 to 6 g in infants and 15 to 20 g in adults.
• Hands should always be washed before and after instilling solution or ointment.
• Not for use with soft contact lenses.
• Weak bacteriostatic, fungistatic agent.
• Patient should not share eye medications. If a family member develops similar symptoms, he should contact the doctor.

No significant interactions.

Special considerations:
• Not for long-term use. Patient should notify doctor if no improvement in 3 days.
• If patient has more than a superficial infection, systemic therapy should be used also.
• Bacteriostatic.
• One of the safest topical ocular antibiotics, especially for endophthalmitis.
• Patient should avoid sharing washcloths and towels with family members.
• Hands should always be washed before and after applying ointment or solution.
• Eye area should always be cleansed of excessive exudate before application.
• Patient should watch for signs of sensitivity, such as itching lids or constant burning. Patient should stop drug and notify doctor immediately.
• Compliance with recommended therapy is important.
• Patient should not touch tip of applicator to eye or surrounding tissue.
• If chloramphenicol drops are to be given every 1 hour then tapered, order should be followed closely to ensure adequate anterior chamber levels.
• Store in tightly closed, light-resistant container.
• Patient should not share eye medications. If a family member develops similar symptoms, he should contact the doctor.

NAMES, INDICATIONS AND DOSAGES	SIDE EFFECTS
chlortetracycline hydrochloride Aureomycin Ophthalmic **Superficial ocular infection:** ADULTS AND CHILDREN: apply 1% ointment to eye q 2 hours or more, p.r.n.	**Eye:** itching and burning. **Other:** overgrowth of nonsusceptible organisms with long-term use, dermatitis.
erythromycin Ilotycin Ophthalmic ♦ **Acute and chronic conjunctivitis, other eye infections:** ADULTS AND CHILDREN: apply 0.5% ointment 1 or more times daily, depending upon severity of infection.	**Eye:** slowed corneal wound healing. **Other:** overgrowth of nonsusceptible organisms with long-term use; hypersensitivity, including itching and burning eye, urticaria, dermatitis, angioedema.
gentamicin sulfate Garamycin Ophthalmic ♦, Genoptic **External ocular infections (conjunctivitis, keratoconjunctivitis, corneal ulcers, blepharitis, blepharoconjunctivitis, meibomianitis, and dacryocystitis) due to susceptible organisms, especially *Pseudomonas aeruginosa, Proteus, Klebsiella pneumoniae, Escherichia coli:*** ADULTS AND CHILDREN: instill 1 to 2 drops in eye q 4 hours. In severe infections, may use up to 2 drops q 1 hour. Apply ointment to lower conjunctival sac b.i.d. to t.i.d.	*Note:* systemic absorption from excessive use may cause systemic toxicities. **Eye:** burning or stinging with ointment, transient irritation from solution. **Other:** hypersensitivity, overgrowth of nonsusceptible organisms with long-term use.
idoxuridine (IDU) Dendrid, Herplex, Stoxil ♦ **Herpes simplex keratitis:** ADULTS AND CHILDREN: instill 1 drop of solution into conjunctival sac q 1 hour during day and q 2 hours at night, or apply ointment to conjunctival sac q 4 hours or 5 times daily, with last dose at bedtime. A response should be seen in 7 days; if not, discontinue and begin alternate therapy. Therapy should not be continued longer than 21 days.	**Eye:** temporary visual haze; irritation, pain, burning, or inflammation of eye; mild edema of eyelid or cornea; photosensitivity; small punctate defects in corneal epithelium; slowed corneal wound healing with ointment. **Other:** hypersensitivity.

INTERACTIONS AND SPECIAL CONSIDERATIONS

No significant interactions.

Special considerations:

- Contraindicated in tetracycline hypersensitivity.
- *Pseudomonas, Proteus,* and *Staphylococcus* resistant to drug. Used mainly for trachoma with oral therapy. Trachoma treatment may continue 2 months or more. Trachoma may cause blindness if untreated or if treated improperly.
- Patient should avoid sharing washcloths and towels with family members.
- Hands should always be washed before and after applying ointment.
- Eye should be cleansed of excessive exudate before application.
- Patient should watch for signs of sensitivity, such as itching lids or constant burning. Patient should stop drug and notify doctor immediately.
- Compliance with recommended therapy is important.
- Patient should not touch tip of tube to eye or surrounding tissue.
- Bacteriostatic.
- Store in tightly closed, light-resistant container.
- Patient should not share eye medications. If a family member develops similar symptoms, he should contact the doctor.

No significant interactions.

Special considerations:

- Bacteriostatic but may be bactericidal in high concentrations or against highly susceptible organisms.
- Has a limited antibacterial spectrum. Should be used only when sensitivity studies show it is effective against infecting organisms. Should not be used in infections of unknown etiology.
- Patient should avoid sharing washcloths and towels with family members.
- Hands should always be washed before and after applying ointment.
- Eye area should be cleansed before and after applying ointment.
- Patient should watch for signs of sensitivity, such as itching lids or constant burning. Patient should stop drug and notify doctor immediately.
- Compliance with recommended therapy is important.
- Patient should not touch tube to eye or surrounding tissue.
- Store at room temperature in tightly closed, light-resistant container.
- Patient should not share eye medications. If a family member develops similar symptoms, he should contact the doctor.

No significant interactions.

Special considerations:

- Contraindicated in aminoglycoside hypersensitivity. Use cautiously in impaired renal function.
- Culture required before drug is taken.
- Importance of following recommended therapy should be stressed. *Pseudomonas* infections can cause complete vision loss within 24 hours if infection is not controlled.
- Patient should avoid sharing washcloths and towels with family members.
- Hands should always be washed before and after applying ointment or solution.
- Eye area should be cleansed of excessive exudate before application.
- Patient should watch for signs of sensitivity, such as itching lids or constant burning. Patient should stop drug and notify doctor immediately.
- Patient should not touch tip of tube or dropper to eye or surrounding tissue.
- Store away from heat.
- Patient should not share eye medications. If a family member develops similar symptoms, he should contact the doctor.

No significant interactions.

Special considerations:

- Contraindicated in deep ulceration.
- Not for long-term use.
- Idoxuridine should not be mixed with other medications.
- Don't use old solution: causes ocular burning and has no antiviral activity.
- Patient should avoid sharing washcloths and towels with family members.
- Hands should always be washed before and after applying ointment or solution.
- Eye area should be cleansed of excessive exudate before application.
- Patient should watch for signs of sensitivity, such as itching lids or constant burning. Patient should stop drug and notify doctor immediately.
- Compliance with recommended therapy should be stressed.
- Tip of tube or dropper should not touch eye or surrounding tissue.
- Idoxuridine 0.1% solution should be refrigerated and stored in tightly closed, light-resistant container.
- Patient should not share eye medications. If a family member develops similar symptoms, he should contact the doctor.

NAMES, INDICATIONS AND DOSAGES	SIDE EFFECTS
natamycin Natacyn **Treatment of fungal keratitis:** ADULTS: initial dosage 1 drop instilled in conjunctival sac q 1 to 2 hours. After 3 to 4 days, reduce dosage to 1 drop 6 to 8 times daily.	**Eye:** ocular edema, hyperemia.
neomycin sulfate Myciguent Ophthalmic **Used alone or in combination with other antibiotics in treating superficial ocular infections involving conjunctiva or cornea:** ADULTS AND CHILDREN: apply ointment to lower conjunctival sac daily to t.i.d.	**Other:** hypersensitivity reactions (itching and burning eye, erythema, dermatitis, urticaria); after long-term use, overgrowth of nonsusceptible organisms.
polymyxin B sulfate Aerosporin♦ **Used alone or in combination with other agents for treating corneal ulcers resulting from *Pseudomonas* infection or other gram-negative organism infections:** ADULTS AND CHILDREN: instill 1 to 3 drops of 0.1% to 0.25% (10,000 to 25,000 units/ml) q 1 hour. Increase interval according to patient response; or up to 10,000 units subconjunctivally daily by doctor.	**Eye:** eye irritation, conjunctivitis. **Other:** overgrowth of nonsusceptible organisms, hypersensitivity (local burning, itching).
silver nitrate 1% **Prevention of gonorrheal ophthalmia neonatorum:** NEONATES: cleanse lids thoroughly; instill 1 drop of 1% solution into each eye.	**Eye:** periorbital edema, temporary staining of lids and surrounding tissue, conjunctivitis (with concentrations greater than 1%).

INTERACTIONS AND SPECIAL CONSIDERATIONS

No significant interactions.

Special considerations:
- Only antifungal available as ophthalmic preparation.
- Treatment of choice for fungal keratitis. May also be used to treat fungal blepharitis and conjunctivitis.
- Therapy should be continued for 14 to 21 days, or until active disease subsides.
- Dosage should be reduced gradually at 4- to 7-day intervals to assure that organism has been eliminated.
- If infection does not improve with 7 to 10 days of therapy, clinical and laboratory reevaluation is recommended.
- Patient should avoid sharing washcloths and towels with family members.
- Hands should always be washed before and after applying ointment or solution.
- Eye area should be cleansed of excessive exudate before application.
- Compliance with recomended therapy should be stressed.
- Tip of dropper should not touch eye or surrounding tissue.
- Patient should not share eye medications. If a family member develops similar symptoms, he should contact the doctor.

No significant interactions.

Special considerations:
- Contraindicated in aminoglycoside hypersensitivity.
- Effective against gram-positive and gram-negative organisms.
- Patient should avoid sharing washcloths and towels with family members.
- Hands should always be washed before and after applying ointment.
- Patient should watch for signs of sensitivity, such as itching lids or constant burning. Patient should stop drug and notify doctor immediately.
- Compliance with recommended therapy should be stressed.
- Patient should not touch tip of tube to eye or surrounding tissue.
- Bactericidal.
- Patient should not share eye medications. If a family member develops similar symptoms, he should contact the doctor.
- For symptoms and treatment of anaphylaxis, see APPENDIX.

No significant interactions.

Special considerations:
- One of the most effective antibiotics against gram-negative organisms, especially *Pseudomonas*.
- Often used in combination with neomycin sulfate.
- Patient should avoid sharing washcloths and towels with family members.
- Hands should always be washed before and after instilling solution.
- Patient should watch for signs of sensitivity, such as itching lids and lashes or constant burning. Patient should stop drug and notify doctor immediately.
- Compliance with recommended therapy should be stressed.
- Patient should not touch tip of dropper to eye or surrounding tissue.
- Bactericidal.
- Not commercially available. Polymyxin B sulfate powder must be reconstituted with sterile water for injection or normal saline solution. Refrigerated solutions stable for 6 months.
- Should be carefully reconstituted to ensure correct drug concentration in solution.
- Patient should not share eye medications. If a family member develops similar symptoms, he should contact the doctor.

Interactions:
BACITRACIN: inactivates silver nitrate. Don't use together.

Special considerations:
- Legally required for neonates in most states.
- Should not be used repeatedly.
- If 2% solution is accidentally used in eye, prompt irrigation with isotonic sodium chloride is advised to prevent eye irritation.
- Instillation may be delayed slightly to allow neonate to bond with mother.
- Hands should always be washed before instilling solution.
- Store wax ampules away from light and heat.
- Bacteriostatic, germicidal, and astringent.
- Eyes should not be irrigated following instillation.

NAMES, INDICATIONS AND DOSAGES	SIDE EFFECTS
sulfacetamide sodium 10% Bleph-10 Liquifilm Ophthalmic♦, Cetamide Ophthalmic♦, 10% Sodium Sulamyd Ophthalmic, Sulf-10 Ophthalmic♦ **sulfacetamide sodium 15%** Isopto Cetamide Ophthalmic♦, Sulfacel-15 Ophthalmic **sulfacetamide sodium 30%** Sodium Sulamyd 30% Ophthalmic♦ **Inclusion conjunctivitis, corneal ulcers, trachoma, prophylaxis to ocular infection:** ADULTS AND CHILDREN: instill 1 to 2 drops of 10% solution into lower conjunctival sac q 2 to 3 hours during day, less often at night; or instill 1 to 2 drops of 15% solution into lower conjunctival sac q 1 to 2 hours initially, increasing interval as condition responds; or instill 1 drop of 30% solution into lower conjunctival sac q 2 hours. Instill ½" to 1" of 10% ointment into conjunctival sac q.i.d. and at bedtime. May use ointment at night along with drops during the day.	**Eye:** slowed corneal wound healing (ointment), pain on instilling eye drop. **Other:** hypersensitivity (including itching or burning), overgrowth of nonsusceptible organisms.
tetracycline hydrochloride Achromycin Ophthalmic♦ ADULTS AND CHILDREN: **Superficial ocular infections and inclusion conjunctivitis:** instill 1 to 2 drops in eye b.i.d., q.i.d., or more often, depending on severity of infection. **Trachoma:** instill 2 drops in each eye b.i.d., t.i.d., or q.i.d. Continue for 1 to 2 months or longer, or use 1% ointment t.i.d. to q.i.d. for 30 days.	**Eye:** itching. **Other:** hypersensitivity (eye itching and dermatitis), overgrowth of nonsusceptible organisms with long-term use.
tobramycin Tobrex **Treatment of external ocular infections caused by susceptible bacteria:** ADULTS AND CHILDREN: In mild-to-moderate infections, instill 1 or 2 drops into the affected eye q 4 hours. In severe infections, instill 2 drops into the infected eye hourly.	**Eye:** burning or stinging upon instillation. **Other:** hypersensitivity.
trifluridine Viroptic Ophthalmic Solution 1% **Primary keratoconjunctivitis and recurrent epithelial keratitis due to herpes simplex virus, types 1 and 2:** ADULTS: 1 drop of solution q 2 hours while patient is awake, to a maximum of 9 drops daily until re-epithelialization of the corneal ulcer occurs; then 1 drop q 4 hours (minimum 5 drops daily) for an additional 7 days.	**Eye:** stinging upon instillation, edema of eyelids.

♦ Available in U.S. and Canada. ♦♦ Available in Canada only.
All other products (no symbol) available in U.S. only. Italicized side effects are common or life-threatening.

INTERACTIONS AND SPECIAL CONSIDERATIONS

Interactions:
LOCAL ANESTHETICS (PROCAINE, TETRACAINE), *P*-AMINOBENZOIC ACID DERIVATIVES: decreased sulfacetamide sodium action. Wait ½ to 1 hour after instilling anesthetic or *p*-aminobenzoic acid derivative before instilling sulfacetamide.

Special considerations:
- Contraindicated in sulfonamide hypersensitivity.
- Often used with systemic tetracycline in treating trachoma and inclusion conjunctivitis.
- Replaced by antibiotics in treating major ocular infections; still used in minor ocular infections.
- Purulent exudate interferes with sulfacetamide action. As much exudate as possible should be removed from lids before instilling sulfacetamide.
- Incompatible with silver preparations.
- Eye drop is painful.
- Patient should avoid sharing washcloths and towels with family members.
- Hands should always be washed before and after applying ointment or solution.
- Patient should watch for signs of sensitivity, such as itching lids or constant burning. Patient should stop drug and notify doctor immediately.
- Compliance with recommended therapy should be stressed.
- Patient should not touch tip of tube or dropper to eye or surrounding tissue.
- Store in tightly closed, light-resistant container away from heat.
- Discolored (dark brown) solution should not be used.
- Patient should not share eye medications. If a family member develops similar symptoms, he should contact the doctor.

No significant interactions.

Special considerations:
- Trachoma therapy should continue for 1 to 2 months or longer. Trachoma may cause blindness if untreated or if not treated properly.
- Gnats and flies are vectors of the trachoma organism. Patient with trachoma should not let them settle around eye area. Infection is spread by direct contact, so handwashing is essential to prevent spread.
- Patient should avoid sharing washcloths and towels with family members.
- Hands should always be washed before and after applying solution.
- Eye area should be cleansed of excessive exudate before application.
- Patient should watch for signs of sensitivity, such as itching lids or constant burning. Patient should stop drug and notify doctor immediately.
- Compliance with recommended therapy should be stressed.
- Patient should not touch tip of dropper to eye or surrounding tissue.
- Store in tightly closed, light-resistant container.
- Patient should not share eye medications. If a family member develops similar symptoms, he should contact the doctor.

Interactions:
TETRACYCLINE-CONTAINING EYE PREPARATIONS: incompatible with tyloxapol, an ingredient in Tobrex. Don't use together.

Special considerations:
- Prolonged use may result in overgrowth of nonsusceptible organisms, including fungi.
- Patient should always wash hands before and after instilling solution.
- Patient should avoid sharing washcloths and towels with family members.
- Patient should report signs of sensitivity (itching lids or constant burning) and discontinue drug.
- Patient should not touch tip of dropper to eye or surrounding tissue.

No significant interactions.

Special considerations:
- Should be prescribed only for those patients with clinical diagnosis of herpetic keratitis.
- Consider another form of therapy if improvement doesn't occur after 7 days' treatment or complete re-epithelialization after 14 days' treatment. Trifluridine shouldn't be used more than 21 days continuously due to potential ocular toxicity.
- Mild local irritation of the conjunctiva and cornea that occurs when solution is instilled is usually temporary.
- Drug should be refrigerated.
- More effective drug than vidarabine with fewer side effects.
- Patient should avoid sharing washcloths and towels with family members.
- Patient should wash hands before and after administration.
- Patient should not touch tip of dropper to eye or surrounding tissue.
- Patient should not share eye medications. If

(continued on following page)

NAMES, INDICATIONS AND DOSAGES	SIDE EFFECTS
trifluridine *(continued)*	
vidarabine Vira-A Ophthalmic♦ **Acute keratoconjunctivitis, superficial keratitis, and recurrent epithelial keratitis resulting from herpes simplex types 1 and 2:** ADULTS AND CHILDREN: instill ½″ ointment into lower conjunctival sac 5 times daily at 3-hour intervals.	**Eye:** temporary visual burning, itching, mild irritation of eye, lacrimation, foreign body sensation, conjunctival injection, superficial punctate keratitis, eye pain, photosensitivity. **Other:** hypersensitivity.

INTERACTIONS AND SPECIAL CONSIDERATIONS

a family member develops the same symptoms, he should contact the doctor.
• Compliance with recommended therapy should be stressed.

No significant interactions.

Special considerations:
• Not for long-term use.
• A relatively new alternative in treating herpes simplex ocular infections.
• Patient should not exceed recommended frequency or duration of dosage.
• Not effective against RNA virus or adenoviral ocular infections, or against bacterial, fungal, or chlamydial infections.
• Patient should avoid sharing washcloths and towels with family members.
• Hands should always be washed before and after applying ointment.
• Patient should watch for signs of sensitivity, such as itching lids or constant burning. Patient should stop drug and notify doctor immediately.
• Patient should not touch tip of tube to eye or surrounding tissue.
• Available in 3% ointment.
• Store in tightly closed, light-resistant container.
• Patient should not share eye medications. If a family member develops similar symptoms, he should contact the doctor.

77

Ophthalmic anti-inflammatory agents

dexamethasone
dexamethasone sodium phosphate
fluorometholone
hydrocortisone
hydrocortisone acetate
medrysone
prednisolone acetate
prednisolone sodium phosphate

These potent corticosteroids are used topically in the eye to treat inflammatory ophthalmic conditions. Their use should be supervised.

Major uses
The drugs are used to treat inflammatory disorders of the eyelids, conjunctiva, cornea, and anterior segment of the globe. They also treat corneal injury from chemical or thermal burns.

Mechanism of action
The drugs decrease the infiltration of leukocytes at the site of inflammation.

Absorption, distribution, metabolism, and excretion
Absorption through the intact corneal membrane is minimal. The drugs available as suspensions are generally absorbed to a greater extent than are the solutions.

Onset and duration
Onset and duration vary. Therapeutic action depends on the inflammation and the drug used.

Combination products
Corticosteroids for ophthalmic use are commonly combined with antibiotics and sulfonamides. See Chapter 76, OPHTHALMIC ANTI-INFECTIVES.

WHEN TO USE CORTICOSTEROID AND ANTIBACTERIAL MIXTURES

Combinations of corticosteroids and antibacterials can be used to treat conditions that require both anti-inflammatory and anti-infective action, such as marginal keratitis secondary to staphylococcal infection, blepharoconjunctivitis, allergic conjunctivitis with chronic bacterial conjunctivitis, phlyctenular keratoconjunctivitis, and selected cases of postoperative inflammation.

These mixtures are not used to treat routine ocular infections or inflammatory disorders because:

- Corticosteroids reduce resistance to infection.
- The antibacterial drug may have an adverse effect on the course of the disease if it's not effective against the invading organism, not present in sufficient concentration, or if nonsusceptible organisms (particularly fungi and viruses) are present.
- Hypersensitivity to the antibacterial may develop but go unnoticed because corticosteroids can mask an allergic response.

PATIENT-TEACHING AID

HOW TO USE EYE DROPS AND EYE OINTMENT

Dear Patient:

To relieve your eye infection or irritation, the doctor has prescribed either eye drops or eye ointment. Here's how to use them.

To instill eye drops

- First, wash your hands thoroughly.
- Hold the bottle to the light and examine it. If the medication is discolored or contains sediment, discard it and have the prescription refilled. If it looks OK, warm the medication to room temperature by holding the bottle between your palms for 2 minutes.
- Next, moisten a cotton ball or tissue with water, and clean all secretions from around your eyes. Use a fresh cotton ball or tissue for each eye, so you don't spread infection.
- Stand or sit before a mirror. Squeeze the bulb of the eyedropper to fill the dropper with medication.
- Tilt your head back slightly and toward the eye you're treating. Pull down your lower eyelid. (Don't pull your upper eyelid, or you'll put unnecessary pressure on your eye.)
- Position the dropper over the area between your lower lid and the white of your eye. Steady your hand by resting two fingers against your cheek or nose.

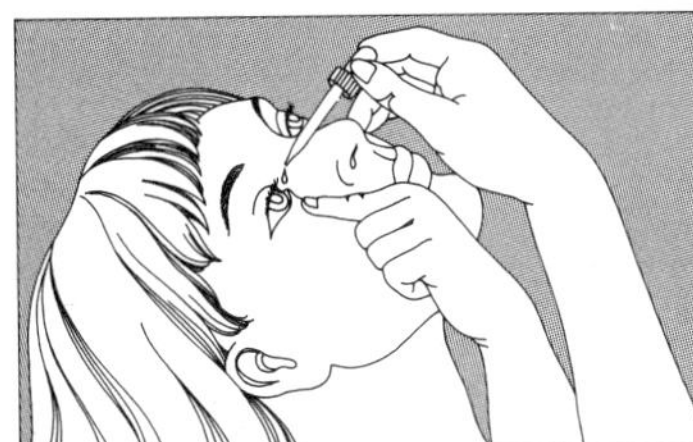

- Look away from the dropper. Then, squeeze the prescribed number of drops into the sac of the lower lid of your eye. (See illustration.) Take care not to drop the medication directly onto your eyeball or touch the dropper to your eye or eyelashes. Wipe away excess medication with a clean tissue.
- Recap the medication. Store the bottle away from light and extreme heat.

To instill eye ointment

- First, cleanse your eyelids and lashes with an irrigating solution.
- Then, remove the cap from the tube, taking care not to contaminate the applicator end by letting it touch anything.

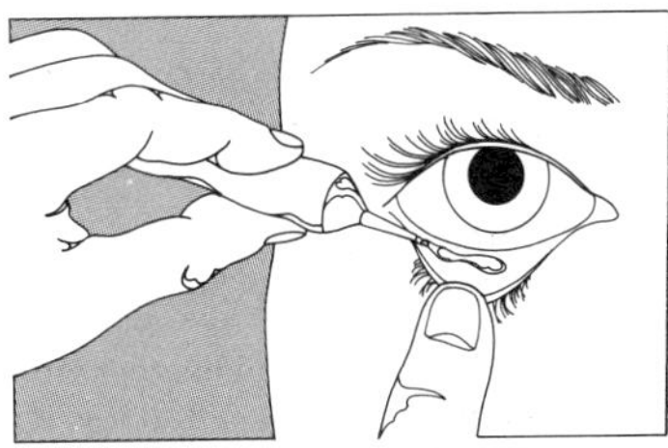

- Squeeze a small ribbon of medication along the inside of your lower eyelid. (See illustration.)
- Keep your eyelids closed for 1 to 2 minutes after application to allow the medication to spread and be absorbed.

You may experience blurred vision for a few minutes after the ointment is applied. This is normal.

A final caution

Never put any medication in your eyes unless the label reads FOR OPHTHALMIC USE or FOR USE IN THE EYES. Call your doctor immediately if you notice such side effects as decreased visual acuity, persistent blurred vision, or unusual redness or irritation when using medication.

NAMES, INDICATIONS AND DOSAGES	SIDE EFFECTS
dexamethasone Maxidex Ophthalmic Suspension♦ **dexamethasone sodium phosphate** Decadron Phosphate Ophthalmic♦, Maxidex Ophthalmic♦, Novadex♦♦, Opto-Methasone♦♦ **Uveitis; iridocyclitis; inflammatory condition of eyelids, conjunctiva, cornea, anterior segment of globe; corneal injury from chemical or thermal burns, or penetration of foreign bodies; allergic conjunctivitis:** ADULTS AND CHILDREN: instill 1 to 2 drops into conjunctival sac. In severe disease, drops may be used hourly, tapering to discontinuation as condition improves. In mild conditions, drops may be used up to 4 to 6 times daily. Treatment may extend from a few days to several weeks.	**Eye:** increased intraocular pressure, especially in elderly patients; thinning of cornea, interference with corneal wound healing, increased susceptibility to viral or fungal corneal infection, corneal ulceration; with excessive or long-term use, glaucoma exacerbations, cataracts, defects in visual acuity and visual field, optic nerve damage. **Other:** systemic effects and adrenal suppression with excessive or long-term use.
fluorometholone FML Liquifilm Ophthalmic♦ **Inflammatory and allergic conditions of cornea, conjunctiva, sclera, anterior uvea:** ADULTS AND CHILDREN: instill 1 to 2 drops q 1 hour for first 1 to 2 days, then b.i.d., t.i.d., or q.i.d.	**Eye:** increased intraocular pressure, especially in elderly patients; thinning of cornea, interference with corneal wound healing, corneal ulceration, increased susceptibility to viral or fungal corneal infections; with excessive or long-term use, glaucoma exacerbations, cataracts, decreased visual acuity, diminished visual field; optic nerve damage. **Other:** systemic effects and adrenal suppression in excessive or long-term use.
hydrocortisone Optef **hydrocortisone acetate** Cortamed♦♦, Hydrocortone♦ **Uveitis, iridocyclitis, inflammatory condition of eyelids, conjunctiva, cornea, anterior segment of globe; to prevent corneal scarring in visual axis; corneal injury from chemical or thermal burns, or penetration of foreign bodies; allergic conjunctivitis:** ADULTS AND CHILDREN: instill 1 to 3 drops into conjunctival sac q 1 hour during the day and q 2 hours during the night in acute situations. May be decreased to 1 drop t.i.d. or q.i.d.; or instill ointment t.i.d. to q.i.d. initially. May decrease to daily or b.i.d.	**Eye:** increased intraocular pressure, especially in elderly patients; thinning of cornea, interference with corneal wound healing, increased susceptibility to viral or fungal corneal infection, corneal ulceration; with excessive or long-term use, glaucoma exacerbations, cataracts, visual acuity and visual field defects, optic nerve damage. **Other:** systemic effects and adrenal suppression with excessive or long-term use.
medrysone HMS Liquifilm Ophthalmic♦ **Allergic conjunctivitis, vernal conjunctivitis, episcleritis, ophthalmic epinephrine sensitivity reaction:** ADULTS AND CHILDREN: instill 1 drop in conjunctival sac b.i.d. to q.i.d. May use q hour during first 1 to 2 days if needed.	**Eye:** thinning of cornea, interference with corneal wound healing, increased susceptibility to viral or fungal corneal infection, corneal ulceration; with excessive or long-term use, glaucoma exacerbations, cataracts, visual acuity and visual field defects, optic nerve damage. **Other:** systemic effects and adrenal suppression with excessive or long-term use.

♦ Available in U.S. and Canada. ♦♦ Available in Canada only.
All other products (no symbol) available in U.S. only. Italicized side effects are common or life-threatening.

INTERACTIONS AND SPECIAL CONSIDERATIONS

No significant interactions.

Special considerations:

• Contraindicated in acute superficial herpes simplex (dendritic keratitis), vaccinia, varicella, or other fungal or viral diseases of cornea and conjunctiva; presence of active diabetes; ocular tuberculosis, or any acute, purulent, untreated infection of the eye. Use cautiously in corneal abrasions, since these may be infected (especially with herpes); and in patients with glaucoma (any form), due to possibility of increasing intraocular pressure (miotic medication drug regimen may need to be increased to compensate).
• Viral and fungal infections of the cornea may be exacerbated by the application of steroids.
• Patient should call doctor immediately and stop drug if visual acuity changes or visual field diminishes.
• Not for long-term use.
• Eye pad may be used with ointment for increased effect.
• Patient may develop corneal ulceration; may require stopping drug.
• Anti-inflammatory effect of dexamethasone is greater than that of dexamethasone sodium phosphate.
• Patient should not use leftover medication for a new eye infection; can cause serious problems.
• Patient should not share eye medications. If a family member develops similar symptoms, he should contact the doctor.

No significant interactions.

Special considerations:

• Contraindicated in vaccinia, varicella, acute superficial herpes simplex (dendritic keratitis), or other fungal or viral eye diseases; ocular tuberculosis; or any acute, purulent, untreated eye infection. Use cautiously in corneal abrasions since they are commonly contaminated (especially with herpes).
• Not for long-term use.
• Less likely to cause increased intraocular pressure with long-term use than other ophthalmic anti-inflammatory drugs (except medrysone).
• Store in tightly covered, light-resistant container.
• Patient should call doctor immediately and stop drug if visual acuity decreases or visual field diminishes.
• Should be shaken before using.
• Patient should not use leftover medication for a new eye infection; can cause serious problems.
• Patient should not share eye medications. If a family member develops similar symptoms, he should contact the doctor.

No significant interactions.

Special considerations:

• Contraindicated in acute superficial herpes simplex (dendritic keratitis), vaccinia, varicella, or other fungal or viral diseases of cornea and conjunctiva; presence of active diabetes; ocular tuberculosis; or any acute, purulent, untreated eye infection. Use cautiously in corneal abrasions since they are commonly contaminated (especially with herpes).
• Viral and fungal infections of the cornea may be exacerbated by the application of steroids.
• Possibility of increasing intraocular pressure.
• Patient should call doctor immediately and stop drug if visual acuity changes or visual field diminishes.
• Not for long-term use.
• Eye pad may be used with ointment for increased effect.
• Patient may develop corneal ulceration; may require stopping drug.
• Patient should not use leftover medication for a new eye infection; can cause serious problems.
• Patient should not share eye medications. If a family member develops similar symptoms, he should contact the doctor.

No significant interactions.

Special considerations:

• Contraindicated in vaccinia, varicella, acute superficial herpes simplex (dendritic keratitis), viral diseases of conjunctiva and cornea, ocular tuberculosis, fungal or viral eye diseases, iritis, uveitis, or any acute, purulent, untreated eye infection. Use cautiously in corneal abrasions since they are commonly contaminated (especially with herpes).
• Should be shaken before using. Should not be frozen.
• Patient should not use leftover medication for a new eye infection; can cause serious problems.
• Patient should not share eye medications. If a family member develops similar symptoms, he should contact the doctor.

NAMES, INDICATIONS AND DOSAGES	SIDE EFFECTS
prednisolone acetate (suspensions) Econopred Ophthalmic, Econopred Plus Ophthalmic, Pred-Forte♦, Pred Mild Ophthalmic♦, Prednicon♦♦, Predulose Ophthalmic **prednisolone sodium phosphate (solutions)** Hydeltrasol Ophthalmic, Inflamase Forte♦, Inflamase Ophthalmic♦, Metreton Ophthalmic, Nova-Pred Forte♦♦ **Inflammation of palpebral and bulbar conjunctiva, cornea, and anterior segment of globe:** ADULTS AND CHILDREN: instill 2 drops in eye. In severe conditions, may be used hourly, tapering to discontinuation as inflammation subsides. In mild conditions, may be used up to 4 to 6 times daily.	**Eye:** increased intraocular pressure, especially in elderly patients; thinning of cornea, interference with corneal wound healing, increased susceptibility to viral or fungal corneal infection, corneal ulceration; with excessive or long-term use, glaucoma exacerbations, cataracts, visual acuity and visual field defects, optic nerve damage. **Other:** systemic effects and adrenal suppression with excessive or long-term use.

♦ Available in U.S. and Canada. ♦♦ Available in Canada only.
All other products (no symbol) available in U.S. only. Italicized side effects are common or life-threatening.

INTERACTIONS AND SPECIAL CONSIDERATIONS

No significant interactions.

Special considerations:

- Contraindicated in acute, untreated, purulent ocular infections, acute superficial herpes simplex (dendritic keratitis), vaccinia, varicella, or other viral or fungal eye diseases, ocular tuberculosis. Use cautiously in corneal abrasions since they are commonly contaminated (especially with herpes).
- Patient on long-term therapy should have frequent tonometric examinations.
- Should be shaken before using and stored in tightly covered container.
- Therapy should not be stopped prematurely.
- Patient should not use leftover medication for a new eye infection; can cause serious problems.
- Patient should not share eye medications. If a family member develops similar symptoms, he should contact the doctor.

78

Miotics

acetylcholine chloride
carbachol
demecarium bromide
echothiophate iodide
isoflurophate
physostigmine salicylate
pilocarpine hydrochloride
pilocarpine nitrate

Miotics are topical drugs that cause pupillary constriction (miosis). They're used in chronic ophthalmic conditions and in surgical procedures for ocular disorders.

Major uses

Miotics are used to treat open-angle and narrow-angle glaucoma. They are also therapeutic in iridectomy, anterior segment surgery, and other ocular surgery. When used with mydriatics, they prevent adhesions after ocular surgery.

Mechanism of action

• Acetylcholine chloride, carbachol, and pilocarpine hydrochloride (cholinergic drugs) cause contraction of the sphincter muscles of the iris, resulting in miosis. They also produce ciliary spasm, deepening of the anterior chamber, and vasodilation of conjunctival vessels of the outflow tract.

• Demecarium bromide, echothiophate iodide, isoflurophate, and physostigmine salicylate (anticholinesterase drugs) inhibit the enzymatic destruction of acetylcholine by inactivating cholinesterase. This leaves acetylcholine free to act on the effector cells of the iridic sphincter and ciliary muscles, causing pupillary constriction and accommodation spasm.

Absorption, distribution, metabolism, and excretion

Although some systemic absorption is possible with all agents except acetylcholine, systemic side effects are unusual. Among all the drugs, demecarium and echothiophate are most likely to produce systemic side effects when used excessively. Drug-related symptoms of significant absorption include hypersalivation, nausea, vomiting, and bronchospasm.

Onset and duration

The accompanying chart summarizes the therapeutic activity of the miotics.

Combination products

E-CARPINE♦: epinephrine bitartrate 0.5% and pilocarpine HCl 1%, 2%, 3%, 4%, or 6%.
E-PILO♦: epinephrine bitartrate 1%; pilocarpine HCl 1%, 2%, 3%, 4%, or 6%.

THERAPEUTIC ACTIVITY OF MIOTICS

DRUG	ONSET	DURATION	ADVANTAGES OR DISADVANTAGES
acetylcholine	10 to 15 sec	15 min	Best for surgery
carbachol	10 to 20 min	4 to 8 hr	Stronger than pilocarpine but doesn't penetrate as well
demecarium	15 to 30 min	12 to 48 hr	May cause prolonged and serious systemic side effects, but a more stable compound than echothiophate
echothiophate	15 to 30 min	1 to 2 wk	May cause prolonged and serious systemic side effects; very unstable
isoflurophate	5 to 10 min	2 to 4 wk	Very unstable
physostigmine	10 to 30 min	24 to 48 hr	Commonly causes headache
pilocarpine	15 min	4 to 8 hr	Tolerance develops; usually strength must be increased

ISOPTO P-ES: pilocarpine HCl 2% and physostigmine salicylate 0.125%.
P_1E_1, P_2E_1, P_3E_1, P_4E_1, P_6E_1: epinephrine bitartrate 1% and pilocarpine HCl 1%, 2%, 3%, 4%, or 6%.

NAMES, INDICATIONS AND DOSAGES	SIDE EFFECTS
acetylcholine chloride Miochol♦ **Anterior segment surgery:** ADULTS AND CHILDREN: doctor instills 0.5 to 2 ml of 1% solution gently in anterior chamber of eye.	None reported with 1% concentration. Iris atrophy possible with higher concentrations.
carbachol (intraocular) Miostat **carbachol (topical)** Carbacel, Isopto Carbachol♦ **Ocular surgery (to produce pupillary miosis):** ADULTS: doctor should gently instill 0.5 ml into the anterior chamber for production of satisfactory miosis. It may be instilled before or after securing sutures. **Open-angle or narrow-angle glaucoma:** ADULTS: instill 1 drop into eye daily, b.i.d., t.i.d., or q.i.d. Ointment form also available with b.i.d. dosage.	**CNS:** headache. **Eye:** accommodative spasm, blurred vision, conjunctival vasodilation, eye and brow pain. **GI:** abdominal cramps, diarrhea. **Other:** sweating, flushing, asthma.
demecarium bromide Humorsol **Glaucoma, postiridectomy:** ADULTS: instill 1 drop 0.125% or 0.25% solution in eyes twice weekly up to b.i.d., depending on intraocular pressure. **Accommodative esotropia:** CHILDREN: instill 1 drop 0.125% solution in each eye daily for 2 to 3 weeks, taper to 1 drop q 2 days for 3 to 4 weeks, then 1 drop twice weekly. Therapy should be discontinued after 4 months if control of condition still requires q other day therapy or if patient shows no response.	**CNS:** headache. **CV:** hypotension, bradycardia. **Eye:** iris cysts (reversible with discontinuation), lens opacity, ciliary or accommodative spasm, blurred vision, eye or brow pain, photosensitivity, eyelid twitching, congestive iritis, iridocyclitis, conjunctival and intraocular hyperemia, ocular pain, photophobia, acute attack of narrow-angle glaucoma. **GI:** nausea, vomiting, abdominal pain, diarrhea, excessive salivation. **GU:** frequent urination. **Skin:** contact dermatitis. **Other:** flushing, bronchial constriction.

INTERACTIONS AND SPECIAL CONSIDERATIONS

No significant interactions.

Special considerations:
• Vial should be shaken gently until clear solution is obtained.
• Should be reconstituted immediately before using.
• Any unused solution should be discarded.
• Complete miosis within seconds.
• Vial should not be gas sterilized. Ethylene oxide may produce formic acid.

No significant interactions.

Special considerations:
• Contraindicated in acute iritis and corneal abrasion. Use cautiously in acute cardiac failure, bronchial asthma, peptic ulcer, hyperthyroidism, GI spasm, urinary tract obstruction, Parkinson's disease.
• A cholinergic agent.
• Used in glaucoma, especially when patient is resistant or allergic to pilocarpine HCl or nitrate.
• Patient should not exceed recommended dosage.
• For single-dose intraocular use only. Premixed; discard unused portions.
• Patient should not touch tip of dropper to eye or surrounding tissue.
• Long-term use may be necessary for glaucoma patients. Compliance should be stressed, and patient should remain under medical supervision for periodic tonometric readings.
• In case of toxicity, atropine should be given parenterally.
• Patient should not drive car for 1 or 2 hours after administration.
• Patient should be shown how to instill medication.

Interactions:
SYSTEMIC ANTICHOLINESTERASE FOR MYASTHENIA GRAVIS: additive effects. Monitor patient for signs of toxicity.
ECHOTHIOPHATE IODIDE: decreased duration of miosis if demecarium bromide is given first. Give echothiophate iodide first.
ORGANOPHOSPHORUS INSECTICIDES: additive effects. Warn patient exposed to insecticides of this danger.
PILOCARPINE: interferes with miosis. Do not use together.
SUCCINYLCHOLINE: respiratory or cardiovascular collapse. Don't use together.

Special considerations:
• Contraindicated in active uveal inflammation, narrow-angle glaucoma, secondary glaucoma resulting from iridocyclitis, ocular hypertension, vasomotor instability, bronchial asthma, spastic GI conditions, peptic ulcer, severe bradycardia, hypotension, recent myocardial infarction, epilepsy, parkinsonism, history of retinal detachment. Use cautiously in patients with myasthenia gravis receiving systemic anticholinesterase therapy and in patients exposed to organophosphorus insecticides.
• Systemic absorption may be minimized by compressing inner canthus of eye for 1 to 2 minutes after instilling drops.
• Dangerous drug capable of producing cumulative systemic side effects. Prescribed concentration and dosage schedule should be followed closely and patient carefully monitored.
• Atropine sulfate given subcutaneously or I.V., and pralidoxine chloride are antidotes of choice.
• Patient should stop drug and report immediately if excessive salivation, diaphoresis, urinary incontinence, diarrhea, or muscle weakness occurs.
• Patient should take at bedtime since drug blurs vision.
• Patient should not exceed recommended dosage.
• Patient should not touch tip of dropper to eye or surrounding tissue.
• Drug should be stopped at least 2 weeks before surgery.
• If solution comes into contact with skin, should be washed promptly with large amount of water.
• Hands should be washed immediately before and after administering medication.
• Patient should be monitored for lenticular opacities every 6 months.
• Close and constant medical supervision is vital.
• Rapid instillation of 1% to 2% epinephrine at 5-minute intervals is recommended for any extraocular pressure changes.
• Antidote for atropine for glaucoma or preglaucoma patients, and to control preoperative and postoperative intraocular pressure tension of glaucoma.
• Store in tightly closed container.
• An extremely potent, long-acting anticholinesterase drug.
• Blurred vision usually diminishes with prolonged use.
• Patient should be shown how to instill medication.

NAMES, INDICATIONS AND DOSAGES	SIDE EFFECTS
echothiophate iodide Echodide, Phospholine Iodide♦ **Open-angle glaucoma, conditions obstructing aqueous outflow, accommodative esotropia:** ADULTS AND CHILDREN: instill 1 drop 0.03% to 0.125% solution into conjunctival sac daily. Maximum 1 drop b.i.d. Use lowest possible dosage to continuously control intraocular pressure.	**CNS:** fatigue, muscle weakness, paresthesias, headache. **CV:** bradycardia, hypotension. **Eye:** ciliary or accommodative spasm, ciliary or conjunctival injection, nonreversible cataract formation (time- and dose-related), reversible iris cysts, pupillary block, blurred or dimmed vision, eye or brow pain, lid twitching, hyperemia, photosensitivity, lens opacities, lacrimation, retinal detachment. **GI:** diarrhea, nausea, vomiting, abdominal pain, intestinal cramps, salivation. **GU:** frequent urination. **Other:** flushing, sweating, bronchial constriction.
isoflurophate Floropryl **Glaucoma:** ADULTS AND CHILDREN: instill ¼" strip 0.025% ointment in conjunctival sac q 8 to 72 hours. **Esotropia uncomplicated by amblyopia or anisometropia:** ADULTS AND CHILDREN: ¼" of ointment every night for 2 weeks.	**CNS:** headache, muscle weakness. **Eye:** moderate conjunctival hyperemia, eye pain, ciliary spasm causing discomfort, iris cysts, cataract formation, retinal detachment, paradoxical increase in intraocular pressure; precipitates attacks of acute narrow-angle glaucoma. **GI:** diarrhea, salivation. **Other:** sweating, bronchial constriction.

INTERACTIONS AND SPECIAL CONSIDERATIONS

Interactions:

ORGANOPHOSPHORUS INSECTICIDES (PARATHION, MALATHION): may have an additive effect that could cause systemic effects. Warn patient exposed to insecticides of this danger.

SUCCINYLCHOLINE: respiratory and cardiovascular collapse. Don't use together.

SYSTEMIC ANTICHOLINESTERASE FOR MYASTHENIA GRAVIS: effects may be additive. Monitor patient for signs of toxicity.

Special considerations:

- Contraindicated in narrow-angle glaucoma, epilepsy, vasomotor instability, parkinsonism, iodide hypersensitivity, active uveal inflammation, ocular hypertension with intraocular inflammatory processes, bronchial asthma, spastic GI conditions, urinary tract obstruction, peptic ulcer, severe bradycardia or hypotension, vascular hypertension, myocardial infarction, history of retinal detachment. Use cautiously in patients routinely exposed to organophosphate insecticides. May cause nausea, vomiting, and diarrhea, progressing to muscle weakness and respiratory difficulty. Use cautiously in patients with myasthenia gravis receiving anticholinesterase therapy.
- Toxicity is cumulative. Toxic systemic symptoms don't appear for weeks or months after initiating therapy.
- Powder should be reconstituted carefully to avoid contamination. Only diluent provided should be used. Refrigerated, reconstituted solution should be discarded after 6 months; solution at room temperature after 1 month.
- Transient brow pain or dimmed or blurred vision is common at first but usually disappears within 5 to 10 days.
- Systemic absorption may be minimized by compressing inner canthus of eye for 1 to 2 minutes after instilling drops.
- Should be instilled at bedtime, since drug causes transient blurred vision.
- Patient should remain under constant medical supervision and not exceed recommended dosage.
- Patient should report salivation, diarrhea, profuse sweating, urinary incontinence, or muscle weakness.
- Drug should be stopped at least 2 weeks before surgery.
- Atropine sulfate (subcutaneously, I.M., or I.V.) is antidote of choice.
- A potent, long-acting, irreversible anticholinesterase.
- Patient should not touch tip of dropper to eye or surrounding tissue.
- Hands should be washed immediately before and after administering medication.
- Patient should be shown how to instill medication.

Interactions:

DEMECARIUM, PHYSOSTIGMINE: competitive action. Decreased duration of miosis if isoflurophate given second. Give isoflurophate first.

PILOCARPINE: interferes with miosis. Use cautiously for ciliary spasm.

SUCCINYLCHOLINE: respiratory or cardiovascular collapse. Don't use together.

SYSTEMIC ANTICHOLINESTERASE FOR MYASTHENIA GRAVIS: additive effects. Monitor patient for signs of toxicity.

Special considerations:

- Contraindicated in hypersensitivity to organophosphorus compounds, peanut oil, and polyethylene mineral oil; in patients with uveal inflammation, narrow-angle glaucoma, ocular hypertension, bronchial asthma, peptic ulcer, severe bradycardia, hypotension, recent myocardial infarction, epilepsy, parkinsonism, or history of retinal detachment. Use cautiously in patients exposed to organophosphate insecticides and in patients with myasthenia gravis receiving concurrent anticholinesterase drugs.
- Patient with glaucoma should use at bedtime, if possible, because of blurred vision and ciliary spasm.
- Tip of tube should not touch eye, surrounding tissues, or any moist surface.
- Close, constant medical supervision is vital. Patient should not exceed prescribed dosage.
- Rapid instillation of 1% to 2% epinephrine at 5-minute intervals should be used to treat paradoxical pressure changes.
- Patient should stop therapy at once and report immediately excessive salivation, diarrhea, sweating, muscle weakness.
- Systemic absorption may be minimized by compressing inner canthus of eye for 1 to 2 minutes after instilling drops.
- Unstable and inactivated in the presence of water.
- Store in refrigerator in a tightly closed container.
- Rapidly absorbed through skin.
- A potent parasympathomimetic, or anticholinesterase, drug.
- Hands should be washed immediately before and after administering medication.
- Patient should be shown how to instill medication.

NAMES, INDICATIONS AND DOSAGES	SIDE EFFECTS
physostigmine salicylate Eserine Salicylate, Isopto Eserine **Atropine mydriasis, acute narrow-angle glaucoma:** ADULTS AND CHILDREN: instill ¼" 0.25% ophthalmic ointment in conjunctival sac, or instill 1 to 2 drops 0.25% to 0.5% solution in conjunctival sac t.i.d. Repeat p.r.n. to obtain miosis.	**CNS:** *headache.* **Eye:** twitching of eyelids, conjunctival irritation, reversible depigmentation of lid skin in Blacks allergic to ointment, eye and brow pain, marked miosis, lacrimation, dimmed or blurred vision, follicular cysts. **Skin:** allergic dermatitis.
pilocarpine hydrochloride Adsorbocarpine♦, Almocarpine, Isopto Carpine♦, Miocarpine♦♦, Nova-Carpine♦♦, Ocusert Pilo♦, Opto-Pilo♦♦, Pilocar, Pilocel, Pilomiotin **pilocarpine nitrate** P.V. Carpine Liquifilm♦ **Chronic open-angle glaucoma, before emergency surgery in acute narrow-angle glaucoma:** ADULTS AND CHILDREN: instill 1 to 2 drops in eye daily b.i.d., t.i.d., q.i.d., or as directed by doctor.	**Eye:** suborbital headache, *myopia,* ciliary spasm, *blurred vision,* conjunctival irritation, lacrimation, changes in visual field, *brow pain.* **GI:** nausea, vomiting, abdominal cramps, diarrhea, salivation. **Other:** bronchiolar spasm, pulmonary edema, hypersensitivity.

♦ Available in U.S. and Canada. ♦♦ Available in Canada only.
All other products (no symbol) available in U.S. only. Italicized side effects are common or life-threatening.

INTERACTIONS AND SPECIAL CONSIDERATIONS

Interactions:
ISOFLUROPHATE: decreased miosis if isoflurophate given second. Give isoflurophate first.
ORGANOPHOSPHORUS INSECTICIDES: additive effect. Warn patient exposed to insecticides of this danger.
PILOCARPINE: prolonged miosis. May be used together therapeutically.
SUCCINYLCHOLINE: additive effect. Don't use together.

Special considerations:
• Contraindicated in inflammatory diseases of iris or ciliary body, asthma, diabetes mellitus, gangrene, cardiovascular disease, mechanical obstruction of intestinal or urogenital tract, vagotonia, secondary glaucoma. Use cautiously in bradycardia, epilepsy, parkinsonism, and in patients exposed to organophosphate insecticides.
• Glaucoma therapy is long-term. Compliance should be stressed. Patient should not exceed dosage.
• Lid twitching, temporarily blurred vision, and difficulty in seeing in the dark are common side effects.
• Irritating to eye. Conjunctivitis or allergic reactions are possible.
• Dropper or tip of tube should not touch eye or surrounding tissue.
• Systemic absorption may be minimized by compressing inner canthus of eye for 1 to 2 minutes after instilling drops.
• Discolored (rusty or pink) solution or ointment should be discarded. Aqueous solutions oxidize on exposure to light or air.
• Anticholinesterase.
• Used in ocular myasthenia gravis.
• May be used alternately with atropine as a miotic to break adhesions between the iris and lens.
• Hands should be washed immediately before and after instilling medication.
• Patient should be shown how to instill medication.

Interactions:
CARBACHOL: additive effect. Do not use together.
PHENYLEPHRINE HCl: decreased dilation by phenylephrine HCl. Don't use together.

Special considerations:
• Contraindicated in acute iritis, acute inflammatory disease of anterior segment of eye, secondary glaucoma. Use cautiously in bronchial asthma and hypertension.
• Vision will be temporarily blurred.
• Transient brow pain and myopia are common at first; usually disappear in 10 to 14 days.
• Patient should not exceed recommended dosage.
• Patient should not touch dropper to eye or surrounding tissue.
• Glaucoma therapy is necessarily prolonged. Compliance should be stressed. Glaucoma can cause blindness.
• Most widely used drug in initial treatment of chronic open-angle glaucoma.
• Systemic absorption may be minimized by compressing inner canthus of eye for 1 to 2 minutes after instilling drops.
• Also used to counteract effects of mydriatics and cycloplegics after surgery or ophthalmoscopic examination.
• May be used alternately with atropine to break adhesions between iris and lens.
• In acute narrow-angle glaucoma before surgery, may be used alone or with physostigmine or mannitol, urea, or glycerol.
• Hands should be washed immediately before and after administering medication.
• Patient should be shown how to instill medication.

79

Mydriatics

atropine sulfate
cyclopentolate hydrochloride
epinephrine bitartrate
epinephrine hydrochloride
epinephryl borate
homatropine hydrobromide
hydroxyamphetamine hydrobromide
phenylephrine hydrochloride
scopolamine hydrobromide
tropicamide

Both anticholinergics (atropine, cyclopentolate, homatropine, scopolamine, and tropicamide) and adrenergics (epinephrine, epinephryl borate, hydroxyamphetamine, and phenylephrine) produce mydriasis (pupillary dilation) when applied topically to the eye. In addition, the anticholinergics produce cycloplegia (paralysis of accommodation).

Major uses

- Atropine, homatropine, and scopolamine are used in acute inflammation of the iris (iritis), or of the iris, ciliary body, and choroid (uveitis).
- Cyclopentolate, hydroxyamphetamine, phenylephrine, and tropicamide are used in diagnostic procedures.
- The epinephrine salts are used with or without miotics to lower intraocular pressure in open-angle glaucoma.

Mechanism of action

- Anticholinergics block acetylcholine, leaving the pupil under the unopposed influence of its sympathetic or adrenergic nerve supply. This causes the pupil to dilate. Relaxation of the ciliary muscle allows the lens to flatten.
- Adrenergics dilate the pupil by contracting the dilator muscle of the pupil.

Absorption, distribution, metabolism, and excretion

- Anticholinergics can be systemically absorbed, causing side effects, particularly in children and elderly persons. (For more information on absorption of anticholinergics, see Chapter 37, CHOLINERGIC BLOCKERS.) Side effects such as dry mouth and tachycardia are most common after instillation of atropine, scopolamine, and cyclopentolate.
- Penetration by adrenergics is heightened during surgical procedures and in the traumatized eye. (For greater detail, see Chapter 38, ADRENERGICS.)
- Adrenergics are systemically absorbed less often than anticholinergics. Repeated instillation of phenylephrine (10% solution) may exacerbate hypertension.

Onset and duration

- Atropine produces mydriasis in 30 to 40 minutes; dilation can last 12 to 14 days before complete recovery. The drug causes cycloplegia within a few hours; this effect lasts 2 weeks or more before complete recovery.
- Cyclopentolate produces mydriasis in 15 to 30 minutes that lasts up to 24 hours. Cyclopentolate produces cycloplegia in 15 to 45 minutes that lasts up to 24 hours
- Epinephrine produces mydriasis within minutes after instillation; dilation lasts several hours. Epinephrine lowers intraocular pressure for variable lengths of time. The maximal interval is 4 to 8 hours; recovery occurs in 12 to 24 or more hours. (Epinephrine also causes, in 5 minutes, vasoconstriction that lasts 1 hour.)
- Homatropine hydrobromide has a shorter duration than atropine. Cycloplegia begins in 30 to 90 minutes, and recovery takes 10 to 48 hours. Maximal cycloplegia occurs

MYDRIATICS FACILITATE EYE EXAMINATION

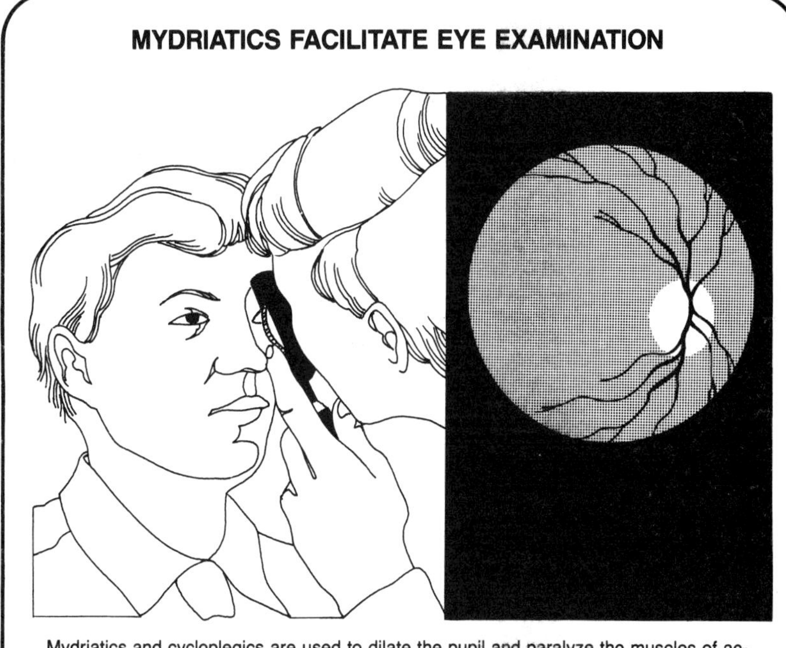

Mydriatics and cycloplegics are used to dilate the pupil and paralyze the muscles of accommodation so that the eyegrounds can be visualized during ophthalmic examination.

within 1 hour; recovery is in 1 to 3 days.

• Hydroxyamphetamine produces maximal dilation within 40 minutes after instillation. The dilation continues for several hours. Cycloplegia begins in 30 to 60 minutes; recovery takes 20 hours for adults and several days for children.

• Phenylephrine (2.5% solution) produces dilation within minutes after instillation. Maximal dilation occurs in 15 to 60 minutes and lasts up to 3 hours.

• Scopolamine produces maximal dilation within 40 minutes after instillation; recovery occurs in 3 to 7 days. Cycloplegia, which begins in 10 to 30 minutes, reaches a maximum within 30 to 45 minutes. Complete recovery may take several days.

• Tropicamide produces maximal dilation in 20 to 25 minutes after application, and cycloplegia that lasts about 20 minutes. Recovery is complete in about 6 hours.

Combination products

CYCLOMYDRIL: cyclopentolate HCl 0.2% and phenylephrine HCl 1%.
MYDRAPRED: prednisolone acetate 0.25% and atropine sulfate 1%

NAMES, INDICATIONS AND DOSAGES	SIDE EFFECTS
atropine sulfate Atropisol, BufOpto Atropine, Isopto Atropine♦, Opto-Tropinal♦♦ **Acute iris inflammation (iritis):** ADULTS: 1 to 2 drops of 1% solution or small amount of ointment 2 to 3 times daily, b.i.d., or t.i.d. CHILDREN: instill 1 to 2 drops of 0.5% solution daily, b.i.d., or t.i.d. **Cycloplegic refraction:** ADULTS: instill 1 to 2 drops of 1% solution 1 hour before refracting. CHILDREN: instill 1 to 2 drops of 0.5% solution to each eye b.i.d. for 1 to 3 days before eye examination and 1 hour before refraction, or instill small amount ointment daily or b.i.d. 2 to 3 days before examination.	**Eye:** increased intraocular pressure, ocular congestion in long-term use, conjunctivitis, contact dermatitis, edema, *blurred vision,* eye dryness, *photophobia*. **Systemic:** flushing, dry skin and mouth, fever, tachycardia, abdominal distention in infants, ataxia, irritability, confusion, somnolence.
cyclopentolate hydrochloride Cyclogyl♦, Mydplegic♦♦, Nova-Cyclo♦♦, Opto-Pentolate♦♦ **Diagnostic procedures requiring mydriasis and cycloplegia:** ADULTS: instill 1 drop 1% solution in eye, followed by 1 more drop in 5 minutes. Use 2% solution in heavily pigmented irises. CHILDREN: instill 1 drop of 0.5%, 1%, or 2% solution in each eye, followed in 5 minutes with 1 drop 0.5% or 1% solution, if necessary. Not recommended for children under 6 years.	**Eye:** burning sensation on instillation, increased intraocular pressure, blurred vision, eye dryness, *photophobia,* ocular congestion, contact dermatitis, conjunctivitis. **Systemic:** flushing, tachycardia, urinary retention, dry skin, fever, ataxia, irritability, confusion, somnolence, convulsions.
epinephrine bitartrate E1, E2, Epitrate♦, Murocoll, Mytrate **epinephrine hydrochloride** Epifrin♦, Glaucon♦ **epinephryl borate** Epinal♦ ADULTS AND CHILDREN: **Intraocular injection:** 0.1 to 0.2 ml of 0.01% or 0.1% epinephrine HCl by doctor. **Open-angle glaucoma:** instill 1 to 2 drops of 1% or 2% bitartrate solution in eye with frequency determined by tonometric readings (once q 2 to 4 days up to q.i.d.), or instill 1 drop 0.5%, 1%, or 2% HCl solution (or 0.25%, 0.5%, or 1% epinephryl borate solution) in eye b.i.d. **During surgery:** 1 or more drops of 0.1% epinephrine HCl up to 3 times.	**Eye:** corneal or conjunctival pigmentation or corneal edema in long-term use; follicular hypertrophy; chemosis; conjunctivitis; iritis; hyperemic conjunctiva; maculopapular rash; severe stinging, burning, and tearing upon instillation; brow pain. **Systemic:** palpitations, tachycardia.
homatropine hydrobromide Homatrocel Ophthalmic, Isopto Homatropine♦ ADULTS AND CHILDREN: **Cycloplegic refraction:** instill 1 to 2 drops 2% or 5% solution in eye; repeat in 5 to 10 minutes. **Uveitis:** instill 1 to 2 drops 2% or 5% solution	**Eye:** eye irritation, *blurred vision, photophobia*. **Systemic:** flushing, dry skin and mouth, fever, tachycardia, ataxia, irritability, confusion, somnolence.

♦ Available in U.S. and Canada. ♦♦ Available in Canada only.
All other products (no symbol) available in U.S. only. Italicized side effects are common or life-threatening.

INTERACTIONS AND SPECIAL CONSIDERATIONS

No significant interactions.

Special considerations:
• Contraindicated in primary glaucoma (shallow anterior chamber or narrow-angle) and in increased intraocular pressure. Use cautiously in infants, children, and in elderly or debilitated patients.
• Vision will be temporarily blurred. Dark glasses should be worn to ease discomfort of photophobia.
• Not for internal use. Drops and ointment should be treated as poison. Physostigmine should be kept available as antidote for poisoning. Signs of poisoning are disorientation and confusion.
• Dropper or tip of tube should not touch eye or surrounding tissue.
• Signs of glaucoma: increased intraocular pressure, ocular pain, headache, progressive blurring of vision.
• Most potent mydriatic and cycloplegic available; long duration of action.
• Patient should not operate machinery or drive car until the temporary visual impairment caused by this drug has worn off.
• Patient should not exceed recommended dosage.
• Systemic absorption may be minimized by compressing inner canthus of eye for 1 to 2 minutes after instilling drops.
• Patient should be shown how to instill medication.
• For symptoms and treatment of toxicity (if ingested), see APPENDIX.

No significant interactions.

Special considerations:
• Contraindicated in narrow-angle glaucoma. Use cautiously in elderly patients.
• Systemic absorption may be minimized by compressing inner canthus of eye for 1 to 2 minutes after instilling drops.
• Container should be closed after each use to avoid contamination.
• Potent drug with mydriatic and cycloplegic effects; superior to homatropine hydrobromide and has shorter duration of action.
• Patient should wear dark glasses to ease discomfort of photophobia.
• Drug will burn when instilled.
• Patient should not operate machinery or drive car until the temporary visual impairment caused by this drug has worn off.
• Patient should be shown how to instill medication.

Interactions:
CYCLOPROPANE OR HALOGENATED HYDROCARBONS: arrhythmias, tachycardia. Use together cautiously, if at all.
TRICYCLIC ANTIDEPRESSANTS, ANTIHISTAMINES (DIPHENHYDRAMINE, DEXCHLORPHENIRAMINE): potentiated cardiac effects of epinephrine. Use together cautiously.

Special considerations:
• Contraindicated in shallow anterior chamber or narrow-angle glaucoma.
• Use cautiously in diabetes mellitus, hypertension, Parkinson's disease, hyperthyroidism, aphakia (eye without lens), cardiac disease, cerebral arteriosclerosis, and in elderly patients or pregnant women.
• May stain soft contact lenses.
• Should be used with pilocarpine: additive effect in lowering intraocular pressure.
• Blood pressure and other systemic effects should be monitored.
• Should be protected from light and heat.
• Darkened solution should not be used.
• Also used during surgery to control local bleeding, or injected into the anterior chamber to produce rapid mydriasis during cataract removal.
• Patient should not touch dropper to eye or surrounding tissue.
• Hands should be washed immediately before and after administration.
• Patient should be shown how to instill medication.

No significant interactions.

Special considerations:
• Contraindicated in primary glaucoma (shallow anterior chamber or narrow-angle). Use cautiously in infants, elderly or debilitated patients, or in patients with hypertension, cardiac disease, or increased intraocular pressure.
• Vision will be temporarily blurred after instillation. Patient should not drive car or operate machinery until this wears off. Dark glasses should be worn to ease discomfort of photophobia.
• Long-term frequent use may produce symp-

(continued on following page)

NAMES, INDICATIONS AND DOSAGES	SIDE EFFECTS

homatropine hydrobromide
(continued)

in eye up to every 3 to 4 hours.

hydroxyamphetamine hydrobromide
Paredrine

Diagnosis of Horner's syndrome:
ADULTS AND CHILDREN OVER 12 YEARS: instill 1 to 2 drops 1% solution into conjunctival sac.

Eye: increased intraocular pressure, blurred vision, *photophobia*.

phenylephrine hydrochloride
Mydfrin, Neo-Synephrine♦

ADULTS AND CHILDREN:
Mydriasis (without cycloplegia): instill 1 drop 2.5% or 10% solution in eye before examination.

Posterior synechia (adhesion of iris): instill 1 drop 10% solution in eye.
Do not use 10% concentration in infants; use cautiously in elderly patients.

Eye: transient burning or stinging on instillation, blurred vision, reactive hyperemia, allergic conjunctivitis, iris floaters, narrow-angle glaucoma, rebound miosis, allergic conjunctivitis, dermatitis.
CNS: headache, brow pain.
CV: *hypertension*, tachycardia, palpitations, premature ventricular contractions.
Other: pallor, trembling, sweating.

scopolamine hydrobromide
Isopto Hyoscine

Cycloplegic refraction:
ADULTS: instill 1 to 2 drops 0.5% to 1% solution in eye 1 hour before refraction.
CHILDREN: instill 1 drop 0.2% or 0.25% solution or ointment b.i.d. for 2 days before refraction.

Iritis:
ADULTS: 1 to 2 drops of 0.1% solution daily, b.i.d., or t.i.d.

Eye: ocular congestion with prolonged use, conjunctivitis, *blurred vision,* eye dryness, increased intraocular pressure, *photophobia,* contact dermatitis.
Systemic: flushing, fever, dry skin and mouth, tachycardia, hallucinations, ataxia, irritability, confusion, delirium, somnolence.

INTERACTIONS AND SPECIAL CONSIDERATIONS

toms of atropine SO_4 poisoning, such as severe dryness of mouth and tachycardia.
• Not for internal use. Should be treated as poison and physostigmine kept available as antidote for poisoning.
• Systemic absorption may be minimized by compressing inner canthus of eye for 1 to 2 minutes after instilling drops.
• Patient should not touch dropper tip to eye or surrounding tissue.
• Hands should be washed immediately before and after administering medication.
• Similar to atropine SO_4 but weaker, with a shorter duration of action.
• Patient should be shown how to instill medication.
• For symptoms and treatment of toxicity (if ingested), see APPENDIX.

No significant interactions.

Special considerations:
• Contraindicated in narrow-angle glaucoma. Use cautiously in hypertension, hyperthyroidism, diabetes mellitus, increased intraocular pressure.
• Patient should wear dark glasses to ease discomfort of photophobia.
• May cause blurred vision. Patient should not drive car or operate machinery until this effect wears off.
• Store in tightly closed container, and discard discolored solution.
• Hands should be washed immediately before and after administering medication.
• If ingested, toxic symptoms include arrhythmias, headache, nausea, vomiting. Doctor should be contacted immediately.

Interactions:
GUANETHIDINE: increased mydriatic and pressor effects of phenylephrine HCl. Use together cautiously.
LEVODOPA (SYSTEMIC): reduced mydriatic effect of phenylephrine HCl. Use together cautiously.
MAO INHIBITORS: may cause arrhythmias due to increased pressor effect. Use together cautiously.
TRICYCLIC ANTIDEPRESSANTS: potentiated cardiac effects of epinephrine. Use together cautiously.

Special considerations:
• Contraindicated in narrow-angle glaucoma and in soft contact lens use. Use cautiously in marked hypertension, cardiac disorders, and in children of low body weight.
• Should be avoided in patients with idiopathic orthostatic hypotension. May produce high blood pressure response.
• Protect from light and heat.
• Patient should not exceed recommended dosage. Systemic effects can result. Blood pressure and pulse should be monitored.
• Patient should not touch dropper tip to eye or surrounding tissue.
• Systemic absorption can be minimized by compressing inner canthus of eye for 1 to 2 minutes after instilling drops.
• Potential for systemic side effects less severe with 2.5% solution.
• Hands should be washed immediately before and after administration.
• May cause blurred vision. Patient should not drive car or operate machinery until this effect wears off.
• Patient should be shown how to instill medication.

No significant interactions.

Special considerations:
• Contraindicated in primary glaucoma (shallow anterior chamber or narrow-angle). Use cautiously in cardiac disease, increased intraocular pressure, and in patients over 40 years.
• Patient may develop systemic effects (disorientation, delirium).
• Vision will be temporarily blurred. Patient should not drive car or operate machinery until this effect wears off.
• Patient should wear dark glasses to ease discomfort of photophobia.
• Not for internal use.
• May be used when patient is sensitive to atropine. Faster acting and has shorter duration of action and fewer side effects.
• Patient should not touch dropper tip to eye or surrounding tissue.
• Hands should be washed immediately before and after administration.
• Systemic absorption may be minimized by compressing inner canthus of eye for 1 to 2 minutes after instilling drops.
• Patient should be shown how to instill medication.
• For symptoms and treatment of toxicity (if ingested), see APPENDIX.

NAMES, INDICATIONS AND DOSAGES	SIDE EFFECTS
tropicamide Mydriacyl♦ ADULTS AND CHILDREN: **Cycloplegic refractions:** instill 1 to 2 drops of 1% solution in each eye; repeat in 5 minutes. Additional drop may be instilled in 20 to 30 minutes. **Fundus examinations:** instill 1 to 2 drops 0.5% solution in each eye 15 to 20 minutes before examination.	**EENT:** *transient stinging on instillation,* increased intraocular pressure (less than with other mydriatic agents because of shorter duration of action), *blurred vision, photophobia,* dry mouth and throat.

♦ Available in U.S. and Canada. ♦♦ Available in Canada only.
All other products (no symbol) available in U.S. only. Italicized side effects are common or life-threatening.

INTERACTIONS AND SPECIAL CONSIDERATIONS

No significant interactions.

Special considerations:

- Contraindicated in narrow-angle and shallow anterior chamber glaucoma. Use cautiously in elderly patients.
- Shortest acting cycloplegic, but mydriatic effect greater than cycloplegic effect.
- Causes transient stinging; vision temporarily blurred. Patient should not drive car or operate machinery until this effect wears off.
- Patient should wear dark glasses if photosensitivity occurs (lasts about 2 hours).
- Should be stored at room temperature in tightly closed container.
- Patient should be shown how to instill medication.

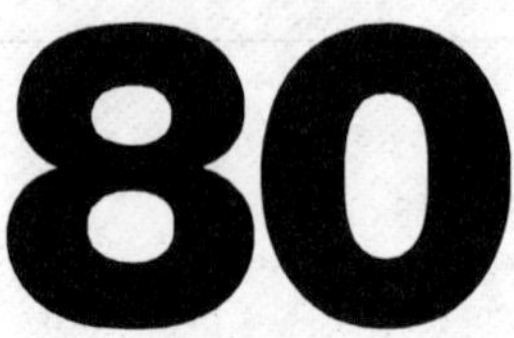

Ophthalmic vasoconstrictors

naphazoline hydrochloride
phenylephrine hydrochloride
tetrahydrozoline hydrochloride
zinc sulfate

Ophthalmic vasoconstrictors relieve the itching and redness of ocular irritations and inflammations. They are available as eye drops, without a prescription.

Major uses

Ophthalmic vasoconstrictors furnish symptomatic relief of ocular congestion, irritation, and itching due to allergic conditions.

Mechanism of action

• Naphazoline, phenylephrine, and tetrahydrozoline produce vasoconstriction by local adrenergic action on the blood vessels of the conjunctiva.
• Zinc sulfate produces astringent action on the conjunctiva.

Absorption, distribution, metabolism, and excretion

• Naphazoline, phenylephrine, and tetrahydrozoline are variably absorbed. The drugs

PATIENT-TEACHING AID

WHEN YOU HAVE RED EYES

Dear Patient:

Irritated red eyes are a symptom of many serious eye diseases. How do you decide when to see a doctor and when to self-medicate with an over-the-counter (OTC) preparation? Consult a doctor if you notice any of the following symptoms:

• your vision is impaired
• your eye is painful
• your eye hurts when exposed to bright light
• your eyelids stick together
• there is any discharge of pus from your eyes
• the redness does not subside after using OTC decongestant eye drops for 2 days
• you suspect you have a foreign body in your eye.

Note: OTC decongestant eye drops should not be used by persons with *narrow-angle* glaucoma or an injured cornea. These preparations make the pupils dilate, which can precipitate a severe glaucoma attack. These attacks can cause blindness. Although the label carries the warning "Do not use in cases of glaucoma," OTC decongestant eye drops can be used by persons with *open-angle* glaucoma.

MATCHING SYMPTOMS WITH CAUSES OF CONJUNCTIVITIS

SYMPTOM	VIRAL	BACTERIAL Purulent	BACTERIAL Nonpurulent	FUNGAL AND PARASITIC	ALLERGIC
Discharge	Minimum	Copious	Minimum	Minimum	Minimum
Tearing	Copious	Moderate	Moderate	Minimum	Moderate
Itching	Minimum	Minimum	None	None	Marked
Localized conjunctival lesions	None	None	Common	Common	None
Preauricular nodes	Common	Uncommon	Common	Common	None
Associated sore throat and fever	Occasionally	Uncommon	None	None	None

Reproduced with permission from Vaughan, D., Asbury, T.: *General Ophthalmology,* 9th ed. Copyright 1980 by Lange Medical Publications, Los Altos, California.

may, however, be absorbed in high enough concentrations to cause systemic side effects, such as transient stinging and irritation, especially in young children.

- Zinc sulfate is not absorbed and has a local effect only.

Onset and duration

- Naphazoline, tetrahydrozoline, and zinc sulfate begin to act within 5 minutes after instillation. Naphazoline acts for as long as 3 to 4 hours; tetrahydrozoline and zinc sulfate are shorter-acting.
- Phenylephrine begins to act within 5 minutes after application; its effect continues for up to 3 hours.

Combination products

BLEPHAMIDE♦: phenylephrine hydrochloride 0.12%, sulfacetamide sodium 10%, and prednisolone acetate 0.2%.
NEOZIN OPHTH: phenylephrine hydrochloride 0.125% and zinc sulfate 0.25%.
PREFRIN-A♦: phenylephrine hydrochloride 0.12%, pyrilamine maleate 0.1%, and antipyrine 0.1%.
PREFIN-Z: phenylephrine hydrochloride 0.12% and zinc sulfate 0.24%.

NAMES, INDICATIONS AND DOSAGES	SIDE EFFECTS
naphazoline hydrochloride 0.012%, 0.1%, 0.02% Albalon Liquifilm Ophthalmic♦, Clear Eyes, Naphcon, Naphcon Forte Ophthalmic♦, Opto-Zoline♦♦, Vasoclear, Vasocon Regular Ophthalmic♦ **Ocular congestion, irritation, itching:** ADULTS: instill 1 to 2 drops in eye q 3 to 4 hours.	**Eye:** transient stinging, pupillary dilation, increased intraocular pressure, irritation.
phenylephrine hydrochloride Isopto Frin, Prefrin, Tear-Efrin **Decongestant, minor eye irritations:** ADULTS AND CHILDREN: 2 drops of 0.12% or 0.25% in affected eye. May repeat in 3 to 4 hours, p.r.n.	**CNS:** headache. **Eye:** transient stinging, iris floaters, narrow-angle glaucoma, blurred vision, reactive hyperemia, brow pain.
tetrahydrozoline hydrochloride Clear & Bright, Soothe, Tetrasine, Visine **Ocular congestion, irritation, and allergic conditions:** ADULTS AND CHILDREN OVER 2 YEARS: instill 1 to 2 drops in eye b.i.d. or t.i.d., or as directed by doctor.	**Eye:** transient stinging, pupillary dilation, increased intraocular pressure, irritation, iris floaters in elderly. **Systemic:** drowsiness, CNS depression, cardiac irregularities, headache, dizziness, tremors, insomnia.
zinc sulfate Bufopto Zinc Sulfate, Eye-Sed Ophthalmic, Op-Thal-Zin **Ocular congestion, irritation:** ADULTS AND CHILDREN: solution 0.2%—instill 1 to 2 drops in eye b.i.d. or t.i.d.	**Eye:** irritation.

♦ Available in U.S. and Canada. ♦♦ Available in Canada only.
All other products (no symbol) available in U.S. only. Italicized side effects are common or life-threatening.

INTERACTIONS AND SPECIAL CONSIDERATIONS

Interactions:
MAO INHIBITORS: hypertensive crisis if naphazoline HCl is systemically absorbed. Use together cautiously.

Special considerations:
• Contraindicated in narrow-angle glaucoma and hypersensitivity to any ingredients. Use cautiously in patients with hyperthyroidism, cardiac disease, hypertension, and diabetes mellitus, and in elderly patients.
• Can produce marked sedation and coma if ingested by child.
• Photophobia may follow pupil dilation if patient is sensitive to drug; it should be reported.
• Patient should not exceed recommended dosage. Rebound congestion and rhinitis may occur with frequent or prolonged use.
• Patient should notify doctor if blurred vision, pain, or lid edema develops.
• Store in tightly closed container.
• Most effective and widely used ocular decongestant.
• Patient should not touch tip of dropper to eye or surrounding tissues.
• Patient should be shown how to instill medication.

Interactions:
MAO INHIBITORS: may cause hypertensive crisis. Don't use together.

Special considerations:
• Contraindicated in narrow-angle glaucoma, in patients taking tricyclic antidepressants or MAO inhibitors, and in hypersensitivity to any ingredient.
• May exacerbate hypertension in hypertensive patients.
• Butacaine drops should not be used as local anesthetic, since phenylephrine and butacaine are incompatible.
• Patient should not exceed prescribed dose.
• Blood pressure and pulse should be monitored; patient should watch for overdosage.
• Solution should be discarded if dark brown or contains precipitate.
• Container should be kept tightly sealed and away from light.
• Patient should not touch tip of dropper to eye or surrounding tissues.
• Patient should not share eye medications.
• Patient should be shown how to instill medication.

Interactions:
MAO INHIBITORS: hypertensive crisis if tetrahydrozoline HCl is systemically absorbed. Don't use together.

Special considerations:
• Contraindicated in patients receiving MAO inhibitors and in those with hypersensitivity to any ingredients or with narrow-angle glaucoma. Use cautiously in patients with hyperthyroidism, cardiac disease, hypertension, diabetes mellitus, and in elderly patients.
• Recommended dosage should not be exceeded. Rebound congestion and rhinitis may occur with frequent or prolonged use.
• Patient should stop drug and notify doctor if relief is not obtained within 48 hours, or if redness or irritation persists or increases.
• Available without prescription.
• Available in 0.05% concentration; less effective than naphazoline hydrochloride 0.1%.
• Patient should not touch dropper tip to eye or surrounding tissue.
• Patient should not share eye medications.
• Patient should be shown how to instill medication.

No significant interactions.

Special considerations:
• Use cautiously in patients with a shallow anterior chamber and in those with predisposition to narrow-angle glaucoma.
• A decongestant astringent.
• Store in tightly closed container.
• Patient should not touch dropper tip to eye or surrounding tissues.
• Patient should not share eye medications.
• Patient should be shown how to instill medication.

81

Topical ophthalmic anesthetics

cocaine hydrochloride
proparacaine hydrochloride
tetracaine hydrochloride

Topical ophthalmic anesthetics are used for various diagnostic and minor surgical procedures. They are not for self-medication and should be used only under a doctor's supervision.

Major uses
The drugs supply anesthesia in tonometric and gonioscopic procedures, suture removal from the cornea, and extraction of a foreign object from the cornea. They are also used as part of emergency management before flushing chemicals from the eye.
• Cocaine hydrochloride is also used to diagnose Horner's syndrome.

Mechanism of action
Topical ophthalmic anesthetics produce anesthesia by preventing initiation and transmission of impulses at the nerve cell membrane.

HOW TO PROTECT THE ANESTHETIZED EYE

After application of topical ophthalmic anesthetics, the patient may need an eye patch to protect his eye from dust, smoke, or other irritants. Here's how to apply it:

1. First, wash your hands. Ask the patient to close both eyes. Then, use as many sterile gauze pads as you need to fill the patients orbital space. Next, grasp the sterile eye patch in the center and place it over the gauze pads, as shown here.

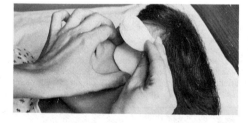

2. Secure the patch with two parallel strips of nonallergenic tape, preferably plastic. Work from the patient's mid-forehead to the cheekbone, as shown here.

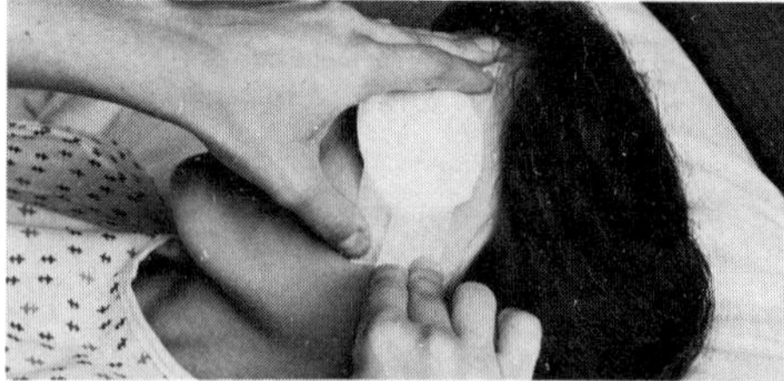

• Cocaine hydrochloride also has an adrenergic action that produces mydriasis and constriction of conjunctival vessels.

Absorption, distribution, metabolism, and excretion

• Proparacaine and tetracaine are not absorbed systemically.
• Cocaine hydrochloride is absorbed systemically, metabolized in the liver, and excreted in urine.

Onset and duration

• Cocaine hydrochloride begins to act within 30 seconds; proparacaine, within 20 seconds; and tetracaine hydrochloride, within 1 minute after administration.
• Proparacaine provides anesthesia up to 15 minutes; tetracaine, up to 20 minutes.
• Cocaine hydrochloride provides complete anesthesia for 10 minutes, moderate anesthesia for another 5 to 10 minutes, and minimal anesthesia for as long as 2 hours.

Combination products

None.

3. For added protection, an eyeshield (or eyecone) may be applied. The eyeshield rests on the bony prominences of the brow, cheek, and nose without touching the underlying dressing. Tape the shield (or cone) in place, as shown here.

When it's time to instill the next dose of medication, remove the patch by loosening the tape from the forehead down. Any drainage on the gauze or the patch should be recorded on the patient's chart.

Replace the gauze pads and patch (if soiled) each time you instill medication.

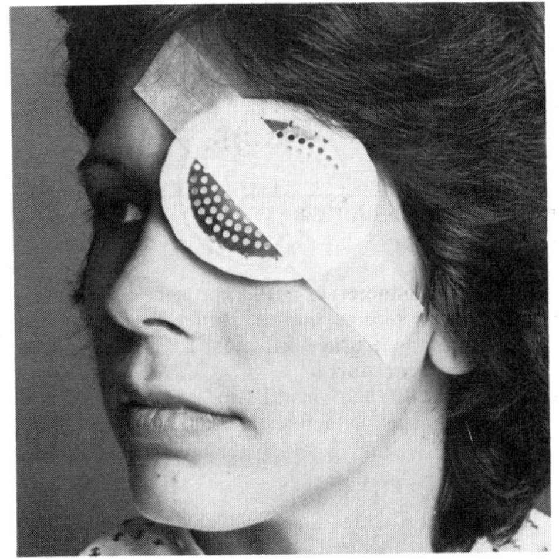

NAMES, INDICATIONS AND DOSAGES	SIDE EFFECTS
cocaine hydrochloride **Diagnosis of Horner's syndrome, topical anesthesia for minor surgery or examinations:** ADULTS AND CHILDREN: instill 1 to 2 drops 4% solution in eye just before procedure or examination.	**Eye:** *blurring*, corneal ulceration or scarring in excessive or long-term use. Varying effects on intraocular pressure. **Systemic:** excitation; nervousness; rapid, shallow respirations; emesis; chills; fever; tachycardia; hypertension; euphoria; anxiety; delirium; convulsions; respiratory and circulatory failure.
proparacaine hydrochloride Alcaine♦, Ophthaine♦, Ophthetic♦ ADULTS AND CHILDREN: **Anesthesia for tonometry, gonioscopy; suture removal from cornea, removal of corneal foreign bodies:** instill 1 to 2 drops 0.5% solution in eye just before procedure. **Anesthesia for cataract extraction, glaucoma surgery:** instill 1 drop 0.5% solution in eye every 5 to 10 minutes for 5 to 7 doses.	**Eye:** occasional conjunctival redness, transient pain. **Other:** hypersensitivity.
tetracaine hydrochloride Anacel, Pontocaine♦ **Anesthesia for tonometry, gonioscopy; removal of corneal foreign bodies, suture removal from cornea; other diagnostic and minor surgical procedures:** ADULTS AND CHILDREN: instill 1 to 2 drops 0.5% solution in eye just before procedure.	**Eye:** transient stinging in eye 30 seconds after initial instillation, epithelial damage in excessive or long-term use. **Other:** sensitization in repeated use (allergic skin rash, urticaria).

♦ Available in U.S. and Canada. ♦♦ Available in Canada only.
All other products (no symbol) available in U.S. only. Italicized side effects are common or life-threatening.

INTERACTIONS AND SPECIAL CONSIDERATIONS

Interactions:
EPINEPHRINE (TOPICAL): increased epinephrine effect. Use together cautiously.

Special considerations:
- Use cautiously and sparingly in patients with known allergies, cardiac disease, hyperthyroidism, or open lesions.
- Patient should be given short-acting barbiturate before administering to avoid CNS stimulation.
- Solutions must be prepared specially by pharmacist. Rarely used.
- Heart rate should be monitored after instillation and patient observed for systemic effects.
- Vision will be blurred for several hours.
- Patient should not rub eye for at least 20 minutes after instillation.
- Protective eye patch recommended following procedure.
- Solution should be pink. Discolored solution should be returned to pharmacy.
- Doesn't require refrigeration.

No significant interactions.

Special considerations:
- Use cautiously in cardiac diseases and hyperthyroidism.
- *Not* for long-term use; may delay wound healing.
- Patient should not rub or touch eye while cornea is anesthetized, since this may cause corneal abrasion and greater discomfort when anesthesia wears off.
- Protective eye patch recommended following procedure.
- Corneal pain is relieved only temporarily in abrasion.
- Systemic reactions unlikely when used in recommended doses.
- Topical ophthalmic anesthetic of choice in diagnostic and minor surgical procedures.
- Discolored solution should not be used.
- Store in tightly closed container.
- Ophthaine brand packaged in bottle that looks similar in size and shape to Hemoccult. Label should be checked carefully when taking bottle from shelf.

Interactions:
SULFONAMIDES: interference with sulfonamide antibacterial activity. Wait ½ hour after anesthesia before instilling sulfonamide.

Special considerations:
- Systemic absorption unlikely in recommended doses.
- Repeated use should be avoided.
- Does not dilate the pupil, paralyze accommodation, or increase intraocular pressure.
- Protective eye patch recommended following procedure.
- Don't use discolored solution. Keep container tightly closed.

82

Artificial tears

artificial tears
eye irrigation solutions

Artificial tears and external eye irrigation solutions are applied topically to relieve eyes that are deficient in or completely devoid of tear production. Among the components that make up these drugs are salts that are isotonic with tears, buffering agents for pH adjustment, viscosity agents to promote length of contact time with the eye, and preservatives to maintain solution integrity. Many of the drugs are available over the counter and without a prescription. The patient may have to try several of the commerically available products before he finds one that suits him.

Major uses

- Artificial tears are instilled in the eye to lubricate, remove debris, and protect against infection when tear production is insufficient.
- External eye irrigation solutions are sterile isotonic preparations used to irrigate the eyes after tonometry, gonioscopy, fluorescein dye examination, foreign body removal, and other procedures. They also soothe minor eye irritation and are used in large quantities for caustic chemical injury.

Mechanism of action

- Artificial tears augment insufficient tear production.
- External irrigation solutions clean the eye.

Absorption, distribution, metabolism, and excretion

The drugs are not systemically absorbed.

HOW TO IRRIGATE THE PATIENT'S EYE

Be sure to wash your hands before instilling eye irrigation. Then:

- Have the patient sit or lie with head tilted toward the affected side. Irrigating solution will flow from the inner canthus of the affected eye toward the outer canthus.
- Place a curved basin at the cheek on the side of the affected eye, to catch irrigating solution.
- Use gentle force to remove secretions as you direct the flow from the inner to the outer canthus. Do not touch any part of the eye with the irrigating tip.
- After irrigation, have the patient close her eyes and wipe excess solution from the lids and lashes.

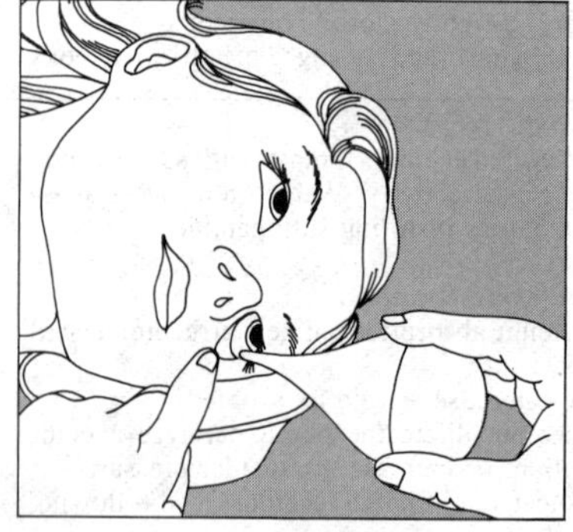

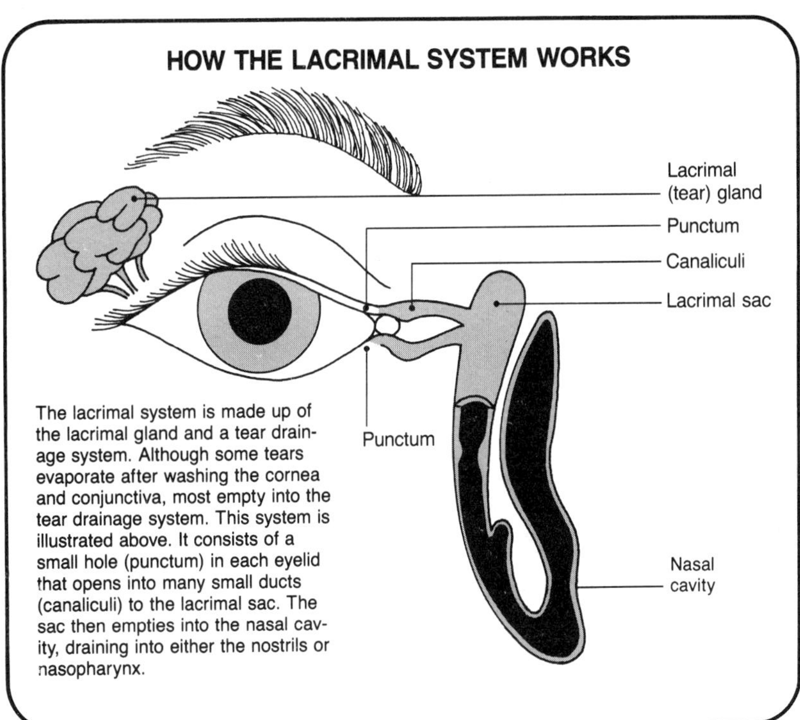

The lacrimal system is made up of the lacrimal gland and a tear drainage system. Although some tears evaporate after washing the cornea and conjunctiva, most empty into the tear drainage system. This system is illustrated above. It consists of a small hole (punctum) in each eyelid that opens into many small ducts (canaliculi) to the lacrimal sac. The sac then empties into the nasal cavity, draining into either the nostrils or nasopharynx.

Onset and duration

The higher the viscosity of the artificial tear products, the longer the action. Duration of some artificial tear products are:

- Adsorbotear: 90 minutes or more
- Isopto Tears: 60 minutes
- Liquifilm Tears: 60 minutes
- Lyteers: 45 minutes
- Tearisol: 40 minutes or more
- Tears Naturale: 90 minutes or more.

Combination products

None.

NAMES, INDICATIONS AND DOSAGES	SIDE EFFECTS
artificial tears Adsorbotear♦, Bro-Lac, Hypotears, Isopto Alkaline, Isopto Plain, Isopto Tears♦, Lacril♦, Liquifilm Forte, Liquifilm Tears, Lyteers, Methulose, Neotears, Tearisol, Tears Naturale♦, Tears Plus, Ultra Tears, Visculose **Insufficient tear production:** ADULTS AND CHILDREN: instill 1 to 2 drops in eye t.i.d., q.i.d., or p.r.n.	**Eye:** discomfort; burning, pain on instillation; blurred vision; crust formation on eyelids and eyelashes in products with high viscosity, such as Adsorbotear, Isopto Tears, and Tearisol.
eye irrigation solutions Blinx, Collyrium Eye Lotion♦, Dacriose, EyeStream, I-Lite Eye Drops, Lauro, Lavoptik Medicinal Eye Wash, Murine Eye Drops, Neo-Flow, Sterile Normal Saline (0.9%) **Eye irrigation:** ADULTS AND CHILDREN: flush eye with 1 to 2 drops t.i.d., q.i.d., or p.r.n.	None reported.

INTERACTIONS AND SPECIAL CONSIDERATIONS

Interactions:
BORATE EXTERNAL IRRIGATION SOLUTIONS: may form gummy deposits on the lid when used with artificial tear products containing polyvinyl alcohol (Liquifilm Forte, Liquifilm Tears). Keep patient's eyelids clean.

Special considerations:
• Contraindicated in hypersensitivity to active product or preservatives.
• Patient should not touch tip of container to eye, surrounding tissue, or other surface, to avoid contamination of solution.
• Product should be used by one person only.

Interactions:
PRODUCTS CONTAINING POLYVINYL ALCOHOL: may form gel and gummy deposits on the eye. Keep eyelids clean.

Special considerations:
• Contraindicated in hypersensitivity to active ingredient or preservatives.
• Patient should not touch tip of container to eye, surrounding tissue, or other surface, to avoid contamination.
• Check date of expiration to make sure solution is potent.
• Store in tightly closed, light-resistant container.
• Should be used by one person only.
• When irrigating, patient should turn his head to the side and irrigate from inner to outer canthus.

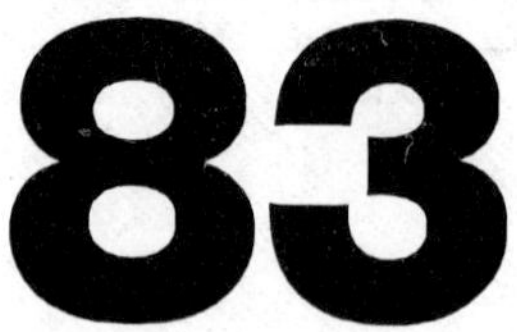

Miscellaneous ophthalmics

alpha-chymotrypsin
dipivefrin
fluorescein sodium
glycerin, anhydrous
isosorbide
sodium chloride, hypertonic
timolol maleate

These drugs are used for various purposes in medical, surgical, and diagnostic procedures.

Major uses

- Alpha-chymotrypsin is a fast-acting proteolytic enzyme that aids cataract extraction.
- Dipivefrin reduces intraocular pressure in chronic open-angle glaucoma.
- Fluorescein is a dye used for various diagnostic procedures.
- Anhydrous glycerin temporarily restores transparency when the cornea is too edematous to permit diagnosis in ophthalmoscopy or gonioscopy.
- Hypertonic sodium chloride reduces edema after surgery and in trauma, bullous keratopathy, and corneal edema associated with excessive use of contact lenses.
- Isosorbide is an oral osmotic agent that reduces intraocular pressure.
- Timolol lowers intraocular pressure in open-angle glaucoma, ocular hypertension, aphakic glaucoma, and secondary glaucoma.

Mechanism of action

- Alpha-chymotrypsin dissolves filaments or zonules holding the lens.
- Dipivefrin is a prodrug of epinephrine (in the eye, dipivefrin is converted to epinephrine). The liberated epinephrine appears to decrease aqueous production and increase aqueous outflow.
- Fluorescein produces an intense green fluorescence in alkaline solution (pH 5.0 or less) or a bright yellow if viewed under cobalt blue illumination.
- Glycerin and sodium chloride remove excess fluid from the cornea.
- Isosorbide acts as an osmotic agent to promote redistribution of water.
- Timolol, classified as a beta blocker, reduces aqueous formation and possibly increases aqueous outflow. It has little or no effect on pupil size.

Absorption, distribution, metabolism, and excretion

- Alpha-chymotrypsin is not absorbed and must be instilled into the posterior chamber. It is removed by irrigation with saline solution.
- Dipivefrin and hypertonic sodium chloride are not absorbed when recommended dosages are used.
- Fluorescein doesn't penetrate an intact corneal epithelium but is distributed to the stroma (assuming a green fluorescence) when the corneal epithelium is broken. After I.V. administration, it is distributed to the skin, causing a yellow discoloration that fades in 6 to 12 hours. It is excreted in urine.

DRUG ALERT

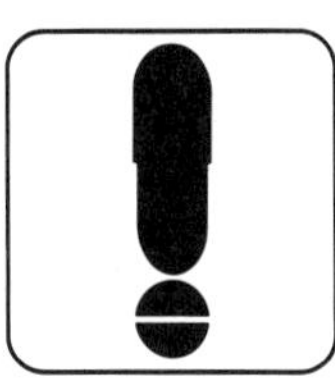

NEW CAUTIONS FOR USING TIMOLOL

Timolol maleate (Timoptic) now carries additional warnings concerning ocular irritations, hypersensitivity reactions, visual disturbances, and precipitation or aggravation of certain cardiovascular and pulmonary disorders.

This beta blocker is absorbed into the systemic circulation and can cause bradycardia, hypotension, syncope, and bronchospasm (mostly in patients with preexisting bronchospastic disease).

FDA reports associate the use of timolol eye drops not only with precipitation and aggravation of bronchospasm, but also with one fatality, that of a patient with status asthmaticus.

- Anhydrous glycerin is not absorbed.
- Isosorbide is rapidly absorbed after oral administration. It is not metabolized and is excreted unchanged in urine.
- Timolol is absorbed systemically in varying amounts. The beta blockade may cause systemic side effects such as bradycardia and bronchospasm.

Onset and duration

- Alpha-chymotrypsin and anhydrous glycerin begin to act within 1 to 2 minutes after they are administered. Both of these drugs have a short duration of action (only minutes).
- Dipivefrin and timolol begin to work within 30 minutes after administration. Maximal effect occurs in 1 hour. Therapeutic action lasts up to 24 hours.
- Fluorescein begins to act immediately after instillation, and its duration is about 30 minutes. After I.V. administration, fluorescein dye appears in the retinal vessels after 13 seconds and remains 20 seconds.
- Hypertonic sodium chloride's effect lasts up to 4 hours.
- Isosorbide begins to act within 30 minutes. Therapeutic effects continue for 5 or 6 hours.

Combination products

FLURESS: sodium fluorescein 0.25% and benoxinate HCl 0.4%.

NAMES, INDICATIONS AND DOSAGES	SIDE EFFECTS
alpha-chymotrypsin Alpha Chymar, Alpha Chymolean♦♦ Catarase♦, Zolyse♦, Zonulyn♦♦ **Zonulysis in cataract surgery:** ADULTS OVER 20 YEARS: 1 to 2 ml instilled into posterior chamber under the iris, by doctor.	**Eye:** transient increase in intraocular pressure (dose-related), moderate uveitis, corneal edema and striation.
dipivefrin Propine **To reduce intraocular pressure in chronic open-angle glaucoma:** ADULTS: for initial glaucoma therapy, 1 drop in eye q 12 hours.	**Eye:** burning, stinging. **CV:** tachycardia, hypertension.
fluorescein sodium Fluorescite, Fluor-I-Strip, Fluor-I-Strip-A.T.♦, Ful-Glo Strips♦, Funduscein Injections **Diagnostic in corneal abrasions and foreign bodies; fitting hard contact lenses; lacrimal patency; fundus photography; applanation tonometry:** TOPICAL: Solution: instill 1 drop of 2% solution followed by irrigation, or moisten strip with sterile water. Touch conjunctiva or fornix with moistened tip. Flush eye with irrigating solution. Patient should blink several times after application. **Indicated in retinal angiography:** ADULTS: 5 ml of 10% solution (500 mg) or 3 ml of 25% solution (750 mg) injected rapidly into antecubital vein, by doctor. CHILDREN: 0.077 ml of 10% solution (7.7 mg/kg body weight) or 0.044 ml of 25% solution (11 mg/kg body weight) injected rapidly into antecubital vein, by doctor.	Topical use: **Eye:** stinging, burning. Intravenous use: **CNS:** headache persisting for 24 to 36 hours. **GI:** nausea, vomiting. **GU:** bright yellow urine (persists for 24 to 36 hours). **Skin:** yellow skin discoloration (fades in 6 to 12 hours). **Local:** extravasation at injection site, thrombophlebitis. **Other:** hypersensitivity, including urticaria and *anaphylaxis*.
glycerin, anhydrous Ophthalgan **Corneal edema before ophthalmoscopy or gonioscopy in acute glaucoma and bullous keratitis:** ADULTS AND CHILDREN: instill 1 to 2 drops glycerin, anhydrous after instilling a local anesthetic.	**Eye:** pain if instilled without topical anesthetic.

♦ Available in U.S. and Canada. ♦♦ Available in Canada only.
All other products (no symbol) available in U.S. only. Italicized side effects are common or life-threatening.

INTERACTIONS AND SPECIAL CONSIDERATIONS

Interactions:
ALCOHOL, SURGICAL DETERGENT: inactivated alpha-chymotrypsin. Rinse off all alcohol or detergents from surgical instruments and syringe with saline solution.

Special considerations:
- Contraindicated in high vitreous pressure with gaping incisional wound; congenital cataract.
- Solutions very unstable. Only freshly reconstituted solution should be used; not recommended for use if it is cloudy or has precipitated. Unused portions should be discarded, including diluent, except for Zonulyn. Retains potency 1 week at room temperature, 1 month when refrigerated.
- Irrigating with intraocular balanced saline solution removes drug.
- Powder or reconstituted solution should not be autoclaved; excess heat will inactivate the enzyme.
- Delayed healing of incision has been reported but not confirmed.

No significant interactions.

Special considerations:
- Contraindicated in narrow-angle glaucoma.
- Use cautiously in patients with aphakia.
- Dipivefrin is a prodrug of epinephrine: converted to epinephrine when it enters the eye.
- May have fewer side effects than conventional epinephrine therapy.
- Often used concomitantly with other antiglaucoma drugs.
- Available as a 0.1% solution in 5-, 10-, and 15-ml dropper bottles.
- Patient should know how to instill.
- Patient should wash hands before and after administration.
- Patient should not touch dropper to eye or surrounding tissue.

No significant interactions.

Special considerations:
- Use with caution in patients with history of allergy or bronchial asthma.
- Topical anesthetic should be used before instilling to partially relieve burning and irritation.
- Aseptic technique required. Easily contaminated by *Pseudomonas*.
- Yellow skin discoloration may persist 6 to 12 hours.
- Urine will be colored bright yellow after I.V. injection.
- Routine urinalysis will be abnormal within 1 hour of I.V. injection.
- A water-soluble dye.
- Should not be frozen but stored below 80° F. (26.7° C.).
- Defects will appear green under normal light, or bright yellow under cobalt blue illumination. Foreign bodies are surrounded by a green ring. Similar lesions of the conjunctiva are delineated in orange-yellow.
- When given parenterally, antihistamine, epinephrine, and oxygen should always be kept available for treatment of anaphylaxis.
- For symptoms and treatment of anaphylaxis, see APPENDIX.

No significant interactions.

Special considerations:
- Topical tetracaine HCl or proparacaine HCl should be used before instilling to prevent discomfort.
- Patient should not touch tip of dropper to eye, surrounding tissues, or tear-film; glycerin will absorb moisture.
- Used to temporarily restore corneal transparency when cornea is too edematous to permit diagnosis.
- Store in tightly closed container.

NAMES, INDICATIONS AND DOSAGES	SIDE EFFECTS
isosorbide Ismotic **Short-term reduction of intraocular pressure due to glaucoma:** ADULTS: Initially, 1.5 g/kg P.O. Usual dosage range is 1 to 3 g/kg.	**CNS:** vertigo, light-headedness, lethargy. **GI:** gastric discomfort, diarrhea, anorexia. **Metabolic:** hypernatremia, hyperosmolality.
sodium chloride, hypertonic Adsorbonac Ophthalmic Solution, Hypersal Ophthalmic Solution, Methylcellulose Ophthalmic Solution, Muro Ointment, Murocoll, Sodium Chloride Ointment 5% **Corneal edema (postoperative) after cataract extraction or corneal transplantation; also in trauma or bullous keratopathy:** ADULTS AND CHILDREN: instill 1 to 2 drops q 3 to 4 hours, or apply ointment at bedtime.	**Eye:** slight stinging. **Other:** hypersensitivity.
timolol maleate Timoptic Solution **Chronic open-angle glaucoma, secondary glaucoma, aphakic glaucoma, ocular hypertension:** ADULTS: initially, instill 1 drop 0.25% solution in each eye b.i.d.; reduce to 1 drop daily for maintenance. If patient doesn't respond, instill 1 drop 0.5% solution in each eye b.i.d. If intraocular pressure is controlled, dosage may be reduced to 1 drop in each eye daily.	**Eye:** minor irritation. Long-term use may decrease corneal sensitivity. **CV:** slight reduction in resting heart rate. **Other:** apnea in infants, *respiratory distress (evidence of beta blockade and systemic absorption).*

♦ Available in U.S. and Canada. ♦♦ Available in Canada only.
All other products (no symbol) available in U.S. only. Italicized side effects are common or life-threatening.

INTERACTIONS AND SPECIAL CONSIDERATIONS

No significant interactions.

Special considerations:
• Contraindicated in anuria due to severe renal disease, severe dehydration, frank or impending acute pulmonary edema, and hemorrhagic glaucoma.
• Repetitive doses should be used cautiously in patients with diseases associated with salt retention, such as congestive heart failure.
• Patient should sip the medication poured over cracked ice. This procedure improves palatability.
• Especially useful when a rapid reduction in intraocular pressure is desired.

No significant interactions.

Special considerations:
• An osmotic agent used to reduce corneal edema when repeated instillation is indicated.
• A few drops of sterile irrigation solution inside bottle cap may be used to prevent caking on tip of dropper bottle.
• Store in tightly closed container.
• Patient should not touch tip of dropper or tube to eye or surrounding tissue.
• Patient should be shown how to instill medication.

Interactions:
PROPRANOLOL HCl, METOPROLOL TARTRATE, OTHER ORAL BETA-ADRENERGIC–BLOCKING AGENTS: increased ocular and systemic effect. Use together cautiously.
MAO INHIBITORS, OTHER ADRENERGIC-AUGMENTING PSYCHOTROPIC DRUGS: hazardous increased effect. Use together cautiously.

Special considerations:
• Use cautiously in bronchial asthma, sinus bradycardia, second- and third-degree heart block, cardiogenic shock, right ventricular failure resulting from pulmonary hypertension, congestive heart failure, severe cardiac disease, and in infants with congenital glaucoma.
• Patient should not touch dropper to eye or surrounding tissue.
• Beta-adrenergic–blocking agent in ophthalmic solution.
• Can be safely used in patients with glaucoma who wear conventional (PMMA) hard contact lenses.
• Patient should lightly press lacrimal sac with finger after drug administration to decrease chance of systemic absorption.
• A systemic form of timolol is currently being investigated (trade name, Blocadren). May reduce the mortality associated with myocardial infarction.
• Patient should be shown how to instill medication.

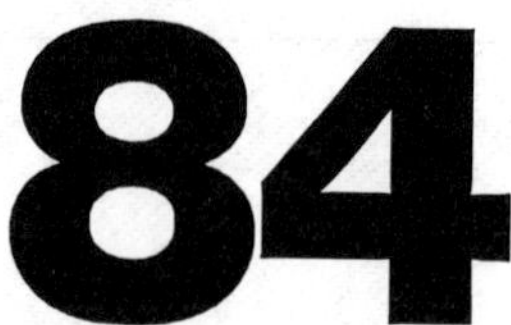

Otics

acetic acid
benzocaine
boric acid
carbamide peroxide
chloramphenicol
colistin B sulfate
dexamethasone sodium phosphate
hydrocortisone
hydrocortisone acetate
methylprednisolone disodium phosphate
neomycin sulfate
oxytetracycline hydrochloride
polymyxin B sulfate
triethanolamine polypeptide oleate-condensate

Most otics act locally; many are combinations of two or more drugs.

Major uses
The otics are used to treat infection, inflammation, and pain of internal or external ear disorders (swimmer's ear, perforation, and otitis media) and are therapeutic adjuncts in surgical procedures (myringotomy and fenestration).
• Carbamide peroxide and triethanolamine also soften impacted cerumen.

Mechanism of action
• Anti-infectives (acetic acid, boric acid, chloramphenicol, colistin B, neomycin, oxytetracycline, and polymyxin B) inhibit or destroy bacteria present in the ear canal.
• Corticosteroids (dexamethasone, hydrocortisone, and methylprednisolone) control inflammation, edema, and pruritus.
• The local anesthetic benzocaine produces analgesic effects.
• Ceruminolytics (carbamide peroxide and triethanolamine) emulsify and disperse accumulated cerumen.

Absorption, distribution, metabolism, and excretion
Long-term use of corticosteroids and certain antibiotics (for example, neomycin) may result in some systemic absorption. The other drugs aren't significantly absorbed systemically.

Onset and duration
• Most otics begin to act within 1 hour, but full therapeutic effect may not be seen for 2 or 3 days.
• The short action of benzocaine requires repeated doses every 2 hours.

Combination products
ADRENOMYXIN♦♦: Each ml contains neomycin SO_4 5 mg, polymyxin B SO_4 10,000 units, and hydrocortisone 10 mg.
COLY-MYCIN S OTIC: Each ml contains neomycin SO_4 5 mg, colistin SO_4 3 mg, hydrocortisone acetate 10 mg, and thonzonium bromide 0.5%.
CORTISPORIN OTIC♦: Each ml contains neomycin SO_4 5 mg, polymyxin B SO_4 10,000 units, and hydrocortisone 1%.
LIDOSPORIN OTIC♦: Each ml contains polymyxin B SO_4 10,000 units and lidocaine HCl 50 mg.
NEO-CORT-DOME OTIC : Each ml contains neomycin SO_4 5 mg, acetic acid 2%, and hydrocortisone 1%.

HOME CARE: USING EAR DROPS CORRECTLY

Dear Patient:

Here's how to administer ear drops safely to yourself or to a child. The general directions apply to both procedures.

General directions

- Wash your hands thoroughly.
- Check the drops for discoloration and sediment. If the drops are in a clear bottle, hold the bottle to the light. If they're in a dark bottle, shake the bottle well, draw some medication into the dropper, and hold the dropper to the light. If the drops are discolored or contain sediment, have the prescription refilled.
- Warm the drops by rolling the bottle between your palms for 2 minutes.
- After instilling the drops, recap the bottle and store it in a cool, dark place.

Giving drops to yourself

- Shake the bottle, if directed, and open it. Fill the dropper and place the bottle within reach.
- Lie on your side so that the ear to be treated is facing up. Then, gently pull the top of your ear up and back to straighten the ear canal.
- Position the dropper above, but not touching the ear, and release the prescribed number of drops.
- To retain the drops in the ear, remain on your side for 10 minutes. If desired, plug the ear with cotton moistened with the ear drops. Don't use dry cotton, because it will absorb the drops.
- If directed, repeat the procedure for the other ear.

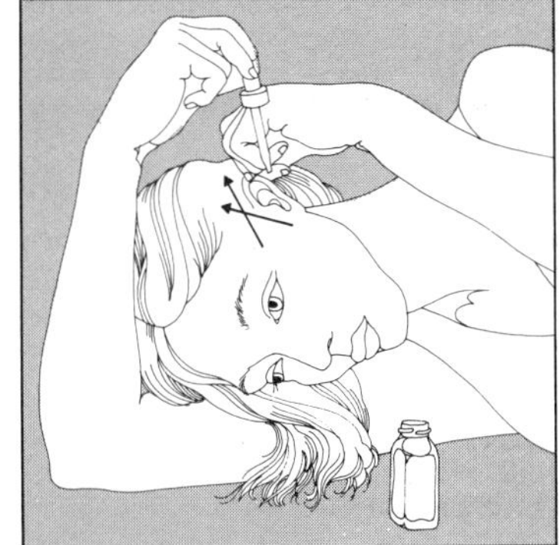

Giving drops to a child

- Lay the child on his side so that the ear to be treated is facing up.
- Gently pull the ear down and back, then slowly release the prescribed number of drops. (Note the difference in the direction the ear is moved for a child. This is due to the immaturity of the child's ear cartilage.)
- If the child has any pain after you've given the drops, notify the doctor.

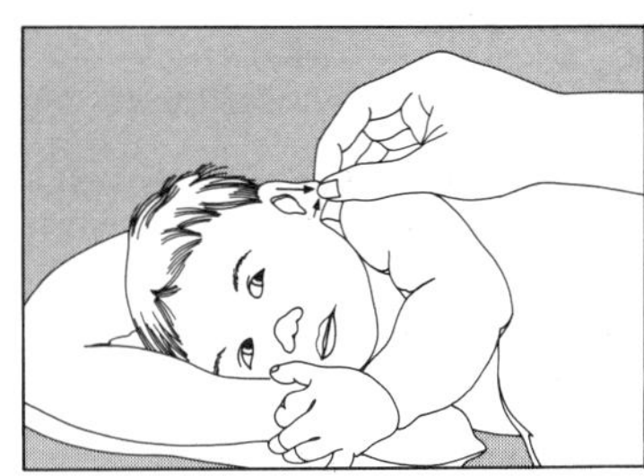

NAMES, INDICATIONS AND DOSAGES	SIDE EFFECTS
acetic acid Domeboro Otic♦, VoSol Otic♦ **External ear canal infection:** ADULTS AND CHILDREN: 4 to 6 drops in ear canal t.i.d. or q.i.d., or insert saturated wick first 24 hours, then continue instillations. **Prophylaxis of swimmer's ear:** ADULTS AND CHILDREN: 2 drops in each ear b.i.d.	**Ear:** irritation or itching. **Skin:** urticaria. **Other:** overgrowth of nonsusceptible organisms.
benzocaine Americaine-Otic, Auralgan♦, Aurasol, Eardro, Myringacaine, Tympagesic **Cerumen removal:** ADULTS AND CHILDREN: fill ear canal t.i.d. for 2 days. **Pain from otitis media:** ADULTS AND CHILDREN: fill ear canal with solution and plug with cotton. May repeat q 1 to 2 hours, p.r.n.	**Ear:** irritation or itching. **Skin:** urticaria. **Other:** edema.
boric acid Ear-Dry, Swim-Ear, Swim 'n Clear **External ear canal infection:** ADULTS AND CHILDREN: fill ear canal with solution and plug with cotton. Repeat t.i.d. or q.i.d.	**Ear:** irritation or itching. **Skin:** urticaria. **Other:** overgrowth of nonsusceptible organisms.
carbamide peroxide Benadyne Ear, Debrox♦ **Impacted cerumen:** ADULTS AND CHILDREN: 5 to 10 drops into ear canal b.i.d. for 3 to 4 days.	None reported.
chloramphenicol Chloromycetin Otic♦, Sopamycetin♦♦ **External ear canal infection:** ADULTS AND CHILDREN: 2 to 3 drops into ear canal t.i.d. or q.i.d.	**Ear:** itching or burning. **Local:** pruritus, burning, urticaria, vesicular or maculopapular dermatitis. **Systemic:** sore throat, angioedema. **Other:** overgrowth of nonsusceptible organisms.
colistin B sulfate available only in combination with neomycin and hydrocortisone (Coly-Mycin-S-Otic♦) **External ear canal infection and otitis media:** ADULTS AND CHILDREN: 3 to 5 drops into ear canal t.i.d. or q.i.d.	**Ear:** ototoxicity in patient with a perforated eardrum and in patient undergoing tympanoplasty; irritation, itching. **Other:** overgrowth of nonsusceptible organisms.
dexamethasone sodium phosphate Decadron♦ **Inflammation of external ear canal:** ADULTS AND CHILDREN: 1 to 2 drops into ear canal t.i.d. or q.i.d.	**Systemic:** adrenal suppression with long-term use. **Other:** masking or exacerbation of underlying infection.

♦ Available in U.S. and Canada. ♦♦ Available in Canada only.
All other products (no symbol) available in U.S. only. Italicized side effects are common or life-threatening.

INTERACTIONS AND SPECIAL CONSIDERATIONS

No significant interactions.

Special considerations:
• Contraindicated in perforated eardrum.
• Has anti-infective, anti-inflammatory, and antipruritic effects.
• *Pseudomonas aeruginosa* particularly sensitive to drug.
• Persistent drainage should be recultured.

No significant interactions.

Special considerations:
• Contraindicated in perforated eardrum.
• Local anesthetic effect only.
• Should be used with antibiotic to treat underlying cause of pain, because use alone may mask more serious condition.
• Patient should call doctor if pain lasts longer than 48 hours.
• Dropper should not touch ear and should not be rinsed.
• Ear should be irrigated gently to remove impacted cerumen.
• Keep container tightly closed and away from moisture.

No significant interactions.

Special considerations:
• Contraindicated in perforated eardrum or excoriated membranes in ear.
• Superinfection (continued pain, inflammation, fever) is possible.
• Weak bacteriostatic action; also fungistatic agent.
• If cotton plug used, should always be moistened with medication.
• Dropper should not touch ear.

No significant interactions.

Special considerations:
• Contraindicated in perforated eardrum.
• Patient should call doctor if redness, pain, or swelling persists.
• Ceruminolytic agent.
• Irrigation of ear may be necessary to aid in removal of cerumen.
• Tip of bottle should not touch ear or ear canal.

No significant interactions.

Special considerations:
• Prolonged use should be avoided.
• History of use and reaction to drug should be obtained.
• Superinfection (continued pain, inflammation, fever) is possible.
• Persistent drainage should be recultured.
• Patient may develop sore throat (early sign of toxicity).
• Bacteriostatic agent.
• Dropper should not touch ear.

No significant interactions.

Special considerations:
• Superinfection (continued pain, inflammation, fever) is possible.
• Persistent drainage should be recultured.
• Patient may develop hearing loss.
• Bactericidal agent.
• Prolonged use should be avoided.
• Should be shaken well before use.
• Dropper should not touch ear.

No significant interactions.

Special considerations:
• Contraindicated in perforated eardrum, fungal infections, herpes or other viral infections.
• Should be used with antibiotic to treat inflammation caused by infection.
• Should be used alone in allergic otitis externa.
• Anti-inflammatory agent.
• Dropper should not touch ear.

NAMES, INDICATIONS AND DOSAGES	SIDE EFFECTS
hydrocortisone **hydrocortisone acetate** Cortamed♦♦, Otall **Inflammation of external ear canal:** ADULTS AND CHILDREN: 3 to 5 drops into ear canal t.i.d. or q.i.d. Available in 0.25%, 0.5%, and 1% concentrations.	**Systemic:** adrenal suppression with long-term use. **Other:** may mask or exacerbate underlying infection.
methylprednisolone disodium phosphate Medrol♦♦ **Inflammation of external ear canal:** ADULTS AND CHILDREN: 2 to 3 drops into ear canal t.i.d. or q.i.d.	**Systemic:** adrenal suppression with long-term use. **Other:** may mask or exacerbate underlying infection.
neomycin sulfate Otobiotic **External ear canal infection:** ADULTS AND CHILDREN: 2 to 5 drops into ear canal t.i.d. or q.i.d.	**Ear:** ototoxicity (in patients undergoing tympanoplasty). **Local:** burning, erythema, vesicular dermatitis, urticaria. **Other:** overgrowth of nonsusceptible organisms.
oxytetracycline hydrochloride available only in combination with polymyxin B sulfate (Terramycin with Polymyxin B) or polymyxin B sulfate and hydrocortisone (Terra-Cortril♦♦) **External ear canal infection:** ADULTS AND CHILDREN: instill ½" of ointment into external ear canal t.i.d. or q.i.d.	**Ear:** irritation, itching, urticaria. **Other:** overgrowth of nonsusceptible organisms.
polymyxin B sulfate Aerosporin♦ **Acute and chronic otitis externa, otitis media if tympanic membrane perforated; otomycosis:** ADULTS AND CHILDREN: 3 to 4 drops t.i.d. or q.i.d.	**Ear:** irritation, itching, urticaria. **Other:** overgrowth of nonsusceptible organisms.
triethanolamine polypeptide oleate-condensate Cerumenex♦ **Impacted cerumen:** ADULTS AND CHILDREN: fill ear canal with solution and insert cotton plug. After 15 to 30 minutes, flush ear with warm water.	**Ear:** erythema, pruritus. **Skin:** severe eczema.

♦ Available in U.S. and Canada. ♦♦ Available in Canada only.
All other products (no symbol) available in U.S. only. Italicized side effects are common or life-threatening.

INTERACTIONS AND SPECIAL CONSIDERATIONS

No significant interactions.

Special considerations:
• Contraindicated in perforated eardrum, fungal infections, herpes or other viral infections.
• Should be used with antibiotic to treat inflammation caused by infection.
• Should be used alone in allergic otitis externa.
• Anti-inflammatory agent.
• Dropper should not touch ear.

No significant interactions.

Special considerations:
• Contraindicated in perforated eardrum, fungal infection, herpes or other viral infections.
• Should be used with antibiotic to treat inflammation caused by infection.
• Should be used alone to treat seborrheic, contact, or uninfected eczematoid dermatitis.
• Anti-inflammatory agent.
• Dropper should not touch ear.

No significant interactions.

Special considerations:
• Contraindicated in perforated eardrum.
• History of use and reaction to neomycin should be obtained.
• Patient may develop hearing loss.
• Superinfection (continued pain, inflammation, fever) is possible.
• Persistent drainage should be recultured.
• Bactericidal agent.
• Best used in combination with other antibiotics.
• Dropper should not touch ear.

No significant interactions.

Special considerations:
• History of reaction to tetracyclines should be obtained.
• Superinfection (continued pain, inflammation, fever) is possible.
• Persistent drainage should be recultured.
• Bacteriostatic agent.

No significant interactions.

Special considerations:
• Superinfection (continued pain, inflammation, fever) is possible.
• Persistent drainage should be recultured.
• Bactericidal agent.
• Best used in combination with other antibiotics.
• Keep container tightly closed and away from moisture.
• Dropper should not touch ear.

No significant interactions.

Special considerations:
• Contraindicated in perforated eardrum, otitis media, and allergies. For patch test, place 1 drop of drug on inner forearm; cover with small bandage. Read in 24 hours. If any reaction (redness, swelling) occurs, don't use drug.
• Drops should not be used more often than prescribed. Ear should be flushed gently with warm water, using soft rubber bulb ear syringe, within 30 minutes after instillation.
• Cerumenolytic agent.
• Cotton plug should be moistened with medication before insertion.
• Keep container tightly closed and away from moisture.
• Dropper should not touch ear.

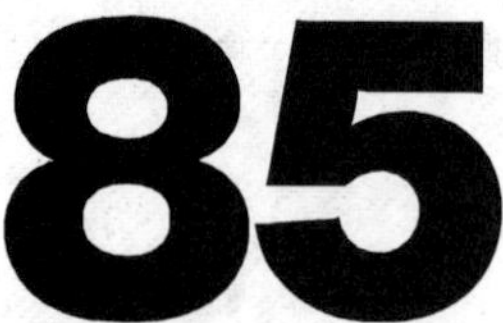

Oral and nasal agents

beclomethasone dipropionate
benzocaine
carbamide peroxide
cocaine hydrochloride
dexamethasone sodium phosphate
ephedrine sulfate
epinephrine hydrochloride
flunisolide
lidocaine hydrochloride
naphazoline hydrochloride
oxymetazoline hydrochloride
phenylephrine hydrochloride
piperocaine hydrochloride
tetrahydrozoline hydrochloride
triamcinolone acetonide
xylometazoline hydrochloride

Oral and nasal agents are used alone or with other drugs to treat conditions affecting the nose and mouth. Many over-the-counter preparations are combinations of these drugs. Combinations for nasal use may also contain antihistamines.

Major uses

- Carbamide peroxide cleans and debrides, provides antimicrobial activity, and is a therapeutic adjunct in oral inflammations.
- Corticosteroids (beclomethasone, dexamethasone, flunisolide, and triamcinolone) reduce inflammation in allergic or inflammatory conditions, such as perennial and seasonal rhinitis, and in nasal polyps. Some are also used to treat stomatitis and traumatic oral lesions.
- Local anesthetics (benzocaine, cocaine hydrochloride, lidocaine, and piperocaine) produce anesthesia for rhinolaryngologic examination, laryngoscopic or bronchoscopic surgical procedures, and endotracheal intubation. They are also used to relieve the pain of dental extractions.
- Sympathomimetic vasoconstrictors (ephedrine, epinephrine, naphazoline, oxymetazoline, phenylephrine, tetrahydrozoline, and xylometazoline) relieve nasal congestion of the common cold, sinusitis, allergy, or chronic or vasomotor rhinitis.

Epinephrine also controls local superficial bleeding.

Mechanism of action

- Carbamide peroxide serves as a source of hydrogen peroxide to produce nascent oxygen, which aids in cleaning and debriding.
- Corticosteroids reduce inflammation and help heal oral ulcers and lesions by interfering with the protein synthesis of various enzymes.
- Local anesthetics block nerve conduction through sensory nerve fibers.
- Sympathomimetic agents produce local vasoconstriction of dilated arterioles to reduce blood flow and nasal congestion.

Absorption, distribution, metabolism, and excretion

Oral and nasal agents are minimally absorbed when they are used in recommended dosages.

Onset and duration

Onset and duration of action vary with the drug, patient response, and conditions being treated. In general, oral and nasal drugs begin to act quickly due to their easy penetration into mucous membranes. The duration of action of local anesthetics depends on the amount of time the drug is in contact with nerve tissue.

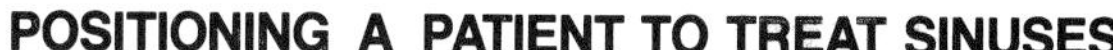

POSITIONING A PATIENT TO TREAT SINUSES

Proetz position

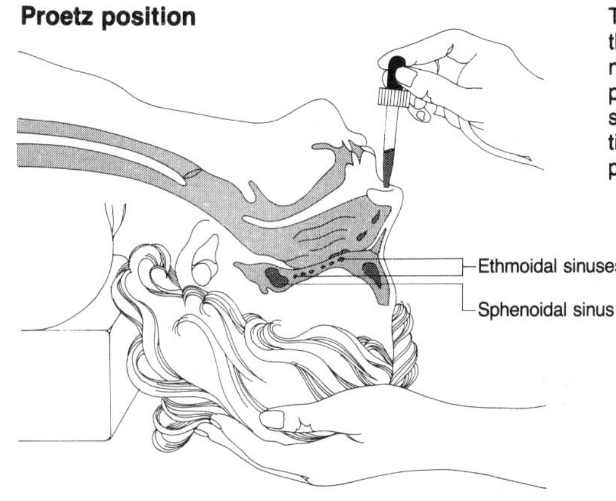

To instill medication in both the ethmoidal and the sphenoidal sinuses, place the patient on his back, with shoulders elevated and head tilted back. This is the Proetz position.

Parkinson position

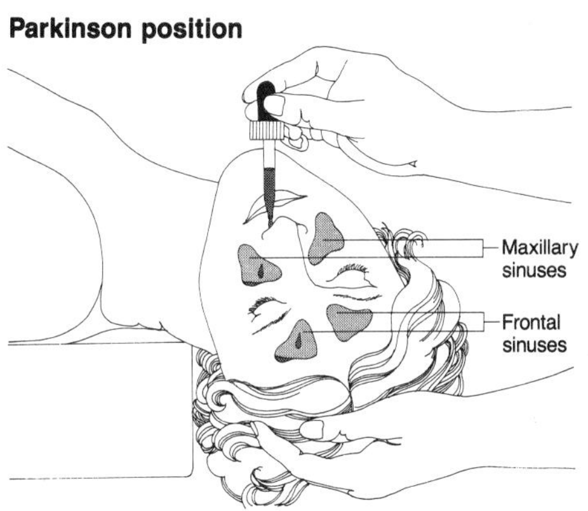

Use the Parkinson position to treat the maxillary and the frontal sinuses, located on each side of the face. As you can see here, this position is like the Proetz position, except the patient's head is tilted to one side instead of straight back.

Important: No matter which position is used, take care not to contaminate the dropper by touching the nostrils.

Combination products

NEO-VADRIN NASAL DECONGESTANT DROPS: phenylephrine hydrochloride 0.15% and phenylpropanolamine hydrochloride 0.4%, with chlorobutanol 0.15% and benzalkonium chloride 0.005%.

NAMES, INDICATIONS AND DOSAGES	SIDE EFFECTS
beclomethasone dipropionate Beconase Nasal Inhaler, Vancenase Nasal Inhaler **Relief of symptoms of seasonal or perennial rhinitis:** ADULTS, AND CHILDREN 12 YEARS OR OLDER: Usual dosage is one spray (42 mcg) in each nostril 2 to 4 times daily (total dosage 168 to 336 mcg daily). Most patients require one spray in each nostil t.i.d. (252 mcg daily). Not recommended for children under age 12.	**CNS:** headache. **EENT:** *mild transient nasal burning and stinging,* nasal congestion, sneezing, epistaxis, watery eyes. **GI:** nausea and vomiting. **Other:** development of local fungal infections.
benzocaine Colrex, Dentition Syrup♦♦, Orabase with Benzocaine, Oracin, Ora-Jel, Spec-T Anesthetic, Trocaine, Tyzomint **Pain from toothache, cold sore, canker sore, oral irritation, minor sore throat:** ADULTS AND CHILDREN: apply syrup or jelly to affected area, or suck lozenges.	**Skin:** hypersensitivity. **Other:** possible tolerance.
carbamide peroxide Cank-aid, Clear Drops, Gly-Oxide♦, Proxigel **Canker sores, herpetic and other lesions, gingivitis, denture irritation, traumatic or surgical wounds:** ADULTS AND CHILDREN OVER 3 YEARS: apply, undiluted, to oral mucosa q.i.d. or p.r.n., leave for several minutes, then expectorate. Don't rinse out mouth.	None reported.
cocaine hydrochloride Controlled Substance Schedule II ADULTS AND CHILDREN: **Acute rhinosinusitis:** use 1% solution with nasal pack. **Diagnostic nasal examination:** apply 4% solution to nasal mucosa. **Local anesthesia of nose or throat:** apply 5% to 10% solution to oral and nasal mucosa.	**CNS:** nervousness, excitation, vasomotor collapse.
dexamethasone sodium phosphate Decadron Phosphate♦, Decadron Phosphate Respihaler, Turbinaire **Allergic or inflammatory conditions, nasal polyps:** ADULTS: 2 sprays in each nostril b.i.d. or t.i.d. Maximum 12 sprays daily. CHILDREN 6 TO 12 YEARS: 1 or 2 sprays in each nostril b.i.d. Maximum 8 sprays daily. Each spray delivers 0.1 mg dexamethasone sodium phosphate equal to 0.084 mg dexamethasone.	**EENT:** nasal irritation, dryness, rebound nasal congestion. **Other:** hypersensitivity, systemic side effects with prolonged use (pituitary-adrenal suppression, sodium retention, congestive heart failure, hypertension, hypokalemia, headaches, convulsions, peptic ulcer, ecchymoses, petechiae, masking of secondary infection).

♦ Available in U.S. and Canada. ♦♦ Available in Canada only.
All other products (no symbol) available in U.S. only. Italicized side effects are common or life-threatening.

INTERACTIONS AND SPECIAL CONSIDERATIONS

No significant interactions.

Special considerations:
• Use cautiously, if at all, in patients with active or quiescent respiratory tract tubercular infections, or in untreated fungal, bacterial, or systemic viral or ocular herpes simplex infections.
• Use cautiously in patients who have recently had nasal septal ulcers or nasal surgery or trauma.
• Recommended dosages will not suppress chypothalamic-pituitary-adrenal (HPA) function. Patient should not exceed this dosage.
• Indicated when conventional treatment (antihistamines, decongestants) fails.
• Beclomethasone is not effective for active exacerbations. Nasal decongestants or oral antihistamines may be needed instead.
• Patient should use drug regularly, as prescribed; its effectiveness depends on regular use.
• The therapeutic effects of this corticosteroid, unlike those of decongestants, are not immediate. Most patients achieve benefit within a few days, but some may need 2 to 3 weeks for maximum benefit.
• If symptoms don't improve within 3 weeks or if nasal irritation persists, patient should stop drug and notify doctor.

No significant interactions.

Special considerations:
• Contraindicated in infants under 1 year. Use cautiously in children under 6 years and in severe oral trauma or sepsis.
• Not intended for use in the presence of infection.
• History of reactions to local anesthetics should be obtained.
• Patient may develop allergic reactions, such as reddening or swelling. If condition persists, patient should stop drug and notify doctor.
• Patient should be shown how to apply.

No significant interactions.

Special considerations:
• Should be used only as adjunct to regular professional care.
• Should not be diluted. Patient should gently massage affected area with medication. He should not drink or rinse his mouth for 5 minutes after use.
• Drug foams in mouth when mixed with saliva.
• Should be used after meals and at bedtime for best results.
• If severe or persistent inflammation continues, patient should notify doctor or dentist.
• Provides chemomechanical cleansing, debriding action, and has nonselective microbial activity.
• An oxygenating agent.
• Store in cool place.
• Only one person should use same dropper bottle or tube.

No significant interactions.

Special considerations:
• Store under lock and key with other controlled drugs.
• Patient should be given a short-acting barbiturate before giving cocaine HCl to prevent excess CNS stimulation or vasomotor collapse.
• Nasal surgery performed with cocaine HCl anesthetic may cause a delayed capillary hemorrhage resulting from capillary dilation. Patient may develop postoperative nasal bleeding when effect of cocaine wears off.
• History of reactions to local anesthetics should be obtained.

No significant interactions.

Special considerations:
• Contraindicated in cutaneous tuberculosis, and in fungal and herpetic lesions. Use cautiously in diabetes mellitus, peptic ulcer, or tuberculosis, as systemic absorption can activate disease.
• Mothers should not breast-feed, as systemic absorption can occur.
• Underlying bacterial infection should be controlled with anti-infectives. Irritation or sensitivity may require stopping drug.
• Should not be broken, incinerated, or stored in extreme heat; contents under pressure.
• Dose should gradually be reduced as nasal condition improves.
• Fluid retention can occur as a result of systemic absorption.
• Patient should be shown how to apply. Only one person should use nasal spray.
• Hypertension and hypokalemia can occur with systemic absorption. Blood pressure and serum potassium should be monitored frequently.
• Should not be used for prolonged periods.

NAMES, INDICATIONS AND DOSAGES	SIDE EFFECTS
ephedrine sulfate Ephedsol-1%, Isofedrol, Nasdro **Nasal congestion:** ADULTS AND CHILDREN: apply 3 to 4 drops 0.5% to 3% solution to nasal mucosa. Use no more frequently than q 4 hours.	**CNS:** nervousness, excitation. **CV:** *tachycardia*. **EENT:** rebound nasal congestion with long-term or excessive use. **Local:** mucosal irritation.
epinephrine hydrochloride Adrenalin Chloride **Nasal congestion, local superficial bleeding:** ADULTS AND CHILDREN: apply 0.1% solution to oral or nasal mucosa.	**CNS:** nervousness, excitation. **CV:** *tachycardia*. **EENT:** rebound nasal congestion, slight sting upon application.
flunisolide Nasalide Nasal Solution **Relief of symptoms of seasonal or perennial rhinitis:** ADULTS: Starting dose is 2 sprays (50 mcg) in each nostril b.i.d. Total daily dose is 200 mcg. If necessary, dose may be increased to 2 sprays in each nostril t.i.d. Maximum total daily dosage is 8 sprays in each nostril (400 mcg daily). CHILDREN 6 TO 14 YEARS: Starting dose is 1 spray (25 mcg) in each nostril t.i.d. or 2 sprays (50 mcg) in each nostril b.i.d. Total daily dose is 150 to 200 mcg. Maximum total daily dose is 4 sprays in each nostril (200 mcg daily). Not recommended for children under 6 years.	**CNS:** heacache. **EENT:** *mild, transient nasal burning and stinging*, nasal congestion, sneezing, epistaxis, watery eyes. **GI:** nausea, vomiting. **Other:** development of local fungal infections.
lidocaine hydrochloride Xylocaine♦, Xylocaine Viscous♦ **Local anesthesia, pain from dental extractions, stomatitis:** ADULTS AND CHILDREN: apply 2% to 5% solution, ointment, or 15 ml of Xylocaine Viscous q 3 to 4 hours to oral or nasal mucosa.	**EENT:** interference with pharyngeal stage of swallowing. **Other:** hypersensitivity (CNS symptoms are excitatory or depressant; CV symptoms are depressant); systemic absorption when used repeatedly.
naphazoline hydrochloride Privine♦ **Nasal congestion:** ADULTS: apply 2 drops or sprays of 0.05% to 0.1% solution to nasal mucosa q 3 to 4 hours. CHILDREN 6 TO 12 YEARS: 1 to 2 drops or sprays of 0.05% solution. Repeat q 3 to 6 hours, p.r.n. Use no longer than 3 to 5 days.	**EENT:** rebound nasal congestion with excessive or long-term use, sneezing, stinging, dryness of mucosa. **Other:** systemic side effects in children after excessive or long-term use; marked sedation.
oxymetazoline hydrochloride Afrin, Duration, Nafrine♦♦, St. Joseph Decongestant for Children **Nasal congestion:** ADULTS AND CHILDREN OVER 6 YEARS: apply 2 to 4 drops or sprays 0.05% solution to nasal mucosa b.i.d.	**CNS:** headache, drowsiness, dizziness, insomnia. **CV:** palpitations. **EENT:** rebound nasal congestion or irritation with excessive or long-term use, dryness of nose and throat, increased nasal discharge, stinging, sneezing. **Other:** systemic side effects in children with

INTERACTIONS AND SPECIAL CONSIDERATIONS	
Interactions: MAO INHIBITORS: may cause hypertensive crisis if ephedrine is absorbed. Don't use together. *Special considerations:* • Use cautiously in hyperthyroidism, coronary artery disease, hypertension, or diabetes mellitus, as systemic absorption can occur.	• Patient should not exceed recommended dose; use only when needed. • Patient should be shown how to apply. Only one person should use dropper bottle or nasal spray.
No significant interactions. *Special considerations:* • Use cautiously in hyperthyroidism, coronary artery disease, hypertension, or diabetes mellitus, as systemic absorption can occur.	• Patient should not exceed recommended dose; use only when needed. • Patient should be shown how to apply. Only one person should use dropper bottle or nasal spray.
No signifcant interactions. *Special considerations:* • Use cautiously, if at all, in patients with active or quiescent respiratory tract tubercular infections or in untreated fungal, bacterial, or systemic viral, or ocular herpes simplex infections. • Use cautiously in patients who have recently had nasal septal ulcers or nasal surgery or trauma. • Recommended dosages will not suppress hypothalamic-pituitary-adrenal (HPA) function. Patient should not exceed this dosage. • Indicated when conventional treatment (antihistamines, decongestants) fails. • Flunisolide is not effective for acute exacerbations. Nasal decongestants or oral antihistamines may be needed instead.	• Patient should use drug regularly, as prescribed; its effectiveness depends on regular use. • The therapeutic effects of this corticosteroid, unlike those of decongestants, are not immediate. Most patients achieve benefit within a few days, but some may need 2 to 3 weeks for maximum benefit. • If symptoms don't improve within 3 weeks or if nasal irritation persists, patient should stop drug and notify doctor.
No significant interactions. *Special considerations:* • Use cautiously in cardiac disease, hyperthyroidism, or severe oral or nasal trauma or sepsis, as systemic absorption can occur. • Chronic, prolonged use for oropharynx anesthesia can lead to systemic absorption and toxicity.	• Xylocaine Viscous should be swished around in the mouth and can be swallowed. Patient should eat or drink cautiously within 60 minutes after oral application, to avoid food aspiration. • History of reactions to local anesthetics should be obtained. • Taste can be improved by adding a drop of oil of peppermint.
No significant interactions. *Special considerations:* • Contraindicated in glaucoma. Use cautiously in hyperthyroidism, heart disease, hypertension, or diabetes mellitus, as systemic absorption can occur. • Patient should not exceed recommended dosage.	• Patient should notify doctor if nasal congestion persists after 5 days. • Patient should be shown how to apply with container held upright. Only one person should use dropper bottle or nasal spray. • Container should not be shaken.
No significant interactions. *Special considerations:* • Use cautiously in hyperthyroidism, cardiac disease, hypertension, or diabetes mellitus, as systemic absorption can occur. • Patient should not exceed recommended dose; use only when needed.	• To apply: bend head forward and sniff spray briskly. Only one person should use dropper bottle or nasal spray.

(continued on following page)

NAMES, INDICATIONS AND DOSAGES	SIDE EFFECTS
oxymetazoline hydrochloride *(continued)* CHILDREN 2 TO 5 YEARS: apply 2 to 3 drops 0.025% solution to nasal mucosa b.i.d. Use no longer than 3 to 5 days. Dosage for younger children has not been established.	excessive or long-term use; possible sedation.
phenylephrine hydrochloride Coricidin Nasal Mist, Neo-Synephrine♦ **Nasal congestion:** ADULTS: 2 to 3 drops or sprays 0.25% to 1% solution; apply jelly or spray to nasal mucosa. CHILDREN 6 TO 12 YEARS: apply 2 to 3 drops or sprays of 0.25% solution. CHILDREN UNDER 6 YEARS: apply 2 to 3 drops or sprays of 0.125% solution. Drops, spray, or jelly given q 4 hours, p.r.n.	**CNS:** headache, tremors, dizziness, nervousness. **CV:** *palpitations, tachycardia,* premature ventricular contractions, hypertension, pallor. **EENT:** transient burning, stinging; dryness of nasal mucosa; rebound nasal congestion may occur with continued use. **GI:** nausea.
piperocaine hydrochloride Metycaine HCl **Anesthetic in dental procedures:** ADULTS AND CHILDREN: apply 5% to 10% solution as a spray or 1% to 2% solution by infiltration to oral or nasal mucosa. **Local anesthetic in rhinolaryngologic examinations:** ADULTS AND CHILDREN: apply 2% solution as a spray to oral or nasal mucosa.	**EENT:** interference with pharyngeal stage of swallowing. **Other:** hypersensitivity.
tetrahydrozoline hydrochloride Tyzine HCl, Tyzine Pediatric **Nasal congestion:** ADULTS AND CHILDREN OVER 6 YEARS: apply 2 to 4 drops 0.1% solution or spray to nasal mucosa q 4 to 6 hours, p.r.n. CHILDREN 2 TO 6 YEARS: 2 to 3 drops 0.05% solution to nasal mucosa q 4 to 6 hours, p.r.n.	**EENT:** transient burning, stinging; sneezing, rebound nasal congestion in excessive or long-term use.
triamcinolone acetonide Kenalog in Orabase **Stomatitis; erosive lichen planus; traumatic oral lesions, including sore denture spots:** ADULTS AND CHILDREN: press ¼" of 0.1% emollient dental paste onto affected area until thin film develops. Repeat b.i.d. or t.i.d. Don't rub in or protection of film will be lost.	**Systemic:** with prolonged use, adrenal insufficiency, altered glucose metabolism, peptic ulcer activation.
xylometazoline hydrochloride 4-Way Long Acting, Neo-Synephrine II **Nasal congestion:** ADULTS AND CHILDREN OVER 12 YEARS: apply 2 to 3 drops or 2 sprays of 0.1% solution to nasal mucosa q 8 to 10 hours. CHILDREN UNDER 12 YEARS: 2 to 3 drops or 1 spray of 0.05% solution q 8 to 10 hours.	**EENT:** rebound nasal congestion or irritation with excessive or long-term use; transient burning, stinging; dryness or ulceration of nasal mucosa; sneezing.

♦ Available in U.S. and Canada. ♦♦ Available in Canada only.
All other products (no symbol) available in U.S. only. Italicized side effects are common or life-threatening.

INTERACTIONS AND SPECIAL CONSIDERATIONS

No significant interactions.

Special considerations:

• Contraindicated in narrow-angle glaucoma. Use cautiously in hyperthyroidism, hypertension, diabetes mellitus, or ischemic cardiac disease, as systemic absorption may occur.

• Patient should not exceed recommended dose; use only when needed.

• To apply: keep head erect to minimize swallowing of medication. Only one person should use dropper bottle or nasal spray.

No significant interactions.

Special considerations:

• Use cautiously in cardiac disease, hyperthyroidism, severe trauma, or sepsis of oral or nasal mucosa, as systemic absorption can occur.

• History of reactions to topical anesthetics should be obtained.

• Patient should not eat or drink within 60 minutes after oral application, to prevent possible food aspiration.

No significant interactions.

Special considerations:

• Contraindicated in glaucoma. Use cautiously in hyperthyroidism, hypertension, diabetes mellitus.

• 0.1% solution should not be used in children under 6 years.

• Patient should not exceed recommended dose; use only as needed.

• Patient should be shown how to apply. Only one person should use dropper or nasal spray.

No significant interactions.

Special considerations:

• Contraindicated in oral herpetic or viral lesions. Use cautiously in diabetes mellitus, peptic ulcer, or tuberculosis, as systemic absorption can occur.

• Should be applied after meals and at bedtime for best results.

No significant interactions.

Special considerations:

• Contraindicated in narrow-angle glaucoma. Use cautiously in hyperthyroidism, cardiac disease, hypertension, diabetes mellitus, and advanced arteriosclerosis, as systemic absorption can occur.

• Patient should not exceed recommended dose.

• Patient should be shown how to apply. Only one person should use dropper bottle or nasal spray.

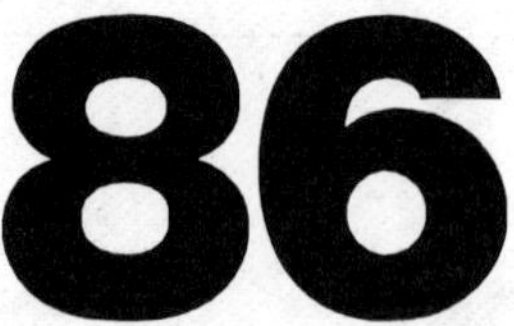

Local anti-infectives

amphotericin B
bacitracin
carbol-fuchsin solution
chloramphenicol
chlortetracycline hydrochloride
clotrimazole
erythromycin
gentamicin sulfate
gentian violet (methylrosaniline chloride)
haloprogin
iodochlorhydroxyquin
mafenide acetate
meclocycline sulfosalicylate
miconazole nitrate 2%
neomycin sulfate
nitrofurazone
nystatin
silver sulfadiazine
tetracycline hydrochloride
tolnaftate
undecylenic acid (zinc undecylenate)

Local anti-infective drugs are widely used in treatment of local bacterial and fungal infections. Bacteriostatic and fungistatic drugs suppress growth of microorganisms; bactericidal antibiotics and fungicidal agents destroy them. *Bacteriostatic* antibiotics include chloramphenicol, chlortetracycline, erythromycin, mafenide, meclocycline, nitrofurazone, tetracycline. *Bactericidal* antibiotics include bacitracin, gentamicin, neomycin.

The effectiveness of the antifungal agents depends on concentration: most of them are fungistatic at low concentrations or against some organisms, but fungicidal at higher concentrations or against other organisms. *Fungistatic* drugs include iodochlorhydroxyquin, nystatin, tolnaftate, and undecylenic acid. The agents that are generally considered *fungicidal* are amphotericin B, carbol-fuchsin, clotrimazole, gentian violet, haloprogin, miconazole, and silver sulfadiazine.

Major uses
- Antibiotics are used to treat bacterial infections that are due to susceptible organisms and responsive to local therapy.
- Antifungal agents are used topically to treat fungal infections.

Mechanism of action
- Amphotericin B and nystatin act mainly by altering the permeability of the cell membrane; the other antifungals act primarily by removing diseased tissue (softening and dissolving the horny layer of the epidermis).
- Bacitracin acts by inhibiting cell wall synthesis; the other antibiotics act primarily by disrupting protein synthesis of bacterial ribosomes.

Absorption, distribution, metabolism, and excretion
Most topical anti-infectives, in the absence of inflammation, undergo minimal systemic absorption; however, absorption increases when they're applied to large areas of denuded or inflamed skin. Applied externally, anti-infectives generally penetrate quickly and easily into the skin.
- Gentamicin and neomycin are systemically absorbed to a greater extent than the other anti-infectives, and special caution is needed with their use. Gentamicin cream may be absorbed more readily than the ointment, with up to 2% to 5% of the drug appearing in urine. Loss of hearing has been reported in persons with normal renal function after topical application of large amounts of neomycin. Large amounts of gentamicin may also cause hearing loss.

DRUG ADVANCES

NEW THREE-DAY CLOTRIMAZOLE REGIMEN FOR VULVOVAGINAL CANDIDIASIS

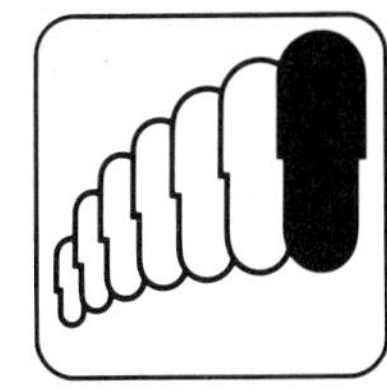

Studies show that a new 3-day regimen of clotrimazole vaginal tablets is just as effective as the standard 7-day regimen for treating vulvovaginal candidiasis in nonpregnant women. The incidence of side effects is comparable with both regimens. But because compliance has been a problem with the 7-day regimen, the shortened dosage schedule represents a significant therapeutic advance.

In the new regimen, two clotrimazole tablets are inserted intravaginally once daily for 3 consecutive days. The 3-day course has *not* proven effective in pregnant women, however. So the 7-day regimen should be used during pregnancy.

Adapted with permission from "Three-day Clotrimazole Regimen Effective in Vulvovaginal Candidiasis," *Drug Therapy*, December 1980.

Onset and duration

• Onset of local anti-infectives is rapid—usually within minutes. The antifungal agents that remove diseased tissue have a more prolonged onset of action than other antifungals. Therapeutic benefit may not appear for 1 to 3 weeks.

• Duration of action of local anti-infectives is limited because they're often inactivated by components of blood, pus, and exudates. They should generally be applied often (three to six times a day) after the skin is cleansed of adherent crusts and debris.

Combination products

AUREOCORT OINTMENT♦♦: triamcinolone acetonide 0.1% and chlortetracycline HCl 3%/15-g tube.

BACIMYCIN OINTMENT: zinc bacitracin 500 units and neomycin sulfate 5 mg/g.

BACIMIN OINTMENT: polymyxin B sulfate 5,000 units, neomycin sulfate 5 mg, and bacitracin 400 units/g.

BIOTRES OINTMENT: polymyxin B sulfate 10,000 units and zinc bacitracin 500 units/g.

CORDRAN-N CREAM, OINTMENT: flurandrenolide 0.05% and neomycin sulfate 0.5%.

CORTISPORIN CREAM: hydrocortisone acetate 0.5%, neomycin sulfate 0.5%, gramicidin 0.25 mg, and polymyxin B sulfate 10,000/g.

CORTISPORIN OINTMENT♦: hydrocortisone 1%, neomycin sulfate 0.5%, bacitracin zinc 400 units and polymyxin B sulfate 5,000 units/g.

MYCITRACIN OINTMENT: polymyxin B sulfate 5,000 units, bacitracin 500 units, and neomycin sulfate 5 mg/g.

MYCOLOG CREAM, OINTMENT: triamcinolone acetonide 0.1%, gramicidin 0.25 mg, nystatin 100,000 units, and neomycin sulfate 0.25%.

TOPICAL THERAPY: MATCHING THE VEHICLE TO THE CONDITION

ACUTE	CLINICAL SIGNS	TYPE OF VEHICLE
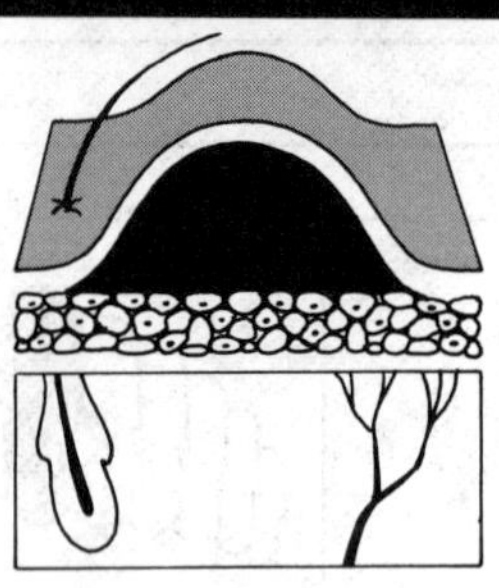	Inflammation is marked. The lesion is erythematous, edematous, and vesicular. To the patient, these often-weepy lesions feel tender, itchy, and hot or burning.	*Apply a wet compress* as often as possible, changing it before it dries. Leave the compress uncovered so as not to impede evaporation, which soothes, cools, and also helps heal through its antipruritic, anti-inflammatory action.
SUBACUTE	**CLINICAL SIGNS**	**TYPE OF VEHICLE**
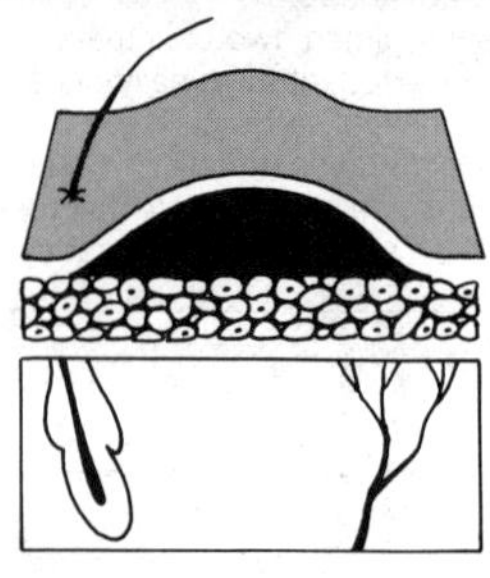	Inflammation is present but is often restricted to the areas immediately surrounding the lesions. Total appearance suggests a drying-out process.	*Apply lotions or creams,* which are protective and lubricating yet not occlusive enough to stop the still-needed evaporation.
CHRONIC	**CLINICAL SIGNS**	**TYPE OF VEHICLE**
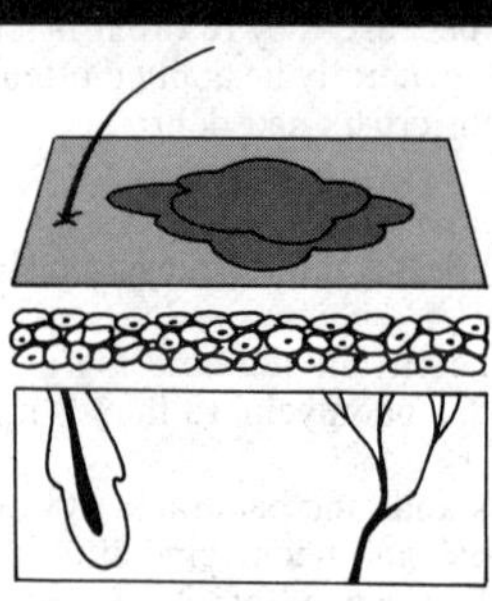	Limited inflammation may still be present. Chronic lesions may assume a scaly, lichenified appearance.	*Apply ointments,* which are occlusive and lubricating, and help the skin to retain moisture and natural skin emollients. At this stage, active medications can be continued in the ointments.

NEO-CORTEF LOTION: hydrocortisone acetate 1% and neomycin sulfate 0.5%.
NEO-CORTEF OINTMENT♦: hydrocortisone acetate 0.5% together with neomycin sulfate 0.5%
NEODECADRON CREAM: dexamethasone phosphate 0.1% and neomycin sulfate 0.5%.
NEO-DELTA-CORTEF OINTMENT: prednisolone acetate 0.5% and neomycin sulfate 0.5%.
NEO-POLYCON OINTMENT: polymyxin B sulfate 5,000 units, neomycin sulfate 5 mg, and zinc bacitracin 400 units/g.
POLYSPORIN CREAM♦♦: polymyxin B sulfate 10,000 units and gramicidin 0.25 mg/g.
POLYSPORIN OINTMENT♦: polymyxin B sulfate 10,000 units, zinc bacitracin 500 units/g.
SOFRAMYCIN OINTMENT♦♦: framycetin sulfate 15 mg, gramicidin 50 mcg, and anhydrous lanolin 10%/g.
SPECTROCIN OINTMENT: neomycin sulfate 3.6 mg and gramicidin 0.25 mg/g.
STERISPRAY♦♦: neomycin sulfate 500 mg, polymyxin B sulfate 165,000 units, and zinc bacitracin 10,000 units/100-g container.
TERRAMYCIN WITH POLYMYXIN B SULFATE OINTMENT♦, POWDER: oxytetracycline HCl 30 mg and polymyxin B sulfate 10,000 units/g.
TRICILONE NNG CREAM: triamcinolone acetonide 0.1%, nystatin 100,000 units, neomycin sulfate 0.25%, and gramicidin 0.25 mg/g.
VALISONE-G CREAM♦♦, OINTMENT♦♦: bethamethasone valerate NF 1.22 mg and gentamicin sulfate 1.67 mg/g.

Combination products
(antifungal combinations)

CORTIN CREAM: iodochlorhydroxyquin 3% and hydrocortisone 0.5% or 1%.
DRENIFORM CREAM♦♦: iodochlorhydorxyquin 3% and flurandrenolide 0.0125%/20-g tube.
KOMED LOTION: sodium thiosulfate 8%, salicylic acid 2%, isopropyl alcohol 25%/g.
LOCACORTEN-VIOFORM CREAM♦♦, OINTMENT♦♦: iodochlorhydroxyquin 3% and flumethasone pivalate 0.02%/g.
MYCOLOG CREAM, OINTMENT: gramicidin 0.25 mg, neomycin sulfate 0.25%, triamcinolone acetonide 0.1%, and nystatin 100,000 units/g.
NEO-POLYCIN HC OINTMENT♦♦: neomycin sulfate 3.5 mg, polymyxin B sulfate 5,000 units, zinc bacitracin 400 units, and hydrocortisone acetate 10 mg/g.
NEOSPORIN CREAM♦♦: polymyxin B sulfate 10,000 units, neomycin sulfate 5 mg, and gramicidin 0.25 mg/g.
NEOSPORIN OINTMENT♦: polymyxin B sulfate 5,000 units, zinc bacitracin 400 units, neomycin sulfate 5 mg/g.
NEOSPORIN-G CREAM: polymyxin B sulfate 10,000 units, neomycin sulfate 5 mg, and gramicidin 0.25 mg/g.
NEO-SYNALAR CREAM♦: fluocinolone acetonide 0.025% and neomycin sulfate 0.5%.
NYSTAFORM OINTMENT♦: nystatin 100,000 units/g and iodochlorhydroxyquin 1%.
NYSTAFORM-HC CREME♦♦, LOTION♦♦, OINTMENT♦: nystatin 100,000 units/g, iodochlorhydroxyquin 3% and hydorcortisone alcohol, 5% or 1%.
P.B.N. OINTMENT: polymyxin B sulfate 5,000 units, neomycin sulfate 5 mg, and bacitracin 400 units/g.
RACET CREAM: iodochlorhydroxyquin 3% and hydrocortisone 0.5%.
TINVER LOTION♦: sodium thiosulfate 25%, salicylic acid 1%, and isopropyl alcohol 10%.
VIOFORM-HYDROCORTISONE CREAM♦, LOTION, OINTMENT♦: iodochlorhydroxyquin 3% and hydrocortisone 1%.
VIOFORM-HYDROCORTISONE MILD CREAM♦, OINTMENT♦: iodochlorhydroxyquin 3% and hydrocortisone 0.5%.
WHITFIELD'S OINTMENT: benzoic acid 12% and salicylic acid 6%.

NAMES, INDICATIONS AND DOSAGES	SIDE EFFECTS
amphotericin B Fungizone Cream, Lotion, Ointment (3% amphotericin B) **Cutaneous or mucocutaneous candidal infections:** ADULTS AND CHILDREN: apply liberally b.i.d., t.i.d., or q.i.d. for 1 to 3 weeks; up to several months for interdigital lesions, paronychias, and onychomycosis (where relapses are frequent).	**Skin:** possible drying, contact sensitivity, erythema, burning, pruritus.
bacitracin Baciguent♦, Bacitin♦♦ **Topical infections, impetigo, abrasions, cuts, minor wounds, seborrheic dermatitis, acne, contact dermatitis, psoriasis:** ADULTS AND CHILDREN: apply thin film b.i.d. or t.i.d. or more often, depending on severity of condition.	**Skin:** rashes and other allergic reactions; itching, burning, swelling of lips or face. **Other:** *possible systemic side effects when used over large areas for prolonged periods: potentially nephrotoxic and ototoxic;* tightness in chest, hypotension.
carbol-fuchsin solution Carfusin, Castaderm, Castellani's Paint **Tinea, dermatophytosis, skin infections:** ADULTS AND CHILDREN: apply liberally 1 or 2 times daily.	**Blood:** possibility of bone marrow hypoplasia with use over long periods or at frequent intervals. **Skin:** *contact dermatitis.*
chloramphenicol Chloromycetin♦ (1% chloramphenicol) **Superficial skin infections caused by susceptible bacteria:** ADULTS AND CHILDREN: after thorough cleansing, apply t.i.d. or q.i.d.	**Skin:** possible contact sensitivity; itching, burning, urticaria, angioneurotic edema in patients hypersensitive to any of the components.
chlortetracycline hydrochloride Aureomycin 3%♦ **Superficial infections of the skin caused by susceptible bacteria:** ADULTS AND CHILDREN: rub into affected area b.i.d. or t.i.d.	**Skin:** *rashes, dermatitis.*
clotrimazole Canesten♦♦, Gyne-Lotrimin, Lotrimin (1% clotrimazole) **Superficial fungal infections (tinea pedis, tinea cruris, tinea versicolor, candidiasis, and tinea corporis):** ADULTS AND CHILDREN: apply thinly and massage into affected and surrounding area, morning and evening, 1 to 8 weeks. **Candidal vulvovaginitis:** ADULTS: insert 1 applicatorful or 1 tablet intravaginally daily for 7 to 14 days at bedtime. Alternatively, insert 2 tablets once daily for 3 consecutive days.	**GU:** *with vaginal use: mild vaginal burning, irritation.* **Skin:** blistering, *erythema,* edema, pruritus, burning, stinging, peeling, urticaria, skin fissures, general irritation.

INTERACTIONS AND SPECIAL CONSIDERATIONS

No significant interactions.

Special considerations:
- Cream or lotion preferred for areas such as folds of groin, armpit, and neck creases.
- Cream discolors skin slightly when rubbed in; lotion or ointment doesn't. Lotion may stain nail lesions.
- Patient should watch for and report signs of local irritation.
- Occlusive dressings and ointments should be avoided.
- Should be stored at room temperature; should not be frozen.
- Well tolerated, even by infants, for long periods.
- A fungistatic agent.
- Patient should continue using medication for full treatment period prescribed, even though condition has improved.

No significant interactions.

Special considerations:
- Contraindicated in hypersensitivity to any of the components and for application in the external ear canal if the eardrum is perforated.
- If used on burns covering more than 20% of body surface, especially if patient suffers impaired renal function, should be applied only once daily.
- If no improvement or if condition worsens, patient should stop using and tell doctor.
- Prolonged use may result in overgrowth of nonsusceptible organisms.
- Excess application should be avoided.
- A bacteriostatic agent.

No significant interactions.

Special considerations:
- Should not be used on large areas or on eroded skin.
- Patient should not continue use after 1 week if no improvement shown.
- Poisonous; should not be swallowed.
- Patient should clean and dry skin thoroughly before applying.
- A fungicidal and bactericidal agent.
- Patient should continue using medication for full treatment period prescribed, even if condition has improved.

No significant interactions.

Special considerations:
- Contraindicated in hypersensitivity to any of the components.
- If no improvement or if condition worsens, patient should stop using and tell doctor.
- Prolonged use may result in overgrowth of nonsusceptible organisms.
- For all but superficial infections, supplement topical use of drug with systemic medication.
- A bacteriostatic agent.
- Discontinue if signs of hypersensitivity develop.
- Use medication for full treatment period prescribed, even if condition has improved.

No significant interactions.

Special considerations:
- Contraindicated in hypersensitivity to any of the components.
- Prolonged use may result in overgrowth of nonsusceptible organisms.
- If no improvement or if condition worsens, patient should stop using and tell doctor.
- A bacteriostatic agent.

No significant interactions.

Special considerations:
- Contraindicated in hypersensitivity to any of the components.
- Not for ophthalmic use.
- Patient should watch for and report irritation or sensitivity. Discontinue use.
- Improvement usually within a week; if none in 4 weeks, diagnosis should be reviewed.
- Shortened dosage schedule with tablets may be used when compliance is a problem.
- A fungicidal agent.
- Should not use occlusive dressing.

NAMES, INDICATIONS AND DOSAGES	SIDE EFFECTS
erythromycin A/T/S, Eryderm, Staticin ♦ **Superficial skin infections due to susceptible organisms:** ADULTS AND CHILDREN: clean affected area; apply t.i.d. or q.i.d.	**Skin:** sensitivity reactions.
gentamicin sulfate Garamycin♦ **Primary and secondary bacterial infections, superficial burns, skin ulcers, infected insect bites and stings, infected lacerations and abrasions, wounds from minor surgery:** ADULTS AND CHILDREN OVER 1 YEAR: rub in small amount gently t.i.d. or q.i.d., with or without gauze dressing.	**Skin:** small percentage of minor skin irritation; possible photosensitivity.
gentian violet (methylrosaniline chloride) Bismuth Violet Solution (1% and 2%), Crystal Violet **Superficial infections of skin; lesions, except ulcerative lesions of face, particularly *Candida albicans:*** ADULTS AND CHILDREN: apply with swab b.i.d. or t.i.d. Keep affected area clean, dry, and exposed to air to prevent spread of infection.	**Skin:** *permanent discoloration if applied to granulation tissue;* ulceration of mucous membranes.
haloprogin Halotex♦ **Superficial fungal infections (tinea pedis, tinea cruris, tinea corporis, tinea manuum, and tinea versicolor):** ADULTS AND CHILDREN: apply liberally b.i.d. for 2 to 3 weeks.	**Skin:** burning sensation, irritation, vesicle formation, increased maceration, *pruritus or exacerbation of preexisting lesions.*
iodochlorhydroxyquin Gentleline, Quinoform, Torofor, Vioform **Inflamed skin conditions, including eczema, athlete's foot, other fungal infections; cutaneous or mucocutaneous mycotic infections caused by *Candida* species *(Monilia):*** ADULTS AND CHILDREN: apply a thin layer b.i.d., t.i.d., q.i.d., or as directed. Continue for 1 week after clinical cure.	**Skin:** *possible burning, itching, acneiform eruptions.* **Systemic:** electrolyte imbalance, adrenal suppression.
mafenide acetate Sulfamylon♦ **Adjunctive treatment of second- and third-degree burns:** ADULTS AND CHILDREN: apply 1/16" daily or b.i.d. to cleansed, debrided wounds.	**Blood:** eosinophilia. **Skin:** pain, *burning sensation,* rash, itching, swelling, hives, blisters, erythema. **Other:** facial edema.

♦ Available in U.S. and Canada. ♦♦ Available in Canada only.
All other products (no symbol) available in U.S. only. Italicized side effects are common or life-threatening.

INTERACTIONS AND SPECIAL CONSIDERATIONS

No significant interactions.

Special considerations:
- Prolonged use may result in overgrowth of nonsusceptible organisms.
- If no improvement or if condition worsens, patient should stop using and tell doctor.
- Usually a bacteriostatic agent, but in high concentrations or against highly susceptible organisms, may be bactericidal.

No significant interactions.

Special considerations:
- Contraindicated in hypersensitivity to any of the components.
- If no improvement or if condition worsens, patient should stop using and tell doctor.
- Use on large skin lesions or over a wide area should be avoided because of possible systemic toxic effects.
- Prolonged use may result in overgrowth of nonsusceptible organisms.
- May clear bacterial infections that have not responded to other antibacterial agents.
- Useful for treating patients who are sensitive to neomycin.
- Useful for infected skin cysts, preceded by incision and draining.
- Store in cool place.
- A bactericidal agent.
- Crusts should be removed before applying gentamicin in impetigo contagiosa.

No significant interactions.

Special considerations:
- Contraindicated in hypersensitivity to any of the components.
- Should not be used on ulcerative lesions of the face.
- Should be applied carefully to avoid undue staining. Will stain skin and clothing.
- Fungistatic.
- When used in infant with oral candidiasis, infant should be face down after application to minimize amount swallowed.
- Should not use occlusive dressings.

No significant interactions.

Special considerations:
- Contraindicated in hypersensitivity to any of the components.
- Diagnosis should be reconsidered if no improvement in 4 weeks.
- Fungistatic and fungicidal.
- Patient should use for full treatment period prescribed, even if condition has improved.

Interactions:
SYSTEMIC CORTICOSTEROIDS: possible increased absorption. Use together cautiously.

Special considerations:
- Contraindicated in hypersensitivity to iodine or iodine-containing preparations. Also contraindicated in tuberculosis, vaccinia, and varicella.
- All side effects and precautions of each component in the combination antifungals should be noted.
- Presence in urine may cause false-positive result for phenylketonuria or inaccurate thyroid function studies. Should be discontinued at least 1 month before thyroid function studies.
- Drug will stain fabric and hair.

No significant interactions.

Special considerations:
- Use with caution in acute renal failure and in known hypersensitivity to mafenide.
- Acid-base balance, especially in the presence of pulmonary and renal dysfunction, should be closely monitored.
- If acidosis occurs, use should be discontinued for 24 to 48 hours.
- Causes pain at application site. Pain and burning should be reported. If other allergic reactions occur, treatment may have to be temporarily discontinued.
- Area should be cleansed before applying. Mafenide washes off with water.
- Accidental ingestion may cause diarrhea.
- Burn areas should be kept medicated at all times.
- Patient should be bathed daily, if possible.

(continued on following page)

NAMES, INDICATIONS AND DOSAGES	SIDE EFFECTS
mafenide acetate *(continued)*	
meclocycline sulfosalicylate Meclan **Treatment of acne vulgaris:** ADULTS AND ADOLESCENTS: apply to affected area b.i.d. morning and evening. Less frequent application may be used depending on patient's response.	**Skin:** *stinging and burning on application,* skin irritation, slight yellowing of treated skin (especially in patients with light complexions). Treated skin areas fluoresce under ultraviolet light.
miconazole nitrate 2% Monistat-Derm Cream and Lotion **Tinea pedis, tinea cruris, tinea corporis, cutaneous candidiasis (moniliasis), infections from common dermatophytes:** ADULTS AND CHILDREN: apply sparingly b.i.d. for 2 to 4 weeks.	**Skin:** isolated reports of irritation, burning, maceration.
neomycin sulfate Herisan Antibiotic♦♦, Mycifradin♦♦, Myciguent♦, Neocin♦♦ **Topical bacterial infections, burns, wounds, skin grafts, following surgical procedure, lesions, pruritus, trophic ulcerations, edema:** ADULTS AND CHILDREN: rub in small quantity gently b.i.d., t.i.d., or as directed.	**Skin:** *rashes.* **Other:** *possible nephrotoxicity, ototoxicity, and neuromuscular blockade; possible systemic absorption when used on extensive areas of the body.*
nitrofurazone Furacin♦, Furazyme **Adjunctive treatment of second- and third-degree burns (especially when resistance to other antibiotics and sulfonamides occurs); skin grafting:** ADULTS AND CHILDREN: apply directly to lesion daily or every few days, depending on severity of burn.	**Skin:** *erythema, pruritus,* burning, edema, severe reactions (vesiculation, denudation, ulceration).
nystatin Mycostatin♦, Nadostine♦♦, Nilstat **Infant eczema, pruritus ani and vulvae, superficial bacterial infections, localized forms of candidiasis:** ADULTS AND CHILDREN: apply and rub into area b.i.d. for 2 weeks.	**Skin:** occasional contact dermatitis from preservatives present in some formulations. **Systemic:** possible nephrotoxicity or ototoxicity with prolonged or frequent use.

♦ Available in U.S. and Canada. ♦♦ Available in Canada only.
All other products (no symbol) available in U.S. only. Italicized side effects are common or life-threatening.

INTERACTIONS AND SPECIAL CONSIDERATIONS

• Safety of use during pregnancy has not yet been established.
• For burns, using reverse isolation technique with sterile gloves and instruments to apply cream prevents further wound contamination.
• Bacteriostatic against several gram-negative and gram-positive organisms.

No significant interactions.

Special considerations:
• Contraindicated in hypersensitivity to any of the components.
• Beneficial response will usually be seen within 2 weeks of start of treatment.
• If condition doesn't improve or worsens, medication should be discontinued and therapy re-evaluated.
• Prolonged use may result in overgrowth of nonsusceptible organisms.
• Patient may continue use of cosmetics.
• Yellow-skin staining is generally worse when excessive amounts are applied.
• To minimize fluorescence under black lights in discotheques, medication should be removed from the skin by washing and reapplied at bedtime.

No significant interactions.

Special considerations:
• For external use only. Should be kept out of eyes.
• Should be discontinued if sensitivity or chemical irritation occurs.
• Fungistatic.
• Patient should continue using for full treatment period prescribed, even if condition has improved.
• Should not use occlusive dressing.

No significant interactions.

Special considerations:
• Contraindicated in hypersensitivity to any of the components, atopy, vaccinia, varicella, fungal or viral lesions.
• If no improvement or if condition worsens, patient should stop using and tell doctor.
• If used on more than 20% of the body surface and on patient with impaired renal function, application should be reduced to once daily.
• Prolonged use may result in overgrowth of nonsusceptible organisms.
• In combination products containing corticosteroids, use of occlusive dressings increases corticosteroid absorption and likelihood of systemic effect.
• Particularly well absorbed on denuded or abraded areas.
• A bactericidal agent.
• Hypersensitivity, contact dermatitis, and ototoxicity may occur.

No significant interactions.

Special considerations:
• Contraindicated in previous hypersensitivity to drug.
• If irritation, sensitization, or infection occurs, use should be stopped.
• When using wet dressing, skin around wound should be protected with zinc oxide.
• Wound should be cleansed as indicated by doctor at each dressing change.
• Adherent dressings should be removed by flushing with solution of nitrofurazone and sterile water, or sterile normal saline solution.
• Store solution in tight, light-resistant containers (brown bottles); avoid exposure of solution to direct light, prolonged heat, and alkaline materials.
• Drug may discolor in light but is still usable because it retains its potency.
• Cloudy solutions should be discarded if warming to 55° to 60° C. (131° to 140° F.) does not restore clarity.
• Use reverse isolation and/or sterile application technique to prevent further wound contamination.

No significant interactions.

Special considerations:
• Contraindicated in viral diseases of the skin (vaccinia and varicella), fungal lesions (except candidiasis), and markedly impaired circulation.
• Generally well tolerated by all age groups, including debilitated infants.
• Preparation does not stain skin or mucous membranes.
• Cream recommended for intertriginous areas, powder for very moist areas, ointment for dry areas.
• Fungistatic and fungicidal.
• Patient should continue using for full treatment period prescribed, even if condition has improved.
• Should not use occlusive dressing.

NAMES, INDICATIONS AND DOSAGES	SIDE EFFECTS
silver sulfadiazine Flamazine♦♦, Silvadene **Prevention and treatment of wound infection for second- and third-degree burns:** ADULTS AND CHILDREN: apply 1/16″ thickness of ointment to cleansed and debrided burn wound, then apply daily or b.i.d.	**Blood:** *neutropenia (in 3% to 5%).* **Skin:** pain, burning, rashes, itching. **Other:** fungal infections.
tetracycline hydrochloride Achromycin♦, Topicycline **Superficial skin infections caused by susceptible bacteria, acne:** ADULTS AND CHILDREN: rub into cleansed affected area b.i.d. or t.i.d. **Acne:** ADULTS: apply Topicycline generously to affected areas b.i.d. until skin is thoroughly wet.	**Skin:** dermatitis with Achromycin; with Topicycline, temporary stinging or burning on application, slight yellowing of treated skin, especially in patients with light complexions; severe dermatitis; treated skin areas fluoresce under ultraviolet light.
tolnaftate Aftate, Tinactin♦ **Superficial fungal infections of the skin, infections due to common pathogenic fungi, tinea pedis, tinea cruris, tinea corporis, tinea manuum, tinea versicolor:** ADULTS AND CHILDREN: 1/4″ to 1/2″ ribbon of cream or 1 or 3 drops of lotion to cover area of one hand; same amount of cream or 2 to 3 drops of lotion to cover the toes and interdigital webs of one foot. Apply and massage gently into skin b.i.d. for 2 or 3 weeks, up to 6 weeks.	None significant.
undecylenic acid (zinc undecylenate) Desenex, Ting, Unde-Jen **Athlete's foot and ringworm of the body exclusive of nails and hairy areas:** ADULTS AND CHILDREN: clean thoroughly. Apply ointment liberally at night and powder during the day. Use regularly to prevent fungal infections.	**Skin:** possible irritation in hypersensitive person.

♦ Available in U.S. and Canada. ♦♦ Available in Canada only.
All other products (no symbol) available in U.S. only. Italicized side effects are common or life-threatening.

INTERACTIONS AND SPECIAL CONSIDERATIONS

Interactions:
TOPICAL PROTEOLYTIC ENZYMES: inactivity of enzymes when used together. Do not use together.

Special considerations:
• Contraindicated for premature and newborn infants during first month of life. (Drug may increase possibility of kernicterus.) Use with caution in hypersensitivity to the drug or sulfonamides.
• Hepatic or renal dysfunction requires possible discontinuation of drug.
• Patient's skin should be inspected daily. Patient should notify doctor if burning or excessive pain develops.
• Should be used only on affected areas. Should be kept medicated at all times.
• For patients with extensive burns, serum sulfa concentrations and renal function should be monitored and urine checked for sulfa crystals.
• Patient should be bathed daily, if possible.
• Darkened cream should be discarded.
• Should be discontinued if infection is suspected.
• Reverse isolation and/or sterile application technique recommended to prevent wound contamination.

No significant interactions.

Special considerations:
• Contraindicated in hypersensitivity to any of the components.
• If no improvement or if condition worsens, patient should stop using and tell doctor.
• Prolonged use may result in overgrowth of nonsusceptible organisms.
• Primarily a bacteriostatic agent.
• Patient may continue normal use of cosmetics.
• Store at room temperature, away from excessive heat.
• Medication to be used by one person only and not shared with family members.
• Should be applied in morning and evening. Drug should be used within 2 months.
• Floating plug in bottle of Topicycline—an inert and harmless result of proper reconstitution of the preparation—shouldn't be removed.
• Serum levels of topical tetracycline HCl are much lower than those for orally administered drug, so systemic effects are unlikely.
• To control flow rate of solution, pressure of the applicator against the skin should be increased or decreased.

No significant interactions.

Special considerations:
• Patient should discontinue if condition worsens, and check with doctor.
• Odorless, greaseless. Won't stain or discolor skin, hair, nails, or clothing.
• Only a small quantity of cream or lotion is needed; area should not be wet with solution when application is completed.
• Fungistatic and fungicidal.
• Commonly available product used to treat athlete's foot (tinea pedis).
• Patient should continue using for full treatment period prescribed, even if condition has improved.

No significant interactions.

Special considerations:
• Use on patient with peripheral neuropathy and peripheral vascular diseases or diabetes should be carefully considered.
• Patient should continue using for full treatment period prescribed, even if condition has improved.

87

Scabicides and pediculicides

benzyl benzoate lotion
copper oleate solution (with tetrahydronaphthalene)
crotamiton
gamma benzene hexachloride (or lindane)
pyrethrins
sulfa (6%) in petrolatum

Scabicides and pediculicides destroy the most common parasitic arthropods that infest man.

Persistent itching after adequate therapy indicates either continued infestation, slow-resolving hypersensitivity, or irritation from the drug. Laundering or dry cleaning all contaminated linens and clothing is essential to eradicate infestations. Commercial sprays can be used to decontaminate furniture or rugs that may harbor the parasites.

Major uses

These drugs eradicate parasitic arthropod infestations such as scabies and pediculosis. They're used against *Sarcoptes scabiei* (scabies), *Pediculus humanus* var. *capitis* (head louse), *Pediculus humanus* var. *corporis* (body louse), and *Phthirus pubis* (crab louse). One application is usually enough to kill adult forms, but repeated applications are necessary to destroy nits.

Mechanism of action

Gamma benzene hexachloride appears to inhibit neuronal membrane function in arthropods.

The mechanism of action of the other agents is unknown.

Absorption, distribution, metabolism, and excretion

Gamma benzene hexachloride is absorbed through intact skin when applied topically. Absorption through skin is usually greatest when drug is applied to face, scalp, neck, axillae, scrotum, or damaged skin. No information is available on systemic absorption of the other drugs.

Gamma benzene hexachloride is stored in body fat, metabolized in the liver, and eliminated in urine and feces.

Onset and duration

Onset of all the drugs is immediate. Duration of action is limited. The drug must be reapplied, if necessary, according to product information.

PARENT-TEACHING AID

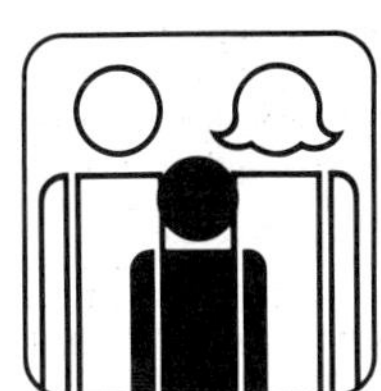

HOW TO GET RID OF HEAD LICE

Dear Parent:

Having head lice is not a disgrace: anyone can get them. They don't necessarily result from poor grooming or bad health habits, but instead can be spread by close contact with those who have lice in schools, locker rooms, buses, and other public places, or by sharing clothing or hairbrushes. Here's how you can relieve your child's itching and help eliminate the lice:

1. Wash your child's hair for 4 minutes with a lindane-medicated shampoo (Kwell), Cuprex shampoo, or pyrinate shampoo. This will destroy lice and nits (lice eggs), but nits will remain attached to hair shafts.
2. Remove nits from hair with a brush or fine-toothed comb dipped in vinegar.
3. Repeat steps #1 and #2 on 2 consecutive days or at weekly intervals.
4. Wash or dry clean all your child's clothing, because nits can survive away from the body for up to 30 days.
5. Spray upholstered furniture and rugs with a pyrethrum spray (R&C). Animals don't become infested, so don't worry about treating family pets.
6. Examine your child's head regularly for recurrent infestation. You can detect head lice and nits with the naked eye. Usually you won't find many adult lice moving through your child's hair. Instead, you'll find nits attached to the hair shafts. Be careful not to mistake hair casts (normal root sheaths that encircle the hair shaft), hair-spray globules, or severe scalp scaling (from psoriasis or seborrhea) for head lice. If you have any questions, consult your child's doctor.

Adapted from Lawrence Charles Parish and Joseph A. Witkowski, "Head Lice: Epidemic in the Schoolroom," *Drug Therapy*, October 1980, with permission from the publisher.

NAMES, INDICATIONS AND DOSAGES	SIDE EFFECTS
benzyl benzoate lotion Scabanca♦♦ **Parasitic infestation (scabies, *Phthirus pubis*):** ADULTS AND CHILDREN: first, scrub entire body with soap and water. Then apply the 25% lotion undiluted over entire body, except the face, while still damp. Be sure to apply around nails. Let dry. Apply second coat on the most involved areas. Bathe after 24 to 48 hours. Adults require 30 ml. Children require 20 ml. **Pediculosis capitis:** ADULTS AND CHILDREN: apply to scalp and leave on overnight; shampoo out in morning. Repeat next night if necessary.	**Skin:** *irritation, itching; contact dermatitis with repeated applications.*
copper oleate solution (with tetrahydronaphthalene) Cuprex **Parasitic infestation (pediculoses capitis and pubis):** ADULTS AND CHILDREN: first, scrub entire body with soap and water. Apply gently and sparingly 3 to 4 tablespoonfuls onto affected areas; after 15 minutes wash off with soap and water.	**Skin:** *irritation with repeated use, or if used on raw or inflamed skin.*
crotamiton Eurax♦ **Parasitic infestation (scabies):** ADULTS AND CHILDREN: scrub entire body with soap and water. Then, apply a thin layer of cream over entire body, from chin down, with special attention to folds, creases, interdigital spaces, genital area. Apply second coat within 24 hours. Wait 48 hours, then wash off. **General itching:** apply locally b.i.d. or t.i.d.	**Skin:** *irritation with repeated use.*
gamma benzene hexachloride (or lindane) GBH♦♦, Kwell, Kwellada♦♦ **Parasitic infestation (scabies, pediculosis):** ADULTS AND CHILDREN: scrub entire body with soap and water. Cream or lotion—apply thin layer over entire skin surface (with special attention to folds, creases, interdigital spaces, genital area) for scabies, or to hairy areas for pediculosis. After 8 to 12 hours, wash off drug. If second application needed for scabies, wait 1 week before repeating. For pediculosis, may be repeated after 7 days but never more than twice in a week.	**Skin:** *irritation with repeated use.*

♦ Available in U.S. and Canada. ♦♦ Available in Canada only.
All other products (no symbol) available in U.S. only. Italicized side effects are common or life-threatening.

INTERACTIONS AND SPECIAL CONSIDERATIONS

No significant interactions.

Special considerations:

• Contraindicated when skin is raw or inflamed. Patient should notify doctor immediately if skin irritation or hypersensitivity develops; discontinue drug; and wash it off skin.
• Should not be applied to face, eyes, mucous membranes, or urethral meatus. If accidental contact with eyes occurs, patient should flush with water and notify doctor.
• Patient should change and sterilize (boil, launder, dry clean, or apply very hot iron) all clothing and bed linen after drug is washed off.
• Itching may continue for several weeks; does not indicate that therapy is ineffective. Itching will cease.
• Tendency to overuse this drug. Amount needed should be estimated.
• Topical corticosteroids may be needed if dermatitis develops from scratching.
• Other family members should be asked about possible infestation.
• After application, a fine comb dipped in white vinegar should be used on hair to remove nits.
• Patient should reapply if washed off (hands, for example) during treatment time.
• Hospitalized patients should be placed in isolation with linen handling precautions until treatment is completed.

No significant interactions.

Special considerations:

• Contraindicated when skin is raw or inflamed, or when there is a severe infection. Patient should notify doctor immediately if skin irritation or hypersensitivity develops; discontinue drug; and wash it off skin.
• Should not be applied more than twice within 48 hours.
• Should not be applied to face, eyes, mucous membranes, or urethral meatus. If contact with eyes occurs, patient should flush with water and notify doctor.
• Patient should change and sterilize (boil, launder, dry clean, or apply very hot iron) all clothing and bed linen after application.
• After application, a fine comb dipped in white vinegar should be used on hair to remove nits.
• Other family members should be asked about possible infestation.
• Tendency to overuse pediculicides. Amount needed should be estimated.
• Hospitalized patients should be placed in isolation with linen handling precautions until treatment is completed.

No significant interactions.

Special considerations:

• Contraindicated when skin is raw or inflamed. Patient should notify doctor immediately if skin irritation or hypersensitivity develops; discontinue drug; and wash it off skin.
• Should not be applied to eyes, mucous membranes, or urethral meatus. If contact with eyes occurs, patient should flush with water and notify doctor.
• Patient should change and sterilize (boil, launder, dry clean, or apply very hot iron) all clothing and bed linen after drug is washed off.
• Topical corticosteroids may be needed if dermatitis develops from scratching.
• Tendency to overuse scabicides. Amount needed should be estimated.
• Other family members should be asked about possible infestation.
• Patient should reapply if washed off (hands, for example) during treatment time.
• Hospitalized patients should be placed in isolation with special linen handling precautions until treatment is completed.

No significant interactions.

Special considerations:

• Contraindicated when skin is raw or inflamed. Patient should notify doctor immediately if skin irritation or hypersensitivity develops; discontinue drug; and wash it off skin. Use cautiously in infants and small children.
• Should not be applied to open areas or acutely inflamed skin, or to face, eyes, mucous membranes, or urethral meatus. If accidental contact with eyes occurs, patient should flush with water and notify doctor.
• Parents should not let infants or children suck their fingers after drug application.
• Repeated use can lead to skin irritation and possible systemic toxicity.
• Itching may continue for several weeks, particularly in scabies.
• Topical corticosteroids may be needed if dermatitis develops from scratching.
• Patient should change and sterilize (boil, launder, dry clean, or apply very hot iron) all clothing and bed linen after drug is washed off.
• After application, fine comb dipped in white vinegar should be used on hair to remove nits.
• Gamma benzene hexachloride shampoo can be used to clean comb or brushes; should be washed thoroughly afterward. Should not use gamma benzene hexachloride as routine shampoo.

(continued on following page)

NAMES, INDICATIONS AND DOSAGES	SIDE EFFECTS
gamma benzene hexachloride *(continued)* Shampoo—apply 30 to 60 ml onto affected area and work into lather for 4 to 5 minutes. Rinse thoroughly and rub with dry towel.	
pyrethrins A-200 Pyrinate, Barc, Pyrin-Aid, Pyrinyl, Rid, TISIT, Triple X **Treatment of infestations of head, body, and pubic (crab) lice and their eggs:** ADULTS AND CHILDREN: apply to hair, scalp, or other infested area until entirely wet. Allow to remain for 10 minutes, but no longer. Wash thoroughly with warm water and soap, or shampoo. Remove dead lice and eggs with fine-toothed comb. Treatment may be repeated, if necessary, but don't exceed 2 applications within 24 hours.	**Skin:** *irritation with repeated use.*
sulfa (6%) in petrolatum **Parasitic infestation (scabies):** ADULTS AND CHILDREN (PREFERRED TREATMENT FOR INFANTS AND PREGNANT WOMEN): after taking a soapy bath, patient should apply drug nightly for 2 to 3 nights consecutively. Patient should take soapy bath 24 hours after last application.	**Skin:** *may produce dermatitis if applied continually for several days.*

♦ Available in U.S. and Canada. ♦♦ Available in Canada only.
All other products (no symbol) available in U.S. only. Italicized side effects are common or life-threatening.

INTERACTIONS AND SPECIAL CONSIDERATIONS

- Other family members should be asked about possible infestation.
- Tendency for overuse. Amount needed should be estimated.
- Patient should reapply if washed off (hands, for example) during treatment time.
- Hospitalized patients should be placed in isolation with special linen handling precautions until treatment is completed.

No significant interactions.

Special considerations:

- Contraindicated when skin is raw or inflamed. Patient should notify doctor immediately if skin irritation develops; discontinue drug; and wash it off skin. Use cautiously in infants and small children.
- Should not be applied to open areas or acutely inflamed skin, or to face, eyes, mucous membranes, or urethral meatus. If accidental contact with eyes does occur, patient should flush with water and notify doctor.
- Parents should not let infants or children suck their fingers after drug application.
- Repeated use can lead to skin irritation and possible systemic toxicity.
- Topical corticosteroids may be needed if dermatitis develops from scratching.
- Patient should change and sterilize (boil, launder, dry clean, or apply very hot iron) all clothing and bed linen after drug is washed off.
- Products containing pyrethrins are available without prescription. Some authorities believe pyrethrins and gamma benzene hexachloride (Kwell) are equally effective for lice infestation.

No significant interactions.

Special considerations:

- Patient should change and sterilize (boil, launder, dry clean, or iron with a very hot iron) all clothing and bed linen after drug is washed off.
- Product has an odor, is messy, and will stain clothing.
- Other members of family should be asked about possible infestation.
- Tendency to overuse scabicides. Amount needed should be estimated.
- Hospitalized patients should be placed in isolation with special linen handling precautions until treatment is completed.

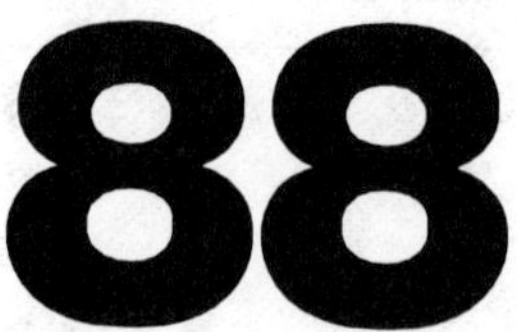

Topical corticosteroids

amcinonide
betamethasone
betamethasone benzoate
betamethasone dipropionate
betamethasone valerate
clocortolone pivalate
desonide
desoximetasone
dexamethasone
dexamethasone sodium phosphate
diflorasone diacetate
flumethasone pivalate
fluocinolone acetonide
fluocinonide
fluorometholone
flurandrenolide
halcinonide
hydrocortisone
hydrocortisone acetate
hydrocortisone valerate
methylprednisolone acetate
prednisolone
triamcinolone acetonide

Topical corticosteroids reduce inflammation, constrict blood vessels, and occasionally relieve itching. Their potency depends on the drug, the method of application, and the degree of penetration. The base or vehicle of the drug may also affect its release and therefore its potency. Ointments furnish most complete penetration of the skin by the drug; gels, creams, and lotions are less penetrating, in descending order. Topical corticosteroids reduce inflammation without curing the underlying disease; use them with caution.

After the drug is applied to the affected site, it may be covered by an occlusive dressing. The dressing facilitates the drug's absorption through the skin. Tape is used to hold the dressing in place. It protects the adjacent unaffected skin from abrasion, rubbing, discoloration, and chemical irritation. It also acts as a mechanical splint for fissured skin and prevents medication from being removed by washing or rubbing against clothing.

Major uses

Topical corticosteroids are used to treat acute and chronic inflammatory dermatoses; psoriasis; atopic and infantile eczemas; pruritus ani and vulvae; neurodermatitis, and contact, seborrheic, and exfoliative dermatitis.

Occlusive dressings are used in the medical management of psoriasis or such resistant conditions as localized neurodermatitis or lichen planus.

Creams are useful for wet lesions; *lotions,* for areas subject to chafing (axillae, feet, or groin); and *ointments,* for dry, scaly lesions.

Mechanism of action

Exactly how these drugs work is unknown. Some investigators believe that corticosteroids attach to tissue receptors, decreasing membrane permeability and inhibiting release of toxins. They may also control the rate of protein synthesis. Their actions on the inflammatory process include inhibition of edema, fibrin deposition, capillary dilation, migration of leukocytes into the inflamed area, and phagocytic activity. They may also moderate later inflammatory developments such as capillary and fibroblast proliferation and deposition of collagen.

Corticosteroid-induced vasoconstriction decreases extravasation of blood, swelling, and itching. The drugs also act as antimitotics, reducing cell multiplication in psoriasis.

DRUG ALERT

BE CAREFUL: TOPICAL STEROIDS CAN BE ABSORBED

If improperly used, topical steroids can be absorbed from local application sites, and if doses are large enough, these drugs may eventually produce adverse systemic effects.

They can be absorbed systemically when administered by these routes:
- ophthalmic
- inhalation (for asthma)
- intranasal (for nasal polyps)
- intrasynovial (for bursitis)
- rectal (for ulcerative colitis)
- intralesional injection (for psoriasis)
- topical (for allergic dermatoses).

Topical steroid absorption may vary at different sites of the body. Hydrocortisone is absorbed **0.14** times as well through the plantar foot arch as it is through the forearm; **0.83** times as well through the palms; **1.7** times as well through the back; **3.5** times as well through the scalp; **6** times as well through the forehead; **13** times as well through the cheeks at the jaw angle; and **42** times as well through scrotal skin.

Although the FDA has approved non-prescription use of hydrocortisone and hydrocortisone acetate as antipruritics in concentrations up to 0.5%, make sure they're *not* used:
- **in children under age 2.** Absorption of these products may cause growth retardation, weight gain, and hypertension.
- **in the eyes.** Activation of viral eye infections, ocular hypertension, glaucoma, and cataract formation may result from unsupervised ophthalmic use.
- **as self-medication therapy for longer than 7 days,** especially in large doses, since systemic absorption occurs even in adults.

Important: Advise patients who use over-the-counter corticosteroid preparations to follow package directions carefully.

Absorption, distribution, metabolism, and excretion

- Corticosteroids are absorbed through the skin, and absorption varies markedly with the area of the body on which the drugs are applied. If the skin is well hydrated, absorption will be increased four to five times. Inflamed or damaged skin also allows increased penetration. Occlusive dressings increase absorption significantly (up to a hundred times). They retain insensible perspiration, causing hydration of the stratum corneum.

  Absorption of these drugs in dressings that occlude extensive areas of skin can lead to adrenal suppression. Adrenal suppression may develop even in the absence of occlusion, if drug use is prolonged.
- These drugs enter the circulation and are metabolized primarily in the liver. The metabolites are excreted in urine. (For greater detail, see Chapter 51, CORTICOSTEROIDS.)

Onset and duration

Topical corticosteroids begin to act within 30 minutes after application. Because their action lasts only 4 to 6 hours, apply 2 to 4 times daily.

Combination products

Corticosteroids are commonly combined with antibiotics, antifungals, and sulfonamides. (See Chapter 16, SULFONAMIDES; Chapter 73, ANTIBIOTIC ANTINEOPLASTIC AGENTS.)

NAMES, INDICATIONS AND DOSAGES	SIDE EFFECTS
amcinonide Cyclocort♦ **Inflammation of corticosteroid-responsive dermatoses:** ADULTS AND CHILDREN: apply a light film to affected areas 2 or 3 times daily. Cream should be rubbed in gently and thoroughly until it disappears.	**Skin:** burning, itching, irritation, dryness, folliculitis, hypopigmentation, striae, acneiform eruptions, perioral dermatitis, hypertrichosis, allergic contact dermatitis. *With occlusive dressings: secondary infection, maceration, atrophy, striae, miliaria.*
betamethasone Celestone♦ **Inflammation of corticosteroid-responsive dermatoses:** ADULTS AND CHILDREN: clean area; apply cream sparingly b.i.d. or t.i.d. Massage gently until it disappears. Apply thick layer with occlusive dressing to manage deep-seated dermatoses, such as neurodermatitis.	**Skin:** burning, itching, irritation, dryness, folliculitis, hypopigmentation, acneiform eruptions, hypertrichosis, allergic contact dermatitis. *With occlusive dressings: secondary infection, maceration, skin atrophy, striae, miliaria.*
betamethasone benzoate Beben♦, Uticort **Inflammation of corticosteroid-responsive dermatoses:** ADULTS AND CHILDREN: clean area; apply cream, lotion, or gel sparingly daily to q.i.d.	**Skin:** burning, itching, irritation, dryness, folliculitis, hypopigmentation, striae, acneiform eruptions, perioral dermatitis, hypertrichosis, allergic contact dermatitis. *With occlusive dressings: secondary infection, maceration, atrophy, striae, miliaria.*

INTERACTIONS AND SPECIAL CONSIDERATIONS

No significant interactions.

Special considerations:

- Use cautiously in viral diseases of skin, such as varicella, vaccinia, herpes simplex; fungal infections; skin tuberculosis; impaired circulation.
- Avoid application in or near eyes. Do not use on face, armpits, groin, or under breasts unless specifically ordered.
- Due to alcohol content of vehicle, gel preparations may cause mild, transient stinging without irritation if used on or near excoriated skin.
- Systemic absorption especially likely with occlusive dressings, prolonged treatment, or extensive body surface treatment.
- Drug should be stopped if patient develops signs of systemic absorption, skin irritation or ulceration, signs of hypersensitivity, infection. (If antifungals or antibiotics are being used with corticosteroids and infection does not respond immediately, corticosteroids should be stopped until infection is controlled.)
- Application tips: first, gently wash skin; to prevent damage to skin, rub in medication gently, leaving a thin coat; when treating hairy sites, part hair and apply directly to lesion; apply lotions to scalp immediately after shampoo, while scalp is still damp.
- Occlusive dressing: apply cream heavily, then cover with a thin, pliable, nonflammable plastic film; seal to adjacent normal skin with hypoallergenic tape. Minimize adverse reactions by using occlusive dressing intermittently.
- For patient with eczematous dermatitis who may develop irritation with adhesive material, dressing may be held in place with gauze, elastic bandages, stockings, or stockinette.
- Occlusive dressing should be removed if body temperature rises.
- Occlusive dressings are generally not used in presence of infections or with weeping or exudative lesions.
- During dressing changes, skin should be inspected for infection, striae, and atrophy. If these occur, drug should be discontinued.
- Treatment should be continued for a few days after clearing of lesions to prevent recurrence.
- Patient should report signs of drug sensitivity.

No significant interactions.

Special considerations:

- Use cautiously in viral diseases of skin, such as vaccinia, varicella, and herpes simplex; fungal infections; skin tuberculosis; impaired circulation.
- Avoid application in or near eyes.
- Systemic absorption especially likely with occlusive dressings, prolonged treatment, or extensive body surface treatment.
- Drug should be stopped if patient develops signs of systemic absorption, skin irritation or ulceration, hypersensitivity, infection. (If antifungals or antibacterials are being used with corticosteroids and infection does not respond immediately, corticosteroids should be stopped until infection is controlled.)
- Application tips: first, gently wash skin; to prevent damage to skin, rub medication in gently, leaving a thin coat.
- Occlusive dressing: apply cream heavily, then cover with a thin, pliable, nonflammable plastic film; seal to adjacent normal skin with hypoallergenic tape. Minimize adverse reactions by using occlusive dressing intermittently.
- For patient with eczematous dermatitis who may develop irritation with adhesive material, dressing may be held in place with gauze, elastic bandages, stockings, or stockinette.
- Occlusive dressing should be removed if body temperature rises.
- Occlusive dressings are generally not used in presence of infection or with weeping or exudative lesions.
- During dressing changes, skin should be inspected for infection, striae, and atrophy. If these occur, drug should be discontinued.
- Treatment should be continued for a few days after clearing of lesions to prevent recurrence.
- Patient should report signs of drug sensitivity.

No significant interactions.

Special considerations:

- Use cautiously in viral diseases of skin, such as varicella, vaccinia, and herpes simplex; fungal infections; skin tuberculosis; impaired circulation.
- Avoid application in or near eyes.
- Due to alcohol content of vehicle, gel preparations may cause mild, transient stinging without irritation if used on or near excoriated skin.
- Systemic absorption especially likely with occlusive dressings, prolonged treatment, or extensive body surface treatment.
- Drug should be stopped if patient develops signs of systemic absorption, skin irritation or ulceration, signs of hypersensitivity, infection. (If antifungals or antibiotics are being used with corticosteroids and infection does not respond immediately, corticosteroids should be stopped until infection is controlled.)
- Application tips: first, gently wash skin; to prevent damage to skin, rub in medication gently, leaving a thin coat; when treating hairy sites, part hair and apply directly to lesion.
- Occlusive dressing: apply cream heavily, then cover with a thin, pliable, nonflammable plastic film; seal to adjacent normal skin with hypoallergenic tape. Adverse reactions may be minimized by using occlusive dressing intermittently.

(continued on following page)

NAMES, INDICATIONS AND DOSAGES	SIDE EFFECTS

betamethasone benzoate
(continued)

betamethasone dipropionate
Diprosone♦

Inflammation of corticosteroid-responsive dermatoses:
ADULTS AND CHILDREN: clean area; apply cream, lotion, or ointment sparingly b.i.d.
Aerosol—direct spray onto affected area from a distance of 6″ for only 3 seconds t.i.d.

Skin: burning, itching, irritation, dryness, folliculitis, hypopigmentation, perioral dermatitis, allergic contact dermatitis, hypertrichosis, acneiform eruptions. *With occlusive dressings: maceration of skin, secondary infection, atrophy, striae, miliaria.*

betamethasone valerate
Betnovate♦♦, Betnovate ½♦♦, Celestoderm-V♦♦, Celestoderm V/2♦♦, Valisone

Inflammation of corticosteroid-responsive dermatoses:
ADULTS AND CHILDREN: clean area; apply cream, lotion, ointment, or aerosol sparingly daily to q.i.d.
Aerosol—shake can well. Direct spray onto affected area from a distance of 6″. Apply for only 3 seconds t.i.d. to q.i.d.
Betnovate 1/2 and Celestoderm V/2 contain less betamethasone.

Skin: burning, itching, irritation, dryness, folliculitis, hypopigmentation, hypertrichosis, acneiform eruptions, perioral dermatitis, allergic contact dermatitis. *With occlusive dressings: maceration of skin, secondary infection, atrophy, striae, miliaria.*

clocortolone pivalate
Cloderm

Inflammation of corticosteroid-responsive dermatoses, such as atopic dermatitis, contact dermatitis, seborrheic dermatitis:
ADULTS AND CHILDREN: apply cream spar-

Skin: burning, itching, irritation, dryness, folliculitis, hypopigmentation, striae, acneiform eruptions, perioral dermatitis, hypertrichosis, allergic contact dermatitis. *With occlusive dressings: secondary infection, maceration, atrophy, striae, miliaria.*

INTERACTIONS AND SPECIAL CONSIDERATIONS

• For patient with eczematous dermatitis who may develop irritation with adhesive material, dressing may be held in place with gauze, elastic bandages, stockings, or stockinette.
• Occlusive dressing should be removed if body temperature rises.
• Occlusive dressings are generally not used in presence of infections or with weeping or exudative lesions.
• During dressing changes, skin should be inspected for infection, striae, and atrophy. If these occur, drug should be discontinued.
• Treatment should be continued for a few days after clearing of lesions to prevent recurrence.
• Patient should report signs of drug sensitivity.

No significant interactions.

Special considerations:
• Use cautiously in viral diseases of skin, such as varicella, vaccinia, and herpes simplex; fungal infections; skin tuberculosis; impaired circulation.
• Avoid application in or near eyes.
• Systemic absorption especially likely with occlusive dressings, prolonged treatment, or extensive body surface treatment.
• Drug should be stopped if patient develops signs of systemic absorption, skin irritation or ulceration, hypersensitivity, infection. (If antifungals or antibiotics are being used with corticosteroids and infection does not respond immediately, corticosteroids should be stopped until infection is controlled.)
• Application tips: first, gently wash skin; to prevent damage to skin, rub in medication gently, leaving a thin coat; when treating hairy sites, part hair and apply directly to lesion.
• Aerosol preparation contains alcohol and may produce irritation or burning in open lesions. When using about the face, cover patient's eyes and warn against inhalation of the spray. To avoid freezing tissues, do not spray longer than 3 seconds or closer than 6″.
• For patient with eczematous dermatitis who may develop irritation with adhesive material, dressing may be held in place with gauze, elastic bandages, stockings, or stockinette.
• Occlusive dressings are generally not used in presence of infection or with weeping or exudative lesions.
• During dressing changes, skin should be inspected for infection, striae, and atrophy. If these occur, drug should be discontinued.
• Patient should report signs of drug sensitivity.

No significant interactions.

Special considerations:
• Use cautiously in viral diseases of skin, such as varicella, vaccinia, and herpes simplex; fungal infections; skin tuberculosis; impaired circulation.
• Avoid application in or near eyes.
• Systemic absorption especially likely with occlusive dressings, prolonged treatment, or extensive body surface treatment.
• Drug should be stopped if patient develops signs of systemic absorption, skin irritation or ulceration, hypersensitivity, infection. (If antifungals or antibiotics are being used with corticosteroids and infection does not respond immediately, corticosteroids should be stopped until infection is controlled.)
• Application tips: first, gently wash skin; to prevent damage to skin, rub in medication gently, leaving a thin coat; when treating hairy sites, part hair and apply directly to lesion.
• Aerosol preparation contains alcohol and may produce irritation or burning in open lesions. When using about the face, cover patient's eyes and warn against inhalation of the spray. To avoid freezing tissues, do not spray longer than 3 seconds or closer than 6″.
• Occlusive dressing: apply cream or ointment heavily, then cover with a thin, pliable, nonflammable plastic film; seal to adjacent normal skin with hypoallergenic tape. Adverse reactions should be minimized by using occlusive dressing intermittently.
• For patient with eczematous dermatitis who may develop irritation with adhesive material, dressing may be held in place with gauze, elastic bandages, stockings, or stockinette.
• Occlusive dressing should be removed if body temperature rises.
• Occlusive dressings are generally not used in presence of infection or with weeping or exudative lesions.
• During dressing changes, skin should be inspected for infection, striae, and atrophy. If these occur, drug should be discontinued.
• Treatment should be continued for a few days after clearing of lesions to prevent recurrence.
• Patient should report signs of drug sensitivity.

No significant interactions.

Special considerations:
• Use cautiously in viral diseases of skin, such as varicella, vaccinia, herpes simplex; fungal infections; skin tuberculosis; impaired circulation.
• Avoid application in or near eyes.
• Systemic absorption especially likely with occlusive dressings, prolonged treatment, or extensive body surface treatment.
• Drug should be stopped if patient develops signs of systemic absorption or hypersensitivity, skin irritation or ulceration, or infection. (If

(continued on following page)

NAMES, INDICATIONS AND DOSAGES	SIDE EFFECTS

clocortolone pivalate
(continued)

ingly to affected areas t.i.d. and rub in gently.

---

desonide
Tridesilon♦

Adjunctive therapy for inflammation in acute and chronic corticosteroid-responsive dermatoses:
ADULTS AND CHILDREN: clean area; apply cream, lotion, or gel sparingly b.i.d. to t.i.d.

Skin: burning, itching, irritation, dryness, folliculitis, hypopigmentation, perioral dermatitis, allergic contact dermatitis, hypertrichosis, acneiform eruptions. *With occlusive dressings: maceration of skin, secondary infection, atrophy, striae, miliaria.*

---

desoximetasone
Topicort♦

Inflammation of corticosteroid-responsive dermatoses:
ADULTS AND CHILDREN: clean area; apply cream sparingly b.i.d.

Skin: burning, itching, irritation, dryness, folliculitis, hypopigmentation, hypertrichosis, acneiform eruptions, perioral dermatitis, allergic contact dermatitis. *With occlusive dressings: maceration of skin, secondary infection, atrophy, striae, miliaria.*

---

dexamethasone
Aeroseb-Dex, Decaderm, Decaspray, Hexadrol♦

Skin: burning, itching, irritation, dryness, folliculitis, hypopigmentation, hypertrichosis, acneiform eruptions, perioral dermatitis, allergic contact dermatitis. *With occlusive dressings:*

INTERACTIONS AND SPECIAL CONSIDERATIONS

antifungals or antibiotics are being used with corticosteroids and infection does not respond immediately, corticosteroids should be stopped until infection is controlled.)
• Application tips: first, gently wash skin; to prevent damage to skin, rub in medication gently, leaving a thin coat; when treating hairy sites, part hair and apply directly to lesion.
• Occlusive dressing: apply cream heavily, then cover with a thin, pliable, nonflammable plastic film; seal to adjacent normal skin with hypoallergenic tape. Minimize adverse reactions by using occlusive dressing intermittently.
• For patient with eczematous dermatitis who may develop irritation with adhesive material, dressing may be held in place with gauze, elastic bandages, stockings, or stockinette.
• Occlusive dressing should be removed if body temperature rises.
• Occlusive dressings are generally not used in presence of infections or with weeping or exudative lesions.
• During dressing changes, skin should be inspected for infection, striae, and atrophy. If these occur, drug should be discontinued.
• Treatment should be continued for a few days after clearing of lesions to prevent recurrence.
• Patient should report signs of drug sensitivity.

No significant interactions.

Special considerations:
• Use cautiously in viral diseases of skin, such as varicella, vaccinia, and herpes simplex; fungal infections; skin tuberculosis; impaired circulation.
• Avoid application in or near eyes.
• Systemic absorption especially likely with occlusive dressings, prolonged treatment, or extensive body surface treatment.
• Drug should be stopped if patient develops signs of systemic absorption, skin irritation or ulceration, hypersensitivity, infection. (If antifungals or antibiotics are being used with corticosteroids and infection does not respond immediately, corticosteroids should be stopped until infection is controlled.)
• Application tips: first, gently wash skin; to prevent damage to skin, rub in medication gently, leaving a thin coat; when treating hairy sites, part hair and apply directly to lesion.
• Occlusive dressing: apply cream or ointment heavily, then cover with a thin, pliable, nonflammable plastic film; seal to adjacent normal skin with hypoallergenic tape. Adverse reactions should be minimized by using occlusive dressing intermittently.
• For patient with eczematous dermatitis who may develop irritation with adhesive material, dressing may be held in place with gauze, elastic bandages, stockings, or stockinette.
• Occlusive dressing should be removed if body temperature rises.
• Occlusive dressings are generally not used in presence of infection or with weeping or exudative lesions.
• During dressing changes, skin should be inspected for infection, striae, and atrophy.
• Treatment should be continued for a few days after clearing of lesions to prevent recurrence.
• Patient should report signs of drug sensitivity.

No significant interactions.

Special considerations:
• Use cautiously in viral diseases of skin, such as varicella, vaccinia, and herpes simplex; fungal infections; skin tuberculosis; impaired circulation.
• Avoid application in or near eyes.
• Systemic absorption especially likely with occlusive dressings, prolonged treatment, or extensive body surface treatment.
• Drug should be stopped if patient develops signs of systemic absorption, skin irritation or ulceration, hypersensitivity, infection. (If antifungals or antibiotics are being used with corticosteroids and infection does not respond immediately, corticosteroids should be stopped until infection is controlled.)
• Application tips: first, gently wash skin; to prevent damage to skin, rub in medication gently, leaving a thin coat; when treating hairy sites, part hair and apply directly to lesion.
• Occlusive dressing: apply cream heavily, then cover with a thin, pliable, nonflammable plastic film; seal to adjacent normal skin with hypoallergenic tape. To minimize adverse reactions, occlusive dressing should be used intermittently.
• For patient with eczematous dermatitis who may develop irritation with adhesive material, dressing may be held in place with gauze, elastic bandages, stockings, or stockinette.
• Occlusive dressing should be removed if body temperature rises.
• Occlusive dressings are generally not used in presence of infection or with weeping or exudative lesions.
• During dressing changes, skin should be inspected for infection, striae, and atrophy. Drug should be discontinued if these occur.
• Treatment should be continued for a few days after clearing of lesions to prevent recurrence.
• Patient should report signs of drug sensitivity.

No significant interactions.

Special considerations:
• Use cautiously in viral diseases of skin, such as varicella, vaccinia, and herpes simplex; fungal infections; skin tuberculosis; impaired circulation.
• Avoid application in or near eyes.

(continued on following page)

NAMES, INDICATIONS AND DOSAGES	SIDE EFFECTS
dexamethasone *(continued)* **Inflammation of corticosteroid-responsive dermatoses:** ADULTS AND CHILDREN: clean area; apply cream, gel, or aerosol sparingly b.i.d. to q.i.d. Aerosol use on scalp—shake can well and apply to dry scalp after shampooing. Hold can upright. Slide applicator tube under hair so that it touches scalp. Spray while moving tube to all affected areas, keeping tube under hair and in contact with scalp throughout spraying, which should take about 2 seconds. Inadequately covered areas may be spot sprayed. Slide applicator tube through hair to touch scalp, press and immediately release spray button. Don't massage medication into scalp or spray forehead or eyes.	maceration of skin, secondary infection, atrophy, striae, miliaria.
dexamethasone sodium phosphate Decadron Phosphate♦ **Inflammation of corticosteroid-responsive dermatoses:** ADULTS AND CHILDREN: clean area; apply cream sparingly b.i.d. to t.i.d.	**Skin:** burning, itching, irritation, dryness, folliculitis, hypopigmentation, hypertrichosis, acneiform eruptions, perioral dermatitis, allergic contact dermatitis. *With occlusive dressings: maceration of skin, secondary infection, atrophy, striae, miliaria.*
diflorasone diacetate Florone, Maxiflor **Inflammation of corticosteroid-responsive dermatoses:** ADULTS AND CHILDREN: clean area; apply ointment daily to t.i.d.; apply cream b.i.d. to q.i.d. Apply sparingly in a thin film.	**Skin:** burning, itching, irritation, dryness, folliculitis, hypopigmentation, perioral dermatitis, hypertrichosis, acneiform eruptions. *With occlusive dressings: maceration, secondary infection, atrophy, striae, miliaria.*

♦ Available in U.S. and Canada. ♦♦ Available in Canada only.
All other products (no symbol) available in U.S. only. Italicized side effects are common or life-threatening.

INTERACTIONS AND SPECIAL CONSIDERATIONS

• Systemic absorption especially likely with occlusive dressings, prolonged treatment, or extensive body surface treatment.
• Drug should be stopped if patient develops signs of systemic absorption, skin irritation or ulceration, signs of hypersensitivity, infection. (If antifungals or antibiotics are being used with corticosteroids and infection does not respond immediately, corticosteroids should be stopped until infection is controlled.)
• Application tips: first, gently wash skin; to prevent damage to skin, rub in medication gently, leaving a thin coat; when treating hairy sites, part hair and apply directly to lesion.
• Occlusive dressing: apply cream heavily and cover with a thin, pliable, nonflammable plastic film; seal to adjacent normal skin with hypoallergenic tape. To minimize adverse reactions, occlusive dressing should be used intermittently.
• For patient with eczematous dermatitis who may develop irritation with adhesive material, dressing may be held in place with gauze, elastic bandages, stockings, or stockinette.
• Occlusive dressing should be removed if body temperature rises.
• During dressing changes, skin should be inspected for infection, striae, and atrophy. Drug should be discontinued if these occur.
• Occlusive dressings are generally not used in presence of infection or with weeping or exudative lesions.
• Aerosol preparation contains alcohol and may produce irritation or burning in open lesions. When using about the face, cover patient's eyes and warn against inhalation of the spray. To avoid freezing tissues, do not spray longer than 3 seconds or closer than 6".
• Treatment should be continued for a few days after clearing of lesions to prevent recurrence.
• Patient should report signs of drug sensitivity.

No significant interactions.

Special considerations:
• Use cautiously in viral diseases of skin, such as varicella, vaccinia, and herpes simplex; fungal infections; skin tuberculosis; impaired circulation.
• Avoid application in or near eyes.
• Systemic absorption especially likely with occlusive dressings, prolonged treatment, or extensive body surface treatment.
• Drug should be stopped if patient develops signs of systemic absorption, skin irritation or ulceration, hypersensitivity, infection. (If antifungals or antibiotics are being used along with corticosteroids and infection does not respond immediately, corticosteroids should be stopped until infection is controlled.)
• Application tips: first, gently wash skin; to prevent damage to skin, rub in medication gently, leaving a thin coat; when treating hairy sites, part hair and apply directly to lesion.
• Occlusive dressing: apply cream heavily, then cover with a thin, pliable, nonflammable plastic film; seal to adjacent normal skin with hypoallergenic tape. To minimize adverse reactions, occlusive dressing should be used intermittently. Occlusive dressings are generally not used in presence of infection or with weeping or exudative lesions.
• For patient with eczematous dermatitis who may develop irritation with adhesive material, dressing may be held in place with gauze, elastic bandages, stockings, or stockinette.
• Occlusive dressing should be removed if body temperature rises.
• During dressing changes, skin should be inspected for infection, striae, and atrophy. Drug should be discontinued if these occur.
• Treatment should be continued for a few days after clearing of lesions to prevent recurrence.
• Patient should report signs of drug sensitivity.

No significant interactions.

Special considerations:
• Use cautiously in viral diseases of skin, such as varicella, vaccinia, and herpes simplex; fungal infections; skin tuberculosis; impaired circulation.
• Avoid application in or near eyes.
• Systemic absorption especially likely with occlusive dressings, prolonged treatment, or extensive body surface treatment.
• Drug should be stopped if patient develops signs of systemic absorption, skin irritation or ulceration, hypersensitivity, infection. (If antifungals or antibiotics are being used along with corticosteroids and infection does not respond immediately, corticosteroids should be stopped until infection is controlled.)
• Application tips: first, gently wash skin; to prevent damage to skin, rub in medication gently, leaving a thin coat; when treating hairy sites, part hair and apply directly to lesion.
• Occlusive dressing: apply cream or ointment heavily, then cover with a thin, pliable, nonflammable plastic film; seal to adjacent normal skin with hypoallergenic tape. Adverse reactions minimized by using occlusive dressing intermittently. Occlusive dressings are generally not used in presence of infection or with weeping or exudative lesions.
• For patient with eczematous dermatitis who may develop irritation with adhesive material, dressing may be held in place with gauze, elastic bandages, stockings, or stockinette.
• Occlusive dressing should be removed if body temperature rises.
• During dressing changes, skin should be inspected for infection, striae, and atrophy. Drug

(continued on following page)

NAMES, INDICATIONS AND DOSAGES	SIDE EFFECTS

diflorasone diacetate
(continued)

flumethasone pivalate
Locacorten♦♦, Locorten

Inflammation of corticosteroid-responsive dermatoses:
ADULTS AND CHILDREN: clean area; apply cream sparingly t.i.d. to q.i.d.

Skin: burning, itching, irritation, dryness, folliculitis, hypopigmentation, hypertrichosis, acneiform eruptions, perioral dermatitis, allergic contact dermatitis. *With occlusive dressings: maceration of skin, secondary infection, atrophy, striae, miliaria.*

fluocinolone acetonide
Fluonid, Synalar♦, Synalar-HP♦, Synamol♦, Synemol

Inflammation of corticosteroid-responsive dermatoses:
ADULTS AND CHILDREN OVER 2 YEARS: clean area; apply cream, ointment, or solution sparingly b.i.d. to q.i.d. Treat multiple or extensive lesions sequentially, applying to only small areas at any one time.

Skin: burning, itching, irritation, dryness, folliculitis, hypopigmentation, hypertrichosis, acneiform eruptions, perioral dermatitis, allergic contact dermatitis. *With occlusive dressings: maceration of skin, secondary infection, atrophy, striae, miliaria.*

fluocinonide
Lidemol♦♦, Lidex♦, Lidex-E, Topsyn♦

Inflammation of corticosteroid-responsive dermatoses:
ADULTS AND CHILDREN: clean area; apply cream, ointment, or gel sparingly t.i.d. to q.i.d.

Skin: burning, itching, irritation, dryness, folliculitis, hypopigmentation, hypertrichosis, acneiform eruptions, perioral dermatitis, allergic contact dermatitis. *With occlusive dressings: maceration of skin, secondary infection, atrophy, striae, miliaria.*

INTERACTIONS AND SPECIAL CONSIDERATIONS

should be discontinued if these occur.
• Patient should report signs of drug sensitivity.
• Diflorasone is often effective with once-daily application.

No significant interactions.

Special considerations:
• Use cautiously in viral diseases of skin, such as varicella, vaccinia, and herpes simplex; fungal infections; skin tuberculosis; impaired circulation.
• Avoid application in or near eyes.
• Systemic absorption especially likely with occlusive dressings, prolonged treatment, or extensive body surface treatment.
• Drug should be stopped if patient develops signs of systemic absorption, skin irritation or ulceration, hypersensitivity, infection. (If antifungals or antibiotics are being used along with corticosteroids and infection does not respond immediately, corticosteroids should be stopped until infection is controlled.)
• Application tips: first, gently wash skin; to prevent damage to skin, rub in medication gently, leaving a thin coat; when treating hairy sites, part hair and apply directly to lesion.
• Occlusive dressing: apply cream heavily, then cover with a thin, pliable, nonflammable plastic film; seal to adjacent normal skin with hypoallergenic tape. To minimize adverse reactions, occlusive dressing should be used intermittently. Occlusive dressings are generally not used in presence of infection or with weeping or exudative lesions.
• For patient with eczematous dermatitis who may develop irritation with adhesive material, dressing may be held in place with gauze, elastic bandages, stockings, or stockinette.
• Occlusive dressing should be removed if body temperature rises.
• During dressing changes, skin should be inspected for infection, striae, and atrophy. Drug should be discontinued if these occur.
• Treatment should be continued for a few days after clearing of lesions to prevent recurrence.
• Patient should report signs of drug sensitivity.

No significant interactions.

Special considerations:
• Use cautiously in viral diseases of skin, such as varicella, vaccinia, and herpes simplex; fungal infections; skin tuberculosis; impaired circulation.
• Avoid application in or near eyes.
• Systemic absorption especially likely with occlusive dressings, prolonged treatment, or extensive body surface treatment.
• Drug should be stopped if patient develops signs of systemic absorption, skin irritation or ulceration, hypersensitivity, infection. (If antifungals or antibiotics are being used with corticosteroids and infection does not respond immediately, corticosteroids should be stopped until infection is controlled.)
• Application tips: first, gently wash skin; to prevent damage to skin, rub in medication gently, leaving a thin coat; when treating hairy sites, part hair and apply directly to lesion.
• Occlusive dressing: apply gently and sparingly to the lesion until cream disappears. Then reapply, leaving a thin coat. Cover with a thin, pliable, nonflammable plastic film; seal to adjacent normal skin with hypoallergenic tape. To minimize adverse reactions, occlusive dressing should be used intermittently. Occlusive dressings are generally not used in presence of infection or with weeping or exudative lesions.
• For patient with eczematous dermatitis who may develop irritation with adhesive material, dressing may be held in place with gauze, elastic bandages, stockings, or stockinette.
• Occlusive dressing should be removed if body temperature rises.
• During dressing changes, skin should be inspected for infection, striae, and atrophy. Drug should be discontinued if these occur.
• Patient should report signs of drug sensitivity.
• Fluonid solution on dry lesions may increase dryness, scaling, or itching; on denuded or fissured areas, may produce burning or stinging. If burning or stinging persists and dermatitis has not improved, solution should be discontinued.

No significant interactions.

Special considerations:
• Use cautiously in viral diseases of skin, such as varicella, vaccinia, and herpes simplex; untreated purulent bacterial skin infections; fungal infections; skin tuberculosis; impaired circulation.
• Avoid application in or near eyes.
• Systemic absorption especially likely with occlusive dressings, prolonged treatment, or extensive body surface treatment.
• Drug should be stopped if patient develops signs of systemic absorption, skin irritation or ulceration, hypersensitivity, infection. (If antifungals or antibiotics are being used with corticosteroids and infection does not respond immediately, corticosteroids should be stopped until infection is controlled.)
• Application tips: first, gently wash skin; to prevent damage to skin, rub in medication gently, leaving a thin coat; when treating hairy sites, part hair and apply directly to lesion.
• Occlusive dressing: apply cream or ointment heavily, then cover with a thin, pliable, nonflammable plastic film; seal to adjacent normal

(continued on following page)

NAMES, INDICATIONS AND DOSAGES	SIDE EFFECTS
fluocinonide *(continued)*	
fluorometholone Oxylone **Inflammation of corticosteroid-responsive dermatoses:** ADULTS AND CHILDREN: clean area; apply cream sparingly daily to t.i.d.	**Skin:** burning, itching, irritation, dryness, folliculitis, hypopigmentation, hypertrichosis, acneiform eruptions, perioral dermatitis, allergic contact dermatitis. *With occlusive dressings: maceration of skin, secondary infection, atrophy, striae, miliaria.*
flurandrenolide Cordran, Cordran SP, Cordran Tape, Drenison♦♦, Drenison ¼♦♦, Drenison Tape♦♦ **Inflammation of corticosteroid-responsive dermatoses:** ADULTS AND CHILDREN: clean area; apply cream, lotion, or ointment sparingly b.i.d. or t.i.d. Apply tape q 12 to 24 hours. Before applying tape, cleanse skin carefully, removing scales, crust, and dried exudates. Allow skin to dry for 1 hour before applying new tape. Shave or clip hair to allow good contact with skin and comfortable removal. If tape ends loosen prematurely, trim off and replace with fresh tape. Lowest incidence of adverse reactions if tape is replaced q 12 hours, but may be left in place for 24 hours if well tolerated and adheres satisfactorily. Drenison ¼—for maintenance therapy of widespread or chronic lesions.	**Skin:** burning, itching, irritation, dryness, folliculitis, hypopigmentation, hypertrichosis, acneiform eruptions, allergic contact dermatitis. *With occlusive dressings: maceration of skin, secondary infection, atrophy, striae, miliaria.* With tape: purpura, stripping of epidermis, furunculosis.
halcinonide Halciderm, Halog♦ **Inflammation of acute and chronic corticosteroid-responsive dermatoses:** ADULTS AND CHILDREN: clean area; apply	**Skin:** burning, itching, irritation, dryness, folliculitis, hypopigmentation, hypertrichosis, acneiform eruptions, allergic contact dermatitis. *With occlusive dressings: maceration of skin, secondary infection, atrophy, striae, miliaria.*

INTERACTIONS AND SPECIAL CONSIDERATIONS

skin with hypoallergenic tape. To minimize adverse reactions, occlusive dressing should be used intermittently. Occlusive dressings are generally not used in presence of infection or with weeping or exudative lesions.
• For patient with eczematous dermatitis who may develop irritation with adhesive material, dressing may be held in place with gauze, elastic bandages, stockings, or stockinette.
• Occlusive dressings should be removed if body temperature rises.
• During dressing changes, skin should be inspected for infection, striae, and atrophy. Drug should be discontinued if these occur.
• Treatment should be continued for a few days after clearing of lesions to prevent recurrence.
• Patient should report signs of drug sensitivity.

No significant interactions.

Special considerations:
• Use cautiously in viral diseases of skin, such as varicella, vaccinia, and herpes simplex; fungal infections; skin tuberculosis; impaired circulation.
• Avoid application in or near eyes.
• Systemic absorption especially likely with occlusive dressings, prolonged treatment, or extensive body surface treatment.
• Drug should be stopped if patient develops signs of systemic absorption, skin irritation or ulceration, hypersensitivity, infection. (If antifungals or antibiotics are being used with corticosteroids and infection does not respond immediately, corticosteroids should be stopped until infection is controlled.)
• Application tips: first, gently wash skin; to prevent damage to skin, rub in medication gently, leaving a thin coat; when treating hairy sites, part hair and apply directly to lesion.
• Occlusive dressing: apply cream heavily, then cover with a thin, pliable, nonflammable plastic film; seal to adjacent normal skin with hypoallergenic tape. To minimize adverse reactions, occlusive dressing should be used intermittently. Occlusive dressings are generally not used in presence of infection or with weeping or exudative lesions.
• For patient with eczematous dermatitis who may develop irritation with adhesive material, dressing may be held in place with gauze, elastic bandages, stockings, or stockinette.
• Occlusive dressing should be removed if body temperature rises.
• During dressing changes, skin should be inspected for infection, striae, and atrophy. Drug should be discontinued if these occur.
• Treatment should be continued for a few days after clearing of lesions to prevent recurrence.
• Patient should report signs of drug sensitivity.

No significant interactions.

Special considerations:
• Use cautiously in viral diseases of skin, such as varicella, vaccinia, and herpes simplex; fungal infections; skin tuberculosis; impaired circulation.
• Tape not advised for exudative lesions or those in intertriginous areas.
• Avoid application in or near eyes.
• Systemic absorption especially likely with occlusive dressings, prolonged treatment, or extensive body surface treatment.
• Drug should be stopped if patient develops signs of systemic absorption, skin irritation or ulceration, hypersensitivity, infection. (If antifungals or antibiotics are being used with corticosteroids and infection does not respond immediately, corticosteroids should be stopped until infection is controlled.)
• Application tips: first, gently wash skin; to prevent damage to skin, rub in medication gently, leaving a thin coat; when treating hairy sites, part hair and apply directly to lesion.
• Occlusive dressing: apply cream heavily, then cover with a thin, pliable, nonflammable plastic film; seal to adjacent normal skin with hypoallergenic tape. To minimize adverse reactions, occlusive dressing should be used intermittently. Occlusive dressings are generally not used in presence of infection or with weeping or exudative lesions.
• For patient with eczematous dermatitis who may develop irritation with adhesive material, dressing may be held in place with gauze, elastic bandages, stockings, or stockinette.
• Occlusive dressing should be removed if body temperature rises.
• During dressing changes, skin should be inspected for infection, striae, and atrophy. Drug should be discontinued if these occur.
• Treatment should be continued for a few days after clearing of lesions to prevent recurrence.
• Patient should report signs of drug sensitivity.

No significant interactions.

Special considerations:
• Contraindicated in viral diseases of skin, such as varicella, vaccinia, and herpes simplex; fungal infections; skin tuberculosis; impaired circulation.
• Avoid application in or near eyes.
• Systemic absorption especially likely with occlusive dressings, prolonged treatment, or extensive body surface treatment.
• Drug should be stopped if patient develops signs of systemic absorption, skin irritation or ulceration, hypersensitivity, infection (if anti-

(continued on following page)

NAMES, INDICATIONS AND DOSAGES	SIDE EFFECTS

halcinonide
(continued)

cream, ointment, or solution sparingly b.i.d. to t.i.d.

---

hydrocortisone
Acticort, Aeroseb-HC♦, Alphaderm, Carmol-HC, Cetacort, Cortaid, Cort-Dome♦, Corticreme♦♦, Cortinal, Cortril♦, Cotacort, Cremesone, Delacort, Dermacort, Dermolate, Durel-Cort, Ecosone, Emo-Cort♦♦, HC Cream, HI-COR-2.5, Hycort, Hycortole, Hydrocortex, Hydro-Cortilean♦♦, Ivocort, Manticor♦♦, Maso-Cort, Microcort♦, Penetrate, Proctocort, Rectocort♦♦, Relecort, Rhus Tox HC, Rocort, Ulcort, Unicort

Inflammation of corticosteroid-responsive dermatoses; adjunctive typical management of seborrheic dermatitis of scalp; may be safely used on face, groin, armpits, and under breasts:

ADULTS AND CHILDREN: clean area; apply cream, lotion, ointment, or aerosol sparingly daily to q.i.d.

Aerosol—shake can well. Direct spray onto affected area from a distance of 6″. Apply for only 3 seconds (to avoid freezing tissues). Apply to dry scalp after shampooing; no need to massage or rub medication into scalp after spraying. Apply daily until acute phase is controlled, then reduce dosage to 1 to 3 times a week as needed to maintain control.

Skin: burning, itching, irritation, dryness, folliculitis, hypopigmentation, hypertrichosis, acneiform eruptions, allergic contact dermatitis. *With occlusive dressings: maceration of skin, secondary infection, atrophy, striae, miliaria.*

---

hydrocortisone acetate
Cortef Acetate, Cortifoam, Cortiprel, Epifoam, Hydrocortisone Acetate, Hydrocortone Acetate, My-Cort Lotion
hydrocortisone valerate
Westcort Cream

Inflammation of corticosteroid-responsive dermatoses:

ADULTS AND CHILDREN: clean area; apply lotion, cream, ointment, or foam (acetate) sparingly daily to q.i.d. Massage gently (valerate) 2 to 3 times daily p.r.n.

Skin: burning, itching, irritation, dryness, folliculitis, hypopigmentation, hypertrichosis, acneiform eruptions, perioral dermatitis, allergic contact dermatitis. *With occlusive dressings: maceration of skin, secondary infection, atrophy, striae, miliaria.*

♦ Available in U.S. and Canada. ♦♦ Available in Canada only.
All other products (no symbol) available in U.S. only. Italicized side effects are common or life-threatening.

INTERACTIONS AND SPECIAL CONSIDERATIONS

fungals or antibiotics are being used with corticosteroids and infection does not respond immediately, corticosteroids should be stopped until infection is controlled).
• Application tips: first, gently wash skin; to prevent damage to skin, rub in medication gently, leaving a thin coat; when treating hairy sites, part hair and apply directly to lesion.
• Occlusive dressing with cream: gently rub small amount into lesion until it disappears. Reapply, leaving a thin coating on lesion, and cover with occlusive dressing. With ointment: apply to lesion and cover with occlusive dressing. Cover with a thin, pliable, nonflammable plastic film; seal to adjacent normal skin with hypoallergenic tape. To minimize adverse reactions, occlusive dressing should be used intermittently; or with extensive lesions, one part of the body should be occluded at a time.
• Good results have been obtained by applying occlusive dressings in the evening and removing them in the morning (for example, 12-hour occlusion). Medication should then be reapplied in the morning, without using the occlusive dressings during the day.
• For patient with eczematous dermatitis who may develop irritation with adhesive material, dressing may be held in place with gauze, elastic bandages, stockings, or stockinette.
• Occlusive dressing should be removed if body temperature rises.
• Occlusive dressings are generally not used in presence of infection or with weeping or exudative lesions.
• During dressing changes, skin should be inspected for infection, striae, and atrophy. Drug should be discontinued if these occur.
• Treatment should be continued for a few days after clearing of lesions to prevent recurrence.
• Patient should report signs of drug sensitivity.

No significant interactions.

Special considerations:
• Use cautiously in viral diseases of skin, such as varicella, vaccinia, and herpes simplex; fungal infections; skin tuberculosis; impaired circulation.
• Avoid application in or near eyes.
• Systemic absorption especially likely with occlusive dressings, prolonged treatment, or extensive body surface treatment.
• Drug should be stopped if patient develops signs of systemic absorption, skin irritation or ulceration, hypersensitivity, infection. (If antifungals or antibiotics are being used with corticosteroids and infection does not respond immediately, corticosteroids should be stopped until infection is controlled.)
• Application tips: first, gently wash skin; to prevent damage to skin, rub in medication gently, leaving a thin coat; when treating hairy sites, part hair and apply directly to lesion.
• Occlusive dressing: apply cream heavily, then cover with a thin, pliable, nonflammable plastic film; seal to adjacent normal skin with hypoallergenic tape. To minimize adverse reactions, occlusive dressing should be used intermittently. Occlusive dressings are generally not used in presence of infection or with weeping or exudative lesions.
• For patient with eczematous dermatitis who may develop irritation with adhesive material, dressing may be held in place with gauze, elastic bandages, stockings, or stockinette.
• Occlusive dressing should be removed if body temperature rises.
• Aerosol preparation contains alcohol and may produce irritation or burning in open lesions. When using about the face, cover patient's eyes and warn against inhalation of the spray. To avoid freezing tissues, do not spray longer than 3 seconds or closer than 6″.
• During dressing changes, skin should be inspected for infection, striae, and atrophy. Drug should be discontinued if these occur.
• Treatment should be continued for a few days following clearing of lesions to prevent recurrence.
• Patient should report signs of drug sensitivity.
• The 0.5% strength is available without prescription.

No significant interactions.

Special considerations:
• Use cautiously in viral diseases of skin, such as varicella, vaccinia, and herpes simplex; fungal infections; skin tuberculosis; impaired circulation.
• Avoid application in or near eyes.
• Systemic absorption especially likely with occlusive dressings, prolonged treatment, or extensive body surface treatment.
• Drug should be stopped if patient develops signs of systemic absorption, skin irritation or ulceration, hypersensitivity, infection. (If antifungals or antibiotics are being used with corticosteroids and infection does not respond immediately, corticosteroids should be stopped until infection is controlled).
• Application tips: first, gently wash skin; to prevent damage to skin, rub in medication gently, leaving a thin coat; when treating hairy sites, part hair and apply directly to lesion.
• Occlusive dressing: apply cream or ointment heavily, then cover with a thin, pliable, nonflammable plastic film; seal to adjacent normal skin with hypoallergenic tape. To minimize ad-

(continued on following page)

NAMES, INDICATIONS AND DOSAGES	SIDE EFFECTS
hydrocortisone *(continued)*	
methylprednisolone acetate Medrol Acetate♦ **Inflammation of corticosteroid-responsive dermatoses:** ADULTS AND CHILDREN: clean area; apply ointment daily to t.i.d.	**Skin:** burning, itching, irritation, dryness, folliculitis, hypopigmentation, hypertrichosis, acneiform eruptions, allergic contact dermatitis. *With occlusive dressings: maceration of skin, secondary infection, atrophy, striae, miliaria.*
prednisolone Meti-Derm **Inflammation of corticosteroid-responsive dermatoses:** ADULTS AND CHILDREN: clean area; apply cream t.i.d. or q.i.d.	**Skin:** burning, itching, irritation, dryness, folliculitis, hypopigmentation, hypertrichosis, acneiform eruptions, perioral dermatitis, allergic contact dermatitis. *With occlusive dressings: maceration of skin, secondary infection, atrophy, striae, miliaria.*
triamcinolone acetonide Aristocort♦, Aristocort A, Kenalog♦, Triamalone♦♦ **Inflammation of corticosteroid-responsive dermatoses:** ADULTS AND CHILDREN: clean area; apply	**Skin:** burning, itching, irritation, dryness, folliculitis, hypopigmentation, hypertrichosis, acneiform eruptions, perioral dermatitis, allergic contact dermatitis. *With occlusive dressings: maceration of skin, secondary infection, atrophy, striae, miliaria.*

INTERACTIONS AND SPECIAL CONSIDERATIONS

verse reactions, occlusive dressings should be used intermittently. Occlusive dressings are generally not used in presence of infection or with weeping or exudative lesions.
• For patient with eczematous dermatitis who may develop irritation with adhesive material, dressing may be held in place with gauze, elastic bandages, stockings, or stockinette.
• Occlusive dressing should be removed if body temperature rises.
• Lotions and foams are not used with occlusive dressings.
• During dressing changes, skin should be inspected for infection, striae, and atrophy. Drug should be discontinued if these occur.
• Treatment should be continued for a few days after clearing of lesions to prevent recurrence.
• Patient should report signs of drug sensitivity.
• The 0.5% strength of hydrocortisone acetate is available without prescription.

No significant interactions.

Special considerations:
• Use cautiously in viral diseases of skin, such as varicella, vaccinia, and herpes simplex; fungal infections; skin tuberculosis; impaired circulation.
• Avoid application in or near eyes.
• Systemic absorption especially likely with occlusive dressings, prolonged treatment, or extensive body surface treatment.
• Drug should be stopped if patient develops signs of systemic absorption, skin irritation or ulceration, hypersensitivity, infection. (If antifungals or antibiotics are being used with corticosteroids and infection does not respond immediately, corticosteroids should be stopped until infection is controlled.)
• Application tips: first, gently wash skin; to prevent damage to skin, rub in medication gently, leaving a thin coat; when treating hairy sites, part hair and apply directly to lesion.
• Occlusive dressing: apply ointment heavily, then cover with a thin, pliable, nonflammable plastic film; seal to adjacent normal skin with hypoallergenic tape. To minimize adverse effects, occlusive dressing should be used intermittently. Occlusive dressings are generally not used in presence of infection or with weeping or exudative lesions.
• For patient with eczematous dermatitis who may develop irritation with adhesive material, dressing may be held in place with gauze, elastic bandages, stockings, or stockinette.
• Occlusive dressing should be removed if body temperature rises.
• During dressing changes, skin should be inspected for infection, striae, and atrophy. Drug should be discontinued if these occur.
• Treatment should be continued for a few days after clearing of lesions to prevent recurrence.
• Patient should report signs of drug sensitivity.

No significant interactions.

Special considerations:
• Use cautiously in viral diseases of skin, such as varicella, vaccinia, and herpes simplex; fungal infections; skin tuberculosis; impaired circulation.
• Avoid application in or near eyes.
• Systemic absorption especially likely with occlusive dressings, prolonged treatment, or extensive body surface treatment.
• Drug should be stopped if patient develops signs of systemic absorption, skin irritation or ulceration, hypersensitivity, infection. (If antifungals or antibiotics are being used with corticosteroids and infection does not respond immediately, corticosteroids should be stopped until infection is controlled.)
• Application tips: first, gently wash skin; to prevent damage to skin, rub in medication gently, leaving a thin coat; when treating hairy sites, part hair and apply directly to lesion.
• Occlusive dressing: apply cream heavily and cover with a thin, pliable, nonflammable plastic film; seal to adjacent normal skin with hypoallergenic tape. To minimize adverse reactions, occlusive dressing should be used intermittently. Occlusive dressings are generally not used in presence of infection or with weeping or exudative lesions.
• For patient with eczematous dermatitis who may develop irritation with adhesive material, dressing may be held in place with gauze, elastic bandages, stockings, or stockinette.
• Occlusive dressing should be removed if body temperature rises.
• During dressing changes, skin should be inspected for infection, striae, and atrophy. Drug should be discontinued if these occur.
• Treatment should be continued for a few days after clearing of lesions to prevent recurrence.
• Patient should report signs of drug sensitivity.

No significant interactions.

Special considerations:
• Use cautiously in viral diseases of skin, such as varicella, vaccinia, and herpes simplex; fungal infections; skin tuberculosis; impaired circulation.
• Avoid application in or near eyes.
• Systemic absorption especially likely with occlusive dressings, prolonged treatment, or extensive body surface treatment.
• Drug should be stopped if patient develops signs of systemic absorption, skin irritation or ulceration, hypersensitivity, infection. (If anti-

(continued on following page)

NAMES, INDICATIONS AND DOSAGES	SIDE EFFECTS
triamcinolone acetonide *(continued)* cream, ointment, lotion, foam, or aerosol sparingly b.i.d. to q.i.d. Aerosol: shake can well. Direct spray onto affected area from a distance of approximately 6″ and apply for only 3 seconds.	

INTERACTIONS AND SPECIAL CONSIDERATIONS

fungals or antibiotics are being used with corticosteroids and infection does not respond immediately, corticosteroids should be stopped until infection is controlled.)

- Application tips: first, gently wash skin; to prevent damage to skin, rub in medication gently, leaving a thin coat; when treating hairy sites, part hair and apply directly to lesion.
- Aerosol preparation contains alcohol and may produce irritation or burning in open lesions. When using about the face, cover patient's eyes and warn against inhalation of the spray. To avoid freezing tissues, do not spray longer than 3 seconds or closer than 6".
- Occlusive dressing: apply cream or ointment heavily, then cover with a thin, pliable, nonflammable plastic film; seal to adjacent normal skin with hypoallergenic tape. To minimize adverse reactions, occlusive dressing should be used intermittently. Occlusive dressings are generally not used in presence of infection or with weeping or exudative lesions.
- For patient with eczematous dermatitis who may develop irritation with adhesive material, dressing may be held in place with gauze, elastic bandages, stockings, or stockinette.
- Occlusive dressing should be removed if body temperature rises.
- During dressing changes, skin should be inspected for infection, striae, and atrophy. Drug should be discontinued if these occur.
- Treatment should be continued for a few days after clearing of lesions to prevent recurrence.
- Patient should report signs of drug sensitivity.

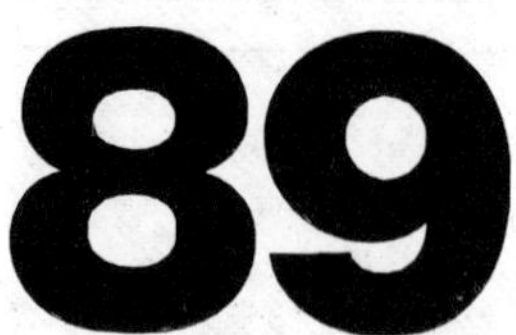

Antipruritics and topical anesthetics

benzocaine
camphor
dibucaine hydrochloride
dimethisoquin hydrochloride
diperodon monohydrate
dyclonine hydrochloride
ethyl chloride
lidocaine
lidocaine hydrochloride
menthol
phenol
pramoxine hydrochloride
tars
tetracaine
tetracaine hydrochloride

These topical drugs are used to produce local anesthesia and relieve discomfort and pruritus. Since they do not penetrate the stratum corneum, their effectiveness on intact skin is limited. But since mucosal surfaces lack a stratum corneum, topical anesthetics can be both effective and useful, as in some oral or anogenital disorders. Because these agents can cause sensitization, leading to contact dermatitis, their use should not be prolonged.

Hypersensitivity is most prevalent in reaction to local anesthetics of the ester type (tetracaine) and commonly develops when chemically related drugs are used. Drugs of the amide type (dibucaine and lidocaine) can usually be given to a patient who is allergic to ester-type drugs because incidence of hypersensitivity is much lower. As an alternative, a compound of a completely different class—such as benzocaine, dyclonine hydrochloride, or pramoxine hydrochloride—might be used.

Major uses

• Antipruritics relieve skin discomfort caused by minor burns, cuts, diaper rash, fungal infections, sunburn, hemorrhoids, insect bites, hives, eczema, skin ulcers, and pruritus ani and vulvae.

• Topical anesthetics anesthetize mucous membranes, as in the rectum, and are commonly used before endoscopic procedures.

Mechanism of action

• The general effect of all these drugs is to block conduction of impulses at the sensory nerve endings by interfering with the cell membrane's permeability to ions.

• Ethyl chloride produces local anesthesia by producing the sensation of cold.

• The specific mechanism of action of the other drugs is largely unknown. Menthol and phenol are general protoplasmic poisons.

Absorption, distribution, metabolism, and excretion

• These agents may be absorbed through mucous membranes and abraded skin, but are poorly absorbed when applied to intact skin.

• Esters such as tetracaine are metabolized extensively in the blood and to a lesser extent in the liver. They are excreted in urine.

• Amides such as dibucaine and lidocaine are metabolized mostly in the liver and excreted in urine.

• The remaining agents follow various routes of metabolism and are excreted in urine.

Onset and duration

Onset is rapid (within minutes). Duration varies according to the specific drug.

APPLYING TOPICAL ANESTHETICS

Take care when applying the topical anesthetics dyclonine hydrochloride (Dyclone) and ethyl chloride (Ethyl Chloride Spray.) If you get any of these preparations on your fingers, you'll experience temporary numbness, which may last up to 45 minutes.

- Benzocaine and pramoxine hydrochloride have a prolonged duration of 2 to 4 hours.
- Dibucaine is one of the most potent and longest-acting of the topical anesthetics, with a duration of 3 hours.
- Dimethisoquin's action lasts 2 to 4 hours.
- Dyclonine is effective for ½ to 1 hour.
- The other drugs have a duration of action from 1 to 3 hours.

Combination products

BALNETAR♦: water-dispersible emollient tar 2.5% in lanolin fraction, mineral oil, and nonionic emulsifiers.
CARMOL HC: urea 10% and hydrocortisone acetate 1%.
CETACAINE LIQUID: benzocaine 14%, tetracaine HCl 2%, benzalkonium chloride 0.5%, butyl aminobenzoate 2%, and cetyl dimethyl ethyl ammonium bromide in a bland water-soluble base.
CETACAINE OINTMENT: benzocaine 14%, tetracaine HCl 2%, butyl aminobenzoate 2%, benzalkonium chloride 0.5%, and cetyl dimethyl ethyl ammonium bromide in a bland water-soluble base.
CHIGGER-TOX LIQUID: benzocaine 2.1% and benzyl benzoate in an isopropanol base.
COR-TAR-QUIN♦: coal tar solution USP 2%, diiodohydroxyquin 1% with hydrocortisone 0.25%, 0.5%, or 1% in an acid-mantle vehicle.
CUTAR BATH OIL EMULSION: coal tar solution 7.5% in liquid petrolatum isopropyl myristate, acetylated lanolin, lanolin alcohols extract, and water.
DERMOPLAST SPRAY: benzocaine 20% and menthol 0.5%.
LAVATAR♦: tar distillate 33.3% in water-miscible emulsion base.
MEDICONE DRESSING (CREAM): benzocaine 0.5%, 8-hydroxyquinoline sulfate 0.05%, cod liver oil 12.5%, zinc oxide 12.5%, and menthol 0.18% with petrolatum, lanolin, talcum, and paraffin.
POLYTAR BATH: polytar 25% (juniper, pine, and coal tars, vegetable oil and solubilized crude coal tar) in water-miscible emulsion base.
PRAGMATAR OINTMENT♦: cetyl alcohol-coal tar distillate 4%, precipitated sulfur 3%, and salicylic acid 3% in an oil-in-water emulsion base.
SEBUTONE♦: tar (equivalent to 0.5% coal tar) in surface-active soapless cleansers and wetting agents, sulfur 2%, and salicylic acid 2%.
TAR DOAK LOTION♦: tar distillate 5% and nonionic emulsifiers.
VANSEB-T♦: coal tar solution USP 5% salicylic acid 1%, sulfur 2% in perfumed base.
ZETAR EMULSION♦: 30% colloidal whole coal tar in polysorbates.
ZETAR SHAMPOO♦: whole coal tar 1% and parachlorometaxylenol 0.5% in foam shampoo base.

NAMES, INDICATIONS AND DOSAGES	SIDE EFFECTS
benzocaine Aerocaine, Americaine, Anbesol, Benzocol, Col-Vi-Nol, Dermoplast, Hurricaine, Morusan, Rhulicream, Rhulihist, Solarcaine **Local anesthetic for pruritic dermatoses, localized idiopathic pruritus, and sunburn:** ADULTS AND CHILDREN: apply locally 2 or 3 times a day. **Hemorrhoids or rectal irritation:** ADULTS AND CHILDREN: apply ointment 2 or 3 times a day. Suppository—insert well into rectum morning, evening, and after each bowel movement.	**Blood:** methemoglobinemia (infants). **Local:** sensitization rash.
camphor **Mild antipruritic and local anesthetic; counterirritant for use in sprains and rheumatic conditions:** ADULTS AND CHILDREN: apply a 1% to 3% lotion or ointment of camphor, as needed.	**Local:** sensitization, rash.
dibucaine hydrochloride D-Caine, Dulzit, Nupercainal Cream♦, Nupercainal Ointment♦, Nupercainal Suppositories, Nuporals (Troches) **Abrasions, sunburn, minor burns, hemorrhoids, and other painful skin conditions:** ADULTS AND CHILDREN: 0.5% to 1% lotion or ointment applied locally several times a day. Suppository—insert rectally morning, evening, and after every bowel movement. Also used as a local anesthetic for mouth and throat.	**Local:** *hypersensitivity.*
dimethisoquin hydrochloride Quotane Cream♦♦, Quotane Ointment **Surface pain and itching:** ADULTS AND CHILDREN: 0.5% ointment or lotion applied topically up to 4 times daily or as directed.	**Skin:** *sensitization and contact dermatitis can develop but incidence is low.*
diperodon monohydrate Diothane Ointment♦, Proctodon **Pain caused by minor burns and cuts (cream); pain caused by anorectal disorders (ointment):** ADULTS AND CHILDREN: apply 3 to 4 times a day.	**Skin:** rash, irritation, and other allergic manifestations.
dyclonine hydrochloride Dyclone **To relieve surface pain and itching caused by minor burns or trauma, surgical wounds, pruritus ani or vulvae, insect bites, and pruritic dermatoses. Also, to anesthetize mucous**	**Local:** *irritation at site of application may occur.*

♦ Available in U.S. and Canada. ♦♦ Available in Canada only.
All other products (no symbol) available in U.S. only. Italicized side effects are common or life-threatening.

INTERACTIONS AND SPECIAL CONSIDERATIONS

No significant interactions.

Special considerations:
- Contraindicated in hypersensitivity to procaine or other para-aminobenzoic acid (PABA) derivatives (often used in topical sun-blocking agents).
- Discontinue if rash develops.
- Avoid contact with eyes.
- Use of spray preparation: hold can 6″ to 12″ from affected area and spray liberally. Avoid inhalation.
- Rectal use: cleanse and thoroughly dry rectal area before applying.

No significant interactions.

Special considerations:
- Extremely toxic if taken orally.
- Avoid contact with eyes.
- Should not be applied to broken skin or mucous membranes.
- Discontinue use if rash develops.

No significant interactions.

Special considerations:
- Avoid contact with eyes.
- Before applying cream or ointment rectally or inserting suppository, rectal area should be cleansed and thoroughly dried.
- Discontinue use if rash develops.

No significant interactions.

Special considerations:
- Useful in patients sensitive to ester- or amide-type agents.
- Should not be applied to extensive areas.
- Avoid contact with eyes.
- Prolonged use should be avoided for patients with chronic conditions.
- Discontinue use if rash develops.

No significant interactions.

Special considerations:
- Before applying cream or ointment rectally, rectal area should be cleansed and thoroughly dried.
- Discontinue use if rash develops.

No significant interactions.

Special considerations:
- Prolonged use in patients with chronic conditions should be avoided.
- May be useful in patients hypersensitive to other local anesthetics because it is a ketone.
- Contraindicated in cystoscopic examinations following an intravenous pyelogram. Iodine-containing contrast material will cause precipitate to form with dyclonine.
- Can be combined with diphenhydramine elixir to provide an effective treatment for stomatitis.
- Accidental contact causes temporary numbness.

(continued on following page)

NAMES, INDICATIONS AND DOSAGES	SIDE EFFECTS
dyclonine hydrochloride *(continued)* **membranes before endoscopic procedures:** ADULTS AND CHILDREN: 0.5% solution or 1% ointment applied 3 or 4 times daily. **Urethral dilation or cystourethroscopy:** ADULTS: 10 ml of 0.5% solution may be instilled into the urethra.	
ethyl chloride Ethyl Chloride Spray **For irritation:** ADULTS AND CHILDREN: hold container about 24″ from skin and spray rhythmically to cover area evenly once or twice. Application may be repeated. **As a local anesthetic in minor operative procedures; relieves pain caused by insect stings and burns, and irritation caused by myofascial and visceral pain syndromes:** ADULTS AND CHILDREN: dosage varies with different procedures. Use smallest dosage needed to produce desired effect. For local anesthesia, hold container about 12″ from area to produce a fine spray. INFANTS: hold a cotton ball saturated with ethyl chloride to injection site, and make injection when site dries.	**Skin:** sensitization; *frostbite and tissue necrosis may occur with prolonged spraying.* **Other:** excessive cooling may increase pain and muscle spasms.
lidocaine **lidocaine hydrochloride** Lida-Mantle Cream, Stanacaine, Xylocaine Jelly (2%), Xylocaine Ointment (2.5%)♦, Xylocaine Ointment (5%)♦, Xylocaine Solution (4%)♦, Xylocaine Viscous Solution (2%) **Local anesthesia of skin or mucous membranes:** ADULTS AND CHILDREN: apply liberally. **In procedures involving the male or female urethra:** ADULTS: instill about 15 ml (male) or 3 to 5 ml (female) into urethra. **Pain, burning, or itching caused by burns, sunburn, or skin irritation:** ADULTS AND CHILDREN: apply liberally.	**Local:** rash, *hypersensitivity.*
menthol **As an antipruritic:** ADULTS AND CHILDREN: apply 0.25% to 2% lotion or ointment, as needed. Often added with phenol to an ointment.	None reported.

♦ Available in U.S. and Canada. ♦♦ Available in Canada only.
All other products (no symbol) available in U.S. only. Italicized side effects are common or life-threatening.

INTERACTIONS AND SPECIAL CONSIDERATIONS

No significant interactions.

Special considerations:
- Should not be applied to broken skin or mucous membranes.
- Skin adjacent to treated area should be protected with petrolatum to avoid tissue sloughing.
- Avoid use near eyes.
- Inhalation should be avoided when spraying.
- Highly flammable; should not be used in areas where open flames or sparks are possible.
- Avoid accidental contact with drug; it produces temporary numbness.

No significant interactions.

Special considerations:
- Use with caution on severely traumatized mucosa or where sepsis is present or for anesthesia of oropharyngeal mucosa, since gag reflex may be suppressed and aspiration may occur.
- The 4% solution can be sprayed or poured onto abrasions to facilitate cleansing and removal of foreign substances (gravel, glass, etc.).
- Discontinue use if rash develops.
- Xylocaine Ointment should be applied carefully to prevent contact with skin; it produces numbness.

No significant interactions.

Special considerations:
- Relieves itching by substituting a cooling effect.
- Avoid contact with eyes.
- Discontinue use if rash develops.

NAMES, INDICATIONS AND DOSAGES	SIDE EFFECTS
phenol **As an antipruritic:** ADULTS AND CHILDREN OVER 6 MONTHS: apply 0.5% to 2% preparations locally several times a day.	None at recommended strengths.
pramoxine hydrochloride Proctofoam, Tronolane, Tronothane♦ **Pain and itching caused by dermatoses, minor burns, surgical wounds, insect bites, and hemorrhoids:** ADULTS AND CHILDREN: apply every 3 to 4 hours.	**Local:** stinging or burning, sensitization.
tars **As an antipruritic:** ADULTS AND CHILDREN: apply preparations 2 or 3 times daily.	**Skin:** irritation, folliculitis, erythema, photosensitivity.
tetracaine **tetracaine hydrochloride** Pontocaine♦ **For relief of pain in hemorrhoids, minor burns, ulcers, sunburn, and poison ivy:** ADULTS AND CHILDREN: apply 5% ointment or 1% cream—no more than 1 oz for adults or ¼ oz for children in 24 hours.	**Local:** *sensitization.*

♦ Available in U.S. and Canada. ♦♦ Available in Canada only.
All other products (no symbol) available in U.S. only. Italicized side effects are common or life-threatening.

INTERACTIONS AND SPECIAL CONSIDERATIONS

No significant interactions.

Special considerations:
• Accidental contact with normal skin should be avoided. If contact occurs, phenol should be removed with alcohol or vegetable oil.
• Tissue necrosis possible with higher than usual concentration or extensive use.
• Avoid contact with eyes.
• Should not be used under occlusive dressings, bandages, or diapers.

No significant interactions.

Special considerations:
• Can be safely used in patients hypersensitive to other local anesthetics.
• May be applied with gauze or sprayed directly on skin. Avoid contact with eyes.
• Rectal area should be cleansed and thoroughly dried before applying ointment or cream, or inserting suppository.

No significant interactions.

Special considerations:
• Caution should be used in applying tar preparations to patients with exacerbation of psoriasis. May precipitate total body exfoliation.
• Should never be used under occlusive dressings.
• Excessive exposure to sunlight should be avoided.
• Darkens color of blond hair when applied to scalp.
• May stain skin and clothing. Use mineral oil to remove from skin, especially if 1% to 5% crude coal tar is used.

No significant interactions.

Special considerations:
• Contraindicated in hypersensitivity to procaine or other para-aminobenzoic acid (PABA) derivatives (often used in topical sun-blocking agents).
• Before applying cream or ointment rectally, rectal area should be thoroughly cleansed and dried.

RELIEVING SUNBURN PAIN

As you know, sunburn results from overexposure to the sun's ultraviolet rays. Unless the burn is severe, it's a benign, self-limiting condition that necessitates no treatment other than application of cool compresses, cool tap water, or local anesthetic preparations to relieve pain.

Among the most popular over-the-counter sunburn pain remedies are preparations containing the -caine derivatives benzocaine, dibucaine, lidocaine, and tetracaine. These products provide local anesthesia by blocking conduction of nerve impulses at sensory nerve endings.

These local anesthetics are available in ointments, creams, solutions, and aerosols. You can help your patient choose an appropriate product by keeping in mind the following considerations:

• Ointments are the least desirable form of local anesthetic because the greasy base may facilitate microbial infection of burns. Also, ointments must be removed before a doctor can examine and treat the sunburn, should this become necessary.
• Creams, solutions, and aerosols are easier to remove than ointments. They also have a cooling effect that may aid in relieving pain.
• Sprays and aerosols are easiest for the patient to use; however, he must be careful to avoid inhaling the fumes or getting the preparation in his eyes, nose, or mouth.

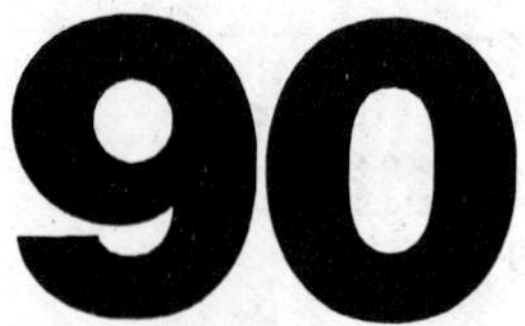

Astringents

acetic acid lotion
aluminum acetate
aluminum sulfate
hamamelis water
tannic acid

Externally applied, astringents are toners, tonics, and comforting agents.

Astringents applied locally cause precipitation of proteins. These drugs have such low cell penetrability that their action is essentially limited to the cell surface and the interstitial spaces. They draw tissues together, cause blanching, reduce inflammation and oozing, and have a soothing effect. Most of them also have antiseptic action (see Chapter 91, ANTISEPTICS AND DISINFECTANTS).

Because most astringents are irritating or caustic in moderate-to-high concentrations, pay strict attention to appropriate concentrations. Long-term use of these agents may result in excessively dry skin.

Major uses

Astringents are used to:

- arrest hemorrhage by coagulating blood (styptic action)
- reduce inflammation of mucous membranes, as in trench mouth, gingivitis, and minor external hemorrhoidal and outer vaginal discomfort
- promote healing and toughen the skin
- treat poison ivy, poison oak, sunburn, heat rash, and minor burns
- treat acute inflammations attended by exudation, oozing, and crusting (in solutions for wet dressings)
- decrease sweating (as an ingredient in many antiperspirants).

Mechanism of action

Astringents precipitate protein, causing tissue to contract. The cement substance of the capillary endothelium is hardened so that transcapillary movement of plasma protein is inhibited. Local edema, inflammation, and exudation are thereby reduced.

Mucus or other secretions may also be reduced so that the affected area becomes drier.

Absorption, distribution, metabolism, and excretion

- Astringents penetrate the cell so poorly that their action is confined to the cell surface.

HOW TO APPLY TANNIC ACID

When treating burns, follow these procedures:

- First, flush the burned areas with water or saline solution.
- Next, apply a thick layer of tannic acid to gauze dressings. Place the dressings on burned areas.
- Later, soak loose adherent gauze with normal or slightly hypertonic saline solution.
- A dark eschar will probably form. Leave it until it loosens and peels off on its own. You may, however, trim or cut away the edges, if hospital policy permits.

Hence, absorption is minimal unless the drugs are applied to large areas of denuded skin.

Tannic acid, when used over large areas of burned tissue, may be absorbed and cause significant hepatic damage. It also causes necrosis of viable tissue in the burned area.

- Distribution of the drugs is generally confined to the area of application.

Onset and duration

Astringents begin to act almost immediately. Their duration of action is limited, and repeated applications may be required for optimal effects.

Combination products

ASTRINGENTS WITH ANESTHETICS, for example, Nupercainal Suppositories.
ASTRINGENTS WITH ANTIPRURITIC/ANTIHISTAMINE, for example, Caladryl, Ziradryl.
ASTRINGENTS WITH ANTIPRURITIC/ANTIHISTAMINE AND ANESTHETIC, for example, Rhulicream, Rhulihist, Rhulispray.
ASTRINGENTS WITH ANTISEPTICS, for example, Tucks Pads, Tanac, Lavoris.
ASTRINGENTS WITH ANTISEPTICS AND ANESTHETICS, for example, Rectal Medicone Suppositories and Unguent, Tanicaine Suppositories and Ointment, Wyanoid Ointment, Pazo Hemorrhoid Suppositories and Ointment.
ASTRINGENTS WITH DEODORANTS, for example, antiperspirant/deodorants.

NAMES, INDICATIONS AND DOSAGES	SIDE EFFECTS
acetic acid lotion (0.1% glacial acetic acid in alcohol) **Superficial fungal or bacterial infection to toughen skin and prevent bedsores:** ADULTS AND CHILDREN: apply and work into area, p.r.n.	**Skin:** burning and irritation of denuded skin and mucous membranes.
aluminum acetate (modified Burow's solution) Acid Mantle Creme and Lotion♦, Buro-sol, Burow's Emulsion, Burow's Lotion **Mild skin irritation from exposure to soaps, detergents, chemicals, diaper rash, acne, scaly skin, eczema:** ADULTS AND CHILDREN: apply p.r.n. **Relieve inflammation of poison ivy, insect bites, athlete's foot:** ADULTS AND CHILDREN: apply as wet dressing, p.r.n. **Ulcerative skin conditions:** ADULTS AND CHILDREN: apply ointment, p.r.n.	**Skin:** irritation; extension of inflammation possible.
aluminum sulfate Bluboro Powder, Domeboro Powder♦, and Tablets♦ **Skin inflammation, insect bites, poison ivy or other contact dermatoses, swelling, athlete's foot:** ADULTS AND CHILDREN: mix powder with 1 pt of lukewarm tap water and apply for 15 to 30 minutes every 4 to 8 hours; bandage loosely.	**Skin:** irritation; extension of inflammation possible.
hamamelis water (witch hazel) Mediconet (wipes), Tucks (Cream, Ointment, Pads) **Anal discomfort, itching, burning, minor external hemorrhoidal or outer vaginal discomfort, diaper rash:** ADULTS AND CHILDREN: apply t.i.d. or q.i.d.	**Skin:** hypersensitivity.
tannic acid Amertan Jelly, Dalidyne Lotion, Tanac **Denture irritation; teething irritation; trench mouth; gingivitis; throat irritation; herpes simplex; oral cavity lesions; adjunctive treatment of second- and third-degree thermal, chemical, or electrical burns:** ADULTS: apply with cotton applicator. As gargle or mouthwash, ½ teaspoon of solution in ½ glass of warm water, p.r.n. **Cold sores, throat irritation, oral cavity lesions, some second- and third-degree burns:** CHILDREN: apply with cotton applicator.	**Local:** stinging. **Other:** large amounts in burn treatment can cause hepatic damage.

♦ Available in U.S. and Canada. ♦♦ Available in Canada only.
All other products (no symbol) available in U.S. only. Italicized side effects are common or life-threatening.

INTERACTIONS AND SPECIAL CONSIDERATIONS

Interactions:
HEAVY METALS: causes precipitation of the metal acetate.

Special considerations:
- Contraindicated under occlusive dressings.
- Acetic acid solutions should never be confused with *glacial* acetic acid solutions. Glacial form is a concentrate.
- Keep away from eyes and mucous membranes.
- Should always be applied to freshly cleansed area, free of other medications.
- Especially good for treating topical infection due to *Pseudomonas aeruginosa*.

No significant interactions.

Special considerations:
- Contraindicated under occlusive dressings.
- Keep away from eyes and mucous membranes.
- Should always be applied to freshly cleansed area, free of other medications.
- May be used in place of boric acid ointment.
- Powder must be diluted in water to prescribed concentration.
- Should be discontinued if irritation develops.
- Clear solution may be stored at room temperature for up to 7 days.

No significant interactions.

Special considerations:
- Contraindicated under occlusive dressings; only open wet dressings used.
- To prepare solution: immediately decant clear portion; discard precipitate; use only clear solution, *not* precipitate, for soaks; never strain or filter solutions. Decanted portion may be stored at room temperature for up to 7 days.
- In general, no more than a third of the body should be treated at any one time, since excessive wet dressings may cause chilling and hypothermia.
- Keep away from eyes and mucous membranes.
- Should be discontinued if irritation develops.

No significant interactions.

Special considerations:
- Should be discontinued if irritation or itching does not improve.
- Pads or wipes should be used after toilet tissue to help prevent pruritus ani and vulvae.
- Cream can be used by breast-feeding mother for nipple care, but area should be washed clean before breast-feeding baby.
- Some products contain potential allergic sensitizers. Allergic reactions may occur.

Interactions:
ORGANIC SALTS OF HEAVY METALS: will precipitate tannate salt of heavy metal. Do not apply.

Special considerations:
- Incompatible with organic salts of heavy metals. Should be applied only to surfaces free of other medication.
- Produces a firm eschar on burned area that helps protect burned tissue from infection and loss of body fluids, and comforts patient.
- Should be applied only after proper debridement of burn.
- Aqueous solutions should be freshly prepared, as they are unstable.
- Light and air cause solution to darken, which reduces potency.
- Avoiding extensive application and prolonged use on denuded tissue decreases possibility of systemic toxicity from absorption.
- Slight stinging on application soon subsides.

91

Antiseptics and disinfectants

alcohol, ethyl
alcohol, isopropyl
benzalkonium chloride
boric acid
chlorhexidine gluconate
formaldehyde
glutaraldehyde
hexachlorophene
hydrogen peroxide
iodine
merbromin
nitromersol
oxychlorosene calcium
oxychlorosene sodium
phenylmercuric nitrate
poloxamer iodine
potassium permanganate
povidone-iodine
silver protein, mild
sodium hypochlorite
thimerosal

Antiseptics inhibit growth of microorganisms; disinfectants destroy them. Antiseptics are used mainly on living tissue, whereas disinfectants are generally applied to inanimate objects. The effectiveness of these drugs depends on their mechanism of action, concentration, the number of microorganisms, the length of time the microorganisms are in contact with the drug, and the temperature and amount of organic matter present.

The antiseptics are boric acid, hexachlorophene, merbromin, oxychlorosene, and potassium permanganate. The rest of the drugs listed in this chapter are disinfectants.

Major uses

These drugs are used to control and prevent infection: antiseptics immobilize and disinfectants destroy pathogens.

• Povidone-iodine, a disinfectant, is especially useful as a preoperative skin disinfectant.

Mechanism of action

These drugs denature protein in microorganisms, changing their chemical structure. They lower surface tension, increasing cell permeability and causing lysis of the cell's contents, and also interfere with cellular metabolic processes.

Absorption, distribution, metabolism, and excretion

Not applicable.

Onset and duration

Onset of all these drugs except alcohol and hexachlorophene is immediate.

• Alcohol, to be effective in reducing bacterial count to 5% of normal, must be left on the skin for at least 2 minutes.

• Hexachlorophene is a chlorinated phenol used as a bacteriostatic cleansing agent. Its

WHAT TO LOOK FOR IN A GOOD ANTISEPTIC OR DISINFECTANT

The ideal antiseptic should:

- be lethal to microorganisms, rather than just inhibit their growth
- have a wide antimicrobial spectrum (although a limited spectrum may be useful in some situations)
- have a low surface tension (if used for topical application)
- retain its activity even in the presence of body fluids, including the exudates in infection
- have a rapid germicidal onset of action
- have a sustained duration of action
- have a wide therapeutic index (effective but nontoxic)
- have a low incidence of hypersensitivity reactions.

The ideal disinfectant should:

- have high germicidal efficacy
- have a wide antimicrobial spectrum
- be rapidly lethal
- be able to penetrate into crevices and cavities
- be germicidal in the presence of blood, sputum, and fecal material
- be compatible with soaps and other chemical substances
- be chemically stable
- be noncorrosive to surgical instruments
- have a pleasant odor and color
- be inexpensive.

Adapted from Stewart C. Harvey, "Antiseptics and Disinfectants; Fungicides; Ectoparasiticides," in *Goodman and Gilman's the Pharmacological Basis of Therapeutics*, 6th Edition, edited by Alfred Goodman Gilman, Louis S. Goodman, and Alfred Gilman (Copyright © 1980 by Macmillan Publishing Co., Inc.), with permission from the publisher.

antibacterial action develops only after repeated daily application. The residual phenol retained on the skin greatly reduces bacterial flora.

Combination products

B.F.I. POWDER: bismuth-formic-iodide, zinc phenosulfonate, amol, potassium alum, bismuth subgallate, boric acid, menthol, eucalyptol, and thymol.

MERCRESIN: secondary-amyltricresols 0.1%, orthohydroxyphenylmercuric chloride 0.1%, acetone 10%, and alcohol 50%.

OBTUNDIA: camphor and metacresol in lanolin-petroleum base.

S.T. 37: hexylresorcinol 0.1% in glycerin aqueous solution.

ZEASORB POWDER: parachlorometaxylenol 0.5%, aluminum dihydroxy allantoinate 0.2%, and microporous cellulose 45%.

NAMES, INDICATIONS AND DOSAGES	SIDE EFFECTS
alcohol, ethyl Alcohol, Ethanol **To disinfect skin, instruments, and ampuls:** disinfect as needed.	**Skin:** dryness.
alcohol, isopropyl isopropyl alcohol 99%, isopropyl rubbing alcohol 70%, isopropyl aqueous alcohol 75% **To disinfect skin, instruments, and ampuls:** disinfect as needed.	**Skin:** dryness.
benzalkonium chloride Benasept, Benzachlor-50♦♦, Benz-All, Drapolex♦♦, Ionax Foam♦♦, Ionax Scrub♦♦, Sabol♦♦, Spensomide, Zalkon, Zalkonium Chloride, Zephiran **Preoperative disinfection of unbroken skin:** apply 1:750 to 1:1,000 tincture or spray. **Disinfection of mucous membranes and denuded skin:** apply 1:10,000 to 1:5,000 aqueous solution. **Irrigation of vagina:** instill 1:5,000 to 1:2,000 aqueous solution. **Irrigation of bladder or urethra:** instill 1:20,000 to 1:5,000 aqueous solution. **Irrigation of deep infected wounds:** instill 1:20,000 to 1:3,000 aqueous solution. **Preservation of metallic instruments, ampuls, thermometers, and rubber articles:** wipe with or soak objects in 1:5,000 to 1:750 solution. **Disinfection of operating room equipment:** wipe with 1:5,000 solution.	**Skin:** hypersensitivity.
boric acid Bluboro, boric acid solution 5%, Borofax♦, Ting **Skin conditions (athlete's foot) as a compress, powder, or ointment (2% to 5%):** ADULTS AND CHILDREN: apply as directed.	Signs of systemic absorption: **CNS:** delirium, convulsions, restlessness, headache. **CV:** *circulatory collapse,* tachycardia. **GI:** irritation, nausea, vomiting, diarrhea. **GU:** renal damage. **Other:** hypothermia.
chlorhexidine gluconate Hibiclens Liquid, Hibistat, Hibitane **Surgical hand scrub, hand wash, hand rinse, skin wound cleanser:** use p.r.n.	**EENT:** irritating to eyes. Causes deafness if instilled into middle ear through perforated eardrum.
formaldehyde Formalin (37% solution of formaldehyde) **Cold sterilization of equipment:** disinfect as needed. **Tissue preservative:** cover tissue.	**EENT:** fumes cause eye, nose, and throat irritation. **Skin:** irritation. **Other:** pungent odor.

♦ Available in U.S. and Canada. ♦♦ Available in Canada only.
All other products (no symbol) available in U.S. only. Italicized side effects are common or life-threatening.

INTERACTIONS AND SPECIAL CONSIDERATIONS

No significant interactions.

Special considerations:
• Effective as fat-solvent germicidal; ineffective against spore-forming organisms, tubercle bacilli, or viruses.
• Alcohol used as 70% solution is known commonly as rubbing alcohol.
• Should not be used on skin before insulin administration. May affect potency of insulin.

No significant interactions.

Special considerations:
• Isopropyl alcohol is slightly more effective than ethyl alcohol as an antibacterial agent, but it also tends to cause more dryness.
• 75% solution for disinfection and storage of thermometers.
• Not effective against spore-forming organisms, tubercle bacilli, or viruses.
• Combined with formaldehyde, makes effective germicide.
• Should not be used in place of ethyl alcohol as skin preparation.

Interactions:
SOAPS: inactivate benzalkonium chloride. Remove soap traces with alcohol.

Special considerations:
• Germicidal for some non–spore-forming organisms and fungi. No effect on tubercle bacilli. Limited viricidal use.
• Used as preservative in ophthalmic solutions.
• Before applying to skin, all traces of soap should be removed with water and 70% alcohol applied.
• Cotton, wool gauze, or sponges should not be stored in solution. They absorb benzalkonium chloride and reduce the strength of the solution.
• Should not be used with occlusive dressings or vaginal packs.
• Should not be stored in bottles with screw caps.
• Incompatible with iodine, silver nitrate, fluorescein, nitrates, peroxide, lanolin, potassium permanganate, aluminum, caramel, kaolin, pine oil, zinc sulfate, zinc oxide, and yellow oxide of mercury.
• To prevent rusting of metallic instruments stored in benzalkonium chloride, add sodium nitrite to final solution. Change solution weekly.
• Available also as 17% concentrate (Zephiran). Even after dilution, this form of Zephiran should be used only on inanimate objects.

No significant interactions.

Special considerations:
• Mild antiseptic and astringent.
• Not absorbed through intact skin, but in high concentrations, may be absorbed through abraded skin or granulating wounds.
• Long-term use should be avoided.
• Ingestion of 5 g (infants) or 20 g (adults) may be fatal.

No significant interactions.

Special considerations:
• Bactericidal. Broad spectrum.
• Can be used many times a day without causing irritation or dryness.
• Low potential for producing skin reactions.
• Skin should be rinsed thoroughly after use.
• Should be kept out of eyes and ears.
• Residual action. Skin should not be cleansed with alcohol after application.

No significant interactions.

Special considerations:
• 0.5% solution germicidal against all forms of microorganisms, including spores, in 6 to 12 hours; 10% solution used to disinfect inanimate objects.
• Not affected by organic matter.
• Used with alcohol and sodium nitrite to disinfect instruments and articles that can't tolerate heat (cold sterilization).
• Skin or mucous membrane contact with solutions greater than 0.5% should be avoided.
• 37% solution should always be diluted.

NAMES, INDICATIONS AND DOSAGES	SIDE EFFECTS
glutaraldehyde Cidex♦ **Cold sterilization of surgical instruments:** cover instruments with 2% solution. **Fumigate hospital and operating rooms:** fog with aerosol.	**Skin:** irritation.
hexachlorophene Germa-Medica "MG," pHisoHex♦, pHisoScrub, Sept-Soft, Septisol Soy-Dome Cleanser, WescoHEX **Surgical scrub, bacteriostatic skin cleanser:** use as directed in 0.25% to 3% concentrations.	*Note:* systemic absorption can cause neurotoxic effects, including irritability, generalized clonic muscular contractions, decerebrate rigidity, convulsions, optic atrophy. (Systemic absorption has occurred only when used on premature infants, mucous membranes, and broken skin and burns.) **Skin:** dermatitis, mild scaling, dryness (especially when combined with excessive scrubbing).
hydrogen peroxide 3% to 6% solution **Cleansing wound:** use 1.5% to 3% solution. **Mouth wash for necrotizing ulcerative gingivitis:** gargle with 3% solution. **Cleansing douche:** use 2% solution.	**EENT:** excessive use as mouthwash causes "hairy tongue."
iodine solution (2% iodine and 2.4% sodium and iodide in water)♦, tincture (2% iodine and 2.4% sodium iodide in diluted alcohol), Sepp Antiseptic Applicators (2% mild iodine tincture), strong iodine tincture (7% iodine and 5% potassium iodide in diluted alcohol) **Preoperative disinfection of skin (small wounds and abraded areas):** apply p.r.n.	**Skin:** irritation, redness, swelling (sign of hypersensitivity).
merbromin Mercurochrome (2% aqueous solution) **General antiseptic and first-aid prophylactic:** ADULTS AND CHILDREN: apply p.r.n. as 1% to 2% solution or tincture.	**Skin:** sensitization.
nitromersol Metaphen **Disinfection of instruments:** soak in 0.04% solution. **Disinfection of skin:** apply 0.2% to 0.5% solution to area p.r.n. **Irrigation of mucous membranes (eye, urethra):** instill 0.01% to 0.02% solution as directed. **Skin antiseptic for abrasions:** apply 0.2% solution to area.	**Skin:** erythematous, papular, or vesicular eruptions indicate hypersensitivity; irritation.

♦ Available in U.S. and Canada. ♦♦ Available in Canada only.
All other products (no symbol) available in U.S. only. Italicized side effects are common or life-threatening.

INTERACTIONS AND SPECIAL CONSIDERATIONS

No significant interactions.

Special considerations:
- Excellent disinfectant; broad spectrum of activity against gram-positive and gram-negative bacteria (vegetative and spores), viruses, and fungi.
- Should be used only on inanimate objects.
- Comes with activator that must be mixed before use to yield active acidic glutaraldehyde.
- Not affected by organic matter.
- Whenever possible, use commercially prepared 2% solution rather than diluting the 25% solution.

No significant interactions.

Special considerations:
- Should be used with caution in infants (especially premature infants) and burn patients. These patients tend to absorb hexachlorophene through the skin and may develop neurotoxic effects.
- Bacteriostatic agent. Spectrum of activity limited to gram-positive organisms, especially staphylococcus.
- Must be used preoperatively for at least 3 days for maximum effectiveness.
- After cleaning area, rinse thoroughly (especially the scrotum and perineum). Do not apply alcohol or organic solvents to cleansed area.

No significant interactions.

Special considerations:
- Germicidal.
- Should not be injected into closed body cavities or abscesses; generated gas can't escape.
- Dilute 1 part concentrate to 4 parts water.
- Useful to remove mucus from inner cannula of tracheostomy tube.
- Store tightly capped in cool, dry place. Protect from light and heat.
- Bottle should not be shaken. This causes decomposition.

No significant interactions.

Special considerations:
- Microbicidal agent effective against bacteria, fungi, viruses, protozoa, and yeasts.
- If skin reaction develops, iodine residue should be removed from skin and use stopped.
- To prevent skin irritation, areas treated with iodine should not be covered.
- Aqueous solution less irritating.
- Sodium thiosulfate renders iodine colorless and is used to remove stains. It is also antidote of choice for accidental ingestion.

No significant interactions.

Special considerations:
- Bacteriostatic.
- Least effective mercurial antiseptic. Its activity is decreased in presence of organic matter.
- Injury should be cleansed with soap and water before applying and let dry.
- Stains may be removed with 2% permanganate solution, followed by 5% oxalic acid solution.
- Solution should never be heated.
- To prepare 1% solution, should be diluted with equal parts water.

No significant interactions.

Special considerations:
- Contraindicated in hypersensitivity to mercury compounds.
- Should not be used when aluminum may come in contact with skin.
- Incompatible with permanganates, strong acids, and heavy metal salts.
- Should be prepared as needed. Solutions tend to precipitate on standing.
- Rings should be removed when working with solution; the mercury component can damage the precious metals in jewelry.

NAMES, INDICATIONS AND DOSAGES	SIDE EFFECTS
oxychlorosene calcium Clorpactin XCB **oxychlorosene sodium** Clorpactin WCS-90 **Topical antiseptic for local infections, preoperative skin cleanser (sodium salt):** apply as spray, soak, wet dressing, or irrigation as a 4% solution. **Ophthalmic and urologic irrigant (sodium salt):** 0.1% to 0.2% solution. **Local irrigation during surgery (calcium salt):** use 0.5% solution.	**Skin:** local irritation.
phenylmercuric nitrate Phe-Mer-Nite **Preoperative disinfection:** apply p.r.n. as a 0.1% to 0.2% solution.	**Skin:** rash.
poloxamer iodine Prepodyne **Preoperative skin preparation and scrub, wound disinfection:** use as directed.	None reported.
potassium permanganate **Topical antiseptic:** apply 1:10,000 to 1:500 solution. **Vaginal douche:** instill 1:5,000 to 1:1,000 solution as directed.	**Skin:** solutions greater than 1:5,000 are irritating to skin.
povidone-iodine ACU-dyne, Aerodine, Betadine♦, BPS, Bridine♦♦, Efodine, Final Step, Frepp, Frepp/Sepp, Isodine, Mallisol, Polydine, Proviodine♦♦, Sepp **Many uses, including preoperative skin preparation and scrub, germicide for surface wounds, postoperative application to incisions, prophylactic application to urinary meatus of catheterized patients, miscellaneous disinfection:** ADULTS: apply p.r.n.	**Skin:** local hypersensitivity reactions.
silver protein, mild Argyrol S.S.♦, Silvol, Solargentum **Topical application for inflammation of eye, nose, throat:** ADULTS AND CHILDREN: apply p.r.n. as a 5% to 25% solution.	**Skin:** argyria in long-term use.

♦ Available in U.S. and Canada. ♦♦ Available in Canada only.
All other products (no symbol) available in U.S. only. Italicized side effects are common or life-threatening.

INTERACTIONS AND SPECIAL CONSIDERATIONS	
No significant interactions. *Special considerations:* • Effective against bacteria, fungi, viruses, yeast, and spores. • Powder reconstituted in saline solution. • Dry crystal should be refrigerated until reconstitution. • Oxychlorosene calcium has a special use as a local irrigating agent during surgery for neoplasms, to destroy loose viable neoplastic cells and thereby prevent iatrogenic metastasis. Oxychlorosene sodium is not used for this purpose.	
No significant interactions. *Special considerations:* • Contraindicated in hypersensitivity to mercury-containing compounds. • Antiseptic and fungicidal.	• Frequent or prolonged use may cause mercury poisoning. • Orange stain removed with soap and water. • Commonly used as a preservative in ophthalmic solutions.
No significant interactions. *Special considerations:* • Contraindicated in hypersensitivity to iodines. • Prolonged germicidal action. • Water-soluble solution releases iodine at predetermined rate, causing prolonged action. • Relatively nonirritating to skin.	
Interactions: IODINE: precipitates iodine salt. Do not use together. *Special considerations:* • Antiseptic astringent with fungicidal properties. • Germicidal effects reduced by organic matter. • Stains caused by potassium permanganate re-	moved with dilute acids (lemon juice, oxalic acid, or dilute hydrochloric acid). • Never mix with charcoal or give charcoal as antidote. May explode.
No significant interactions. *Special considerations:* • Use as a vaginal antiseptic should be discouraged during pregnancy. • Germicidal activity of iodine without irritation to skin and mucous membranes. • Thought to be superior to soap as a disinfectant; less effective than aqueous or alcoholic solutions of iodine. • Treated areas may be bandaged or taped. • Germicidal activity reduced if area cleansed with alcohol or other organic solvents after application of povidone-iodine.	• Prolonged, excessive use may lead to systemic absorption and toxicity.
No significant interactions. *Special considerations:* • Store in amber glass bottles; protect from light.	

NAMES, INDICATIONS AND DOSAGES	SIDE EFFECTS
sodium hypochlorite 5% solution (instruments, swimming pools), 0.5% aqueous solution for wounds, Modified Dakin's solution **Athlete's foot, wound irrigation, disinfection of walls and floors:** apply as directed.	**Skin:** irritation.
thimerosal Aeroaid Thimerosal, Merthiolate **Preoperative disinfection of skin; antiseptic for open wounds:** apply or instill to affected area daily, b.i.d., or t.i.d. as a 0.1% solution or tincture.	**Skin:** erythematous, vesicular, papular eruptions (indicate hypersensitivity); irritation with tincture.

INTERACTIONS AND SPECIAL CONSIDERATIONS

No significant interactions.

Special considerations:
- Germicidal and weakly fungicidal.
- Interferes locally with thrombin formation, delaying blood clotting. Dissolves necrotic tissue.
- Unstable in solution. Make fresh solution and use immediately.
- Contact with hair should be avoided due to its bleaching properties.

No significant interactions.

Special considerations:
- Contraindicated in hypersensitivity to mercury-containing compounds.
- Should not be used when aluminum may come in contact with skin.
- Incompatible with permanganate, strong acids, and salts of heavy metals.
- Wound should be cleansed thoroughly before applying tincture.
- To prevent skin irritation, tincture should be allowed to dry completely before applying dressing.
- Can be instilled into body cavities.
- Store in amber glass container.

HOW TO WASH YOUR HANDS PROPERLY

Proper handwashing is the key to medical asepsis. Before administering medications, remove your rings and watch, then wash your hands.

- Using warm running water, lather well for 30 to 60 seconds; be sure to clean your fingernails and interdigital spaces well.
- Rinse your hands; dry with a paper towel.
- Turn faucet off with a clean, dry paper towel.

Note: Don't lean against sink or splash water.

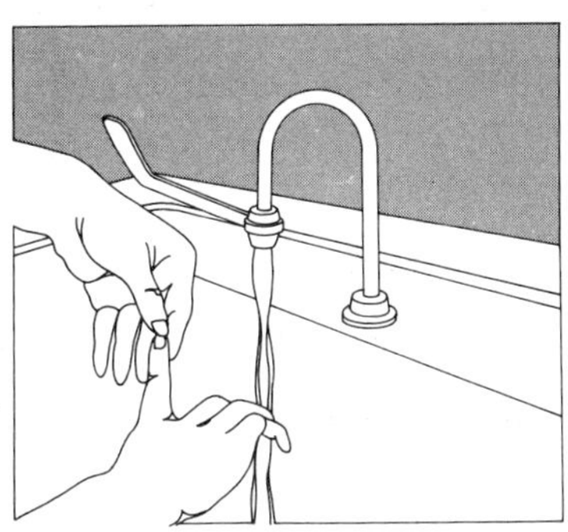

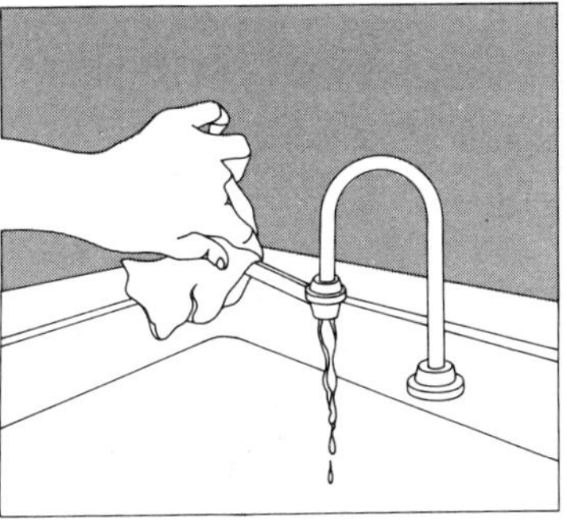

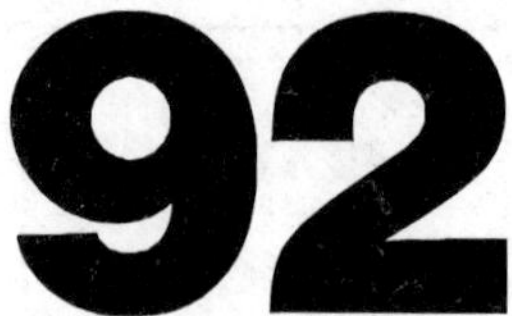

Emollients, demulcents, and protectants

aluminum paste
calamine
collodion, USP
collodion, flexible
compound benzoin tincture
dexpanthenol
glycerin
hydrophilic lotion
hydrophilic ointment
hydrophilic petrolatum
hydrous wool fat
hydrous wool fat and castor oil
liquid petrolatum
methyl salicylate
oatmeal
para-aminobenzoic acid
petrolatum
silicone
starch
talc (magnesium silicate)
urea or carbamide
vitamins A and D ointment
zinc gelatin

These preparations not only serve as vehicles for other drugs but are also used alone. *Emollients* protect and soften skin and mucous membranes; *demulcents* soothe inflamed or abraded skin and mucous membranes; *protectants* occlude and protect skin, ulcers, and wounds.

Major uses

These preparations are used to treat burns, wounds, itching, insect bites, poison ivy, rashes, skin irritation and dryness, mild eczema, sunburn, rheumatic pains, muscle soreness, low back pain, cutaneous ulcers, and varicose veins.

Mechanism of action

- Emollients soften dry skin by preventing evaporation of perspiration.

Methyl salicylate is a counterirritant that increases circulation to the area of application. This causes localized redness and warmth and helps reduce muscle soreness and stiffness.

- Demulcents have analgesic properties to soothe irritation and cool inflammation. Some (such as starch) absorb moisture when secretions are excessive, helping to dry skin.
- Protectants promote healing by reducing irritation and friction.

Talc and other dusting powders are not completely biologically inert and may cause irritation, granulomas, fibrosis, or adhesion.

Flexible collodion is collodion USP, a protectant to which castor oil has been added to improve pliability.

Absorption, distribution, metabolism, and excretion

- Absorption of most of the preparations is confined to the skin: penetration is usually limited to the outer layers. The preparations do not generally reach the systemic circulation.

Methyl salicylate can be absorbed through the skin and, if used in excess, can cause toxicity.

- The preparations are distributed only to the affected areas, and they're usually removed topically.

Onset and duration

Onset is generally rapid. Duration depends on the preparation and length of contact with the affected areas.

PATIENT-TEACHING AID

HOW TO CLEAN AND DRESS YOUR WOUND

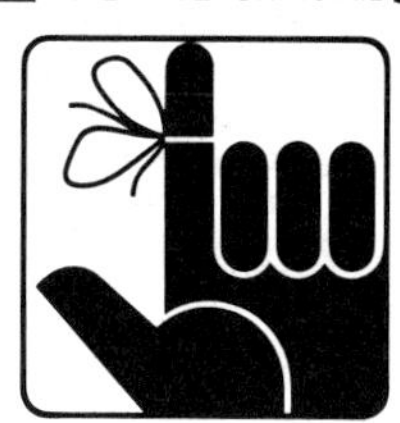

Dear Patient:

To ensure the proper healing of your wound or incision, change the dressing as often as your doctor suggested. But if you notice some drainage before the next scheduled change, apply a new dressing immediately. Follow these procedures:

- Before you begin, collect all the materials you'll need and place them within reach: sterile forceps, sterile gloves, sterile dressings, nonperfumed soap, water, and tape.
- If your doctor has asked you to maintain sterile technique, wear sterile gloves, use sterile equipment, and avoid touching the part of the bandage that will cover the wound. In any case, wash your hands carefully before handling the dressings; then handle them carefully and as little as possible.
- Remove soiled dressings and discard carefully in a waterproof bag. Don't contaminate the outside of the bag with soiled dressings.
- If dressings stick to the wound, moisten them with sterile water or hydrogen peroxide before attempting to remove them.
- With a sterile gauze pad, clean the wound with a single circular motion; always wipe from inside to out. Discard the pad after each single circular motion.
- If an ointment was used on the wound, remove it with nonperfumed soap and water; rinse well. Again, always clean and rinse in an in-to-out direction.
- If ordered, apply ointment or other medication to dressing; then apply the dressing to the wound or incision.
- If ordered, apply a protective ointment to the surrounding area.
- If the wound or incision is to be covered, apply a sterile dressing, being careful to handle only the outer top surface of the dressing.
- Secure the dressing with nonallergenic tape, not adhesive tape.
- If you note any changes in the wound, such as redness, swelling, foul odors or pus, notify the doctor immediately.

Combination products

CALADRYL LOTION: diphenhydramine hydrochloride 1%, calamine, camphor, alcohol 2%.
CALADRYL CREAM: diphenhydramine hydrochloride 1% with calamine.
GER-O-FOAM AEROSOL: methyl salicylate 30%, benzocaine 3%, in oil emulsion.
PANALGESIC: methyl salicylate 50%, aspirin 8%, menthol and camphor 4%, emollient oils 20%, alcohol 18%.

NAMES, INDICATIONS AND DOSAGES	SIDE EFFECTS
aluminum paste (10% aluminum in zinc oxide ointment with liquid petrolatum) **Emollient and protectant: colostomy area or other surgical sites:** apply p.r.n.	None.
calamine liniment (15% calamine), lotion (8% calamine), ointment (17% calamine), Rhulihist (3% calamine), Rhulispray (1% calamine) **Topical astringent and protectant: itching, poison ivy and poison oak, nonpoisonous insect bites, mild sunburn, minor skin irritations:** apply p.r.n.	**Skin:** transient light stinging, irritation, dry skin.
collodion, USP (5% pyroxylin in 1 part alcohol, 3 parts ether) **collodion, flexible** (5% pyroxylin in 1 part alcohol, 3 parts ether plus 20% camphor, 30% castor oil) **Protectant; vehicle for other medicinal agents; and sealant for small wounds:** apply to dry skin, p.r.n., or use flexible collodion when a flexible noncontracting film is desired.	None.
compound benzoin tincture (10% benzoin in alcohol mixed with glycerin and water) Benzoin Spray **Demulcent and protectant: cutaneous ulcers, bedsores, cracked nipples, fissures of lips and anus:** apply locally once daily or b.i.d.	None.
dexpanthenol Panthoderm Cream♦ (dexpanthenol 2% in a water-miscible cream base), Panthoderm Lotion (dexpanthenol 2%, menthol 0.1%, and camphor 0.1%) **Epithelial-bed stimulator in emollient base: itching, wounds, insect bites, poison ivy, poison oak, diaper rash, chafing, mild eczema, decubitus ulcers, dry lesions:** apply topically, p.r.n.	None.

INTERACTIONS AND SPECIAL CONSIDERATIONS

Interactions:
TOPICAL ENZYMES: aluminum may inactivate preparations used to debride wounds. Don't use together.

Special considerations:
• Zinc oxide paste can be used as an alternative.
• Inflammation or infection may occur since protectants are occlusive layers that retain moisture, exclude air, and trap cutaneous bacteria.
• Skin should be cleaned daily or more often, as needed.
• Emollients and protectants may be used alone, as vehicles for medications, or with other topical medications.

No significant interactions.

Special considerations:
• Contraindicated in hypersensitivity to any of the components.
• Sensitivity reactions to calamine may develop. Preparations containing antihistamines may cause sensitivity.
• Cotton will absorb the solute; instead, gauze sponge should be used to apply.
• Should not be applied to blistered, raw, or oozing areas of the skin.
• Toxic if taken internally.
• May irritate and dry skin.
• Inflammation or infection may occur since protectants are occlusive layers that retain moisture, exclude air, and trap skin bacteria.
• Skin should be cleaned daily or more often as needed.
• Emollients, demulcents, and protectants may be used alone, as vehicles for medications, or with other topical medications.
• Highly flammable; never use near flame. Shake well before use.
• Container should be kept tightly closed so solvent won't evaporate.

No significant interactions.

Special considerations:
• Inflammation or infection may occur since protectants are occlusive layers that retain moisture, exclude air, and trap cutaneous bacteria.
• Skin should be cleaned daily or more often as needed.
• Protectants may be used alone, as vehicles for medications, or with other topical medications.
• Camphor in flexible collodion is weakly antiseptic and antipruritic; may irritate and dry skin.
• Highly flammable; should never be used near flame.
• Container should be kept tightly closed so solvent won't evaporate.
• Toxic if taken internally.
• Excessive inhalation of vapors should be avoided.

No significant interactions.

Special considerations:
• Should not be applied to acutely inflamed areas.
• Inflammation or infection may occur since protectants are occlusive layers that retain moisture, exclude air, and trap cutaneous bacteria.
• Skin should be cleaned daily or more often as needed.
• Protectants may be used alone, as vehicles for medications, or with other topical medications.
• For demulcent and expectorant action in laryngitis or croup, should be used in boiling water; patient inhales vapors.
• Spray is not intended for use as inhalant.
• Can be mixed with magnesium-aluminum hydroxide and applied on bedsores.

No significant interactions.

Special considerations:
• Contraindicated in wounds of hemophilia patients.
• Before each new application, affected area should *always* be thoroughly cleansed, removing all traces of previously applied medication. Inflammation or infection may develop.
• Dry lesions respond better than oozing lesions.
• May heal skin lesions in mild eczema and dermatoses.

NAMES, INDICATIONS AND DOSAGES	SIDE EFFECTS
glycerin Corn Huskers Lotion (tragacanth 1 g, glycerin 30 ml, propylene glycol 10 ml) **Emollient and lubricant: rectal tubes and catheters; dry skin, hands:** apply p.r.n.	None.
hydrophilic lotion (white petrolatum 4.2 g, stearyl alcohol 4.2 g, methylparaben 0.004 g, propylparaben 0.002 g, sodium lauryl sulfate 0.167 g, propylene glycol 2 ml, perfume q.s., purified water) **Protectant and emollient: dry skin, irritation:** apply p.r.n.	None.
hydrophilic ointment Cetaphil, Heb Cream Base, Multibase, Neobase, Unibase, Vanibase (methylparaben 0.025 g, propylparaben 0.015 g, stearyl alcohol 25 g, white petrolatum 25 g, propylene glycol 12 g, sodium lauryl sulfate 1 g, purified water) **Protectant and emollient: dry skin, oozing lesions:** apply p.r.n.	None.
hydrophilic petrolatum Aquaphor, Hydrosort, Plastibase Hydrophilic, Polysort (cholesterol 3 g, stearyl alcohol 3 g, white wax 8 g, white petrolatum 86 g) **Protectant and emollient: dry skin, eczema, or psoriasis:** mix with other medicinal ingredients as ordered, and apply p.r.n.	None.
hydrous wool fat Lanolin Lotion (stearic acid 2 g, triethanolamine 0.8 ml, light liquid petrolatum 10 ml, propylparaben 0.2 g, rose water) **hydrous wool fat and castor oil** (hydrous wool fat 25 g, castor oil 25 g, ceresin wax 5 g, polysorbate 60 5 g, white petrolatum) **Protectant and emollient:** apply hydrous wool fat p.r.n. **Protection against hydrocarbons, solvents, and cutting oils:** apply hydrous wool fat and castor oil before exposure.	**Skin:** allergic rash.
liquid petrolatum Liquid Petrolatum, USP; Light Liquid Petrolatum, NF; Mineral Oil **Protectant and emollient:** apply locally, full strength, or diluted.	None.

♦ Available in U.S. and Canada. ♦♦ Available in Canada only.
All other products (no symbol) available in U.S. only. Italicized side effects are common or life-threatening.

INTERACTIONS AND SPECIAL CONSIDERATIONS

No significant interactions.

Special considerations:
- Applied undiluted to inflamed, dehydrated skin. Paradoxically, excessive use may dry the skin.
- Diluted with rose water, glycerin is useful for irritated or dry lips.

No significant interactions.

Special considerations:
- Inflammation or infection may occur since protectants are occlusive layers that retain moisture, exclude air, and trap skin bacteria.
- Skin should be cleaned daily or more often as needed.
- Emollients and protectants may be used alone, as vehicles for medications, or with other topical medications.

No significant interactions.

Special considerations:
- Easily removed with water.
- Should be used when little penetration of medicinal agent is desired.
- Inflammation or infection may occur since protectants are occlusive layers that retain moisture, exclude air, and trap skin bacteria.
- Skin should be cleaned daily or more often as needed.
- Emollients and protectants may be used alone, as vehicles for medications, or with other topical medications.
- This nongreasy ointment is especially suited for application to hairy areas.

No significant interactions.

Special considerations:
- Not water-soluble; greasy.
- Inflammation or infection may occur since protectants are occlusive layers that retain moisture, exclude air, and trap skin bacteria.
- Skin should be cleaned daily or more often as needed.
- Emollients and protectants may be used alone, as vechicles for medications, or with other topical medications.

No significant interactions.

Special considerations:
- Contraindicated in hypersensitivity to lanolin.
- Should not be confused with anhydrous wool fat, which will dry skin if applied alone.
- Inflammation or infection may occur since protectants are occlusive layers that retain moisture, exclude air, and trap skin bacteria.
- Skin should be cleaned daily or more often as needed.
- Emollients and protectants may be used alone, as vehicles for medications, or with other topical medications.

No significant interactions.

Special considerations:
- Occasionally used with other drugs.
- Available in two forms: light mineral oil and heavy mineral oil.
- Heavy mineral oil can be used internally as a laxative. Light mineral oil should never be used as a laxative. Mineral oil used as nose drops can cause lipid pneumonia.
- Inflammation or infection may occur since protectants are occlusive layers that retain mois-

(continued on following page)

NAMES, INDICATIONS AND DOSAGES	SIDE EFFECTS
liquid petrolatum *(continued)*	
methyl salicylate Banalg, Baumodyne Gel and Ointment, Betula Oil, Gaultheria Oil, Sweet Birch Oil, Wintergreen Oil **Counterirritant: minor pains of osteoarthritis, rheumatism, sprains, muscle and tendon soreness and tightness, lumbago, sciatica:** ADULTS: apply with gentle massage several times daily. Not recommended for children.	**Skin:** rash, irritation, burning, blistering.
oatmeal Aveeno Colloidal, Aveeno Oilated Bath (with liquid petrolatum and hypoallergenic lanolin) **Emollient and demulcent: local irritation:** use as a lotion; 1 level tablespoon to a cup of warm water. **Skin irritation, pruritus, common dermatoses, sunburn, dry skin:** ADULTS: 1 packet in tub of warm water. CHILDREN: 1 to 2 rounded tablespoons in 3″ to 4″ of bath water. INFANTS: 2 or 3 level teaspoons, depending on size of bath.	None.
para-aminobenzoic acid PABA♦, Pabagel♦, Pabanol♦, Pre-Sun♦, PreSun Gel, RV Paba Lipstick **Topical protectant: sunburn protection, sun-sensitive skin, slow tanning:** ADULTS: apply evenly to dry skin; follow directions on various products for number and time of application, which vary from 2 to 6 hours; reapply after swimming. Not recommended for children.	**Local:** allergic reaction, irritation, sensitization. **Skin:** photocontact dermatitis.
petrolatum Vaseline **Topical protectant and emollient:** use alone or with other drugs, as directed.	None.
silicone Silicone and Zinc Oxide Compound **Topical protectant: dermatoses, diaper rash, decubitus ulcers:** apply b.i.d. or t.i.d. in ointment. **Protection against water and corrosive chemicals:** apply before exposure.	None.

♦ Available in U.S. and Canada. ♦♦ Available in Canada only.
All other products (no symbol) available in U.S. only. Italicized side effects are common or life-threatening.

INTERACTIONS AND SPECIAL CONSIDERATIONS

ture, exclude air, and trap skin bacteria.
• Skin should be cleaned daily or more often as needed.
• Emollients and protectants may be used alone, as vehicles for medications, or with other topical medications.

No significant interactions.

Special considerations:
• Should never be applied directly, undiluted, to skin.
• *Warning:* as little as 4 ml ingested by children can cause fatal toxicity; in adults, as little as 30 ml. Since GI absorption may be delayed, treat such ingestion with emetic lavage, then a saline cathartic. Continue lavage until no odor of methyl salicylate can be detected in the washings.
• Absorbed through skin; prolonged increased application can cause toxicity. Toxic effects include hyperpnea leading to respiratory alkalosis, nausea, vomiting, tinnitus, hyperpyrexia, and convulsions.
• Should be discontinued if rash or redness occurs. Patient should consult doctor if pain or redness persists more than 10 days.
• Avoid use near eyes, open wounds, and mucous membranes.
• Should not be used on sunburned membranes.
• Treated area should not be wrapped or bandaged.
• Store in tightly closed container.

No significant interactions.

Special considerations:
• Not to be ingested. Should not be confused with oatmeal as food.
• Patient should exercise caution to avoid slipping in tub.
• Contact with eyes should be avoided.

No significant interactions.

Special considerations:
• Contraindicated in hypersensitivity to any of the components and for persons with damaged or diseased skin.
• Should be discontinued if skin rash occurs.
• Encourage slow tanning and short exposure to sun.
• Avoid contact with eyes and lids.
• Avoid contact with open flame.
• May stain clothing.
• Inflammation or infection may occur since protectants produce an occlusive layer that retains perspiration, excludes air, and traps cutaneous bacteria, producing sites for anaerobic infections.

No significant interactions.

Special considerations:
• Stable, does not become rancid.
• Inflammation or infection may occur since protectants are occlusive layers that retain moisture, exclude air, and trap skin bacteria.
• Skin should be cleaned daily or more often as needed.
• Emollients and protectants may be used alone, as vehicles for medications, or with other topical medications.

No significant interactions.

Special considerations:
• Protect eyes against spray.
• Very difficult to remove from skin; resistant to water and soap.
• Will not protect against oils or solvents.
• Inflammation or infection may occur since protectants are occlusive layers that retain moisture, exclude air, and trap cutaneous bacteria.
• Skin should be cleaned daily or more often as needed.
• Protectants may be used alone, as vehicles for medications, or with other topical medications.

NAMES, INDICATIONS AND DOSAGES	SIDE EFFECTS
starch **Demulcent: minor skin irritations, pruritus associated with common dermatoses:** mix 2 cups of starch with 4 cups of water, add to tub of water, and soak affected area for 30 minutes.	None.
talc (magnesium silicate) **Topical lubricant, protectant, drying agent, absorbent dusting powder: irritation such as intertrigo prickly heat:** sprinkle on affected areas p.r.n. for soothing and lubrication.	None.
urea or carbamide Aquacare Dry Skin Cream and Lotion♦, Aquacare/HP Cream and Lotion♦, Aqua Lacten, Artra Ashy Skin Cream, Carmol Ten, Carmol Twenty, Gormel Cream, Nutraplus♦, Rea-Lo, Ultra-Mide, Uremol♦♦, Urtex♦♦ **Emollient: hard, dry skin on hands, elbows, or knees:** ADULTS: apply to affected area b.i.d. or t.i.d., particularly after exposure to sun or wind. Not recommended for children.	**Skin:** transient stinging when applied to irritated or fissured skin.
vitamins A and D ointment A&D, Balmex, Caldesene Medicated, Clocream, Comfortine, Desitin, Primaderm **Emollient, demulcent, and epithelial-bed stimulant: superficial burns, sunburn, abrasions, slow-healing lesions, chapped skin, diaper rash, skin care of infants or bedridden patients:** apply several times a day.	**Skin:** irritation.
zinc gelatin Dome-Paste, Unna's Boot **Protectant: varicosities, lesions or injuries of lower legs or arms:** heat in hot bath till liquefied, clean skin, dust with talc, and apply gel with paint brush; make three layers, with gauze between each layer; retain 2 weeks. Dome-Paste, in 3″ and 4″ bandages, can be applied directly to arm or leg.	None.

INTERACTIONS AND SPECIAL CONSIDERATIONS

No significant interactions.

Special considerations:
• Patient should exercise caution to avoid slipping in tub.
• Use of cornstarch in intertriginous areas may promote or accelerate a yeast infection since yeast can feed on the sugar.

No significant interactions.

Special considerations:
• Should not be used on surgical gloves; causes granulation and adhesions in open wounds.
• Dust entering eyes or inhalation of talc dust should be avoided.
• Should not be used on open, weeping surfaces; it cakes and crusts.

No significant interactions.

Special considerations:
• Contraindicated in viral skin diseases or in impaired circulation. Should be used cautiously on face or broken skin.
• Skin should be wet before application. If irritation persists, should be discontinued.
• Contact with eyes should be avoided.
• Emollients produce an occlusive layer that retains perspiration, excludes air, and traps cutaneous bacteria, producing sites for anaerobic infections. Before each new application, affected area should *always* be thoroughly cleansed, removing all traces of previously applied medication. Inflammation or infection may develop.

No significant interactions.

Special considerations:
• Should be discontinued if skin condition persists or irritation develops.
• Inflammation or infection may occur since emollients and demulcents are occlusive layers that retain moisture, exclude air, and trap cutaneous bacteria.
• Skin should be cleaned daily or more often as needed.
• Emollients and demulcents may be used alone, as vehicles for medications, or with other topical medications.

No significant interactions.

Special considerations:
• Inflammation and infection may occur since protectants produce an occlusive layer that retains perspiration, excludes air, and traps cutaneous bacteria, producing sites for anaerobic infections. Before each new application, affected area should *always* be thoroughly cleansed, removing all traces of previously applied medication.
• Zinc gelatin boot can be removed by unwinding outer bandage and soaking leg or arm in warm water until dressing floats off. Patient should not shower or take tub bath with zinc gelatin boot on leg.

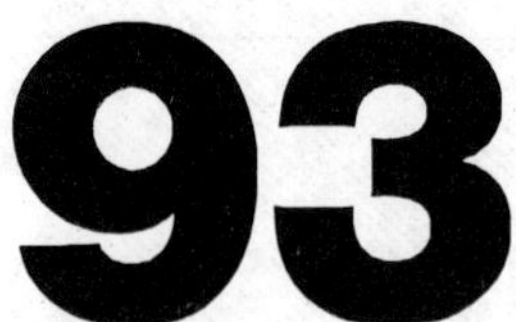

Keratolytics and caustics

cantharidin
dichloroacetic acid
podophyllum resin
resorcinol
resorcinol monoacetate
salicylic acid
silver nitrate
sulfur
sulfurated lime solution

Keratolytic agents loosen the tightly packed cell products, cell wall, and protein (keratin) that constitute the outer, protective layer (stratum corneum) of the epidermis. They are used in the treatment of benign skin growths and other dermatologic disorders.

By cauterizing tissue at the site of application, caustic agents can destroy moles and warts. Take care when using these agents, however, to protect adjacent skin from their harmful effects.

Major uses

- Keratolytics (cantharidin, resorcinol, salicylic acid, sulfur, and sulfurated lime solution) are used to treat dermatophytosis, warts, corns, and certain acneiform and eczematous dermatoses. In addition, they are used to control fungal infections.
- Caustics (dichloroacetic acid, podophyllum resin, and silver nitrate) destroy warts, condylomata, keratoses, certain types of moles, and hyperplastic tissue.

Mechanism of action

- Keratolytics soften keratin and loosen cornified epithelium, causing even viable cells to swell, soften, and dissolve.
- Caustics except podophyllum precipitate cell proteins, causing formation of a scab that eventually sloughs off.

Podophyllum inhibits cell division and other cellular processes, leading to the death of the cell.

Absorption, distribution, metabolism, and excretion

Most of these agents are not appreciably absorbed.

- Cantharidin can be absorbed and may cause severe genitourinary tract irritation.
- Podophyllum can be absorbed through mucous membranes and cause significant toxicity due to cerebral vasoconstriction. For this reason, the use of podophyllum-coated tampons for the treatment of vaginal warts should be discouraged.

Onset and duration

These agents begin to act immediately upon application.

Duration of action and necessity for re-treatment depend on the specific agent and the condition.

BEWARE OF TOXICITY FROM PODOPHYLLUM THERAPY

Topical application of podophyllum resin can cause increased side effects and severe systemic toxicity *when an accelerated treatment schedule produces a high cumulative dose.*

Leukopenia and thrombocytopenia developed rapidly in a 15-year-old girl who received three applications of the drug, in combination with benzoin tincture, in 24 hours, to treat condylomata acuminata (genital warts). In a patient undergoing similarly aggressive treatment, dizziness, nausea, vomiting, abdominal pain, oliguria, anuria, fever, confusion, peripheral neuropathy, lethargy, tachycardia, and tachypnea are possible.

To prevent toxic complications, podophyllum resin should be applied only to small target areas of unbroken skin, and left in contact for no longer than 1 hour. The drug should be withdrawn at the first sign of toxic reaction.

Adapted with permission from Gary P. Stoehr, et al., "Systemic Complications of Local Podophyllin Therapy," *Annals of Internal Medicine,* 89:3:362, September 1978.

Combination products

ACNE-AID CREAM: sulfur 2.5%, resorcinol 1.25%, and parachlorometaxylenol 0.375% in a microporous cellulose base.

ACNE-DOME: colloidal sulfur 4% and resorcinol monoacetate 2% in an acid-mantle vehicle.

ACNOMEL CAKE♦: sulfur 4% and resorcinol 1% in a washable base.

ACNOMEL CREAM♦: sulfur 8%, resorcinol 2%, and alcohol 11% in a greaseless base.

BENSULFOID LOTION: fusion of finely divided sulfur (33% by weight) onto colloidal bentonite 6%, resorcinol 2%, zinc oxide 6%, thymol 0.5%, and alcohol 12% in a greaseless base.

CLEARASIL CREAM: benzoyl peroxide 10% and bentonite.

COMPOUND W WART REMOVER: salicylic acid 14%, acetic acid 11%, in castor oil, alcohol, ether, and collodion.

DUOFILM♦: salicylic acid 16.7% and lactic acid 16.7% in flexible collodion.

EXZIT: colloidal sulfur 4% and resorcinol monoacetate 2%.

FOSTEX CAKE♦: sulfur 2% and salicylic acid 2%.

FREEZONE CORN AND CALLUS REMOVER: salicylic acid 13.6%, zinc chloride 2.17%, in castor oil, and collodion, alcohol, and ether.

REZAMID LOTION♦: sulfur 5%, resorcinol 2%, parachlorometaxylenol 0.5%, and alcohol 28.5% in a hydroalcoholic lotion base.

SULFORCIN BASE CREAM: sulfur 4% and resorcinol monoacetate 1.5%.

NAMES, INDICATIONS AND DOSAGES	SIDE EFFECTS
cantharidin Cantharone ADULTS AND CHILDREN: **Molluscum contagiosum:** coat each lesion. Repeat in a week on new or remaining lesions, this time covering with occlusive tape. Remove tape in 6 to 8 hours. **Palpebral warts:** apply, and leave lesion uncovered. **Plantar warts:** pare away keratin, apply generously to affected area, allow to dry, apply protective padding, cover with nonporous tape for a week, then debride. Repeat 3 times, if necessary, on large lesions. **Removal of ordinary and periungual warts and other benign epithelial growths:** apply directly to lesion and cover completely. Allow to dry, then cover with nonporous adhesive tape. Remove tape in 24 hours (or less if extreme pain) and replace with loose bandage. Reapply, if necessary.	**Skin:** annular warts, burning, tingling, extreme tenderness, inflammation.
dichloroacetic acid Bichloracetic Acid **All types of verrucae; calluses, corns; xanthelasma; ingrown toenails; cysts and benign erosion of the cervix; sebaceous adenoma; infectious granuloma; tattoo marks; epistaxis; spider nevi; tonsil tabs:** ADULTS: applied only by doctor at his discretion.	**Local:** irritation, inflammation of normal skin.
podophyllum resin Podoben **Venereal warts and granuloma inguinale:** ADULTS: apply podophyllum resin preparation to the lesion, cover with waxed paper, and bandage. Leave covered for 8 to 12 hours, then wash lesion to remove medication. Repeat at weekly intervals.	**Blood:** thrombocytopenia, leukopenia when systemically absorbed. **Local:** irritation of normal skin. **Other:** peripheral neuropathy when systemically absorbed.
resorcinol **resorcinol monoacetate** Euresol, Resorcin **Acute eczema, urticaria, and other inflammatory skin diseases (1% or 2% concentration in alcohol); acne or seborrhea (5% lotion or 10% soap liniment for scalp); chronic eczema, psoriasis (2% to 10% ointment); acne scarring (45% peeling paste):** ADULTS AND CHILDREN: apply as directed.	**Skin:** irritation, moderate erythema or scaling. **Other:** darkening of light hair (resorcinol only).
salicylic acid Calicylic, Keralyt♦, Salactic Liquifilm, Salonil **Superficial fungal infections, acne, psoriasis, seborrheic dermatitis, other scaling dermatoses, hyperkeratosis, calluses, warts:** ADULTS AND CHILDREN: apply to affected	**Skin:** irritation, drying. **Other:** salicylism with percutaneous absorption.

♦ Available in U.S. and Canada. ♦♦ Available in Canada only.
All other products (no symbol) available in U.S. only. Italicized side effects are common or life-threatening.

INTERACTIONS AND SPECIAL CONSIDERATIONS

No significant interactions.

Special considerations:
• If dropped on normal skin: remove immediately with acetone, alcohol, or tape remover; scrub with warm, soapy water; and rinse well, as blistering of skin may result.
• If dropped on mucous membranes or in eyes: flush well with water to remove precipitated collodion; then continue to flush with water for 15 minutes.
• Only one or two lesions should be treated initially to test patient's sensitivity.
• Treatment should be stopped if severe inflammation develops.
• If application causes burning, tenderness, or tingling: remove tape and soak area in cool water for 10 to 15 minutes; repeat, if necessary.
• If annular warts develop: assure patient that lesions are superficial; re-treat, or substitute another procedure.
• Does not affect tissue layers below the epidermis, and leaves no scar.
• Treatment should be supervised by a doctor.

No significant interactions.

Special considerations:
• Contraindicated for treatment of malignant or premalignant lesions.
• Adjacent areas should be protected with petrolatum, especially when using 50% solutions.
• Sodium bicarbonate is local antidote.
• Area should be thoroughly dried before application.
• Once solution is applied, treated area will turn from white to red in about 4 hours.
• Peeling of skin usually is noticed in 4 days and is completed in a week.
• If acid comes in contact with normal skin, area should be wiped off with cotton gauze and flushed with water.

Interactions:
OTHER KERATOLYTICS: may cause extensive damage to the skin. Do not use together.

Special considerations:
• Resin is irritating and cytotoxic, and should not be applied to normal skin. Petrolatum can be applied to adjacent areas to protect them during treatment.
• Should be applied only by a doctor because of toxicity.
• Should not be used on extensive areas or for prolonged therapy; may be absorbed systemically.
• Soreness from local irritation may develop 12 to 48 hours after treatment.

No significant interactions.

Special considerations:
• Do not use preparations on or near eyes.
• If skin irritation persists, medication should be discontinued.
• Lotion should be applied with cotton ball to affected area.
• When applying the peeling paste, close observation of the patient and site of application is necessary until paste is removed.
• Careful use with topical acne preparations necessary because of local irritation.

No significant interactions.

Special considerations:
• Use with caution in patients with diabetes or peripheral vascular disease. The skin inflammation that may result is difficult to treat. Use for children under 12 years should not exceed 1 oz in 24 hours.
• Avoid contact with eyes and mucous membranes.
• Application of bland cream or lotion is recommended if excessive skin drying or irritation occurs.
• Hands should be rinsed after application (un-

(continued on following page)

NAMES, INDICATIONS AND DOSAGES	SIDE EFFECTS

salicylic acid
(continued)

area and place under occlusion at night.

silver nitrate

Cauterization of mucous membranes, fissures, aphthous lesions (5% to 10% solution); cauterization of granulomatous tissues and warts (solid form):
ADULTS AND CHILDREN: applied only by doctor at his discretion.

Local: *argyria (permanent silver discoloration of skin).*

sulfur
Acne-Aid♦, Acnomead, Bensulfoid, EpiClear, Liquimat, Postacne♦, Transact, Xerac

Acne, ringworm, psoriasis, seborrheic dermatitis, chigger infestation, scabies, favus, staphylococcal folliculitis:
ADULTS AND CHILDREN: apply preparation to affected areas b.i.d., t.i.d., or as directed.

Local: excessive drying of skin, blackheads, contact dermatitis.

sulfurated lime solution
Vlem-Dome, Vleminckx's solution

Acne vulgaris, seborrhea:
ADULTS AND CHILDREN: dilute 1 packet in 1 pt hot water and apply as hot dressing for 15 to 20 minutes daily.

Generalized furunculosis:
ADULTS AND CHILDREN: add 30 to 60 ml solution to bath water.

Local: may cause excessive drying of skin.

INTERACTIONS AND SPECIAL CONSIDERATIONS	
less they are being treated). • Skin should be hydrated for at least 5 minutes before treatment and should be washed the morning after treatment. • Most preparations are occlusive, which increases percutaneous absorption. Should not be used on large surface areas for prolonged periods.	• Not for use on broken, inflamed, or ulcerated areas.
No significant interactions. *Special considerations:* • May cause burns. Avoid accidental contact with skin and eyes. If accidental contact with skin: flush with water for at least 15 minutes; if accidental contact with eyes: call doctor at once. • If ingested (may cause altered respiration, coma, convulsions, paralysis, and even death): give 1 tablespoon salt in warm water, and repeat until emesis is clear; or have patient drink milk or beaten egg whites mixed in warm water; keep patient warm and lying down. • Silver nitrate stains skin and clothing.	• Silver nitrate pencils must be moistened with water before use.
No significant interactions. *Special considerations:* • Prolonged use may cause severe contact dermatitis. • Should be used sparingly for patients with sensitive skin. • Avoid contact with eyes. If accidental contact occurs, flush with water. • Skin should be washed thoroughly before application. Tingling sensation may be felt upon application. • Skin is more reactive to drug in cold, dry climates, so decrease frequency of application; in hot, humid climates, increase frequency of application. • Not for use on same area with topical acne preparation or preparations containing a peeling agent (for example, benzoyl peroxide); may cause severe irritation.	• Not for use on same area with any mercury-containing preparation; may cause a foul odor, irritate the skin, or stain skin black.
No significant interactions. *Special considerations:* • Use should be discontinued if excessive drying or skin irritation develops. • Contact with jewelry, metallic objects, or clothing should be avoided. • Getting solution in eyes, nose, or mouth should be avoided. • Fumes are irritating and malodorous (rotten eggs). Ventilate adequately. • Not for use in same area with topical acne preparations; may cause severe irritation. • Not for use in same area with mercury-containing preparations; may cause a foul odor, irritate skin, or turn skin black.	

94

Miscellaneous dermatomucosal agents

ammoniated mercury
anthralin
benzoyl peroxide
collagenase
dextranomer
fluorouracil
hydroquinone
methoxsalen
scarlet red
selenium sulfide
streptokinase-streptodornase
sutilains
tretinoin (vitamin A acid, retinoic acid)

Miscellaneous topical drugs include acne and burn products, irritants, rubefacients, antiseptics, enzymes, antimetabolites, and preparations that affect skin pigmentation.

Major uses

- Ammoniated mercury, anthralin, and selenium sulfide relieve psoriasis, atopic dermatitis, chronic dermatitis and eczema, seborrhea, pruritus, ringworm, and other skin conditions.
- Benzoyl peroxide and tretinoin are used to treat acne vulgaris.
- Collagenase, dextranomer, scarlet red, streptokinase-streptodornase, and sutilains clean, debride, and heal burns, surgical wounds, and ulcerative and pyogenic lesions.
- Fluorouracil is used to treat superficial forms of skin cancer.
- Hydroquinone is used to treat problems of skin hyperpigmentation.
- Methoxsalen accelerates pigmentation.

Mechanism of action

- Ammoniated mercury inhibits sulfhydryl enzymes and combines with amino and other chemical groups.
- Anthralin acts as a local antieczematous irritant.
- Benzoyl peroxide has antimicrobial and keratolytic activity.
- Collagenase is an enzymatic debriding agent that digests undenatured collagen fibers in necrotic tissue and removes substrates for bacterial proliferation. It facilitates access to infected areas by antibiotics, antibodies, and leukocytes.
- Dextranomer is a synthetic polymer that aids in granulation.
- Fluorouracil acts as an antimetabolite. It interferes with DNA synthesis by inhibiting thymidylate synthetase.
- Hydroquinone inhibits tyrosinase, preventing the conversion of tyrosine to melanin.
- Methoxsalen is a potent photosensitizer of the skin that promotes melanin formation by facilitating the action of ultraviolet light. It does not promote pigmentation in the absence of light.
- Scarlet red stimulates proliferation of the basal layer of the skin.
- Selenium sulfide has irritant, antibacterial, and antifungal properties.
- Streptokinase-streptodornase are enzymes produced during growth of certain strains of hemolytic streptococci. Streptokinase stimulates plasminogen activator; streptodornase

APPLYING TOPICAL DRUGS TO BURNS

Apply topical drugs after hydrotherapy or debridement. Using sterile technique, apply ointment and creams as follows:
• Apply a layer 2 to 4 mm thick directly to the burn eschar and leave it open to air. Reapply as necessary to keep the eschar covered.
• Apply the topical medication to the gauze and then apply the medicated gauze to the burn. Place dry gauze over the dressing, and cover with a stockinette or net dressing, such as Surgifix. Change dressings one to three times a day.

Drug solutions are used in all stages of burn care. Apply in one of the following ways:
• *Wet to dry.* Soak dressings in the solution and apply them to the burn. Apply a dry dressing over them.
• *Wet.* Prepare and apply dressings as described above, but keep them wet by frequent irrigations with the topical solution. Change dressings at least daily. Monitor the patient's temperature for hypothermia due to the cooling effect produced by evaporation from dressings.

hydrolyzes deoxyribonucleoprotein.
• Sutilains is a proteolytic enzyme that selectively digests necrotic tissue.
• Tretinoin (vitamin A acid) is a potent drying and peeling agent.

Absorption, distribution, metabolism, and excretion
These topical drugs may be absorbed systemically if they're used for long periods or applied to large areas of the body.

Onset and duration
These agents begin to act immediately upon application. The duration of action and the necessity for re-treatment depend not only on the specific agent but also on the condition being treated.

Combination products
LOROXIDE♦: benzoyl peroxide 5.5% and chlorhydroxyquinoline 0.25%.
LOROXIDE HC♦: benzoyl peroxide 5.5%, chlorhydroxyquinoline 0.25%, and hydrocortisone 0.5%.
SULFOXYL REGULAR: benzoyl peroxide 5% and sulfur 2%.
SULFOXYL STRONG: benzoyl peroxide 10% and sulfur 5%.
VANOXIDE♦: benzoyl peroxide 5% and chlorhydroxyquinoline 0.25%.
VANOXIDE-HC♦: benzoyl peroxide 5%, chlorhydroxyquinoline 0.25%, and hydrocortisone 0.5%.

NAMES, INDICATIONS AND DOSAGES	SIDE EFFECTS
ammoniated mercury Mercuronate 5% Ointment **Psoriasis, seborrheic dermatitis, impetigo contagiosa, tinea capitis, and favus:** ADULTS AND CHILDREN: apply to affected area b.i.d. or t.i.d.	None reported.
anthralin Anthra-Derm♦ **Psoriasis, chronic dermatitis:** ADULTS AND CHILDREN: apply thinly daily or b.i.d. Concentrations range from 0.1% to 1%; start with lowest and increase, if necessary.	**GU:** possible renal toxicity. **Skin:** erythema on healthy skin.
benzoyl peroxide Benoxyl♦, Benzac, Benzagel♦, Clear by Design, Dermodex, Desquam-X♦♦, Dry and Clear, Epi-Clear Antiseptic, Oxy-5, Oxy-10, Panoxyl♦, Persadox, Persadox HP, Persa-Gel, Xerac BP **Adjunctive treatment of acne:** ADULTS AND CHILDREN: apply once daily or b.i.d.	**Skin:** transient stinging on application, feeling of warmth, painful irritation.
collagenase Biozyme-C, Santyl♦ **Debridement of dermal ulcers and severely burned areas:** ADULTS AND CHILDREN: apply ointment (250 units/g) to lesion daily or every other day.	**Skin:** slight erythema of surrounding area, especially if ointment is not confined to lesion. **Other:** hypersensitivity reactions.
dextranomer Debrisan **To clean secreting wounds, such as venous stasis and decubitus ulcers, infected surgical wounds, and burns:** ADULTS AND CHILDREN: apply to affected area daily, b.i.d., or more often, p.r.n. Apply to ⅛" or ¼" thickness, and cover with sterile gauze pad.	**Skin:** temporary pain.

♦ Available in U.S. and Canada. ♦♦ Available in Canada only.
All other products (no symbol) available in U.S. only. Italicized side effects are common or life-threatening.

INTERACTIONS AND SPECIAL CONSIDERATIONS

No significant interactions.

Special considerations:
• Patient should not apply to large areas of body or use for extended periods of time. Mercury poisoning could result.
• Patient should not apply to highly inflamed skin, sunburn, open wounds.
• Has no odor. Doesn't stain.
• Patient should not use in same area with topical preparations containing sulfur; may cause foul odor or skin irritation, or may stain skin black.

No significant interactions.

Special considerations:
• Contraindicated in renal damage. Should not be used on acute or inflammatory eruptions.
• Partial excretion in urine may cause renal irritation, casts, and albuminuria. Urine should be checked weekly.
• Should be discontinued if allergic reaction, pustular folliculitis, or renal irritation occurs.
• Avoid contact with eyes. May cause conjunctivitis, keratitis, or corneal opacity.
• Patient should wear plastic gloves to apply anthralin; hands should be washed thoroughly after using.
• May cause a temporary yellow-brown discoloration to hair, skin, and alkaline urine. May stain clothing.
• Patient should avoid applying medication to normal skin by coating the area surrounding the lesion with petrolatum.

Interactions:
TRETINOIN: reduced effectiveness of benzoyl peroxide. Do not use together.

Special considerations:
• Contraindicated in sensitivity to any of the ingredients.
• Patient should not use on eyelids, mucous membranes, denuded or highly inflamed skin.
• Dryness, redness, and peeling should occur 3 to 4 days after starting treatment. If these common reactions cause considerable discomfort, patient should discontinue temporarily until they subside.
• If painful irritation develops, should be discontinued.
• Cleanser (4%) may cause bleaching of hair or colored fabric.

Interactions:
DETERGENTS, HEXACHLOROPHENE, ANTISEPTICS (ESPECIALLY THOSE CONTAINING HEAVY METAL IONS SUCH AS MERCURY OR SILVER), IODINE, SOAKS OR ACIDIC SOLUTIONS CONTAINING METAL IONS SUCH AS ALUMINUM ACETATE (BUROW'S SOLUTION): decreased enzymatic activity. Do not use together.

Special considerations:
• Use with caution in debilitated patients, since debriding enzymes may increase risk of bacteremia; systemic infection may occur.
• Before application: cleanse lesion with gauze saturated in normal saline, neutral buffer solution, or hydrogen peroxide; use topical antibacterial agent (such as neomycin-bacitracin-polymyxin B) if infection is present; apply to lesion in powder form before using collagenase; if infection does not respond, discontinue collagenase until infection is healed. Application tips: confine collagenase ointment to area of lesion (Lassar's paste may protect surrounding skin); apply ointment in thin layers to assure contact with necrotic tissue and complete wound coverage; apply collagenase ointment with tongue depressor on deep wounds; with gauze on shallow wounds; remove any debris that comes off easily; remove excess ointment, and cover wound with sterile gauze pad.
• Should be discontinued when sufficient debridement has occurred.
• Appearance of granulation may indicate effectiveness. Inflammation or color of drainage may indicate spread of infection.
• Symptoms of protein sensitization (long-term therapy) may occur.
• If enzymatic action must be stopped for any reason, Burow's solution should be applied.
• Avoid getting ointment in eyes. If this occurs, flush with water at once.
• Protect drug from heat.

No significant interactions.

Special considerations:
• Before application, wound should be cleansed with sterile water, saline, or other appropriate solution. Should not be dried.
• Cratered wounds should be packed with beads, allowing room for expansion of beads. A dressing should be applied to hold beads in place.
• When saturated, medication turns gray-yellow and should be removed.
• To remove, wound should be irrigated with sterile water, saline, or other cleansing solution.
• Dextranomer beads are not effective in cleaning nonsecreting wounds. When the wound has healed to the point where it is no longer exuding, treatment should be discontinued.
• Dextranomer beads are hydrophilic; each gram of bead can absorb 4 ml of exudate.
• Should be stored away from moisture, in

(continued on following page)

NAMES, INDICATIONS AND DOSAGES	SIDE EFFECTS
dextranomer *(continued)*	
fluorouracil Efudex♦, Fluoroplex♦ **Multiple actinic or solar keratoses; superficial basal cell carcinoma:** ADULTS AND CHILDREN: apply cream (5%) or solution (2% or 5%) b.i.d.	**Skin:** erythema, pain, burning, scaling, pruritus, hyperpigmentation, dermatitis, soreness, suppuration, swelling.
hydroquinone Artra Skin Tone Cream, Derma-Blanch, Eldopaque♦, Eldopaque-Forte♦, Eldoquin♦, Eldoquin Forte♦, Esoterica Medicated Cream, Golden Peacock, HQC Kit, Melanex, Quinnone **Bleaching of blemished skin, lentigo, chloasma, freckles, old-age spots, and other skin conditions due to increased melanin:** ADULTS AND CHILDREN 12 YEARS AND OVER: apply 2% to 4% concentration daily or b.i.d.	**Skin:** mild irritation, sensitization, rash.
methoxsalen Oxsoralen♦ **Protect against sunburn, enhance pigmentation, and induce repigmentation in vitiligo:** ADULTS AND CHILDREN OVER 12 YEARS: for small, well-defined lesions, apply topically weekly or less often and expose to ultraviolet A light gradually, as directed.	**CNS:** nervousness, insomnia, depression. **GI:** discomfort, nausea, diarrhea. **Hepatic:** hepatic toxicity. **Skin:** edema, erythema, painful blistering, burning, peeling, *photosensitivity*.
scarlet red Decubitex Ointment (also contains peruvian balsam, zinc oxide, starch, castor oil, petrolatum, xantham gum, sodium propionate, methylparaben, propylparaben, propylene glycol, and water) **Aid in management of decubitus ulcers:** ADULTS AND CHILDREN: pour a small amount of 3% hydrogen peroxide or normal saline solution on the affected area. Cleanse thoroughly and apply ointment. Cover with dry sterile gauze.	None reported.
selenium sulfide Exsel♦, Iosel 250, Selsun♦, Selsun Blue, Sul-Blue	**Skin:** oily or dry scalp and hair, hair discoloration, hair loss, sensitivity reactions.

♦ Available in U.S. and Canada. ♦♦ Available in Canada only.
All other products (no symbol) available in U.S. only. Italicized side effects are common or life-threatening.

INTERACTIONS AND SPECIAL CONSIDERATIONS

tightly closed container.
• Avoid contact with eyes.
• Care should be taken not to spill beads onto floor, as the resultant slipperiness can be a safety hazard.

No significant interactions.

Special considerations:
• Hands should be washed immediately after handling medication.
• Avoid using with occlusive dressings.
• Patient should avoid prolonged exposure to sunlight or ultraviolet light.
• Apply with caution near eyes, nose, and mouth.
• Treated area may be unsightly during therapy and for several weeks after therapy is stopped. Complete healing may not occur until 1 or 2 months after treatment is stopped.
• Ingestion and systemic absorption may cause leukopenia, thrombocytopenia, stomatitis, diarrhea, or GI ulceration, bleeding, and hemorrhage.
• Topical application to large ulcerated areas may cause systemic toxicity.
• For basal cell carcinoma, 5% strength should be used.

No significant interactions.

Special considerations:
• Contraindicated in patients with prickly heat, sunburn, irritated skin, or as depilatory.
• Don't use near eyes.
• Rash or irritation requires discontinuation of therapy.
• Sensitivity can be tested by applying a small amount of low-concentration medication on skin before treatment is started. Allergic reactions should appear within 24 hours.
• Doesn't cause permanent depigmentation.
• Opaque sunscreen should be used when outdoors since sun can darken lesions faster than hydroquinone can lighten them.

Interactions:
PHOTOSENSITIZING AGENTS: do not use together.

Special considerations:
• Contraindicated in hepatic insufficiency, porphyria, acute lupus erythematosus, hydromorphic and polymorphic light eruptions. Use with caution in familial history of sunlight allergy, GI diseases, or chronic infection.
• Therapy should be regulated carefully. Overdosage or overexposure to light can cause serious burning or blistering.
• Topical treatment should be directly supervised by a doctor.
• When applied topically to face or hands, patient should protect area from light (except during treatment exposure) for 24 hours after therapy.
• Eyes and lips should be protected during light-exposure treatments.
• Monthly liver function studies should be done on patients with vitiligo (especially at beginning of therapy).
• Significant changes require 6 to 9 months of therapy.

No significant interactions.

Special considerations:
• Dressing should be changed twice daily, especially where seeping and secretions are present.
• Ointment should be in contact with newly forming tissue for maximum therapeutic results. Wound should be allowed to "breathe" by being loosely covered.
• Using excess ointment or covering the wound completely will retard wound healing.
• Ointment should be used until healing is complete.
• In advanced decubitus ulcers, normal saline solution should be used, rather than hydrogen peroxide.

No significant interactions.

Special considerations:
• Contraindicated in sulfur hypersensitivity.
• Use with caution around areas of acute inflammation or exudation to avoid increased absorption.
• If sensitivity reactions occur, use should be discontinued.
• Thorough rinsing after treatment reduces or

(continued on following page)

NAMES, INDICATIONS AND DOSAGES	SIDE EFFECTS
selenium sulfide *(continued)* **Dandruff, seborrheic scalp dermatitis:** ADULTS AND CHILDREN: massage 1 to 2 teaspoonfuls into clean, wet scalp. Leave on for 2 to 3 minutes. Rinse thoroughly, and repeat application. Apply twice weekly for 2 weeks, then once a week for 2 weeks, or as often as needed to maintain control.	
streptokinase-streptodornase Varidase♦ **Adjunctive treatment of suppurative surface tissues, including ulcers, radiation necrosis, infected wounds, burns, surgical incisions, skin grafts, and whenever clotted blood, or fibrinous or purulent accumulations are undesirable:** ADULTS AND CHILDREN: apply on individual basis, depending on area treated and doctor's instructions.	**Systemic:** fever.
sutilains Travase♦ **Debridement of second- and third-degree burns, adjunctive debridement of decubitus ulcers, pyogenic wounds, or ulcers resulting from peripheral vascular disease:** ADULTS AND CHILDREN: apply thinly to area extending ¼" to ½" beyond area to be debrided. Cover with loose wet dressing t.i.d. or q.i.d.	**CNS:** local paresthesias. **Skin:** mild pain, bleeding, transient dermatitis.
tretinoin (vitamin A acid, retinoic acid) **Acne vulgaris (especially grades I, II, and III):** ADULTS AND CHILDREN: cleanse affected area and lightly apply solution once daily at bedtime.	**Skin:** *feeling of warmth, slight stinging, local erythema, peeling at site,* chapping and swelling, blistering and crusting, temporary hyperpigmentation or hypopigmentation.

♦ Available in U.S. and Canada. ♦♦ Available in Canada only.
All other products (no symbol) available in U.S. only. Italicized side effects are common or life-threatening.

INTERACTIONS AND SPECIAL CONSIDERATIONS

prevents hair discoloration.
• Avoid contact with eyes.
• Highly toxic if ingested.
• Hands should be washed carefully after handling.
• Protect from heat.

Interactions:
DETERGENTS, ANTI-INFECTIVES (SUCH AS BENZALKONIUM CHLORIDE, HEXACHLOROPHENE, IODINE): decreased enzymatic activity. Do not use together.

Special considerations:
• Contraindicated in areas of active hemorrhage.
• Exudates should be removed carefully and frequently, especially from closed areas, to avoid pyogenesis.
• Not effective on fibrous tissue, mucoproteins, or collagens.
• Refrigerated solution stable for 2 weeks. Room temperature solution stable for 24 hours.
• Rubber dams, or gauze or nylon dressing should be used to keep medication in constant contact with lesion.
• Prolonged use may result in a high antienzyme titer. Dosage may need to be increased.
• Solution or jelly. Mix to dilution ordered.
• Protect drugs from heat.
• To make jelly, add 5 ml sterile water for injection or sterile physiological saline to 125,000-unit vial streptokinase-streptodornase (SK-SD); mix with 15 ml jar of carboxymethyl cellulose jelly 4.5%. The resulting mixure contains 5,000 IU SK and 1,250 IU SD/ml or g.
• Wound area should be thoroughly cleansed and irrigated with sterile normal saline or water before treatment to remove antiseptics, detergents, and heavy metal antibacterials, which can decrease enzyme activity.
• Treatment tips: moisten wound area for optimal enzymatic activity; dress wound if necessary, but remove waste products frequently; observe wound to monitor progress of therapy. Appearance of granulation tissue may indicate effectiveness. Inflammation or color of drainage may indicate spread of infection.
• Avoid getting solution in eyes. If this occurs, flood with water at once.

Interactions:
DETERGENTS, ANTI-INFECTIVES (SUCH AS BENZALKONIUM CHLORIDE, HEXACHLOROPHENE, IODINE, AND NITROFURAZONE), AND COMPOUNDS CONTAINING METALLIC IONS (SUCH AS SILVER NITRATE AND THIMEROSAL): adversely affected enzymatic activity. Do not use together.

Special considerations:
• Contraindicated in wounds involving major body cavities or containing exposed nerves or nerve tissue, fungating neoplastic ulcers, wounds in women of childbearing age, persons having limited cardiac or pulmonary reserves.
• If accidental contact with eyes occurs, eyes should be flushed repeatedly with large amounts of normal saline solution or sterile water.
• Before application, affected area should be cleansed and irrigated with normal saline or sterile water solution to remove antiseptic or heavy metal antibacterial agents.
• Mild analgesic may be given to reduce painful reactions, but drug should be discontinued if pain is severe or if bleeding or dermatitis occurs.
• Keep affected area moist for best response.
• In concomitant use of topical antimicrobial agent, sutilains should be applied first.
• Store at 2° to 10° C. (35.6° to 50° F.). Check expiration date.

No significant interactions.

Special considerations:
• Contraindicated in hypersensitivity to any tretinoin component. Use with caution in eczema.
• If severe local irritation develops, solution should be discontinued temporarily and dosage readjusted when application is resumed.
• Some redness and scaling are normal.
• Beneficial effects should be seen within 6 weeks of treatment. When treatment is stopped, relapses generally occur within 3 to 6 weeks.
• Wash face with mild soap no more than 2 or 3 times a day. Avoid strong or medicated cosmetics, soaps, or other skin cleansers.
• Exposure to sunlight or ultraviolet rays should be minimal during treatment. In sunburned patient, therapy should be delayed until sunburn subsides.
• Avoid contact with eyes, mouth, nose, and mucous membranes. Apply to dry skin only.
• Not for use with topical products containing alcohol, astringents, spices, and lime. These may interfere with action of tretinoin.

95

Local anesthetics

bupivacaine hydrochloride
chloroprocaine hydrochloride
dibucaine hydrochloride
etidocaine hydrochloride
lidocaine hydrochloride
mepivacaine hydrochloride
piperocaine hydrochloride
prilocaine hydrochloride
procaine hydrochloride
tetracaine hydrochloride

Local anesthetics block nerve conduction when they're injected locally into nerve tissue in appropriate concentrations. They can act on any part of the central nervous system (CNS) and on any type of nerve cell. First they affect the small, nonmyelinated autonomic fibers; then those mediating cold, warmth, pain, and touch; and finally those mediating motor function. Nerve function is regained in reverse order.

Local anesthetics can be divided into two groups, amides and esters, depending on which type of chemical bond is in the molecule. Amide-derived drugs are bupivacaine, dibucaine, etidocaine, lidocaine, mepivacaine, and prilocaine. Ester derivatives are chloroprocaine, piperocaine, procaine, and tetracaine.

The amide or ester bond affects certain pharmacologic properties such as the duration of action, which, with these agents, can be considered a determinant of toxicity. Dosage varies greatly according to the procedure to be performed, level of anesthesia required, number of neuronal segments to be blocked, tissue vascularity, and patient response. The smallest dose and lowest concentration needed to produce the desired anesthesia should be used.

Major uses

Local anesthetics are used in dental or minor surgical procedures (biopsy, for example). In addition, they furnish regional (nerve block) anesthesia, including spinal, caudal, and epidural anesthesia (in tubal ligation or hernia repair, for example).

Mechanism of action

Local anesthetics block depolarization by interfering with sodium-potassium exchange across the nerve cell membrane, preventing generation and conduction of the nerve impulse.

When local anesthetics are combined with epinephrine, anesthesia is prolonged because

MONITORING THE PATIENT WHO'S RECEIVED A NERVE BLOCK

After receiving a nerve block with a local anesthetic, the patient needs special attention. Be sure to:

- Watch the patient for anaphylaxis or other reactions to the drug used. These may include hives, rash, or seizure activity.
- Protect the extremity in which the drug was given. For example, pad the side rails of the bed, or position and support the arm or leg with pillows.
- Frequently check the patient's circulation and level of sensation (every 15 to 30 minutes) until the block is reversed.

PREVENTING ROUTE SIDE EFFECTS

Sometimes the route by which a regional anesthetic is administered precipitates complications or side effects. For example, local anesthetics are often injected into the epidural space—commonly in the lumbar area—within the vertebral canal. The epidural route affords easy administration, minimal trauma to the spinal cord, and widespread sympathetic blockade. And because it doesn't puncture the dural space, patients seldom suffer a spinal headache. However, because the epidural space is highly vascular, a high dosage may cause systemic toxic effects. Signs of toxicity, such as CNS disturbances, rising blood pressure, and a rapid pulse are possible.

When a local anesthetic is injected directly into the cerebrospinal fluid (CSF), it produces sympathetic blockade. The patient who is anesthetized by the *spinal route* may suffer a spinal headache, caused by CSF leaking around the dural puncture site. He may even experience diplopia and tinnitus. If the patient sits up, CSF pressure may be reduced, causing side effects.

The patient should be kept in a horizontal position and, unless contraindicated, he should be well hydrated. Mild analgesics should be given p.r.n. If the patient's headache is severe, normal saline solution may be injected into the epidural space to prevent further CSF leakage.

the rate of absorption decreases. The vasoconstriction produced by the epinephrine also helps control local bleeding.

Absorption, distribution, metabolism, and excretion

- Absorption varies according to dose, site of injection, and vasodilation produced by the drug. Epinephrine combined with a local anesthetic decreases absorption.
- The drugs are distributed to all body tissues.
- Esters are hydrolyzed (metabolized) rapidly and almost completely by blood cholinesterases. The remaining drug is metabolized by the liver, and the metabolites are excreted in urine.
- Amides are metabolized primarily in the liver, and the metabolites are excreted in urine.

Onset and duration

The drugs begin to act in less than 15 minutes after application, but duration of action varies.

Epinephrine prolongs duration of effect.

- Bupivacaine, dibucaine, etidocaine, and tetracaine have long durations (3 to 6 hours).
- Chloroprocaine and procaine have short durations (30 to 60 minutes).
- Lidocaine, mepivacaine, piperocaine, and prilocaine provide anesthesia for 1 to 3 hours.

Combination products

None, although epinephrine is added to some solutions to prolong effect.

NAMES, INDICATIONS AND DOSAGES	SIDE EFFECTS

bupivacaine hydrochloride

Marcaine♦

Available with or without epinephrine. Dosages given are for drug *without* epinephrine.

Epidural:

Sol.	*Vol. (ml)*	*Dose (mg)*
0.75%	10 to 20	75 to 150
0.50%	10 to 20	50 to 100
0.25%	10 to 20	25 to 50

Caudal:

Sol.	*Vol. (ml)*	*Dose (mg)*
0.50%	15 to 30	75 to 150
0.25%	15 to 30	37.5 to 75

Peripheral nerve block:

Sol.	*Vol. (ml)*	*Dose (mg)*
0.50%	5 to 80	25 to 400 (max.)

May repeat dose q 3 hours. Dose and interval may be increased with epinephrine. Maximum 400 mg daily.

Skin: dermatologic reactions.
Other: edema, status asthmaticus, or *anaphylaxis* and anaphylactoid reactions.
Side effects of local anesthetics generally result from high blood levels of the drug. Examples of these are:
CNS: anxiety, apprehension, nervousness, convulsions followed by drowsiness, unconsciousness, and *respiratory arrest.*
CV: myocardial depression, *arrhythmias, cardiac arrest.*
EENT: blurred vision.
GI: nausea, vomiting.

chloroprocaine hydrochloride

Nesacaine (for infiltration and regional anesthesia), Nesacaine-CE (for caudal and epidural anesthesia)

Available only without epinephrine.

Infiltration and nerve block:

Sol.	*Vol. (ml)*	*Dose (mg)*
1%	3 to 20	30 to 200
2%	2 to 40	20 to 400

Caudal and epidural:

Sol.	*Vol. (ml)*	*Dose (mg)*
2% to 3%	15 to 25	300 to 750

May repeat with smaller doses q 40 to 50 minutes. Dose and interval may be increased with epinephrine. Maximum adult dose 800 mg, or 1 g when mixed with epinephrine.

Skin: dermatologic reactions.
Other: edema, status asthmaticus, or *anaphylaxis* and anaphylactoid reactions.
Side effects of local anesthetics generally result from high blood levels of the drug. Examples of these are:
CNS: anxiety, apprehension, nervousness, convulsions followed by drowsiness, unconsciousness, and *respiratory arrest.*
CV: myocardial depression, *arrhythmias, cardiac arrest.*
EENT: blurred vision.
GI: nausea, vomiting.

dibucaine hydrochloride

Nupercaine

Available only without epinephrine.

Spinal anesthesia:

Perineum and lower limbs

Sol.	*Vol. (ml)*	*Dose (mg)*
0.5%	0.5 to 1	2.5 to 5

Lower abdomen

Sol.	*Vol. (ml)*	*Dose (mg)*
0.5%	1 to 1.5	5 to 7.5

Upper abdomen

Sol.	*Vol. (ml)*	*Dose (mg)*
0.5%	2	10

Spinal anesthesia:

Lower extremities as high as pelvis

Sol.	*Vol. (ml)*	*Dose (mg)*
1:1,500	6	4

Skin: dermatologic reactions.
Other: edema, status asthmaticus, or *anaphylaxis* and anaphylactoid reactions.
Side effects of local anesthetics generally result from high blood levels of the drug. Examples of these are:
CNS: anxiety, apprehension, nervousness, convulsions followed by drowsiness, unconsciousness, and *respiratory arrest.*
CV: myocardial depression, *arrhythmias, cardiac arrest.*
EENT: blurred vision.
GI: nausea, vomiting.

INTERACTIONS AND SPECIAL CONSIDERATIONS

Interactions:
CHLOROFORM, HALOTHANE, CYCLOPROPANE, TRICHLOROETHYLENE, AND RELATED DRUGS: cardiac arrhymias may occur when used with bupivacaine *with* epinephrine. Use with extreme caution.
MAO INHIBITORS, TRICYCLIC ANTIDEPRESSANTS: severe, sustained hypertension may occur when used with bupivacaine *with* epinephrine. Use with extreme caution.

Special considerations:
• Contraindicated in children under 12 years and for spinal, paracervical block, or topical anesthesia. Use cautiously in debilitated, elderly, or acutely ill patients; severe hepatic disease; drug allergies.
• Solutions with epinephrine should be used cautiously in cardiovascular disorders and in body areas with limited blood supply (ears, nose, fingers, toes).
• Resuscitative equipment and drugs should be kept available.
• Don't use solution with preservatives for caudal or epidural block.
• Onset in 4 to 17 minutes; duration 3 to 7 hours.
• Causes less fetal depression than other local anesthetics.
• Discard partially used vials without preservatives.

No significant interactions.

Special considerations:
• Contraindicated in hypersensitivity to procaine, tetracaine, or other *p*-aminobenzoic acid derivatives, and for spinal or topical anesthesia. Epidural and caudal contraindicated in CNS disease. Use cautiously in children, and in debilitated, elderly, or acutely ill patients; drug allergies; paracervical block; cardiovascular disease.
• A 3-ml test dose should be injected at least 10 minutes before giving total dose to check for intravascular or subarachnoid injection. Motor paralysis and extensive sensory anesthesia indicate subarachnoid injection.
• Test dose should be repeated if patient moves in a way that might displace the epidural catheter.
• At least 5 minutes should elapse after each test before proceeding further.
• Do not use solution with preservatives for caudal or epidural block.
• Discolored solution should not be used.
• Resuscitative equipment and drugs should be kept available.
• Duration 30 to 60 minutes.
• Discard partially used vials without preservatives.

No significant interactions.

Special considerations:
• Contraindicated in cerebrospinal disease, septicemia, pernicious anemia with spinal cord symptoms, arthritis, pyogenic skin infection in puncture area. Use cautiously in hysteria, chronic backache, headache of long duration, migraine, shock, hypotension, leaking spinal fluid, cardiac decompensation, pleural effusions, increased abdominal pressure, possibility of hemorrhage.
• Low spinal solution contraindicated in cesarean section or in presence of blood when doing lumbar puncture. Low spinal solutions should be used cautiously in cardiac or neurologic disease, back problems, uncooperative or hysterical patients.
• Solutions with epinephrine should be used cautiously in cardiovascular disorders and in body areas with limited blood supply (ears, nose, fingers, toes).
• Resuscitative equipment and drugs should be kept available.
• Contraindicated for nerve block or infiltration.
• Discolored solution should not be used.
• Used primarily for spinal block and as topical anesthetic.
• Onset in 10 to 15 minutes; duration 6 hours.
• Discard partially used vials without preservatives.

(continued on following page)

NAMES, INDICATIONS AND DOSAGES | SIDE EFFECTS

dibucaine hydrochloride
(continued)

Lower abdomen

Sol.	*Vol. (ml)*	*Dose (mg)*
1:1,500	10 to 15	6.67 to 10

Upper abdomen

Sol.	*Vol. (ml)*	*Dose (mg)*
1:1,500	15 to 18	10 to 12

etidocaine hydrochloride
Duranest

Available with or without epinephrine. Doses cited are for drug *with* epinephrine.

Dose and interval may be decreased without epinephrine.

Infiltration:

Sol.	*Vol. (ml)*	*Dose (mg)*
0.5%	1 to 80	5 to 400

Peripheral nerve block:

Sol.	*Vol. (ml)*	*Dose (mg)*
0.5%	5 to 80	25 to 400
1%	5 to 40	50 to 400

Central neural block:

Lower limbs, cesarean section, lumbar peridural

Sol.	*Vol. (ml)*	*Dose (mg)*
1%	10 to 30	100 to 300
1.5%	10 to 20	150 to 300

Vaginal

Sol.	*Vol. (ml)*	*Dose (mg)*
0.5%	10 to 30	50 to 150
1%	5 to 20	50 to 200

Caudal:

Sol.	*Vol. (ml)*	*Dose (mg)*
0.5%	10 to 30	50 to 150
1%	10 to 30	100 to 300

Skin: dermatologic reactions.
Other: edema, status asthmaticus, or *anaphylaxis* and anaphylactoid reactions.
Side effects of local anesthetics generally result from high blood levels of the drug. Examples of these are:
CNS: anxiety, apprehension, nervousness, convulsions followed by drowsiness, unconsciousness, and *respiratory arrest.*
CV: myocardial depression, *arrhythmias, cardiac arrest.*
EENT: blurred vision.
GI: nausea, vomiting.

lidocaine hydrochloride
Ardecaine, Canocaine, Dilocaine, Dolicaine, L-Caine, Nervocaine, Norocaine, Rocaine, Ultracaine, Xylocaine Hydrochloride♦

Available with or without epinephrine. Doses cited are for drug *without* epinephrine except where indicated.

Caudal *(obstetric use)* **or epidural** *(thoracic):*

Sol.	*Vol. (ml)*	*Dose (mg)*
1%	20 to 30	200 to 300

Caudal *(surgery):*

Sol.	*Vol. (ml)*	*Dose (mg)*
1.5%	15 to 20	225 to 300

Epidural *(lumbar anesthesia):*

Sol.	*Vol. (ml)*	*Dose (mg)*
1.5%	15 to 20	225 to 300
2%	10 to 15	200 to 300

Maximum dose 200 to 300 mg/hour.

Skin: dermatologic reactions.
Other: edema, status asthmaticus, or *anaphylaxis* and anaphylactoid reactions.
Side effects of local anesthetics generally result from high blood levels of the drug. Examples of these are:
CNS: anxiety, apprehension, nervousness, convulsions followed by drowsiness, unconsciousness, and *respiratory arrest.*
CV: myocardial depression, *arrhythmias, cardiac arrest.*
EENT: blurred vision.
GI: nausea, vomiting.

INTERACTIONS AND SPECIAL CONSIDERATIONS

Interactions:
CHLOROFORM, HALOTHANE, CYCLOPROPANE, TRICHLOROETHYLENE, AND RELATED DRUGS: cardiac arrhythmias may occur when used with etidocaine *with* epinephrine. Use with extreme caution.
MAO INHIBITORS, TRICYCLIC ANTIDEPRESSANTS, PHENOTHIAZINES: severe, sustained hypertension or hypotension may occur when used with etidocaine solution *with* epinephrine. Use with extreme caution.

Special considerations:
- Contraindicated in inflammation or infection in puncture region, children under 14 years, septicemia, severe hypertension, spinal deformities, neurologic disorders, and spinal block. Use cautiously in debilitated, elderly, or acutely ill patients; severe shock; heart block; epidural block in obstetrics; general drug allergies; hepatic and renal disease.
- Solutions with epinephrine should be used cautiously in cardiovascular disease and in body areas with limited blood supply (nose, ears, fingers, toes).
- Solution with preservatives contraindicated for caudal or epidural block.
- Resuscitative equipment and drugs should be kept available.
- Onset in 2 to 8 minutes, duration 4.5 to 13 hours.
- For symptoms and treatment of anaphylaxis, see APPENDIX.

Interactions:
CHLOROFORM, HALOTHANE, CYCLOPROPANE, TRICHLOROETHYLENE, AND RELATED DRUGS: cardiac arrhythmias may occur when used with lidocaine *with* epinephrine. Use with extreme caution.
MAO INHIBITORS, TRICYCLIC ANTIDEPRESSANTS: severe, sustained hypertension may occur when used with lidocaine *with* epinephrine. Use with extreme caution.

Special considerations:
- Contraindicated in inflammation or infection in puncture region, septicemia, severe hypertension, spinal deformities, neurologic disorders. Use cautiously in debilitated, elderly, or acutely ill patients; in severe shock; heart block; in obstetrics; general drug allergies; and paracervical block.
- Solutions with epinephrine should be used cautiously in cardiovascular disorders and in body areas with limited blood supply (nose, ears, fingers, toes).
- Resuscitative equipment and drugs should be kept available.
- A 2- to 5-ml test dose should be injected at least 5 minutes before giving total dose to check for intravascular or subarachnoid injection. Motor paralysis and extensive sensory anesthesia indicate subarachnoid injection.
- Solutions containing preservatives should not be used for spinal, epidural, or caudal block.
- Discard partially used vials without preservatives.
- For symptoms and treatment of anaphylaxis, see APPENDIX.

(continued on following page)

NAMES, INDICATIONS AND DOSAGES | SIDE EFFECTS

lidocaine hydrochloride
(continued)

For anesthesia other than spinal: maximum single adult dose 4.5 mg/kg or 300 mg.
With epinephrine for anesthesia other than spinal: maximum single adult dose 7 mg/kg or 500 mg. Don't repeat dose more often than q 2 hours.

Spinal surgical anesthesia:

Sol.	*Vol. (ml)*	*Dose (mg)*
5% with 7.5% dextrose	1.5 to 2	75 to 100

Dose and interval may be increased with epinephrine.

mepivacaine hydrochloride
Carbocaine♦, Cavacaine, Isocaine

Available with or without levonordefrin (vasoconstrictor). Doses cited are for drug *without* levonordefrin.

Nerve block:

Sol.	*Vol. (ml)*	*Dose (mg)*
1%	5 to 20	50 to 200
2%	5 to 20	100 to 400

Transvaginal block or infiltration *(maximum dose):*

Sol.	*Vol. (ml)*	*Dose (mg)*
1%	40	400

Paracervical block *(obstetric use):*

Sol.	*Vol. (ml)*	*Dose (mg)*
1%	10	100

Give on each side (200 mg total) per 90-minute period.

Caudal and epidural:

Sol.	*Vol. (ml)*	*Dose (mg)*
1%	15 to 30	150 to 300
1.5%	10 to 25	150 to 375
2%	10 to 20	200 to 400

Therapeutic block *(pain management):*

Sol.	*Vol. (ml)*	*Dose (mg)*
1%	1 to 5	10 to 50
2%	1 to 5	20 to 100

ADULTS: maximum single dose 7 mg/kg up to 550 mg. Don't repeat more often than q 90 minutes. Maximum total dose 1,000 mg daily.

CHILDREN: maximum dose 5 to 6 mg/kg. In children under 3 years or weighing less than 14 kg, use 0.5% or 1.5% solution only. Dose and interval may be increased with levonordefrin.

Side effects:

Skin: dermatologic reactions.
Other: edema, status asthmaticus, or *anaphylaxis* and anaphylactoid reactions.
Side effects of local anesthetics generally result from high blood levels of the drug. Examples of these are:
CNS: anxiety, apprehension, nervousness, convulsions followed by drowsiness, unconsciousness, and *respiratory arrest.*
CV: myocardial depression, *arrhythmias, cardiac arrest.*
EENT: blurred vision.
GI: nausea, vomiting.

piperocaine hydrochloride
Metycaine

Caudal block *(obstetric use in women with*

Side effects:

Skin: dermatologic reactions.
Other: edema, status asthmaticus, *anaphylaxis* and anaphylactoid reactions.
Side effects of local anesthetics generally result

♦ Available in U.S. and Canada. ♦♦ Available in Canada only.
All other products (no symbol) available in U.S. only. Italicized side effects are common or life-threatening.

INTERACTIONS AND SPECIAL CONSIDERATIONS

Interactions:
CHLOROFORM, HALOTHANE, CYCLOPROPANE, TRICHLOROETHYLENE, AND RELATED DRUGS: cardiac arrhythmias may occur when used with mepivacaine *with* levonordefrin. Use with extreme caution.
MAO INHIBITORS, TRICYCLIC ANTIDEPRESSANTS: severe, sustained hypertension may occur when used with mepivacaine *with* levonordefrin. Use with extreme caution.

Special considerations:
- Contraindicated in sensitivity to methylparaben, in heart block, or for spinal anesthesia. Use cautiously in debilitated, elderly, or acutely ill patients, or for paracervical block.
- Solutions with levonordefrin should be used cautiously in cardiovascular disease and in body areas with limited blood supply (nose, ears, fingers, toes).
- Fetal heart rate should be monitored when paracervical block used in delivery.
- Resuscitative equipment and drugs should be kept available.
- Solutions with preservatives contraindicated for caudal or epidural block.
- Onset in 15 minutes; duration 3 hours.
- Discard partially used vials without preservatives.

No significant interactions.

Special considerations:
- Contraindicated in hypersensitivity to procaine, tetracaine, or other *p*-aminobenzoic acid derivatives, CNS diseases, spinal deformity, infection at injection site, profound anemia, spinal block, in extremely obese patients, and in highly

(continued on following page)

NAMES, INDICATIONS AND DOSAGES	SIDE EFFECTS

piperocaine hydrochloride
(continued)

normal-sized pelvic canals):

Sol.	*Vol. (ml)*	*Dose (mg)*
1.5%	30	450

May give additional 20 ml doses (300 mg) q 30 to 40 minutes, p.r.n.

Infiltration *(maximum dose):*

Sol.	*Vol. (ml)*	*Dose (mg)*
0.5%	200	1,000
1%	80	800

For dental infiltration, use a 1% to 2% solution.

For peripheral or sympathetic nerve block, use 0.5% to 2% solution.

from high blood levels of the drug. Examples of these are:
CNS: anxiety, apprehension, nervousness, convulsions followed by drowsiness, unconsciousness, and *respiratory arrest.*
CV: myocardial depression, *arrhythmias, cardiac arrest.*
EENT: blurred vision.
GI: nausea, vomiting.

prilocaine hydrochloride
Citanest♦, Propitocaine

Infiltration:

Sol.	*Vol. (ml)*	*Dose (mg)*
1% to 2%	20 to 30	200 to 600

Peripheral nerve block *(intercostal or paravertebral):*

Sol.	*Vol. (ml)*	*Dose (mg)*
1% to 2%	3 to 5	30 to 100

Peripheral nerve block *(sciatic [femoral or brachial plexus] or caudal nerve block [surgery])*

Sol.	*Vol. (ml)*	*Dose (mg)*
2%	20 to 30	400 to 600
3%	15 to 20	450 to 600

Caudal nerve block *(obstetric use):*

Sol.	*Vol. (ml)*	*Dose (mg)*
1%	20 to 30	200 to 300

Epidural:

Sol.	*Vol. (ml)*	*Dose (mg)*
1%	20 to 30	200 to 300
2%	20 to 30	400 to 600
3%	15 to 20	450 to 600

Maximum single adult dose 8 mg/kg up to 600 mg. In continuous caudal or epidural anesthesia, don't give maximum dose more often than q 2 hours.

Skin: dermatologic reactions.
Other: edema, status asthmaticus, or *anaphylaxis* and anaphylactoid reactions.
With 4% solution: swelling and paresthesia of lips and mouth.
At maximum dose: methemoglobinemia.
Side effects of local anesthetics generally result from high blood levels of the drug. Examples of these are:
CNS: anxiety, apprehension, nervousness, convulsions followed by drowsiness, unconsciousness, and *respiratory arrest.*
CV: myocardial depression, *arrhythmias, cardiac arrest.*
EENT: blurred vision.
GI: nausea, vomiting.

procaine hydrochloride
Novocain♦, Unicaine

Spinal anesthesia:

Before using, dilute 10% solution with 0.9% NaCl injection, sterile distilled water, or cerebrospinal fluid.

For hyperbaric technique, use dextrose solution.

Perineum: use 0.5 ml 10% solution and 0.5 ml diluent injected at fourth lumbar interspace.

Perineum and lower extremities: use 1 ml 10%

Skin: dermatologic reactions.
Other: edema, status asthmaticus, or *anaphylaxis* and anaphylactoid reactions.
Side effects of local anesthetics generally result from high blood levels of the drug. Examples of these are:
CNS: anxiety, apprehension, nervousness, convulsions followed by drowsiness, unconsciousness, and *respiratory arrest.*
CV: myocardial depression, *arrhythmias, cardiac arrest.*
EENT: blurred vision.
GI: nausea, vomiting.

INTERACTIONS AND SPECIAL CONSIDERATIONS

nervous women.
• Solutions with preservatives contraindicated for caudal block.
• Resuscitative equipment and drugs should be kept available.
• Effect peaks in 20 to 30 minutes, then begins to decrease over next 10 minutes. Duration up to 3 hours.
• 2% solutions should be diluted to 0.5% or 1% with NaCl injection or Ringer's injection. Sterile water for injection should not be used.
• An 8-ml dose of anesthetic solution should be injected a few minutes before giving total dose to check for subarachnoid injection. Motor paralysis and extensive sensory anesthesia indicate subarachnoid injection.
• Discard partially used vials that do not contain preservatives.

No significant interactions.

Special considerations:
• Contraindicated in methemoglobinemia, severe shock, heart block, infection at injection site, or for spinal block. Use cautiously in debilitated, elderly, or acutely ill patients; children under 10 years; and in general drug sensitivities.
• Epidural and caudal blocks contraindicated in CNS disease, spinal deformities, septicemia, severe hypertension, and in children.
• Resuscitative equipment and drugs should be kept available.
• Duration 1 to 3 hours.
• Solutions with preservatives contraindicated for caudal or epidural block.
• Discard partially used vials without preservatives.
• A 5-ml test dose should be injected at least 5 minutes before giving total dose to check for intravascular or subarachnoid injection. Motor paralysis and extensive sensory anesthesia indicate subarachnoid injection.
• For symptoms and treatment of anaphylaxis, see APPENDIX.

Interactions:
ECHOTHIOPHATE IODIDE: reduced hydrolysis of procaine. Use together cautiously.

Special considerations:
• Contraindicated in traumatized urethra and in hypersensitivity to chloroprocaine, tetracaine, or other *p*-aminobenzoic acid derivatives. Use cautiously in CNS diseases, infection at puncture site, shock, profound anemia, cachexia, sepsis, hypertension, hypotension, hyperexcitable patients, GI hemorrhage, bowel perforation or strangulation, peritonitis, cardiac decompensation, massive pleural effusions, and increased intra-abdominal pressure.
• Contraindications to obstetric use: pelvic disproportion, placenta previa, abruptio placentae, floating fetal head, intrauterine manipulation.
• Resuscitative equipment and drugs should be kept available.
• A 1- to 5-ml test dose should be given 5 to 15 minutes before total epidural dose to check for intravascular or subarachnoid injection. Motor paralysis and extensive sensory anesthesia indicate subarachnoid injection.
• Solution without preservatives should be used

(continued on following page)

NAMES, INDICATIONS AND DOSAGES	SIDE EFFECTS

procaine hydrochloride
(continued)

solution and 1 ml diluent injected at third or fourth lumbar interspace.

Up to costal margin: use 2 ml 10% solution and 1 ml diluent injected at second, third, or fourth lumbar interspace.

Epidural block:

Sol.	*Vol. (ml)*	*Dose (mg)*
1.5%	25	375

Peripheral nerve block:

Sol.	*Vol. (ml)*	*Dose (mg)*
1%	50	250
2%	25	500

Infiltration: use 250 to 600 mg 0.25% to 0.5% solution. Maximum initial dose 1 g. Dose and interval may be increased with epinephrine.

tetracaine hydrochloride
Pontocaine♦

Low spinal (saddle block) in vaginal delivery: Give 2 to 5 mg as hyperbaric solution (in 10% dextrose). Maximum dose 15 mg.

Perineum and lower extremities: give 5 to 10 mg.

Prolonged spinal anesthesia (2 to 3 hours): dilute 1% solution with equal volume of cerebrospinal fluid, or dissolve 5 mg powdered drug in 1 ml cerebrospinal fluid immediately before giving. Give 1 ml/5 seconds.

Up to costal margin: give 15 to 20 mg.

Skin: dermatologic reactions.

Other: edema, status asthmaticus, or *anaphylaxis* and anaphylactoid reactions.

Side effects of local anesthetics generally result from high blood levels of the drug. Examples of these are:

CNS: anxiety, apprehension, nervousness, convulsions followed by drowsiness, unconsciousness, and *respiratory arrest.*

CV: myocardial depression, *arrhythmias, cardiac arrest.*

EENT: blurred vision.

GI: nausea, vomiting.

INTERACTIONS AND SPECIAL CONSIDERATIONS

for epidural block.

- Onset in 2 to 5 minutes; duration 60 minutes.
- Discard partially used vials without preservatives.

No significant interactions.

Special considerations:

- Contraindicated in infection at injection site, serious CNS diseases, and in hypersensitivity to procaine, chloroprocaine, tetracaine, or other *p*-aminobenzoic acid derivatives. Use cautiously in shock, profound anemia, cachexia, hypertension, hypotension, peritonitis, cardiac decompensation, massive pleural effusion, increased intracranial pressure, infection, and in highly nervous patients.
- Saddle block contraindicated in cephalopelvic disproportion, placenta previa, abruptio placentae, intrauterine manipulation, floating fetal head.
- Cloudy, discolored, or crystallized solutions should not be used.
- Resuscitative equipment and drugs should be kept available.
- 10 times as strong as procaine HCl.
- Onset in 15 minutes; duration up to 3 to 6 hours.
- When cerebrospinal fluid is added to powdered drug or drug solution during spinal anesthesia, solution may be cloudy.
- Protect from light; store in refrigerator.

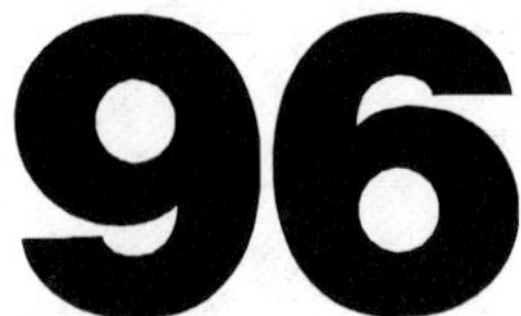

General anesthetics

fentanyl citrate with droperidol
ketamine hydrochloride
methohexital sodium
thiamylal sodium
thiopental sodium

General anesthetics (two types: inhalation and parenteral) are CNS depressants that induce varying degrees of analgesia, depression of consciousness, skeletal muscle relaxation, and reduced reflex activity. Except for ketamine and fentanyl with droperidol, these agents are ultra–short-acting barbiturates. They're potent anesthetics, generally given I.V., that cause loss of consciousness in seconds and allow pleasant recovery.

Ketamine is a short-acting nonbarbiturate that may be given I.V. or I.M. It induces a state of dissociative anesthesia that is characterized by sedation, immobility, amnesia, and marked analgesia. The patient seems awake but is really unconscious.

Fentanyl, a narcotic analgesic, is chemically related to meperidine. It's used in combination with droperidol, a neuroleptic derivative of haloperidol. The combination can be given either I.V. or I.M. and produces neuroleptanalgesia, a state that resembles the dissociative anesthesia caused by ketamine.

Major uses

Parenteral general anesthetics induce anesthesia before administration of inhalation anesthetics. They're also used alone for short-term procedures or for basal anesthesia in children.

- Thiopental sodium is also used to control postanesthetic convulsive states.

Mechanism of action

- Barbiturate anesthetics (methohexital, thiamylal, and thiopental) act by depressing CNS. They inhibit firing rate of neurons within ascending reticular activating system.
- Ketamine appears to interrupt association pathways in the brain, causing dissociative anesthesia, a feeling of dissociation from the environment.
- Fentanyl with droperidol acts as a CNS depressant to produce reduced motor activity and analgesia.

Absorption, distribution, metabolism, and excretion

- All barbiturate anesthetics are given by the I.V. route. They are well distributed to body tissues, metabolized in the liver, and excreted in urine.
- Fentanyl with droperidol is well absorbed from I.M. injection sites and distributed widely to body tissues. It is metabolized in the liver and eliminated in urine and in feces.
- Ketamine is well absorbed after I.M. injection, widely distributed to body tissues, and metabolized in the liver. The metabolite is excreted primarily in urine, with smaller amounts eliminated in feces.

Onset and duration

- Barbiturate anesthetics have an onset within 30 to 60 seconds after administration. Duration is usually 10 to 30 minutes after the last I.V. dose.

  Methohexital furnishes anesthesia for 5 to 15 minutes.

  Thiamylal, when administered rectally, produces maximal effects within 30 minutes; its duration of action is about 1 hour.
- Fentanyl begins to work in seconds; its duration of action is 30 to 60 minutes. Onset

STAGES AND SIGNS IN ANESTHESIA

STAGE	PLANES AND CHARACTERISTICS		SITE OF DEPRESSION ON CNS	THIOPENTAL EFFECTS	BARBITURATE EFFECTS
	Analgesia	**Amnesia**			
I **Analgesia and amnesia** (conscious)	1. None 2. Partial effect 3. Total effect	None Total effect Total effect	Slight-to-moderate depression of cortex	Euphoria, loss of discrimination and inability to interact with the environment	Intercostal and diaphragmatic breathing slows immediately. Patient *may* be quiet or euphoric.
II **Dream** (unconscious)	Unpredictable reactions; irregular breathing		Predominant control by subcortex	Loss of consciousness	No delirium
III **Surgical** Light	1. Rhythmical breathing		Moderate depression of subcortex	Hypoactivity to painful stimulus	Vigilance to airway important; assisted respiration indicated
Medium	2. Sensory loss (pauses after expiration grow longer)		Predominant control by midbrain	Loss of somatic response to pain	Same as for light stage
	3. Level of progressive intercostal paralysis				
Deep	4. Level of diaphragmatic breathing (intercostal paralysis complete)		Moderate depression of midbrain	Loss of visceral response to pain	Same as for light stage
IV **Medullary paralysis**	Respiratory arrest		Moderate depression of pons	Fall in pulse pressure	If continued, cardiac arrest will occur.

Adapted from Etsten and Himwich, *Anesthesiology*, vol. 7 (Philadelphia: J.B. Lippincott Co., 1946) and Possati, et al., *Anesthesia and Analgesia Current Researchers*, vol. 32 (Cleveland: International Anesthesia Research Society, 1953). Used with permission of the publishers.

of droperidol occurs in 3 to 10 minutes; duration is 2 to 4 hours.

- Ketamine has an onset within 30 seconds after I.V. or I.M. administration. Duration, when the drug is given I.V., is 5 to 10 minutes. Duration after I.M. induction is 12 to 25 minutes.

NAMES, INDICATIONS AND DOSAGES	SIDE EFFECTS

fentanyl citrate with droperidol

Controlled Substance Schedule II
Innovar (Each ml contains [in a 1:50 ratio] fentanyl 0.05 mg as a citrate and droperidol 2.5 mg.)

Doses vary depending on application, use of other agents, and patient's age, body weight, and physical status.

ADULTS:
Premedication to anesthesia: 0.5 to 2 ml I.M. 45 to 60 minutes before surgery.
Adjunct to general anesthetic: Induction: 1 ml/20 to 25 lb body weight by slow I.V. to produce neuroleptanalgesia.

Maintenance: not indicated as sole agent for maintenance of surgical anesthesia. Used in combination with other measures. To prevent excessive accumulation of the relatively long-acting droperidol component, fentanyl alone should be used in increments of 0.025 to 0.05 mg (0.5 to 1 ml) for maintenance of analgesia. However, during prolonged surgery, additional 0.5- to 1-ml amounts of Innovar may be given with caution.
Diagnostic procedures: 0.5 to 2 ml I.M. 45 to 60 minutes before procedure. In prolonged procedure, give 0.5 to 1 ml I.V. with caution and without a general anesthetic.
Adjunct in regional anesthesia: 1 to 2 ml I.M. or slow I.V.

CHILDREN:
Premedication: 0.25 ml/20 lb body weight I.M. 45 to 60 minutes before surgery.
Adjunct to general anesthetic:
0.5 ml/20 lb body weight (total combined dose for induction and maintenance). Following induction with Innovar, fentanyl alone in a dose of 1/4 to 1/3 of adult dose should be used to avoid accumulation of droperidol. However, during prolonged surgery, additional amounts of Innovar may be administered with caution. Safety of use in children under 2 years has not been established.

CNS: emergence delirium and hallucinations, postoperative drowsiness.
CV: vasodilation, *hypotension*, decreased pulmonary arterial pressure, bradycardia, or tachycardia.
EENT: blurred vision, *laryngospasms*.
GI: *nausea, vomiting*.
Respiratory: *respiratory depression, apnea*, or *arrest*.
Other: drug dependence, muscle rigidity, chills, *shivering*, twitching, diaphoresis.

ketamine hydrochloride

Ketaject, Ketalar♦

Induce anesthesia for procedures, especially short-term diagnostic or surgical, not requiring skeletal muscle relaxation; before giving other general anesthetics or to supplement low-potency agents, such as nitrous oxide:

ADULTS AND CHILDREN: 1 to 4.5 mg/kg I.V., administered over 60 seconds; or 6.5 to 13 mg/kg I.M. To maintain anesthesia, repeat in increments of half to full initial dose.

CNS: *tonic and clonic movements resembling convulsions, respiratory depression, apnea when administered too rapidly*.
CV: *increased blood pressure and pulse rate*, hypotension, bradycardia.
EENT: diplopia, nystagmus, slight increase in intraocular pressure, *laryngospasms, salivation*.
GI: mild anorexia, nausea, vomiting.
Skin: transient erythema, measleslike rash.
Other: *dreamlike states, hallucinations, confusion, excitement*, irrational behavior, psychic abnormalities.

INTERACTIONS AND SPECIAL CONSIDERATIONS

Interactions:

CNS DEPRESSANTS (SUCH AS BARBITURATES, TRANQUILIZERS, NARCOTICS, AND GENERAL ANESTHETICS): additive or potentiating effect. Dosage should be reduced.

MAO INHIBITORS: severe and unpredictable potentiation of Innovar. Do not use together or within 2 weeks of MAO inhibitor therapy.

Special considerations:

• Contraindicated in intolerance to either component. Use with caution in elderly and debilitated patients, and in those with head injuries and increased intracranial pressure, chronic obstructive pulmonary disease, hepatic and renal dysfunction, bradyarrhythmias.

• Hypotension is a common side effect. However, if blood pressure drops, hypovolemia should also be considered as a possible cause. Appropriate parenteral fluids help restore blood pressure.

• Vital signs should be monitored frequently.

• Respiratory depression, muscular rigidity of respiratory muscles, and respiratory arrest can occur. Narcotic antagonist and CPR equipment should be kept available.

• Airway should be maintained.

• Postoperative EEG pattern may return to normal slowly.

• Postoperatively, if narcotic analgesics are required, should be used initially in reduced doses, as low as ¼ to ⅓ those usually recommended.

• When Innovar is given for anesthesia induction, fentanyl (Sublimaze) should be used for maintenance analgesia during the procedure.

• Premedication with Innovar has sometimes been associated with patient agitation and refusal of surgery. Administration of diazepam may relieve this.

• For symptoms and treatment of toxicity, see APPENDIX.

Interactions:

THYROID HORMONES: may elevate blood pressure and cause tachycardia. Give cautiously.

Special considerations:

• Contraindicated in history of cerebrovascular accident; severe hypertension; severe cardiac decompensation; surgery of the pharynx, larynx, or bronchial tree, unless used with muscle relaxants; and in patients who would be endangered by a significant rise in blood pressure. Use with caution in chronic alcoholism, alcohol-intoxicated patients, and in patients with cerebrospinal fluid pressure elevated before anesthesia.

• Patient should receive nothing by mouth for at least 6 hours before elective surgery.

• Because of rapid induction, patient should be physically supported during administration.

• Barbiturates and ketamine HCl should not be injected from same syringe, as they are chemically incompatible.

• Vital signs should be monitored before, during, and after anesthesia.

• Cardiac function should be checked in patients with hypertension or cardiac depression.

• Airway should be maintained.

• Resuscitation equipment should be available and ready for use.

• Supportive respiration required if respiratory depression occurs. Mechanical support should be used rather than administering analeptics.

(continued on following page)

NAMES, INDICATIONS AND DOSAGES	SIDE EFFECTS

ketamine hydrochloride
(continued)

methohexital sodium
Controlled Substance Schedule IV
Brevital Sodium, Brietal Sodium♦♦

General anesthetic for short-term procedures (oral surgery, gynecologic and genitourinary examinations); reduction of fractures; before electroconvulsive therapy; for prolonged anesthesia when used with gaseous anesthetics:

ADULTS AND CHILDREN: 5 to 12 ml 1% solution (50 to 120 mg) I.V. at 1 ml/5 seconds. Dose required for induction may vary from 50 to 120 mg or more; average about 70 mg. Induction dose provides anesthesia for 5 to 7 minutes. Maintenance—intermittent injection: 2 to 4 ml 1% solution (20 to 40 mg) q 4 to 7 minutes; continuous I.V. drip: administer 0.2% solution (1 drop/second).

CNS: *muscular twitching*, headache, emergence delirium.
CV: *temporary hypotension, tachycardia*, circulatory depression, *peripheral vascular collapse*.
GI: excessive salivation, *nausea, vomiting*.
Skin: tissue necrosis with extravasation.
Local: pain at injection site, injury to nerves adjacent to injection site.
Respiratory: *laryngospasm, bronchospasm, respiratory depression, apnea*.
Other: hiccups, coughing, acute allergic reactions, *twitching*. Extended use may cause cumulative effect.

thiamylal sodium
Controlled Substance Schedule III
Surital♦

General anesthetic for short-term procedures; anesthetic before administering other general anesthetics (dosage individualized to patient's response):

ADULTS: 3 to 6 ml 2.5% solution I.V. at 1 ml/5 seconds. Additional intermittent injections of 0.5 to 1 ml. Maximum dose 1 g (40 ml 2.5% solution).

Rectal administration before diagnostic procedures:

CHILDREN: 800 mg to 1 g 5% solution/22.5 kg body weight.

Supplemental anesthetic:

ADULTS: 0.2% or 0.3% solution continuous I.V. drip. Recovery occurs within 20 to 30 minutes after last injection.

CNS: excitement, headache, emergence delirium.
CV: hypotension, *circulatory depression*, thrombophlebitis, *hypoxia*.
GI: nausea, vomiting, excessive salivation.
Skin: rash, urticaria, tissue necrosis with extravasation.
Respiratory: *laryngospasm, bronchospasm, respiratory depression, apnea*.
Local: pain at injection site, injury to nerves adjacent to injection site.
Other: hiccups. Extended use can cause cumulative effects.

thiopental sodium
Controlled Substance Schedule III
Pentothal Sodium♦
(injection and rectal suspension)

Induce anesthesia before administering other anesthetics:

210 to 280 mg (3 to 4 ml/kg) usually required for average adult (70 kg).

General anesthetic for short-term procedures:

ADULTS: 2 to 3 ml 2.5% solution (50 to

CNS: *prolonged somnolence*, retrograde amnesia.
CV: *myocardial depression, arrhythmias*.
Skin: tissue necrosis with extravasation.
Respiratory: *respiratory depression (momentary apnea following each injection is typical), bronchospasm, laryngospasm*.
Local: pain at injection site.
Other: sneezing, coughing, *shivering*.

♦ Available in U.S. and Canada. ♦♦ Available in Canada only.
All other products (no symbol) available in U.S. only. Italicized side effects are common or life-threatening.

INTERACTIONS AND SPECIAL CONSIDERATIONS	
• Keep verbal, tactile, and visual stimulation at a minimum during recovery phase to reduce incidence of emergent reactions. • Hallucinations and excitement can occur on emergence from anesthesia; they can be abated by administering diazepam.	• A potent hallucinogen that can readily produce dissociative anesthesia (patient feels detached from environment). Dissociative effect and hallucinatory side effects have made this a popular drug of abuse among young people.
No significant interactions. *Special considerations:* • Contraindicated in severe hepatic dysfunction, hypersensitivity to barbiturates, or porphyria; in shock or impending shock; and in patients for whom general anesthetics would be hazardous. Use with caution in debilitated patients, and in patients with asthma, respiratory obstruction, severe hypertension or hypotension, myocardial disease, congestive heart failure, severe anemia, or extreme obesity. • Pulmonary ventilation should be maintained. • Extravascular or intra-arterial injections should be avoided. • Vital signs should be monitored before, during, and after anesthesia. • Resuscitative equipment and drugs should be available.	• Fasting before administration reduces postoperative nausea. • Incompatible with silicone. Contact with rubber stoppers or parts of syringes that have been treated with silicone should be avoided. • Incompatible with lactated Ringer's solution. • Should not be mixed with acid solutions such as atropine sulfate. • Solvents recommended are 5% glucose solution or isotonic (0.9%) sodium chloride instead of distilled water. • Rate of flow must be individualized for each patient. • Solutions may be stored and used as long as they remain clear and colorless. Solutions cannot be heated for sterilization. • Has potential for abuse.
No significant interactions. *Special considerations:* • Contraindicated in hepatic dysfunction or disease, traumatic or impending shock, porphyria, hypersensitivity to barbiturates, and in patients for whom general anesthetics would be hazardous. Use with caution in respiratory disease or obstruction, obesity, marked disturbance of arterial tension, cardiac failure, anemia, status asthmaticus, endocrine or renal dysfunction, and in debilitated patients. • Airway should be maintained. • Resuscitative equipment and drugs should be available. • Vital signs should be monitored before, during, and after anesthesia. • Extravascular or intra-arterial injection should be avoided. • Incompatible with lactated Ringer's solution or with solutions containing bacteriostatic or buffer agents, which tend to cause precipitation.	• Air should not be injected into solution: may cause cloudiness. • Sterile water is the preferred solvent for injections. For drip maintenance, use of 5% glucose or isotonic sodium chloride avoids extreme hypotonicity. • Solutions of atropine sulfate, *d*-tubocurarine, or succinylcholine may be given concurrently but should not be mixed together. • Solutions should not be heated for sterilization. Solutions should be stored in refrigerator and used within 6 days; at room temperature, within 24 hours. • Has potential for abuse.
No significant interactions. *Special considerations:* • Contraindicated in absence of suitable veins for intravenous administration, hypersensitivity to barbiturates, status asthmaticus, porphyria, respiratory depression or obstruction, decompensated cardiac disease, severe anemia, hepatic cirrhosis, shock, renal dysfunction, increased intracranial pressure, myxedema. • Test dose (1 to 3 ml 2.5% solution) should be given to assess reaction to drug. • When used as general anesthetic, atropine sulfate should be given as premedication to diminish laryngeal reflexes and to prevent spastic abduction of vocal cords.	• Resuscitative equipment and oxygen should be kept available. • Extravasation and intra-arterial injection should be avoided. • Airway should be maintained. • Vital signs should be monitored before, during, and after anesthesia. • Solutions of atropine sulfate, *d*-tubocurarine, or succinylcholine may be given concurrently but should not be mixed together.

(continued on following page)

NAMES, INDICATIONS AND DOSAGES	SIDE EFFECTS

thiopental sodium
(continued)

75 mg) administered I.V. only at intervals of 20 to 40 seconds, depending on reaction. Dose may be repeated with caution, if necessary.
Convulsive states following anesthesia: 75 to 125 mg (3 to 5 ml of 2.5% solution) immediately.
Psychiatric disorders (narcoanalysis, narcosynthesis): 100 mg/minute (4 ml/minute 2.5% solution) until confusion occurs and before sleep. Maximum dose 50 ml/minute.

Basal anesthesia by rectal administration:
ADULTS AND CHILDREN: administer up to 1 g/22.5 kg (50 lb) body weight, or 0.5 ml 10% solution/kg body weight. Maximum 1 to 1.5 g (children weighing 34 kg or more) and 3 to 4 g (adults weighing 91 kg or more).
Note: Thiopental is rarely administered rectally for basal sedation or anesthesia because of variable absorption from the rectum.

INTERACTIONS AND SPECIAL CONSIDERATIONS

• Do not heat solutions for sterilization. Store solutions in refrigerator and use within 6 days; at room temperature, within 24 hours.
• Has potential for abuse.

97

Vitamins and minerals

vitamin A
- oleovitamin A

vitamin B complex
- cyanocobalamin (B_{12})
- cyanocobalamin hydroxocobalamin (B_{12a})
- folic acid (B_9)
- leucovorin calcium
- niacin (B_3)
- niacinamide
- pyridoxine hydrochloride (B_6)
- riboflavin (B_2)
- thiamine hydrochloride (B_1)

vitamin C
- ascorbic acid

vitamin D
- cholecalciferol (D_3)
- ergocalciferol (D_2)

vitamin E

vitamin K analogs
- menadione/menadiol sodium diphosphate (K_3)
- phytonadione (K_1)

multivitamins

sodium fluoride

trace elements
- chromium
- copper
- iodine
- manganese
- zinc
- zinc sulfate

Vitamins are organic dietary constituents that are necessary for health. Supplied in small amounts, they're important components of enzyme systems that catalyze metabolic reactions. Diseases now known to be caused by vitamin deficiencies include night blindness (vitamin A deficiency), beriberi (thiamine deficiency), pellagra (niacin deficiency), scurvy (ascorbic acid deficiency), and rickets (vitamin D deficiency). Vitamins have been categorized as water-soluble (B complex and C) and fat-soluble (A, D, E, and K).

Trace elements are inorganic substances needed in small quantities to maintain homeostasis.

Major uses

- Vitamins are used to prevent or treat selective or multiple vitamin deficiencies. They're essential to the proper synthesis and metabolism of body protein.
- Trace elements are used to prevent or treat dietary deficiencies and other clinical problems that result from these deficiencies.

Zinc sulfate is also a therapeutic adjunct for various skin disorders, acrodermatitis enteropathica, rheumatoid arthritis, and hypogeusia (reduced sense of taste) when these disorders coexist with low serum zinc levels.

Chromium enhances intracellular transport of insulin and glucose.

Copper is essential for the synthesis of ceruloplasmin, which aids the normal flow of iron from cells to plasma and catalyzes the oxidation of iron from the ferrous to the ferric state.

Iodine aids in the synthesis of the thyroid hormones thyroxine and triiodothyronine.

Manganese is used by enzymes involved in polysaccharide synthesis.

- Sodium fluoride is used to retard tooth decay and may be beneficial in bone disorders.

Mechanism of action

• Vitamins act as coenzymes or coenzyme precursors to catalyze protein, fat, and carbohydrate metabolism, and to facilitate energy-producing and anabolic reactions.

• Trace elements may act in metalloenzyme units. Trace elements participate in synthesis and stabilization of proteins and nucleic acids in subcellular and membrane transport systems.

• Sodium fluoride's mechanism is unknown; however, the compound may catalyze bone remineralization.

Absorption, distribution, metabolism, and excretion

• Vitamins are readily absorbed and distributed in the body tissues. Excretion rates of water-soluble vitamins vary with metabolic status, stress, disease, and requirements for tissue repair. Excess water-soluble vitamins (B and C) are generally metabolized in the liver and rapidly excreted in urine. Fat-soluble vitamins (A, D, E, and K), which require bile and adequate pancreatic secretions for absorption, are stored for longer periods.

• Vitamins A and E are metabolized largely in the liver and eliminated mainly through the bile in feces.

• Vitamin D has a complex metabolism. Cholecalciferol and ergocalciferol are metabolized in the liver to more active metabolites (25-hydroxy derivatives). In the kidneys, these forms are metabolized to their 1,25-dihydroxy derivatives, which are even more active. Eventually, all vitamin D metabolites are eliminated mainly through the bile in feces.

• Vitamin K's metabolism and excretion are unknown.

• Trace minerals are readily absorbed after oral or parenteral administration and distributed throughout the body. They are excreted largely unchanged in urine.

Onset and duration

Most vitamin and trace element deficiencies respond quickly to therapeutic doses. Duration of action depends on the patient's total metabolic needs.

Combination products

Vitamin A and D combinations
B vitamin combinations
B complex vitamins
B complex with vitamin C
Multivitamins
Multivitamins with B_{12}
Calcium and vitamin products
Fluoride with vitamins
B complex vitamins with iron
Miscellaneous vitamins and minerals
Geriatric supplements with multivitamins and minerals
Multivitamins and minerals with hormones

NAMES, INDICATIONS AND DOSAGES	SIDE EFFECTS

oleovitamin A

Acon, Afaxin♦♦, Alphalin, Aquasol A♦, Dispatabs, Natola

Severe vitamin A deficiency with xerophthalmia:

ADULTS AND CHILDREN OVER 8 YEARS: 500,000 IU P.O. daily for 3 days, then 50,000 IU P.O. daily for 14 days, then maintenance with 10,000 to 20,000 IU P.O. daily for 2 months, followed by adequate dietary nutrition and RDA vitamin A supplements.

Severe vitamin A deficiency:

ADULTS AND CHILDREN OVER 8 YEARS: 100,000 IU P.O. or I.M. daily for 3 days, then 50,000 IU P.O. or I.M. daily for 14 days, then maintenance with 10,000 to 20,000 IU P.O. daily for 2 months, followed by adequate dietary nutrition and RDA vitamin A supplements.

CHILDREN 1 TO 8 YEARS: 17,500 to 35,000 IU I.M. daily for 10 days.

INFANTS UNDER 1 YEAR: 7,500 to 15,000 IU I.M. daily for 10 days.

Maintenance only:

CHILDREN 4 TO 8 YEARS: 15,000 IU I.M. daily for 2 months, then adequate dietary nutrition and RDA vitamin A supplements.

CHILDREN UNDER 4 YEARS: 10,000 IU I.M. daily for 2 months, then adequate dietary nutrition and RDA vitamin A supplements.

Side effects are usually seen only with toxicity (hypervitaminosis A).

Blood: hypoplastic anemia, leukopenia.

CNS: irritability, headache, increased intracranial pressure, fatigue, lethargy, malaise.

EENT: miosis, papilledema, exophthalmos.

GI: anorexia, epigastric pain, diarrhea.

GU: hypomenorrhea.

Hepatic: jaundice, hepatomegaly.

Skin: alopecia; drying, cracking, scaling of skin; pruritus; lip fissures; massive desquamation; increased pigmentation; night sweating

Other: skeletal—slow growth, decalcification of bone, fractures, hyperostosis, painful periostitis, premature closure of epiphyses, migratory arthralgia, cortical thickening over the radius and tibia, bulging fontanelles; splenomegaly.

cyanocobalamin (vitamin B_{12})

Anacobin♦♦, Bedoce, Bedoz♦♦, Berubigen, Betalin-12, Bio-12♦♦, Crystimin, Cyanabin♦♦, Cyanocobalamin, Cyano-Gel, DBH-B_{12}, Dodex, Kaybovite, Pernavite, Poyamin, Redisol♦, Rubesol, Rubion♦♦, Rubramin♦, Ruvite, Sigamine, Vibedoz, Vi-Twel

cyanocobalamin, hydroxocobalamin (vitamin B_{12a})

Alpha Redisol, Alpha-Ruvite, Codroxomin, Droxomin, Neo-Betalin 12, Rubesol-LA, Sytobex-H

Vitamin B_{12} deficiency due to inadequate diet, subtotal gastrectomy, or any other condition, disorder, or disease except malabsorption related to pernicious anemia or other gastrointestinal disease:

ADULTS: 25 mcg P.O. daily as dietary supplement, or 30 to 100 mcg S.C. or I.M. daily for 5 to 10 days, depending on severity of deficiency. Maintenance dose: 100 to 200 mcg I.M. once monthly. For subsequent prophylaxis, advise adequate nutrition and daily RDA vitamin B_{12} supplements.

CHILDREN: 1 mcg P.O. daily as dietary supplement, or 1 to 30 mcg S.C. or I.M. daily for 5 to 10 days, depending on severity of deficiency. Maintenance: at least 60 mcg/month I.M. or

CV: peripheral vascular thrombosis.

GI: transient diarrhea.

Skin: itching, transitory exanthema, urticaria.

Local: pain, burning at S.C. or I.M. injection sites.

Other: *anaphylaxis*, anaphylactoid reactions.

♦ Available in U.S. and Canada. ♦♦ Available in Canada only.
All other products (no symbol) available in U.S. only. Italicized side effects are common or life-threatening.

INTERACTIONS AND SPECIAL CONSIDERATIONS

Interactions:
MINERAL OIL, CHOLESTYRAMINE RESIN: reduced GI absorption of fat-soluble vitamins. If needed, give mineral oil at bedtime.

Special considerations:
• Oral administration contraindicated in presence of malabsorption syndrome; if malabsorption is due to inadequate bile secretion, oral route may be used with concurrent administration of bile salts (dehydrocholic acid). Also contraindicated in hypervitaminosis A. Intravenous administration contraindicated except for special water-miscible forms intended for infusion with large parenteral volumes. Intravenous push of vitamin A of any type is also contraindicated (anaphylaxis or anaphylactoid reactions and death have resulted).
• *Caution:* Evaluate intake from fortified foods, dietary supplements, self-administered drugs, and prescription drug sources.
• In pregnant women, doses should not exceed 6,000 IU daily.
• To avoid toxicity, patient self-administration of megavitamin doses should be discouraged without specific indications. Also, prescribed vitamins should not be shared with family or others. Family member who feels vitamin therapy may be of value should contact his doctor.
• Side effects may occur if dosage is high.
• Acute toxicity has resulted from single doses of 25,000 IU/kg of body weight; 350,000 IU in infants and over 2,000,000 IU in adults have also proved acutely toxic.
• Chronic toxicity in infants (3 to 6 months) has resulted from doses of 18,500 IU daily for 1 to 3 months. In adults, chronic toxicity has resulted from doses of 50,000 IU daily for over 18 months; 500,000 IU daily for 2 months; and 1,000,000 IU daily for 3 days.
• Patient should be monitored closely during vitamin A therapy for skin disorders, since high dosages may induce chronic toxicity.
• Liquid preparations available if nasogastric administration is needed.
• Eating and bowel habits should be monitored.
• Adequate vitamin A absorption requires suitable protein intake, bile (give supplemental salts if necessary), concurrent RDA doses of vitamin E; and zinc (multivitamins usually supply zinc, but supplements may be necessary in long-term hyperalimentation).
• Absorption is faster and more complete with water-miscible preparations, intermediate with emulsions, and slowest with oil suspensions.
• In severe hepatic dysfunction, diabetes, and hypothyroidism, vitamin A should be used rather than carotenes for vitamin therapy, because the vitamin itself is more easily absorbed and the diseases adversely affect conversion of carotenes into vitamin A. If carotenes are prescribed, dosage should be doubled.
• Protect from light.

Interactions:
PARA-AMINOSALICYLIC ACID AND SALTS, NEOMYCIN, COLCHICINE, CHLORAMPHENICOL: malabsorption of vitamin B_{12}. Don't use together.

Special considerations:
• Parenteral administration contraindicated in hypersensitivity to vitamin B_{12} or cobalt. Alternate use of large oral doses of vitamin B_{12} is controversial and should not be considered routine; combined with intrinsic factor increases risk of hypersensitive reactions and should be avoided. Therapeutic dose contraindicated before proper diagnosis; B_{12} therapy may mask folate deficiency.
• I.V. administration may cause anaphylactic reactions. Should be used cautiously and only if other routes are ruled out.
• Use cautiously in anemic patients with coexisting cardiac, pulmonary, or hypertension problems; in patients with early Leber's disease; in patients with severe B_{12}-dependent deficiencies, especially those receiving cardiac glycosides (patient should be monitored closely the first 2 to 3 days for hypokalemia, fluid overload, pulmonary edema, congestive heart failure, and hypertension); and in patients with gouty conditions (monitor serum uric acid levels for hyperuricemia).
• Parenteral liquids should not be mixed in same syringe with other medication.
• Protect from light.
• Repository forms add cost without extra effectiveness and may stimulate antibody formation.
• Infection, tumors, or renal, hepatic, and other debilitating diseases may reduce therapeutic response.
• Deficiencies more common in strict vegetarians and their breast-fed infants.
• Patients with pernicious anemia should return for monthly injections. Although total body stores may last 3 to 6 years, anemia will recur if not treated monthly.
• May cause false-positive intrinsic factor antibody test.
• B_{12a} is approved for I.M. use only. Only advantage of B_{12a} over B_{12} is longer duration.
• 50% to 98% of injected dose may appear in urine within 48 hours. Major portion is excreted within the first 8 hours.
• Close observation for serum potassium needed the first 48 hours and potassium given if necessary.
• Serum uric acid and CBC should be monitored.
• Physically incompatible with dextrose solutions, alkaline or strongly acidic solutions, oxidizing and reducing agents, and many other

(continued on following page)

NAMES, INDICATIONS AND DOSAGES	SIDE EFFECTS

cyanocobalamin
(continued)

S.C. For subsequent prophylaxis, advise adequate nutrition and daily RDA vitamin B_{12} supplements.

Pernicious anemia or vitamin B_{12} malabsorption:
ADULTS: initially, 100 to 1,000 mcg I.M. daily for 2 weeks, then 100 to 1,000 mcg I.M. once monthly for life. If neurologic complications are present, follow initial therapy with 100 to 1,000 mcg I.M. once every 2 weeks before starting monthly regimen.
CHILDREN: 1,000 to 5,000 mcg I.M. or S.C. given over 2 or more weeks in 100-mcg increments; then 60 mcg I.M. or S.C. monthly for life.

Methylmalonic aciduria:
NEONATES: 1,000 mcg I.M. daily for 11 days with a protein-restricted diet.

Diagnostic test for vitamin B_{12} deficiency without concealing folate deficiency in patients with megaloblastic anemias:
ADULTS AND CHILDREN: 1 mcg I.M. daily for 10 days with diet low in vitamin B_{12} and folate. Reticulocytosis between days 3 and 10 confirms diagnosis of vitamin B_{12} deficiency.

Schilling test flushing dose:
ADULTS AND CHILDREN: 1,000 mcg I.M. in a single dose.

folic acid (vitamin B_9)
Folvite♦, Novofolacid♦♦

Megaloblastic or macrocytic anemia secondary to folic acid or other nutritional deficiency, hepatic disease, alcoholism, intestinal obstruction, excessive hemolysis:
PREGNANT AND LACTATING WOMEN: 0.8 mg P.O., S.C., or I.M. daily.
ADULTS AND CHILDREN OVER 4 YEARS: 1 mg P.O., S.C., or I.M. daily for 4 to 5 days. After anemia secondary to folic acid deficiency is corrected, proper diet and RDA supplements are necessary to prevent recurrence.
CHILDREN UNDER 4 YEARS: up to 0.3 mg P.O., S.C., or I.M. daily.

Prevention of megaloblastic anemia of pregnancy and fetal damage:
WOMEN: 1 mg P.O., S.C., or I.M. daily throughout pregnancy.

Nutritional supplement:
ADULTS: 0.1 mg P.O., S.C., or I.M. daily.
CHILDREN: 0.05 mg P.O. daily.

SIDE EFFECTS (folic acid):

Skin: allergic reactions (rash, pruritus, erythema).
Other: *allergic bronchospasms,* general malaise.

♦ Available in U.S. and Canada. ♦♦ Available in Canada only.
All other products (no symbol) available in U.S. only. Italicized side effects are common or life-threatening.

INTERACTIONS AND SPECIAL CONSIDERATIONS

drugs.
• For treatment of anaphylaxis, see APPENDIX.

Interactions:
CHLORAMPHENICOL: antagonism of folic acid. Monitor for decreased folic acid effect. Use together cautiously.

Special considerations:
• Contraindicated in normocytic, refractory, or aplastic anemias; as sole agent in treatment of pernicious anemia (since it may mask neurologic effects); in treatment of methotrexate, pyrimethamine, or trimethoprim overdose; and in undiagnosed anemia (since it may mask pernicious anemia).
• Patients with small bowel resections and intestinal malabsorption may require parenteral administration routes.
• Should not be mixed with other medications in the same syringe for I.M. injections.
• Protect from light.
• Concurrent folic acid and vitamin B_{12} therapy may be used if supported by diagnosis.
• Proper nutrition is necessary to prevent recurrence of anemia.
• Peak folate activity occurs in the blood in 30 to 60 minutes.
• Hematologic response to folic acid in patients receiving chloramphenicol concurrently with folic acid should be carefully monitored.

(continued on following page)

NAMES, INDICATIONS AND DOSAGES	SIDE EFFECTS

folic acid
(continued)

Treatment of tropical sprue:
ADULTS: 3 to 15 mg P.O. daily.

Test of megaloblastic anemia patients to detect folic acid deficiency without masking pernicious anemia:
ADULTS AND CHILDREN: 0.1 to 0.2 mg P.O. or I.M. for 10 days while maintaining a diet low in folate and vitamin B_{12}.
(Reticulosis, reversion to normoblastic hematopoiesis, and return to normal hemoglobin indicate folic acid deficiency.)

---

leucovorin calcium (citrovorum factor or folinic acid)
Calcium Folinate

Overdose of folic acid antagonist:
ADULTS AND CHILDREN: P.O., I.M., or I.V. dose equivalent to the weight of the antagonist given.

Leucovorin rescue after high methotrexate dose in treatment of malignancy:
ADULTS AND CHILDREN: dose at doctor's discretion within 6 to 36 hours of last dose of methotrexate.

Toxic effects of methotrexate used to treat severe psoriasis:
ADULTS AND CHILDREN: 4 to 8 mg I.M. 2 hours after methotrexate dose.

Hematologic toxicity due to pyrimethamine therapy:
ADULTS AND CHILDREN: 5 mg P.O. or I.M. daily.

Hematologic toxicity due to trimethoprim therapy:
ADULTS AND CHILDREN: 400 mcg to 5 mg P.O. or I.M. daily.

Megaloblastic anemia due to congenital enzyme deficiency:
ADULTS AND CHILDREN: 3 to 6 mg I.M. daily, then 1 mg P.O. daily for life.

Folate-deficient megaloblastic anemias:
ADULTS AND CHILDREN: up to 1 mg of leucovorin I.M daily. Duration of treatment depends on hematologic response.

Skin: allergic reactions (rash, pruritus, erythema).
Other: *allergic bronchospasms.*

---

niacin (vitamin B_3, nicotinic acid)
niacinamide (nicotinamide)
Diacin, Lipo-Nicin, Niac, Nico400, Nicobid, Nicocap, Nicolar, Nico-Span, Ni-Span, Vasotherm

Most side effects are dose-dependent.
CNS: dizziness, transient headache.
CV: *excessive peripheral vasodilation.*
GI: *nausea, vomiting, diarrhea,* possible activation of peptic ulcer, epigastric or substernal pain.
Hepatic: hepatic dysfunction.

INTERACTIONS AND SPECIAL CONSIDERATIONS

No significant interactions.

Special considerations:
• Contraindicated in treatment of undiagnosed anemia, since it may mask pernicious anemia. Use cautiously in pernicious anemia; a hemolytic remission may occur while neurologic manifestations remain progressive.
• Leucovorin (folinic acid) should not be confused with folic acid.
• Leucovorin rescue schedule and protocol should be followed closely to maximize therapeutic response. Generally, leucovorin should not be administered simultaneously with systemic methotrexate.
• Overdosage of folic acid antagonists should be treated within 1 hour if possible; treatment usually ineffective after 4-hour delay.
• Protect from light, especially reconstituted parenteral preparations.
• Since allergic reactions have been reported with folic acid, the possibility of allergic reactions to leucovorin should be kept in mind.

Interactions:
ANTIHYPERTENSIVE DRUGS OF THE SYMPATHETIC BLOCKING TYPE: may have an additive vasodilating effect and cause postural hypotension. Use together cautiously. Warn patient about postural hypotension.

Special considerations:
• Contraindicated in hepatic dysfunction, active peptic ulcer disease, severe hypotension, arterial hemorrhage. Use with caution in patients with gallbladder disease, diabetes mellitus, or gout.
• Hepatic function and blood glucose should be

(continued on following page)

NAMES, INDICATIONS AND DOSAGES	SIDE EFFECTS
niacin *(continued)* **Pellagra:** ADULTS: 10 to 20 mg P.O., S.C., I.M., or I.V. infusion daily, depending on severity of niacin deficiency. Maximum daily dose recommended, 500 mg; divide into 10 doses, 50 mg each. CHILDREN: up to 300 mg P.O. or 100 mg I.V. infusion daily, depending on severity of niacin deficiency. After symptoms subside, adequate nutrition and RDA supplements prevent recurrence. **Hyperlipoproteinemia types III, IV, and V, and as secondary agent in type II:** ADULTS: up to 1 g 3 or 4 times a day. **Peripheral vascular disease and circulatory disorders:** ADULTS: 250 to 800 mg P.O. daily in divided doses.	**Metabolic:** hyperglycemia, hyperuricemia. **Skin:** *flushing*, pruritus, dryness.
pyridoxine hydrochloride (vitamin B_6) Bee six, Hexa-Betalin♦, Hexacrest **Dietary vitamin B_6 deficiency:** ADULTS: 10 to 20 mg P.O., I.M., or I.V. daily for 3 weeks, then 2 to 5 mg daily as a supplement to a proper diet. CHILDREN: 100 mg P.O., I.M., or I.V. to correct deficiency, then an adequate diet with supplementary RDA doses to prevent recurrence. **Seizures related to vitamin B_6 deficiency or dependency:** ADULTS AND CHILDREN: 100 mg I.M. or I.V. in single dose. **Vitamin B_6-responsive anemias or dependency syndrome (inborn errors of metabolism):** ADULTS: up to 600 mg P.O., I.M., or I.V. daily until symptoms subside, then 50 mg daily for life. CHILDREN: 100 mg I.M. or I.V., then 2 to 10 mg I.M. or 10 to 100 mg P.O. daily. **Prevention of vitamin B_6 deficiency during isoniazid therapy:** ADULTS: 25 to 50 mg P.O. daily. CHILDREN: at least 0.5 to 1.5 mg daily. INFANTS: at least 0.1 to 0.5 mg daily. If neurologic symptoms develop in pediatric patients, increase dosage as necessary. **Treatment of vitamin B_6 deficiency secondary to isoniazid:** ADULTS: 100 mg P.O. daily for 3 weeks, then 50 mg daily. CHILDREN: titrate dosages.	**CNS:** drowsiness, paresthesias.

INTERACTIONS AND SPECIAL CONSIDERATIONS

monitored early in therapy.

- Should be given with meals to minimize GI side effects.
- Timed-release niacin or niacinamide may avoid excessive flushing effects with large doses. Should be given slowly I.V. Patient should know flushing syndrome is harmless.
- Medication used to treat hyperlipoproteinemia or to dilate peripheral vessels not "just a vitamin." Adhering to therapeutic regimen is important.

No significant interactions.

Special considerations:

- Contraindicated in hypersensitivity to parenteral pyridoxine and in doses larger than 5 mg for patients also receiving levodopa. Patient should check dosage, especially in multivitamins.
- Protect from light. Injection solution should not be used if it contains a precipitate. Slight darkening is acceptable.
- Excessive protein intake increases daily pyridoxine requirements.
- If sodium bicarbonate is required to control acidosis in isoniazid toxicity, should not be mixed in same syringe with pyridoxine.
- If prescribed for maintenance therapy to prevent deficiency recurrence, compliance and good nutrition are important. Pyridoxine in combination therapy with isoniazid has a specific therapeutic purpose and is not "just a vitamin." Adhering to therapeutic regimen is necessary.
- Patients receiving levodopa alone (not with carbidopa) shouldn't take pyridoxine.

NAMES, INDICATIONS AND DOSAGES	SIDE EFFECTS

riboflavin (vitamin B_2)

Riboflavin deficiency or adjunct to thiamine treatment for polyneuritis or cheilosis secondary to pellagra:

ADULTS AND CHILDREN OVER 12 YEARS: 5 to 50 mg P.O., S.C., I.M., or I.V. daily, depending on severity.

CHILDREN UNDER 12 YEARS: 2 to 10 mg P.O., S.C., I.M., or I.V. daily, depending on severity.

For maintenance, increase nutritional intake and supplement with vitamin B complex.

GU: high doses make urine bright yellow.

thiamine hydrochloride (vitamin B_1)

Apatate Drops, Betaline S, Betaxin♦♦, Megamin♦♦, Thia

Beriberi:

ADULTS: 10 to 500 mg, depending on severity, I.M. t.i.d. for 2 weeks, followed by dietary correction and multivitamin supplement containing 5 to 10 mg daily thiamine for 1 month.

CHILDREN: 10 to 50 mg, depending on severity, I.M. daily for several weeks with adequate dietary intake.

Anemia secondary to thiamine deficiency; polyneuritis secondary to alcoholism, pregnancy, or pellagra:

ADULTS: 100 mg P.O. daily.

CHILDREN: 10 to 50 mg P.O. daily in divided doses.

Wernicke's encephalopathy:

ADULTS: up to 500 mg to 1 g I.V. for crisis therapy, followed by 100 mg b.i.d. for maintenance.

"Wet beriberi," with myocardial failure:

ADULTS AND CHILDREN: 100 to 500 mg I.V. for emergency treatment.

CNS: restlessness.
CV: *hypotension after rapid I.V. injection,* angioneurotic edema, cyanosis.
EENT: tightness of throat (allergic reaction).
GI: nausea, hemorrhage, diarrhea.
Skin: feeling of warmth, pruritus, urticaria, sweating.
Other: *anaphylactic reactions,* weakness, pulmonary edema.

ascorbic acid (vitamin C)

Adenex♦♦, Ascorbajen, Ascorbicap, Ascorbineed, Ascoril♦♦, Best-C, Cecon, Cemill, Cenolate, Cetane, Cevalin, Cevi-Bid, Ce-Vi-Sol♦, Cevita, C-Ject, C-Long, C-Syrup-500, Megascorb♦♦, Redoxon♦♦, Saro-C, Solucap C, Vitacee, Viterra C

Frank manifestations of scurvy and subclinical scurvy:

ADULTS: 100 mg to 2 g, depending on severity, P.O., S.C., I.M., or I.V. daily, then at least 50 mg daily for maintenance.

CHILDREN: 100 to 200 mg, depending on severity, P.O., S.C., I.M., or I.V. daily, then at least 35 mg daily for maintenance.

INFANTS: 50 to 100 mg P.O., I.M., I.V., or S.C. daily.

Extensive burns, delayed fracture or wound

CNS: faintness or dizziness with fast I.V. administration.
GI: diarrhea, epigastric burning.
GU: acid urine, oxaluria, renal calculi.
Skin: discomfort at injection site.

♦ Available in U.S. and Canada. ♦♦ Available in Canada only.
All other products (no symbol) available in U.S. only. Italicized side effects are common or life-threatening.

INTERACTIONS AND SPECIAL CONSIDERATIONS

No significant interactions.

Special considerations:
• Protect from light.
• Proper nutritional habits are important to avoid recurrence of deficiency.
• Riboflavin deficiency usually accompanies other B complex deficiencies and may require multivitamin therapy.

No significant interactions.

Special considerations:
• Contraindicated in hypersensitivity to thiamine products. I.V. push contraindicated, except when treating life-threatening myocardial failure in "wet beriberi." Use with caution in I.V. administration of large doses (to avoid anaphylactic reactions); patients with history of hypersensitivity should have skin test before therapy. Have epinephrine on hand to treat anaphylaxis should it occur after a large parenteral dose.
• Parenteral administration should be used only when oral route is not feasible.
• Clinically significant deficiency can occur in approximately 3 weeks of totally thiamine-free diet. Thiamine deficiency usually requires concurrent treatment for multiple deficiencies.
• Doses larger than 30 mg t.i.d. may not be fully utilized. After tissue saturation with thiamine, it is excreted in urine as pyrimidine.
• If beriberi occurs in a breast-fed infant, both mother and child should be treated with thiamine.
• Unstable in alkaline solutions; should not be used with materials that yield alkaline solutions.
• For treatment of anaphylaxis, see APPENDIX.

No significant interactions.

Special considerations:
• Use cautiously in G-6-PD deficiency to avoid possibility of hemolytic anemia.
• Rapid I.V. administration should be avoided.
• Protect solution from light.
• Self-administration for colds should be discouraged; harmful side effects possible.
• I.V. form used investigationally as adjunct to treat some forms of cancer.

(continued on following page)

NAMES, INDICATIONS AND DOSAGES	SIDE EFFECTS

ascorbic acid
(continued)

healing, postoperative wound healing, severe febrile or chronic disease states:
ADULTS: 200 to 500 mg S.C., I.M., or I.V. daily.
CHILDREN: 100 to 200 mg P.O., S.C., I.M., or I.V. daily.

Prevention of vitamin C deficiency in those with poor nutritional habits or increased requirements:
ADULTS: at least 45 to 50 mg P.O., S.C., I.M., or I.V. daily.
PREGNANT OR LACTATING WOMEN: at least 60 mg P.O., S.C., I.M., or I.V. daily.
CHILDREN: at least 40 mg P.O., S.C., I.M., or I.V. daily.
INFANTS: at least 35 mg P.O., S.C., I.M., or I.V. daily.

Potentiation of methenamine in urine acidification:
ADULTS: 4 to 12 g daily in divided doses.

Preoperatively before gastrectomy:
ADULTS: 1 g daily for 4 to 7 days.

---

vitamin D
(cholecalciferol: vitamin D_3; ergocalciferol: vitamin D_2)
Calciferol, Deltalin, Drisdol♦, Radiostol♦♦, Radiostol Forte♦♦

Rickets and other vitamin D deficiency diseases:
ADULTS: 12,000 IU P.O. or I.M. daily initially, increased as indicated by response up to 500,000 IU daily in most cases and up to 800,000 IU daily for vitamin D–resistant rickets.
CHILDREN: 1,500 to 5,000 IU P.O. or I.M. daily for 2 to 4 weeks, repeated after 2 weeks, if necessary. Alternatively, a single dose of 600,000 IU.
Monitor serum calcium daily to guide dosage. After correction of deficiency, maintenance includes adequate dietary nutrition and RDA supplements.

Hypoparathyroidism:
ADULTS AND CHILDREN: 50,000 to 200,000 IU P.O. or I.M. daily, with 4 g calcium supplement.

Side effects listed are usual only in vitamin D toxicity.
CNS: headache, dizziness, ataxia, weakness, somnolence, decreased libido, overt psychosis, convulsions.
CV: calcifications of soft tissues, including the heart.
EENT: dry mouth, metallic taste, rhinorrhea, conjunctivitis (calcific), photophobia, tinnitus.
GI: anorexia, nausea, constipation, diarrhea.
GU: polyuria, albuminuria, hypercalciuria, nocturia, impaired renal function, renal calculi.
Metabolic: hypercalcemia, hyperphosphatemia.
Skin: pruritus.
Other: bone and muscle pain, bone demineralization, weight loss.

---

vitamin E
Aquasol E♦, D-Alpha-E, Daltose♦♦, Eprolin, Epsilan-M, Hy-E-Plex, Kell-E, Lethopherol, Maxi-E, Pertropin, Solucap E, Tocopher-Caps, Tokols, Viterra E

Vitamin E deficiency in premature infants

None reported.

INTERACTIONS AND SPECIAL CONSIDERATIONS

Interactions:
MINERAL OIL, CHOLESTYRAMINE RESIN: inhibited GI absorption of oral vitamin D. Space doses. Use together cautiously.

Special considerations:
- Contraindicated in hypercalcemia, hypervitaminosis A, renal osteodystrophy with hyperphosphatemia.
- If I.V. route is necessary, only water-miscible solutions intended for dilution in large-volume parenterals should be used. Use cautiously in cardiac patients, especially if they are receiving glycosides.
- Eating and bowel habits should be monitored for indications of toxicity.
- Patients with hyperphosphatemia require dietary phosphate restrictions and binding agents to avoid metastatic calcifications and renal calculi.
- Dosage range between therapeutic and toxic effects is narrow. When high therapeutic doses are used, frequent serum and urinary calcium, potassium, and urea determinations should be made.
- Malabsorption due to inadequate bile or hepatic dysfunction may require addition of exogenous bile salts to oral vitamin D.
- Protect solution from light.
- This vitamin is fat soluble. Patient should be warned of the dangers of increasing dosage without consulting the doctor. Also, drug should not be shared: it is not "just a vitamin" and can have serious toxic effects.
- Patients taking vitamin D should restrict their intake of magnesium-containing antacids.

Interactions:
MINERAL OIL, CHOLESTYRAMINE RESIN: inhibited GI absorption of oral vitamin E. Space doses. Use together cautiously.

Special considerations:
- Water-miscible forms more completely absorbed in GI tract than other forms.
- Adequate bile is essential for absorption.
- Requirements increase with rise in dietary polyunsaturated acids.
- May protect other vitamins against oxidation.
- Used for a variety of disorders with mixed successes and failures. Dosages not established.

(continued on following page)

NAMES, INDICATIONS AND DOSAGES	SIDE EFFECTS

vitamin E
(continued)

and in patients with impaired fat absorption:
ADULTS: 60 to 75 IU, depending on severity, P.O. or I.M. daily. Maximum 300 IU daily.
CHILDREN: 1 mg equivalent per 0.6 g of dietary unsaturated fat P.O. or I.M. daily.

menadione/menadiol sodium diphosphate (vitamin K_3)
Kappadione, Synkavite♦♦, Synkayvite

Hypoprothrombinemia secondary to vitamin K malabsorption or drug therapy, or when oral administration is desired and bile secretion is inadequate:
ADULTS: 2 to 10 mg menadione P.O. or 5 to 15 mg menadiol sodium diphosphate P.O. or parenterally, titrated to patient's requirements.

Side effects:
CNS: headache, kernicterus.
GI: nausea, vomiting.
Skin: allergic rash, pruritus, urticaria.
Local: pain, hematoma at injection site.

phytonadione (vitamin K_1)
AquaMephyton♦, Konakion♦, Mephyton♦

Hypoprothrombinemia secondary to vitamin K malabsorption, drug therapy, or excess vitamin A:
ADULTS: 2 to 25 mg, depending on severity, P.O. or parenterally, repeated and increased up to 50 mg, if necessary.
CHILDREN: 5 to 10 mg P.O. or parenterally.
INFANTS: 2 mg P.O. or parenterally.
I.V. injection rate for children and infants should not exceed 3 mg/m^2/minute or a total of 5 mg.

Hypoprothrombinemia secondary to effect of oral anticoagulants:
ADULTS: 2.5 to 10 mg P.O., S.C., or I.M., based on prothrombin time, repeated, if necessary, 12 to 48 hours after oral dose or 6 to 8 hours after parenteral dose. In emergency, give 10 to 50 mg slow I.V., rate not to exceed 1 mg/minute, repeated q 4 hours, as needed.

Prevention of hemorrhagic disease in neonates:
NEONATES: 0.5 to 1 mg S.C. or I.M. immediately after birth, repeated in 6 to 8 hours, if needed, especially if mother received oral anticoagulants or long-term anticonvulsant therapy during pregnancy.

Side effects:
CNS: dizziness, convulsive movement.
CV: transient hypotension after I.V. administration, rapid and weak pulse, cardiac irregularities.
GI: nausea, vomiting.
Skin: sweating, flushing, erythema.
Local: pain, swelling, and hematoma at injection site.
Other: bronchospasms, dyspnea, cramplike pain, *anaphylaxis and anaphylactoid reactions, usually after rapid I.V. administration.*

INTERACTIONS AND SPECIAL CONSIDERATIONS

- Megadoses can cause thrombophlebitis.
- This vitamin is fat soluble. Patient should be discouraged from self-medication with megadoses, as they can cause undesirable side effects.

Interactions:

MINERAL OIL, CHOLESTYRAMINE RESIN: inhibited GI absorption of oral vitamin K. Space doses. Use together cautiously.

Special considerations:

- Contraindicated in treatment of oral anticoagulant overdose or heparin-induced bleeding; in treatment for hereditary hypoprothrombinemia (because vitamin K_3 can paradoxically worsen it); or in patients with hepatocellular disease, unless it is caused by biliary obstruction. Use cautiously during last weeks of pregnancy to avoid toxic reactions in newborns and in G-6-PD deficiency to avoid hemolysis. In severe bleeding, other measures, such as giving fresh frozen plasma or whole blood, should not be delayed. Use large doses cautiously in severe hepatic disease.
- Failure to respond to vitamin K_3 may indicate coagulation defects.
- Excessive use of vitamin K_3 may temporarily defeat oral anticoagulant therapy. Higher doses of oral anticoagulant or interim use of heparin may be required.
- Protect parenteral products from light.
- When I.V. route must be used, rate shouldn't exceed 1 mg/minute.
- Effects of I.V. injections more rapid but shorter-lived than subcutaneous or I.M. injections.
- Prothrombin time should be monitored to determine dosage effectiveness.
- Side effects may occur.
- Bulk menadione powder is irritating to the skin and respiratory tract and should be handled with caution.
- Leafy vegetables are high in vitamin K content. May alter warfarin needs.
- This vitamin is fat soluble.

Interactions:

MINERAL OIL, CHOLESTYRAMINE RESIN: inhibited GI absorption of oral vitamin K. Use together cautiously.

Special considerations:

- Contraindicated in hereditary hypoprothrombinemia; bleeding secondary to heparin therapy or overdose; hepatocellular disease, unless it is caused by biliary obstruction (vitamin K can paradoxically worsen the hypoprothrombinemia). Oral administration contraindicated if bile secretion is inadequate, unless supplemented with bile salts. Use cautiously, if at all, during last weeks of pregnancy to avoid toxic reactions in newborns and in G-6-PD deficiency to avoid hemolysis. Use large doses cautiously in severe hepatic disease.
- Failure to respond to vitamin K may indicate coagulation defects.
- In severe bleeding, other measures, such as giving fresh frozen plasma or whole blood, should not be delayed.
- Protect parenteral products from light. Containers and tubing should be wrapped in foil during infusion.
- Effects of I.V. injections more rapid but shorter-lived than subcutaneous or I.M. injections.
- Prothrombin time should be monitored to determine dosage effectiveness.
- Side effects may occur.
- Phytonadione therapy for hemorrhagic disease in infants causes fewer adverse reactions than do other vitamin K analogs.
- Trade name labels should be checked for administration route restrictions.
- Should be administered I.V. by slow infusion and mixed in normal saline solution, dextrose 5% in water, or dextrose 5% in normal saline. Flushing, weakness, tachycardia, and hypotension are possible; may progress to shock.
- Leafy vegetables are high in vitamin K content. May alter warfarin needs.
- This vitamin is fat soluble.
- For treatment of anaphylaxis, see APPENDIX.

(continued on following page)

NAMES, INDICATIONS AND DOSAGES	SIDE EFFECTS

phytonadione
(continued)

Differentiation between hepatocellular disease or biliary obstruction as source of hypoprothrombinemia:
ADULTS AND CHILDREN: 10 mg I.M. or S.C.

Prevention of hypoprothrombinemia related to vitamin K deficiency in long-term parenteral nutrition:
ADULTS: 5 to 10 mg S.C. or I.M. weekly.
CHILDREN: 2 to 5 mg S.C. or I.M. weekly.

Prevention of hypoprothrombinemia in infants receiving less than 0.1 mg/liter vitamin K in breast milk or milk substitutes:
INFANTS: 1 mg S.C. or I.M. monthly.

---

multivitamins
Available by many brand names. Contain vitamins A, B complex, C, D, and E in varying amounts.

Prevention of vitamin deficiencies in patients with inadequate diets or increased daily requirements; treatment of multiple vitamin deficiencies and prevention of recurrence; additions to parenteral nutrition solutions to meet patient's normal or increased requirements:
ADULTS AND CHILDREN: dosage depends on nature and severity of deficiencies and composition of multivitamin preparation.

Side effects: None reported.

---

sodium fluoride
Flo-Tabs, Fluor-A-Day ♦♦, Fluoritabs, Flura-Drops, Karidium♦, Luride Lozi-Tabs, Pediaflor

Aid in the prevention of dental caries:
Oral:
CHILDREN 3 YEARS AND UNDER: 0.5 mg daily.
CHILDREN OVER 3 YEARS: 1 mg daily.
Topical:
CHILDREN 6 TO 12 YEARS: 5 ml.
ADULTS AND CHILDREN OVER 12 YEARS: 10 ml. Use once daily after thoroughly brushing teeth and rinsing mouth. Rinse around and between teeth for 1 minute, then spit out.

Side effects:
CNS: headaches, weakness.
GI: gastric distress.
Skin: hypersensitivity reactions such as atopic dermatitis, eczema, and urticaria.

---

trace elements
chromium, copper, iodine (as iodide), manganese, zinc

Side effects: None reported.

INTERACTIONS AND SPECIAL CONSIDERATIONS

Interactions:
Refer to each component of the multivitamin combination.

Special considerations:
• A single discovered vitamin deficiency usually coexists with others. After initial deficiencies are corrected, need for adequate nutrition and multivitamin supplements should be stressed, if appropriate.
• Precautions should be taken to avoid problems of possible interactions of vitamins in combinations.
• Patient should follow doctor's orders regarding daily dosages and follow-up therapy.
• Excessive use of large-volume parenteral solutions of multivitamin supplements containing fat-soluble vitamins could cause hypervitaminosis. I.V. solutions of water-soluble multivitamins may be used more freely.
• Chewable flavored multivitamins available for children. These drugs should not be used as candy.
• Liquid preparations may contain varying percentages of alcohol. Label should be checked for content.
• Patient should eat a well-balanced diet and avoid overdosing. Self-administered megadoses of vitamins can be hazardous. These medications are drugs, not just harmless vitamins.
• Multivitamin preparations with ordinary doses of each component are usually nontoxic.
• Megavitamin combinations may promote significant accumulation of fat-soluble vitamins, with resultant toxicity.
• Multivitamins containing therapeutic doses of folic acid may mask pernicious anemia. Unless prescribed otherwise by doctor, patient should avoid folic acid in undiagnosed but suspected pernicious anemia.
• Other side effects depend on specific components and concentrations in each multivitamin preparation.
• Store vitamins in a cool place in light-resistant containers to limit loss of potency.

No significant interactions.

Special considerations:
• Contraindicated when fluoride intake from drinking water exceeds 0.7 ppm and in patients on sodium-restricted diets.
• Chronic toxicity (fluorosis) may result from prolonged use of higher than recommended doses.
• Patient should notify dentist if tooth mottling occurs.
• Tablets may be dissolved in mouth, chewed, or swallowed whole.
• Drops may be administered orally undiluted or mixed with fluids or food.
• Topical forms (rinses and gels) should not be swallowed. Most effective when used immediately after brushing teeth.
• Patient should dilute drops or rinses in plastic containers rather than glass.
• Used investigationally in the treatment of osteoporosis.

No significant interactions at recommended dosages.

Special considerations:
• Trace element serum levels of patients who have received total parenteral nutrition for 2 months or longer should be checked and sup-

(continued on following page)

NAMES, INDICATIONS AND DOSAGES	SIDE EFFECTS
trace elements *(continued)* **Prevention of individual trace element deficiencies in patients receiving long-term hyperalimentation:** *Chromium:* ADULTS: 10 to 15 mcg I.V. daily. CHILDREN: 0.14 to 0.20 mcg/kg I.V. daily. *Copper:* ADULTS: 0.5 to 1.5 mg I.V. daily. CHILDREN: 0.05 to 0.2 mg/kg I.V. daily. *Iodine:* ADULTS: 1 mcg/kg I.V. daily. *Manganese:* ADULTS: 1 to 3 mg I.V. daily. *Zinc:* ADULTS: 2 to 4 mg I.V. daily. CHILDREN: 0.05 mg/kg I.V. daily.	
zinc sulfate Orazinc **Treatment of zinc deficiency or adjunct to treatment of disorders related to low serum zinc levels, including oral and decubitus leg ulcers, acne, granulomata of the ear, rheumatoid arthritis, idiopathic hypogeusia, anosmia; also, as adjunct to vitamin A therapy when patient fails to respond to vitamin A alone and in acrodermatitis enteropathica:** ADULTS: 200 to 220 mg P.O. t.i.d. (equivalent to 135 to 150 mg elemental zinc daily, 9 times the adult RDA of 15 mg daily). CHILDREN: dosages not established. RDA is 0.3 mg/kg daily.	**GI:** distress and irritation, nausea, vomiting with high doses.

INTERACTIONS AND SPECIAL CONSIDERATIONS

plement given, if necessary.
- Serum copper and zinc levels are inversely proportional.
- Normal serum levels are 0.07 to 0.15 mg/ml copper; 0.05 to 0.15 mg/100 ml zinc; 4 to 20 mcg/100 ml manganese.
- Solutions of trace elements are compounded by pharmacy for addition to total parenteral nutrition solutions according to various formulas. One common trace element solution is Shil's solution, which contains copper 1 mg/ml, iodide 0.06 mg/ml, manganese 0.4 mg/ml, and zinc 2 mg/ml.

No significant interactions.

Special considerations:
- Beneficial only if patient is zinc-deficient.
- Normal serum levels may not reliably show absence of zinc deficiency.
- Results may not appear for 6 to 8 weeks in zinc-depleted patients.
- Decreasing dosage to 100 mg b.i.d. may ease nausea or other GI side effects; zinc is believed to irritate gastric mucosa.
- Brown bread and dairy products may interfere with zinc absorption.

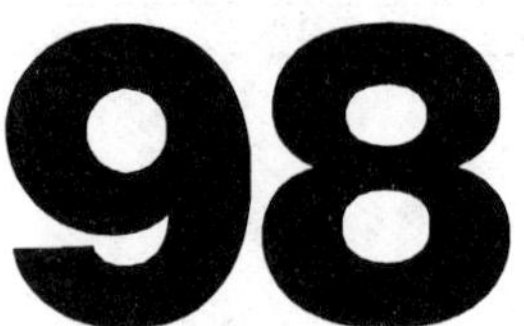

Calorics

amino acid solution
corn oil
dextrose (D-glucose)
essential crystalline amino acid solution
fat emulsions
fructose (levulose)
invert sugar
medium-chain triglycerides

Calorics are nutrients that furnish calories for metabolic energy, promote protein synthesis, and prevent essential fatty acid deficiency.

Major uses

Calorics supply calories to establish a positive nitrogen balance. Each caloric component provides energy for the patient's basal metabolic expenditure.

- Amino acids are used to supply protein for the protein-depleted patient.
- Carbohydrates (dextrose, fructose, and invert sugar) are a source of energy for central nervous system functions, hematopoiesis, and renal metabolism.

  Fructose and invert sugar also furnish partial fluid replacement.
- Fat emulsions contain the essential fatty acids linoleic and linolenic acids. These are useful both as calorie sources and as treatment of essential fatty acid deficiency. Linoleic acid also prevents dermatologic scaling.

  Medium-chain triglycerides are used as an oral calorie source in patients who suffer from fat malabsorption.

Mechanism of action

- Amino acids are used for protein synthesis of the viscera and skeletal muscle in the protein-depleted patient.
- I.V. carbohydrates minimize glyconeogenesis and promote anabolism in patients who can't receive sufficient oral caloric intake. I.V. solutions of dextrose, fructose, and invert sugar supply the energy equivalent of 3.4 kcal/g.
- Fat emulsions, administered I.V., contribute essential fatty acids and a denser calorie source (1.1 kcal/ml) than proteins or carbohydrates.

  Medium-chain triglycerides provide a denser oral calorie source than proteins or carbohydrates in the patient who absorbs fat poorly.

Absorption, distribution, metabolism, and excretion

Calorics are rapidly absorbed and utilized by the body.

- Carbohydrates are, as the renal threshold is exceeded, excreted in the urine.
- The essential fatty acids are metabolized to water and carbon dioxide and are excreted through the urine and perspiration.
- Amino acids are not excreted as such. The nitrogen portion of the amino acid molecule, however, is excreted in urine as urea nitrogen.

Onset and duration

- Anabolism may develop 1 to 5 days after initiation of total parenteral nutrition, which is meant to exceed the patient's basal energy expenditure. Daily replenishment will ensure continued anabolism.

DRUG ALERT

I.V. LIPIDS CAN THREATEN PREMATURE INFANTS

The risks of I.V. lipids can equal and even outweigh potential benefits for premature infants. Because several infants have died following this treatment, each patient must be carefully evaluated before receiving these emulsions.

Evidence indicates that I.V. lipids sharply increase susceptibility to infection, a particular hazard for the unstable premature infant. I.V. lipids also appear to cause life-threatening fat buildup in the pulmonary capillaries, even when infusion rates are well under the recommended maximum and when serum tests show no lipemia.

Infants who are preterm and small for gestational age have diminished ability to metabolize lipids and shouldn't receive more than the recommended dosage of 4 g/kg/day. To decrease the chance of I.V. fat overload, less than this maximum recommended dose may be prescribed. Infusion should be as slow as possible, not exceeding the recommended rate of 1 g/kg/4 hours (0.25 g/kg/hour).

Throughout such infusions, the infant should be watched closely for signs of acute hypersensitivity: dyspnea, tachypnea, wheezing, palpitations, cyanosis, fever, shivering, and vomiting. If any of these side effects occur, the infusion should be stopped.

The infant's serum triglycerides and plasma free fatty acid levels should be carefully monitored to determine whether infused fat is being eliminated from the infant's circulation. Lipemia should clear before the next infusion is to be administered. Premature infants with a bilirubin level greater than 5 mg/100 ml shouldn't receive I.V. fat emulsions.

Combination products

DEXTROSE 2½%, 5%, 10% and sodium chloride 0.45%.

DEXTROSE 2½%, 5%, 10% and sodium chloride 0.9%.

DEXTROSE 3⅓% and sodium chloride 0.3%.

DEXTROSE 5% and sodium chloride 0.11%, 0.2%, 0.33%.

POTASSIUM CHLORIDE 10 mEq, 20 mEq, 27 mEq, 30 mEq, 40 mEq, in 5% dextrose in water.

POTASSIUM CHLORIDE 10 mEq, 20 mEq, 30 mEq, 40 mEq in 5% dextrose, and 0.2% sodium chloride.

POTASSIUM CHLORIDE 10 mEq, 20 mEq, 30 mEq, 40 mEq in 5% dextrose, and 0.45% sodium chloride.

DEXTROSE 5% WITH ELECTROLYTE #75: 50 g/L dextrose, 40 mEq/L Na^+, 35 mEq/L K^+, 40 mEq/L Cl^-, 15 mEq/L phosphate, and 20 mEq/L lactate.

ISOLYTE M WITH 5% DEXTROSE: 50 g/L dextrose, 40 mEq/L Na^+, 35 mEq/L K^+, 40 mEq/L Cl^-, 15 mEq/L phosphate, and 20 mEq/L acetate.

ISOLYTE G WITH 5% DEXTROSE: 50 g/L dextrose, 63 mEq/L Na^+, 17 mEq/L K^+, and 150 mEq/L Cl^-.

IONOSOL G IN 10% DEXTROSE: 100 g/L dextrose, 63 mEq/L Na^+, 17 mEq/L K^+, and 151 mEq/L Cl^-.

ISOLYTE G WITH 10% DEXTROSE: 100 g/L dextrose, 63 mEq/L Na^+, 17 mEq/L K^+, and 150 mEq/L Cl^-.

NAMES, INDICATIONS AND DOSAGES / SIDE EFFECTS

amino acid solution

(crystalline amino acid solution)
Aminosyn, Travasol♦, Veinamine

Total, supportive, or supplemental and protein-sparing parenteral nutrition when gastrointestinal system must rest during healing, or when patient can't, shouldn't, or won't eat at all or eat enough to maintain normal nutrition and metabolism:

ADULTS: 1 to 1.5 g/kg I.V. daily.

CHILDREN: 2 to 3 g/kg I.V. daily. Individualize dosage to metabolic and clinical response as determined by nitrogen balance and body weight corrected for fluid balance. Add electrolytes, vitamins, and nonprotein caloric solutions as needed.

CNS: mental confusion, unconsciousness, headache, dizziness.
CV: hypervolemia related to congestive heart failure (in susceptible patients), *pulmonary edema,* exacerbation of hypertension (in predisposed patients).
GI: nausea, vomiting.
GU: glycosuria, osmotic diuresis.
Hepatic: fatty liver.
Metabolic: *rebound hypoglycemia* (when long-term infusions are abruptly stopped), *hyperglycemia,* metabolic acidosis, alkalosis, hypophosphatemia, *hyperosmolar syndrome, hyperosmolar-hyperglycemic-nonketotic syndrome,* hyperammonemia, *electrolyte imbalances,* and dehydration (if hyperosmolar solutions used).
Skin: chills, flushing, feeling of warmth.
Local: tissue sloughing at infusion site due to extravasation, *catheter sepsis, thrombophlebitis, thrombosis.*
Other: allergic reactions.

corn oil

Lipomul♦

As energy source:

ADULTS: 45 ml P.O. b.i.d. to q.i.d. after or between meals, alone or with proteins, milk, or other energy sources.

CHILDREN: 30 ml P.O. daily to q.i.d. after or between meals, alone or with proteins, milk, or other energy sources.

GI: nausea, vomiting, diarrhea.

dextrose (D-glucose)

Fluid replacement and caloric supplementation in patient who can't maintain adequate oral intake or who is restricted from doing so:

ADULTS AND CHILDREN: dosage depends on fluid and caloric requirements. Use peripheral I.V. infusion of 2.5%, 5%, or 10% solution, central I.V. infusion of 20% solution for minimal fluid needs. Use 50% solution to treat insulin-induced hypoglycemia. Solutions from 40% to 70% are used diluted in admixtures, normally with amino acid solutions, for total parenteral nutrition given through a central vein.

CNS: mental confusion, unconsciousness in hyperosmolar syndrome.
CV: (with fluid overload) pulmonary edema, exacerbated hypertension, and congestive heart failure in susceptible patients. *Prolonged or concentrated infusions may cause phlebitis, sclerosis of vein, especially with peripheral route of administration.*
GU: glycosuria, osmotic diuresis.
Metabolic: (with rapid infusion of concentrated solution or prolonged infusion) hyperglycemia, hypervolemia, hyperosmolarity. Rapid termination of long-term infusions may cause hypoglycemia from rebound hyperinsulinemia.
Skin: sloughing and tissue necrosis, if extravasation occurs with concentrated solutions.

essential crystalline amino acid solution

Aminosyn-RF, Nephramine

Management of potentially reversible renal decompensation:

CNS: mental confusion, dizziness, unconsciousness, headache.
CV: hypervolemia related to congestive heart failure (in susceptible patients), *pulmonary edema,* exacerbation of hypertension (in predisposed patients).

INTERACTIONS AND SPECIAL CONSIDERATIONS

No significant interactions.

Special considerations:

• Contraindicated in patients with severe uncorrected electrolyte or acid/base imbalances, in hyperammonemia, and in decreased circulating blood volume. Use cautiously in renal insufficiency or failure, cardiac disease, and hepatic impairments. Long-term use not advised for infants and children.

• Serum electrolytes, magnesium, glucose, BUN, renal and hepatic function should be monitored. Serum calcium levels should be checked frequently to avoid bone demineralization in children.

• Trace element and vitamin supplements may be ordered if long-term therapy is needed. Overuse of fat-soluble vitamins A and D can cause toxic hypervitaminosis.

• Refrigerate solution until half hour before ready to use.

• Pharmacist should be consulted before mixing any medication—except electrolytes, vitamins, and trace elements—with hyperalimentation solution.

• Infusion rate should be controlled carefully with infusion pump.

• If infusion rate falls behind, doctor should be notified.

• Infusion site should be checked frequently for irritation, tissue sloughing, necrosis, and phlebitis. I.V. sites should be changed periodically to prevent irritation and infection; usually given by I.V. catheter into subclavian vein.

• Fluid overload may develop.

• Some crystalline amino acid solutions contain large amounts of acetates and lactates; should be used cautiously in alkalosis or hepatic insufficiency.

• Most side effects are due to mixing amino acid with hypertonic dextrose solutions.

• Fractional urines should be checked every 6 hours for glycosuria. (If present, insulin coverage may be ordered.)

• Body temperature should be assessed every 4 hours; elevation may indicate sepsis and infection.

• I.V. tubing and bottle should be replaced and sent to the laboratory to be cultured if patient has chills, fever, or other signs of sepsis.

Interactions:

GRISEOFULVIN: increased GI absorption of griseofulvin. Space doses.

Special considerations:

• Contraindicated in gallbladder calculi or complete GI obstructions. Use cautiously in steatorrhea, partial GI obstruction, enterostomies, hepatic cirrhosis, portacaval shunts.

• More frequent, smaller doses taken with meals or mixed with milk minimize nausea, diarrhea, and vomiting.

No significant interactions.

Special considerations:

• Contraindicated in hyperglycemia, diabetic coma, intracranial or intraspinal hemorrhage, delirium tremens. Use cautiously in cardiac or pulmonary disease, hypertension, renal insufficiency, urinary obstruction, or hypovolemia.

• Infusion rate should be controlled carefully. Maximal rate for dextrose infusion is 0.5 g/kg/hour. Infusion pump should be used when infusing dextrose with amino acids for total parenteral nutrition.

• Concentrated solutions should never be infused rapidly.

• Serum glucose should be monitored carefully. Prolonged therapy with 5% dextrose can cause depletion of pancreatic insulin production and secretion.

• Should never be stopped abruptly. If necessary, 10% dextrose should be available to prevent rebound hyperinsulinemia and resulting hypoglycemia.

• Extravasation should be avoided, and infusion site checked frequently to prevent irritation, tissue sloughing, necrosis, and phlebitis.

• Patient should be watched closely for signs of fluid overload, especially if fluid intake is restricted.

• Intake and output should be monitored carefully, especially in impaired renal function.

• Vital signs should be checked frequently. Side effects possible.

• Dextrose solutions should not be given without saline with blood transfusions; may cause clumping of red blood cells.

No significant interactions.

Special considerations:

• Contraindicated in severe uncorrected electrolyte or acid/base imbalances, hyperammonemia, and decreased circulating blood volume.

• Serum electrolytes, magnesium, glucose, BUN, renal and hepatic function should be monitored. Serum calcium levels should be checked frequently to avoid bone demineralization in children.

• Trace element and vitamin supplements may

(continued on following page)

NAMES, INDICATIONS AND DOSAGES / SIDE EFFECTS

essential crystalline amino acid solution
(continued)

ADULTS: 0.3 to 0.5 g/kg I.V., up to 26 g total daily (250 ml with 500 ml 70% dextrose injection), and infuse through central I.V. line at initial rate of 20 to 30 ml/hour, increased in steps of 10 ml/hour every 24 hours, to a maximum of 60 to 100 ml/hour. Individualize dose and infusion rate to tolerance for glucose, fluid, and nitrogen. Add electrolytes and vitamins as needed.

CHILDREN: up to 1 g/kg daily, individualized to patient's tolerance for glucose, fluid, and nitrogen. Add electrolytes, trace elements, and vitamins as needed.

GI: nausea, vomiting.
GU: glycosuria, osmotic diuresis.
Metabolic: *rebound hypoglycemia* (when long-term infusions are abruptly stopped), *hyperglycemia*, metabolic acidosis, alkalosis, hypophosphatemia, hyperosmolar syndrome, *hyperosmolar-hyperglycemic-nonketotic syndrome*, hyperammonemia, *electrolyte imbalances*, and dehydration (if hyperosmolar solutions used).
Skin: chills, flushing, feeling of warmth.
Local: tissue sloughing at infusion site due to extravasation, *catheter sepsis*, *thrombophlebitis*.
Other: allergic reactions.

fat emulsions
Intralipid♦, Liposyn

Intralipid:

Source of calories adjunctive to total parenteral nutrition:

ADULTS: 1 ml/minute I.V. for 15 to 30 minutes. If no adverse reactions, increase rate to deliver 500 ml over 4 hours. Infuse only 1,500-ml unit the first day. Total daily dose should not exceed 2.5 g/kg (25 ml/kg 10% emulsion).

CHILDREN: 0.1 ml/minute for 10 to 15 minutes. If no adverse reactions, increase rate to deliver 10 ml/kg over 4 hours. Daily dose should not exceed 4 g/kg (40 ml/kg 10% emulsion). Equals 60% of daily caloric intake. Protein-carbohydrate hyperalimentation should supply remaining 40%.

Fatty acid deficiency:

ADULTS AND CHILDREN: 8% to 10% of total caloric intake I.V.

Liposyn:

Prevention of fatty acid deficiency:

ADULTS: 500 ml I.V. twice weekly. Infuse initially at a rate of 1 ml/minute for 30 minutes. Rate may be increased but should not exceed 500 ml over 4 to 6 hours.

CHILDREN: 5 to 10 ml/kg I.V. daily. Infuse initially at a rate of 0.1 ml/minute for 30 minutes. Rate may be increased but should not exceed 100 ml/hour.

Early reactions of fat overload:
Blood: hyperlipemia, hypercoagulability, rarely thrombocytopenia in neonates.
CNS: headache, sleepiness, dizziness.
EENT: pressure over eyes.
GI: nausea, vomiting.
Skin: flushing, diaphoresis.
Local: irritation at infusion site.
Other: fever, dyspnea, chest and back pains, cyanosis, allergic reactions, deposition of I.V. fat.
Delayed reactions:
Blood: thrombocytopenia, leukopenia, leukocytosis.
CNS: focal seizures.
CV: shock.
Hepatic: transient increased liver function test, hepatomegaly.
Other: fever, splenomegaly.

fructose (levulose)

Source of carbohydrate calories primarily when fluid replacement is also indicated and as a dextrose substitute for patients with diabetes:

ADULTS AND CHILDREN: dosage depends on caloric needs. I.V. infusion rate should not ex-

CV: increased pulse rate, precipitation or exacerbation of congestive heart failure in susceptible patients, *pulmonary edema*.
Hepatic: hepatomegaly.
Metabolic: metabolic acidosis, hypervolemia.
Local: extravasation at infusion site may cause sloughing of skin, thrombophlebitis.
Other: increased respiratory rate.

INTERACTIONS AND SPECIAL CONSIDERATIONS

be ordered in long-term therapy. Overuse of fat-soluble vitamins should be avoided.
• Refrigerate solution until half hour before it will be infused.
• Pharmacist should be consulted before mixing any medication—except electrolytes, vitamins, and trace elements—with hyperalimentation solution.
• Infusion rate should be controlled carefully with infusion pump.
• Infusion site should be checked frequently for irritation, tissue sloughing, necrosis, and phlebitis. I.V. sites should be changed periodically to prevent irritation; usually given by I.V. catheter into subclavian vein.
• Fluid overload may develop.
• Essential amino acid solution is used identically to other crystalline amino acid solutions, except that it contains only the essential amino acids. By controlling amino acid content, patients with impaired renal function have decreases in blood urea nitrogen level, minimized deterioration of serum potassium, magnesium, and phosphorus balances. May lead to earlier return of renal function in patients with potentially reversible acute renal failure and may decrease morbidity associated with acute renal failure.
• Most side effects are due to mixing essential crystalline amino acid solution with hypertonic dextrose solutions.
• Fractional urines should be checked every 6 hours for glycosuria. (If present, insulin coverage may be ordered.)
• Body temperature should be assessed every 4 hours; elevation may indicate sepsis and infection.
• I.V. tubing and bottle should be replaced and sent to the laboratory to be cultured if patient has chills, fever, or other signs of sepsis.

No significant interactions.

Special considerations:
• Contraindicated in hyperlipemia, lipoid nephrosis, and acute pancreatitis accompanied by hyperlipemia. Use cautiously in severe hepatic disease, pulmonary disease, anemia, blood coagulation disorders, or in patients with possible danger of fat embolism.
• Never dilute or mix with electrolyte or other nutrient products. Infusion may be piggybacked into another I.V. line, but additives should not be placed in the fat emulsion bottle.
• An in-line filter should not be used when administering this drug because the fat particles are larger than the 0.22-micron cellulose filter.
• Fat emulsion should be discarded if it separates or becomes oily. Intralipid may be refrigerated, although refrigeration is not essential. Liposyn needs no refrigeration.
• Rapid infusion should be avoided and infusion pump used to regulate rate.
• Infusion site should be checked daily for signs of inflammation or infection.
• Side effects may occur, especially during first half hour of infusion.
• Serum lipids should be monitored closely when patient is receiving fat emulsion therapy. Lipemia must clear between dosing.
• Platelet count should be checked frequently in neonates receiving fat emulsions I.V.
• Hepatic function should be monitored carefully in long-term use.
• Intralipid and liposyn differ mainly by their fatty acid components.

No significant interactions.

Special considerations:
• Contraindicated in hereditary fructose intolerance or in patients receiving therapy for hypoglycemia. Use cautiously in cardiac disease, hypertension, pulmonary disease, hypervolemia, renal insufficiency, or urinary tract obstructions.
• Infusion rate should be controlled carefully. Rate should not exceed 1 g/kg/hour in infants.
• Infusion sites should be changed frequently to avoid irritation with prolonged therapy. Extravasation should be avoided.
• Fluid overload, pulmonary edema, or congestive heart failure may occur. Blood pressure

(continued on following page)

NAMES, INDICATIONS AND DOSAGES	SIDE EFFECTS
fructose *(continued)* ceed 1 g/kg/hour. Single liter 10% solution yields 375 calories.	
invert sugar Travert **Nonelectrolyte fluid replacement and caloric supplementation solution:** ADULTS AND CHILDREN: dosage depends on patient's age, weight, clinical need. I.V. infusion rate should not exceed 1 g/kg/hour. Single liter 5% invert sugar yields 375 calories.	**CNS:** mental confusion. **CV:** increased pulse rate, precipitation or exacerbation of congestive heart failure in susceptible patients, *pulmonary edema,* hypertension. **GU:** glycosuria, osmotic diuresis. **Metabolic:** metabolic acidosis, hypervolemia, hyperglycemia, hypoglycemia. **Local:** extravasation at infusion site may cause sloughing of skin, thrombophlebitis. **Other:** increased respiratory rate.
medium-chain triglycerides M.C.T. Oil♦ **Inadequate digestion or absorption of food fats:** ADULTS: 15 ml P.O. t.i.d. to q.i.d.	**CNS:** reversible coma and precoma in susceptible patients. **GI:** *nausea, vomiting, diarrhea.*

♦ Available in U.S. and Canada. ♦♦ Available in Canada only.
All other products (no symbol) available in U.S. only. Italicized side effects are common or life-threatening.

INTERACTIONS AND SPECIAL CONSIDERATIONS

should be monitored frequently.
- May be safely used in patients with diabetes.

No significant interactions.

Special considerations:
- Contraindicated in hereditary fructose intolerance, hyperglycemia, diabetic coma, intracranial or intraspinal hemorrhage, or delirium tremens. Use cautiously in cardiac disease, hypertension, pulmonary disease, hypervolemia, renal insufficiency, or urinary tract obstructions.
- Infusion rate should be carefully controlled. Rate should not exceed 1 g/kg/hour in infants.
- Infusion sites should be changed frequently to avoid irritation with prolonged therapy. Extravasation should be avoided.
- Fluid overload, pulmonary edema, or congestive heart failure may occur. Blood pressure should be monitored.
- May be safely used in patients with diabetes.
- Serum glucose should be monitored closely. Prolonged therapy can cause depletion of pancreatic insulin production and secretion.
- Should not be stopped abruptly. If necessary, 10% dextrose should be available to prevent rebound hyperinsulinemia and subsequent hypoglycemia.
- Intake and output should be monitored closely, especially if renal function is impaired.
- Vital signs should be checked frequently. Side effects may occur.

No significant interactions.

Special considerations:
- Contraindicated in advanced hepatic disease.
- To minimize GI side effects, smaller doses should be taken more frequently with meals or mixed with fruit juice or salad dressing.
- More easily absorbed than long-chain fats.
- Rapid metabolism provides quick energy.
- May be useful in obesity control and in lowering cholesterol levels. Also used in patients with short-bowel syndrome.

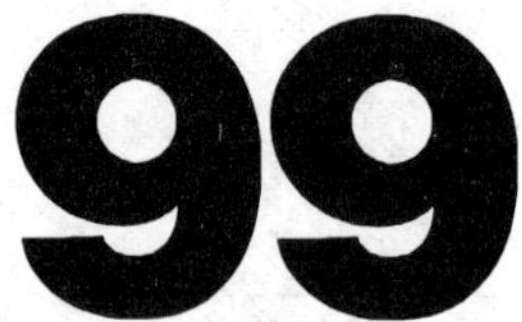

Immune serums

antirabies serum, equine
hepatitis B immune globulin, human
immune serum globulin
rabies immune globulin, human
Rh_0 (D) immune globulin, human
tetanus immune globulin, human

Immune serums provide passive immunity against various infectious diseases or suppress antibody formation, as in Rh incompatibility. Immune serum globulins are obtained from hyperimmunized human or animal donors, or pooled plasma. These products are then purified and standardized. Immune serums are effective only for prophylaxis.

Major uses
Immune serums prevent various infectious diseases; they may relieve symptoms after suspected exposure (postexposure prophylaxis). They also prevent formation of active antibodies, as in Rh_0-negative, D^u-negative mothers who deliver Rh_0-positive or D^u-positive infants, or in transfusion accidents.

Mechanism of action
Immune serums contain preformed protective substances (antibodies) from the serum of human beings or animals, especially horses, that have been immunized by injection with the organisms or toxins of diseases. These antibodies, therefore, combat specific diseases.

Absorption, distribution, metabolism, and excretion
Not applicable.

Onset and duration
Onset of passive immunity is immediate but duration is temporary, generally lasting about 3 to 4 weeks after immunization.

Combination products
None.

THE FACTS ABOUT RH ISOIMMUNIZATION

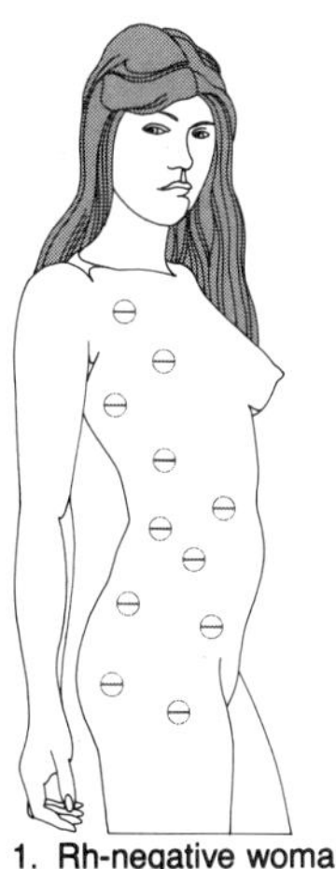

1. Rh-negative woman prepregnancy.

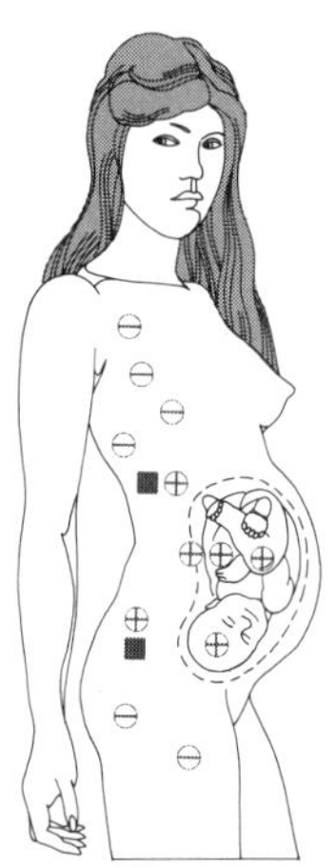

2. First pregnancy with Rh-positive fetus.

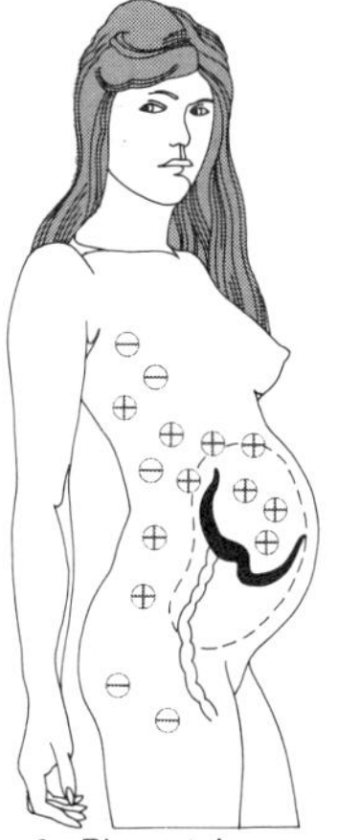

3. Placental separation.

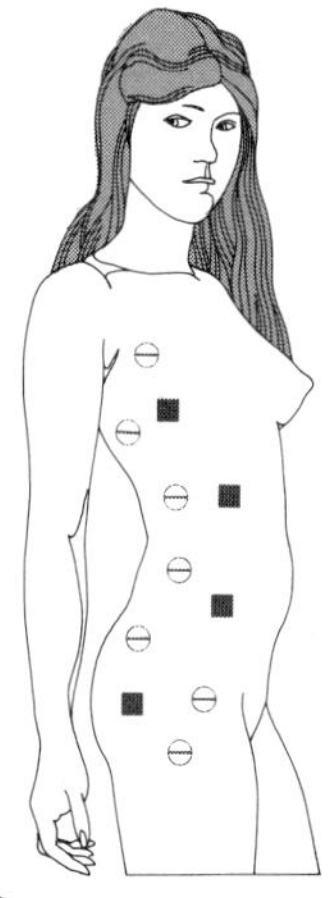

4. Postdelivery, mother becomes sensitized to Rh-positive blood and develops anti-Rh-positive antibodies (darkened squares).

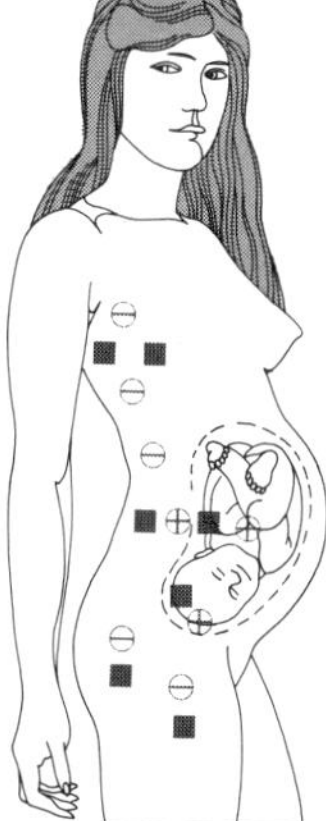

5. During next pregnancy with Rh-positive fetus, maternal anti-Rh-positive antibodies enter fetal circulation, attach to Rh-positive RBCs, and subject them to hemolysis.

NAMES, INDICATIONS AND DOSAGES	SIDE EFFECTS
antirabies serum, equine **Rabies exposure:** ADULTS AND CHILDREN: 40 to 55 units/kg at time of first dose of rabies vaccine. Use half dose to infiltrate wound area. Give remainder I.M. Don't give rabies vaccine and antirabies serum in same syringe or at same site.	**Local:** pain at injection site. **Systemic:** within 6 to 12 days serum sickness occurs in 15% to 25% of patients. Symptoms are skin eruptions, arthralgia, pruritus, lymphadenopathy, fever, headache, malaise, abdominal pain, *anaphylaxis*.
hepatitis B immune globulin, human H-BIG, Hep-B-Gammagee, HyperHep **Hepatitis B exposure:** ADULTS AND CHILDREN: 0.06 ml/kg I.M. within 7 days after exposure. Repeat 28 days after exposure.	**Systemic:** *anaphylaxis*.
immune serum globulin Gamastan, Gammar, Immu-G, Immuglobin **Agammaglobulinemia or hypogammaglobulinemia:** ADULTS: 30 to 50 ml I.M. monthly. CHILDREN: 20 to 40 ml I.M. monthly. **Hepatitis A exposure:** ADULTS AND CHILDREN: 0.02 to 0.04 ml/kg I.M. as soon as possible after exposure. Up to 0.1 ml/kg may be given after prolonged or intense exposure. **Serum hepatitis post-transfusion:** ADULTS AND CHILDREN: 10 ml I.M. within 1 week after transfusion and 10 ml I.M. 1 month later. **Measles exposure:** ADULTS AND CHILDREN: 0.02 ml/kg within 6 days after exposure. **Modification of measles:** ADULTS AND CHILDREN: 0.04 ml/kg I.M. within 6 days after exposure. **Measles vaccine complications:** ADULTS AND CHILDREN: 0.02 to 0.04 ml/kg I.M. **Poliomyelitis exposure:** ADULTS AND CHILDREN: 0.3 to 0.4 ml/kg I.M. within 7 days after exposure. **Chickenpox exposure:**	**Skin:** urticaria. **Local:** pain, erythema, muscle stiffness. **Systemic:** angioedema, headache, malaise, fever, nephrotic syndrome, *anaphylaxis*.

INTERACTIONS AND SPECIAL CONSIDERATIONS

No significant interactions.

Special considerations:
- In hypersensitivity to equine serum: use rabies immune globulin, human, instead; if unavailable, desensitize before giving. Consult doctor or pharmacist.
- Do sensitivity test on all patients before giving: dilute serum 1:100 or 1:1,000 with 0.9% sodium chloride for injection; inject intradermally on inner forearm; inject other arm with 0.1 ml 0.9% sodium chloride for injection intradermally as control; read within 20 minutes. Positive reaction: wheal 10 mm or more and erythematous flare 20 x 20 mm.
- Should be used only when rabies immune globulin, human, not available.
- History of animal bite, allergies (especially to equine serum and to eggs), and reaction to immunization should be obtained.
- Epinephrine solution 1:1,000 should always be available when administering this drug.
- This immune serum provides immediate passive immunity (short-term).
- This drug should not be confused with rabies vaccine, which is a suspension of attenuated or killed microorganisms used to confer long-term active immunity. These two drugs are often administered together prophylactically after exposure to known or suspected rabid animals.
- Patient should report last tetanus immunization; a booster may be ordered at this time.
- For treatment of anaphylaxis, see APPENDIX.

No significant interactions.

Special considerations:
- Buttocks or deltoid areas preferred injection sites.
- Immunization recommended after exposure to hepatitis B (for example, needle-stick or direct contact).
- History of allergies and reaction to immunization should be obtained.
- For treatment of anaphylaxis, see APPENDIX.

No significant interactions.

Special considerations:
- History of allergies and past reaction to immunization should be obtained.
- Drugs should be available for anaphylactic reaction.
- Dose of more than 10 ml should be divided and injected into different sites, preferably buttocks. No more than 3 ml should be injected per injection site.
- Should not be given for hepatitis A exposure if 6 weeks or more have elapsed since exposure, or after onset of clinical illness.
- For treatment of anaphylaxis, see APPENDIX.

(continued on following page)

NAMES, INDICATIONS AND DOSAGES	SIDE EFFECTS
immune serum globulin *(continued)* ADULTS AND CHILDREN: 0.2 to 1.3 ml/kg I.M. as soon as exposed. **Rubella exposure in first trimester of pregnancy:** WOMEN: 0.2 to 0.4 ml/kg I.M. as soon as exposed.	
rabies immune globulin, human Hyperab **Rabies exposure:** ADULTS AND CHILDREN: 20 IU/kg at time of first dose of rabies vaccine. Use half dose to infiltrate wound area. Give remainder I.M. Don't give rabies vaccine and rabies immune globulin in same syringe or at same site.	**Local:** pain, redness, induration at injection site. **Other:** slight fever, *anaphylaxis.*
Rh_O (D) immune globulin, human Gamulin R, HypRho-D, MICRhoGAM, RhoGam **Rh exposure:** WOMEN POSTABORTION, POSTMISCARRIAGE, ECTOPIC PREGNANCY, OR POSTPARTUM: transfusion unit or blood bank determines fetal packed red blood cell volume entering woman's blood, then gives one vial I.M. if fetal packed RBC volume is less than 15 ml. More than one vial I.M. may be required if there is large fetomaternal hemorrhage. Must be given within 72 hours after delivery or miscarriage. **Transfusion accidents:** ADULTS AND CHILDREN: consult blood bank or transfusion unit at once. Must be given within 72 hours. **Postabortion or postmiscarriage to prevent Rh antibody formation:** WOMEN: consult transfusion unit or blood bank. Ideally should be given within 3 hours, but may be given up to 72 hours after abortion or miscarriage.	**Local:** discomfort at injection site. **Other:** slight fever.
tetanus immune globulin, human Homo-Tet, Hu-Tet, Hyper-Tet, Immu-Tetanus **Tetanus exposure:** ADULTS AND CHILDREN: 250 units I.M. **Tetanus treatment:** ADULTS AND CHILDREN: single doses of 3,000 to 6,000 units have been used, but optimal dosage schedules not established. Do not give at same site as toxoid.	**Local:** pain, stiffness, erythema. **Other:** slight fever, allergy, *anaphylaxis.*

INTERACTIONS AND SPECIAL CONSIDERATIONS

No significant interactions.

Special considerations:

- Repeated doses contraindicated once rabies vaccine started.
- Used only with rabies vaccine and immediate local treatment of wound. Given regardless of interval between exposure and initiation of therapy.
- History of animal bite, allergies, and past reaction to immunization should be obtained.
- Corticosteroids decrease resistance to infection and antibody response to vaccine. Corticosteroids should be stopped after possible rabies exposure.
- This immune serum provides passive immunity.
- This drug should not be confused with rabies vaccine, which is a suspension of attenuated or killed microorganisms used to confer active immunity. These two drugs are often used together prophylactically after exposure to known or suspected rabid animals.
- Patient should report last tetanus immunization; a booster may be ordered at this time.
- For treatment of anaphylaxis, see APPENDIX.

No significant interactions.

Special considerations:

- Contraindicated in Rh_o (D)-positive or D_u-positive patients and those previously immunized to Rh_o (D) blood factor.
- Immediately after delivery, infant's cord blood should be sent to laboratory for type and crossmatch. Confirm mother is Rh_o (D) negative and D_u negative. Infant must be Rh_o (D) positive or D_u positive.
- Should be given only to postpartum mother, not infant.
- History of allergies and past reaction to immunization should be obtained.
- MICRhoGAM recommended for every woman undergoing abortion or miscarriage up to 12 weeks' gestation unless she is Rh_o (D) positive or D_u positive, has Rh antibodies, or the father and/or fetus is Rh negative.
- For I.M. use only.
- Store at 36° to 46° F. (2° to 8° C.). Do not freeze.
- This immune serum provides passive immunity to the woman exposed to Rh_o-positive fetal blood during pregnancy. Prevents formation of maternal antibodies (active immunity), which would endanger future Rh_o-positive pregnancies.
- Drug protects future Rh_o-positive infants.

No significant interactions.

Special considerations:

- Tetanus immune globulin should be used only if wound is over 24 hours old or patient has had less than 2 previous tetanus toxoid injections.
- History of injury, past tetanus immunizations, last tetanus toxoid injection, allergies, and past reaction to immunization should be obtained.
- All foreign matter should be thoroughly cleansed and removed from wound.
- This immune serum provides passive immunity. Antibodies remain at effective levels for 3 weeks or longer, which is several times the duration of antitoxin-induced antibodies. Protects the patient for the incubation period of most tetanus cases.
- Human globulin is not a substitute for tetanus toxoid, which should be given at the same time to produce active immmunization.
- Don't confuse this drug with tetanus toxoid.
- For treatment of anaphylaxis, see APPENDIX.

100

Vaccines and toxoids

BCG vaccine
cholera vaccine
diphtheria and tetanus toxoids, adsorbed
diphtheria and tetanus toxoids and pertussis vaccine (DPT)
diphtheria toxoid, adsorbed, pediatric
influenza virus vaccine, trivalent
measles, mumps, and rubella virus vaccine, live
measles (rubeola) and rubella virus vaccine, live attenuated
measles (rubeola) virus vaccine, live attenuated
meningitis vaccines
mumps virus vaccine, live
plague vaccine
pneumococcal vaccine, polyvalent
poliovirus vaccine, live, oral, trivalent
rabies vaccine (duck embryo), dried, killed virus
rabies vaccine, human diploid cell (HDCV)
rubella and mumps virus vaccine, live
rubella virus vaccine, live attenuated (RA 27/3)
smallpox vaccine
tetanus toxoid adsorbed
tetanus toxoid fluid
typhoid vaccine
yellow fever vaccine

Vaccines and toxoids provide active immunity against certain bacterial and viral diseases. Vaccines contain killed or attenuated living microorganisms that stimulate the formation of antibodies. Toxoids contain exotoxins (heat-labile, proteinaceous toxins formed by bacteria and secreted outside the bacterial cell). These substances are chemically changed to make them nontoxic, but they retain the ability to stimulate antitoxin (antibody) formation.

Major uses

Vaccines and toxoids prevent certain infectious diseases and childhood diseases. They also prevent diseases that are transmitted through injury or animal bite, such as tetanus and rabies.

Mechanism of action

Vaccines and toxoids initiate formation of specific antibodies by stimulating the host's antigen-antibody mechanism, providing active, acquired immunity. (Active immunity can be induced by exposure to an infectious disease or to one of its antigens, or by vaccination.)

Absorption, distribution, metabolism, and excretion

Not applicable.

Onset and duration

Onset of active immunity is not immediate. Antibody production doesn't reach immunity-providing levels for a few days to a few weeks. Duration of immunity is long, lasting for years.

Combination products

None.

PATIENT-TEACHING AID

IMMUNIZATIONS FOR TRAVELERS

Dear Patient:

When planning a trip abroad, you need to know which immunizations are required by countries you'll visit. Here are some general guidelines:

VACCINE	WHO SHOULD RECEIVE
Tetanus and diphtheria	Everyone, whether traveling or not, should have a booster injection every 10 years.
Polio	Travelers not previously immunized should receive primary immunization series; previously immunized travelers to rural/remote areas of tropical or developing countries should receive one additional dose of vaccine.
Measles	Persons born after 1957 who haven't received vaccine and don't have a history of infection
Hepatitis A	Travelers to developing countries who are going beyond normal tourist routes or staying 3 months or longer
Yellow fever	Travelers to infected areas (check with local health department); some countries require vaccination for travelers from infected areas.
Typhoid	Travelers to rural areas of tropical countries and any area of outbreak
Plague	Travelers to interior regions of Vietnam, Democratic Kampuchea, and the Lao People's Democratic Republic
Typhus	Travelers to remote highland areas of Bolivia, Ecuador, Guatemala, Mexico, Peru, Burundi, Ethiopia, and Rwanda, or mountainous areas of Asia
Rabies	Travelers anticipating contact with possibly infected animals
Cholera	Not generally recommended for tourists, but some countries require it for travelers from infected areas
Smallpox	Many countries require evidence of vaccination for entry.
Malaria chemoprophylaxis	Travelers to malarious areas should make sure adequate chemoprophylaxis is available.

For more information write for Health Information for International Travel, *by the Center for Disease Control (U.S. Government Printing Office, Washington, D.C. 20402).*

Adapted with permission from *The Medical Letter,*® No. 14, July 13, 1979, pp. 57 and 60.

NAMES, INDICATIONS AND DOSAGES	SIDE EFFECTS
BCG vaccine **Tuberculosis exposure, cancer immunotherapy:** ADULTS AND CHILDREN: 0.1 ml intradermally. NEWBORNS: 0.05 ml intradermally.	**Local:** lymphangitis, lymph node and skin abscess, ulceration at site of injection (2 to 3 weeks after injection), lupus reaction. **Other:** urticaria of trunk and limbs, *anaphylaxis.*
cholera vaccine **Primary immunization:** ADULTS AND CHILDREN OVER 10 YEARS: 2 doses of 0.5 ml I.M. or 1 ml S.C., 1 week to 1 month before traveling in cholera area. Booster: 0.5 ml q 6 months as long as protection is needed. CHILDREN 5 TO 10 YEARS: 0.3 ml I.M. or S.C. CHILDREN 6 MONTHS TO 4 YEARS: 0.2 ml I.M. or S.C. Boosters of same dose should be given q 6 months as long as protection needed.	**Systemic:** malaise, fever, flushing, urticaria, tachycardia, hypotension, headache, *anaphylaxis.* **Local:** erythema, swelling, pain, induration.
diphtheria and tetanus toxoids, adsorbed **Primary immunization:** ADULTS AND CHILDREN 7 YEARS AND OVER: use adult strength; 0.5 ml I.M. 4 to 6 weeks apart for 2 doses and a third dose 1 year later. Booster: 0.5 ml I.M. q 10 years. CHILDREN UNDER 7 YEARS: use pediatric strength; 0.5 ml I.M. 4 to 8 weeks apart for 2 doses and a third dose 6 to 12 months later. Booster: 0.5 ml when starting school.	**Systemic:** chills, fever, malaise, *anaphylaxis.* **Local:** stinging, edema, erythema, pain, induration.
diphtheria and tetanus toxoids and pertussis vaccine (DPT) Tri-Immunol, Triple Antigen **Primary immunization:** CHILDREN 6 WEEKS TO 6 YEARS: 0.5 ml I.M. 2 months apart for 3 doses and a fourth dose 1 year later. Booster: 0.5 ml I.M. when starting school. Not advised for adults, or children over 6 years.	**Systemic:** slight fever, chills, malaise, *convulsions, encephalopathy, anaphylaxis.* **Local:** soreness, redness, expected nodule remaining several weeks.
diphtheria toxoid, adsorbed, pediatric **Diphtheria immunization:** CHILDREN UNDER 6 YEARS: 0.5 ml I.M. 6 to 8 weeks apart for 2 doses and a third dose	**Systemic:** fever, malaise, urticaria, tachycardia, flushing, pruritus, hypotension, aches and pains, *anaphylaxis.* **Local:** erythema, pain, induration, expected nodule persistent for several weeks.

INTERACTIONS AND SPECIAL CONSIDERATIONS

Interactions:
ISONIAZID (INH): inhibited multiplication of BCG. Avoid using together.

Special considerations:
• Contraindicated in patients with hypogammaglobulinemia, positive tuberculin reaction (when meant for use as immunoprophylactic after exposure to tuberculosis), immunosuppression, fresh smallpox vaccination, burns, and in those receiving corticosteroid therapy. Use cautiously in chronic skin disease. Should be injected in area of healthy skin only.
• History of allergies and past reaction to immunization should be obtained.
• Vaccine is of no value in patients with positive tuberculin test.
• Epinephrine 1:1,000 should be available to treat anaphylaxis.
• Recommended injection site is over insertion of deltoid muscle.
• Vial should not be shaken after reconstitution.
• Expected lesion forms in 7 to 10 days.
• Live vaccine: destroy by autoclaving or formalin solution before disposal.
• Patient should have tuberculin skin test 2 to 3 months after BCG vaccination to determine success of vaccine.
• Use of BCG has shown some value in treatment of various cancers such as leukemia, malignant melanoma, multiple myeloma, some lung cancers, and some breast tumors. Currently, researchers are trying to find ways of augmenting the immune system's response to cancer. They hope to stimulate the body to destroy tumor cells.
• For treatment of anaphylaxis, see APPENDIX.

No significant interactions.

Special considerations:
• Contraindicated in corticosteroid therapy or in immunosuppression. Should be deferred in acute illness.
• History of allergies and past reaction to immunization should be obtained.
• Epinephrine 1:1,000 should be available.
• May be given intradermally, but I.M. and subcutaneous routes give higher levels of protection.
• For treatment of anaphylaxis, see APPENDIX.

No significant interactions.

Special considerations:
• Contraindicated in immunosuppression, radiation, or corticosteroid therapy. Should be deferred in respiratory illness or polio outbreaks, or acute illness except in emergency. Single antigen should be used during polio risks. In children under 6 years, should be used only when diphtheria, tetanus, and pertussis toxoid combination is contraindicated because of pertussis component.
• Strength (pediatric or adult) of toxoid used should be verified.
• Hot or cold compresses should not be used; may increase severity of local reaction.
• History of allergies and past reaction to immunization should be obtained.
• Epinephrine 1:1,000 should be available.
• Should be given in site not previously used for vaccines or toxoids.
• For treatment of anaphylaxis, see APPENDIX.

No significant interactions.

Special considerations:
• Contraindicated in corticosteroid therapy or immunosuppression. Should be deferred in acute illness.
• Immunization should be stopped if CNS disorder occurs. Immunization may be continued with diphtheria and tetanus toxoids without pertussis component at doses of 0.05 to 0.1 ml.
• DPT injection may be given at same time as trivalent oral polio vaccine (TOPV).
• History of allergies and past reaction to immunization should be obtained.
• Epinephrine 1:1,000 should be available.
• Not to be used for active infection.
• Should not be given subcutaneously.
• Vial should be shaken well before using. Store in refrigerator.
• For treatment of anaphylaxis, see APPENDIX.

No significant interactions.

Special considerations:
• Contraindicated in immunosuppression, radiation or corticosteroid therapy, and in children under 12 months with cerebral damage. Should be deferred in acute illness or polio outbreak, except in emergency.
• Hot or cold compresses should not be used; may intensify local reaction.

(continued on following page)

NAMES, INDICATIONS AND DOSAGES	SIDE EFFECTS
diphtheria toxoid, adsorbed, pediatric *(continued)* 1 year later. Booster: 0.5 ml I.M. at 5- to 10-year intervals. Not advised for adults or for children over 6 years; instead, use adult strength of diphtheria toxoid (usually combined with tetanus toxoid).	
influenza virus vaccine, trivalent types A & B (whole virus) Fluax♦♦, Fluzone-Connaught **influenza virus vaccine, trivalent types A & B (split virus)** Fluogen ♦ **Brazil, Bangkok, and Singapore influenza prophylaxis:** ADULTS 29 YEARS AND OLDER: 0.5 ml whole or split virus I.M. YOUTHS AND ADULTS 13 TO 28 YEARS: 0.5 ml whole or split virus I.M. Repeat dose in 4 weeks. Those who received the 1978 to 1979, 1979 to 1980, or 1980 to 1981 vaccine require only 1 dose. CHILDREN 3 TO 12 YEARS: give 0.5 ml split virus I.M. Repeat dose in 4 weeks unless child received 1978 to 1979, 1979 to 1980, or 1980 to 1981 vaccine. CHILDREN 6 TO 35 MONTHS: 0.25 ml split virus I.M. Repeat dose in 4 weeks unless child received 1978 to 1979, 1979 to 1980, 1980 to 1981 vaccine. Recommendations are for 1981 to 1982 only. Must check yearly for new recommendations.	**Systemic:** *fever, malaise, myalgia, Guillain-Barré syndrome, anaphylaxis.* **Local:** erythema, induration. Side effects occur most often in children and in others not exposed to influenza viruses.
measles, mumps, and rubella virus vaccine, live M-M-R-II♦ **Immunization:** CHILDREN 12 MONTHS TO PUBERTY: 1 vial (1,000 units) S.C.	**Systemic:** fever, rash, regional lymphadenopathy, urticaria, *anaphylaxis.* **Local:** erythema.
measles (rubeola) and rubella virus vaccine, live attenuated M-R-Vax-II **Immunization:** CHILDREN 15 MONTHS TO PUBERTY: 1 vial (1,000 units) S.C.	**Systemic:** fever, rash, lymphadenopathy, *anaphylaxis.*

♦ Available in U.S. and Canada. ♦♦ Available in Canada only.
All other products (no symbol) available in U.S. only. Italicized side effects are common or life-threatening.

INTERACTIONS AND SPECIAL CONSIDERATIONS

• History of allergies and past reaction to immunization should be obtained.
• Epinephrine 1:1,000 should be available to treat anaphylaxis.
• Vial should be shaken well before using. Store in refrigerator.

No significant interactions.

Special considerations:
• Contraindicated in hypersensitivity to eggs. Should be deferred in acute respiratory or other active infection, or when there is risk of poliomyelitis infection.
• History of allergies, especially to eggs, and past reaction to immunization should be obtained.
• Injections should be given into deltoid or midlateral thigh.
• Epinephrine 1:1,000 should be available.
• Recommended for patients with chronic disease, metabolic disorders, and those over age 65.
• Influenza vaccine available as whole virus and split virus preparations. Split virus vaccines cause somewhat fewer side effects than whole virus in children.
• Fever, malaise, and myalgia begin 6 to 12 hours after vaccination and persist 1 to 2 days.
• Allergic reactions, which occur immediately, are extremely rare.
• Paralysis associated with Guillain-Barré syndrome is uncommon, but patients should be made aware of risk as compared with risk of influenza and its complications.
• For treatment of anaphylaxis, see APPENDIX.

Interactions:
IMMUNE SERUM GLOBULIN, WHOLE BLOOD, PLASMA: antibodies in serum may interfere with immune response. Don't use vaccine within 3 months of transfusion.

Special considerations:
• Contraindicated in immunosuppression; cancer; blood dyscrasias; corticosteroid or radiation therapy; gamma globulin disorders; fever; active, untreated tuberculosis. Use cautiously in hypersensitivity to neomycin, chickens, ducks, eggs, or feathers. Immunization should be deferred in acute illness.
• Presence of maternal antibodies may prevent response in children under 12 months.
• Fever should be treated with antipyretics.
• Store in refrigerator and protect from light. Solution may be used if red, pink, or yellow but must be clear.
• Only diluent supplied should be used and vaccine discarded 8 hours after reconstituting.
• History of allergies, especially to ducks, rabbits, and antibiotics, and past reaction to immunization should be obtained.
• Should be injected in outer aspect of upper arm. Should not be given I.V.
• Epinephrine 1:1,000 should be available.
• For treatment of anaphylaxis, see APPENDIX.

Interactions:
IMMUNE SERUM GLOBULIN, WHOLE BLOOD, PLASMA: antibodies in serum may interfere with immune response. Don't use vaccine within 3 months of transfusion.
TUBERCULIN SKIN TEST: may temporarily decrease response to test. Defer skin testing.

Special considerations:
• Contraindicated in immunosuppression; cancer; blood dyscrasias; corticosteroid or radiation therapy; gamma globulin disorders; fever; active, untreated tuberculosis. Use cautiously in hypersensitivity to neomycin, chickens, ducks, eggs, or feathers, and when there is a history of febrile seizures or in cerebral injury. Defer immunization in acute illness.
• Should not be given within 1 month of other live virus vaccines, except oral poliovirus vaccine.

(continued on following page)

NAMES, INDICATIONS AND DOSAGES	SIDE EFFECTS
measles (rubeola) and rubella virus vaccine, live attenuated *(continued)*	
measles (rubeola) virus vaccine, live attenuated Attenuvax♦ **Immunization:** ADULTS AND CHILDREN 15 MONTHS OR OVER: 0.5 ml (1,000 units) S.C.	**Systemic:** fever, rash, lymphadenopathy, *anaphylaxis,* febrile convulsions in susceptible children, anorexia, leukopenia. **Local:** erythema, swelling, tenderness.
meningitis vaccines Meningovax-A/C, Menomune-A, Menomune-C, Menomune-A/C **Meningococcal meningitis prophylaxis:** ADULTS AND CHILDREN OVER 2 YEARS: 0.5 ml S.C. Use vaccine group C or A, except in highly endemic areas; in these areas use A/C combination. CHILDREN 3 MONTHS TO 2 YEARS: 0.5 ml S.C. Use vaccine group A.	**Systemic:** headache, malaise, chills, fever, cramps, *anaphylaxis.* **Local:** pain, erythema, induration.
mumps virus vaccine, live Mumpsvax♦ **Immunization:** ADULTS AND CHILDREN OVER 12 MONTHS: 1 vial (5,000 units) S.C.	**Systemic:** *slight fever,* rash, malaise, mild allergic reactions.
plague vaccine **Primary immunization and booster:** ADULTS AND CHILDREN OVER 11 YEARS: 1 ml I.M. followed by 0.2 ml in 1 to 3 months, then 0.2 ml 3 to 6 months after second injection. Booster: 0.1 to 0.2 ml q 6 months while in plague area.	**Systemic:** malaise, headache, slight fever, lymphadenopathy, *anaphylaxis.* **Local:** swelling, induration, erythema.

INTERACTIONS AND SPECIAL CONSIDERATIONS

- Store in refrigerator and protect from light. Solution may be used if red, pink, or yellow but must be clear (with no precipitation).
- Use only diluent supplied; discard vaccine 8 hours after reconstituting.
- Should be injected in outer aspect of upper arm. Should not be injected I.V.
- For treatment of anaphylaxis, see APPENDIX.

Interactions:
IMMUNE SERUM GLOBULIN, WHOLE BLOOD, PLASMA: antibodies in serum may interfere with immune response. Don't use vaccine within 3 months of transfusion.
TUBERCULIN SKIN TEST: may temporarily decrease response to test. Defer skin testing.

Special considerations:
- Contraindicated in immunosuppression; cancer; blood dyscrasias; corticosteroid or radiation therapy; gamma globulin disorders; active, untreated tuberculosis; fever. Use with caution in hypersensitivity to neomycin, chickens, eggs, or feathers. Defer in acute illness or after administration of blood or plasma.
- Patient should avoid pregnancy for 3 months after vaccination.
- Should not be given I.V.
- History of allergies, especially to eggs, and past reaction to immunization should be obtained.
- Epinephrine 1:1,000 should be available.
- Store in refrigerator and protect from light. Solution may be used if red, pink, or yellow but must be clear (with no precipitation).
- Use only diluent supplied; discard vaccine 8 hours after reconstituting.
- May be given with oral polio vaccine.
- For treatment of anaphylaxis, see APPENDIX.

No significant interactions.

Special considerations:
- Contraindicated in immunosuppression. Should be deferred in acute illness.
- Patient should avoid pregnancy for 3 months after vaccination.
- History of allergies and past reaction to immunization should be obtained.
- Should not be given I.V.
- Epinephrine 1:1,000 should be available.
- For treatment of anaphylaxis, see APPENDIX.

Interactions:
IMMUNE SERUM GLOBULIN, WHOLE BLOOD, PLASMA: antibodies in serum may interfere with immune response. Don't use vaccine within 3 months of transfusion.
TUBERCULIN SKIN TEST: may temporarily decrease response to test. Defer skin testing.

Special considerations:
- Contraindicated in immunosuppression; cancer; blood dyscrasias; corticosteroid or radiation therapy; gamma globulin disorders; active, untreated tuberculosis. Use cautiously in hypersensitivity to neomycin, chickens, ducks, eggs, or feathers. Should be deferred in acute illness and for 3 months after transfusions or immune serum globulin.
- Avoiding pregnancy for 3 months after immunization should be stressed, and, if necessary, contraceptive information provided.
- Fever should be treated with antipyretics.
- Should not be given within 1 month of other live virus vaccines except oral poliovirus vaccine.
- Store in refrigerator and protect from light. Solution may be used if red, pink, or yellow but must be clear.
- Only diluent supplied should be used and vaccine discarded 8 hours after reconstituting. Should not be given I.V.
- History of allergies, especially to antibiotics, and past reaction to immunization should be obtained.
- Administration of other live virus vaccines should be separated by at least 1 month if possible.
- Epinephrine 1:1,000 should be available.
- For treatment of anaphylaxis, see APPENDIX.

No significant interactions.

Special considerations:
- Contraindicated in immunosuppression. Should be deferred in respiratory infection.
- Deltoid area preferred injection site. History of allergies and past reaction to immunization should be obtained.
- Epinephrine 1:1,000 should be available.
- For treatment of anaphylaxis, see APPENDIX.

(continued on following page)

NAMES, INDICATIONS AND DOSAGES	SIDE EFFECTS
plague vaccine *(continued)* CHILDREN UNDER 1 YEAR: ⅕ adult primary or booster dose. CHILDREN 1 TO 4 YEARS: ⅖ adult primary or booster dose. CHILDREN 5 TO 10 YEARS: ⅗ adult primary or booster dose.	
pneumococcal vaccine, polyvalent Pneumovax♦, Pnu-Imune **Pneumococcal immunization:** ADULTS AND CHILDREN 2 YEARS OR OVER: 0.5 ml I.M. or S.C. Not recommended for children under 2 years.	**Systemic:** *slight fever, anaphylaxis.* **Local:** severe local reaction can occur when revaccination takes place within 3 years.
poliovirus vaccine, live, oral, trivalent Orimune **Poliovirus immunization:** ADULTS AND CHILDREN OVER 6 WEEKS: two drops or 0.5 ml P.O. in 5 ml of water or simple syrup, or on sugar cube. Repeat dose in 8 weeks. Give third dose at 18 months. Booster: two drops or 0.5 ml P.O.	None reported.
rabies vaccine (duck embryo), dried, killed virus **Postexposure immunization for domestic animal bite:** ADULTS AND CHILDREN: 1 ml S.C. daily for 14 days in the abdomen on alternate sides. **Postexposure immunization for wild animal bite:** ADULTS AND CHILDREN: 2 ml S.C. daily for 7 days, then 1 ml daily for 7 more days. Supplemental doses may be needed after initial therapy. **Preexposure immunization (for patients constantly exposed to rabies):** ADULTS AND CHILDREN: 1 ml S.C. weekly for 3 weeks, then fourth dose 6 months later; or 1 ml S.C. 1 month apart for 2 doses, then third dose 7 months after second. Booster (for patients constantly exposed to rabies): 1 ml q 1 to 2 years.	**Systemic:** peripheral neuritis, dorsolumbar myelitis, acute idiopathic polyneuritis, acute encephalomyelitis, fever, weakness, stiff neck, respiratory distress, *anaphylaxis.* **GI:** *nausea, vomiting, diarrhea, abdominal cramps.* **Skin:** urticaria. **Local:** *stinging, pain, erythema, induration,* lymphadenopathy.
rabies vaccine, human diploid cell (HDCV) **Postexposure antirabies immunization:** ADULTS AND CHILDREN: 5 1-ml doses of HDCV I.M. (for example, in the deltoid region). Give first dose as soon as possible after expo-	**Systemic:** headache, nausea, abdominal pain, muscle aches, dizziness. **Local:** *pain, erythema, swelling or itching at injection site.*

INTERACTIONS AND SPECIAL CONSIDERATIONS

No significant interactions.

Special considerations:
• Immunization history needs careful checking to avoid revaccination within 3 years.
• Should be injected in deltoid or midlateral thigh; should not be injected I.V.
• Keep refrigerated. Reconstitution or dilution not necessary.
• Fever should be treated with mild antipyretics.
• Protects against 14 pneumococcal types, which account for 80% of pneumococcal disease.
• History of allergies and past reaction to immunization should be obtained.
• Epinephrine 1:1,000 should be available.
• For treatment of anaphylaxis, see APPENDIX.

Interactions:
IMMUNE SERUM GLOBULIN, WHOLE BLOOD, PLASMA: antibodies in serum may interfere with immune response. Don't use vaccine within 3 months of transfusion.

Special considerations:
• Contraindicated in immunosuppression, cancer, immunoglobulin abnormalities, radiation, or corticosteroid therapy. Should be deferred in acute illness, vomiting, or diarrhea.
• Keep frozen until used. Once thawed, if unopened, may store refrigerated up to 30 days. Opened vials may be refrigerated up to 7 days.
• Should be discarded if vaccine color changes from red or pink to yellow.
• History of allergies and past reaction to immunization should be obtained.
• Not for parenteral use.
• Administration of other live virus vaccines should be separated by at least 1 month if possible.

No significant interactions.

Special considerations:
• Contraindicated in corticosteroid therapy. Corticosteroids should be discontinued during immunization period.
• When postexposure immunization is indicated, pregnancy is not a contraindication.
• Immediate, thorough cleaning of wound is best way to prevent rabies.
• In serious reaction to duck embryo component, state health department and Center for Disease Control in Atlanta, Georgia, can advise on experimental alternatives.
• Rabies immune globulin may be given at time of first vaccine dose to provide immediate protection.
• 23G or 24G, ½" to ¾" needle should be used.
• History of allergies, especially to eggs, ducks, or proteins, and past reaction to immunization should be obtained.
• Epinephrine 1:1,000 should be available.
• For treatment of anaphylaxis, see APPENDIX.

No significant interactions.

Special considerations:
• Corticosteroids should be discontinued during immunization period.
• When postexposure immunization is indicated, pregnancy is not a contraindication.
• Persons with a history of hypersensitivity should be given rabies vaccine with caution. Persons allergic to duck embryo vaccine are less likely to be allergic to HDCV.
• Epinephrine 1:1,000 should be available to manage possible anaphylaxis.
• HDCV is the preferred rabies vaccine because

(continued on following page)

NAMES, INDICATIONS AND DOSAGES	SIDE EFFECTS
rabies vaccine, human diploid cell *(continued)* sure; give an additional dose on each of days 3, 7, 14, and 28 after first dose.	
rubella and mumps virus vaccine, live Biavax-II **Measles and mumps immunization:** ADULTS AND CHILDREN OVER 12 MONTHS: 1 vial (1,000 units) S.C.	**Systemic:** fever, rash, thrombocytopenic purpura, urticaria, arthritis, arthralgia, polyneuritis, *anaphylaxis.* **Local:** pain, erythema, induration, lymphadenopathy.
rubella virus vaccine, live attenuated (RA 27/3) Meruvax-II♦ **Measles immunization:** ADULTS AND CHILDREN 12 MONTHS OR OVER: 1 vial (1,000 units) S.C.	**Systemic:** fever, rash, thrombocytopenic purpura, urticaria, arthritis, arthralgia, polyneuritis, *anaphylaxis.* **Local:** pain, erythema, induration, lymphadenopathy.
smallpox vaccine Dryvax **Immunization:** ADULTS: deposit drop of vaccine on cleansed site and make series of multiple pressures with sharp needle through drop. Use only for laboratory personnel working with virus.	**Systemic:** encephalopathy, transverse myelitis, acute infection, polyneuritis, eczema vaccinatum, eye infection, rash, *anaphylaxis,* fever. **Local:** necrosis, pustule (expected), infection.

INTERACTIONS AND SPECIAL CONSIDERATIONS

of its presumed greater efficacy and because fewer adverse reactions are known to be associated with it.
• Contact state health department or Merieux Institute (1-800-327-8387) on vaccine availability.

Interactions:
IMMUNE SERUM GLOBULIN, WHOLE BLOOD, PLASMA: antibodies in serum may interfere with immune response. Don't give vaccine within 3 months of transfusion.
TUBERCULIN SKIN TEST: may temporarily decrease response to test. Defer skin testing.

Special considerations:
• Contraindicated in immunosuppression; cancer; blood dyscrasias; corticosteroid or radiation therapy; gamma globulin disorders; active, untreated tuberculosis; fever; pregnancy. Use with caution in hypersensitivity to neomycin, chickens, ducks, eggs, or feathers. Should be deferred in acute illness and after administration of immune serum globulin, blood, or plasma.
• Avoiding pregnancy for 3 months after immunization should be stressed, and, if necessary, contraceptive information provided.
• Store in refrigerator and protect from light. Solution may be used if red, pink, or yellow but must be clear.
• Only diluent supplied should be used and vaccine discarded 8 hours after reconstituting.
• History of allergies, especially to ducks, rabbits, and antibiotics, and past reaction to immunization should be obtained.
• Should be injected into outer aspect of upper arm. Should not be injected I.V.
• Epinephrine 1:1,000 should be available.
• For treatment of anaphylaxis, see APPENDIX.

Interactions:
IMMUNE SERUM GLOBULIN, WHOLE BLOOD, PLASMA: antibodies in serum may interfere with immune response. Don't use vaccine within 3 months of transfusion.
TUBERCULIN SKIN TEST: may temporarily decrease response to test. Defer skin testing.

Special considerations:
• Contraindicated in immunosuppression; cancer; blood dyscrasias; corticosteroid or radiation therapy; gamma globulin disorders; active, untreated tuberculosis; fever. Use cautiously in hypersensitivity to neomycin, chickens, ducks, eggs, or feathers.
• Avoiding pregnancy for 3 months after immunization should be stressed, and, if necessary, contraceptive information provided.
• Store in refrigerator and protect from light. Solution may be used if red, pink, or yellow but must be clear.
• Only diluent supplied should be used and vaccine discarded 8 hours after reconstituting.
• History of allergies, especially to ducks and rabbits, and past reaction to immunization should be obtained.
• Should be injected into outer aspect of upper arm. Should not be injected I.V.
• Epinephrine 1:1,000 should be available.
• For treatment of anaphylaxis, see APPENDIX.

Interactions:
IMMUNE SERUM GLOBULIN, WHOLE BLOOD, PLASMA: antibodies in serum may interfere with immune response. Don't use vaccine within 3 months of transfusion.
METHOTREXATE: may interfere with immune response. Don't use together.

Special considerations:
• Contraindicated in wounds or burns, skin disorders (for example, eczema), immunosuppression, antimetabolite and radiation therapy, and pregnancy. Also contraindicated in patients with direct contact with smallpox virus, and in those with leukemia, lymphomas, or other malignant neoplasms affecting the bone marrow or lymphatic system. Weigh risks against benefits. Use cautiously in hypersensitivity to eggs, chickens, or feathers, or to neomycin or other antibiotic preservatives in this vaccine (polymyxin B, streptomycin, chlortetracycline).
• Site should not be exposed to direct sunlight for several days, or water for 2 hours. Site should not be covered initially. In pustular stage, loose dressing may be applied. Touching site may spread lesion and cause secondary infection.
• History of allergies, especially to chickens or beef, antibiotics, and past reaction to immunization should be obtained.
• Should not be injected.
• Reconstituted solution may be kept for 3 months under refrigeration.
• A successful primary vaccination shows a typical jennerian vesicle. If none is observed, vaccination procedures should be checked and vaccination repeated with a different lot of vaccine until a successful result is obtained.
• After revaccination, two responses are possible. A major reaction is the formation of a vesicular or pustular lesion of an area of definite

(continued on following page)

NAMES, INDICATIONS AND DOSAGES	SIDE EFFECTS
smallpox vaccine *(continued)*	
tetanus toxoid, adsorbed **tetanus toxoid fluid** **Primary immunization:** ADULTS AND CHILDREN: 0.5 ml (adsorbed) I.M. 4 to 6 weeks apart for 2 doses, then third dose 1 year after the second. **Primary immunization:** ADULTS AND CHILDREN: 0.5 ml (fluid) I.M. or S.C. 4 to 8 weeks apart, for 3 doses, then fourth dose of 0.5 ml 6 to 12 months after third dose. Booster: 0.5 ml I.M. at 10-year intervals.	**Systemic:** slight fever, chills, malaise, aches and pains, flushing, urticaria, pruritus, tachycardia, hypotension, *anaphylaxis.* **Local:** erythema, induration, nodule.
typhoid vaccine **Primary immunization:** ADULTS AND CHILDREN OVER 10 YEARS: 0.5 ml S.C.; repeat in 4 weeks. Booster: same dose as primary immunization q 3 years. CHILDREN 6 MONTHS TO 10 YEARS: 0.25 ml S.C.; repeat in 4 weeks. Booster: same dose as primary immunization q 3 years.	**Systemic:** *fever,* malaise, headache, nausea, *anaphylaxis.* **Local:** swelling, pain, inflammation.
yellow fever vaccine **Primary vaccination:** ADULTS AND CHILDREN OVER 6 MONTHS: 0.5 ml S.C. Booster: repeat 0.5 ml S.C. q 10 years.	**Systemic:** fever, malaise, *anaphylaxis.*

INTERACTIONS AND SPECIAL CONSIDERATIONS

palpable induration, which indicates virus multiplication has most likely taken place and revaccination is successful. Any other reaction is regarded as equivocal. When an equivocal reaction is observed, revaccination procedures should be checked and revaccination repeated with another lot of vaccine.
- Epinephrine 1:1,000 should be available.
- For treatment of anaphylaxis, see APPENDIX.

No significant interactions.

Special considerations:
- Contraindicated in immunosuppression and immunoglobulin abnormalities. Should be deferred in acute illness and polio outbreaks, except in emergencies.
- For prevention, not treatment, of tetanus infections.
- Date of last tetanus immunization should be checked.
- Hot or cold compresses should not be used; may increase severity of local reaction.
- History of allergies and past reaction to immunization should be obtained.
- Epinephrine 1:1,000 should be available.
- Adsorbed form produces longer duration of immunity. Fluid form provides quicker booster effect in patients actively immunized previously.
- This drug should not be confused with tetanus immune globulin, human.

No significant interactions.

Special considerations:
- Contraindicated in corticosteroid therapy. Should be deferred in acute illness.
- Fever should be treated with antipyretics.
- Should not be given intradermally.
- History of allergies and past reaction to immunization should be obtained.
- Epinephrine 1:1,000 should be available.
- Store at 2° to 10° C. (35.6° to 50° F.).
- Should be shaken thoroughly before withdrawal from vial.
- For treatment of anaphylaxis, see APPENDIX.

No significant interactions.

Special considerations:
- Contraindicated in gamma globulin deficiency, immunosuppression, cancer, corticosteroid or radiation therapy, hypersensitivies to chickens or eggs, and in pregnancy. Also contraindicated in infants under 6 months except in high-risk areas.
- Reconstitute with sodium chloride injection that contains no preservatives (preservatives decrease potency of vaccine).
- Store in freezer; shake well before using; use within 1 hour following reconstitution; discard remainder.
- History of allergies, especially to eggs, and past reaction to immunization should be obtained.
- Should not be given within 1 month of other live virus vaccines.
- Epinephrine 1:1,000 should be available.
- For treatment of anaphylaxis, see APPENDIX.

101

Antitoxins and antivenins

black widow spider antivenin
botulism antitoxin, bivalent equine
crotaline antivenin, polyvalent
diphtheria antitoxin, equine
***Micrurus fulvius* antivenin**
tetanus antitoxin (TAT), equine

Antitoxins and antivenins bind to and neutralize toxins and venoms. The preparations are made from blood of horses inoculated with specific toxins.

Major uses
- Antitoxins are used to prevent and treat bacterial toxin infections.
- Antivenins are used to treat symptoms of insect and spider bites, and snakebites.

Mechanism of action
- Antitoxins provide passive immunity. This type of immunity is acquired by inoculation with purified, concentrated antibodies formed in the blood of horses immunized by specific toxins.
- Toxins and venoms are bound to and neutralized by the specific antitoxin or antivenin.

Absorption, distribution, metabolism, and excretion
Not applicable.

Onset and duration
Onset is immediate, but duration of immunity hasn't been determined.

Combination products
None.

PATIENT-TEACHING AID

HOW TO USE AN EMERGENCY ANAPHYLAXIS KIT

Dear Patient:

This emergency anaphylaxis kit contains all you need to combat an allergic reaction from an insect bite or sting: prefilled syringe with two doses of epinephrine, alcohol swabs, tourniquet, and antihistamine tablets. If you've been stung:

1. Notify the doctor immediately.
2. Remove the insect's stinger. Don't push, pinch, squeeze, or drive the stinger farther into the skin. If you can't remove the stinger quickly, go immediately to step 3.

A

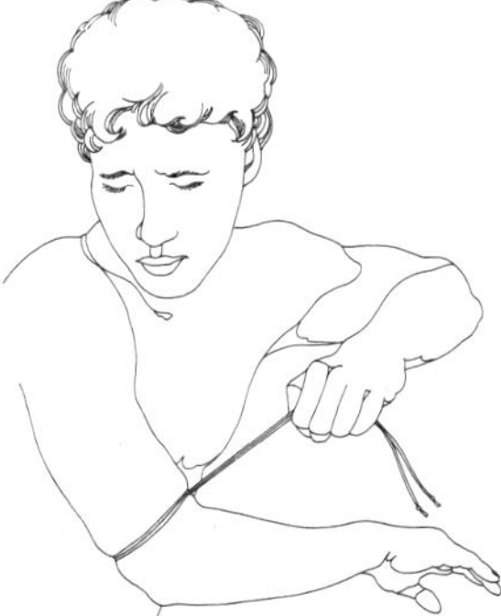

3. If you were stung on the arm or leg, apply the tourniquet between the sting and your torso, and tighten it (A). *(Note:* Loosen the tourniquet slightly every 10 minutes to maintain circulation.) If you were stung on the face, neck, or a place where you can't apply a tourniquet, apply ice to the affected area.
4. Use an alcohol swab to clean a 4″ area of skin above the tourniquet.
5. Remove the needle cover from the prefilled syringe. Expel air from the syringe by pointing the needle upward and carefully pushing the plunger until a bead of liquid forms on the needle tip.
6. Insert the whole needle straight down into the cleaned area and pull back on the plunger (B). If blood enters the syringe, the needle's in a blood vessel. Withdraw the needle, insert it in another site within the cleaned area, and retest for blood.

B

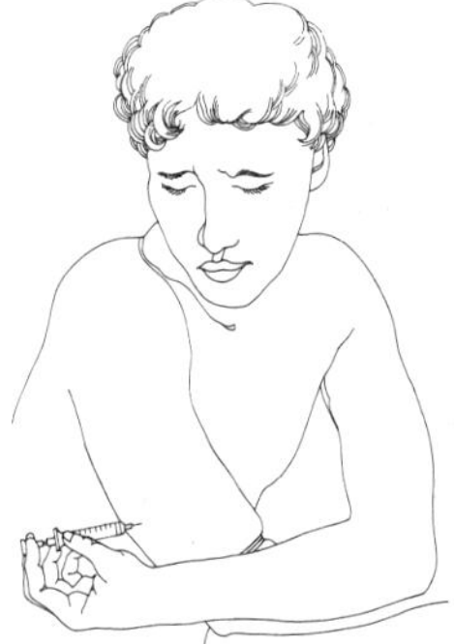

7. When you're sure the needle's not in a blood vessel, depress the plunger and inject the prescribed dose of epinephrine. Guidelines: Adults, and children over age 12—up to 0.5 ml; children ages 7 to 12—0.2 ml; children ages 2 to 6—0.15 ml; infants to age 2—0.05 to 0.1 ml.
8. Chew and swallow antihistamine tablets. Guidelines: Adults, and children over age 12—4 tablets; children under age 12—2 tablets.
9. Apply ice or meat tenderizer to the affected area, if available. Keep warm. Avoid exertion.
10. If you see no improvement in 10 minutes, prepare the syringe for a second injection. Rotate the plunger one quarter turn to the right, to align with the rectangular slot in the syringe. Repeat steps 4 through 7.
11. See the doctor or go to your hospital emergency department as soon as you finish this procedure.

NAMES, INDICATIONS AND DOSAGES	SIDE EFFECTS
black widow spider antivenin Antivenin *(Latrodectus mactans)*♦ **Black widow spider bite:** ADULTS AND CHILDREN: 2.5 ml I.M. in deltoid. Second dose may be needed.	**Systemic:** hypersensitivity, *anaphylaxis, neurotoxicity*.
botulism antitoxin, bivalent equine **Botulism:** ADULTS AND CHILDREN: 1 vial I.V. stat and q 4 hours, p.r.n., until patient's condition improves. Dilute antitoxin 1:10 in 5% or 10% dextrose in water or normal saline solution before giving. Give first 10 ml of dilution over 5 minutes; after 15 minutes, rate may be increased.	**Systemic:** hypersensitivity, *anaphylaxis,* serum sickness (urticaria, pruritus, fever, malaise, arthralgia) may occur in 5 to 13 days.
crotaline antivenin, polyvalent **Crotalid (rattlesnake) bites:** ADULTS AND CHILDREN: initially, 10 to 50 ml or more I.M. or S.C., depending on severity of bite and patient's response. If large amount of venom, 70 to 100 ml I.V. directly into superficial vein. Subsequent doses based on patient's response; may give 10 ml q ½ to 2 hours, p.r.n. If bite is in extremity, inject part of initial dose at various sites around limb above swelling; don't inject in finger or toe. The smaller the patient, the larger the initial dose.	**Systemic:** hypersensitivity, *anaphylaxis*.
diphtheria antitoxin, equine **Diphtheria prevention:** ADULTS AND CHILDREN: 1,000 to 5,000 units I.M. **Diphtheria treatment:** ADULTS AND CHILDREN: 20,000 to 80,000 units or more slow I.V. Additional doses may be given in 24 hours. I.M. route may be used in mild cases.	**Systemic:** hypersensitivity, *anaphylaxis,* serum sickness (urticaria, pruritus, fever, malaise, arthralgia) may occur in 7 to 12 days.
***Micrurus fulvius* antivenin** **Eastern and Texas coral snake bite:** ADULTS AND CHILDREN: 3 to 5 vials slow I.V. through running I.V. of 0.9% normal saline solution. Give first 1 to 2 ml over 3 to 5 minutes, and watch for signs of allergic reaction. If no signs develop, continue injection. Up to 10 vials may be needed. Not effective for Sonoran or Arizona coral snake bites.	**Systemic:** hypersensitivity, *anaphylaxis*.

♦ Available in U.S. and Canada. ♦♦ Available in Canada only.
All other products (no symbol) available in U.S. only. Italicized side effects are common or life-threatening.

INTERACTIONS AND SPECIAL CONSIDERATIONS

No significant interactions.

Special considerations:
- If possible, patient should be hospitalized.
- Patient should be immobilized and the bitten extremity splinted to prevent spread of venom.
- Sensitivity test required before giving.
- Epinephrine 1:1,000 should be available in case of adverse reaction.
- Venom is neurotoxic and may cause respiratory paralysis and convulsions. Patient should be watched carefully for 2 to 3 days.
- Accurate patient history of allergies, especially to horses, and past reaction to immunization should be obtained.
- Earliest possible use of the antivenin is recommended for best results.
- Antivenin may also be given I.V. in severe cases (as when the patient is in shock). Drug is given in 10 to 15 ml of saline solution over a 15-minute period.
- For treatment of anaphylaxis, see APPENDIX.

No significant interactions.

Special considerations:
- Sensitivity test required before giving.
- Epinephrine 1:1,000 should be available in case of adverse reaction. Bivalent antitoxin contains antibodies against types A and B *Clostridium botulinum*. Antitoxins against other types available only from Center for Disease Control in Atlanta, Georgia.
- Accurate patient history of allergies, especially to horses, and past reaction to immunization should be obtained.
- Earliest possible use of the antitoxin is recommended for best results.
- For treatment of anaphylaxis, see APPENDIX.

Interactions:
ANTIHISTAMINES: enhanced toxicity of crotaline venoms. Don't use together.

Special considerations:
- Sensitivity test required before giving.
- Patient should be immobilized immediately and bitten extremity splinted.
- Epinephrine 1:1,000 should be available in case of adverse reaction.
- Type and crossmatch as soon as possible since hemolysis from venom prevents accurate crossmatching.
- Early use of antivenin recommended for best results.
- Patient should be watched carefully for delayed allergic reaction or relapse.
- Because children have less resistance and less body fluid to dilute venom, they may need twice the adult dose.
- Accurate patient history of allergies, especially to horses, and past reaction to immunization should be obtained.
- Unused reconstituted drug should be discarded.
- For treatment of anaphylaxis, see APPENDIX.

No significant interactions.

Special considerations:
- Sensitivity test required before giving.
- Epinephrine 1:1,000 should be available in case of adverse reaction.
- Accurate patient history of allergies, especially to horses, and past reaction to immunization should be obtained.
- Therapy should be started immediately, without waiting for culture and sensitivity reports, if patient has clinical symptoms of diphtheria (sore throat, fever, tonsillar membrane).
- Refrigerate antitoxin at 35.6° to 50° F. (2° to 10° C.). May be warmed to 90° to 95° F. (32.2° to 35° C.), never higher.
- For treatment of anaphylaxis, see APPENDIX.

No significant interactions.

Special considerations:
- Patient should be tested for sensitivity before giving.
- Patient should be immobilized or bitten limb splinted to prevent spread of venom.
- Patient should be hospitalized if possible.
- Early use of antivenin recommended for best results.
- Patient should be watched carefully for 24 hours. Venom is neurotoxic and may cause respiratory paralysis, requiring supportive measures. Epinephrine 1:1,000 should be available in case of adverse reaction.
- Accurate patient history of allergies, especially to horses, and past reaction to immunization should be obtained.
- For treatment of anaphylaxis, see APPENDIX.

NAMES, INDICATIONS AND DOSAGES	SIDE EFFECTS
tetanus antitoxin (TAT), equine **Tetanus prophylaxis:** PATIENTS OVER 29.5 KG: 3,000 to 5,000 units I.M. or S.C. PATIENTS UNDER 29.5 KG: 1,500 to 3,000 units I.M. or S.C. **Tetanus treatment:** ALL PATIENTS: 10,000 to 20,000 units injected into wound. Give additional 40,000 to 200,000 units I.V. Start tetanus toxoid at same time but at different site and with a different syringe.	**Local:** pain, numbness, skin eruptions. **Systemic:** joint pain, hypersensitivity, *anaphylaxis*.

♦ Available in U.S. and Canada. ♦♦ Available in Canada only.
All other products (no symbol) available in U.S. only. Italicized side effects are common or life-threatening.

INTERACTIONS AND SPECIAL CONSIDERATIONS

No significant interactions.

Special considerations:
- Patient should be tested for sensitivity before giving.
- Should be used only when tetanus immune globulin (human) not available.
- Accurate patient history of allergies, especially to horses, and past reaction to immunization should be obtained. If respiratory difficulty develops, 0.4 ml of 1:1,000 solution epinephrine HCl should be given.
- Preventative dose should be given to patients who have had 2 or fewer injections of tetanus toxoid and who have tetanus-prone injuries more than 24 hours old.
- For treatment of anaphylaxis, see APPENDIX.

TEST FOR HYPERSENSITIVITY

Antitoxin and antivenin preparations frequently cause hypersensitivity. All patients, therefore, should receive a test dose of the drug either intradermally or ophthalmically, regardless of past history of negative sensitivity.

Intradermal test
- Dilute serum 1:10 with 0.9% sodium chloride for injection. Inject 0.02 ml of diluted serum intradermally on inner aspect of forearm. As a control, inject the other arm with 0.02 ml of 0.9% sodium chloride for injection.
- Observe for 20 minutes. If a wheal 10 mm or larger develops at the test site, surrounded by an erythematous flare 20 mm × 20 mm, the test is positive for hypersensitivity.
- If the skin test is positive, give an ophthalmic test.

Ophthalmic test
- Dilute serum 1:10 with 0.9% sodium chloride for injection. Instill one drop of dilution into conjunctival sac.
- Observe for 20 minutes. Hyperemia and congestion of the mucous membranes are a positive test for hypersensitivity.
- If the skin test is positive and the eye test is negative, the patient may be desensitized before antitoxin or antivenin is administered.

Note: Always have epinephrine 1:1,000 on hand when administering antitoxins or antivenins, even though test dose results are negative. The patient can develop hypersensitivity at any time during therapy.

102

Acidifiers and alkalinizers

Acidifiers
ammonium chloride
dilute hydrochloric acid

Alkalinizers
sodium bicarbonate
sodium lactate
tromethamine

Acidifiers and alkalinizers may correct acid-base imbalances in metabolic disorders. In severe metabolic alkalosis, acidifiers may be given to lower blood pH. In metabolic acidosis, alkalinizers raise blood pH.

Major uses

- Acidifiers are used to treat metabolic alkalosis. Ammonium chloride also acidifies the urine.
- Alkalinizers are used to treat metabolic acidosis. Sodium bicarbonate and sodium acetate may also alkalinize the urine. This blocks tubular reabsorption of acidic drugs and increases their excretion. Alkalinizing the urine can be part of the treatment of aspirin or phenobarbital overdose.

Mechanism of action

- Acidifiers increase free hydrogen ion (H^+) concentration.
- Alkalinizers decrease free hydrogen ion concentration. Sodium bicarbonate restores the buffering capacity of the body. Sodium lactate is metabolized to sodium bicarbonate before it can produce a buffering effect. Tromethamine combines with hydrogen ions and associated acid anions; the resulting salts are excreted by the kidneys.

Absorption, distribution, metabolism, and excretion

- Ammonium chloride and sodium bicarbonate are rapidly and well absorbed orally. Sodium lactate, dilute hydrochloric acid, and tromethamine are administered I.V. Ammonium chloride and sodium bicarbonate can be administered either orally or I.V.
- Ammonium chloride and sodium lactate are metabolized in the liver.
- Ammonium chloride is excreted in urine.
- Tromethamine is not metabolized and is excreted in urine.

Onset and duration

Onset is rapid after oral administration and immediate after I.V. administration. Duration of action varies, depending on use and underlying disease.

Combination products

None.

THE REGULATORS OF BLOOD pH

The body regulates its pH through three mechanisms, as shown here:

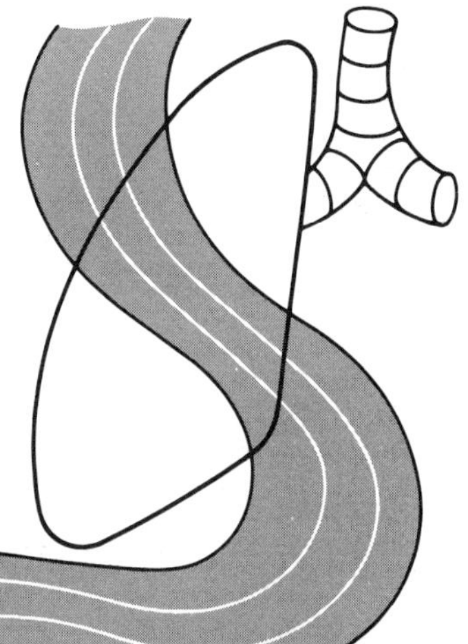

- *The lungs* act within minutes to regulate the volatile carbonic acid in the blood through exhalation or retention of carbon dioxide. If there is an excess of H^+ and the blood is too acidic, the patient may *hyper*ventilate to get rid of excess acid. If there is an inadequate amount of H^+ and blood is too alkaline, the patient may *hypo*ventilate to store CO_2 (which forms carbonic acid) and restore the pH to normal.

- *Blood buffers* neutralize excess acids or alkalies that form as a result of metabolic processes. In plasma, pH is determined by the ratio of bicarbonate to carbonic acid—the principal buffer pair. The ratio of carbonic acid to base bicarbonate is usually 1:20, but this ratio changes as one shifts into the other to help offset changes in hydrogen ion concentration.

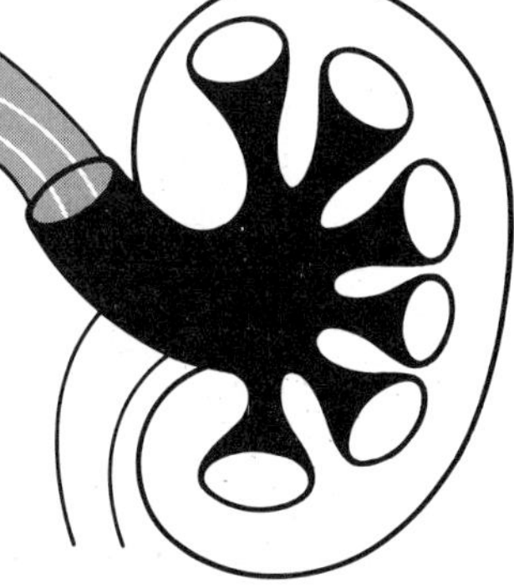

- *The kidneys* take hours or days to play their part in acid-base regulation, but they secrete or retain hydrogen or bicarbonate ions until the pH balance is exactly normal.

Remember that you cannot effectively evaluate serum electrolytes without knowing the blood pH. This is because small changes in pH greatly affect the movement of electrolytes across the cell membrane and cause dramatic changes in the serum levels. Normal blood pH is 7.35 to 7.45.

NAMES, INDICATIONS AND DOSAGES	SIDE EFFECTS
ammonium chloride **Metabolic alkalosis:** ADULTS AND CHILDREN: 4 mEq/kg slow I.V. or calculated by amount of chloride deficit. Infusion rate: 0.9 to 1.3 ml/minute 2.14% solution. Do not exceed 2 ml/minute. Hypodermoclysis has been used in infants and young children. One half calculated volume should be given, then patient should be reassessed. **As an acidifying agent:** 4 to 12 g P.O. daily in divided doses.	Side effects usually result from ammonia toxicity or too rapid I.V. administration. **CNS:** headache, confusion, progressive drowsiness, excitement alternating with coma, hyperventilation, *calcium-deficient tetany, twitching, hyperreflexia, EEG abnormalities.* **CV:** bradycardia. **GI:** (with oral dose) *gastric irritation, nausea, vomiting,* thirst, anorexia, retching. **GU:** glycosuria. **Metabolic:** *acidosis, hyperchloremia, hypokalemia,* hyperglycemia. **Skin:** rash, pallor. **Local:** pain at injection site. **Other:** irregular respirations with periods of apnea.
dilute hydrochloric acid **Metabolic alkalosis:** Pharmacy prepares (0.1 normal HCl solution in sterile water) 100 mEq hydrogen and 100 mEq chloride/liter.	None confirmed.
sodium bicarbonate **Cardiac arrest:** ADULTS AND CHILDREN: as a 7.5% or 8.4% solution, 1 to 3 mEq/kg I.V. initially; may repeat in 10 minutes. Further doses based on blood gases. If blood gases unavailable, use 0.5 mEq/kg q 10 minutes until spontaneous circulation returns. INFANTS UP TO 2 YEARS: 4.2% solution, I.V. infusion. Rate not to exceed 8 mEq/kg/day. **Metabolic acidosis:** ADULTS AND CHILDREN: dose depends on blood CO_2 content, pH, and patient's clinical condition. Generally, 2 to 5 mEq/kg I.V. infused over 4- to 8-hour period. **Systemic or urinary alkalinization:** ADULTS: 325 mg to 2 g P.O. q.i.d.	**GI:** gastric distention, belching, flatulence. **GU:** renal calculi or crystals. **Metabolic:** (with overdose) alkalosis, hypernatremia, hyperkalemia, hyperosmolarity.
sodium lactate **Alkalinize urine:** ADULTS: 30 ml of a ⅙ molar solution/kg of body weight given in divided doses over 24 hours. **Metabolic acidosis:** ADULTS: usually given as ⅙ molar injection (167 mEq lactate/liter). Dosage depends on degree of bicarbonate deficit.	**Metabolic:** (with overdose) alkalosis, hypernatremia, hyperkalemia, hyperosmolarity.
tromethamine Tham♦ **Metabolic acidosis (associated with cardiac bypass surgery or with cardiac arrest):** ADULTS: dose depends on bicarbonate deficit.	**CNS:** respiratory depression. **Metabolic:** hypoglycemia, hyperkalemia (with decreased urinary output). **Local:** venospasm; intravenous thrombosis; inflammation, necrosis, and sloughing if extravasation occurs.

INTERACTIONS AND SPECIAL CONSIDERATIONS

Interactions:
SPIRONOLACTONE: systemic acidosis. Use together cautiously.

Special considerations:
• Contraindicated in severe hepatic or renal dysfunction. Use cautiously in pulmonary insufficiency or cardiac edema and in infants.
• Should be given after meals to decrease GI side effects. Enteric-coated tablets may also minimize GI symptoms but are absorbed erratically.
• Pain of I.V. injection may be lessened by decreasing rate of infusion.
• CO_2 combining power and serum electrolytes should be determined before and during therapy.
• Urine pH and output should be monitored. Diuresis normal for first 2 days.
• Concentrated solutions (21.4%, 26.75%) should be diluted to 2.14% before giving.
• Rate and depth of respiration should be monitored frequently.
• Hypodermoclysis should be into lateral aspect of thigh. Infusion should be stopped immediately if pain occurs.

No significant interactions.

Special considerations:
• Not available commercially; prepared in pharmacy.
• I.V. solution should be administered slowly through a central venous line.
• PH, blood gases, and electrolytes should be monitored at 4- to 6-hour intervals.

No significant interactions.

Special considerations:
• No contraindications for use in life-threatening emergencies. Contraindicated in hypertension, in patients with tendency toward edema, in patients who are losing chlorides by vomiting or from continuous GI suction, in patients receiving diuretics known to produce hypochloremic alkalosis, and in patients on salt restriction or with renal disease.
• May be added to other I.V. fluids.
• Parenteral bicarbonate solutions will precipitate calcium salts. Should not be mixed in same infusion fluid. I.V. bolus injections should be given only through running I.V. lines free of calcium salts.
• To avoid risk of alkalosis, blood pH, PO_2, PCO_2, and electrolytes should be determined.
• Patient should not take with milk; may cause hypercalcemia, alkalosis, and possibly renal calculi.
• Because sodium bicarbonate inactivates catecholamines such as epinephrine and levarterenol, should not be mixed with I.V. solutions of these agents.

No significant interactions.

Special considerations:
• Contraindicated in severe hepatic disease, respiratory alkalosis, and in acidosis associated with congenital heart disease with persistent cyanosis.
• Monitor serum electrolytes to avoid alkalosis and hyperkalemia.

No significant interactions.

Special considerations:
• Contraindicated in anuria, uremia, chronic respiratory acidosis, pregnancy (except acute, life-threatening situations). Use cautiously in renal disease or poor urinary output. Monitor EKG and serum K^+ in these patients.
• To prevent blood pH from rising above normal, dose should be adjusted carefully.
• Should be given slowly through large needle (18G to 20G) into largest antecubital vein or by

(continued on following page)

NAMES, INDICATIONS AND DOSAGES	SIDE EFFECTS

tromethamine
(continued)

Calculate as follows: ml of 0.3 M tromethamine solution required = wt in kg × bicarbonate deficit (mEq/liter). Additional therapy based on serial determinations of existing bicarbonate deficit.

CHILDREN: calculate dose as above. Give slowly over 3 to 6 hours. Additional therapy based on degree of acidosis. Total 24-hour dose should not exceed 33 to 40 ml/kg.

INTERACTIONS AND SPECIAL CONSIDERATIONS

Foley catheter.

- Before, during, and after therapy: determine blood pH; carbon dioxide tension; bicarbonate, glucose, and electrolyte levels.
- Mechanical ventilation should be available and used when giving drug to patient with associated respiratory acidosis.
- Except in life-threatening situations, should not be used longer than 1 day.
- If I.V. extravasates, area should be infiltrated with 1% procaine and hyaluronidase 150 units; may reduce vasospasm and dilute remaining drug in local area.
- Concentration of tromethamine should not exceed 0.3 M.

103

Uricosurics

probenecid
sulfinpyrazone

Uricosurics are renal tubular blocking agents. By inhibiting active reabsorption of uric acid at the proximal convoluted tubule, they promote excretion of uric acid. This action then lowers uric acid levels in the blood. (For information on allopurinol and colchicine, which are not uricosuric agents but are used in gout, see Chapter 110, UNCATEGORIZED DRUGS.)

Major uses
Both uricosurics are used for maintenance therapy in chronic gouty arthritis and tophaceous gout.
• Probenecid is used as an adjunct in penicillin antibiotic therapy by increasing antibiotic blood concentrations.
• Sulfinpyrazone also inhibits platelet aggregation. Some studies have found it useful for patients with myocardial infarction.

Mechanism of action
Uricosurics block renal tubular reabsorption of uric acid, increasing excretion. They also inhibit active renal tubular secretion of many weak organic acids (for example, penicillins and cephalosporins).

Absorption, distribution, metabolism, and excretion
• The drugs are rapidly and completely absorbed from the gastrointestinal tract after oral administration.
• Probenecid is 95% bound to plasma proteins; sulfinpyrazone is 98% bound to plasma proteins.
• Probenecid and sulfinpyrazone are metabolized in the liver and excreted in urine. A small amount of sulfinpyrazone is also eliminated in feces.

Onset and duration
• Onset (appearance in blood and uric acid clearance) occurs 30 minutes after oral administration.
• Probenecid's effect on penicillin begins after 2 hours. Blood levels peak 2 to 4 hours after administration.
The drug's duration of action is 4 to 10 hours.
• Sulfinpyrazone blood levels peak 1 to 2 hours after ingestion. Duration of action is also 4 to 10 hours.

Combination products
COLBENEMID: probenecid 500 mg and colchicine 0.5 mg.
PROBEN-C: probenecid 500 mg and colchicine 0.5 mg.

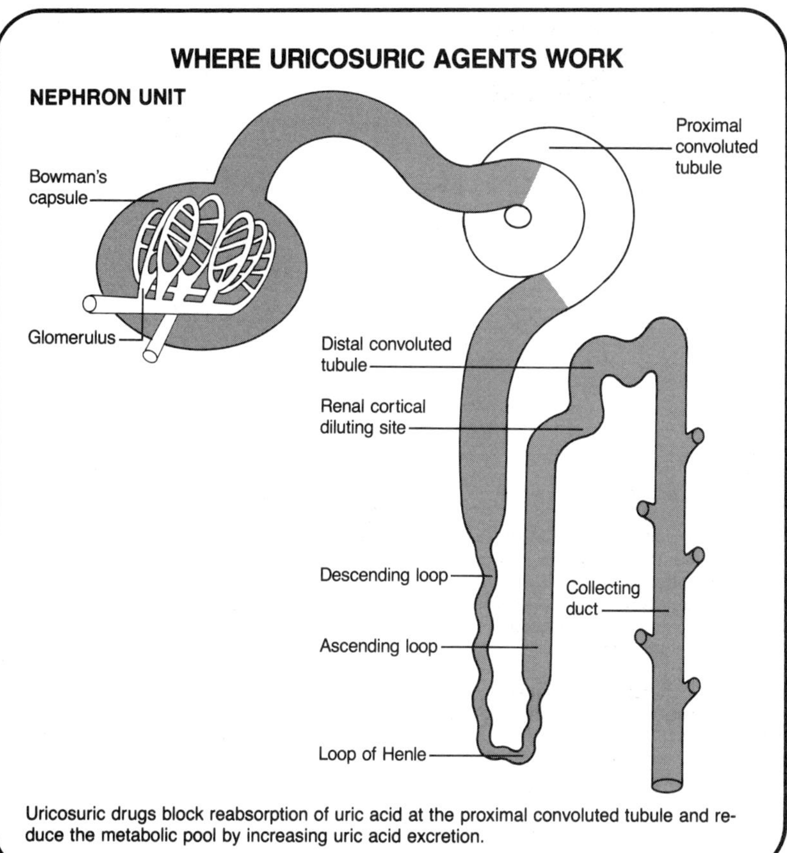

Uricosuric drugs block reabsorption of uric acid at the proximal convoluted tubule and reduce the metabolic pool by increasing uric acid excretion.

NAMES, INDICATIONS AND DOSAGES	SIDE EFFECTS
probenecid Benemid♦, Benn, Benuryl♦♦, Probalan, Probenimead, Robenecid, SK-Probenecid **Adjunct to penicillin or cephalosporin therapy:** ADULTS AND CHILDREN OVER 50 KG: 500 mg P.O. q.i.d. CHILDREN 2 TO 14 YEARS (UNDER 50 KG): initially, 25 mg/kg P.O., then 40 mg/kg divided q.i.d. **Single-dose treatment of gonorrhea:** ADULTS: 3.5 g ampicillin P.O. with 1 g probenecid P.O. given together; or 1 g probenecid P.O. 30 minutes before dose of 4.8 million units of aqueous penicillin G procaine I.M., injected at 2 different sites. **Treatment of hyperuricemia of gout, gouty arthritis:** ADULTS: 250 mg P.O. b.i.d. for first week, then 500 mg b.i.d., to maximum of 2 g daily. Maintenance: 500 mg daily for 6 months.	**Blood:** *hemolytic anemia.* **CNS:** headache, dizziness. **CV:** hypotension. **GI:** anorexia, nausea, vomiting, *gastric distress.* **GU:** urinary frequency. **Skin:** dermatitis, pruritus. **Other:** flushing, sore gums, fever.
sulfinpyrazone Anturan♦♦, Anturane **Inhibition of platelet aggregation, increase of platelet survival time in treatment of thromboembolic disorders, angina, myocardial infarction, transient cerebral ischemic attacks, peripheral arterial atherosclerosis:** ADULTS: 200 mg P.O. q.i.d. **Maintenance therapy for common gout: reduction, prevention of joint changes and tophi formation:** ADULTS: 100 to 200 mg P.O. b.i.d. first week, then 200 to 400 mg P.O. b.i.d. Maximum 800 mg daily.	**GI:** *nausea, dyspepsia,* epigastric pain, blood loss, reactivation of peptic ulcers. **Skin:** rash.

INTERACTIONS AND SPECIAL CONSIDERATIONS

Interactions:
SALICYLATES: inhibited uricosuric effect of probenecid, causing urate retention. Do not use together.

Special considerations:
- Contraindicated in blood dyscrasias; acute gout attack; penicillin therapy in presence of known renal impairment; gouty nephropathy; urinary tract stones or obstruction; azotemia or hyperuricemia secondary to cancer chemotherapy, radiation, or myeloproliferative neoplastic diseases. Use cautiously with peptic ulcer or renal impairment.
- Usually preferred over sulfinpyrazone because probenecid produces fewer, less severe GI and hematologic side effects.
- Contains no analgesic or anti-inflammatory agent and is of no value during acute gout attacks.
- Suitable for long-term use; no cumulative effects or tolerance.
- Not effective with chronic renal insufficiency (glomerular filtration rate less than 30 ml/minute).
- Periodic BUN and renal function studies recommended in long-term therapy.
- May increase frequency, severity, and length of acute gout attacks during first 6 to 12 months of therapy. Prophylactic colchicine is given during first 3 to 6 months.
- Alcohol should be avoided; increases urate level.
- Force fluids to maintain daily output of 2 to 3 liters minimum. Sodium bicarbonate or potassium citrate may be ordered to akalinize urine. These measures will prevent hematuria, renal colic, urate stone development, and costovertebral pain.
- Should be given with milk, food, or antacids to minimize GI distress. Continued disturbances might indicate need to lower dose.
- Foods high in purine should be restricted: anchovies, liver, sardines, kidneys, sweetbreads, peas, lentils.
- Drug must be taken regularly as ordered or gout attacks may result. Blood levels should be monitored regularly and dosage adjusted if necessary. Lifelong therapy may be required in patients with hyperuricemia.
- May have false-positive glucose tests with Benedict's solution or Clinitest, but not with the glucose oxidase method (Clinistix, Diastix, Tes-Tape).
- Decreases urinary excretion of 17-ketosteroids, phenolsulfonphthalein, bromsulphalein, aminohippuric acid, and iodine-related organic acids, interfering with laboratory procedures.
- For symptoms and treatment of anaphylaxis, see APPENDIX.

Interactions:
PROBENECID: inhibited renal excretion of sulfinpyrazone. Use together with caution.
SALICYLATES: inhibited uricosuric effect of sulfinpyrazone. Do not use together.

Special considerations:
- Contraindicated in hypersensitivity to pyrazole derivatives (including oxyphenbutazone and phenylbutazone); active peptic ulcer; gouty nephropathy; urolithiasis or urinary obstruction; bone marrow depression; azotemia or hyperuricemia secondary to cancer chemotherapy, radiation, or myeloproliferative neoplastic diseases; and during or within 2 weeks after gout attack. Use cautiously with diminished hepatic or renal function.
- Use for treating thromboembolic conditions is investigational and is most often directed at prevention of myocardial infarction recurrence.
- Recommended for patients unresponsive to probenecid. Suitable for long-term use; no cumulative effects or tolerance.
- Contains no analgesic or anti-inflammatory agent and is of no value during acute gout attacks.
- Periodic BUN, CBC, and renal function studies advised during long-term therapy.
- May increase frequency, severity, and length of acute gout attacks during first 6 to 12 months of therapy; prophylactic colchicine is given during first 3 to 6 months.
- Therapy, especially at start, may lead to renal colic and formation of uric acid stones. Until acid levels are normal (about 6 mg/100 ml), intake and output should be monitored closely.
- Force fluids to maintain daily output of 2 to 3 liters minimum. Sodium bicarbonate or other agent may be ordered to alkalinize urine.
- Should be given with milk, food, or antacids to minimize GI disturbances.
- Foods high in purine should be restricted: anchovies, liver, sardines, kidneys, sweetbreads, peas, lentils.
- Drug must be taken regularly as ordered or gout attacks may result. Blood levels should be monitored regularly and dosage adjusted if necessary.
- Decreases urinary excretion of aminohippuric acid and phenolsulfonphthalein interfering with laboratory procedures.
- Alkalinizing agents are used therapeutically to increase sulfinpyrazone activity, preventing urolithiasis.
- Patient should not take any aspirin-containing medications.
- Patients taking oral hypoglycemic agents should be monitored; these drugs' effects may be potentiated by sulfinpyrazone, causing hypoglycemia.

104

Enzymes

bromelains
chymotrypsin
fibrinolysin and desoxyribonuclease
hyaluronidase
papain
streptokinase-streptodornase
trypsin

Enzymes are complex proteins that induce chemical changes without being changed themselves. Although several enzyme groups are used therapeutically, only those that reduce inflammation or debride necrotic tissue are described in this chapter.

Enzymes can be given orally, topically, locally, subcutaneously, or intramuscularly. They work best in a moist environment but are destroyed by heat or cold. They are also inactivated by detergents, antiseptics, and heavy metal compounds. Enzymes furnish adjunctive therapy only, so other medical or surgical management is necessary to cure or alleviate underlying causes of tissue necrosis and inflammation.

Major uses

- Bromelains, chymotrypsin, papain, and trypsin (proteolytic enzymes) are used as adjunctive therapy for inflammation and edema from accidental or surgical trauma.
- Fibrinolysin and desoxyribonuclease—in topical applications only—remove necrotic debris and exudate from wounds.
- Hyaluronidase increases absorption and dispersion of infusions and locally injected drugs such as anesthetics.
- Streptokinase-streptodornase (a mixture of bacterial enzymes) dissolves blood clots and the fibrinous portion of exudate.

Mechanism of action

Enzymes reverse the decreased tissue permeability that develops with inflammation and edema. In this way, they restore flow of blood and other body fluids, and facilitate drainage and tissue repair.

They degrade protein of blood clots, necrotic tissue, and purulent exudate, which may block free flow of body fluids and impede resolution of inflammation and edema.

They digest protein matter, cleaning wounds by liquefaction and dissolution.

Absorption, distribution, metabolism, and excretion

The extent of absorption of these enzymes cannot be measured. Their distribution, metabolism, and excretion are unknown.

Onset and duration

Unknown.

PROMOTING EFFECTIVE ENZYME THERAPY FOR DECUBITUS ULCERS

Proteolytic enzymes are used primarily for debridement of necrotic tissue from wounds of decubitus ulcers. Their main effect is a gradual appearance of granulation tissue around the site and gradual decrease in the depth of the crater as deeper tissue generates new cells.

Enzyme therapy has many limitations. Because enzymes are proteins, they need a high degree of purification before administration. Even then, they may be antigenic and cause toxic reactions. Another drawback is that protein-digesting enzymes of the gastrointestinal tract tend to inhibit proteolytic enzyme activity. Despite these limitations, enzymes have been proven useful.

However, effective treatment with enzymes requires certain supportive measures, depending on the underlying cause—stasis, trauma, or infection.

- Sterile technique should be used in treating decubitus ulcers.
- A heat lamp and air exposure should be used between dressings to promote drying and increase the blood supply to the ulcerated area.
- Oxygen saturation should be provided by inserting an oxygen catheter through a paper-cup tent over decubitus ulcers. This promotes healing by producing a drying effect.
- Enzymes should be used carefully according to the progress of the wound or decubitus area. Denuding necrotic areas may expose capillaries and cause bleeding at the site.
- The patient should be placed on a flotation pad to protect pressure points on the body.
- The patient should be turned frequently.
- Back rubs should be given regularly and all pressure areas of the body massaged gently.
- Food and fluid intake should be monitored to speed recovery.

Combination products

CHYMORAL ENTERIC-COATED TABLETS: 50,000 units enzymatic activity; trypsin and chymotrypsin in ratio of 6:1.

CHYMORAL-100: 100,000 units enzymatic activity; trypsin and chymotrypsin in ratio of 6:1.

GRANULEX AEROSOL: trypsin 0.1 mg, balsam Peru 72.5 mg, and castor oil 650 mg/ 0.82 ml.

ORENZYME BITABS ENTERIC-COATED TABLETS: 100,000 units trypsin and 8,000 units chymotrypsin.

NAMES, INDICATIONS AND DOSAGES	SIDE EFFECTS
bromelains Ananase **Adjunct to reduce inflammation and edema, ease pain, and speed tissue repair of traumatic injuries (contusions, sprains, strains, dislocations), cellulitis, furunculosis, ulcerations:** ADULTS: initially, 100,000 units P.O. q.i.d., then 50,000 units t.i.d. or q.i.d. for maintenance.	**Blood:** bleeding tendencies. **GI:** mild diarrhea, nausea, vomiting. **GU:** menorrhagia, metrorrhagia. **Other:** fever, hypersensitivity reactions (rash, urticaria).
chymotrypsin Avazyme **Adjunct in general, rectal, oral, and dental surgery:** ADULTS: preoperatively, 2,500 units I.M.; then 2,500 units once or twice daily, as indicated. **Adjunct in treatment of respiratory conditions (asthma, bronchitis, rhinitis, sinusitis):** ADULTS: 2,500 to 5,000 units I.M. once or twice weekly; more often if needed. CHILDREN: ½ adult dose. **Chronic or recurrent inflammation (peptic ulcer, ulcerative colitis, phlebitis, thrombophlebitis, dermatologic conditions):** ADULTS: 2,500 to 5,000 units I.M. once or twice weekly. Tablet containing 10,000 units may be given buccally q.i.d. alone or in conjunction with I.M. therapy. **Relief of episiotomy symptoms:** ADULTS: 5,000 units I.M. repeated twice at 12-hour intervals. Tablet containing 20 mg (20,000 units) may be given P.O. q.i.d. **Pelvic inflammatory diseases:** ADULTS: 2,500 units daily for 7 days; repeat course if needed.	**Blood:** increased bleeding tendencies. **GI:** nausea, vomiting, diarrhea with oral administration. **GU:** hematuria, albuminuria, menorrhagia. **Local:** pain, induration at injection site. **Other:** chills, dizziness, fever, rapid dissolution of animal-origin sutures, *hypersensitivity reactions (rash, urticaria, itching, anaphylaxis).*
fibrinolysin and desoxyribonuclease Elase♦ **Debridement of inflammatory and infected lesions (surgical wounds, ulcerative lesions, second- and third-degree burns, circumcision, episiotomy, cervicitis, vaginitis, abscesses, fistulas, and sinus tracts):** *Intravaginally:* 5 ml ointment may be inserted using applicator supplied, once daily for vaginitis or cervicitis. *Topical use:* apply ointment 30 units fibrinolysin, 20,000 units desoxyribonuclease/30 g at intervals as long as enzyme action is desired. **Irrigating agent for infected wounds, empyema cavities, abscesses, otorhinolaryngologic wounds, subcutaneous hematomas:** Dilution for irrigation depends on extent and	**Local:** hyperemia with high doses.

♦ Available in U.S. and Canada. ♦♦ Available in Canada only.
All other products (no symbol) available in U.S. only. Italicized side effects are common or life-threatening.

INTERACTIONS AND SPECIAL CONSIDERATIONS

Interactions:
ALKALINE SOLUTIONS, ANTACIDS: dissolve enteric coating of tablet. Do not use within 1 hour of bromelains.

Special considerations:
• Contraindicated in hypersensitivity to pineapple or pineapple products. Use cautiously with anticoagulant therapy and in patients with blood-clotting abnormalities, including hemophilia, hepatic or renal disease, and systemic infection.
• History of allergies needed. Hypersensitivity reactions possible; drug should be discontinued immediately if any occur.
• Destruction of enteric coating may decrease effectiveness. Tablets must be swallowed whole, not crushed or broken.
• Appearance of granulation tissue may indicate effectiveness of therapy. Inflammation or color of drainage may indicate spread of infection.
• Protect from heat.

Interactions:
ALKALINE SOLUTIONS, ANTACIDS: dissolve enteric coating of tablet. Do not use within 1 hour of oral administration of chymotrypsin.

Special considerations:
• Contraindicated in hypersensitivity to trypsin or to sesame oil (injectable form), septicemia, severe generalized or localized infection, and blood coagulation disorders such as hemophilia. Use with caution in severe hepatic or renal disease.
• Parenteral administration: do not give I.V. Test for sensitivity before giving. Inject deep into gluteal muscle; rotate sites. Watch for hypersensitivity reactions, including changes in blood pressure and pulse. Watch for pain and induration at injection site. Stop if reaction occurs.
• Contact with eyes should be avoided. After accidental contact, flush eyes with water immediately.
• Protect from heat.
• For treatment of anaphylaxis, see APPENDIX.

No significant interactions.

Special considerations:
• Contraindicated for parenteral use.
• Dense, dry eschar must be removed surgically before enzymatic debridement. Enzyme must be in constant contact with substrate. Accumulated necrotic debris must be removed periodically.
• Treatment: clean wound with water or peroxide and dry gently; cover with thin layer of Elase. Cover with nonadhering dressing. Change dressing at least once a day. Flush away necrotic debris and reapply ointment.
• Solution as wet dressing: mix 1 vial of Elase powder with 10 to 50 ml saline solution; saturate strips of fine gauze with solution. Pack ulcerated area with Elase gauze. Allow the gauze to dry in contact with the ulcerated lesion for about 6 to 8 hours. Remove dried gauze and repeat 3 to 4 times daily.
• Solution as irrigant: drain cavity and replace Elase every 6 to 10 hours to reduce amount of by-product accumulation and to minimize loss of enzyme activity. Although parenteral use is contraindicated, Elase is used as an irrigant in certain specific conditions.
• Solution should be prepared just before use and discarded after 24 hours.

(continued on following page)

NAMES, INDICATIONS AND DOSAGES	SIDE EFFECTS
fibrinolysin and desoxyribonuclease *(continued)* severity of wound: 25 units fibrinolysin powder, 15,000 units desoxyribonuclease per 30-ml vial.	
hyaluronidase Wydase♦ **Adjunct to increase absorption and dispersion of other injected drugs:** ADULTS AND CHILDREN: 150 units to injection medium containing other medication. **Hypodermoclysis:** ADULTS AND CHILDREN OVER 3 YEARS: 150 units injected S.C. before clysis or injected into clysis tubing near needle for each 1,000 ml clysis solution. **Subcutaneous urography:** ADULTS AND CHILDREN: with patient prone, give 75 units S.C. over each scapula, followed by injection of contrast medium at same sites.	**Skin:** rash, urticaria. **Local:** irritation.
papain Panafil, Papase♦ **Prevention of inflammation and edema in surgical procedures:** ADULTS AND CHILDREN: 10,000 to 20,000 units P.O. or buccally 1 to 2 hours before surgery, then 20,000 units q.i.d. for up to 5 days. **Treatment of inflammation and burns, enzymatic debridement, promotion of normal healing and deodorization of surface lesions, particularly in local infection, necrosis, fibrinous or purulent debris, sloughing:** ADULTS AND CHILDREN: apply ointment 10% directly to lesion 1 to 2 times daily. Cover with gauze.	**Blood:** increased bleeding tendencies. **GI:** nausea, vomiting, diarrhea with oral administration. **Local:** tingling at site of buccal absorption, occasional itching or stinging with first application of ointment. **Other:** fever, hypersensitivity reactions (rash, urticaria, pruritus).
streptokinase-streptodornase Varidase♦ **Anti-inflammatory agent to relieve pain, swelling, tenderness, erythema; management of edema and localized extravasation of blood from infection, trauma, certain dental conditions:** Dose and route of administration determined by patient's response, location of lesion, ease of drainage or aspiration, size of cavity, ability of cavity to expand. Higher doses than those stated may be advisable in severe cases. ADULTS AND CHILDREN: 1 tablet containing 10,000 IU streptokinase (SK) and 2,500 IU streptodornase (SD) q.i.d. for 4 to 6 days; 0.5 ml P.O. of injectable solution (5,000 IU SK) I.M. b.i.d.	**GI:** nausea, vomiting, diarrhea with oral administration. **Skin:** rash, urticaria.

♦ Available in U.S. and Canada. ♦♦ Available in Canada only.
All other products (no symbol) available in U.S. only. Italicized side effects are common or life-threatening.

INTERACTIONS AND SPECIAL CONSIDERATIONS

Interactions:
LOCAL ANESTHETICS: increased potential for toxic local reaction. Use together cautiously.

Special considerations:
• Use with caution in blood-clotting abnormalities and in severe hepatic or renal disease.
• Should not be injected into acutely inflamed or cancerous areas.
• In hypodermoclysis, dose, rate of injection, and type of solution should be adjusted to patient response.
• Administration precautions: skin-test for sensitivity. Avoid injecting into diseased areas (may spread infection). Observe injection site for local reactions.
• Contact with eyes should be avoided. After accidental contact, flush eyes with water at once.
• Protect from heat. Cloudy or discolored solution should not be used.

Interactions:
WITH TOPICAL USE, DETERGENTS AND ANTISEPTICS (BENZALKONIUM CHLORIDE, HEXACHLOROPHENE, IODINE, HYDROGEN PEROXIDE): decreased enzymatic activity. Do not use together.

Special considerations:
• Contraindicated in hypersensitivity to papaya fruit. Oral administration contraindicated in anticoagulant therapy; blood-clotting abnormalities, including hemophilia; and systemic infections. Use cautiously in severe hepatic or renal disease.
• Patient should know proper route to be used. Oral tablets may be swallowed with water or chewed.
• Treatment: thoroughly cleanse and irrigate wound area with sterile normal saline or water to remove antiseptics, detergents, and heavy metal antibacterials, which can decrease enzyme activity; don't use hydrogen peroxide, as it inactivates topical papain; moisten area for optimal enzymatic activity; apply ointment in thin layers to assure contact with necrotic tissue; cover with gauze.
• Lesion should be irrigated with mild cleansing solution (not hydrogen peroxide) at each redressing.
• Appearance of granulation tissue may indicate effectiveness of therapy. Inflammation or color of drainage may indicate spread of infection.
• Contact with eyes should be avoided. After accidental contact, flush eyes with water at once.
• Protect drug from heat.

No significant interactions.

Special considerations:
• Contraindicated in active hemorrhage; decreased level of fibrinogen; acute cellulitis without suppuration; or risk of reopening preexisting bronchopleural fistulas, especially in active tuberculosis. Use oral and I.M. forms with caution in severe renal disease, depressed hepatic function or hepatic disease, or abnormalities of blood-clotting mechanism.
• Should not be given I.V.
• Concomitant antimicrobial therapy with compatible agent, such as tetracycline, penicillin, streptomycin, should be considered if infection present.
• I.M. use: add 2 ml sterile water for injection or sterile physiologic saline solution to 25,000-unit vial streptokinase-streptodornase (result is solution of 5,000 IU SK per 0.5 ml). Inject deep I.M., preferably into gluteal muscle. Store remaining solution for 2 weeks in refrigerator or 24 hours at room temperature.
• Contact with eyes should be avoided. After accidental contact, flush eyes with water at once.
• Protect from heat.
• Streptokinase and streptodornase are antigenic; antienzymes may develop following prolonged therapy or acute hemolytic streptococcal infections. High antienzyme titer apparently not harmful, but dosage may have to be increased to overcome its effect.

NAMES, INDICATIONS AND DOSAGES	SIDE EFFECTS
trypsin **In general and oral surgical procedures to reduce inflammation, accelerate reabsorption of edema, facilitate restoration of local tissue circulation; to reduce inflammation and edema of bronchial mucosa; as adjunct in treatment of phlebothrombosis, thrombophlebitis, iritis, iridocyclitis, chorioretinitis, cutaneous ulcerative conditions:** ADULTS: 50,000 to 100,000 units P.O. q.i.d.; or 12,500 units I.M. daily or for severe conditions b.i.d. for 1 to 2 days, then 12,500 units daily. *Solution for wet dressings:* 10,000 units in each ml normal saline solution or water for injection. Apply new dressings when dry. *Ointment:* 5,000 units/g once daily or b.i.d. *Inhalation:* 125,000 units dissolved in 3 ml saline solution or water inhaled at least once daily.	**Blood:** increased bleeding tendencies. **CNS:** dizziness, fainting. **EENT:** rhinorrhea, sneezing, with aerosol inhalation. **GI:** nausea, vomiting, diarrhea, abdominal pain. **GU:** albuminuria, hematuria. **Skin:** rash, pruritus, urticaria. **Local:** pain and induration, local irritation. **Other:** febrile reactions, angioneurotic edema, rapid dissolution of sutures of animal origins, *anaphylaxis.*

INTERACTIONS AND SPECIAL CONSIDERATIONS

Interactions:

WITH TOPICAL USE, DETERGENTS AND ANTISEPTICS (BENZALKONIUM CHLORIDE, HEXACHLOROPHENE, IODINE, HYDROGEN PEROXIDE): decreased enzymatic activity. Do not use together.

Special considerations:

- Contraindicated in history of allergic reactions to parenteral enzyme therapy. Use with extreme caution in severe hepatic or renal disease and in abnormalities of blood-clotting mechanism.
- Before I.M. administration: test for possible hypersensitivity reactions. Observe for 30 minutes after I.M. administration. Have epinephrine 1:1,000 available.
- Should not be applied to actively bleeding areas, ocular lesions, or to ulcerated carcinomas.
- Should not be given I.V.
- Enteric-coated tablets must be swallowed whole; should not be crushed or broken.
- Should be given deep I.M. in gluteal muscle, alternating sites. I.M. route not recommended in infants or children.
- Nasal inhalation should be followed with water or saline spray. Patient should take several swallows of water to remove large droplets from oropharynx.
- Store in tight container. Protect from heat.

105

Oxytocics

carboprost tromethamine
dinoprost tromethamine
dinoprostone
ergonovine maleate
methylergonovine maleate
oxytocin citrate, buccal
oxytocin, synthetic injection
oxytocin, synthetic nasal
sodium chloride 20% solution

Oxytocics stimulate the smooth muscle of the uterus during childbirth. They are especially useful in the last stage of labor (stage III), in which the placenta is sloughed and expelled. Generally, oxytocics should be avoided in stages I and II since they increase the risk of uterine rupture.

Major uses

- Carboprost, dinoprost, dinoprostone, and sodium chloride induce therapeutic abortion in the second trimester.
- Ergonovine and methylergonovine correct postpartum uterine atony.
- Ergonovine, methylergonovine, and oxytocins control postpartum bleeding.
- Oxytocins induce labor or intensify uterine contractions at term.
- Oxytocin, synthetic nasal preparation, stimulates contraction of the myoepithelium in the mammary glands, facilitating milk ejection in lactating females.

Mechanism of action

- Carboprost, dinoprost, and dinoprostone (prostaglandins) produce strong, prompt contractions of uterine smooth muscle, possibly mediated by calcium and cyclic 3',5'-adenosine monophosphate. Endocrine levels also influence contractions. These drugs promote cervical dilation and softening, and exert uterine effects by direct stimulation of the myometrium.
- Ergonovine and methylergonovine (ergot alkaloids) increase motor activity of the uterus by direct stimulation. A gravid uterus responds markedly even to small doses.
- Oxytocin may act as a hormone in potent and selective stimulation of uterine and mammary gland smooth muscle. It produces uterine contractions of the same intensity, duration, and frequency as those in spontaneous labor. Oxytocin may stimulate contractions of uterine smooth muscle by increasing the sodium permeability of uterine myofibrils.
- Sodium chloride 20% solution may damage decidual cells, causing release of prostaglandins and leading to fetal death and abortion.

Absorption, distribution, metabolism, and excretion

- Carboprost, dinoprost, and dinoprostone diffuse slowly into maternal blood after administration and are widely distributed in maternal and fetal tissues. They concentrate in fetal liver and are rapidly metabolized in maternal lungs and liver. They're excreted within 24 hours, mainly in urine.
- Ergonovine and methylergonovine are rapidly absorbed after oral or I.M. administration and are slowly metabolized in the liver. Metabolism in neonates may be prolonged.
- Oxytocin is inactivated by trypsin in the gastrointestinal tract; tissue peptidases inactivate most of the drug when it is administered buccally. It is distributed to extracellular fluid, and small amounts may reach the fetal circulation. The drug has a short half-life (3 to 5 minutes), which is reduced late in pregnancy and in lactation. The liver and

WHEN OXYTOCIN IS USED TO INDUCE LABOR

The hormone oxytocin stimulates uterine contractions and initiates labor naturally. But when *synthetic* oxytocin is used to induce labor, the contractions are, in many cases, stronger and longer, with shorter relaxation periods between. Thus, synthetic oxytocin should only be used when medically indicated and *not* for the convenience of the doctor or the mother. Unfortunately, oxytocin is used to induce labor in 40% to 50% of deliveries, yet it may be needed in less than 2%.

These problems may occur when using synthetic oxytocin to induce labor:

• The baby may be stressed before its first breath. Frequent strong contractions diminish the baby's ability to restore its supply of oxygen between contractions because uterine blood flow is shut off during each strong contraction. Be especially alert for signs of fetal distress.

• Studies show that when oxytocin is given to women in labor, 25% show some asphyxiation patterns. When oxytocin and epidural anesthetic are used together, 50% of the women show asphyxiation patterns.

• The need for pain-killing drugs or anesthetic is probably higher with oxytocin, because the contractions are stronger.

• Oxytocin's rate of success is only 85%. Thus, labor sometimes stops abruptly, leaving the mother with a partially dilated cervix. This is a disappointing and potentially frightening experience for the woman who is sent home in this condition and told to return when labor begins normally. Such patients require extra health teaching and emotional support.

Adapted from Dr. Silvia Feldman, *Choices in Childbirth* (New York: Grosset & Dunlap, 1978), with permission from the publisher.

kidneys destroy most of the drug. Small amounts are excreted unchanged in urine.

• Sodium chloride undergoes little or no systemic absorption. It appears to concentrate in the decidual and fetal parts of the placenta. Some of the drug diffuses into the maternal blood and is excreted in urine.

Onset and duration

• Carboprost, dinoprost, and dinoprostone begin to act promptly. Their action is dose-dependent, with sensitivity increasing at term. Contractions usually begin within 10 to 15 minutes after administration and may continue 10 to 30 minutes after the drug is stopped. In most patients, abortion occurs within 30 hours.

• Ergonovine and methylergonovine produce uterine contractions immediately after I.V. administration and within 5 to 15 minutes after oral or I.M. administration. Contractions may continue 3 or more hours after oral or I.M. administration, and 45 minutes after I.V. administration. Small doses produce increased contractions followed by a normal degree of relaxation; larger doses produce more forceful contractions but increase resting tonus.

• Oxytocin produces uterine contractions within several minutes; they continue 2 to 3 hours.

• A sodium chloride 20% solution that produces a sodium concentration in amniotic fluid of at least 2.2 mEq/ml usually induces abortion within 50 hours. Instillation may be repeated in 48 hours. If the patient fails to respond to the second dose, other abortifacient methods should be tried.

NAMES, INDICATIONS AND DOSAGES	SIDE EFFECTS
carboprost tromethamine Prostin/M15 **Abort pregnancy between 13th and 20th weeks of gestation:** Initially, 250 mcg is administered deep I.M. Subsequent doses of 250 mcg should be administered at intervals of 1½ to 3½ hours, depending on uterine response. Increments in dosage may be increased to 500 mcg if contractility is inadequate after several 250 mcg doses. Total dose should not exceed 12 mg.	**GI:** *vomiting, diarrhea.* **Other:** *fever.*
dinoprost tromethamine Prostin F_2 Alpha **Abort second trimester pregnancy:** 1 ml of amniotic fluid is withdrawn by transabdominal intra-amniotic catheter. If no blood is present in tap, 40 mg of dinoprost is injected directly into amniotic sac. Initially, 5 mg is given very slowly (1 mg/minute), and patient is watched for adverse reactions. Then, remainder is injected. If abortion not completed in 24 hours, another 10 to 40 mg may be given. Uterine activity may continue 10 to 30 minutes after drug is stopped.	**CNS:** dizziness, fainting. **GI:** *nausea, vomiting, diarrhea,* abdominal cramps, epigastric pain. **Other:** bronchospasms, wheezing.
dinoprostone Prostin E_2♦ **Abort second trimester pregnancy, evacuate uterus in cases of missed abortion, intrauterine fetal deaths up to 28 weeks of gestation, or benign hydatidiform mole:** Insert 20 mg suppository high into posterior vaginal fornix. Repeat q 3 to 5 hours until abortion is complete.	**CNS:** *headache.* **CV:** hypotension (in large doses). **GI:** *nausea, vomiting, diarrhea.* **GU:** vaginal pain, vaginitis. **Other:** fever, shivering, chills.
ergonovine maleate Ergotrate Maleate♦ **Prevent or treat postpartum and postabortion hemorrhage due to uterine atony or subinvolution:** 0.2 mg I.M. q 2 to 4 hours, maximum 5 doses; or 0.2 mg I.V. (only for severe uterine bleeding or other life-threatening emergency) over 1 minute while blood pressure and uterine contractions are monitored. I.V. dose may be diluted to 5 ml with 0.9% sodium chloride injection. After initial I.M. or I.V. dose, may give 0.2 to 0.4 mg P.O. q 6 to 12 hours for 2 to 7 days. Decrease dose if severe uterine cramping occurs.	**CNS:** dizziness, headache. **CV:** hypertension, chest pain. **EENT:** tinnitus. **GI:** *nausea, vomiting.* **GU:** uterine cramping. **Other:** sweating, dyspnea, hypersensitivity.

INTERACTIONS AND SPECIAL CONSIDERATIONS

No significant interactions.

Special considerations:
• Contraindicated in patients with pelvic inflammatory disease or active cardiac, pulmonary, renal, or hepatic disease. Use cautiously in patients with a history of asthma; hypertension; cardiovascular, renal, or hepatic disease; anemia; jaundice; diabetes; epilepsy.
• I.M. injection of this drug is technically less difficult and poses fewer potential risks than other prostaglandin abortifacients.
• Carboprost can be used without concern that expulsion of vaginal suppositories may occur in the presence of profuse vaginal bleeding.
• Live birth may result.
• Should be used only in a hospital setting by trained personnel.

Interactions:
ALCOHOL (I.V. INFUSIONS OF 500 ML OF 10% OVER 1 HOUR): inhibited uterine activity.
I.V. OXYTOCIN: cervical perforation, especially in primigravida patients or in those with inadequately dilated cervices. Use with caution.

Special considerations:
• Contraindicated in patients with pelvic inflammatory disease. Use with caution in cardiovascular, renal, or hypertensive disease; asthma; glaucoma; or epilepsy.
• Character and amount of vaginal bleeding should be monitored.
• Live birth may result.
• Other measures may be needed if dinoprost fails to terminate pregnancy completely. Utilization of hypertonic saline should be delayed until uterine contractions stop.
• Vital signs should be monitored. Rapid fall in blood pressure or hypertonic uterine contractions may occur.
• Patient should remain in prone position.
• After abortion, patient should be checked frequently for cervical injuries.
• Store at 2° to 8° C. (35.6° to 46.4° F.). Discard 24 months after manufacture date.
• Should be used only in hospital setting.

No significant interactions.

Special considerations:
• Contraindicated in patients with pelvic inflammatory disease or history of pelvic surgery, incisions, uterine fibroids, or cervical stenosis. Use with caution in asthma; epilepsy; anemia; diabetes; hypertension or hypotension; jaundice, or cardiovascular, renal, or hepatic disease.
• Live birth may result.
• Dinoprostone suppositories should be warmed in their wrapping to room temperature.
• After insertion, patient should stay supine for 10 minutes.
• Store suppositories at temperature no higher than −20° C. (−4° F.).
• Should be used only when critical care facilities are readily available.
• Dinoprostone-induced fever is self-limiting and transient. Should be treated with water or alcohol sponging and increased fluid intake rather than with aspirin, which has not proved effective.
• Abortion should be complete within 30 hours.

Interactions:
REGIONAL ANESTHETICS, DOPAMINE, I.V. OXYTOCIN: excessive vasoconstriction. Use together cautiously.

Special considerations:
• Contraindicated for induction or augmentation of labor; before delivery of placenta; in threatened spontaneous abortion; in patients with allergy or sensitivity to ergot preparations. Use cautiously in hypertension, cardiac disease, venoatrial shunts, mitral value stenosis, obliterative vascular disease, sepsis, or hepatic or renal impairment.
• Blood pressure, pulse, and uterine response should be monitored. Sudden changes in vital signs and character and amount of bleeding, or frequent periods of uterine relaxation may occur.
• Hypocalcemia may decrease patient response. If patient is not also taking digitalis, cautious administration of calcium gluconate I.V. may produce desired oxytocic action.
• Contractions begin 5 to 15 minutes after oral administration; immediately following I.V. injection. May continue 3 hours or more after oral or I.M. administration; 45 minutes after I.V. injection.
• Store in tightly closed, light-resistant containers. Discard if discolored.
• Store I.V. solutions below 8° C. (46.4° F.). Daily stock may be kept at cool room temperature for 60 days.
• Patient should be kept warm.
• Drug should be ready for immediate use if it is to be given postpartum.
• I.V. bolus doses of ergonovine are used to diagnose coronary artery spasm.

NAMES, INDICATIONS AND DOSAGES	SIDE EFFECTS
methylergonovine maleate Methergine **Prevent and treat postpartum hemorrhage due to uterine atony or subinvolution:** 0.2 mg I.M. q 2 to 5 hours for maximum of 5 doses; or I.V. (excessive uterine bleeding or other emergencies) over 1 minute while blood pressure and uterine contractions are monitored. I.V. dose may be diluted to 5 ml with 0.9% sodium chloride injection. Following initial I.M. or I.V. dose, may give 0.2 to 0.4 mg P.O. q 6 to 12 hours for 2 to 7 days. Dose may be decreased if severe cramping occurs.	**CNS:** dizziness, headache. **CV:** hypertension, transient chest pain, dyspnea, palpitation. **EENT:** tinnitus. **GI:** *nausea, vomiting.* **Other:** sweating, hypersensitivity.
oxytocin citrate, buccal Pitocin Citrate♦ **Induction of labor:** 1 tablet (200 USP units) in alternate cheeks until firm, regular uterine contractions, 40 to 60 seconds long, q 3 minutes, are achieved. Repeat q 30 minutes until 15 tablets (3,000 units) have been given over 24 hours, or until delivery is imminent or anesthetic is administered. Average dose to complete labor, 1,700 units; same number of tablets are used to maintain labor once induced.	*Maternal* **CV:** hypertension; premature ventricular contractions; hypotension; increase in heart rate, venous return, cardiac output; *arrhythmias in large doses.* **GI:** nausea, vomiting. **GU:** uterine hypertonicity, spasm, tetanic contraction or rupture, postpartum hemorrhage. **Local:** parabuccal irritation. *Fetal* **CV:** bradycardia, cardiac arrhythmias. **Hepatic:** jaundice. **Other:** hypoxia, intracranial hemorrhage due to overstimulation of uterus during labor, birth canal trauma.
oxytocin, synthetic injection Oxytocin♦, Pitocin♦, Syntocinon♦, Uteracon **Induction or stimulation of labor:** Initially, 1 ml (10 units) ampul in 1,000 ml of 5% dextrose injection or 0.9% sodium chloride solution I.V. infused at 1 to 2 milliunits/minute. Increase rate at 15- to 30-minute intervals until normal contraction pattern is established. Maximum 1 to 2 ml (20 milliunits)/minute. Decrease rate when labor is firmly established. **Reduction of postpartum bleeding after expulsion of placenta:** 10 to 40 units added to 1,000 ml of 5% dextrose in water or 0.9% sodium chloride solution infused at rate necessary to control bleeding.	*Maternal* **Blood:** afibrinogenemia; may be related to increase in postpartum bleeding. **CNS:** subarachnoid hemorrhage resulting from hypertension; *convulsions or coma resulting from water intoxication.* **CV:** hypotension; increased heart rate, systemic venous return, and cardiac output; arrhythmia. **GI:** nausea, vomiting. **Other:** hypersensitivity, tetanic contractions, abruptio placentae, impaired uterine blood flow, and increased uterine motility. *Fetal* **Blood:** increased risk of hyperbilirubinemia. **CV:** bradycardia, tachycardia, premature ventricular contractions. **Other:** *anoxia, asphyxia.*

♦ Available in U.S. and Canada. ♦♦ Available in Canada only.
All other products (no symbol) available in U.S. only. Italicized side effects are common or life-threatening.

INTERACTIONS AND SPECIAL CONSIDERATIONS

Interactions:
REGIONAL ANESTHETICS, DOPAMINE, I.V. OXYTOCIN: excessive vasoconstriction. Use together cautiously.

Special considerations:
• Contraindicated for induction of labor; before delivery of placenta; in patients with hypertension, toxemia, or sensitivity to ergot preparations; in threatened spontaneous abortion. Use with caution in sepsis, obliterative vascular disease, hepatic or renal problems, hypertension, cardiac disease, venoatrial shunts, mitral value stenosis.
• Blood pressure, pulse, and uterine response should be monitored. Sudden changes in vital signs and character and amount of vaginal bleeding, or frequent periods of uterine relaxation are possible.
• Contractions begin 5 to 15 minutes after oral administration; 2 to 5 minutes after I.M. injection; immediately following I.V. injection. May continue 3 hours or more after oral or I.M. administration; 45 minutes after I.V. injection.
• Store in tightly closed, light-resistant containers. Discard if discolored.
• Store below 8° C. (46.4° F.). Daily stock may be kept at room temperature for 60 to 90 days.

Interactions:
CYCLOPROPANE ANESTHETICS: increased risk of hypotension or bradycardia. Use together cautiously.
THIOPENTAL ANESTHETICS: delayed induction time. Adjust dose.
VASOCONSTRICTORS (VASOPRESSORS): severe hypertension if oxytocin is used within 3 to 4 hours of vasoconstrictor. Monitor patient closely.

Special considerations:
• Contraindicated in control and management of third stage of labor; to expel placenta; to control postpartum bleeding; in management of inevitable, incomplete, or missed abortion, abruptio placenta, placenta previa, fetal distress, or other obstetrical emergencies and in unconscious or postpartum patients. Use cautiously in prematurity, previous major cervical or uterine surgery (including cesarean section), grand multiparity, invasive cervical carcinoma, overdistention of uterus, history of uterine sepsis.
• In eclampsia, if delivery isn't imminent within 12 hours after oxytocin is started, cesarean section is recommended.
• Used to induce or reinforce labor only when pelvis is known to be adequate, when fetal maturity is assured, when fetal position is favorable, and when vaginal delivery is indicated.
• May be hazardous in patients with cardiac disease or in those receiving spinal or epidural anesthetic.
• Should be given only in hospital setting under qualified supervision.
• Buccal administration is more difficult to control than I.M. or I.V. route; can be given by different routes sequentially but never at same time.
• Uterine contractions, heart rate, blood pressure, intrauterine pressure, and character and volume of blood loss should be monitored.
• Fetal heart beat should be monitored.
• Patient may rinse mouth with cold water before tablet is placed in parabuccal space. For maximum buccal absorption, patient should avoid disturbing tablet. A tablet swallowed accidentally is not harmful, but the digestive process destroys its oxytocic action.
• Contractions measured by electronic monitor may exceed 50 mmHg.
• Store at temperature lower than 25° C. (77° F.).
• For treatment of anaphylaxis, see APPENDIX.

Interactions:
CYCLOPROPANE ANESTHETICS: less pronounced bradycardia; more severe hypotension than occurs with oxytocin alone. Use together cautiously.
THIOPENTAL ANESTHETICS: delayed induction reported. May require dosage adjustment.
VASOCONSTRICTORS: severe hypertension if oxytocin is given within 3 to 4 hours of vasoconstrictor in patient receiving caudal block anesthetic. Monitor patient closely.

Special considerations:
• Contraindicated in cases of cephalopelvic disproportion or where delivery requires conversion, as in transverse lie; fetal distress, when delivery isn't imminent, severe toxemia, and other obstetric emergencies. Use cautiously in history of cervical or uterine surgery, grand multiparity, uterine sepsis, traumatic delivery, or overdistended uterus and primipara over 35 years. Use with extreme caution during first and second stages of labor, since cervical laceration, uterine rupture, and maternal and fetal death have been reported.
• Used to induce or reinforce labor only when pelvis is known to be adequate, when vaginal delivery is indicated, when fetal maturity is assured, and when fetal position is favorable. Should be used only in hospital where critical care facilities and doctor are immediately available.
• Oxytocin should never be given simultaneously by more than one route.
• Incompatible with fibrinolysis, levarterenol bitartrate, prochlorperazine edisylate, protein hydrolysate, and warfarin sodium. Compatibility with other I.V. infusion fluids may be influenced by drug concentration, temperature, pH, and other factors. Rotate bottle gently to dis-

(continued on following page)

NAMES, INDICATIONS AND DOSAGES	SIDE EFFECTS
oxytocin, synthetic injection *(continued)* **Facilitate threatened abortion:** 10 to 40 units (1 to 4 ml) oxytocin added to 1,000 ml of 5% dextrose in water, normal saline solution, or other nonhydrating solution; infused at rate necessary to control uterine atony.	
oxytocin, synthetic nasal **To promote initial milk ejection; may be useful in relieving postpartum breast engorgement:** One spray or three drops into one or both nostrils 2 or 3 minutes before breast-feeding or pumping breasts.	None reported.
sodium chloride 20% solution **To induce fetal death and abortion in second trimester of pregnancy (beyond 16th week of gestation):** After transabdominal tap of amniotic sac, at least 1 ml of fluid is withdrawn and examined. If no blood is found, 250 ml of amniotic fluid may be aspirated and 250 ml (maximum dose) of sodium chloride solution instilled over 20 to 30 minutes, while patient is observed for adverse reactions. Sodium chloride instillation may be repeated in 48 hours if membranes are still intact. I.V. infusion of oxytocin or intra-amniotic dinoprost tromethamine may be given to patients who fail to respond to second dose after oxytocic action of saline solution has ceased.	**Blood:** mild, self-limiting disseminated intravascular coagulation; coagulation changes, including decreased platelet count, hematocrit, fibrinogen, and factors V and VIII; increased plasma volume, fibrin levels, and thrombin, prothrombin, and partial thromboplastin times. Occur within first 12 to 24 hours. **CV:** *pulmonary embolism,* pneumonia. **GU:** *cortical necrosis of kidneys,* cervical laceration and perforation, cervicovaginal fistula, and uterine rupture reported in primigravida patients receiving concomitant I.V. oxytocin before cervix is adequately dilated. **Local:** infection at injection site. **Other:** fever, flushing.

INTERACTIONS AND SPECIAL CONSIDERATIONS

tribute drug in diluted solution.
- Uterine contractions, heart rate, blood pressure, intrauterine pressure, fetal heart rate, character and volume of blood loss should be monitored.
- Store at temperature below 25° C. (77° F.), but do not freeze.
- Oxytocin may produce antidiuretic effect; fluid intake and output should be monitored.
- If contractions occur less than 2 minutes apart and if contractions above 50 mmHg are recorded, or if contractions last 90 seconds or longer, infusion should be stopped and patient turned on her side.
- Oxygen administration may be necessary.
- Not recommended for I.M. use.

No significant interactions.

Special considerations:
- Patient should clear nasal passages first. With patient's head in vertical position, squeeze bottle should be held upright and solution ejected into patient's nostril.
- Patient's wish to breast-feed should be supported with quiet, nonstressful environment and encouragement.

Interactions:
INDOMETHACIN: may prolong abortion if used within 4 to 6 hours after intra-amniotic instillation of sodium chloride solution. Defer indomethacin dose.
OXYTOCIN: intense uterine contractions and increased risk of uterine rupture or cervical laceration. Don't use together.

Special considerations:
- Contraindicated in blood disorders or in actively contracting or hypertonic uterus. Use with extreme caution in cardiac disease, hypertension, epilepsy, renal impairment, uterine incision, pelvic adhesions, or in history of pelvic surgery.
- Should be done only by doctors trained in amniocentesis when critical care facilities are immediately available.
- Should be monitored constantly for signs of accidental intravascular, endometrial, or intraperitoneal injection. Procedure usually painless. If patient complains of pain, burning, feeling of heat, thirst, severe headache, mental confusion, distress, tinnitus, numbness of fingertips, or anxiety, instillation should be stopped at once. Inadvertent I.V. injection can cause hypernatremia, myometrial necrosis, with secondary vomiting, cerebral blood clots, cardiovascular collapse, and death.
- Patient should drink at least 2 liters of water on day of procedure to improve salt excretion.
- General anesthetics or sedatives should not be used during administration of hypertonic saline.

106

Spasmolytics

aminophylline or theophylline ethylenediamine
dyphylline
flavoxate hydrochloride
oxtriphylline
oxybutynin chloride
theophylline
theophylline sodium glycinate

Spasmolytics check or relieve smooth muscle spasms. The xanthine derivatives (theophylline and its salts, and dyphylline) are direct-acting bronchodilators; that is, they act directly on the smooth muscle of the respiratory tract. The theophylline salts include oxtriphylline, theophylline, theophylline ethylenediamine (aminophylline), and theophylline sodium glycinate.

These drugs are mainstays of therapy for chronic obstructive pulmonary disease and especially acute bronchial asthma. They are usually combined with various sympathomimetics in a total treatment program. In addition to exerting bronchodilating actions, they also act as mild diuretics.

Flavoxate and oxybutynin, unlike the xanthine derivatives, act on the genitourinary system rather than the respiratory system.

Major uses

• Flavoxate and oxybutynin relieve symptoms of certain bladder disorders, including uninhibited neurogenic bladder.

• Xanthine derivatives relieve acute bronchial asthma and reverse bronchospasm associated with asthma, bronchitis, and emphysema.

Mechanism of action

• Flavoxate has a direct spasmolytic effect on smooth muscles of the urinary tract. It also provides some local anesthesia and analgesia.

• Oxybutynin has both a direct spasmolytic effect and an atropine-like effect on urinary tract smooth muscles; it has little or no effect on smooth muscles of blood vessels. It increases urinary bladder capacity and provides local anesthesia and analgesia.

• Of the xanthine derivatives, theophylline and its salts competitively inhibit phosphodiesterase, the enzyme that degrades cyclic adenosine monophosphate (AMP). This increases intracellular cyclic AMP, which in turn causes relaxation of the smooth muscle of the bronchial airways and pulmonary blood vessels. This action relieves bronchospasm and increases vital capacity.

Dyphylline presumably has the same mechanism of action as theophylline, but this has not been proven.

Absorption, distribution, metabolism, and excretion

- Flavoxate's metabolism has not been determined, but the drug is excreted by the kidneys.
- Oxybutynin is metabolized probably by the liver. Its metabolites are excreted by the kidneys.
- Xanthine derivatives have delayed absorption after oral administration if there is food in the stomach. Absorption is delayed and incomplete when the drugs are given by rectal suppository.

They are distributed to body fluids and tissues, metabolized in the liver, then excreted in urine.

The drugs may accumulate in elderly patients and in those with hepatic dysfunction, cor pulmonale, and congestive heart failure.

Onset and duration

- Onset of flavoxate and oxybutynin takes place 30 to 60 minutes after administration. Blood levels peak in 3 to 6 hours, and duration of action is 6 to 10 hours.
- Because xanthine derivatives vary widely in onset and duration, individual responses must be carefully observed. Blood levels of 10 to 20 mcg/ml are usually needed to produce optimal bronchodilation. I.V. administration supplies the highest and most rapid concentration. Blood levels usually peak about 1 to 2 hours after administration of capsules or uncoated tablets; extended-release forms, about 4 hours; retention enemas, 1 to 2 hours; and rectal suppositories, 3 to 5 hours.

Combination products

None.

NAMES, INDICATIONS AND DOSAGES	SIDE EFFECTS
aminophylline or theophylline ethylenediamine Aminodur Dura-Tab, Aminophyl♦♦, Aminophyllin, Corophyllin♦♦, Lixaminol, Phyllocontin, Somophyllin, Somophyllin-DF **For treatment of acute and chronic bronchial asthma, bronchospasm; also used for Cheyne-Stokes respiration, pulmonary vasodilator:** *Oral:* ADULTS: 500 mg stat; then 250 to 500 mg q 6 to 8 hours. CHILDREN: 7.5 mg/kg stat; then 3 to 6 mg/kg q 6 to 8 hours. I.V.: inject very slowly, minimum time 4 to 5 minutes; do not exceed 25 mg/minute infusion rate. Loading dose: 5.6 mg/kg over 30 minutes. *Maintenance dose:* ADULTS: 0.3 to 0.9 mg/kg/hour I.V. by continuous infusion. CHILDREN LESS THAN 9 YEARS: 1 mg/kg/hour. *I.M.:* ADULTS: 500 mg. Painful. Not recommended. *Rectal:* ADULTS: 500 mg suppository or by retention enema q 6 to 8 hours.	**CNS:** *restlessness, dizziness,* headache, *insomnia,* light-headedness, *convulsions.* **CV:** *palpitations, sinus tachycardia,* extrasystoles, flushing, marked hypotension, increase in respiratory rate. **GI:** *nausea, vomiting, anorexia,* bitter aftertaste, dyspepsia, heavy feeling in stomach. **Skin:** urticaria. **Local:** *rectal suppositories may cause irritation.*
dyphylline Airet, Air-Tabs, Brophylline, Coeurophylline♦♦, Dilin♦, Dilor, Dyflex, Dylline, Emfabid, Lufyllin, Neothylline, Protophylline♦♦ **For relief of acute and chronic bronchial asthma and reversible bronchospasm associated with chronic bronchitis and emphysema:** ADULTS: 200 to 800 mg P.O. q 6 hours; or 250 to 500 mg I.M. injected slowly at 6-hour intervals. CHILDREN OVER 6 YEARS: 4 to 7 mg/kg P.O. daily, in divided doses.	**CNS:** *restlessness, dizziness,* headache, *insomnia,* light-headedness, *convulsions.* **CV:** *palpitations, sinus tachycardia,* extrasystoles, flushing, marked hypotension, increase in respiratory rate. **GI:** *nausea, vomiting, anorexia,* bitter aftertaste, dyspepsia, heavy feeling in stomach. **Skin:** urticaria.

♦ Available in U.S. and Canada. ♦♦ Available in Canada only.
All other products (no symbol) available in U.S. only. Italicized side effects are common or life-threatening.

INTERACTIONS AND SPECIAL CONSIDERATIONS

Interactions:

ALKALI-SENSITIVE DRUGS: reduced activity. Do not add to I.V. fluids containing aminophylline.

PROPRANOLOL AND NADOLOL: antagonism. Propranolol and nadolol may cause bronchospasm in sensitive patients. Use together cautiously.

TROLEANDOMYCIN, ERYTHROMYCIN: decreased hepatic clearance of theophylline; elevated theophylline levels. Monitor for signs of toxicity.

BARBITURATES: enhanced metabolism and decreased theophylline blood levels. Monitor for decreased aminophylline effect.

Special considerations:

- Contraindicated in hypersensitivity to xanthine compounds (caffeine, theobromine) and in preexisting cardiac arrhythmias, especially tachyarrhythmias. Use cautiously in young children; in elderly patients with congestive heart failure or other cardiac or circulatory impairment, cor pulmonale, or hepatic disease; in patients with active peptic ulcer, since it may increase volume and acidity of gastric secretions; and in hyperthyroidism or diabetes mellitus.
- Individuals metabolize xanthines at different rates. Dose should be adjusted by monitoring response, tolerance, pulmonary function, and theophylline plasma levels: therapeutic level = 10 to 20 mcg/ml; toxicity seen over 20 mcg/ml.
- Plasma clearance may be decreased in patients with congestive heart failure, hepatic dysfunction, or pulmonary edema. Smokers show accelerated clearance. Dose adjustments necessary.
- I.V. drug administration can cause burning; should be diluted with dextrose in water solution.
- Vital signs and intake and output should be monitored. Expected clinical effects include improvement in quality of pulse and respiration.
- Dizziness is common side effect for elderly patients at start of therapy.
- GI symptoms may be relieved by taking oral drug with full glass of water at meals, although food in stomach delays absorption. Enteric-coated tablets may also delay and impair absorption. No evidence that antacids reduce GI side effects.
- Suppositories slowly and erratically absorbed; retention enemas may be absorbed more rapidly. Rectally administered preparations can be given when patient cannot take drug orally. Should be scheduled following evacuation, if possible; may be retained better if given before meal. Patient advised to remain recumbent 15 to 20 minutes following insertion.
- Patient should report other drugs used. Over-the-counter remedies may contain ephedrine in combination with theophylline salts; excessive CNS stimulation may result. Patient should check with doctor before taking *any* other medications.
- Whether or not patient has had recent theophylline therapy should be checked before giving loading dose.
- Instructions for home care and dosage schedule should be supplied. Some patients may require round-the-clock dosage schedule.
- Exposure to allergens may exacerbate bronchospasm in patients with allergies.
- For symptoms and treatment of toxicity, see APPENDIX.

No significant interactions.

Special considerations:

- Contraindicated in hypersensitivity to xanthine compounds (caffeine, theobromine) and in preexisting cardiac arrhythmias, especially tachycardias. Use cautiously in young children; in elderly patients with congestive heart failure, any impaired cardiac or circulatory function, cor pulmonale, renal or hepatic disease; in patients with peptic ulcer, hyperthyroidism, or diabetes mellitus.
- I.V. use not recommended.
- Dyphylline is metabolized faster than theophylline; dosage intervals may have to be decreased to ensure continual therapeutic effect. Higher daily doses may be needed.
- Dose should be decreased in renal insufficiency.
- Vital signs and intake and output should be monitored. Expected clinical effects include improvement in quality of pulse and respiration.
- Dizziness is a common side effect for elderly patients.
- Gastric irritation may be relieved by taking oral drug after meals; no evidence that antacids reduce this side effect. May produce less gastric discomfort than theophylline.
- Discard dyphylline ampule if precipitate is present. Protect from light.
- Patient should be asked about other drugs used. Over-the-counter remedies may contain ephedrine in combination with theophylline salts; excessive CNS stimulation may result. Patient should check with doctor before taking *any* other medications.
- Instructions for home care and dosage schedule should be supplied.
- For symptoms and treatment of toxicity, see APPENDIX.

NAMES, INDICATIONS AND DOSAGES	SIDE EFFECTS
flavoxate hydrochloride Urispas **Symptomatic relief of dysuria, frequency, urgency, nocturia, incontinence, and suprapubic pain associated with urologic disorders:** ADULTS AND CHILDREN OVER 12 YEARS: 100 to 200 mg P.O. q.i.d.	**CNS:** *mental confusion* (especially in elderly), nervousness, dizziness, headache, drowsiness, difficulty with concentration. **CV:** tachycardia, palpitations. **EENT:** *dry mouth and throat, blurred vision,* disturbed eye accommodation. **GI:** abdominal pain, constipation (with high doses), nausea, vomiting. **Skin:** urticaria, dermatoses. **Other:** fever.
oxtriphylline Choledyl♦, Theophylline Choline♦♦ **To relieve acute bronchial asthma and reversible bronchospasm associated with chronic bronchitis and emphysema:** ADULTS AND CHILDREN OVER 12 YEARS: 200 mg P.O. q 6 hours. CHILDREN 2 TO 12 YEARS: 4 mg/kg P.O. q 6 hours. Increase as needed to maintain therapeutic levels of theophylline (10 to 20 mcg/ml).	**CNS:** *restlessness, dizziness,* headache, *insomnia,* light-headedness, *convulsions.* **CV:** *palpitations, sinus tachycardia,* extrasystoles, flushing, marked hypotension, increase in respiratory rate. **GI:** *nausea, vomiting, anorexia,* bitter aftertaste, dyspepsia, heavy feeling in stomach. **Skin:** urticaria.
oxybutynin chloride Ditropan **Antispasmodic for neurogenic bladder:** ADULTS: 5 mg P.O. b.i.d. to t.i.d. to maximum of 5 mg q.i.d. CHILDREN OVER 5 YEARS: 5 mg P.O. b.i.d. to maximum of 5 mg t.i.d.	**CNS:** *drowsiness,* dizziness, insomnia, *dry mouth,* flushing. **CV:** *palpitations, tachycardia.* **EENT:** *transient blurred vision,* mydriasis, cycloplegia. **GI:** nausea, vomiting, *constipation,* bloated feeling. **GU:** impotence, suppression of lactation, *urinary hesitance or retention.* **Skin:** urticaria, severe allergic reactions in patients sensitive to anticholinergics. **Other:** decreased sweating, fever.
theophylline Accurbron, Adophyllin, Aerolate, Asthmophylline♦♦, Bronkodyl, Bronkodyl S-R, Elixicon, Elixophyllin♦, Labid, Lanophyllin, Liquophylline, Norophylline, Optiphyllin, Oralphyllin, Physpan, Quibron BID, Slo-Phyllin, Somophyllin♦, Theo-dur, Theo-Lix, Theo II, Theobid, Theocap, Theoclear, Theolair♦, Theolixir♦, Theolline, Theon, Theophyl♦, Theo-Span, Theostat, Theotal, Theovent **theophylline sodium glycinate** Acet-Am♦♦, Panophylline Forte, Synophylate, Theocyne♦♦, Theo-tort **Prophylaxis and symptomatic relief of bron-**	**CNS:** *restlessness, dizziness,* headache, *insomnia,* light-headedness, *convulsions.* **CV:** *palpitations, sinus tachycardia,* extrasystoles, flushing, marked hypotension, increase in respiratory rate. **GI:** *nausea, vomiting, anorexia,* bitter aftertaste, dyspepsia, heavy feeling in stomach. **Skin:** urticaria.

♦ Available in U.S. and Canada. ♦♦ Available in Canada only.
All other products (no symbol) available in U.S. only. Italicized side effects are common or life-threatening.

INTERACTIONS AND SPECIAL CONSIDERATIONS

No significant interactions.

Special considerations:
• Contraindicated in pyloric or duodenal obstruction, obstructive intestinal lesions or ileus, achalasia, GI hemorrhage, obstructive uropathies of lower urinary tract. Use cautiously in patients with glaucoma.
• History of other drug use should be checked before giving drugs with anticholinergic side effects.
• Drowsiness, mental confusion, and blurred vision may occur.
• Patient should report adverse effects or lack of response to drug.
• For symptoms and treatment of toxicity, see APPENDIX.

Interactions:
ERYTHROMYCIN, TROLEANDOMYCIN: decreased hepatic clearance of theophylline; increased plasma level. Monitor for signs of toxicity.
BARBITURATES: enhanced metabolism and decreased theophylline blood levels. Monitor for decreased effect.
PROPRANOLOL AND NADOLOL: antagonism. May cause bronchospasms in sensitive patients. Use together cautiously.

Special considerations:
• Contraindicated in hypersensitivity to xanthines (caffeine, theobromine).
• Patient should report GI distress, palpitations, irritability, restlessness, nervousness, or insomnia; may indicate excessive CNS stimulation.
• Drug should be administered after meals and at bedtime.
• Store at 15° to 30° C. (59° to 86° F.). Protect elixir from light and tablets from moisture.
• Equivalent to 80% anhydrous theophylline.
• Therapy should be monitored carefully.
• Combination products that contain ephedrine not recommended; excessive CNS stimulation may result.
• For symptoms and treatment of toxicity, see APPENDIX.

No significant interactions.

Special considerations:
• Contraindicated in myasthenia gravis, GI obstruction, adynamic ileus, megacolon, severe or ulcerative colitis; in elderly or debilitated patients with intestinal atony; and in patients with obstructive uropathy. Use cautiously in elderly patients; in patients with autonomic neuropathy, reflux esophagitis, or hepatic or renal disease.
• May aggravate symptoms of hyperthyroidism, coronary heart disease, congestive heart failure, cardiac arrhythmias, tachycardia, hypertension, or prostatic hypertrophy.
• Therapy should be stopped periodically to determine whether patient can get along without it. Minimizes tendency toward tolerance.
• Rapid onset of action; peaks at 3 to 4 hours; lasts 6 to 10 hours.
• Neurogenic bladder should be confirmed by cystometry before oxybutynin is given. Patient response to therapy should be evaluated periodically by cystometry.
• Partial intestinal obstruction should be ruled out in patients with diarrhea, especially those with colostomy or ileostomy, before giving oxybutynin.
• If urinary tract infection is present, patient should receive antibiotics concomitantly.
• Drug may impair alertness or vision.
• Since oxybutynin suppresses sweating, its use during very hot weather may precipitate fever or heatstroke.
• Store in tightly closed containers at 15° to 30° C. (59° to 86° F.).
• For symptoms and treatment of toxicity, see APPENDIX.

Interactions:
ERYTHROMYCIN, THIABENDAZOLE, TROLEANDOMYCIN: decreased hepatic clearance of theophylline; increased plasma levels. Monitor for signs of toxicity.
BARBITURATES: enhanced metabolism and decreased theophylline blood levels. Monitor for decreased effect.
PROPRANOLOL AND NADOLOL: antagonism. May cause bronchospasms in sensitive patients. Use together cautiously.
INFLUENZA VACCINATION: metabolism of theophylline is impaired. Monitor for higher theophylline blood levels.

Special considerations:
• Contraindicated in hypersensitivity to xanthine compounds (caffeine, theobromine) and in preexisting cardiac arrhythmias, especially tachyarrhythmias. Use cautiously in young children; in elderly patients with congestive heart failure or other circulatory impairment, cor pulmonale, renal or hepatic disease; and in patients with peptic ulcer, hyperthyroidism, or diabetes mellitus.
• Individuals metabolize xanthines at different rates; dose should be determined by monitoring response, tolerance, pulmonary function, and theophylline plasma levels: therapeutic level = 10 to 20 mcg/ml.

(continued on following page)

NAMES, INDICATIONS AND DOSAGES	SIDE EFFECTS

theophylline
(continued)

chial asthma, bronchospasm of chronic bronchitis and emphysema:
ADULTS: 100 to 200 mg P.O. q 6 hours; or 250 to 500 mg rectally q 8 to 12 hours.
CHILDREN: 50 to 100 mg P.O. q 6 hours, not to exceed 10 to 12 mg/kg/24 hours, in divided doses q 8 to 12 hours.
Oral timed-release form given q 8 to 12 hours.

Symptomatic relief of bronchial asthma, pulmonary emphysema, and chronic bronchitis:
ADULTS: 330 to 660 mg (sodium glycinate) P.O. q 6 to 8 hours, after meals.
CHILDREN OVER 12 YEARS: 220 to 330 mg (sodium glycinate) P.O. q 6 to 8 hours.
CHILDREN 6 TO 12 YEARS: 330 mg (sodium glycinate) P.O. q 6 to 8 hours.
CHILDREN 3 TO 6 YEARS: 110 to 165 mg (sodium glycinate) P.O. q 6 to 8 hours.
CHILDREN 1 TO 3 YEARS: 55 to 110 mg (sodium glycinate) P.O. q 6 to 8 hours.

♦ Available in U.S. and Canada. ♦♦ Available in Canada only.
All other products (no symbol) available in U.S. only. Italicized side effects are common or life-threatening.

WHAT YOU SHOULD KNOW ABOUT AMINOPHYLLINE

The usual loading dose for aminophylline is 5 to 6 mg/kg, followed by an infusion of 0.4 to 0.6 mg/kg/hour. The patient's history should be kept in mind as the prescribed dose is checked to be sure it's within the proper range.

Since the patient may suffer convulsions if the drug infuses too fast, an I.V. infusion pump should be used to administer it. If a pump isn't available, a minidripper should be used.

A total daily aminophylline dose should never be placed in a single 24-hour I.V. container. As a safety measure, the dose should be divided into separate containers, for example, four infusions of 6 hours each. This minimizes potential toxic reactions if the contents accidentally infuse too fast.

The patient will respond to the drug almost immediately. Since both the drip rate and the patient's reaction to the drug

FLOW RATES FOR AMINOPHYLLINE INFUSIONS

DOSE (every 6 hr)	FLOW RATE*
100 mg	9 ml/hr
150 mg	14 ml/hr
200 mg	19 ml/hr
250 mg	23 ml/hr
300 mg	28 ml/hr
350 mg	33 ml/hr
400 mg	37 ml/hr

*1 g/500 ml *or* 2 g/1,000 ml

Courtesy of Temple University Hospital, Philadelphia, Pa.

INTERACTIONS AND SPECIAL CONSIDERATIONS

- Vital signs and intake and output should be monitored. Expected clinical effects include improvement in quality of pulse and respiration.
- Dizziness is common side effect at start of therapy for elderly patients.
- GI symptoms may be relieved by taking oral drug with full glass of water after meals, although food in stomach delays absorption.
- Patient should be asked about other drugs used. Over-the-counter remedies may contain ephedrine in combination with theophylline salts; excessive CNS stimulation may result. Patient should check with doctor before taking *any* other medications.
- Instructions for home care and dosage schedule should be supplied.
- Daily dosage should be decreased in patients with congestive heart failure or hepatic disease, or in elderly patients, since metabolism and excretion may be decreased. Should be monitored carefully, using serum levels, observation, examination, and interview. Drug should be given around the clock, using sustained-release product at bedtime.
- Sustained-release dosage forms should not be confused with standard-release dosage forms.

can be monitored, side effects can be easily observed:

- Pulse rate and blood pressure should be checked.
- Heart rate should be monitored to detect cardiac arrhythmias. If arrhythmias are detected, the infusion should be stopped.
- The patient's fluid intake and output should be recorded. Since aminophylline has a diuretic effect, the patient could become dehydrated.

The usual therapeutic blood levels of aminophylline are between 10 and 20 mcg/ml. If the patient's blood levels rise above 20 mcg/ml, he may exhibit symptoms of drug toxicity—anorexia, nausea, vomiting, abdominal pain, and nervousness. The patient's blood levels should be monitored after the first hour of administration, then after 12 hours and 24 hours, and finally, once every 3 days. If the patient demonstrates a toxic symptom, his blood levels should be checked immediately.

Another caution: Since the patient's breathing difficulty will make him restless, the I.V. site should be checked frequently; his restlessness may dislodge the I.V.

After 3 days of I.V. aminophylline, most patients improve enough to proceed to oral drug therapy.

Suppositories unreliable

In special, short-term situations and when the oral form of the drug is poorly tolerated or impossible to administer, suppositories can be used. However, recent studies indicate that absorption of aminophylline in suppository form is slow and unreliable. The patient would have to retain the suppository at least 6 hours to achieve maximum absorption! Blood concentrations of the drug fall below the therapeutic level desired. And rectal suppositories take longer than oral forms to attain maximum blood concentrations.

107

Heavy metal antagonists

deferoxamine mesylate
dimercaprol
edetate calcium disodium
edetate disodium
D-penicillamine

Heavy metal antagonists prevent or reverse formation of complexes that heavy metals make with organic compounds in the body. Heavy metals such as antimony, arsenic, cadmium, copper, iron, lead, mercury, and thallium can form insoluble metal complexes that interfere with normal functions, poisoning the central nervous system, gastrointestinal tract, and various organs, especially the kidneys. By combining with the heavy metals, the antagonists neutralize their toxic effects.

Major uses

- Deferoxamine is used in treatment of acute iron intoxication, chronic iron poisoning, and iron storage diseases.
- Dimercaprol is used to treat heavy metal poisoning such as Wilson's disease.
- Edetate calcium disodium is effective for symptoms of heavy metal poisoning.
- Edetate disodium is used to treat heavy metal poisoning and hypercalcemia.
- D-penicillamine relieves Wilson's disease and rheumatoid arthritis. It also prevents formation of kidney stones in cystinuria.

Mechanism of action

Heavy metal antagonists act as chelating agents to react with and neutralize calcium, cysteine, and heavy metals such as iron and copper. These substances bind more easily to heavy metal antagonists than to body tissues. The resulting complex (chelate) is stable, soluble, and easily excreted in urine.

- D-penicillamine's action on rheumatoid arthritis is unknown but is probably due to inhibited collagen formation.

CARING FOR PATIENTS WITH CYSTINURIA: SOME GUIDELINES

To prevent the formation of calculi:
Make sure the patient drinks large amounts of fluid during the day. Suggest that he drink 16 oz (approximately 500 ml) of fluid before he goes to bed and another 16 oz if he awakes during the night, since urine tends to be most concentrated and acidic at this time.

To lessen the risk of calculi formation:
Advise the patient to avoid foods containing methionine. These include rich meat soups and broths, milk, eggs, cheese, and peas. Methionine is a major forerunner of cystine.
Note: Because of its low protein content, this diet is not recommended for children and pregnant women.

To determine whether the patient has calculi:
The patient should have X-rays taken regularly.

PATIENT-TEACHING AID

WHAT YOU SHOULD KNOW ABOUT WILSON'S DISEASE

Dear Patient:

In addition to the medication your doctor has prescribed, here are some ways you can help control your condition:

- Avoid foods that contain copper, such as chocolate, nuts, shellfish, mushrooms, liver, molasses, broccoli, and cereals enriched with copper. Read product labels for contents, especially if these foods have minerals added or are fortified.
- Use distilled or demineralized water if your drinking water contains more than 0.1 mg of copper/liter. (You can get this information from the local water authority or public health agency.)
- Except when you're taking supplemental iron, take sulfurated potash or Carbo-Resin with your meals to minimize your absorption of copper.
- Make sure any vitamin preparations you take are copper-free.
- Continue your medication therapy as ordered. It may take 1 to 3 months before your neurologic symptoms begin to subside. This is normal, so don't be discouraged or stop therapy before the benefits have a chance to occur.

Absorption, distribution, metabolism, and excretion

- D-penicillamine is the only drug that's well absorbed when given orally. The others must be given parenterally.
- All the drugs are distributed to all body tissues, except edetate calcium disodium, which doesn't penetrate cerebrospinal fluid or red cells.
- All the drugs are excreted primarily unchanged in urine, exception dimercaprol and D-penicillamine. These two drugs are metabolized in the liver and then eliminated in urine and feces.

Onset and duration

- Onset of action for deferoxamine and for edetate disodium hasn't been determined.
- Dimercaprol begins to act 30 to 60 minutes after I.M. administration.
- Edetate calcium disodium takes effect approximately 1 hour after I.V. administration.
- D-penicillamine, when given orally, begins to work after about 1 hour.
- Duration of action varies with the ratio of heavy metal antagonist to metal present and also with renal function.

NAMES, INDICATIONS AND DOSAGES	SIDE EFFECTS
deferoxamine mesylate Desferal♦ **Acute iron intoxication:** ADULTS AND CHILDREN: 1 g I.M. or I.V. followed by 500 mg I.M. or I.V. for two doses, q 4 hours; then 500 mg I.M. or I.V. q 4 to 12 hours. Infusion rate shouldn't exceed 15 mg/kg/hour. **Chronic iron overload and in patients requiring multiple transfusions:** ADULTS AND CHILDREN: 500 mg to 1 g I.M. daily and 2 g slow I.V. infusion in separate solution along with each unit of blood transfused. Maximum dose 6 g daily. I.V. infusion rate shouldn't exceed 15 mg/kg/hour. S.C.: 1 to 2 g administered q 8 to 24 hours.	**Local:** pain and induration at injection site. *After rapid I.V. administration: erythema, urticaria, hypotension.* **With long-term use:** sensitivity reaction (cutaneous wheal formation, pruritus, rash, *anaphylaxis), diarrhea, leg cramps, fever, tachycardia, blurred vision, dysuria, abdominal discomfort.*
dimercaprol BAL in Oil♦ ADULTS AND CHILDREN: **Severe arsenic or gold poisoning:** 3 mg/kg deep I.M. q 4 hours for 2 days, then q.i.d. on 3rd day, then b.i.d. for 10 days. **Mild arsenic or gold poisoning:** 2.5 mg/kg deep I.M. q.i.d. for 2 days, then b.i.d. on 3rd day, then once daily for 10 days. **Mercury poisoning:** 5 mg/kg deep I.M. initially, then 2.5 mg/kg daily or b.i.d. for 10 days. **Acute lead encephalopathy or lead level more than 100 mcg/ml:** 4 mg/kg deep I.M. injection, then q 4 hours with edetate calcium disodium (12.5 mg/kg I.M.). Use separate sites. Maximum dose 5 mg/kg/dose.	**CNS:** pain or tightness in throat, chest, or hands; headache; paresthesias; muscle pain or weakness. **CV:** *transient increase in blood pressure, returns to normal in 2 hours; tachycardia.* **EENT:** blepharospasm, conjunctivitis, lacrimation, rhinorrhea, excessive salivation. **GI:** halitosis; nausea; vomiting; burning sensation in lips, mouth, and throat. **GU:** renal damage if alkaline urine not maintained. **Metabolic:** decreased iodine uptake. **Local:** sterile abscess, pain at injection site. **Other:** fever (especially in children), sweating, pain in teeth.
edetate calcium disodium Calcium Disodium Versenate♦, Calcium EDTA **Lead poisoning:** ADULTS: 1 g/250 to 500 ml of 5% dextrose in water or 0.9% normal saline solution I.V. over 1 to 2 hours daily or q 12 hours for 3 to 5 days; repeat after 2 days if indicated. Maximum dose 50 mg/kg daily. CHILDREN: 35 mg/kg I.M. daily divided q 8 to 12 hours. Maximum dose 50 mg/kg daily. **Acute lead encephalopathy or lead levels above 100 mcg/ml:** ADULTS AND CHILDREN: 12.5 mg/kg with dimercaprol 4 mg/kg deep I.M. after initial dose of dimercaprol 4 mg deep I.M. Use separate sites. After first dose, reduce to 3 mg/kg for 2 to 7 days.	**CNS:** headache, paresthesias, numbness. **CV:** cardiac arrhythmias, hypotension. **GI:** anorexia, nausea, vomiting. **GU:** *proteinuria, hematuria; nephrotoxicity with renal tubular necrosis leading to fatal nephrosis in excessive dose.* **Other:** arthralgia, myalgia, hypercalcemia. **4 to 8 hours after infusion:** sudden fever and chills, fatigue, excessive thirst, sneezing, nasal congestion.
edetate disodium Disodium EDTA, Disotate, Endrate, Sodium Versenate	**CNS:** circumoral paresthesias, numbness, headache, malaise, fatigue, muscle pain or weakness. **CV:** hypertension, thrombophlebitis. **GI:** nausea, vomiting, diarrhea, anorexia, abdominal cramps.

♦ Available in U.S. and Canada. ♦♦ Available in Canada only.
All other products (no symbol) available in U.S. only. Italicized side effects are common or life-threatening.

INTERACTIONS AND SPECIAL CONSIDERATIONS

No significant interactions.

Special considerations:

• Contraindicated in severe renal disease or anuria. Use cautiously in impaired renal function.
• Intake and output should be monitored carefully.
• I.M. route preferred.
• I.V. should be used only when patient has cardiovascular collapse or shock. For I.V. use, dissolve as for I.M. use; dilute in normal saline, 5% dextrose in water, or lactated Ringer's solution.
• If given I.V., should be changed to I.M. as soon as possible.
• For reconstitution, add 2 ml sterile water for injection to each ampule. Make sure drug is completely dissolved. Reconstituted solution good for 1 week at room temperature. Protect from light.
• Urine may be red.
• Epinephrine 1:1,000 should be available in case of allergic reaction.
• For symptoms and treatment of anaphylaxis, see APPENDIX.

Interactions:

^{131}I UPTAKE THYROID TESTS: decreased; don't schedule patient for this test during course of dimercaprol therapy.

IRON: formed toxic metal complex; concurrent therapy contraindicated.

Special considerations:

• Contraindicated in hepatic dysfunction (except postarsenical jaundice) and acute renal insufficiency.
• Should not be used for iron, cadmium, or selenium toxicity. Complex formed is highly toxic, even fatal.
• Ephedrine or antihistamine may prevent or relieve mild side effects.
• Ineffective in arsine gas poisoning.
• Solution with slight sediment is usable.
• Urine should be kept alkaline to prevent renal damage. Oral $NaHCO_3$ bicarbonate may be ordered.
• Should not be given I.V.; instead should be given deep I.M. route only. The injection site can be massaged after drug is given.
• Drug has an unpleasant, garliclike odor.
• Drug should not come in contact with skin when being prepared and administered, as it may cause a skin reaction.

No significant interactions.

Special considerations:

• Contraindicated in severe renal disease or anuria.
• I.V. use contraindicated in lead encephalopathy; may increase intracranial pressure. I.M. route should be used instead.
• Fluids should be forced to facilitate lead excretion in all patients except those with lead encephalopathy.
• Intake and output, urinalysis, BUN, and EKG should be monitored.
• Use with dimercaprol avoids toxicity.
• Oral form available but ineffective because of poor GI absorption; often used ineffectively as prophylaxis against lead exposure; can even increase lead absorption from GI tract.
• Procaine HCl may be added to I.M. solutions to minimize pain. Local reactions may develop.
• Rapid I.V. infusions should be avoided. I.M. route preferred.
• Drug should not be confused with edetate disodium, which is used for the emergency treatment of hypercalcemia.

No significant interactions.

Special considerations:

• Contraindicated in anuria, known or suspected hypocalcemia, or significant renal disease; active or healed tubercular lesions; history of seizures or intracranial lesions; generalized arteriosclerosis associated with aging. Use cautiously in limited cardiac reserve, incipient congestive failure, hypokalemia, diabetes.

(continued on following page)

NAMES, INDICATIONS AND DOSAGES	SIDE EFFECTS
edetate disodium *(continued)* **Hypercalcemic crisis:** ADULTS AND CHILDREN: 15 to 50 mg/kg slow I.V. infusion. Dilute in 500 ml of 5% dextrose in water or 0.9% normal saline solution. Give over 3 to 4 hours. Maximum adult dose 3 g/day; maximum children's dose 70 mg/kg/day.	**GU:** in excessive doses—nephrotoxicity with urgency, nocturia, dysuria, polyuria, proteinuria, renal insufficiency and failure, tubular necrosis. **Metabolic:** *severe hypocalcemia,* decreased magnesium. **Local:** pain at site of infusion, erythema, dermatitis.
D-penicillamine Cuprimine♦, Depen **Wilson's disease:** ADULTS: 250 mg P.O. q.i.d. before meals. Adjust dose to achieve urinary copper excretion of 0.5 to 1 mg daily. CHILDREN: 20 mg/kg daily P.O. divided q.i.d. before meals. Adjust dose to achieve urinary copper excretion of 0.5 to 1 mg daily. **Cystinuria:** ADULTS: 250 mg P.O. q.i.d. before meals. Adjust dose to achieve urinary cystine excretion of less than 100 mg daily when renal calculi present, or 100 to 200 mg daily when no calculi present. Maximum adult dose is 5 g daily. CHILDREN: 30 mg/kg daily P.O. divided q.i.d. before meals. Adjust dose to achieve urinary cystine excretion of less than 100 mg daily when renal calculi present, or 100 to 200 mg daily when no calculi present. **Rheumatoid arthritis:** ADULTS: 250 mg P.O. daily initially, with increases of 250 mg q 2 to 3 months if necessary. Maximum dose 1 g daily.	**Blood:** *leukopenia, eosinophilia, thrombocytopenia, monocytosis, granulocytopenia,* elevated sedimentation rate, lupus erythematosus–like syndrome. **EENT:** tinnitus. **GU:** *nephrotic syndrome, glomerulonephritis.* **Hepatic:** hepatotoxicity. **Metabolic:** *decreased pyridoxine (may cause optic neuritis),* decreased zinc and mercury. **Skin:** friability, especially at pressure spots; wrinkling; erythema; urticaria; ecchymoses. **Other:** reversible taste impairment, especially of salts and sweets; hair loss. *About 1/3 of patients develop allergic reactions (rash, pruritus, fever), arthralgia, lymphadenopathy.* With long-term use, myasthenia gravis syndrome.

INTERACTIONS AND SPECIAL CONSIDERATIONS

• Rapid I.V. infusion should be avoided; profound hypocalcemia may occur.
• EKG should be monitored, and renal function tested often.
• Serum calcium levels should be obtained after each dose.
• I.V. calcium should be kept available.
• Patient should remain in bed for 15 minutes after infusion to avoid postural hypotension.
• Don't use to treat lead toxicity; use edetate calcium disodium instead.
• I.V. site should be recorded and repeated use of same site avoided to decrease likelihood of thrombophlebitis.
• Generalized systemic reactions may occur 4 to 8 hours after drug administration and should be reported; these include fever, chills, back pain, emesis, muscle cramps and urinary urgency. Treatment is usually supportive. Symptoms generally subside within 12 hours.
• Drug should not be confused with edetate calcium disodium, which is used to treat lead poisoning.
• Edetate disodium not currently drug of choice for treatment of hypercalcemia; other treatments are safer and more effective.

Interactions:
ORAL IRON: decreased effectiveness of D-penicillamine. If used together, give at least 2 hours apart.

Special considerations:
• Contraindicated in pregnant women with cystinuria. Use cautiously in penicillin allergy; cross-sensitivity may occur.
• Fever or other allergic reactions may occur.
• Patient should receive pyridoxine daily.
• Patients should be handled carefully to avoid skin damage.
• Dose should be given on empty stomach.
• Patient should drink large amounts of fluid, especially at night.
• Therapeutic effect may be delayed up to 3 months.
• CBC, and renal and hepatic function should be monitored regularly throughout therapy (every 2 weeks for the first 6 months, then monthly).
• Drug should be held and doctor notified if WBC falls below 3,500/mm^3 and/or platelet count falls below 100,000/mm^3 (these are indications to stop drug). A progressive decline in platelet or WBC in three successive blood tests may necessitate temporary cessation of therapy, even if these counts are within normal limit.
• Fever, sore throat, chills, bruising, increased bleeding time may be early signs of granulocytopenia.
• Appropriate health teaching for patients with Wilson's disease and cystinuria should be provided.

108

Gold salts

aurothioglucose
gold sodium thiomalate

Gold, the precious metal, has been used in the treatment of arthritis since 1929. Since the early 1960s, numerous studies have confirmed the effectiveness of gold therapy (also known as chrysotherapy), so its use has been increasing.

The drugs are actually gold *salts* that contain about 50% gold; the gold is attached to sulphur molecules.

Although the drugs can retard juvenile and adult rheumatoid arthritis in the early stages, they have little value in advanced stages of the disease. Unfortunately, gold therapy often produces serious side effects and must be discontinued.

Although gold salts do not possess analgesic properties, they can produce remissions. Many rheumatologists believe that gold salts constitute the drugs of choice after aspirin. These drugs may also retard the advance of new erosive lesions.

In patients who can tolerate gold injections without developing severe toxic reactions, about 75% show symptomatic improvement; 20% to 25% of these show disease remission.

Major uses

Gold salts are used to treat active rheumatoid arthritis that has not responded adequately to salicylates, penicillamine, rest, and physical therapy.

Mechanism of action

The exact mechanism of action is unknown. Anti-inflammatory effects in the active stage of rheumatoid arthritis are probably due to inhibition of sulfhydryl systems, which alters cellular metabolism. Gold salts may also alter enzyme function and immune response, and suppress phagocytic activity.

Absorption, distribution, metabolism, and excretion

- Aurothioglucose, in oil suspension, is absorbed slowly and irregularly after I.M. injection.
- Gold sodium thiomalate is well absorbed after I.M. injection.
- Gold salts are widely distributed to body tissues but concentrate in arthritic joints, which contain two to two and a half times as much gold as uninvolved joints.
- The metabolism of gold salts is unclear. In all likelihood, however, the compounds are *not* reduced to the element gold.
- The drugs are excreted slowly, mostly in urine. A small amount, however, is eliminated in feces. After a cumulative dose of 1 g, urinary excretion of gold can be detected for as long as 1 year.

Onset and duration

Although action may not begin for 8 to 12 weeks after administration, it may last long after therapy is stopped, depending on the patient's response.

Combination products

None.

ABOUT RHEUMATOID ARTHRITIS

Rheumatoid arthritis (RA), which is often treated with gold compounds, is a chronic systemic disease characterized by a fluctuating, progressive inflammation and destruction of the joints.

CLINICAL FEATURES	TREATMENT	PATIENT TEACHING
• History of persistent painful morning stiffness that may last for hours (in other forms of arthritis, stiffness may last only a short while) • Spindle-shaped joint swelling • Subcutaneous nodules (small non-tender masses over pressure points) • Swelling of ulnar side of the wrist • Signs of muscle wasting, weight loss, erythema of palms, malaise • Fatigue occurring at same time each day regardless of previous activity level • Elevated erythrocyte sedimentation rate • Presence of rheumatoid factor in the serum (in about 30% of patients with RA)	Long-term management aims to relieve pain, arrest the inflammatory process, and prevent further joint damage by means of: • *Team evaluation* (nurse, doctor, physical therapist, social worker, dietitian) • *Drug therapy:* Teach patient to watch for and report side effects of salicylates, anti-inflammatory agents, corticosteroids, antimalarial agents, cytotoxic and immunosuppressive agents, chelating agents, and gold compounds. • *Specialized physical and occupational therapy:* Teach the importance of continuing prescribed ranges-of-motion and specialized exercises. Assess tolerance for physical activities, including activities of daily living. • *Prescribed rest:* 8 to 12 hours of sleep a night and a rest period during the day (total body rest or rest of the involved joints). To achieve correct resting and sleeping positions, patient should use a firm mattress; a small pillow, to avoid flexion contractures of the neck; and a footboard, to avoid footdrop. He should avoid using pillows under the knees. • *Diets:* For weight reduction or increased protein intake. • *Orthopedic appliances:* Special shoes, splints, and soft collars can ease pain, prevent fatigue, and provide proper alignment.	Some specific advice for patients with RA: • Avoid fatigue: Try to rest 5 to 10 minutes out of each hour. Plan your work. Work slowly but at an even pace. Sit whenever possible. Alternate sitting and standing tasks. Use good posture. • Avoid undue stress on the joints: Use the largest joint available for a given task. Support weak or painful joints. Avoid holding objects for long periods; hold objects parallel to knuckles. Use hands toward the center of the body. Slide—don't lift—objects. Avoid bending and climbing. • Use aids for dressing—long-handled shoehorn, reacher, elastic shoelaces. Whenever possible, sit to dress. Use a zipper-pull for long or difficult zippers; avoid back zippers. Use a button hook for manipulating buttons. Arrange closets efficiently. Keep like items and items usually worn together, hanging together. • Be skeptical of anyone offering cures. Arthritis quacks defraud patients of millions of dollars annually in the United States.

NAMES, INDICATIONS AND DOSAGES	SIDE EFFECTS
aurothioglucose Solganal **gold sodium thiomalate** Myochrysine♦ **Rheumatoid arthritis:** ADULTS: initially, 10 mg (aurothioglucose) I.M., followed by 25 mg for second and third doses at weekly intervals. Then, 50 mg weekly until 1 g has been given. If improvement occurs without toxicity, continue 25 to 50 mg at 3- to 4-week intervals indefinitely as maintenance therapy. CHILDREN 6 TO 12 YEARS: ¼ usual adult dose. Alternatively, 1 mg/kg I.M. once weekly for 20 weeks. **Rheumatoid arthritis:** ADULTS: initially, 10 mg (gold sodium thiomalate) I.M., followed by 25 mg in 1 week. Then, 50 mg weekly until 14 to 20 doses have been given. If improvement occurs without toxicity, continue 50 mg q 2 weeks for 4 doses; then, 50 mg q 3 weeks for 4 doses; then, 50 mg q month indefinitely as maintenance therapy. If relapse occurs during maintenance therapy, resume injections at weekly intervals. CHILDREN: 1 mg/kg/week I.M. for 20 weeks. If response is good, may be given q 3 to 4 weeks indefinitely.	Adverse reactions to gold are considered severe and potentially life-threatening. Report any side effect to the doctor at once. **Blood:** *thrombocytopenia* (with or without purpura), *aplastic anemia, agranulocytosis,* leukopenia, eosinophilia. **CNS:** *dizziness,* syncope, sweating. **CV:** bradycardia. **EENT:** corneal gold deposition, corneal ulcers. **GI:** *metallic taste, stomatitis,* difficulty swallowing, nausea, vomiting. **GU:** *albuminuria, proteinuria, nephrotic syndrome,* nephritis, acute tubular necrosis. **Hepatic:** hepatitis, jaundice. **Skin:** *rash and dermatitis in 20% of patients. (If drug is not stopped, may lead to fatal exfoliative dermatitis.)* **Other:** *anaphylaxis,* angioneurotic edema.

INTERACTIONS AND SPECIAL CONSIDERATIONS

No significant interactions.

Special considerations:

- Contraindicated in patients with severe, uncontrollable diabetes, renal disease, hepatic dysfunction, marked hypertension, heart failure, systemic lupus erythematosus, Sjögren's syndrome skin rash, and drug hypersensitivities. Use cautiously with other drugs that cause blood dyscrasias.
- Indicated only in active rheumatoid arthritis that has not responded adequately to salicylates, D-penicillamine, rest, and physical therapy.
- Should be administered only under constant supervision of a doctor who is thoroughly familiar with the drug's toxicities and benefits.
- Most side effects are readily reversible if drug is stopped immediately.
- All gold salts should be administered intramuscularly, preferably intragluteally. Color of drug is pale yellow; should not be used if it darkens.
- Possibility of anaphylactic reaction requires observation of patient for 30 minutes after administration.
- Benefits of therapy may not appear for 6 to 8 weeks or longer.
- Gold therapy may alter liver function studies.
- Aurothioglucose is a suspension. Vial should be immersed in warm water and shaken vigorously before injecting.
- When patient is given gold sodium thiomalate, he should lie down and remain recumbent for 10 minutes following injection.
- CBCs including platelet estimation should be performed before every second injection for the duration of therapy.
- Dermatitis is the most common side effect of these drugs. Skin rashes or other problems may occur. Pruritus often precedes dermatitis and should be considered a warning of impending skin reactions. Any pruritic skin eruption while a patient is receiving gold therapy should be considered a reaction until proven otherwise. Therapy is stopped until reaction subsides.
- Stomatitis is the second most common side effect of gold therapy. Stomatitis is often preceded by a metallic taste. This warning should be reported to the doctor immediately.
- Close medical follow-up and the need for frequent blood and urine tests are important during therapy.
- Urine should be analyzed for protein and sediment changes before each injection.
- Platelet counts should be performed if patient develops purpura or ecchymoses.
- If side effects are mild, some rheumatologists resume gold therapy after 2- to 3-weeks' rest.
- Dimercaprol (BAL) should be kept on hand to treat acute toxicity.

AN IMPORTANT ADVANCEMENT: ORAL GOLD

Auranofin, oral gold, may be a possible alternative for patients with rheumatoid arthritis on gold therapy.

Until now, all gold compounds have been administered I.M. Patients receiving gold therapy require a painful weekly injection of 50 mg. This large dose can cause major side effects, such as damage to the kidneys.

Auranofin is more convenient than I.M. gold therapy: administered orally, it's taken daily in a smaller dose. So far, only minor side effects, such as diarrhea and skin irritations, have been observed. Investigations are now under way to determine whether oral gold has any long-term adverse effects.

Preliminary studies show that oral gold may have other benefits over injectable gold. For example, patients who don't respond to I.M. gold therapy may improve with oral gold. This suggests auranofin may work by a different mechanism than parenteral gold.

109

Diagnostic skin tests

histoplasmin
Old tuberculin
tuberculin purified protein derivative

Diagnostic skin tests are used to assess immunocompetence. They contain bacterial, fungal, or viral antigens not previously encountered by a patient (new antigens) that evaluate primary immune response. The tests also use common antigens previously encountered by a patient (recall antigens) to evaluate his secondary immune response.

When antigens combine with previously formed antibodies to cause an antigen-antibody response, they produce an immediate hypersensitivity (anaphylactic) reaction. Diagnostic skin tests indicate delayed hypersensitivity reactions. Delayed hypersensitivity reactions are mediated by T cells reacting to the antigen.

Reactions are read as significant positive or negative according to size of induration (varies with specific test). Positive reactions (erythema and induration in 24 to 48 hours, followed by resolution of the reactions) may indicate an intact cellular immune response due to past or possibly active infection, or a nonspecific inflammatory response.

Negative reactions mean active infection is highly unlikely. False-positive and false-negative reactions may occur, so skin tests alone are not diagnostic.

A patient's inability to react to a battery of common antigens (anergy) suggests that he is immunodeficient.

Major uses

Skin tests are used to:

- diagnose and differentiate infectious diseases
- determine immunity to infectious diseases
- help evaluate a patient's response to immunotherapy
- identify diminished or delayed hypersensitivity or anergy in a patient.

Purified protein derivative is one of the substances used to assess immunocompetence in patients with cancer.

Mechanism of action

Skin tests cause antigen-antibody reactions and nonspecific inflammatory reactions.

Absorption, distribution, metabolism, and excretion

Not applicable.

Onset and duration

Not applicable.

Combination products

None.

HOW TO PERFORM AND INTERPRET THE MANTOUX (PPD) TEST FOR TUBERCULOSIS

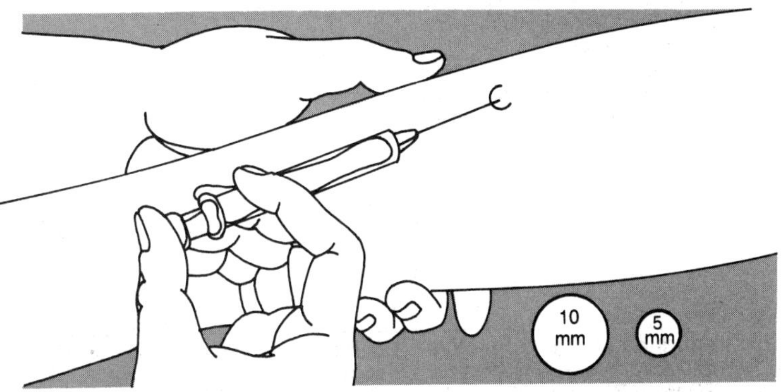

1. Check the label of the PPD vial for drug strength and expiration date. (PPD is available in three strengths, containing 1, 5, or 250 tuberculin units. The intermediate strength, containing 5 tuberculin units, is the one most often used for diagnostic testing.)
2. Use an easy-to-read tuberculin syringe with a 25G needle.
3. After you draw the PPD into the syringe, administer it within 5 minutes (it can be absorbed by glass and plastic).
4. After cleansing the site with alcohol, allow the skin to dry and then inject the PPD in the upper third of the patient's ventral forearm, just beneath the skin's surface (intradermal injection). Be sure the needle bevel is facing up.
5. A wheal—a pale elevation of skin—6 to 10 mm in diameter should appear immediately.
6. If no wheal forms, the injection may have been too deep. Reinject the PPD at a site at least 2" (5 cm) from the first site, or on the other arm.
7. To interpret the skin test, measure the area of induration (hardening or thickening of tissues) at 48 and 72 hours. *(Note:* Erythema isn't generally considered evidence of an active or dormant infection.)

An induration of 10 mm or greater indicates a significant reaction. (This was formerly called a positive reaction.) Significance of a reaction is determined not only by the size of the reaction but by circumstances. For example, a reaction of 5 mm or more may be considered significant in a person who has an immediate family member with tuberculosis.
8. Results should be recorded.

Note: A significant PPD reaction usually results in patients previously vaccinated with bacille Calmette-Guérin (BCG) vaccine. If you know a patient has received BCG vaccine, don't administer the PPD test. Also, a false-negative reaction can occur in an anergic patient (who can't react to any skin tests) or in an immunosuppressed patient.

Tuberculosis diagnosis must be confirmed by chest X-ray and/or positive sputum smear.

Source: Center for Disease Control criteria, and American Thoracic Surgeons Society statement on tuberculosis skin test reactions, August 1981

NAMES, INDICATIONS AND DOSAGES	SIDE EFFECTS
histoplasmin♦ **Suspected histoplasmosis:** ADULTS AND CHILDREN: 0.1 ml of 1:100 dilution intradermally on inner forearm. Use tuberculin syringe with 26G or 27G, ⅜" needle.	**Local:** urticaria, ulceration or necrosis in highly sensitive patients. **Other:** shortness of breath, sweating, *anaphylaxis.*
Old tuberculin Old Tuberculin Test♦; Old Tuberculin Tine Test; Tuberculin, Mono-Vacc Test **Diagnosis of tuberculosis:** ADULTS AND CHILDREN: 10 tuberculin units (0.1 ml of 1:1,000) Old tuberculin intradermally on inner forearm. In suspected tuberculosis, use 1 tuberculin unit first. Use tuberculin syringe with 26G or 27G, ⅜" needle. Multiple-puncture test: cleanse skin thoroughly with alcohol; make skin taut on inner forearm; press points firmly into selected site.	**Local:** hypersensitivity (vesiculation, ulceration, necrosis). **Other:** *anaphylaxis.*
tuberculin purified protein derivative Aplisol, Aplitest, Sclavo test-PPD, Sterneedle, Tuberculin PPD-Heaf, Tuberculin PPD-Stabilized, Tubersol **Diagnosis of tuberculosis, evaluation of immunocompetence in patients with cancer:** ADULTS AND CHILDREN: 5 tuberculin units (0.1 ml) intradermally on inner forearm. Suspected sensitivity dose is 1 tuberculin unit. Patients failing to react to 5 tuberculin units should be tested with 250 tuberculin units. First strength equals 1 tuberculin unit/0.1 ml; intermediate strength, 5 tuberculin units/0.1 ml. Second strength equals 250 tuberculin units/0.1 ml. Use tuberculin syringe with 26G or 27G, ⅜". Multiple-puncture test: cleanse skin thoroughly with alcohol; make skin taut on inner forearm; press points firmly into selected site.	**Local:** pain, pruritus, vesiculation, ulceration, necrosis. **Other:** *anaphylaxis.*

♦ Available in U.S. and Canada. ♦♦ Available in Canada only.
All other products (no symbol) available in U.S. only. Italicized side effects are common or life-threatening.

INTERACTIONS AND SPECIAL CONSIDERATIONS

No significant interactions.

Special considerations:
- Read test at 24 to 48 hours. Induration of 5 mm or more is positive.
- Reaction may be depressed in patients with malnutrition or immunosuppression.
- Cross-reaction may occur with other fungi (for example, *Candida albicans, Blastomyces dermatitides*).
- History of allergies and past reactions to skin tests should be obtained.
- Epinephrine 1:1,000 should be available.
- Cold packs or topical corticosteroids may relieve pain and itching if severe reaction occurs.
- For treatment of anaphylaxis, see APPENDIX.

No significant interactions.

Special considerations:
- Contraindicated in known tuberculin-positive reactors.
- False-positive reaction can occur in sensitive patients.
- Reaction may be depressed in malnutrition or in immunosuppression.
- Read test in 48 to 72 hours. Induration of 10 mm or more is positive; 5 to 9 mm, doubtful; less than 5, negative. Amount of induration determines whether a reaction is positive or negative, not amount of redness at site.
- Multiple-puncture test: 1 to 2 mm induration is positive.
- Old Tuberculin Tine Test equals 5 tuberculin units purified protein derivatives.
- Accurate history of allergies, especially to acacia (contained in tine test as stabilizer), and past reactions to skin tests should be obtained.
- Epinephrine 1:1,000 should be available.
- Subcutaneous injection invalidates test results. Bleb must form on skin upon injection.
- Corticosteroids and other immunosuppressants may suppress skin test reaction.
- Cold packs or topical corticosteroids may relieve pain and itching if severe reaction occurs.
- For treatment of anaphylaxis, see APPENDIX.

No significant interactions.

Special considerations:
- Contraindicated in known tuberculin-positive reactors; severe reactions may occur. Use cautiously with active tuberculosis.
- Read test in 48 to 72 hours. Induration of 10 mm or more is positive; 5 to 9 mm, doubtful; less than 5 mm, negative. Amount of induration determines whether the test is positive or negative, not amount of redness at the site.
- Multiple-puncture test: vesiculation is positive reaction; induration of less than 2 mm without vesiculation is negative.
- 1 tuberculin unit may give false-negative test; 250 tuberculin units may give false-positive test.
- History of allergies and past reactions to skin tests should be obtained.
- Reaction may be depressed in malnutrition, immunosuppression, or viral infections (up to 4 weeks' postinfection).
- Antigen adsorbed by plastic. Should be used at once after drawing into plastic syringe.
- Epinephrine 1:1,000 should be available.
- Subcutaneous injection invalidates test results. Bleb must form on skin upon injection.
- Cold packs or topical corticosteroids may relieve pain and itching if severe reaction occurs.
- Initial test should never be given with second test strength (250 tuberculin units).
- A tine test is available for rapid screening.
- Corticosteroids and other immunosuppressants may suppress skin test reaction.
- Positive response at the injection site in patients with cancer indicates immunocompetence (the patient can respond to a challenge of his immune system). These patients have a better chance of responding to immunotherapy than those with negative responses.
- For treatment of anaphylaxis, see APPENDIX.

110

Uncategorized drugs

adenosine phosphate
allopurinol
alprostadil
amantadine hydrochloride
bromocriptine mesylate
clomiphene citrate
colchicine
cromolyn sodium
diazoxide, oral
dimethyl sulfoxide 50% (DMSO)
disulfiram
levodopa
levodopa-carbidopa
methoxsalen
pralidoxime chloride
ritodrine hydrochloride

These drugs, with diverse uses, don't fall into the preceding classes of drugs.

Major uses

- Adenosine phosphate is a therapeutic adjunct for varicose veins and thrombophlebitis; it is also used to treat symptoms of bursitis, tendinitis, tenosynovitis, intractable pruritus, and multiple sclerosis.
- Allopurinol lowers blood and urine uric acid levels in primary gout.
- Alprostadil is used to maintain patency of the ductus arteriosus until corrective heart surgery can be performed.
- Amantadine alleviates idiopathic parkinsonism, parkinsonian syndrome, and drug-induced extrapyramidal reactions.
- Bromocriptine is used in short-term treatment of amenorrhea or galactorrhea associated with hyperprolactinemia. It also prevents postpartum galactorrhea.
- Clomiphene induces ovulation in anovulatory women who want to become pregnant.
- Colchicine relieves attacks of gouty arthritis.
- Cromolyn is a therapeutic adjunct for severe, chronic bronchial asthma.
- Oral diazoxide is used to treat hypoglycemia, particularly in infants and children.
- Dimethyl sulfoxide is instilled into the urinary bladder for symptomatic relief of interstitial cystitis.
- Disulfiram is an adjunct in the treatment of chronic alcoholism.
- Levodopa and levodopa-carbidopa are therapeutic for symptoms of idiopathic parkinsonism and parkinsonian syndrome resulting from encephalitis lethargica, carbon monoxide poisoning, chronic manganese poisoning, and cerebral arteriosclerosis.
- Methoxsalen is effective in the repigmentation of idiopathic vitiligo.
- Pralidoxime is an antidote for poisoning by pesticides and organophosphorus chemicals. It is also used to treat overdose of anticholinesterase drugs given in myasthenia gravis.
- Ritodrine is used in the management of preterm labor.

Mechanism of action

- Adenosine phosphate may correct biochemical imbalance or deficiency at the cellular level. Therapeutic effects may also result from the drug's vasodilation and ability to reduce tissue edema and inflammation.
- Allopurinol reduces uric acid production by inhibiting the biochemical reactions preceding its formation.
- Alprostadil is a prostaglandin derivative that relaxes the smooth muscle of the ductus arteriosus, maintaining adequate blood oxygenation.
- Amantadine increases dopamine release in animal brain, but its exact mechanism of action in humans is unknown.

PATIENT-TEACHING AID

PREVENTING ANTABUSE-ALCOHOL REACTIONS

Dear Patient:

The doctor has prescribed Antabuse (disulfiram) to help you stop drinking alcoholic beverages. Most patients tolerate the drug well, but you may suffer such side effects as drowsiness, fatigue, impotence, headache, skin eruptions, and metallic aftertaste. These effects will disappear after about 2 weeks of therapy, as your body adjusts to the drug.

Antabuse interferes with the breakdown of alcohol in your body. Should you take a drink, toxic levels of acetaldehyde will accumulate and produce a rapid, intense, and unpleasant reaction. *Caution: A severe reaction could be fatal.* Be aware of the hidden alcohol content of common substances. Don't use alcohol in food, sauces, or vinegar; apply alcohol-containing shampoos, liniments, or lotions (such as after-shave); or take alcohol-containing medications, such as Paregoric, Comtrex, Nyquil, Nervine, or liquid vitamins. Metronidazole and paraldehyde may also cause a reaction. If you have a reaction, you may experience severe nausea and vomiting, hypotension, rapid pulse rate and respirations, flushed face, bloodshot eyes, throbbing in the head and neck, sweating, thirst, weakness, confusion, and blurred vision.

An Antabuse reaction may last as long as there's alcohol in the blood. You may have an Antabuse-alcohol reaction up to 2 weeks after you've stopped taking the drug.

If you're undergoing Antabuse therapy, always carry an identification card in case of an emergency. It should state that you're receiving Antabuse; the symptoms and treatment of an Antabuse-alcohol reaction; and your doctor's name, address, and phone number.

• Bromocriptine inhibits secretion of prolactin. It acts as a dopamine-receptor antagonist by activating postsynaptic dopamine receptors.
• Clomiphene appears to stimulate release of pituitary gonadotropins, follicle-stimulating hormone, and luteinizing hormone. This results in maturation of the ovarian follicle, ovulation, and development of the corpus luteum.
• Colchicine inhibits migration of granulocytes to an area of inflammation. It decreases lactic acid production associated with phagocytosis and interrupts the cycle of urate crystal deposition and inflammatory response.
• Cromolyn inhibits the degranulation of sensitized mast cells that occurs after a patient's exposure to specific antigens. It also inhibits release of histamine and slow-reacting substance of anaphylaxis (SRS-A).
• Oral diazoxide inhibits release of insulin from the pancreas and decreases peripheral utilization of glucose.
• Dimethyl sulfoxide acts nonspecifically as an anti-inflammatory agent. Its exact mechanism of action is unknown.
• Disulfiram blocks oxidation of alcohol at the acetaldehyde stage. Excess acetaldehyde produces a highly unpleasant reaction in the presence of even small amounts of alcohol.

THERAPEUTIC ACTIVITY

THERAPEUTIC ACTIVITY OF UNCATEGORIZED DRUGS

DRUG	ONSET	DURATION
adenosine phosphate	5 to 30 minutes	1 to 2 hours
allopurinol	30 to 60 minutes	Blood and urine uric acid levels fall within 2 to 3 days, but full effect may not be seen for 1 week. Uric acid returns to pretreatment levels slowly.
alprostadil	Immediate	Throughout infusion
amantadine	10 to 15 minutes	Up to 24 hours; acidification of urine increases excretion rate.
bromocriptine	2 hours	4 to 5 hours
clomiphene	Unknown	Unknown
colchicine	Pain alleviated within 12 hours after P.O. administration and completely gone usually within 24 to 48 hours after P.O. and 4 to 12 hours after I.V. administration.	Blood levels fall 1 to 2 hours after oral dose, then rise due to recycling; drug found in leukocytes 9 days after single I.V. dose.
cromolyn	Immediately on inhalation	3 to 4 hours
diazoxide	Within 1 hour	8 hours
dimethyl sulfoxide	Unknown	Unknown
disulfiram	Rapidly absorbed from gastrointestinal tract, but full effect may not be seen for 12 hours.	Slowly eliminated; about 20% remains in body after 1 week; sensitization to alcohol may last 6 to 12 days after last dose.
levodopa and levodopa-carbidopa	Rapidly absorbed (10 to 15 minutes), especially when stomach is empty.	5 to 24 hours
methoxsalen	1 hour; peaks in 2 hours	8 hours
pralidoxine	2 to 5 minutes	Short-acting; repeated doses every 3 to 4 hours may be needed.
ritodrine	I.V.: immediate P.O.: 30 minutes	Depends on amount of uterine activity (generally 2 to 6 hours)

• Levodopa and levodopa-carbidopa act as follows: Levodopa is decarboxylated to dopamine, countering depletion of striatal dopamine in extrapyramidal centers, which is thought to produce parkinsonism. Carbidopa inhibits peripheral decarboxylation of levodopa without affecting levodopa's metabolism within the central nervous system. Therefore, more levodopa is available to be decarboxylated to dopamine in the brain.
• Methoxsalen may enhance melanogenesis, either directly or secondarily, to an inflammatory process.
• Pralidoxime reactivates cholinesterase that has been inactivated by organophosphorus pesticides and related compounds. It permits degradation of accumulated acetylcholine and facilitates normal functioning of neuromuscular junctions.
• Ritodrine is a beta-receptor agonist that stimulates the $beta_2$-adrenergic receptors in uterine smooth muscle, inhibiting contractility.

Absorption, distribution, metabolism, and excretion
• Allopurinol is well absorbed orally from the gastrointestinal (GI) tract. Most of it is metabolized in the liver to the active metabolite oxypurinol. This metabolite, as well as some unchanged drug, is excreted in urine.
• Alprostadil is administered intravenously and is rapidly metabolized by the liver. The metabolites are excreted largely by the kidney.
• Amantadine is well absorbed from the GI tract. It is largely excreted unchanged in urine.
• Bromocriptine is poorly absorbed from the GI tract. Metabolized by the liver, it is eliminated in urine and—through the bile—in feces.
• Clomiphene is well absorbed from the GI tract and metabolized largely in the liver. About 50% of the drug is eliminated in feces within 5 days; the remaining unchanged drug and metabolites are either recirculated in the enterohepatic vascular network or stored in body fat.
• Colchicine is well absorbed from the GI tract when given orally. It is metabolized in the liver and eliminated in both urine and feces.
• Cromolyn is absorbed into the systemic circulation after its inhalation into the lungs. The drug is excreted unchanged in urine and bile. Small amounts are swallowed and eliminated in feces.
• Oral diazoxide is well absorbed from the GI tract. Most of it is excreted unchanged in urine.
• Dimethyl sulfoxide's absorption is unknown. It is metabolized in the liver to dimethyl sulfone and dimethyl sulfide. Dimethyl sulfone is excreted in urine and feces; dimethyl sulfide is excreted in the breath and through the skin.
• Disulfiram is well absorbed from the GI tract. It is metabolized in the liver and excreted slowly in urine. About 20% of the drug remains in the body for 1 week or longer.
• Levodopa and levodopa-carbidopa are well absorbed from the GI tract. Levodopa's penetration into the CNS is enhanced when carbidopa is administered concurrently. Levodopa is metabolized (decarboxylated) to dopamine in the peripheral tissues and the GI tract. Eventually dopamine itself is metabolized in the liver and excreted in urine. Carbidopa is not extensively metabolized; most of it is excreted unchanged in urine.
• Methoxsalen is well absorbed from the GI tract, metabolized in the liver, and excreted in urine.
• Pralidoxime is variably and incompletely absorbed from the GI tract and after I.M injection. It is largely metabolized in the liver and excreted in urine both as a metabolite and as the unchanged compound.
• Ritodrine is poorly absorbed orally but is completely bioavailable after I.V. infusion. The drug is excreted in urine within 24 hours.

Onset and duration
The chart on the opposite page summarizes the therapeutic activity of the drugs described in this chapter.

Combination products
COLBENEMID: probenecid 500 mg and colchicine 0.5 mg.
PROBENECID WITH COLCHICINE: probenecid 500 mg and colchicine 0.5 mg.

NAMES, INDICATIONS AND DOSAGES	SIDE EFFECTS
adenosine phosphate Adenocrest, Adenyl, Cobalasine, My-B-Den **To relieve edema, pruritus, dermatitis, and erythema of varicose veins; symptomatic treatment of bursitis, tendinitis, intractable pruritus, and multiple sclerosis:** ADULTS: 20 to 100 mg I.M. (extended-release) daily for 3 or 4 days, reduced to same dosage every other day. Depending on patient response, reduce dose to 20 mg once or twice weekly; or 20 mg I.M. daily to t.i.d. (simple aqueous solution); or every hour for 5 doses for first 3 days, followed by 20 mg daily as needed; or 100 mg in aqueous solution injected as single dose daily for 3 days, followed by 100 mg on alternate days as needed. **Sublingual dose to supplement I.M. injection:** ADULTS: 20 mg sublingually q hour, 5 to 7 doses/day for 4 to 7 days. Maintenance dose: 40 to 100 mg daily sublingually, adjusted to patient response.	**CNS:** dizziness, headache. **CV:** *palpitations, hypotension, dyspnea.* **GI:** epigastric discomfort, nausea, diarrhea. **Skin:** erythema, flushing. **Other:** *anaphylaxis; local reaction at injection site; may increase symptoms of bursitis or tendinitis.*
allopurinol Lopurin, Zyloprim♦ **Gout, primary or secondary to hyperuricemia; secondary to diseases such as acute or chronic leukemia, polycythemia vera, multiple myeloma, and psoriasis:** Dosage varies with severity of disease; can be given as single dose or divided, but doses larger than 300 mg should be divided. ADULTS: mild gout, 200 to 300 mg P.O. daily; severe gout with large tophi, 400 to 600 mg P.O. daily. Same dose for maintenance in secondary hyperuricemia. **Hyperuricemia secondary to malignancies:** CHILDREN 6 TO 10 YEARS: 300 mg P.O. daily. CHILDREN UNDER 6 YEARS: 150 mg P.O. daily. **Impaired renal function:** ADULTS: 200 mg P.O. daily if creatinine clearance is 10 to 20 ml/minute; 100 mg P.O. daily if creatinine is less than 10 ml/minute; 100 mg P.O. more than 24 hours apart if clearance is less than 3 ml/minute. **To prevent acute gouty attacks:** ADULTS: 100 mg P.O. daily; increase at weekly intervals by 100 mg without exceeding maximum dose (800 mg), until serum uric acid level falls to 6 mg/100 ml or less. **To prevent uric acid nephropathy during cancer chemotherapy:** ADULTS: 600 to 800 mg P.O. daily for 2 to 3 days, with high fluid intake.	**Blood:** *agranulocytosis*, anemia, *aplastic anemia.* **CNS:** drowsiness. **EENT:** cataracts, retinopathy. **GI:** nausea, vomiting, diarrhea, abdominal pain. **Hepatic:** altered liver function studies. **Skin:** *rash, usually maculopapular; exfoliative,* urticarial, and purpuric lesions; erythema multiforme; severe furunculosis of nose; ichthyosis, *toxic epidermal necrolysis.*

INTERACTIONS AND SPECIAL CONSIDERATIONS

No significant interactions.

Special considerations:

- Contraindicated in myocardial infarction and cerebral hemorrhage. Use cautiously in patients with history of allergy or asthma; treatment should be kept available. History of allergies should be obtained before first dose.
- Anaphylactoid reactions have occurred following use of gelatin I.M. solution. Should be discontinued if patient complains of dyspnea or tightness in chest.
- Should not be given I.V.
- Sublingual tablets should be placed under tongue. Patient should not mix with food or water, or swallow excessively until dissolved.
- I.M. extended-release in gelatin vehicle: warm solution before using. Inject into gluteal muscle, using 22G to 20G needle, 1″ to 1½″ long.
- Patient should be assessed for reduction of edema and inflammation.

Interactions:

URICOSURIC AGENTS: additive effect; may be used to therapeutic advantage.

Special considerations:

- Contraindicated in hypersensitivity and in patients with idiopathic hemochromatosis or in those who have developed reactions to it. Use cautiously in hepatic or renal disease.
- Accurate patient history should be obtained; before first dose, possible allergies with other drug use should be noted.
- Should be discontinued at first sign of skin rash, which may precede severe hypersensitivity reaction, or any other adverse reaction. Patient should report all side effects immediately.
- Intake and output should be monitored; daily urinary output of at least 2 liters and maintenance of neutral or slightly alkaline urine are desirable. Patient should be encouraged to drink plenty of fluids while taking this drug unless otherwise contraindicated.
- CBC, and hepatic and renal function should be checked periodically, especially at start of therapy.
- Acute gouty attacks may occur in first 6 weeks of therapy; concurrent use of colchicine may be prescribed prophylactically.
- GI side effects may be minimized by giving with meals or immediately after.
- Serum uric acid levels may be used to evaluate effectiveness. Goal is to lower serum level to 6 mg/100 ml, usually within 7 to 10 days; to gradually reduce size of tophi, with no new deposits within 6 months; and to relieve joint pain and increase mobility.
- Allopurinol may predispose patient to ampicillin-induced skin rash.
- Allupurinol may cause rash even weeks after discontinuation.
- Since drug may cause drowsiness, patient should not drive car or perform tasks requiring mental alertness until CNS response to drug is known.

NAMES, INDICATIONS AND DOSAGES	SIDE EFFECTS
alprostadil Prostin VR Pediatric **Palliative therapy for temporary maintenance of patency of ductus arteriosus until surgery can be performed:** INFANTS: 0.1 mcg/kg/minute by I.V. infusion. When therapeutic response is achieved, reduce infusion rate to give lowest dosage that will maintain response. Maximum dosage is 0.4 mcg/kg/minute. Alternatively, administer through umbilical artery catheter placed at ductal opening.	**Blood:** disseminated intramuscular coagulation. **CNS:** seizures. **CV:** *flushing,* bradycardia, hypotension, tachycardia. **GI:** diarrhea. **Other:** *apnea, fever, sepsis.*
amantadine hydrochloride Symmetrel♦ **To treat drug-induced extrapyramidal reactions:** ADULTS: 100 mg P.O. b.i.d., up to 300 mg daily in divided doses. Patient may benefit from as much as 400 mg daily, but doses over 200 mg must be closely supervised. **To treat idiopathic parkinsonism, parkinsonian syndrome:** ADULTS: 100 mg P.O. b.i.d.; in patients who are seriously ill or receiving other antiparkinsonism drugs, 100 mg daily for at least 1 week, then 100 mg b.i.d., p.r.n.	**CNS:** depression, fatigue, confusion, *dizziness,* psychosis, hallucinations, anxiety, irritability, *ataxia, insomnia,* weakness, headache. **CV:** peripheral edema, *orthostatic hypotension,* congestive heart failure. **GI:** anorexia, nausea, constipation, vomiting, dry mouth. **GU:** urinary retention. **Skin:** *livedo reticularis,* dermatitis.
bromocriptine mesylate Parlodel♦ **To treat amenorrhea and galactorrhea associated with hyperprolactinemia:** 2.5 mg P.O. b.i.d. or t.i.d. with meals for 14 days, but for no longer than 6 months. **Prevention of postpartum lactation:** 2.5 mg P.O. b.i.d. with meals for 14 days. Treatment may be extended for up to 21 days, if necessary.	**CNS:** *dizziness,* headache, fatigue, mania, delusions, nervousness. **EENT:** nasal congestion, tinnitus, blurred vision. **GI:** *nausea,* vomiting, abdominal cramps, constipation, diarrhea.
clomiphene citrate Clomid♦ **To induce ovulation:** 50 to 100 mg P.O. daily for 5 days, starting any time; or 50 to 100 mg P.O. daily starting on day 5 of menstrual cycle (first day of menstrual flow is day 1). Repeat until conception occurs or until 3 courses of therapy are completed.	**CNS:** headache, restlessness, insomnia, dizziness, light-headedness, depression, fatigue, tension. **CV:** hypertension. **EENT:** blurred vision, diplopia, scotoma, photophobia (signs of impending visual toxicity). **GI:** nausea, vomiting, bloating, distention, increased appetite, weight gain. **GU:** urinary frequency and polyuria; ovarian enlargement and cyst formation, which regress spontaneously when drug is stopped. **Metabolic:** hyperglycemia.

♦ Available in U.S. and Canada. ♦♦ Available in Canada only.
All other products (no symbol) available in U.S. only. Italicized side effects are common or life-threatening.

INTERACTIONS AND SPECIAL CONSIDERATIONS

No significant interactions.

Special considerations:
- Contraindicated in neonatal respiratory distress syndrome.
- Because drug inhibits platelet aggregation, use cautiously in neonates with bleeding tendencies.
- Arterial pressure should be monitored by umbilical artery catheter, auscultation, or Doppler transducer. Rate of infusion should be slowed if arterial pressure falls significantly.
- In infants with restricted pulmonary bloodflow, blood oxygenation should be monitored to measure drug's effectiveness. In infants with restricted systemic bloodflow, systemic blood pressure and blood pH should be monitored to measure drug's effectiveness.
- Drug must be diluted before being administered. Fresh solution must be prepared daily, and any solution more than 24 hours old should be discarded.
- Apnea and bradycardia may signal drug overdose. If the signs occur, infusion should be stopped immediately.

No significant interactions.

Special considerations:
- Use cautiously in epilepsy or seizures, with congestive heart failure, renal impairment, peripheral edema, hepatic disease, eczematoid dermatitis, uncontrolled psychosis, or severe psychoneurosis.
- Should not be stopped abruptly, since this might precipitate a parkinsonian crisis; drug should be tapered off gradually.
- Elderly patients may experience orthostatic hypotension. They should change position slowly, dangle legs before getting up, and lie down if they feel faint or dizzy. Elderly males should sit down to urinate, especially at night.
- Last daily dose should be given as early as possible to avoid insomnia.
- Drug may produce dizziness, blurred vision, and impaired coordination; activities requiring mental alertness should be resumed gradually.
- Patient should report any decrease in drug's effectiveness to doctor.

No significant interactions.

Special considerations:
- Contraindicated in hypersensitivity to ergot derivatives.
- Patient should be examined carefully for pituitary tumor (Forbes-Albright syndrome). Use of Parlodel will not affect tumor size (cause tumor to regress) although it may alleviate amenorrhea or galactorrhea.
- May lead to early postpartum conception. Patient should be tested for pregnancy every 4 weeks or whenever period is missed once menses are reinitiated.
- Patient should use contraceptive methods other than oral contraceptive during treatment.
- Safe use of bromocriptine during pregnancy has not been established; therefore, this drug is not indicated in treatment of infertility.
- First-dose phenomenon occurs in 1% of patients. Sensitive patients may collapse for 15 to 60 minutes but can usually tolerate subsequent treatment without ill effects.
- Incidence of adverse effects is high (68%); however, most are mild to moderate, and only 6% of patients discontinue drug for this reason. Nausea is the most common side effect.
- Recurrence rates when used to treat amenorrhea or galactorrhea associated with hyperprolactinemia are high (70% to 80%).
- Menses should be reinstated and galactorrhea should be suppressed in 6 to 8 weeks.
- Should be given with meals.
- Giving last daily dose at bedtime with a snack may help decrease nausea and dizziness.
- Has been used investigationally in management of parkinsonism.

No significant interactions.

Special considerations:
- Contraindicated in thrombophlebitis, thromboembolic disorders, or history of these conditions; cancer of breast or reproductive organs; undiagnosed abnormal genital bleeding; ovarian cyst; hepatic disease or dysfunction. Use cautiously in hypertension, mental depression, migraines, seizures, diabetes mellitus, or gonadotropin sensitivity. Development or worsening of these conditions may require stopping drug.
- Patient with visual disturbances should report symptoms to doctor immediately.
- Possibility of multiple births exists with this drug. Risk increases with higher doses.
- Patient should learn how to take basal body temperature and chart on graph to ascertain whether ovulation has occurred.
- Drug should be discontinued and doctor notified immediately if abdominal symptoms or pain occurs because these indicate ovarian enlargement or ovarian cyst.
- Response (ovulation) generally occurs after

(continued on following page)

NAMES, INDICATIONS AND DOSAGES	SIDE EFFECTS
clomiphene citrate *(continued)*	**Skin:** urticaria, rash, dermatitis. **Other:** *hot flashes,* reversible alopecia, *breast discomfort.*
colchicine Colchicine, Novocolchine♦♦ **To prevent acute attacks of gout as prophylactic or maintenance therapy:** ADULTS: 0.5 or 0.6 mg P.O. daily; or 1 to 1.8 mg P.O. daily for more severe cases. **To prevent attacks of gout in patients undergoing surgery:** ADULTS: 0.5 to 0.6 mg P.O. t.i.d. 3 days before and 3 days after surgery. **To treat acute gout, acute gouty arthritis:** ADULTS: initially, 1 to 1.2 mg P.O., then 0.5 or 0.6 mg q hour, or 1 to 1.2 mg q 2 hours until pain is relieved or until nausea, vomiting, or diarrhea ensues. Or 2 mg I.V. followed by 2 mg I.V. in 12 hours if necessary. Total I.V. dose over 24 hours not to exceed 4 mg. *Note:* Give I.V. by slow I.V. push over 2 to 5 minutes. Avoid extravasation. Don't dilute colchicine injection with 0.9% sodium chloride or 5% dextrose injection, or any other fluid that might change pH of colchicine solution. If lower concentration of colchicine injection needed, dilute with sterile water for injection. However, if diluted solution becomes turbid, don't inject.	**Blood:** *aplastic anemia and agranulocytosis with prolonged use;* nonthrombocytopenic purpura. **CNS:** peripheral neuritis. **GI:** *nausea, vomiting, abdominal pain, diarrhea.* **Skin:** urticaria, dermatitis. **Local:** severe local irritation if extravasation occurs. **Other:** alopecia.
cromolyn sodium Intal, Intal P♦♦, Rynacrom♦♦ **Adjunct in treatment of severe perennial bronchial asthma:** ADULTS AND CHILDREN OVER 5 YEARS: contents of 20-mg capsule inhaled q.i.d. at regular intervals.	**CNS:** dizziness, headache. **EENT:** *irritation of the throat and trachea, cough, bronchospasm following inhalation of dry powder; esophagitis;* nasal congestion; pharyngeal irritation; wheezing. **GI:** nausea. **GU:** dysuria, urinary frequency. **Skin:** rash, urticaria. **Other:** joint swelling and pain, lacrimation, swollen parotid gland, angioedema.
diazoxide, oral Proglycem **Management of hypoglycemia due to a variety of conditions resulting in hyperinsulinism:** ADULTS AND CHILDREN: 3 to 8 mg/kg/day P.O., divided into 3 equal doses q 8 hours. INFANTS AND NEWBORNS: 8 to 15 mg/kg/day P.O., divided into 2 or 3 equal doses q 8 to 12 hours.	**Blood:** *leukopenia, thrombocytopenia.* **CV:** *cardiac arrhythmias.* **EENT:** diplopia. **GI:** nausea, vomiting. **Metabolic:** sodium and fluid retention, ketoacidosis and hyperosmolar nonketotic coma, hyperuricemia. **Other:** *severe hypertrichosis (hair growth) in 25% of adults and higher percentage of children.*

♦ Available in U.S. and Canada. ♦♦ Available in Canada only.
All other products (no symbol) available in U.S. only. Italicized side effects are common or life-threatening.

INTERACTIONS AND SPECIAL CONSIDERATIONS

the first course of therapy. If pregnancy does not occur, course of therapy may be repeated twice.
• Since drug may cause dizziness or visual disturbances, patient should not perform hazardous tasks until her response to the drug is known.
• Patient should stop drug and contact doctor immediately if she suspects she is pregnant (drug may have teratogenic effect).

No significant interactions.

Special considerations:
• Use cautiously in hepatic dysfunction, cardiac disease, renal disease, GI disorders, and in aged or debilitated patients.
• Dosage should be reduced if weakness, anorexia, nausea, vomiting, or diarrhea appears. First sign of acute overdosage may be GI symptoms, followed by vascular damage, muscle weakness, ascending paralysis. Delirium and convulsions may occur without patient losing consciousness.
• Should not be administered I.M. or subcutaneously; severe local irritation occurs.
• As maintenance therapy, should be given with meals to reduce GI effects. May be used with uricosuric agents.
• Baseline laboratory studies, including CBC, should precede therapy and be repeated periodically.
• Fluid intake and output should be monitored, and output maintained at 2,000 ml daily.
• Store in tightly closed, light-resistant container.
• Needle should be changed before making direct I.V. injection.

No significant interactions.

Special considerations:
• Contraindicated in acute asthma attacks and status asthmaticus.
• Not to be taken orally; capsule should be inserted into inhaler provided and manufacturer's directions followed.
• Recurrence of asthmatic symptoms is possible when dosage is decreased, especially when corticosteroids are also used.
• Should be used only when acute episode has been controlled, airway is cleared, and patient is able to inhale.
• Patient considered for cromolyn therapy should have pulmonary function studies to show significant bronchodilator-reversible component to his airway obstruction.
• Correct use of inhaler: insert capsule in device properly, exhale completely before placing mouthpiece between lips, then inhale deeply and rapidly with steady, even breath; remove inhaler from mouth, hold breath a few seconds, and exhale. Repeat until all powder has been inhaled.
• Store capsules at room temperature in tightly closed containers; protect from moisture and temperatures higher than 40° C. (104° F.).
• Avoid excessive handling of capsule.
• Esophagitis may be relieved by antacids or a glass of milk.

Interactions:
THIAZIDE DIURETICS: may potentiate hyperglycemic, hyperuricemic, and hypotensive effects. Monitor appropriate laboratory values.

Special considerations:
• Contraindicated in thiazide hypersensitivity and functional hypoglycemia.
• Oral diazoxide does not significantly lower blood pressure.
• A nondiuretic congener of thiazide diuretics.
• Most important use is in management of hypoglycemia due to hyperinsulinism in infants and children.
• Urine should be monitored regularly for glucose and ketones.
• If not effective after 2 or 3 weeks, drug should be stopped.
• Hair growth on arms and forehead is a common side effect that will subside when drug treatment is completed.
• Available in capsules and oral suspension.

NAMES, INDICATIONS AND DOSAGES	SIDE EFFECTS
dimethyl sulfoxide 50% (DMSO) Rimso-50 **Symptomatic relief of interstitial cystitis:** ADULTS: instill 50 ml directly into bladder with catheter or syringe; allow to remain for 15 minutes. Repeat every 2 weeks until maximum symptomatic relief is obtained. Thereafter, intervals between therapy may be increased.	**Other:** *garliclike taste in mouth*, hypersensitivity.
disulfiram Antabuse♦, Cronetal, Ro-Sulfiram **Adjunct in management of chronic alcoholism:** ADULTS: maximum of 500 mg q morning for 1 to 2 weeks. Can be taken in evening if drowsiness occurs. Maintenance: 125 to 500 mg daily (average dose 250 mg) until permanent self-control is established. Treatment may continue for months or years.	**CNS:** drowsiness, headache, fatigue, delirium, depression, neuritis. **EENT:** optic neuritis. **GI:** metallic or garliclike aftertaste. **GU:** impotence. **Skin:** acneiform or allergic dermatitis. **Other:** disulfiram reaction, which may include flushing, throbbing headache, dyspnea, nausea, copious vomiting, sweating, thirst, chest pain, palpitations, hyperventilation, hypotension, syncope, anxiety, weakness, blurred vision, confusion. In severe reactions, respiratory depression, cardiovascular collapse, arrhythmias, myocardial infarction, acute congestive heart failure, convulsions, unconsciousness, and even death can occur.
levodopa Dopar, Larodopa♦, Levopa♦, Parda, Rio-Dopa **Treatment of idiopathic parkinsonism and parkinsonian syndrome resulting from encephalitis lethargica; carbon monoxide and chronic manganese intoxication; and cerebral arteriosclerosis:** Administered orally with food in dosages carefully adjusted to individual requirements, tolerance, response. ADULTS: initially, 0.5 to 1 g P.O. daily, given b.i.d., t.i.d., or q.i.d. with food; increase by	**Blood:** hemolytic anemia, leukopenia. **CNS:** *choreiform, dystonic, dyskinetic movements; involuntary grimacing, head movements, myoclonic body jerks, ataxia, tremors, muscle twitching; bradykinetic episodes; psychiatric disturbances, memory loss, nervousness, anxiety, disturbing dreams, euphoria, malaise, fatigue; severe depression, suicidal tendencies, dementia, delirium, hallucinations (may necessitate reduction or withdrawal of drug).* **CV:** *orthostatic hypotension*, cardiac irregularities, flushing, hypertension, phlebitis. **EENT:** blepharospasm, blurred vision, diplo-

INTERACTIONS AND SPECIAL CONSIDERATIONS

No significant interactions.

Special considerations:
- Chronic use of DMSO has been associated with ophthalmic changes. Eyes should be examined periodically.
- After retention of Rimso-50 for 15 minutes, it's expelled by spontaneous voiding.
- Administration of oral analgesics or opium and belladonna suppositories before instillation can reduce bladder spasm in sensitive patients.
- Lidocaine jelly or similar local anesthetic should be applied to urethra before insertion of catheter to avoid spasm.
- Patient may experience some discomfort as the drug is introduced into the bladder; this generally subsides with repeated administration.
- Patient may experience a garliclike taste several minutes after administration, which may persist for several hours.
- Not for I.M. or I.V. injection.
- Patients on DMSO therapy should have liver and kidney function studies and CBC every 6 months while receiving drug.
- Safety of DMSO in pregnancy has not been established. Use only if potential maternal benefits outweigh potential risks to fetus.
- Safety and effectiveness of DMSO in children not yet established.
- Used investigationally as a topical treatment for arthritis-inflamed joints.

Interactions:
ISONIAZID (INH): ataxia or marked change in behavior. Avoid use.
METRONIDAZOLE: psychotic reaction. Do not use together.
PARALDEHYDE: toxic levels of the acetaldehyde. Do not use together.
ALCOHOL: disulfiram reaction.

Special considerations:
- Contraindicated in alcohol intoxication, psychoses, myocardial disease, coronary occlusion, or in patients receiving metronidazole, paraldehyde, alcohol, or alcohol-containing preparations. Use cautiously in diabetes mellitus, hypothyroidism, epilepsy, cerebral damage, nephritis, hepatic cirrhosis or insufficiency, abnormal EEG, multiple drug dependence.
- Should be used only under close medical and nursing supervision. Patient should clearly understand consequences of disulfiram therapy and give permission. Drug should be used only in patients who are cooperative, well motivated, and are receiving supportive psychiatric therapy.
- Complete physical examination and laboratory studies, including CBC, SMA-12, and transaminase, should precede therapy and be repeated regularly.
- If compliance is questionable, tablets should be crushed and mixed with juice or other liquid; patient should be observed.
- Patient should avoid all sources of alcohol: sauces and cough syrups. Even external application of liniments, shaving lotion, and back-rub preparations may precipitate disulfiram reaction. Alcohol reaction may occur as long as 2 weeks after single dose of disulfiram; the longer patient remains on drug, the more sensitive he will become to alcohol.
- Patient should wear a bracelet or carry a card supplied by drug manufacturer identifying him as disulfiram user. Cards may be obtained from Ayerst Laboratories, 685 Third Avenue, New York, N.Y. 10017.

Note: Mild reactions may occur in sensitive patients with blood alcohol level of 5 to 10 mg/100 ml; symptoms are fully developed at 50 mg/100 ml; unconsciousness usually occurs at 125 to 150 mg/100 ml level. Reaction may last ½ hour to several hours, or as long as alcohol remains in blood.
- Disulfiram should never be given to patient without his knowledge; severe reaction or death could result if such a patient then ingested alcohol.
- Disulfiram side effects, such as drowsiness, fatigue, impotence, headache, peripheral neuritis, and metallic- or garliclike taste, subside after about 2 weeks of therapy.

Interactions:
ANTICHOLINERGIC DRUGS, TRICYCLIC ANTIDEPRESSANTS, BENZODIAZEPINES, CLONIDINE, PAPAVERINE, PHENOTHIAZINES AND OTHER ANTIPSYCHOTICS, PHENYTOIN: watch for decreased levodopa effect.
PYRIDOXINE: reduced efficacy of levodopa. Examine vitamin preparations for content of vitamin B_6 (pyridoxine).
ANTACIDS, PROPRANOLOL: may increase levodopa effect. Use together cautiously.

Special considerations:
- Contraindicated in narrow-angle glaucoma, melanoma, or undiagnosed skin lesions. Use cautiously in cardiovascular, renal, hepatic, and pulmonary disorders; in patients with peptic ulcer, psychiatric illness, myocardial infarction with residual arrhythmias; and in patients with bronchial asthma, emphysema, and endocrine disease.
- Patients also receiving antihypertensive medication and hypoglycemic agents should be carefully monitored. MAO inhibitors should be stopped at least 2 weeks before therapy is begun.

(continued on following page)

NAMES, INDICATIONS AND DOSAGES	SIDE EFFECTS
levodopa *(continued)* no more than 0.75 g daily q 3 to 7 days, until usual maximum of 8 g is reached. Larger dose requires close supervision.	pia, mydriasis or miosis, widening of palpebral fissures, activation of latent Horner's syndrome, oculogyric crises, nasal discharge. **GI:** *nausea, vomiting, anorexia;* weight loss may occur at start of therapy; constipation; flatulence; diarrhea; epigastric pain; hiccups; sialorrhea; dry mouth; bitter taste. **GU:** urinary frequency, retention, incontinence; darkened urine; excessive and inappropriate sexual behavior; priapism. **Hepatic:** hepatotoxicity. **Other:** dark perspiration, hyperventilation.
levodopa-carbidopa (combination) Sinemet♦ **Treatment of idiopathic Parkinson's disease, postencephalitic parkinsonism, and symptomatic parkinsonism; carbon monoxide and manganese intoxication:** ADULTS: 3 to 6 tablets of 25 mg carbidopa/250 mg levodopa daily given in divided doses. Do not exceed 8 tablets of 25 mg carbidopa/250 mg levodopa a day. Optimum daily dosage must be determined by careful titration for each patient.	**Blood:** hemolytic anemia. **CNS:** *choreiform, dystonic, dyskinetic movements; involuntary grimacing, head movements, myoclonic body jerks, ataxia,* tremors, muscle twitching; bradykinetic episodes; psychiatric disturbances, memory loss, nervousness, anxiety, disturbing dreams, euphoria, malaise, fatigue; severe depression, suicidal tendencies, dementia, delirium, hallucinations (may necessitate reduction or withdrawal of drug). **CV:** *orthostatic hypotension,* cardiac irregularities, flushing, hypertension, phlebitis. **EENT:** blepharospasm, blurred vision, diplopia, mydriasis or miosis, widening of palpebral fissures, activation of latent Horner's syndrome, oculogyric crises, nasal discharge. **GI:** nausea, vomiting, anorexia, weight loss may occur at start of therapy; constipation; flatulence; diarrhea; epigastric pain; hiccups; sialorrhea; dry mouth; bitter taste. **GU:** urinary frequency, retention, incontinence; darkened urine; excessive and inappropriate sexual behavior; priapism. **Hepatic:** hepatotoxicity. **Other:** dark perspiration, hyperventilation.

INTERACTIONS AND SPECIAL CONSIDERATIONS

• Dosage should be adjusted according to patient's response and tolerance, and vital signs monitored, especially while adjusting dose. Significant changes should be reported.
• Patient should report adverse reactions and therapeutic effects.
• Possible dizziness and orthostatic hypotension, especially at start of therapy. Patient should change position slowly and dangle legs before getting out of bed. Elastic stockings may control this side effect in some patients.
• Muscle twitching and blepharospasm (twitching of eyelids) may be an early sign of drug overdosage; should be reported immediately.
• Patients on long-term use should be tested regularly for diabetes and acromegaly; blood tests, and liver and kidney function studies should be repeated periodically.
• Multivitamin preparations, fortified cereals, and certain over-the-counter medications may contain pyridoxine (vitamin B_6), which can reverse the effects of levodopa.
• If therapy is interrupted for long period, drug should be adjusted gradually to previous level.
• Therapeutic response usually occurs after each dose and disappears within 5 hours, but varies considerably.
• Patient who must undergo surgery should continue levodopa as long as oral intake is permitted, generally 6 to 24 hours before surgery. Drug should be resumed as soon as patient is able to take oral medication.
• Protect from heat, light, moisture. If preparation darkens, it has lost potency and should be discarded.
• Coombs' test occasionally becomes positive during extended use. Uric acid elevations expected with colorimetric method, but not with uricase method.
• Alkaline phosphatase, SGOT, SGPT, LDH, bilirubin, BUN, and PBI show transient elevations in patients receiving levodopa; WBC, hemoglobin, and hematocrit show occasional reduction.
• A doctor-supervised period of drug discontinuance (called a drug holiday) may reestablish the effectiveness of a lower dose regimen.
• Combination of levodopa-carbidopa usually reduces amount of levodopa needed by 75%, thereby reducing incidence of side effects.
• Pills may be crushed and mixed with applesauce or baby food fruits for patients who have difficulty swallowing pills.
• Patient and family should not increase drug dose without doctor's orders (they may be tempted to do this as disease symptoms of parkinsonism progress). Daily dose should not exceed 8 g.

Interactions:

PAPAVERINE, DIAZEPAM, CLONIDINE, PHENOTHIAZINES: may antagonize anti-Parkinson actions. Use together cautiously.

Special considerations:

• Contraindicated in narrow-angle glaucoma, melanoma, or undiagnosed skin lesions. Use cautiously in cardiovascular, renal, hepatic, and pulmonary disorders; in history of peptic ulcer, psychiatric illness, myocardial infarction with residual arrhythmias; and in bronchial asthma, emphysema, and endocrine disease.
• Patients also receiving antihypertensive medication and hypoglycemic agents should be carefully monitored. MAO inhibitors should be discontinued at least 2 weeks before therapy is begun.
• Dosage is adjusted according to patient's response and tolerance to drug. Therapeutic and adverse reactions occur more rapidly with levodopa-carbidopa than with levodopa alone. Vital signs should be monitored, especially while dosage is being adjusted.
• Patient should report adverse reactions and therapeutic effects.
• Possible dizziness and orthostatic hypotension, especially at start of therapy. Patient should change position slowly and dangle legs before getting out of bed. Elastic stockings may control this side effect in some patients.
• Muscle twitching and blepharospasm (twitching of eyelids) may be early signs of drug overdosage; should be reported immediately.
• Patients on long-term therapy should be tested regularly for diabetes and acromegaly; blood tests, and liver and kidney function studies should be repeated periodically.
• Treatment with levodopa should be discontinued at least 8 hours before starting Sinemet.
• This combination drug usually reduces the amount of levodopa needed by 75%, thereby reducing the incidence of side effects.
• Pyridoxine (B_6) does not reverse the beneficial effects of Sinemet. Multivitamins can be taken without fear of losing control of symptoms.
• If therapy is interrupted temporarily, the usual daily dosage may be given as soon as patient resumes oral medication.
• Available as tablets with carbidopa-levodopa in a 1 to 10 ratio (Sinemet 10/100 and Sinemet 25/250); also in a 1:4 ratio (Sinemet 25/100).
• Sinemet 25/100 may reduce many side effects seen with 1:10 ratio strengths.
• Carbidopa (Lodosyn) as a single agent is available from Merck Sharp & Dohme on doctor's request.
• Dose should not be increased without doctor's orders.

NAMES, INDICATIONS AND DOSAGES	SIDE EFFECTS
methoxsalen Oxsoralen♦ **To induce repigmentation in vitiligo:** ADULTS AND CHILDREN OVER 12 YEARS: 20 mg P.O. daily, 2 to 4 hours before carefully timed exposure to ultraviolet light.	**CNS:** nervousness, insomnia, depression. **GI:** *discomfort, nausea, diarrhea.* **Skin:** edema, erythema, painful blistering, burning, peeling.
pralidoxime chloride Protopam♦ **Antidote for organophosphate poisoning:** ADULTS: I.V. infusion of 1 to 2 g in 100 ml of saline solution over 15 to 30 minutes. If pulmonary edema is present, give drug by slow I.V. push over 5 minutes. Repeat in 1 hour if muscle weakness persists. Additional doses may be given cautiously. I.M. or S.C. injection can be used if I.V. is not feasible; or 1 to 3 g P.O. q 5 hours. CHILDREN: 20 to 40 mg/kg I.V. **To treat cholinergic crisis in myasthenia gravis:** ADULTS: 1 to 2 g I.V., followed by increments of 250 mg I.V. q 5 minutes.	**CNS:** dizziness, headache, drowsiness, excitement, and manic behavior following recovery of consciousness. **CV:** tachycardia. **EENT:** blurred vision, diplopia, impaired accommodation, laryngospasm. **GI:** nausea. **Other:** muscular weakness, muscle rigidity, hyperventilation.
ritodrine hydrochloride Yutopar **Management of preterm labor:** *I.V. therapy:* dilute 150 mg (3 ampuls) in 500 ml of fluid, yielding a final concentration of 0.3 mg/ml. Usual initial dose is 0.1 mg/minute, to be gradually increased according to the results by 0.05 mg/minute q 10 minutes until desired result obtained. Effective dosage range usually lies between 0.15 and 0.35 mg/minute. *Oral maintenance:* 1 tablet (10 mg) may be given approximately 30 minutes before termination of I.V. therapy. Usual dosage for first 24 hours of oral maintenance is 10 mg q 2 hours. Thereafter, usual dose is 10 to 20 mg q 4 to 6 hours. Total daily dose should not exceed 120 mg.	*Intravenous* **CNS:** nervousness, anxiety, headache. **CV:** *dose-related alterations in blood pressure, palpitations,* EKG changes. **GI:** nausea, vomiting. **Other:** erythema. *Oral* **CNS:** tremors. **CV:** palpitations. **GI:** nausea, vomiting. **Skin:** rash.

♦ Available in U.S. and Canada. ♦♦ Available in Canada only.
All other products (no symbol) available in U.S. only. Italicized side effects are common or life-threatening.

INTERACTIONS AND SPECIAL CONSIDERATIONS

Interactions:
PHOTOSENSITIZING AGENTS: do not use together. May increase toxicity.

Special considerations:
• Contraindicated in hepatic insufficiency, porphyria, acute lupus erythematosus, hydromorphic and polymorphic light eruptions. Use with caution in familial history of sunlight allergy, GI diseases, or chronic infection.
• Therapy should be regulated carefully. Overdosage or overexposure to light can cause serious burning or blistering.
• Drug should be taken orally with meals or milk.
• Eyes and lips should be protected during light exposure treatments.
• Monthly liver function studies should be done on patients with vitiligo (especially at beginning of therapy).

No significant interactions.

Special considerations:
• Contraindicated in poisoning with Sevin, a carbamate insecticide, since it increases drug's toxicity. Use with extreme caution in renal insufficiency or myasthenia gravis (overdosage may precipitate myasthenic crisis); also in patients with history of asthma or peptic ulcer.
• Use in hospitalized patients only; have respiratory and other supportive measures available; obtain accurate medical history and chronology of poisoning if possible; give as soon as possible after poisoning.
• I.V. preparation should be given slowly, as dilute solution.
• Initial measures should include removal of secretions, maintenance of patient airway, artificial ventilation if needed.
• Drug relieves paralysis of respiratory muscles but is less effective in relieving depression of respiratory center.
• Atropine along with pralidoxime should be given I.V., 2 to 4 mg, if cyanosis is not present. If cyanosis is present, atropine should be given I.M. Atropine should be given every 5 to 10 minutes until signs of atropine toxicity appear (flushing, tachycardia, dry mouth, blurred vision, excitement, delirium, hallucinations); atropinization should be maintained for at least 48 hours.
• Should be diluted with sterile water without preservative.
• Not effective against poisoning due to phosphorus, inorganic phosphates, or organophosphates with no anticholinesterase activity.
• Difficult to distinguish toxic effects produced by atropine or organophosphate compounds and those resulting from pralidoxime. Patient should be observed for 48 to 72 hours if poison ingested. Delayed absorption may occur from lower bowel.
• Patients treated for organophosphate poisoning should avoid contact with insecticides for several weeks.
• Patients with myasthenia gravis treated for overdose of cholinergic drugs should be observed closely for signs of rapid weakening. These patients can pass quickly from a cholinergic crisis to a myasthenic crisis, and require more cholinergic drugs to treat the myasthenia. Edrophonium (Tensilon) should be available in such situations for establishing differential diagnosis.

Interactions:
CORTICOSTEROIDS: may produce pulmonary edema in mother. When these drugs are used concomitantly, monitor closely.

Special considerations:
• Contraindicated before 20th week of pregnancy and in the following conditions: antepartum hemorrhage, eclampsia, intrauterine fetal death, chorioamnionitis, maternal cardiac disease, pulmonary hypertension, maternal hyperthyroidism, uncontrolled maternal diabetes mellitus.
• Because cardiovascular responses are common and more pronounced during I.V. administration, cardiovascular effects—including maternal pulse rate and blood pressure, and fetal heart rate—should be closely monitored.
• Amount of fluids administered intravenously should be monitored to prevent circulatory overload.
• Ritodrine decreases intensity and frequency of uterine contractions.
• Ritodrine I.V. should not be used if solution is discolored or contains a precipitate.

Drug toxicities

Drug toxicity—unlike anaphylaxis, which results from hypersensitivity—follows overdosage, or ingestion of a drug meant for external use. Cumulative toxicity may result from long-term use of a drug that is slowly excreted. The information that follows tells you how to identify, treat, and reverse toxic reactions with specific antidotes; and how to relieve their symptoms with other drugs or with supportive measures. Generally, the doses cited are recommended for adults. With some exceptions, children's doses should be calculated individually. (Supportive treatment of toxicity is covered in the tabular information for each drug.)

Anaphylaxis

Anaphylaxis is an immediate allergic reaction that occurs within 1 hour—though usually within minutes—after administration of a drug to a patient who is hypersensitive to it. Anaphylaxis may also occur in susceptible persons after ingestion of certain foods and after insect stings.

Symptoms to watch for:

Rapidly falling blood pressure, sweating, weakness, anxiety, dizziness, thready pulse; nausea, vomiting, abdominal cramps, diarrhea; urticaria, erythema, angioedema, and pruritus; dyspnea, wheezing, choking, airway obstruction, cyanosis. *Note:* Symptoms may progress rapidly to cardiovascular respiratory arrest.

What to do:

Stop drug. Maintain an open airway. Assess the patient's breathing. If he develops a sudden airway obstruction (from laryngeal edema), give mouth-to-mouth resuscitation, or insert an oral airway and apply mechanical ventilation. Keep an emergency tray on hand in case a tracheotomy may be necessary.

Administer 0.2 to 1 ml epinephrine 1:1,000 I.M. or subcutaneously. If needed, repeat the dose four or five times at 3- to 5-minute intervals. Vigorously massage the injection site to increase absorption. Epinephrine may produce complete reversal of the patient's symptoms. Give 50 to 100 mg diphenhydramine (Benadryl) P.O., I.M., or I.V., depending on patient's condition, size, and age. Giving an antihistamine with epinephrine may be the last treatment step the patient needs.

If symptoms of shock continue, start an I.V. with lactated Ringer's solution, using a large-bore catheter. This will support the patient's jeopardized circulatory system. The large-bore catheter makes it easier to give medications I.V.

Check blood pressure regularly. If the patient's blood pressure drops rapidly, administer a vasopresser (such as norepinephrine) I.V. to constrict the vessels. *Recommended dosage:* 4 ml of the commercially prepared solution added to 1 liter of 5% dextrose in water. *Caution:* Watch the injection site carefully for signs of drug infiltration (redness and swelling) to prevent tissue necrosis.

Note: If the reaction's severe, aminophylline may be used to combat bronchospasms. *Recommended dosage:* 5.6 mg/kg (usually 250 to 500 mg in 500 ml of 5% dextrose in water). Infusion rate shouldn't exceed 50 mg/minute. After loading dose, begin continuous infusion of 0.6 to 0.9 mg/kg/hour.

For persistent bronchospasm, give hydrocortisone sodium phosphate or hydrocortisone sodium succinate, I.V., 100 mg, repeated every 6 hours.

Important: *Keep emergency drugs/equipment handy in either a crash cart or an emergency box.*

Acetaminophen

Symptoms to watch for:

In the first 3 to 4 hours after ingestion: nausea, vomiting, anorexia, and sweating are likely, but some patients have no symptoms; 24 to 36 hours after ingestion, the patient may still be asymptomatic; liver enzyme levels may begin to rise. Hepatic toxicity may develop 2 to 5 days after ingestion. Watch for vomiting; right upper quadrant tenderness; elevated SGOT, SGPT, and serum bilirubin levels; and increased prothrombin time (PT). Hypoglycemia is possible.

How to confirm toxicity:
• Monitor SGOT, SGPT, and serum bilirubin levels, and PT.
• Monitor serum acetaminophen levels. Levels over 300 mcg/ml 4 hours after ingestion are associated with severe hepatic damage; levels under 120 mcg/ml 4 hours after ingestion usually mean hepatic damage is unlikely.
What to do:
Stop drug. Induce emesis with 15 to 30 ml of ipecac syrup or perform gastric lavage. **Important:** Do not give ipecac syrup if the patient is unconscious. Supportive measures include parenteral fluids, fresh frozen plasma, or clotting factors. Immediately begin therapy with acetylcysteine (Mucomyst), the direct antidote to acetaminophen overdose: Give 140 mg/kg P.O. of the 20% acetylcysteine (Mucomyst) solution; then give 70 mg/kg P.O. q 4 hours for a total of 17 doses (total dosage, 1,330 mg/kg). Acetylcysteine solution may be diluted to a 5% concentration with a soft drink (such as cola and ginger ale) to make it more palatable.

Anticholinergics (including tricyclic antidepressants)

Anisotropine methylbromide, atropine sulfate, belladonna leaf, benztropine mesylate, biperiden hydrochloride, biperiden lactate, chlorphenoxamine hydrochloride, clidinium bromide, cycrimine hydrochloride, dicyclomine hydrochloride, diphemanil methylsulfate, ethopropazine hydrochloride, flavoxate hydrochloride, glycopyrrolate, hexocyclium methylsulfate, homatropine methylbromide, hyoscyamine sulfate, isopropamide iodide, mepenzolate bromide, methantheline bromide, methixene hydrochloride, methscopolamine bromide, orphenadrine hydrochloride, oxybutynin chloride, oxyphencyclimine hydrochloride, oxyphenonium bromide, procylidine hydrochloride, propantheline bromide, scopolamine hydrobromide, thiphenamil hydrochloride, tridihexethyl chloride, trihexyphenidyl hydrochloride. Diphenoxylate hydrochloride with atropine sulfate may cause anticholinergic as well as narcoticlike toxicity. *Remember:* Other drugs, such as antihistamines and phenothiazines, also have secondary anticholinergic actions.
Symptoms to watch for:
Confusion, excitement, convulsions, coma; increased heart rate, dilated pupils, blurred vision, increased intraocular tension, and dry mouth (all may occur with therapeutic doses); dysphagia; urinary retention; hot, dry, and red skin; rapid respirations, muscle stiffness, and fever
What to do:
Stop drug. Maintain airway and respirations. Induce emesis with 15 to 30 ml of ipecac syrup or do gastric lavage. **Important:** Don't give ipecac syrup if patient is unconscious. Give activated charcoal 5 to 50 g, or 5 to 10 times estimated weight of ingested drug. Give saline laxative (e.g., 200 ml of magnesium citrate).

Give antidote: physostigmine salicylate can reverse life-threatening central and peripheral effects of anticholinergics. Dilute each mg in 5 ml of normal saline solution. Give 0.5 to 4 mg I.M. or I.V. slowly q 2 hours. Keep atropine sulfate available for treating possible physostigmine salicylate toxicity (symptoms are bradycardia, convulsions, and severe bronchoconstriction). Physostigmine is contraindicated in hypotension. Monitor EKG. If the patient has fever, sponge with wet towels. If the patient shows excitement, delirium, or convulsions, give small doses of short-acting barbiturate (sodium pentobarbital). Catheterize patient unable to void. Darken room, or use pilocarpine eye drops for dilated pupils.

Barbiturates and primidone

Amobarbital, amobarbital sodium, aprobarbital, barbital, butabarbital sodium, hexobarbital, mephobarbital, metharbital, pentobarbital, pentobarbital sodium, phenobarbital, phenobarbital sodium, secobarbital, secobarbital sodium, talbutal. Primidone is not a barbiturate, but symptoms and treatment of primidone toxicity are similar to those of barbiturate toxicity.
Symptoms to watch for (all indicate acute toxicity):
Headache, confusion, ataxia, CNS depression ranging from sleepiness to coma (may be preceded by excitement and hallucinations); hypotension; crystalluria (in primidone toxicity),

low urinary output; ptosis, miosis, mydriasis in severe poisoning; cyanosis, especially in earlobes, nose, or fingers; occasional blisters or bullous lesions; slow, shallow breathing; flaccid muscles; hypothermia, hyperthermia; and shock

How to confirm toxicity:

- Positively identify ingested drug.
- Measure and identify barbiturates in blood, urine, or gastric contents.
- Monitor for potentially lethal blood levels:
  —phenobarbital, 80 mcg/ml or higher
  —amobarbital and butabarbital, 50 mcg/ml or higher
  —secobarbital and pentobarbital, 30 mcg/ml or higher.

What to do:

Stop drug. Maintain adequate airway. Perform endotracheal suction every hour unless pulmonary edema develops (in which case endotracheal suction is contraindicated). Maintain adequate oxygen intake and carbon dioxide removal. Begin gastric lavage (most effective when started within 2 hours of ingestion). Use cuffed endotracheal tube.

Delay absorption with activated charcoal. Dose: 5 to 10 times estimated weight of ingested drug. Barbiturate toxicity has no specific antidote. Don't give analeptic drugs, such as caffeine. Maintain blood pressure by infusing 5% plasma or low-molecular–weight dextran I.V. Monitor central venous pressure. If fluid infusion doesn't maintain blood pressure, give metaraminol or levarterenol. Elevate patient's head 15 degrees to help prevent cerebral edema. Give up to 40 ml/kg fluids daily if renal function is adequate. Maintain daily urine output at 15 to 30 ml/kg. Monitor sodium, potassium, and chloride levels daily. In phenobarbital toxicity, forced alkaline diuresis with sodium bicarbonate and osmotic diuretic may be useful. Dialysis is indicated in severe barbiturate poisoning or inadequate renal function. Treat hypothermia by applying blankets, but avoid warming the patient too rapidly. Frequently monitor the patient's pulse rate, temperature, color of skin, reflexes, and response to painful stimuli. Turn the patient regularly, at least every 2 hours.

Benzodiazepines

Chlordiazepoxide hydrochloride, diazepam, lorazepam, prazepam, oxazepam

Symptoms to watch for:

Confusion, coma, diminished reflexes; possibly hypotension and depression

What to do:

Stop drug. Maintain airway; promote oxygen intake and carbon dioxide removal. Monitor respirations, pulse, and blood pressure. Induce emesis with 15 to 30 ml of ipecac syrup or perform gastric lavage. **Important:** Do not give ipecac syrup if the patient is unconscious. Delay absorption with activated charcoal. Dose: 5 to 10 times estimated weight of ingested drug or 1 g/kg of patient's body weight.

Bethanechol chloride

Symptoms to watch for:

Headache; circulatory collapse, hypotension, and cardiac arrest after I.M. or I.V. administration; substernal pressure or pain, transient complete heart block, orthostatic hypotension; bloody diarrhea after I.M. or I.V. administration; abdominal cramps, nausea, and vomiting; flushed skin; shock after I.M. or I.V. administration; salivation, sweating, fainting, bronchoconstriction

What to do:

Stop drug immediately. Give 0.4 to 0.6 mg of atropine sulfate subcutaneously or I.V. q 4 to 6 hours. For severe cardiovascular reactions or bronchoconstriction, give 0.2 to 1 ml of epinephrine 1:1,000.

Cardiotonic glycosides

Deslanoside, digitalis leaf, digitoxin, digoxin, gitalin, lanatoside, ouabain

Symptoms to watch for:

Headache, weakness, lassitude, fatigue, somnolence, memory loss, dizziness, ataxia, confusion, aphasia, neuralgias, paresthesias, muscle pain and weakness, fainting, seizures, stupor, coma, apathy, depression, personality changes, irritability, restlessness, insomnia, nightmares, euphoria, mania, giddiness, excitement, agitation, belligerence, violent behavior, delusions, hallucinations, psychosis, delirium; premature ventricular beats (most common in adults), paroxysmal and nonparoxysmal nodal rhythms, atrioventricular dissociation; paroxysmal atrial tachycardia with AV block (most common in children)

How to confirm toxicity:

- Monitor EKG. Watch for premature ventricular contractions, paroxysmal atrial tachycardia with AV block, nonparoxysmal AV nodal tachycardia, sinus bradycardia, atrial fibrillation, ventricular tachycardia or fibrillation, sinus arrest, SA block, premature atrial contraction, premature AV nodal contraction, and junctional tachycardia with escape rhythms.
- Monitor blood levels: 2 ng/ml of digoxin and 35 ng/ml of digitoxin may indicate toxicity.

What to do:

Stop drug. Treat arrhythmias. If patient has marked hypokalemia and atrial, junctional, or ventricular tachycardia, give potassium chloride: adults, 40 mEq/liter of 5% dextrose in water, maximum 20 mEq/hour; children, potassium chloride 0.5 mEq/kg in 5% dextrose in water. Don't use potassium in patients with hyperkalemia, impaired kidney function, second and third degree AV block, or SA block. Throughout, monitor EKG to end the potassium infusion promptly when hypokalemia is corrected and to avoid overcorrection to hyperkalemia by watching for signs of potassium toxicity (peaking T waves).

If patient is not hypokalemic, use *phenytoin.* The loading dose is up to 15 mg/kg I.V. at 50 mg/minute; maintenance, 5 to 7 mg/kg I.V. q 12 hours at a rate not to exceed 50 mg/minute. Don't use phenytoin in patients with second and third degree AV block, SA block, or marked sinus bradycardia. If phenytoin is contraindicated, infuse 1 mg/kg lidocaine hydrochloride as an I.V. bolus, at 25 to 50 mg/minute followed by constant infusion of 1 to 4 mg/minute. Use lidocaine hydrochloride with caution in patients with congestive heart failure. Lidocaine is contraindicated in patients with second and third degree AV block, SA block, and marked sinus bradycardia.

In patients with atrial tachycardia with AV block and premature ventricular contractions, give 1 to 3 mg of propranolol by slow I.V. infusion (1 mg/minute). Repeat after 2 minutes, if needed. Wait 4 hours before giving subsequent doses. Propranolol is contraindicated in patients with asthma, marked sinus bradycardia, SA block, second and third degree AV block, cardiogenic shock, heart failure, or pulmonary hypertension. Occasionally, quinidine and procainamide are also useful. The patient with second or third degree AV block, SA block, and marked sinus bradycardia may need an artificial pacemaker.

Remember, all patients with cardiotonic glycoside toxicity need constant EKG monitoring. Keep in mind that many of the arrhythmias that cardiotonic glycosides effectively treat closely resemble the arrhythmias that result from cardiotonic glycoside toxicity, and that patients with congestive heart failure often complain of nausea and vomiting. So whenever you see these symptoms in a patient receiving cardiotonic glycosides, and you can't positively rule out toxicity, withhold the drug temporarily if the patient's clinical condition permits.

Cholinergic (parasympathetic) drugs

Ambenonium chloride, edrophonium chloride, neostigmine bromide, neostigmine methylsulfate, physostigmine salicylate, and pyridostigmine bromide

Symptoms to watch for (all indicate cholinergic crisis):

Incoordination, blurred vision, weakness, fasciculation, paralysis; agitation and restlessness with extreme overdosage of neostigmine bromide, neostigmine methylsulfate, and pyridostigmine bromide; agitation, restlessness, dizziness, and mental confusion with extreme overdosage of ambenonium chloride; hypotension, cardiospasm, bradycardia, and tachycardia; miosis, and lacrimation; nausea, vomiting, diarrhea; salivation, sweating, muscle cramps, bronchospasm, and dyspnea

What to do:

Stop drug. Maintain adequate respirations; if necessary, use mechanical ventilation with repeated bronchial aspiration. Give atropine sulfate I.V. Atropine should be used in adequate doses to reverse the cholinergic effects of these drugs. Adequate atropinization is indicated by complete clearing of bronchial and pulmonary rales. Dosage: adults, 2 to 5 mg I.V.; children, 0.05 mg/kg. To reduce ganglionic and skeletal side effects of physostigmine salicylate, may give slow infusion of pralidoxime chloride I.V. Dosage: adults, 1 to 2 g in 100 ml of normal saline solution over 15 to 30 minutes; children, 20 to 40 mg/kg.

Heparin sodium

Symptoms to watch for:
Bleeding, especially in elderly women, postoperative patients, or after recent trauma
How to recognize it:
• Watch for partial thromboplastin time or activated clotting time greater than 2½ times control value accompanied by signs of bleeding.
• Monitor for decreased red blood cell count, hematocrit, or hemoglobin.
What to do:
Stop heparin immediately. If necessary, give heparin antagonist protamine sulfate by slow I.V. injection over 1 to 3 minutes. Usually, 1 mg of protamine sulfate neutralizes 90 units of heparin. Protamine sulfate doses may have to be repeated, based on clotting tests. However, repeat protamine doses cautiously, because large doses may act as an anticoagulant. Don't exceed 50 mg of protamine sulfate in a 10-minute period.

Insulin and oral hypoglycemic agents (antidiabetic drugs)

Acetohexamide, chlorpropamide, insulin (all forms), tolazamide, and tolbutamide
Symptoms to watch for (all indicate hypoglycemia):
Parasympathetic phase—hunger, nausea, belching, bradycardia, mild hypotension; decreased cerebral function phase—lethargy, frequent yawning, decreased spontaneity of conversation, and inability to do simple calculations; sympathetic phase—increased systolic and mean blood pressure, sweating, and tachycardia; coma with or without convulsions
Confirming diagnostic measures:
• Monitor blood for hypoglycemia (serum glucose level less than 50 mg/100 ml).
What to do:
• For mild hypoglycemia, if patient is alert, give 120 ml (4 oz) of an oral carbohydrate, such as orange juice or other sweetened juices, cola, or ginger ale, q 5 to 10 minutes until symptoms of hypoglycemia disappear. Alternately may give 0.5 to 2 mg of glucagon I.M. For comatose patients or those not responding to or refusing oral carbohydrates, give 50 ml of 50% dextrose I.V., or 0.5 to 2 mg of glucagon I.M. if not used previously. Keep airway open. Prevent tongue-biting. If patient doesn't respond, repeat 50% dextrose dose twice; then start 10% dextrose by continuous I.V. infusion (at rate of 20 drops/minute). Monitor blood glucose level.

Lithium carbonate, lithium citrate

Symptoms to watch for:
Seizures, impaired consciousness, transitory neurologic asymmetries similar to those produced by cerebral hemorrhage; tremors, fasciculations, stiff neck, ataxia, seizures, restlessness, confusion, stupor, and coma; arrhythmias, pulse deficit, and hypotension; widely opened eyes, transient vertical nystagmus, and tinnitus; dry mouth; urinary incontinence; irregular or deep respirations; gasping and grunting with hyperextension of arms and legs, allergic vasculitis, and fecal incontinence
What to do:
Stop drug. Use gastric suction. Monitor lithium serum levels (should not exceed 2 mEq/liter in acute treatment phase; or 1.5 mEq/liter in maintenance phase). Replace fluids and electrolytes as necessary. Increase lithium excretion by forced osmotic diuresis, using up to 200 g of mannitol I.V. (5% to 10% solution). Maintain urinary output of 100 to 500 ml/hour and a positive fluid balance; by alkalization of urine with 325 mg to 2 g sodium bicarbonate P.O. q.i.d., or 30 ml/kg sodium lactate by slow I.V. infusion daily; and by administration of caffeine, aminophylline, and sometimes acetozolamide.

Methaqualone

Symptoms to watch for:
Nasal or GI bleeding; hypertonia, hyperreflexia, muscle twitching, convulsions, coma, and delirium; tachycardia; dilated pupils; vomiting; renal insufficiency; pulmonary and cutaneous edema, shock, and hepatic damage
What to do:
Stop drug. If patient is not convulsing, induce emesis with 15 to 30 ml of ipecac syrup or perform gastric lavage. **Important:** Do not give ipecac syrup if the patient is unconscious. Delay absorption with activated charcoal. Dose: 5 to 10 times estimated weight of ingested drug or 1 g/kg of patient's body weight.
- Adults: For prolonged convulsions, give a neuromuscular blocker, such as tubocurarine, 1 unit/kg of body weight I.V. slowly over 60 to 90 seconds. Initial dose should be 20 units (3 mg) less than dose calculated by body weight. Assist respirations.
- Hemodialysis may be useful.

Methyprylon

Symptoms to watch for:
Coma, excitation, convulsions, delirium, hallucinations, somnolence, and confusion; hypotension; constricted pupils; fever, hypothermia, and respiratory depression
What to do:
Stop drug. Induce emesis with 15 to 30 ml of ipecac syrup or perform gastric lavage. **Important:** Do not give ipecac syrup if patient is unconscious. Delay drug absorption with administration of activated charcoal. Dose: 5 to 10 times estimated weight of ingested drug or 1 g/kg of patient's body weight. Provide supportive measures. Give norepinephrine 8 to 12 mcg/minute by I.V. infusion adjusted to maintain normal blood pressure. To dilute, add 4 mg of levarterenol to 1 liter of 5% dextrose in water. To treat convulsions and excitation, administer short-acting barbiturate, such as thiopental sodium, 75 to 124 mg I.V. Severe overdosage may require treatment with hemodialysis.

Narcotics

Phenanthrene derivatives: codeine, codeine phosphate, codeine sulfate, hydrocodone bitartrate, hydromorphone hydrochloride, hydromorphone sulfate, levorphanol tartrate, morphine sulfate, opium alkaloids (concentrated), oxycodone, oxymorphone hydrochloride. Morphine sulfate is the prototype of this class.

Phenylpiperidine derivatives: anileridine hydrochloride, fentanyl citrate, and meperidine hydrochloride. Meperidine hydrochloride is the prototype of this class.

Diphenoxylate hydrochloride with atropine sulfate may cause meperidine-like toxicity as well as anticholinergic toxicity.

Symptoms to watch for:
Respiratory depression, which may progress to Cheyne-Stokes respiration; apnea; CNS depression, ranging from stupor to profound coma; muscle tremors and twitches; delirium; disorientation; hallucinations; bradycardia; hypotension; cyanosis; circulatory collapse; cardiac arrest; miosis (with morphine derivatives and methadone); cold, clammy skin; hypothermia; flaccid skeletal muscles; and (with meperidine derivatives) occasional grand mal seizures, possibly tachycardia, mydriasis, and dry mouth.
Confirming diagnostic measures:
- Make a positive identification of ingested drug, if possible.
- Note symptoms:
  —coma, pinpoint pupils, and depressed respirations indicative of morphine derivative and methadone toxicity. Keep in mind that in terminal narcosis or severe hypoxia, morphine and methadone toxicity may cause mydriasis.
  —coma, dilated pupils, depressed respirations indicative of meperidine derivative toxicity.
- Analyze urine, blood, gastric contents, or all three body fluids for narcotics.

What to do:
Stop drug. Establish airway; ventilate as needed. Induce emesis with 15 to 30 ml of ipecac syrup or perform gastric lavage, especially within first 2 hours of ingestion. **Important:** Do not give ipecac syrup if the patient is unconscious or shows signs of CNS depression.

Give naloxone (Narcan). Dosage: in adults, 0.4 mg I.V., I.M., or subcutaneously repeated after 2 to 3 minutes up to 3 times, as needed; in children, 0.01 mg/kg I.V., I.M., or subcutaneously repeated after 2 to 3 minutes up to 3 times, as needed. Keep in mind that a narcotic antagonist (naloxone, for example) may precipitate acute withdrawal syndrome in patients who are physically addicted to narcotics.

Maintain body warmth and adequate fluid intake. Treat shock with oxygen, I.V. fluids, and vasopressors as needed. Monitor vital signs and level of consciousness frequently.

Oral anticoagulants

Anisindione, dicumarol, phenindione, phenprocoumon, warfarin potassium, and warfarin sodium

Symptoms to watch for:
Minor bleeding, such as purpura, hematoma, epistaxis, hematuria. Red-orange discoloration of urine with anisindione and phenindione may be mistaken for hematuria. Major bleeding, such as GI or intracranial, intrapulmonary, adrenal, or retroperitoneal bleeding; hemarthroses and bleeding into pericardial space are also possible but less common. Skin necrosis and the sudden onset of painful ecchymoses, usually on the lower half of the body or on the breast, may occur with coumarin derivatives.

How to confirm toxicity:
- Watch for PT greater than twice control value.
- Monitor for decreased red blood cell count, hematocrit, or hemoglobin.
- Test for blood in stools (Hematest, Hemoccult).

What to do:
Stop anticoagulant and control bleeding immediately. Give antidote, vitamin K_1 (phytonadione) 2.5 to 10 mg I.M., subcutaneously, or by slow I.V. injection. Repeat in 6 to 8 hours if necessary. If patient is not bleeding but has elevated PT, you may give 2.5 to 10 mg of phytonadione P.O. May repeat in 12 to 48 hours. In emergency, you may give 10 to 50 mg by slow I.V.; maximum rate 1 mg/minute. Repeat q 4 hours as needed. You may give fresh frozen plasma or fresh whole blood to replace clotting factors. In major bleeding, fresh frozen plasma is necessary because onset of phytonadione begins after 6 to 8 hours.

Phenothiazines

Acetophenazine maleate, butaperazine maleate, carphenazine maleate, chlorpromazine hydrochloride, dimethothiazine mesylate, fluphenazine decanoate, fluphenazine enanthate, fluphenazine hydrochloride, mesoridazine besylate, methdilazine hydrochloride, perphenazine, piperacetazine, prochlorperazine, prochlorperazine edisylate, prochlorperazine maleate, promazine hydrochloride, promethazine hydrochloride, thiethylperazine maleate, thioridazine, trifluoperazine, triflupromazine, trimeprazine tartrate

Symptoms to watch for:
Restlessness, confusion, excitement in early or mild intoxication; convulsions; depression ranging from drowsiness to coma; areflexia; parkinsonianlike extrapyramidal symptoms (tremors, rigidity, akinesia, shuffling gait, postural abnormalities, pill-rolling movements, masklike facies, and excessive salivation); dystonic and dyskinesic extrapyramidal symptoms; dystonia most common in children; dyskinesia most common in adults (disordered tonicity of muscles and torsion spasms, opisthotonos, drooping of the head, protrusion of tongue, mandibular tics, and stiff neck); difficult swallowing and breathing (accompanied by profuse sweating, pallor, and fever); akathisia (extreme motor restlessness; and continual moving of hands, mouth, and body); hypotension, tachycardia, EKG changes, cardiac arrhythmias, cyanosis, and vasomotor collapse; miosis; dry mouth; hypothermia, and sudden apnea

What to do:
Stop drug. Maintain airway; promote adequate ventilation. Gastric lavage is effective up to

several hours after drug is ingested. Delay absorption with activated charcoal. Dose: 5 to 10 times estimated weight of ingested drug or 1 g/kg of patient's body weight. Don't induce emesis; dystonic reactions may cause aspiration of vomitus.

Treat severe dystonia and dyskinesia with 2 mg of benztropine mesylate I.V. followed by 1 to 2 mg P.O. b.i.d. to prevent recurrence; or diphenhydramine hydrochloride 25 to 50 mg deep I.M. or I.V. Treat parkinsonian reactions with benztropine mesylate 0.5 to 6 mg P.O. daily; with trihexyphenidyl hydrochloride 2.5 mg P.O. daily to t.i.d.; with biperiden hydrochloride or lactate 2 mg t.i.d. to q.i.d.; or with 2 to 2.5 mg procyclidine hydrochloride P.O. t.i.d., increased to 60 mg daily, if necessary. Don't use levodopa. Attempt to treat akathisia with anti-Parkinson drugs as above; treatment is often ineffective. If stimulants are needed, use amphetamines, ephedrine, or caffeine and sodium benzoate. Don't use pentylenetetrazol or other stimulants, which may cause convulsions.

Observe patient for orthostatic hypotension; monitor blood pressure in supine and standing positions. Instruct ambulatory patient to rise from bed slowly and dangle feet for a few minutes before standing. Treat severe hypotension with slow I.V. infusion of norepinephrine 8 to 12 mcg/minute. Adjust to maintain normal blood pressure. To dilute, add 4 mg of norepinephrine to 1 liter of 5% dextrose in water. Or use phenylephrine hydrochloride 0.1 to 0.5 mg added to 500 ml of 5% dextrose in water, at a rapid rate initially, then slowed to maintain blood pressure at desired level. Do not use epinephrine; it may paradoxically lower blood pressure. Stay with patient and give reassurance that symptoms will subside.

Propoxyphene salts

Symptoms to watch for:
Stupor, coma, and convulsions; EKG abnormalities, and circulatory collapse; miosis; nephrogenic diabetes insipidus; respiratory depression, pulmonary edema, and cyanosis
Confirming diagnostic measures:
- Watch for EKG abnormalities.

What to do:
Stop drug. Maintain airway. Give antidote, naloxone hydrochloride (Narcan). Dosage: in adults, 0.4 mg I.V., I.M., or subcutaneously repeated after 2 to 3 minutes up to 3 times, as needed; in children, 0.01 mg/kg I.V. or I.M. Doses may be repeated in 2 to 3 minutes. Induce emesis with 15 to 30 ml of ipecac syrup or perform gastric lavage. **Important:** Do not give ipecac syrup if the patient is unconscious. Delay absorption with activated charcoal. Dose: 5 to 10 times estimated weight of ingested drug or 1 g/kg of patient's body weight. Use supportive measures as needed (oxygen, I.V. fluids, and vasopressors).

Salicylates

Symptoms to watch for:
Mild toxicity—burning pain in mouth, throat, or abdomen; slight to moderate hyperpnea; lethargy; vomiting; tinnitus; hearing loss; and dizziness. Moderate toxicity—ecchymoses, restlessness, incoordination, dehydration, fever, sweating, delirium, excitability, marked lethargy, and severe hyperpnea. Severe toxicity—sodium, potassium, and bicarbonate loss and metabolic acidosis in young children; coma; convulsion; cyanosis; oliguria; uremia; pulmonary edema; respiratory failure; and severe hyperpnea. Small doses of methyl salicylate are potentially fatal in children.
Confirming diagnostic measures:
- Monitor blood salicylate levels for 6 hours after ingestion. (*Note:* Salicylamide is not determined by serum salicylate analysis.) Look for the following salicylate levels in adults:

—no intoxication: less than 45 mg/dl
—mild intoxication: 45 to 65 mg/dl
—moderate intoxication: 65 to 90 mg/dl
—severe intoxication: 90 to 120 mg/dl. (Blood levels above 120 mg/dl are usually fatal.)
Blood levels may continue to rise for 6 to 10 hours after overdose.
What to do:
Stop drug. Induce emesis with 15 to 30 ml of ipecac syrup. **Important:** Don't give ipecac to

unconscious patient. If patient shows CNS depression, perform gastric lavage and protect airway. Delay absorption with activated charcoal. Dose: 5 to 10 times estimated weight of drug or 1 g/kg body weight. Give a saline cathartic (e.g., magnesium citrate 200 ml). For hypotension, give I.V. fluids according to the acid-base and electrolyte status. For respiratory depression, give artificial respiration with oxygen. For hypoglycemia, give dextrose I.V.

Maintain fluid balance with 5% dextrose in water with sodium chloride. Begin management with the following dosages, adjusting according to results of physical and laboratory examinations. In mild salicylate intoxication, give 100 ml/kg of fluids P.O.; in severe intoxication, give 400 ml of 5% dextrose in water/m^2 body surface area, with 5 mEq sodium chloride/dl and 2.5 mEq sodium bicarbonate/dl; when adequate urine flow is established, decrease sodium dose by 50% and add potassium chloride.

For acidosis, initially give 2 to 5 mEq sodium bicarbonate/kg by slow I.V. infusion over 24 to 48 hours. For bleeding due to hypoprothrombinemia give phytonadione (vitamin K_1), 25 mg/day I.M. or I.V. For impaired renal function, use dialysis to remove salicylates. For hyperpyrexia, sponge patient with tepid water. Don't use alcohol. Continue monitoring serum sodium, potassium, glucose, blood gases, and salicylate levels.

Spasmolytics

Aminophylline, dyphilline, oxtriphylline, papaverine, theophylline, theophylline sodium glycinate

Symptoms to watch for:

Headache, insomnia, irritability, restlessness, convulsions (especially in infants and small children), hyperreflexia, fasciculations, coma, and fainting; tachycardia, marked hypotension, and circulatory failure; tinnitus and flashing lights; nausea, vomiting, epigastric pain, hematemesis, and diarrhea; albuminuria and microhematuria; cyanosis; dehydration, extreme thirst, tachypnea, respiratory arrest, and fever

What to do:

Stop drug. Induce emesis with 15 to 30 ml of ipecac syrup or perform gastric lavage. **Important:** Do not give ipecac syrup if the patient is unconscious. Delay absorption with activated charcoal. Dose: 5 to 10 times estimated weight of ingested drug or 1 g/kg of patient's body weight. Give I.V. fluids and oxygen. Prevent hypotension, maintain fluid and electrolyte balance, and monitor serum levels until drug concentration is below 20 mcg/ml.

Index

A

B

B

C

D

D

E

F

G

G

H

I

J

K

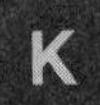

L

M

N

O

P

R

S

S

T

T

U

V

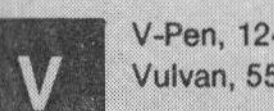

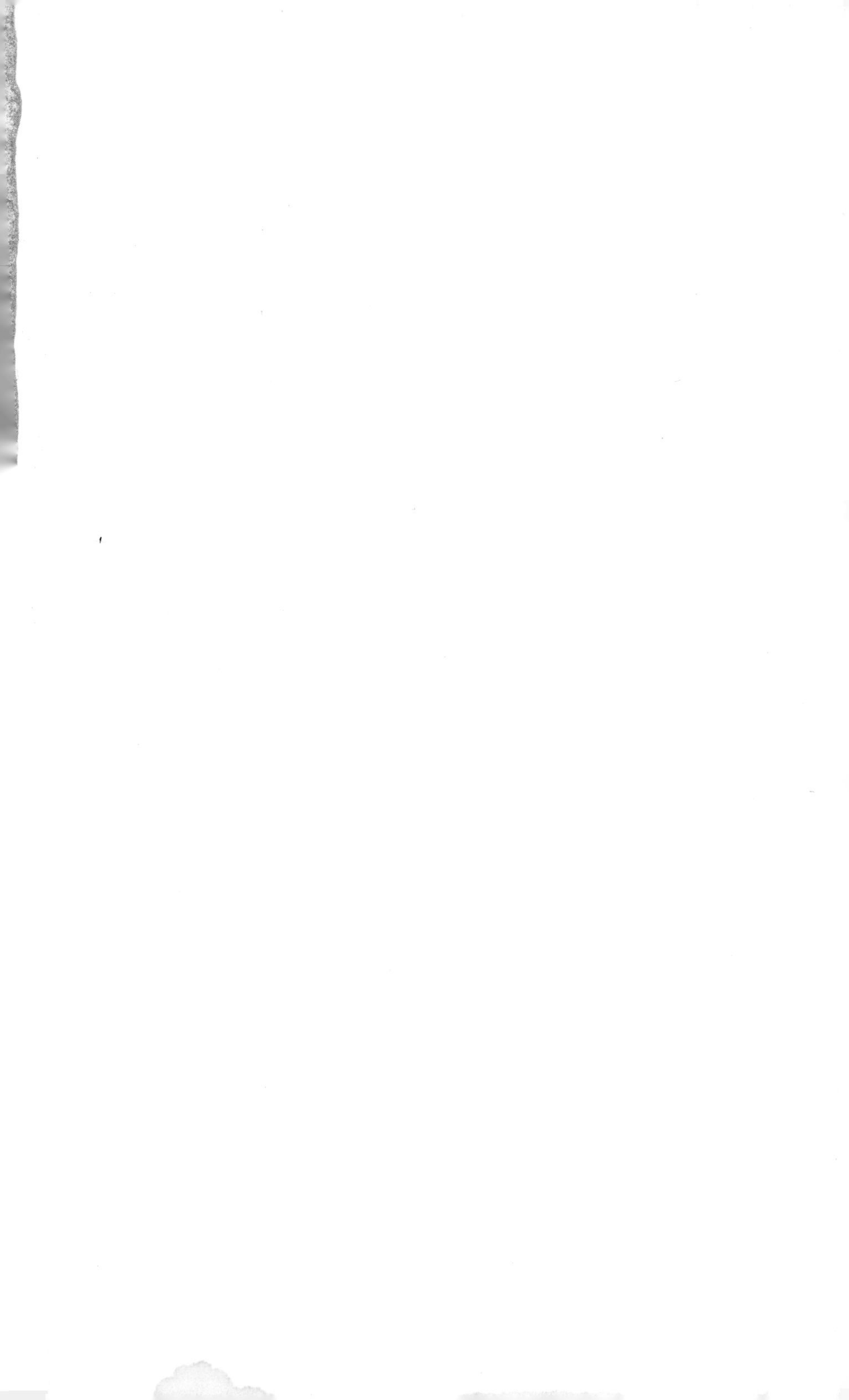

POISON & DRUG Information Centers

All offer 24-hour service unless otherwise noted.

ALABAMA
Southeast Alabama Medical Ctr.
Ashford Highway
Dothan 36302
(205) 793-8800

West Alabama Poison Control Ctr.
Druid City Hospital
809 University Boulevard
Tuscaloosa 35404
(205) 345-0600

ALASKA
Fairbanks Mem. Hospital
1605 Cowles
Fairbanks 99701
(907) 456-7182

Providence Hospital
3200 Providence Drive
Anchorage 99504
(907) 274-6535
(907) 274-6536

ARIZONA
St. Luke's Hospital
525 N. 18th Street
Phoenix 85006
(602) 253-3334

College of Pharmacy
University of Arizona
Arizona Health Science Ctr.
Tucson 85724
(602) 626-6016
(800) 362-0101

ARKANSAS
University of Arkansas Medical Ctr.
4301 W. Markham Street
Little Rock 72201
(501) 661-6161

CALIFORNIA
Los Angeles Co. Medical Association
Regional Poison Information Ctr.
1925 Wilshire Boulevard
Los Angeles 90057
(213) 484-5151

San Francisco Bay Area Poison Control Ctr.
San Francisco Gen. Hospital
Room 1E86
1001 Potrero Avenue
San Francisco 94110
(415) 666-2845

COLORADO
Rocky Mountain Poison Ctr.
West 8th Avenue and Cherokee Street
Denver 80204
(303) 629-1123

CONNECTICUT
Connecticut Poison Ctr.
University of Connecticut Health Ctr.
Farmington 06032
(203) 674-3456

DELAWARE
Delaware Poison Information Service, Inc.
501 W. 14th Street
Wilmington 19899
(302) 655-3389

DISTRICT OF COLUMBIA
National Capital Poison Ctr.
Georgetown Hospital
3800 Reservoir Road, N.W.
Washington 20007
(202) 652-3333

FLORIDA
Jackson Mem. Hospital
1611 N.W. 12th Avenue
Miami 33136
(305) 325-7429

Poison Control Ctr.
Shands Hospital
Box J316
Gainesville 32610
(904) 392-3389

GEORGIA
Athens Gen. Hospital
1199 Prince Avenue
Athens 30613
(404) 543-5215

Georgia Poison Control Ctr.
Box 26066
80 Butler Street, S.E.
Atlanta 30335
(404) 588-4400
teletype line for the deaf
(404) 525-3323

HAWAII
Hawaii Poison Ctr.
1319 Punahou Street
Honolulu 96826
(808) 941-4411

IDAHO
St. Anthony Hospital
650 N. 7th Street
Pocatello 83201
(206) 232-2733

ILLINOIS
Cook Co. Children's Hospital
700 S. Wood Street
Chicago 60612
(312) 633-7777

INDIANA
Indiana Poison Control Ctr.
1001 W. 10th Street
Indianapolis 46202
(317) 630-7351

Methodist Hospital of Ind., Inc.
1604 N. Capitol Avenue
Indianapolis 46202
(317) 927-3033

IOWA
University of Iowa Hospital and Clinics
Iowa City 52240
(319) 356-2922

KANSAS
University of Kansas Medical Ctr.
39th and Rainbow Boulevard
Kansas City 66103
(913) 588-6633

KENTUCKY
Central Baptist Hospital
1740 S. Limestone
Lexington 40503
(606) 278-3411
8 a.m. to 9 p.m.

Kentucky Poison Control Ctr.
Norton-Kosair Children's Hospital
200 E. Chestnut Street
Louisville 40202
(502) 589-8222

LOUISIANA
Charity Hospital
1532 Tulane Avenue
New Orleans 70140
(504) 568-5222

MAINE
Maine Medical Ctr.
Emergency Division
22 Bramhall Street
Portland 04102
(207) 871-0111
(800) 442-6305

MARYLAND
University of Maryland School of Pharmacy
636 W. Lombard Street
Baltimore 21201
(301) 528-7701
(800) 492-2414

MASSACHUSETTS
Massachusetts Poison Control Systems
300 Longwood Avenue
Boston 02115
(617) 232-2120
(800) 682-9211

MICHIGAN
University Hospital
1405 E. Ann Street
Ann Arbor 48104
Poison Ctr. (313) 764-5102
Drug Info. (313) 763-0243

Western Michigan Poison Ctr.
1840 Wealthy, S.E.
Grand Rapids 49506
(616) 774-7854
(800) 632-2727